ASSOCIATION OF PEDIATRIC ONCOLOGY NURSES

*N*ursing Care
OF CHILDREN *AND*
ADOLESCENTS
WITH CANCER

Third Edition

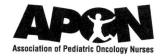

Association of Pediatric Oncology Nurses

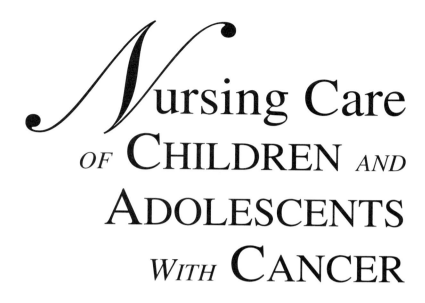

*N*ursing Care
OF CHILDREN *AND*
ADOLESCENTS
WITH CANCER

Third Edition

CHRISTINA RASCO BAGGOTT, RN-CS, MN, PNP, CPON
Pediatric Nurse Practitioner
Hematology/Oncology
Lucile Packard Children's Hospital at Stanford
Palo Alto, California

KATHERINE PATTERSON KELLY, RN, MN, CPON
Clinical Nurse Specialist
Pediatric Hematology/Oncology
Children's Hospital
University of Missouri Health Care
Columbia, Missouri

DIANNE FOCHTMAN, RN, MN, CPNP, CPON
Pediatric Oncology Nurse Practitioner
Kapiolani Medical Center for Women and Children
Honolulu, Hawaii;
Clinical Associate Professor
School of Nursing
University of Hawaii
Honolulu, Hawaii

GENEVIEVE V. FOLEY, RN, MSN, OCN, CNAA
Vice President, Patient Care Services
St. Jude Children's Research Hospital
Memphis, Tennessee

SAUNDERS
An Imprint of Elsevier Science

SAUNDERS
An Imprint of Elsevier Science
The Curtis Center
Independence Square West
Philadelphia, PA 19106

Library of Congress Cataloging-in-Publication Data

Nursing care of children and adolescents with cancer / Association of Pediatric Oncology Nurses ; volume editors, Christina Rasco Baggott ... [et al.].—3rd ed.
    p. ; cm.
Includes bibliographical references and index.
ISBN 0-7216-8718-0
    1. Cancer in children—Nursing. 2. Tumors in adolescence—Nursing. I. Baggott, Christina Rasco. II. Association of Pediatric Oncology Nurses (U.S.) III. Nursing care of the child with cancer.
    [DNLM: 1. Neoplasms—nursing—Adolescence. 2. Neoplasms—nursing—Child. 3. Neoplasms—nursing—Infant. WY 156 N9727 2001]
RC281.C4 N87 2001
610.73'698—dc21

2001049143

Vice President and Nursing Editorial Director: Sally Schrefer
Executive Editor: Barbara Nelson Cullen
Managing Editor: Sandra Clark Brown
Developmental Editor: Eric Ham
Project Manager: John Rogers
Senior Production Editor: Mary Turner
Designer: Kathi Gosche
Cover Art: Kathi Gosche

NURSING CARE OF CHILDREN AND ADOLESCENTS WITH CANCER   0-7216-8718-0

Printed in the United States of America

Last digit is the print number: 9   8   7   6   5   4   3   2   CL/MV

To the children and their families

and

To past, present, and future pediatric oncology nurses

CONTRIBUTORS

ARLENE L. ANDROKITES, MSN, RN, CPNP, CPON
Pediatric Oncology Nurse Practitioner
Dana Farber Cancer Institute
Children's Hospital
Boston, Massachusetts
Wilms Tumor

CHRISTINA RASCO BAGGOTT, RN-CS, MN, PNP, CPON
Pediatric Nurse Practitioner
Hematology/Oncology
Lucile Packard Children's Hospital at Stanford
Palo Alto, California
Management of Disease and Treatment-Related Complications; Interdisciplinary Collaboration

HOLLY BAGNALL-REEB, RN, MN
Clinical Nurse Specialist
Pediatric Hematology/Oncology
Baystate Medical Center
Springfield, Massachusetts
Surgery

KATHY L. BERTOLONE, RN, MSN, CFNP, CPON
Pediatric Oncology Nurse Practitioner
Kosair Children's Hospital
Louisville, Kentucky
Acute Lymphoblastic Leukemia

DONNA L. BETCHER, RN, MS, CPNP, CPON
Oncology Clinical Nurse Specialist;
Pediatric Nurse Practitioner
Pediatric Oncology
Mayo Clinic
Rochester, Minnesota
Bone Tumors

DANA M. BOND, RN, MN, CPNP
Pediatric Oncology Nurse Practitioner
Children's Medical Center of Dallas
Center for Cancer and Blood Disorders
Dallas, Texas
Chemotherapy

ROSALIND BRYANT, MN, RN-CS, PNP
Pediatric Nurse Practitioner
Pediatric Hematology
Texas Children's Cancer Center and Hematology Service
Houston, Texas
Blood Component Deficiencies

SUSAN L. COHN, MD
Associate Professor of Pediatrics
Division of Hematology/Oncology
Northwestern University
Chicago, Illinois
Langerhans Cell Histiocytosis

MICHAEL COMEAU, RN, MS, AOCN, CPON
Coordinator for Clinical Trials in Nursing
Dana Farber Cancer Institute
Boston, Massachusetts
Management of Disease and Treatment-Related Complications

KELLY D. COYNE, MSN, CPNP
Pediatric Nurse Practitioner
Children's Memorial Hospital
Chicago, Illinois
Hematopoietic Stem Cell Transplantation

PATSY McGUIRE CULLEN, RN, MS, CPNP, CPON
Pediatric Nurse Practitioner
Childhood Hematology-Oncology Associates
Rocky Mountain Children's Cancer Center
Denver, Colorado
Radiation Therapy

GAYE DADD, RN, BSc
Clinical Manager
Hematology/Oncology
Princess Margaret Hospital for Children
Perth, Western Australia
Australia
Neuroblastoma

JOYCE D. DERRICKSON, RN, BSN, CPON
Nurse Coordinator
Radiation Oncology Program
Childrens Hospital Los Angeles
Los Angeles, California
Radiation Therapy

ROSEMARY DRIGAN, MSN, MEd, RN, CPNP, CPON
Pediatric Nurse Practitioner;
Oncology Consultant
Children's Health Services
John C. Lincoln Hospital
Phoenix, Arizona
Wilms Tumor

SUSAN DULCZAK, MSN, RN-CS, PNP
Clinical Nurse Specialist/Oncology
The Children's Hospital of Philadelphia
Philadelphia, Pennsylvania
Retinoblastoma

DANITA DUMAS, RN
Clinical Resource Nurse
Pediatric Neuro-Oncology
University of California–Davis
Sacramento, California
Langerhans Cell Histiocytosis

JANET M. DUNCAN, BSN, RN, CPON
Clinical Educator, Oncology Program
Children's Hospital
Boston, Massachusetts
*Management of Disease and Treatment-Related
Complications*

ALICE G. ETTINGER, RN, MSN, CPNP, CPON
Program Coordinator
Division of Pediatric Hematology-Oncology
Saint Peter's University Hospital
New Brunswick, New Jersey
Chemotherapy

JEAN H. FERGUSSON, RN, EdD, CRNP
Research Fellow, Psychosocial Oncology
School of Nursing
University of Pennsylvania
Philadelphia, Pennsylvania
History, Issues, and Trends

MAURA A. FITZGERALD, MS, RN, C
Clinical Nurse Specialist
Integrative Medicine and Cultural Care
Children's Hospital and Clinics
Minneapolis, Minnesota
Complementary and Alternative Treatments

DIANNE FOCHTMAN, RN, MN, CPNP, CPON
Pediatric Oncology Nurse Practitioner
Kapiolani Medical Center for Women and Children
Honolulu, Hawaii;
Clinical Associate Professor
School of Nursing
University of Hawaii
Honolulu, Hawaii
Palliative Care

GENEVIEVE V. FOLEY, RN, MSN, OCN, CNAA
Vice President, Patient Care Services
St. Jude Children's Research Hospital
Memphis, Tennessee
History, Issues, and Trends

KATHY FORTE, RN, MS, CPNP
Advanced Practice Nurse
AFLAC Cancer Center and Blood Disorders Service
Children's Healthcare of Atlanta
Atlanta, Georgia
Ethical Issues

SHARON FRIERDICH, RN, MSC
Pediatric Hematology-Oncology Nurse Practitioner
University of Wisconsin Children's Hospital
Madison, Wisconsin
Home Care

BARBARA FROTHINGHAM, MSN, FNP, CPON
Nurse Practitioner
Legacy Emanuel Children's Cancer Program
Portland, Oregon
Retinoblastoma

VALERIE GROBEN, RN, BSN, CPON
Pediatric Oncology Nurse
St. Jude Children's Research Hospital
Memphis, Tennessee
*Management of Disease and Treatment-Related
Complications*

JEANNE HARVEY, RN, MSN, CS, PNP, CPON
Formerly, Nurse Practitioner
David B. Perini Quality of Life Clinic
Dana Farber Cancer Institute
Boston, Massachusetts;
School Nurse
Westborough High School
Westborough, Massachusetts
Care of Survivors

MAUREEN S. HAUGEN, RN, MS, CPNP
Pediatric Nurse Practitioner
Children's Memorial Hospital
Chicago, Illinois
Hematopoietic Stem Cell Transplantation

SUE P. HEINEY, PhD, RN, CS, FAAN
Manager, Psychosocial Oncology
South Carolina Cancer Center of Palmetto Health
Columbia, South Carolina
Family-Centered Psychosocial Care

PAMELA S. HINDS, PhD, RN, CS
Director of Nursing Research
St. Jude Children's Research Hospital
Memphis, Tennessee
Research

WENDY HOBBIE, RN, MSN, CRNP
Coordinator, Follow-Up Program
The Children's Hospital of Philadelphia;
Associate Program Director
Pediatric Oncology Nurse Practitioner Program
University of Pennsylvania
School of Nursing
Philadelphia, Pennsylvania
Care of Survivors

MARILYN J. HOCKENBERRY, PhD, RN-CS, PNP, FAAN
Professor of Pediatrics
Baylor College of Medicine;
Director of Nurse Practitioners
Texas Children's Cancer Center
Texas Children's Hospital
Houston, Texas
Research

M. MAUREEN HUBBELL, RN, MSN
Advanced Practice Nurse
Children's Memorial Hospital
Chicago, Illinois
Hematopoietic Stem Cell Transplantation

MARGARET RYAN HUSSONG, RN, MS, PNP
Advanced Practice Nurse/Clinical Associate
Pediatric Hematology/Oncology
University of Rochester Medical Center
Children's Hospital at Strong
Rochester, New York
Non-Hodgkin's Lymphoma

DEBRA P. HYMOVICH, PhD, RN, FAAN
Professor Emeritus
University of North Carolina at Charlotte
Naples, Florida
Family-Centered Psychosocial Care

KATHERINE PATTERSON KELLY, RN, MN, CPON
Clinical Nurse Specialist
Pediatric Hematology/Oncology
Children's Hospital
University of Missouri Health Care
Columbia, Missouri
Interdisciplinary Collaboration

NANCY E. KLINE, PhD, RN, CPNP
Assistant Professor of Pediatrics
Baylor College of Medicine;
Pediatric Nurse Practitioner
Texas Children's Hospital
Houston, Texas
Prevention and Treatment of Infections

CAROL ZINGER KOTSUBO, RN, MPH, MS, OCN, CPON
Clinical Nurse Specialist, Pediatric Oncology
Kapiolani Medical Center for Women and Children
Honolulu, Hawaii
Rhabdomyosarcoma

KAREN MARIE KRISTOVICH, RN, MSN, PNP
Pediatric Nurse Practitioner
Hematopoietic Stem Cell Transplantation
Lucile Packard Children's Hospital at Stanford
Palo Alto, California
Hematopoietic Stem Cell Transplantation

WENDY LANDIER, RN, MSN, CPNP, CPON
Pediatric Nurse Practitioner
City of Hope National Medical Center
Duarte, California;
Assistant Clinical Professor
UCLA School of Nursing
Los Angeles, California
Myeloid Diseases

MARCIA LEONARD, RN, PNP
Pediatric Nurse Practitioner
Division of Pediatric Hematology/Oncology
University of Michigan
Ann Arbor, Michigan
Diagnostic Evaluations and Staging Procedures

PATRICIA LIEBHAUSER, RN, MSN
Clinical Nurse Specialist
Hughes Spalding Children's Hospital
Grady Health System
Atlanta, Georgia
Hodgkin's Disease

KIM M. McHARD, RN, MSN, CPNP
Orthopaedic Oncology Nurse Practitioner
Private Practice
Dallas, Texas
Bone Tumors

IDA M. (KI) MOORE, RN, DNS, FAAN
Professor and Director
Division of Nursing Practice
College of Nursing
The University of Arizona
Tucson, Arizona
Care of Survivors

ROBBIE NORVILLE, RN, MSN, CPON
Clinical Specialist—Bone Marrow Transplant
Texas Children's Cancer Center and Hematology Service
Houston, Texas
Blood Component Deficiencies

JILL E. BRACE O'NEILL, MS, RN-CS, PNP

Coordinator of Clinical Research and Nurse Practitioner
Hematology, Oncology, and Stem Cell Transplant
Children's Hospital and Dana Farber Cancer Institute
Boston, Massachusetts
Rare Tumors

CHERYL PANZARELLA, MS, RN, CPON

Per Diem Nurse
Dana Farber Cancer Institute
Boston, Massachusetts
Management of Disease and Treatment-Related Complications

SHIRLEY PERRY, RN, MScN

Nurse Practitioner
Pediatric Oncology
Stollery Children's Health Center
University of Alberta Hospital
Edmonton, Alberta, Canada
Surgery

MARY MCELWAIN PETRICCIONE, RN, MSN, CPNP

Pediatric Nurse Practitioner of the Pediatric Neuro-Oncology
Service
Memorial Sloan-Kettering Cancer Center
New York, New York
Central Nervous System Tumors

JANICE POST-WHITE, RN, PhD, FAAN

Associate Professor
American Cancer Society Professor of Oncology Nursing
University of Minnesota School of Nursing
Minneapolis, Minnesota
Complementary and Alternative Treatments

JENNIFER A. POTTER, MSN, RN-CS, PNP

Pediatric Nurse Practitioner
Division of Neuro-Oncology
St. Jude Children's Research Hospital
Memphis, Tennessee
Radiation Therapy

KATHY RUCCIONE, RN, MPH

Center Nursing Administrator;
Co-Director, Health Promotions and Outcomes Program
Children's Center for Cancer & Blood Diseases
Childrens Hospital Los Angeles;
Associate Professor of Clinical Nursing
USC Department of Nursing;
Associate Professor of Clinical Pediatrics
USC Keck School of Medicine
University of Southern California
Los Angeles, California
*Biologic Basis of Cancer in Children and Adolescents;
Care of Survivors*

LYDIA GONZALEZ RYAN, MSN, PNP

Clinical Director, Hematology/Oncology/Stem Cell
Transplantation
Children's Healthcare of Atlanta
Atlanta, Georgia
Hematopoietic Stem Cell Transplantation

JANIS RYAN-MURRAY, RN, MSN, CPNP, CPON

Pediatric Nurse Practitioner
Division of Pediatric Hematology/Oncology
Duke University Medical Center
Durham, North Carolina
Central Nervous System Tumors

LISA SCHUM, BA

Professional Oncology Education Student
St. Jude Children's Research Hospital
Memphis, Tennessee
Research

SUSAN F. SENCER, MD

Director, Integrative Cancer Care
Children's Hospitals and Clinics
Minneapolis/St. Paul, Minnesota
Complementary and Alternative Treatments

SANDY SENTIVANY-COLLINS, RN, MS

Clinical Nurse Specialist
Pediatric Pain Management
Lucile Packard Children's Hospital at Stanford
Palo Alto, California
Treatment of Pain

THERESA D. SIEVERS, RN, MS

Administrative Director
North Shore Children's Hospital
Salem, Massachusetts
Chemotherapy

PAMELA J. SIMON, BSN, MSN, CPNP

Oncology Pediatric Nurse Practitioner
Lucile Packard Children's Hospital at Stanford
Palo Alto, California;
Formerly, Oncology Pediatric Nurse Practitioner
University of Nebraska Medical Center
Omaha, Nebraska
Bone Tumors

JANET L. STEWART, MN, RN, CPON

Doctoral Candidate
School of Nursing
University of North Carolina at Chapel Hill
Chapel Hill, North Carolina
Management of Disease and Treatment-Related Complications

JACQUIE M. TOIA, RN, MS, ND, CPNP
Pediatric Nurse Practitioner
Hematology/Oncology
Children's Memorial Hospital
Chicago, Illinois
Langerhans Cell Histiocytosis

CAROLYN L. WALKER, PhD, RN, CPON
Professor
San Diego State University
San Diego, California
Family-Centered Psychosocial Care

LINDA MATHIS WELLS, MA, RN, CNA, FAAN
Nurse Manager
Children's Center for Cancer and Blood Disorders
South Carolina Cancer Center
Columbia, South Carolina
Family-Centered Psychosocial Care

SUSAN K. WESTLAKE, PhD, RN, CPON
Clinical Nurse Specialist for Oncology Services
Children's Hospital of Wisconsin
Milwaukee, Wisconsin
Acute Lymphoblastic Leukemia

KARLA D. WILSON, RN, MSN, FNP, CPON
Clinical Nurse Specialist/Nurse Practitioner
Childrens Hospital Los Angeles
Los Angeles, California
Oncologic Emergencies

DEBBIE A. WOODS, MSN, RN, CPNP, CPON
Inpatient Advanced Practice Nurse
Sutter Memorial Hospital
Sacramento, California
Management of Disease and Treatment-Related Complications

MYRA WOOLERY-ANTILL, RN, MN
Pediatric Clinical Nurse Specialist
Clinical Center Nursing Department
National Institutes of Health
Bethesda, Maryland
Biotherapy

PREFACE

On April 15, 1976, the Association of Pediatric Oncology Nurses (APON) was formally incorporated in the state of Tennessee. APON's silver anniversary in 2001 provides an opportunity to look back at the accomplishments and ahead to future challenges.

When APON was founded, pediatric oncology nursing was a fledgling specialty. The organization quickly adopted the goal of improving care for children and adolescents with cancer and their families. Enhancing the nurse's knowledge base became a key strategy to achieving better patient outcomes. In that effort, the publication of a textbook devoted to pediatric oncology nursing became essential.

The first edition of *Nursing Care of the Child With Cancer,* published in 1982, had 12 chapters filling 380 pages. The approach was factual and straightforward, with emphasis on the fundamental issues of diseases, treatments, and physical and psychosocial care. By the time the second edition was published in 1993, the book had grown to 18 chapters. Clearly evident were the enormous strides that had been made in increasing survival, improving the understanding of cancer's basic causes, and expanding treatment modalities. For the first time, specific chapters on bone marrow transplantation and biologic response modifiers were included. Application of research findings was evident. For example, a new chapter on the biologic basis of childhood cancers examined the research on cancer causation, and the psychosocial chapter looked at the results of studies on the impact of cancer on the entire family, including siblings. Outcomes of care were emphasized with chapters dedicated to the terminally ill child and late effects in long-term survivors. The development of the specialty of pediatric oncology nursing was highlighted through historical review and an assessment of emerging roles.

The third edition of the book, *Nursing Care of Children and Adolescents With Cancer,* builds on the previous editions but goes well beyond them. All of the previously published chapters have been revised. Additional sections have been developed. In this text, 33 chapters respond to the complexity that now distinguishes pediatric oncology nursing in these important areas: the disease and its treatment, the child's stressors, and the roles and responsibilities of the pediatric oncology nurse.

Advances in the basic sciences have led to revolutionary insights into the origin, life, and death of cancer cells. Although it is still unclear why any one child develops a malignancy, much more is now known about the genetic and cellular factors that favor the development of cancers. Translational research has started to bring those basic scientific findings out of the laboratory and into the clinical setting much more quickly than in the past. Improvements in staging and greater precision in cell type identification have already begun to affect treatment.

The society in which children and adolescents with cancer live is very different from the society of 25 years ago. Indeed, most pioneers in the specialty would cite changing family values, diminished social supports, and reduced material resources, sometimes to the point of poverty, as key transformations over the last quarter century. For some families, the oncology team becomes their primary source of caring and support. For most families, the pediatric oncology nurse must anticipate and deal with interpersonal and community challenges that severely test the adaptation and coping skills of the entire family.

Challenges on the scientific and technologic side, coupled with more complicated social and family systems, necessitate more depth and breadth in the role of the pediatric oncology nurse. In recognition of these expanded responsibilities additional emphasis has been placed on providing exceptional physical and emotional care, anticipating and dealing with treatment complications, and engaging families in the process of patient education. New chapters on complementary and alternative treatments, nursing research, and ethics highlight the nurse's broad responsibilities for patient advocacy. Throughout the text emphasis has been added on the nurse's role as a key member of the multidisciplinary care team.

In its own way, the development of a book of this scope and size is an arduous labor of love. Neither the authors nor the editors received monetary compensation for their efforts. Time and talents were generously shared. Particular thanks are due to the chapter authors who worked diligently to provide the latest, most accurate, relevant information. Their intelligence, dedication, and good humor made a difficult job easier. To the expert reviewers, both physicians and nurses, who contributed thoughtful comments to several chapters, special words of appreciation are due.

The staff of Harcourt Health Sciences offered support, encouragement, guidance, and always gentle nudging. Second edition editor Thomas Eoyang provided valuable initial advice and guidance to the editors and helped us smoothly transition to the third edition publication team of Sandra Brown, Managing Editor, and Eric Ham, Developmental Editor. Under the direction of Mary Turner, Senior Production Editor, a dedicated staff of copy editors worked to satisfy four perfectionist editors. To these individuals and to those behind the scenes at Harcourt, our heartfelt thanks.

The APON presidents and board members involved with this endeavor were unfailing sources of support. Particular thanks to Robbie Norville and Alice Ettinger for their leadership. To the APON central office staff in Chicago, our appreciation for their assistance with logistics.

We are deeply indebted to our families and friends for their understanding and support. They were unusually patient with the limited time we had available for them, forgiving of our physical absences and mental lapses caused by preoccupation with the book, and resourceful with helping us juggle family responsibilities. Without their sustaining caring, we could not have persisted.

Our co-workers, likewise, were often inconvenienced as we attempted to balance the needs of the workplace with our writing and editing duties. We are grateful to all of them, particularly to Sheila Gardner in Memphis, for the roles they played indirectly in bringing this professional resource to reality.

Finally, the pioneer editors, Dianne and Gen, thank Tina and Kathy for their scholarship, dedication, and superb computer skills! This edition of *Nursing Care of Children and Adolescents With Cancer* represents the linking of two eras in the history of the book. It is our fondest hope that a third generation of editors will be unnecessary, so successful will be our efforts to prevent and treat pediatric cancers. Until that time comes, we wish for all our readers the satisfaction that comes from a job well done in the care of children and adolescents with cancer and their families.

Christina Rasco Baggott
Katherine Patterson Kelly
Dianne Fochtman
Genevieve V. Foley

CONTENTS

I

Foundations

History, Issues, and Trends

Genevieve V. Foley
Jean H. Fergusson

". . . I believe there is merit in looking at the past in order to have a perspective of accomplishments, challenges, trends and future needs. Moreover, I think it can give us courage and determination to pursue our ideas and ideals."[58]

The history of pediatric oncology nursing as a distinct subspecialty began soon after the end of World War II. The complex factors prompting its emergence are rooted in the histories of oncology, pediatrics, and nursing. This chapter describes the mosaic of traditions, beliefs, values, and practices that influenced the past, shaped the present, and suggest the future of pediatric oncology nursing. It also portrays how historical forces continue to influence attitudes and behaviors related to pediatric cancer.

Has pediatric cancer always existed?

Hippocrates (460-370 BC) was the first to use the term *karkinos,* or *crab,* to describe a cancer. It was an imprecise term characterizing a variety of conditions, some of which correspond to the present definition of malignant neoplasm.[63] Hippocrates mentions neck growths in children, but it is not known whether these growths were cancers.[28] Often a swelling was considered a cancer if the patient died.[76] Thus, although true malignancies did exist during this time, paleo-pathology studies suggest that cancer was an uncommon occurrence.[14,25,76,89]

For centuries, little note was made of cancer in children, in part because it was not a significant health problem, in part because cancer was not well understood and misdiagnosis was common. The first documented account of cancer in children appeared in 1809 when James Wardrop described 24 cases of malignant eye tumors, 20 of which occurred in children less than 12 years of age. This report represents the first collection of childhood cancer cases.[29] In 1876 C.J. Duzan published a tabulation of 182 pediatric malignancies reported in the literature between 1832 and 1875. Duzan's work represents the first publication devoted exclusively to cancer in children.[28] Determining the incidence and prevalence of childhood malignancies has been a difficult task. Procedures for collecting and reporting cancer statistics were not clarified and organized until the twentieth century. In the United States, for example, the incidence and mortality of cancers for persons less than 30 years of age were presented in a single age category. James Ewing, the pathologist for whom Ewing's sarcoma is named, objected strongly to that reporting system. He believed that juvenile cancers "are so peculiar that properly they may not be compared with any adult tumors, and that this entire subject deserves to be treated as a special department in the descriptive history of neoplastic disease."[37]

The leading causes of death in children 1 to 14 years of age in 1936, 1966, and 1998 are compared in Table 1-1. Leukemia and Hodgkin's disease were included with other cancers in the 1936 statistics, thus providing a more accurate picture of cancer deaths in children. Differences in the causes of death between 1936 and 1966 were also due to advances in general pediatric care, particularly the control of infectious disease. Sydney Farber (1903-1973) believed that these advances "unmasked" the problem of pediatric cancer. Indeed, by the end of World War II, cancer was identified as the leading cause of death from disease in the 1- to 15-year-old age-group,[38] a position it still holds.

What causes cancer?

Throughout the centuries mankind has struggled to understand the complex entity known as cancer. The theories suggested in each era reflected how diseases were understood. Although some of the theories seem outlandish, ill conceived, even silly, remnants of them persist in some form even today, providing the basis for misconceptions and concerns in patients and families.[24] The earliest explanations for the cause of cancers come from Hippocrates (460-370 BC) and Galen (130-200 AD), who defined health as a balance among the body's four humors: blood, phlegm, yellow bile, and black

TABLE 1-1	LEADING CAUSES OF DEATH IN THE UNITED STATES IN 1936, 1966, AND 1998 FOR CHILDREN 1 TO 14 YEARS: RATE PER 100,000						
Rank	Cause	1936	Cause	1966	Cause	1998
1	Accidents	40.1	Accidents	23.7	Accidents	21.0
2	Pneumonia	38.6	Cancer	7.0	Cancer	5.0
3	Diarrhea and enteritis	16.1	Congenital malformations	4.9	Congenital anomalies	4.6
4	Influenza	11.0	Influenza and pneumonia	4.5	Homicide	3.8
5	Appendicitis	10.6	Meningitis	0.8	Heart diseases	2.2
6	Tuberculosis	9.7	Heart diseases	0.8	Influenza and pneumonia	1.3
7	Heart diseases	8.8	Homicide	0.8	Suicide	0.8
8	Diphtheria	7.6	Gastritis	0.7	Cerebrovascular	0.6
9	Cancer	5.3	Cerebral hemorrhage (stroke)	0.7	Septicemia	0.6
10	Scarlet fever	5.1	Meningococcal infections	0.7	Benign neoplasms	0.5

From "Vital Statistics of the United States," Washington, D.C.: U.S. Government Printing Office.

bile. Hippocrates suggested that cancer was caused by an excess of black bile, or melanchole,[99] a view reaffirmed and elaborated on by Galen, who described an unhealthy swelling arising from a single or multiple humor as "oncos."[63] Galen, the medical authority of the Western world for the next 13 centuries, listed cancer among tumors contrary to nature. Ulcers, fistulas, and carbuncles also were so classified.[99] Both these men believed that cancer was a systemic disease and that advanced cancer was best left alone.

The opinions of Hippocrates and Galen were unchallenged for nearly 2000 years. During the Renaissance many aspects of the theory were abandoned. Koten maintains, however, that compelling aspects of the humoral theory persisted, particularly that cancer is related to internal imbalances and that individuals have a constitutional tendency for certain diseases.[68]

In the fifteenth and sixteenth centuries the idea of cancer being caused by an external factor, often manifesting itself locally rather than systemically, was proposed. Over the next 200 years the idea emerged that bacterial and viral infections were that cause. In the sixteenth century the theory of irritation contended that cancer is the result of an inappropriate physical stimulus. This concept was useful in early explanations of chemical and environmental factors leading to the development of cancer. Thus awareness of occupational and environmental carcinogens developed relatively early. In 1700 Bernardini Ramazzini published *Diseases of Tradesmen* (English translation), the first systematic compilation of occupational diseases. He noted that nuns had a high incidence of breast cancer and postulated that this was due to their celibate lifestyle. This association between an occupation and a specific cancer is considered the first of its kind. Contributions related to the environment include John Hill's association in 1761 between the use of snuff and nasal cancer and Samuel von Soemmering's identification in 1795 of the correlation between pipe smoking and lip cancer. Percivall Pott in 1775 documented the first occupational exposure to carcinogenic materials resulting in clinical disease when he linked cancer of the scrotum with the occupation of chimney sweep.[8,99]

Understanding metastasis was an especially difficult problem. According to the humoral theory cancer was a systemic disease. Later, the generally held belief was that cancer was a local disease caused by external factors, often either infectious agents or irritants of some type. Scientific discoveries that emerged in one era but did not fit with prevailing thought often were ignored. For example, Henri Francais Le Dran (1685-1770) postulated that cancer began as a local disease that spread through the lymphatic system to the lymph nodes and then to the general circulation. Decades later, in 1829, Joseph Claude Anselme Récamier (1774-1852) used the term *metastasis* to describe what he believed were secondary tumors in the brain of a woman with breast cancer.[25,99]

The current understanding of what causes cancer in general is an interesting amalgam of the historical concepts prevalent for centuries.[34] The individual disease chapters that follow describe what is currently known about the specific factors leading to cancers in children. The fact remains, however, that why cancer strikes a particular child is still incompletely understood and that the theories of internal imbalance, family tendency, and infectious origin all influence contemporary thought.

What was the influence of pediatrics on childhood cancer?

For centuries children were considered miniature adults.[105] Pediatrics struggled to establish itself as a separate discipline, to broaden its scope of practice beyond newborns and infants. The development of separate facilities for children was an important milestone. Children began to be admitted to hospitals during the sixteenth century in France.[45] Specialized facilities for children came into existence first in Europe when l'Hopital des Enfants Malades opened in Paris in 1802, followed by The Hospital for Sick Children in Great Ormond Street, London, in 1852.[4] The Children's Hospital of Philadelphia, the first hospital in the United States devoted exclusively to children, was established in 1955.[54]

In 1880 pediatrics became a specialty when the American Medical Association (AMA) established a section on diseases of children and named Abraham Jacobi (1830-1919) president of the section.[22] Eight years later the first medical specialty society in the United States, the American Pediatric Society, was founded.[86]

L. Emmett Holt's (1855-1924) milestone textbook *The Diseases of Infancy and Childhood* contributed to pediatrics what Osler's *Principles and Practice of Medicine* gave to internal medicine.[87] With funds from the Rockefeller Foundation, Holt developed a laboratory at Babies Hospital in New York that used the biochemical methods then known to study diseases of children. John Howland (1873-1926) shared Holt's funding to implement physical and chemical measurements of children treated at the Harriett Lane Home of the Johns Hopkins University Hospital, Baltimore. These activities were pioneering efforts in the use of quantitative research in pediatrics.[80]

Jacobi, Holt, and Howland were influenced by medical schools in Germany and Vienna, Austria, that used autopsy to confirm clinical evaluations and diagnosis. This acceptance of pediatric autopsy was an important element in the advancement of pediatrics in the United States,[80] including pediatric oncology.

The introduction of sulfonamides and penicillin and key discoveries pertaining to the fluid and electrolyte disorders of children combined to change childhood morbidity and mortality rates in the 1940s and 1950s.[54] New and perhaps more difficult challenges emerged, engendered by chronic illnesses such as cancer, social diseases, and psychologic problems resulting from changes in the child's and adolescent's environments.

A key philosophical bond between pediatrics and pediatric oncology is advocacy. Across cultures and throughout the centuries, the fate of children has been linked with the major societal values and problems of the time. In virtually all cases, whatever the societal malady, the impact on children is more adverse than on other groups.[45,69] In response to the realities of children's needs, it has been customary for many of those caring for children to assume a broad mandate.[18] In the United States the American Academy of Pediatrics has been a role model in this regard.[22] Pediatrics has been concerned not only with the ill child but also with health education, preventive health guidance, and child-rearing practices. To better the lives of children, advocacy and social activism have been accepted elements of pediatric practice for almost two centuries.[69] This heritage emerges in pediatric oncology in wide-ranging efforts such as preventing youth smoking and ensuring access to care.

What historical forces helped cancer treatments to develop?

Throughout much of oncology's history, surgery stood virtually alone as a treatment for cancer. From the time of Hippocrates, superficial external lesions were treated with caustic pastes and various herbal preparations, excision, or cautery.[90] Deeper tumors posed considerable problems. Surgeons were limited by the difficulties of operating on a conscious patient struggling in pain as the surgeon worked.[106] The introduction of anesthesia in 1846,[36] coupled with the slowly advancing doctrines on antiseptic surgery of Joseph Lister,[6] enabled surgeons to excise internal cancers. Since surgery was the only effective treatment available for cancer at the time, the expanded possibilities for surgery were critical to improved patient outcomes.[13]

Radiation therapy was the second modality to emerge, with the discovery of x-rays by Wilhelm Conrad Roentgen and the identification of radium by Pierre and Marie Curie.[26] For decades little was understood about the powerful effects of this modality. Unknowingly, pioneers did nothing to protect themselves from the radiation source, often exposing themselves to radiation hazards. Marie Curie, who succumbed to anemia and bone marrow suppression, is but one example of an early leader who most likely died as a consequence of long-term exposure to radiation.[106] Before that time the radiation given was the amount that caused skin reddening or irritation; that is, the therapeutic amount was the dose that caused erythema.[65]

Insufficient radium sources slowed the early development of radiation therapy. The first division of radium therapy was established at the Memorial Hospital in New York City in 1916.[23] The radium source for the facility was donated by bereaved parent James Douglas, a physician and philanthropist who tried unsuccessfully to have his daughter treated in the United States with radium. In her memory Douglas established a mining operation in Colorado that yielded a significant supply of uranium. Clinical uses for radium expanded quickly, leading the way for recognition of radiation therapy as an important treatment option. Over the years improvement in the techniques, technologies, and delivery systems of radiation therapy has ensured advancement of the specialty.

Cancer chemotherapy has played a pivotal role in saving the lives of many children with cancer. Yet its beginnings are rooted in the Great Wars of the twentieth century.[114] Nitrogen mustard gas had been used with lethal effect during World War I. In 1919 E.B. Khrumbaar noted bone marrow aplasia and lymph tissue destruction among the deleterious attributes of the gas. Interest in the potential of nitrogen mustard gas reemerged during World War II. As part of a classified, chemical-warfare-type project, a group of investigators at Yale University in New Haven, Connecticut, Louis Goodman, Alfred Gilman, T.F. Dougherty, and Fredrick S. Philips, demonstrated that the nitrogen analogue of the gas was capable of shrinking lymphoma in laboratory animals.[99] Clinical trials were authorized at Yale, the University of Chicago, and Memorial Sloan-Kettering Hospital in New York. In 1946, after the war had ended, the results of these studies were declassified and published. The subsequent introduction of other antineoplastic medications reinforced the usefulness of chemotherapy to improve outcomes.[13]

Developing chemotherapy as an effective modality for children was complicated by a lack of fundamental information on normal hematologic values of infants and children and techniques designed to deliver care safely to the pediatric population. For example, determining the life span of fetal and mature red blood cells took from 1919 to the 1950s, and studying bone marrow directly was not widely accepted. It took until the late 1940s to develop the techniques of marrow aspiration, including sternal aspirations, and to establish the marrow characteristics in a variety of diseases.[32] Technical limitations were common. Small-caliber butterfly needles were not available in the 1940s.[88] Blood transfusions were uncommon,[115] partially because blood group subtypes were unknown, resulting in transfusion reactions with some frequency and intensity. Transfusions often were administered in the operating room, both for safety and for ensuring freshness of the blood. Louis Diamond developed the technique of umbilical artery catheterization in the late 1940s. Modern blood administration techniques were commonplace only after World War II.

The contributions of Sydney Farber and his colleagues at Boston Children's Hospital pioneered the era of chemotherapy as an effective primary and adjuvant therapy. Their work with folic acid

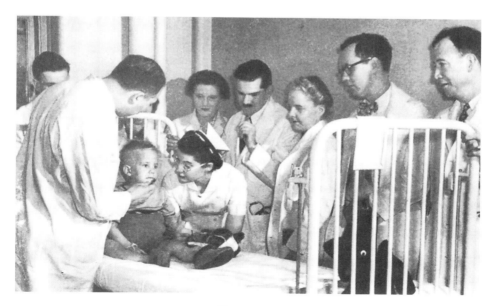

Figure 1-1

At Boston Children's Hospital the small patient's soft toys are laid aside as he is visited by nurse Lisa Blumenthal and Dr. Sydney Farber and his staff. (Copyright 1951 by the Saturday Evening Post. Reprinted with permission.)

antagonists was a milestone in the history of pediatric cancer (Figure 1-1). As other advances were made, the need to establish specialized clinical facilities was identified.[107] The first children's cancer unit, a four-bed ward, was established in 1934 at Memorial Hospital in New York City. It was enlarged to 26 beds in the early 1950s (Figure 1-2). St. Jude Children's Research Hospital, founded in 1962 in Memphis, was the first hospital devoted exclusively to pediatric malignancies.

Surgery, radiation, chemotherapy, and advances in supportive care such as blood transfusions and antibiotics have provided the foundation for improving cure rates in children with cancer. Other modalities such as hematopoietic stem cell transplant (HSCT),[1] biologic response modifiers,[51,77,83] and gene therapy[57,104] are playing increasingly important roles. These modalities are discussed in later chapters. Table 1-2 identifies selected milestones in the history of oncology.

TABLE 1-2 SELECTED MILESTONES—MATURATION OF ONCOLOGY	
Milestone	**Date**
The New York Cancer Hospital is established (later called Memorial Hospital)—first private facility in the United States treating cancer patients.	1884
Wilhelm Conrad von Roentgen discovers x-rays.	1895
Pierre and Marie Sklodowska Curie identify and isolate radium.	1898
Bertillon classification of the causes of death is issued for international use. U.S. Death Registration System is set up, with 10 states participating.	1900
Rockefeller Institute for Medical Research is established in New York City (first of its kind). Karl Landsteiner discovers blood types.	1901
American Association for Cancer Research (AACR) is established. Compiling cancer statistics is major priority.	1907
F. Peyton Rous describes a filterable substance that causes chicken sarcoma (now called Rous sarcoma virus).	1911
American Society for the Control of Cancer and the American College of Surgeons are founded.	1913
Journal of Cancer Research begins publication as official journal of AACR.	1916
U.S. Public Health Service sets up Office of Cancer Investigations, which issued public Health Bulletin 155.	1922
Appreciable 20-year increase in cancer deaths is documented.	1925
Connecticut sets up first population-based tumor registry in United States. International Union Against Cancer is established.	1935
National Cancer Institute of Act of 1937 is passed, authorizing National Cancer Institute (NCI).	1937
First Phase I study of bone marrow transplantation is reported.	1939
Journal of the National Cancer Institute begins publication.	1940
American Society for the Control of Cancer is reorganized and renamed the American Cancer Society.	1944
Cancer begins publication.	1948
Austin Hill and Richard Doll report cancer-cigarette connection.	1956
Results of first prospective randomized clinical trial in oncology is published by Freireich et al.	1958
The surgeon general issues landmark report "Smoking and Health."	1964
International Society of Pediatric Oncology (SIOP) is formed.	1969
National Cancer Act of 1971 guarantees bypass budget approval to NCI.	1971
Certifying examination for physicians in pediatric hematology/oncology is given (first in the world).	1974
Society of Surgical Oncology is established.	1975
Knudson proposes two-mutation theory as probable model for retinoblastoma.	1975
The p53 protein is identified.	1979
IFN-alpha is introduced into clinical trials to treat human malignancies.	1979
American Journal of Pediatric Hematology/Oncology begins publication.	1979
The p53 protein is determined to be a tumor-suppressor gene.	1989

Data from California, University of at Los Angeles School of Public Health. (1979). *A history of cancer control in the United States 1946-1971: Book two, A history of programmatic developments in cancer control.* Washington, DC: Department of Health, Education and Welfare; *Closing in on Cancer.* (1987). Washington, DC: U.S. Department of Health and Human Services; Foundations of clinical cancer research: Perspective for the 21st century. (1997). *Clinical Cancer Research, 3,* 2551-2553; Pochedly, C. P. (1985). Emergence of pediatric hematology/oncology as an independent specialty. *American Journal of Pediatric Hematology/Oncology, 7,* 183-190; Raven, R. W. (1990). *The theory and practice of oncology: Historical evolution and present principles.* Park Ridge, NJ: Parthenon; Ross, W. (1987). *Crusade: The official history of the American Cancer Society.* New York: Arbor House; Shimkin, M. B. (1977). *Contrary to nature.* Washington, DC: U.S. Department of Health, Education and Welfare.

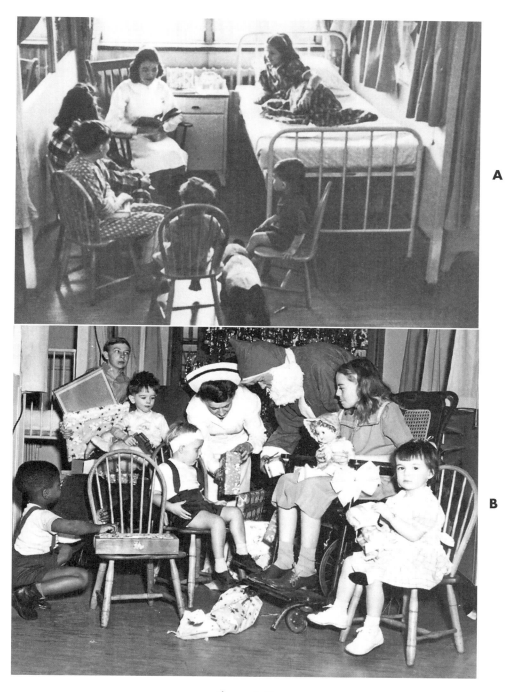

Figure 1-2

A, Story hour in Children's Ward, Memorial Hospital, New York City, 1939. For many years only surgery and radiation were available to treat childhood cancers. Nurses monitored the effects of these treatments while focusing on providing care and comfort. **B,** Christmas party, Children's Ward, Memorial Hospital, New York City, 1945. Even during holiday times, parental visitation was limited. (Courtesy Memorial Sloan-Kettering Cancer Center, New York.)

What role did cancer research have in helping treatment advance?

Unlike today, cancer research did not always enjoy public support, an understandable situation given the priorities of controlling infectious diseases and improving sanitation.[16] Support for research came initially from the private sector and voluntary organizations. Their efforts encouraged government participation in cancer research. An early leader in philanthropic giving was John D. Rockefeller, who established the Rockefeller Institute. The American Society for the Control of Cancer was founded in 1913 to educate the public.[85] Support for research was accomplished through influencing public policy and legislation. The society played a key role in securing passage of the National Cancer Institute Act of 1937 authorizing establishment of the National Cancer Institute (NCI) and a National Advisory Cancer Council. Physician reaction to these initiatives was mixed, with concern expressed about governmental intrusion into research.[17]

In 1944, under the leadership of Mary Lasker, the society was reorganized as the American Cancer Society (ACS). Although a strong emphasis on education and patient services was maintained, a financial commitment to research was made[94] (Figure 1-3).

Undoubtedly the most important piece of legislation affecting cancer in the latter decades of the twentieth century was the National Cancer Act of 1971,[17] which upgraded the National Advisory Cancer Council to the National Cancer Board and which guaranteed by-pass budget approval, a special privilege enjoyed by no other component of the National Institutes of Health. The National Cancer Act also provided for the development of regional cancer centers, a critical element in enhancing availability of optimal treatment to all citizens, and reaffirmed cancer control activities as part of the national agenda.

Although many advances in cancer research, care, and treatment have been made in the United States, it would be an error to assume leadership by the United States alone.[90] Significant contributions have been made by scientists worldwide. Through the efforts of the International Union for Cancer Control (UICC) and other international agencies, global achievements and advances are shared on a regular basis.

An important component of the worldwide effort to advance treatment through research has been the randomized clinical trial. A prospective randomized trial of streptomycin for the control of tuberculosis was published in 1948, the first such contribution to the literature.[43] In oncology, the first randomized clinical trial involved a comparison of two combination chemotherapy regimens. The study was conducted by Emil J. Freireich and

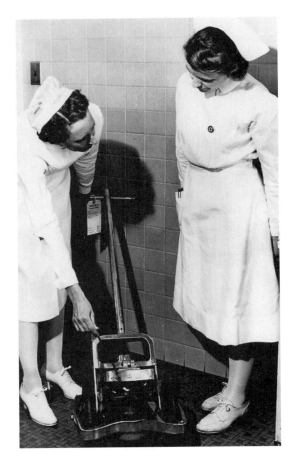

Figure 1-3

Katherine Nelson of Columbia University, New York City, received an American Cancer Society grant in the late 1940s for continuing education of nurses caring for cancer patients. Here she instructs a nurse about transporting radium. (Courtesy Memorial Sloan-Kettering Cancer Center, New York).

his colleagues and was reported in 1958.[46] Acceptance of randomized trials has been variable. Currently less than 10% of adult oncology patients take part in clinical trials.[113] In pediatric oncology the opposite is true, with participation in clinical trials being the rule rather than the exception. Indeed, this acceptance of clinical trials is often identified as the major reason for the enormous strides made in improving childhood cancer outcomes.[11,52]

The factors promoting pediatric oncology clinical trials are both pragmatic and philosophical. Fortunately, pediatric cancer is rare. No one institution cares for sufficient numbers of patients to answer the multiple questions needing resolution for outcomes to improve. This reality becomes more important as disease incidence decreases.

In the mid-1950s two groups were formed that began the development of the cooperative group now in existence.[96,107] The Acute Leukemia Chemotherapy Cooperative Group A led in 1974 to the Children's Cancer Study Group. In 1992 the name of that pediatric group was changed to the Children's Cancer Group (CCG).

The Cancer and Leukemia Group B was the second group started in the 1950s. It was made up of adult and pediatric cancer specialists. The Southwest Oncology Group was originally established as a pediatric group in 1958, although it later became an adult patient group. The pediatric members of these two groups joined forces and asked for recognition as a separate entity. The National Cancer Institute agreed, and in 1980 the Pediatric Oncology Group (POG) came into existence.

Two other groups are important to mention as examples of disease-specific entities dealing with less common pediatric cancers. The National Wilms Tumor Study Group (NWTSG) was established in 1969, the Intergroup Rhabdomyosarcoma Study Group (IRSG) in 1972.

The most recent step in the evolution of the pediatric groups came in 1998, when the leaders of CCG, POG, NWTSG, and IRSG agreed to form a single entity. The unified group, named the Children's Oncology Group (C.O.G.), came into being in part to respond to NCI initiatives aimed at streamlining processes, reducing duplication, and responding to the managed care environment. Other important factors, however, were a growing realization that merger would enhance opportunities for dialogue, research possibilities, quicker accrual of patients, and possibly more rapid answers to some clinical questions.

The philosophical underpinnings of pediatric oncology have been key elements in enhancing cooperation. As a specialty, pediatric oncology welcomed the contributions of various medical specialties from the time of Dr. James Ewing. As noted previously, Dr. Sydney Farber's team at Boston Children's Hospital in the 1940s included nurses and other disciplines. This ability to focus on the needs of patients and families and to welcome all disciplines needed for that care has been a tradition. Like all traditions, in some places and at some times the tradition was honored more fully than others. Yet the basic outlook remains: to guide the specialty through the next set of challenges.

How did nursing respond to the needs of children?

Little documentation exists about the beginnings of nursing.[3,31,61] Evidence from diverse sources indicates that the roles of caretaker of the sick, re-liever of suffering, and conservator of health existed from mankind's earliest days. These roles were implemented in homes, usually by women, as part of everyday life. Another common role was that of wet nurse or caretaker of children. Early Greek literature, for example, contains numerous references to nurses who were primarily children's nurses and not attendants of the sick.[3] The advent of Christianity was a critical event in the history of nursing,[33,35] for it provided the altruistic basis needed to extend caring and service beyond the home, the neighborhood, and the tribe. Christianity elevated care of the sick, homeless, and imprisoned to acts of nobility. Men and women, some wealthy and well-educated for the time, joined religious organizations or communities dedicated to the care of the sick and suffering. No longer were such activities commonplace and unworthy of notice.

Ensuing centuries witnessed the rise of military nursing orders and the formation of several Catholic and Protestant religious communities that provided the finest nursing care for centuries.[33] The Reformation, and later the Industrial Revolution, fostered societal changes that altered the role of religion, the status of women, and attitudes toward children.[31] The care of the sick, the young, and the poor was most adversely affected by these changes.[35] Most hospitals were dirty, overcrowded, and poorly ventilated. Nursing was an undesirable occupation, and those women employed as attendants to the sick were poorly paid, lacked education, and often were of disreputable character.[61] Florence Nightingale (1829-1910) responded to the pressing need to reform nursing. Nightingale was born into an upperclass English family. Well-educated and devoutly religious, Nightingale felt called to care for the sick from her teen years. Because nursing was not suitable for a woman of her social class and moral character, her father refused her permission to become a nurse.[98] Finally she prevailed by going to Kaisersworth Institute for the Training of Deaconesses in Germany. The institute was a model center for learning at that time and taught what was then known about care of the sick.[97]

Almost single-handedly Florence Nightingale addressed key barriers to establishing nursing as a profession. She established a system of education for nurses, used specific measures of patient outcome to demonstrate the correctness of her interventions, and implemented systems of record keeping. A gifted writer, she used prose and statistics to document her many accomplishments.[82,97] The care of children was not Nightingale's main concern, although she wrote regularly about their welfare. She understood the special problems of children and commented that ". . . [they] are much more susceptible than grown people to all noxious influences. They are affected by the same things, but much more quickly and seriously. . . ."[82]

With the establishment of children's hospitals, specialty nursing started to develop. One of the earliest pediatric nursing textbooks, *How to Nurse Sick Children,* was published in London in 1855. It reflected the nurse's predominant role of child caretaker, concerned with maintaining physical care and comfort.[79] Toward the end of the nineteenth century Harvard University in Cambridge, Massachusetts, established the nation's first Department of Pediatrics. Academic pediatrics entered a new era, a development that supported the need for special preparation for nurses to care for children.[111]

The roles assumed by nurses caring for children reflected the needs of the times. As the twentieth century began, most pediatric nurses were experts in infectious diseases. These nurses cared for children in many settings, including the floating hospitals, ships anchored at some distance from the shore that often served as isolation centers.[33]

Care of well children was the prime responsibility of the public health nurse. Many Nightingale schools were located in the large cities of the East, which often had active public health departments. Lillian Wald, founder of the Henry Street Settlement House, and other socially conscious nurses were active participants in the struggle to improve sanitation, decrease morbidity and mortality, and improve the infant mortality rate.[15,35]

The segregation of patients by disease entities began in the 1920s and encouraged the emergence of staff dedicated to a specific clinical problem.[33] The explosion of knowledge and technology that occurred after World War II further hastened the trend toward specialization. Although the roles of nurse midwife and nurse anesthetist had existed since the early part of the century, other expanded and extended roles gradually developed as specialization increased.

Resistance to undergraduate and graduate education for nurses prevented these early efforts from gaining momentum. A parallel issue was the struggle to develop a knowledge base for nursing through nursing research.[81] Without nurses educationally prepared in institutions of higher learning, nursing research could not flourish. Although Florence Nightingale used clinical research to improve patient outcomes, it has taken more than 100 years for nursing research to establish itself firmly.[48]

Collegiate education for nurses, specialization of nursing practice, and nursing research have provided the impetus for sustained progress of the profession of nursing. Table 1-3 highlights selected milestones in the maturation of nursing in the United States.

How did pediatric oncology nursing develop?

The emergence of pediatric oncology nursing as a distinct subspecialty occurred in the late 1940s. At that time the diagnosis of cancer in childhood was a metaphor for death. Nursing care consisted of providing comfort measures and skillfully using analgesics. Keeping a child clean, comfortable, and out of pain was the primary nursing goal. In contrast to the present, complete disclosure was not the norm. Protecting the children from the knowledge of their diagnosis was mandatory, as was supporting the family's denial. It was a time of strained silences and incomplete communication that was difficult for staff and families.[39]

In the 1940s care for children with cancer was provided by private duty nurses as "specials." Most often nurses gained skill and expertise through self-instruction and on-the-job training. Educational opportunities were limited.[27,73] There was little in the literature to inform the specialist nurse. Continuing education as it is known today did not exist.

In the late 1940s children began receiving chemotherapy. At that time the treatment was directed by a tumor therapist, now called a pediatric oncologist, who worked in association with a tumor therapy nurse. Many of the clinical functions of the tumor therapy nurse—administration of chemotherapy, teaching about the disease and treatment, coordinating hospital services for families, home visiting, school visiting, and involvement in research—are similar to ones performed today. Triage skills were taught and monitored by the tumor therapist. Patient management decisions were based on joint decisions about treatment. In sum, most of the earlier nurse's "advanced clinical practice skills" were developed through clinical practice and close association with the tumor therapist who treated children with cancer. Jean Fergusson, an early pioneer in oncology nursing, worked with Dr. Sydney Farber and his associates at Children's Hospital in Boston and helped develop one of the first tumor therapy clinics in the United States for children with cancer. From 1948 to 1953, working both full- and part-time, she enjoyed a clinical practice that included all of the aforementioned responsibilities.

Much of the history of pediatric oncology nursing during the 1950s is lost. A generation of nurses provided undocumented, unheralded care during what was one of the most difficult eras of pediatric oncology. In those days administering chemotherapy to children was considered cruel by some because the remissions were brief, the side effects

TABLE 1-3	SELECTED MILESTONES—MATURATION OF NURSING IN THE UNITED STATES	
Milestone		**Date**
American Society of Superintendents of Training Schools for Nurses forms (eventually known as National League for Nursing).		1893
American Journal of Nursing begins publication.		1900
North Carolina, New Jersey, New York, and Virginia adopt licensing requirements for nursing.		1903
M. Adelaide Nutting is appointed the United States' first Professor of Nursing, Teacher's College, New York.		1907
National Association of Colored Graduated Nurses is established.		1908
University of Minnesota offers first university-based nursing program.		1909
American Nurses Association (ANA) is founded.		1911
National Organization for Public Health Nursing is established.		1912
Sigma Theta Tau, national honor society of nursing, is founded at Indiana University.		1922
The Goldmark Report is released (calls for upgrading of nursing education).		1923
Teacher's College, Columbia University, offers Doctor of Education for nurses preparing to teach at the college level.		1924
Sigma Theta Tau begins funding nursing research.		1936
Esther Lucile Brown publishes *Nursing for the Future,* and recommends collegiate education for nursing.		1948
Nursing Research begins publication.		1952
American Nurses Foundation is established.		1955
Lysaught Report is issued (urges funding for nursing research).		1970
Department of Nursing Research is established within ANA.		1972
Center for Nursing Research is established.		1983
National Center for Nursing Research is set up within the National Institutes of Health.		1985
Title of National Center for Nursing Research is changed to National Institute for Nursing Research.		1993

Data from Deloughery, G. L. (1977). *History and trends of professional nursing* (8th ed.). St. Louis: C. V. Mosby; Dolan, J. A. (1978). *Nursing in society: A historical perspective.* Philadelphia: W. B. Saunders; Kelly, L. Y. (1985). *Dimensions of professional nursing* (5th ed.). New York: Macmillan; Niewsiadomy, R. M. (1987). *Foundations of nursing research.* Norwalk, CT: Appleton & Lange.

devastating, and the supportive interventions limited. Family-centered care was almost unknown. Stringent hospital policies prevented parents from visiting their children more than a few hours per week unless the child was critically ill, and siblings were forgotten (Figure 1-4).

By the 1960s physical outcomes for the child began to improve substantially. More effective treatment strategies were developed, and advances in blood banking, infection control, and pediatric intensive care provided essential supportive care. Psychosocial care became more family centered,[67] partially in response to research findings and partially because of consumer pressure for change. Pediatric oncology nurses established new relationships with parents, which included more emphasis on parent and family participation and education.

In the 1960s pediatric oncology nurses began to assume new roles. Physician mentorship was a key factor in educating nurses for these roles.[42] Once a cadre of nurses was established, continuing education programs often led by these nurses provided the necessary instruction and support. As the roles matured, preparation for them moved into academic institutions.

Research and practice roles followed this general pattern. In the 1960s nurses were recruited to assist with clinical research in pediatric oncology. They received on-the-job training that included physical assessment skills and basic knowledge about medical research methodology. This training was conducted by a pediatric oncologist who was primarily interested in cancer research and who needed a nurse to assist with data collection and patient evaluation. Initially many of these nurses were employed by the Clinical Cancer Research Branch of the National Institutes of Health. Today almost all pediatric oncology nurses play a vital role with pediatric oncologists in the management of medical research protocols. In addition, some nurses design and implement nursing research studies.

The 1960s also were an important period for the development of advanced practice roles. The role of pediatric nurse practitioner developed early and exerted a significant influence on pediatric oncology nursing. The first pediatric nurse practitioner program was established at the University of Colorado in Denver by Dr. Henry Silver, a pediatrician, and Dr. Loretta Ford, a nurse educator.[41,101] This continuing education program prepared candidates

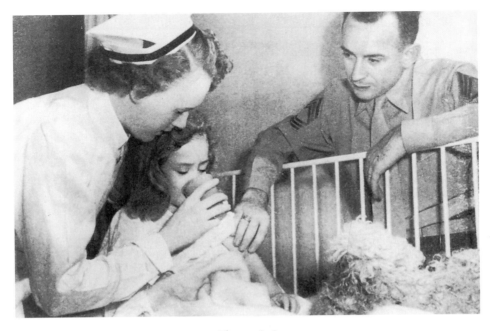

Figure 1-4

Great care was taken in the 1950s to keep the children unaware of what was wrong with them. This father must avoid betraying his feelings to his daughter, who is being given a drink by nurse Lois Jenkins, Head Nurse, Inpatient Tumor Therapy Service, Children's Hospital, Boston.   (Copyright 1951 by the Saturday Evening Post. Thanks to Thomas Coates, MD, an oncologist from the Division of Oncology at Childrens Hospital of Los Angeles [CHLA], who found this issue of the Saturday Evening Post in a thrift shop in Big Bear, California. He brought it back to Kathy Ruccione at CHLA, who sent it east to Jean Fergusson, who will treasure it forever.)

to provide comprehensive well-child care, manage common disorders of childhood, and support age-appropriate development. The program modeled the realignment of the functions performed by pediatric nurses and pediatricians. The nurse practitioner program at the University of Colorado came to the attention of Dr. Donald Pinkel, the first medical director of St. Jude Children's Research Hospital in Memphis. Dr. Pinkel and other physician leaders at St. Jude adapted the Colorado model and provided selected nurses with training in physical assessment skills and advanced technical skills such as bone marrow aspirations and spinal taps.[103] First Andi Wood, then Ellen Shanks, Clara Mason, and Shirley Stagner became nurse practitioners through this program. These women were pioneers in oncology nursing.[49]

The nurse practitioner program at St. Jude was in place when Robbie Simpson, a much-respected staff nurse, died of hepatitis.[50] In her honor the Robbie Simpson Fellowship was created in 1972. The program focused on assessment and advanced technical skills, which were taught through direct participation in care and through educational conferences, seminars, and/or symposia offered by the institution. Those completing the fellowship were

awarded a certificate from St. Jude and were called nurse practitioners in pediatric oncology. Trish Greene, later the first president of the Association of Pediatric Oncology Nurses (APON), was the initial graduate of the program.

The nurse practitioner program at St. Jude Children's Research Hospital and the Robbie Simpson Fellowship influenced the development of pediatric oncology nursing throughout the country. The early leaders of the program emphasized nursing as the central component of the role. These nurses stressed a tradition of nurse mentorship that has characterized the specialty.[95,103]

Jean Fergusson took the next step in the maturation process. In 1976 Fergusson, who was prepared as a nurse practitioner by Northeastern University in Boston, designed a two-semester educational program in pediatric oncology at Children's Hospital of Philadelphia (CHOP). The program offered continuing education for pediatric oncology nurses seeking advanced clinical practice skills, particularly in the ambulatory care setting. Curriculum for the program followed the guidelines developed by the American Nurses Association (ANA) and the American Academy of Pediatrics (AAP), with didactic and clinical focus in pediatric oncology. The

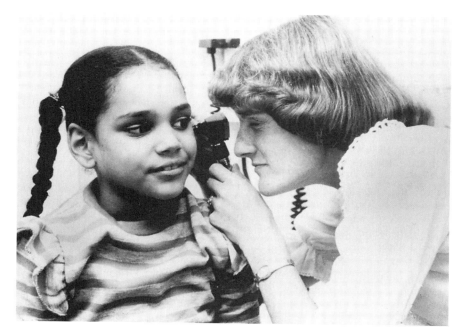

Figure 1-5

The Pediatric Nurse Practitioner program developed by Jean Fergusson at Children's Hospital of Philadelphia educated a cadre of advanced practitioners who provided pediatric oncology nursing throughout the country.   (Photograph of Judie Lea courtesy Jean Fergusson, RN, and Children's Hospital of Philadelphia.)

first two students in the program were Mary Waskerwitz from Mott Children's Hospital in Ann Arbor, Michigan, and Betsy Becker from CHOP. Within a year this pioneering program was approved by the National Association of Pediatric Nurse Associates and Practitioners (NAPNAP) and the Pennsylvania State Board of Nursing.

The CHOP program provided a select group of pediatric oncology nurses with practitioner skills and knowledge about the most recent advances in pediatric oncology. Eventually the program became associated with Widener University Graduate School of Nursing in Chester, Pennsylvania, and was changed from continuing education to graduate education, with ongoing sponsorship by the cancer center at CHOP. The influence of the CHOP program was enormous. Ninety-four nurses completed the program, and most are practicing in cancer centers throughout this nation and Canada, with many becoming leaders in pediatric oncology nursing (Figure 1-5).

By the mid-1980s continuing education programs to prepare nurses as practitioners were phased out. Education for the role became part of graduate nursing programs that award a master's degree and enable graduates to obtain specific practitioner licensure in those states requiring it.

Pediatric oncology nursing was a pioneer in the development and use of expanded nursing roles.[49] The idea that nurse practitioners could provide ambulatory care for chronically ill children was tested and validated in pediatric oncology. That contribution is part of the specialty's lasting legacy. Other advanced roles such as nurse clinician[40] and clinical nurse specialist[56] have contributed to the development of pediatric oncology nursing. These roles have been based primarily in the inpatient setting. Each role has been characterized by the ability to use advances in medical and nursing research and in clinical practice, to exhibit a high level of professional accountability, and to function both independently and interdependently with other providers.[53] Individuals in these advanced roles understand that accountability flows from an adequate knowledge base and a lifelong commitment to learning.[84]

Advanced nursing practice is a dynamic, evolving entity. In some settings the roles of pediatric nurse practitioner and clinical nurse specialist are coming together to provide care for hospitalized pediatric patients.[47] This trend may represent an opportunity to expand the definition of nursing practice. Nurse practitioner care of chronically ill children was a development of the role beyond well-child care. Having nurse practitioners care for children sick enough to require hospitalization may be another plateau. The nurse practice act of each state may or may not accommodate such a change, but testing of that limit is likely.

As cancer prevention strategies mature, pediatric oncology nurses will assume more visible roles in educating young people about avoiding the cancers of adulthood. Prime opportunities involve informing young people about positive measures they can take to control their health. Areas of particular emphasis include use of sunscreens, prevention of obesity, selection of low-fat, high-roughage foods, and moderate use of alcohol. Of special importance are behaviors that support avoidance of tobacco in all its deleterious forms. In these and other areas of cancer prevention, the most basic role of the pediatric oncology nurse is that of exemplar (Figure 1-6).

In the evolution of oncology nursing, nursing research has played a vital role.[74] The concept of research as the foundation for oncology nursing practice developed in the 1970s, relatively early in the specialty, but its actualization awaited the formation of the Oncology Nursing Society (ONS) and APON. The small band of doctoral-prepared nurse researchers flourished once opportunities for collabo-

ration, education, and improved funding emerged. Efforts of these national oncology nursing associations also helped to influence the development of key ACS programs. In the 1980s, under the leadership of Trish Greene, then National Vice President for Patient Services, the society established scholarships for nurses at the master's and doctoral levels and a program of ACS Professors of Oncology Nursing.

Collaborations between specialty nursing and voluntary organizations were critical to the development of the specialty. The ACS's National Nursing Advisory Committee, established in 1951, provided the sole national forum for cancer nurses for decades.[58] APON quickly established ties with the National Nursing Advisory Committee, and in the process APON began to identify itself as a leader in cancer care.[55] Trish Greene and Gen Foley were the first APON representatives to the committee. They and other pediatric oncology nurses made significant and varied contributions to ACS throughout its organizational structure.

As oncology nursing developed and specialized, more specific opportunities for networking and education were needed.[5] APON met this challenge and established formal relationships with other nursing organizations, particularly ONS, ANA, and

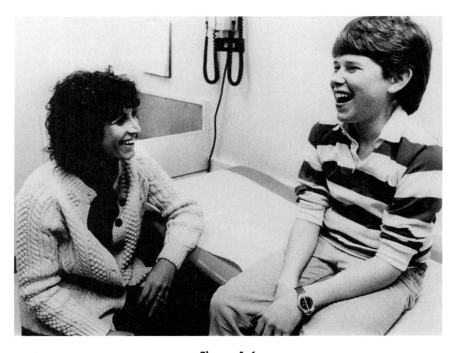

Figure 1-6

Physical and psychosocial evaluation of childhood cancer survivors is an important new role for the pediatric oncology nurse. (Photograph of Wendy Hobbie courtesy Jean Fergusson, RN, and Children's Hospital of Philadelphia.)

the Federation of Nursing Specialty Organizations. Strong ties with the national parent support group, Candlelighters, and other parent groups have matured throughout the years and constitute a significant source of support for both groups. Improvements in physical and psychosocial aspects of care have been facilitated by these relationships.

The contributions made by pediatric oncology nurses, through professional and voluntary organizations and with consumer groups, were matched in significance by the contributions made to the pediatric cooperative groups.[96] Dr. Denman Hammond, chair of the Children's Cancer Group, directed that a nursing committee be formed. Gail Perin took up the challenge, becoming nursing committee chair in February 1979. Over the years the role of nursing matured so that most study committees included nurses. The contributions of these nurses has been broad, from review of protocol design and recommendations about frequency of laboratory tests to writing selected protocol sections and studying the process of informed consent.

POG used a different model, in part because the nursing leaders (Geri Van-Wezel, Pat Klopovich, Debra Gaddy, and Ann Pumphrey) who requested a nursing committee in 1981 focused on nursing research. The POG Nursing Research Committee formed with ambivalent support from POG physician leaders. As a result original goals were not fully attained, and reorganization occurred in 1989. The newly revamped Nursing Committee was divided into Administration, Education, and Research subcommittees, with resultant expansion of opportunities for nurses. Nursing began participating in core POG committees concerned with protocol development and review, patient and professional education, and initiation and review of research activities. The new role of nursing in POG was acknowledged formally when the Nursing Discipline chair, Kathy Patterson Kelly, was fully funded to participate in the group's competitive renewal site visit in 1995.

With the establishment of C.O.G., new opportunities have been identified. Pediatric oncology nurses are in an ideal position to assist the transition of CCG and POG into a unified group. Most nurse members of each group have worked together through APON, ACS, or disease-specific and consumer-led groups. As the multidisciplinary C.O.G. moves the pediatric cancer agenda forward, the expectation is that pediatric oncology nursing is ready and able to play critical roles and meet future challenges.

Pediatric oncology nurses are proud of their historical contributions to the care of children and families, the multidisciplinary team, the profession of nursing in general, and cancer nursing in particular. They have facilitated advances in the biologic and social sciences by their own scholarship and research and by participation in the scholarly and research activities of other professionals. These accomplishments provide a strong foundation from which to face future challenges. Table 1-4 presents selected milestones in the history of pediatric oncology nursing.

What are the issues and trends?

What are the actual and potential issues and trends that will test pediatric oncology nursing in the years ahead; influence practice, education, and research; compel the establishment or renewal of alliances; and require the assessment and development of more effective strategies for action? Although prediction is always a risky business, it is likely that the following will be of importance:

Managing the impact of changes in family life

General societal trends in the United States related to family composition and structure will continue to exert an important influence on young people in the United States as children and adolescents seek to establish long-term emotional ties with significant adults. Key demographic variables for marriage, nonmarital child-bearing, divorce, and cohabitation all indicate that many children and teens will experience being in a single-parent family, having parents divorce, or living in a household where the adults are cohabitating.[110]

Beginning in the mid-1960s and continuing through 1999, there was a clear trend for women to remain unmarried.[110] As might be expected, with such significant numbers of women of childbearing age unmarried, nonmarital childbearing rose steadily with dramatic increases in the late 1970s through the 1980s to a peak in 1990 (Figure 1-7). The number of births to unmarried women rose sharply in the 1980s, averaging a 6% increase per year. The number of births to unmarried women increased an average of 1% per year between 1990 and 1999. The birth rate shows a similar pattern, with a return to close to 1990 values (43.8 births per 1000 unmarried women age 14 to 44 years) by the end of that decade. Finally the percent of births to unmarried women has followed a similar course, with stable percentages in the 32% to 33% range.[110]

Two other demographic facts of importance are the age shift for unmarried mothers and a decline in childbearing for those who are married. The typical age for an unmarried mother increased between 1970 and 1999. In 1970 half of all unmarried births were to teens. Since 1985 women in their twenties make up half of all unmarried births, with teens accounting for about a third (Figure 1-8). Youth Risk Behavior Surveys, conducted by the Centers for Disease Control and Prevention (CDC), indicate more effective use of contraceptives and a rise in abstinence behaviors. The leveling off of teenage women even having sexual intercourse reverses a 2-decade upward trend from the 1970s and 1980s.

There was a 40% decrease in birth rates for married women from the 1960s to the late 1980s (Figure 1-9). The causes for the decline are not well defined, but later age at marriage, economic and career demands, and responsibilities for aging family members are all possible factors.[110]

Divorce statistics provide another data point to consider. From a 1960 low of 9.2 divorces per 1000 married woman 15 years of age and older, the rate of divorce rose steadily. Since 1975 the national divorce rate has been in a range from 20.3 to 22.8 divorces per 1000 married woman 15 years of age and older. Although state-by-state variations in rates occur, the general trend mirrors national data.[9]

From 1950 to 1988 the median years of marriage before divorce fluctuated from 5.8 years to 7.1 years. As might be anticipated, large numbers of young people were impacted by the dissolution of marriages in this range of years married. In that period the number of children under 18 involved in divorce each year rose from 299,000 in 1950 to 1,044,000 in 1988.[10] In addition, older adolescents have experienced the repercussions of recent increases in dissolution of marriages lasting 25 to 30 years.[2] Cumulative figures of children involved in or affected by divorce are not available.

Cohabitation is a demographic variable that has emerged as an important societal trend. The Center

TABLE 1-4	SELECTED MILESTONES IN PEDIATRIC ONCOLOGY NURSING	
Milestone	**Date**
Pediatric Oncology Nurse Practitioner role is created at St. Jude Children's Research Hospital. Andi Wood, Ellen Shanks, Clara Mason, and Shirley Stagner are first to implement role.	1969
Candlelighters forms under leadership of Grace Powers Monaco.	1970
Eugenia Waechter publishes landmark study on children's awareness of fatal illness.	1971
St. Jude Hospital institutes Robbie Simpson Memorial Traineeship. Patricia E. Greene is first graduate.	1972
American Cancer Society's First National Cancer Nursing Conference is held. Session on childhood cancer nursing is included. Association of Pediatric Oncology Nurses (APON) is founded.	1973
Trish Greene is elected first APON president.	1974
Oncology Nursing Society (ONS) is incorporated in the state of Illinois.	July 1, 1975
APON is incorporated in the state of Tennessee.	April 15, 1976
Jean Fergusson develops pediatric nurse practitioner (PNP) in oncology program at Children's Hospital of Philadelphia.	1976
Liaison is established with ONS.	1978
Ida Martinson publishes pioneer research on home care for children dying of cancer.	1978
Standards of Care is published; provides first subspecialty standards in oncology nursing.	1979
First textbook of pediatric oncology nursing is published, with Dianne Fochtman and Genevieve Foley as editors.	1982
Journal of the Association of Pediatric Oncology Nursing (JAPON) is established, with Dianne Fochtman as editor.	1984
Marilyn Hockenberry and Deborah Coody publish *Pediatric Oncology and Hematology: Perspectives on Care.*	1986
First issue of the *Journal of Pediatric Oncology Nursing (JOPON)* is published by W.B. Saunders, with Dianne Fochtman continuing as editor.	1989
Certification for pediatric oncology nursing begins.	1993
Core Curriculum is published by APON.	1998
State of the Science in Pediatric Oncology Nursing Research Summit is held.	2000

Data from Ferguson, J. (1991). Pediatric oncology nursing: A historical perspective. Fifteenth Annual APON Conference: Keynote Address. Boston; Greene, P. (1983). The Association of Pediatric Oncology Nurses: The first ten years. *Oncology Nursing Forum, 10,* 59-63; Heiney, S.P., & Wiley, F.M. (1996). Historical beginnings of a professional nursing organization dedicated to the care of children and adolescents with cancer and their families: The Association of Pediatric Oncology Nursing from 1974-1993. *Journal of Pediatric Oncology Nursing, 13,* 196-203; Hilkemeyer, R. (1982). A historical perspective in cancer nursing. *Oncology Nursing Forum, 9,* 47.

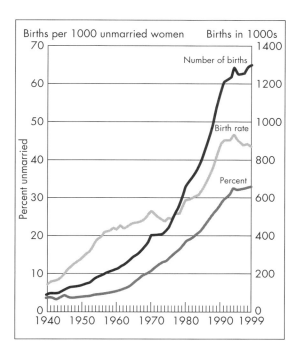

Figure 1-7

Number of births, birth rate, and percent of births to un-married women: United States, 1940-1999.

for Law and Social Policy[93] indicates that between 1970 and 1994 the number of unmarried couples living together went from approximately 500,000 to almost 3.7 million. In 1994 35% of those cohabiting households included children under the age of 15. In 1990 one in seven children residing with a cohabiting couple were officially defined as being in a single-parent situation. Neither gender nor ethnicity is a significant variable in the rate of living in a cohabiting family situation, although cohabitation is more likely among those without a high school education and those who have experienced marital instability.

About 40% of cohabiting relationships end before marriage. Typically, there is a 2-year period of cohabitation that precedes either marriage or the conclusion of the relationship. The longer a couple lives together, the less likely they will marry. About 10% of nonmarried cohabitants will have a long-term relationship.

Taken together, these demographic factors indicate a continuous and substantial need to support children and adolescents attempting to cope with changing family environments. Even if these demographics begin to trend toward greater family stability, an unlikely prospect given the consistency of these trends, millions of children and teens have been impacted.

In assessing the implications of these trends, the pediatric oncology nurse must understand that in

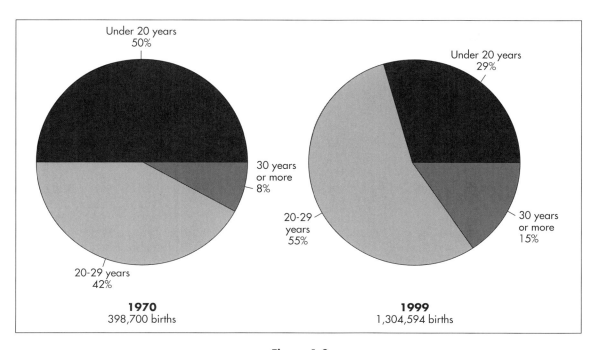

Figure 1-8

Distribution of nonmarital births by age: United States, 1970 and 1999.

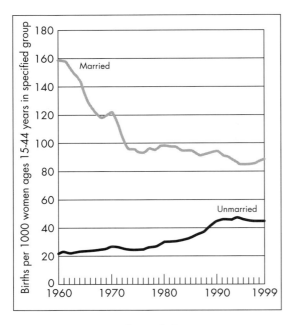

Figure 1-9

Birth rates for married and unmarried women: United States, 1960-1999.

periods of rapid social change, the problem of adjustment is especially great and leads to increasing signs of personal and family stress.[72] A significant stressor for children is that fewer children today know the benefits of lifelong dependable ties between themselves and their parents. In addition, nontraditional living patterns, although not necessarily detrimental to the child, do require extra attention by the adults in the child's world to mitigate negative consequences. One potentially positive development is the increased life expectancy in the United States, such that the norm is becoming the three-generation family.[112] Healthy, involved elders may be able to assume roles of consistent nurturer, supporter, and advocate.

Another suggested consequence of these trends is increased family isolation. Greater efforts must also be made to decrease isolation experienced by families as they try to maintain cohesion and stability. In those efforts, the child's parents or caretakers often turn to health and social agencies, their local religious and civic communities, and their extended families. A new initiative developed by the Annie E. Casey Foundation seeks to reframe the lens through which families, especially poor families, are viewed. The foundation is stressing the importance of family connections, inclusion in economic opportunities, and stronger ties to social networks. Particular emphasis is being placed on

faith institutions, for so long a stabilizing force but now many times an overwhelmed resource, and on restoring social networks and human connections. Such ambitious efforts must be supported.[64]

The diagnosis of cancer strains the most stable marriage and the strongest family. The pediatric oncology nurse likely will encounter more complex, less stable family situations, requiring greater theoretic knowledge and more sophisticated skills. Knowledge of community resources will be ever more essential to assist growing numbers of single adult families taking on the complex care needs of pediatric oncology patients.

Another emerging issue from an assessment of demographic data is how this information pertains to cancer survivors. Traditional measures such as age at marriage or whether ever married have been used to gauge the emotional health of survivors. Social scientists and researchers must take societal trends into account, lest a false picture be created. In the history of pediatric oncology, such a situation has occurred already. Early studies on divorce among couples came from a state with a divorce rate higher than the national average.[62] Later work verified that years married and state of residence should be factored into research methodology.[70]

These scholarly endeavors will be hampered by a 1996 decision that the National Center for Health Statistics (NCHS) would no longer keep comprehensive, detailed data on marriage and divorce. Although some nongovernment sources are planning to fill the void created by the NCHS, it remains likely that the process of obtaining data, analyzing trends, and forming appropriate social policy interventions will be more difficult.[21]

Maintaining and improving outcomes of care

The therapies of the last 50 years have resulted in significant advances in lives saved. Since 1973 overall survival has improved yearly. For specific pediatric cancers, an upward survival curve has existed even longer.[78,92] So dramatic are these improvements that currently it is estimated that 1 in 900 persons 15 to 45 years of age is a survivor of childhood cancer.[11] Despite this substantial progress, more must be done, for the average years of life lost to pediatric cancer remains unacceptably high.[91] Three factors are likely to be important in improving outcomes of care: changes in treatment, improvement in care delivery systems, and advocacy for special populations.

James Ewing once likened the struggle against cancer to a marathon.[60] Indeed the history of oncology demonstrates that progress has been uneven, with times of rapid progress alternating with languid or stagnant periods.[68] To move patient outcomes for the diseases such as neuroblastoma and brain tumors, new ideas are needed. Where will these ideas come from? The hope is that the insights gained from the mapping of the human genome and the development of therapies targeted to alter basic cellular processes will provide that new energy and innovation. Technical problems abound, however, and the pace of progress may be slower than hoped.

A related issue concerns the nature of clinical trials. In some quarters there is frustration with the current reliance on prospective, randomized clinical trials as the only way to advance outcomes.[44,59] In the decade ahead, it is possible that other strategies will be employed to improve outcomes, especially in bleak clinical situations. The acquired immuno-deficiency syndrome (AIDS) advocacy community has demonstrated the benefits of selectively fast-tracking treatment alternatives. This model may be of use in certain pediatric cancers.

Largely in response to the era of managed care, the new discipline of outcomes management has emerged to systematically assess changes in health care delivery systems.[71] New federal initiatives have emerged, and a growing body of literature has developed. Although the nursing profession's contribution to improved patient outcomes is not an important aspect of outcomes research at present, nursing organizations have begun to develop outcome indicators reflective of quality nursing practice.[74] It is essential that these efforts be supported by the nursing community. Identifying populations at risk for not participating in cancer care improvements is an important task. Concerns remain that adolescents are an underserved population. Most pediatric statistics end after 14 years of age, some extend to 19 years of age, and others group 15- to 24-year-olds together. Obtaining accurate data describing cancer in the teen years is important for several reasons. Recent Surveillance, Epidemiology, and End Results (SEER) data demonstrate an increasing cancer incidence in 15- to 19-year-olds.[102] Evidence suggests that some adolescents are not receiving state-of-the-art physical and psychosocial care.[19] Adolescents apparently are not entered in either pediatric or adult cooperative group trials; therefore they less frequently receive the benefits of multidisciplinary involvement in planning and carrying out treatment strategies.[12] Adolescents may receive care on adult units from staff members who are not aware of the appropriate spectrum of psychosocial supports and interventions required. The ACS maintains that adolescent care outcomes require further study and action if outcomes of care are suboptimal. Pediatric oncology nurses need to assist in the fact-finding effort, offer consultation services to adult units caring for

adolescents, and advocate adolescent registration in clinical trials.

Attention must be paid to a broad range of concerns. Thus two other significant areas involved in maintaining and improving outcomes of care are psychosocial wellness and late effects of cancer and its treatment, both of which are covered in specific chapters of this book. The concept of the truly cured child[109] is a goal for all pediatric oncology patients.

Economics and access to care

The United States is one of the world's wealthiest countries, yet data from a United Nations (UN) study indicate that child poverty in the United States is the highest of 17 developed countries.[64] Data gathered in the United States reveal that the percentage of children in poverty worsened by 5% in 1998. Between 1976 and 1998 there was an increase of 2.3 million children among the ranks of the poor. A shift has occurred in that most of the increase took place among the "working poor." Over the last 20 years the number of children living in welfare-dependent families has steadily declined.[64]

An issue closely linked to child poverty is availability of health care resources and the ability to access those resources. In general, access to well-child care among children and adolescents is uneven and in some cases inadequate.[100] Among children living in central cities in 1998, 11% of those in affluent communities did not have health insurance. In neighborhoods with high poverty rates the uninsured child rate rose to 17%.[64]

Availability of health insurance is often tied to job benefits. The phenomenon of companies' diminishing health benefits has been somewhat softened by the shrinking labor pool and competition to attract qualified workers. Efforts to enhance job training, provide computer education, and improve schools all impact marketability and, indirectly, access to health insurance. In 1998 in high poverty neighborhoods 84% of households with children did not have a computer; indeed 17% did not even have a telephone. This is in contrast to 35% in low poverty neighborhoods being without a computer in 1998 and 4% without telephone service.[64]

Also influencing availability of health insurance is variability in state "safety net" programs. State eligibility criteria for inclusion in Medicaid programs, the degree of state participation in the Children's Health Insurance Program (CHIP), and elimination of benefits previously used by welfare-dependent families have all caused gaps in the safety net constructed to protect the nation's most vulnerable citizens, its children.

The impact of managed care was alluded to earlier. There certainly are positive aspects of managed care, such as the emphasis on prevention and early detection for cancers, support of smoking cessation programs, and lowered health premiums for some individuals and businesses.

On the negative side there are institutional and individual examples. One of the most well-known, yet in some ways perplexing, outcomes of the managed care environment occurred in Boston. The Harvard Joint Center for Radiation Therapy was established in 1968 as a model of collaborative, inter-hospital ventures. A group of Harvard teaching hospitals agreed not to duplicate services, to focus on patient needs, and to conduct high-quality research. Despite great success, this model could not withstand the pressures of the managed care environment. Beginning in late 1996 a process of mergers began that increased competition and weakened the cooperation and mutual trust on which the Joint Center rested. In 1999 the Joint Center's 31-year history came to an end.[20]

On a day-in, day-out level, families and health care institutions devote considerable time, effort, and emotional energy to securing needed services. Efforts to pass a national Patient's Bill of Rights have failed despite strong support by patient advocate groups and national cancer organizations. While the previously offered bills may have been flawed in some respects, the concept of holding managed care companies accountable for their part in patient outcomes is likely to gain momentum as the baby boomer generation needs more services.

Awareness of economic factors is essential for the pediatric oncology nurse. Also vital is knowledge of the resources available and missing in the child's particular community. Close working relationships with social workers and the personnel of community agencies are critical. Finally alliances must be formed with those concerned with improving access. Organizations such as the American Academy of Pediatrics, Candlelighters, the National Association of Children's Hospitals and Related Institutions (NACHRI), and the Children's Defense Fund have advocacy programs for children. The pediatric oncology nurse, individually and through APON and ANA, must work to forge improvements in children's health.

Creating and strengthening alliances

The problems facing children with cancer and their families will be increasingly complex and will require new strategies. Alliances among the current pediatric team must be strengthened to provide the child and family with optimal care. Also important will be strengthening ties within pediatric nursing. As the pediatric community has become increas-ingly concerned about over-subspecialization, there has been a call for renewed cooperation within pediatrics. Nurses caring for children with other chronic illnesses may be a valuable resource in areas such as adherence to treatment regimens, integration of growth and development concepts in psychosocial care and patient teaching, and bereavement interventions.

The creation of nurse-to-nurse networks with colleagues in adult nursing will be of greater importance. The emergence of a large group of pediatric cancer survivors will compel dialogue with nurses in college infirmaries, internal medicine practices, obstetric practices, and gynecology facilities. Such collaboration is essential to enhance understanding of late consequences of treatment and to ensure optimal care for the "pediatric graduate."[66,75]

Pediatric oncology nurses must also broaden their role to encompass public and social advocacy. The time and energy required to provide nursing care to the children and families are extensive. Yet without a commitment to participate in legislative and public policy change, the work of the pediatric oncology nurse cannot achieve its full potential.

Retaining nursing focus on humanizing the cancer experience

A key role of the pediatric oncology nurse is to humanize the cancer experience[3]—to connect with the child and family in such a way that the dignity, uniqueness, and strengths of the child and family are enhanced. Technology is a potential force for dehumanization, and pediatric oncology is a technology-intense specialty. To focus beyond the disease, beyond the technology, is a constant challenge for the nurse.

Although there are many possible concerns, those relating to ethics are especially important.[7,30,108] Integrating ethical principles into nursing practice and research requires that the nurse be knowledgeable about specific issues relating to the care of minors. Consent for treatment, particularly if it is of limited or no benefit to the child, the need to obtain the child's assent for participation in research studies, and limits on parental decision making are all areas of special importance. Pediatric oncology first challenged existing ethical thought by using investigational agents on terminally ill children. Now broad ethical issues involve genetic engineering, whether it is ethical to conceive a child to be a transplant donor, and conflicts between parent and child about termination of treatment. It is clear that technology will continue to become available before society has reached consensus on the ethical issues involved. The long tradition of advocacy and social activism that has characterized pediatrics will demand that pediatric oncology nurses contribute to the societal dialogue and assist in achieving resolution.

REFERENCES

1. Armitage, J. O. (1997). *The development of bone marrow transplantation as a treatment for patients with lymphoma.* 20th Richard and Hinds Rosenthal Foundation Award Lecture, *Clinical Cancer Research 3,* 829-836.
2. Arp, D., & Arp, C. (1997). *The second half of marriage.* Grand Rapids, MI: Zondervan.
3. Austin, A. L. (1957). *History of nursing source book.* New York: G. P. Putnam's Sons.
4. Ballabriga, A. (1991). One century of pediatrics in Europe. In B. L. Nichols, A. Ballabriga, & N. Kretchmer (Eds.), *Nestle nutrition workshop series* (Vol. 22, pp. 1-21). New York: Raven Press.
5. Barckley, V. (1982). The best of times and the worst of times: Historical reflections from an American Cancer Society national nursing consultant. *Oncology Nursing Forum, 9,* 54-56.
6. Bender, G. A. (1961). *Great moments in medicine.* Detroit, MI: Parke-Davis.
7. Benjamin, M., & Cures, J. (1992). *Ethics in nursing* (3rd ed.). New York: Oxford Press.
8. Bett, W. R. (1957). Historical aspects of cancer. In R. W. Raven (Ed.), *Cancer* (Vol. 1). London: Butterworth & Co.
9. Births, marriages, divorces, and deaths: provisional data for October 1999. (September 6, 2000). *National Vital Statistics Reports, 48,* 15.
10. Births, marriages, divorces, and deaths: provisional data for November 1999. (October 31, 2000). *National Vital Statistics Reports, 48,* 17.
11. Bleyer, W. A. (1990). The impact of childhood cancer on the United States and the world. *CA: A Cancer Journal for Clinicians, 40,* 355-367.
12. Bleyer, W., Tejada, H., Murphy, S. et al. (1997). National cancer clinical trials: Children have equal access; adolescents do not. *Journal of Adolescent Health, 2,* 366-373.
13. Bordley, J. III, & McGehee, H. A. (1976). *Two centuries of American medicine.* Philadelphia: W. B. Saunders.
14. Brothwell, D. (1967). The evidence for neoplasms. In D. Brothwell, & A. T. Sanderson (Eds.) *Diseases in antiquity.* Springfield, IL.: Charles C. Thomas.
15. Buhler-Wilkerson, K. (1991). Lillian Wald: Public health pioneer, *Nursing Research, 40,* 316-317.
16. California, University of, at Los Angeles School of Public Health. (1979). *A history of cancer control in the United States 1946-1971: Introductory materials.* Washington, DC: Department of Health, Education and Welfare.
17. California, University of, at Los Angeles School of Public Health. (1979). *A history of cancer control in the United States 1946-1971: Book two, A history of programmatic developments in cancer control.* Washington, DC: Department of Health, Education and Welfare.
18. Charney, E. (1990). The field of pediatrics. In F. A. Oski, C. D. De Angelis, R. D. Feigin et al. (Eds.), *Principles and practice of pediatrics* (pp. 4-10). Philadelphia: J. B. Lippincott.
19. Children and adolescents with cancer: Report of an American Cancer Society workshop. (1992). Atlanta: American Cancer Society.
20. Coleman, C. N., Govern, F. S., Svensson, G. et al. (2000). The Harvard Joint Center for Radiation Therapy, 1968-1999: A unique concept and its relationship to the prevailing times in academic medicine. *International Journal Radiation Oncology Biology Physics, 47,* 1357-1369.
21. Concerned Woman for America. (1999). Marriages no longer count: Government stops collecting marriage/divorce data. (http://cwfa.org/library/family/1999-06-18 marriage-stats.shtml).
22. Cone, T. E., Jr. (1979). *History of American pediatrics.* Boston: Little, Brown.
23. Considine, B. (1959). *That many may live.* New York: Memorial Center for Cancer & Allied Diseases.
24. Copeland, E. M. (1999). Surgical oncology: A specialty in evolution. *Annals of Surgical Oncology, 6,* 424-432.
25. Cox, J. D. (1999). Oncology at the end of the century. Signed editorial. *International Journal of Radiation Oncology Biology Physics, 45,* 1095-1096.
26. Cox, J. D. (1999). The science and art of radiation oncology after a century. Signed editorial. *International Journal of Radiation Oncology Biology Physics, 43,* 1-2.
27. Craytor, J. K. (1982). Highlights in education for cancer nursing. *Oncology Nursing Forum, 9,* 51-59.
28. Dargeon, H. W. (1940). Malignant tumors in childhood. In H. W. Dargeon (Ed.), *Cancer in childhood* (pp. 21-30). St. Louis: C. V. Mosby.
29. Dargeon, H. W. (1960). *Tumors of childhood: A clinical treatise.* New York: Paul B. Hoeber.
30. Davis, A. J., & Aroskar, M. A. (1991). *Ethical dilemmas and nursing practice* (3rd ed.). Norwalk, CT: Appleton & Lange.
31. Deloughery, G. L. (1977). *History and trends of professional nursing* (8th ed.). St. Louis: C. V. Mosby.
32. Diamond, L. K. (1989). Foreword. In D. R. Miller, R. Baehner, & L. P. Miller (Eds.), *Blood diseases of infancy and childhood* (pp. 9-13). St. Louis: C. V. Mosby.
33. Dolan, J. A. (1978). *Nursing in society: A historical perspective.* Philadelphia: W. B. Saunders.
34. Doll, R. (1999). Nature and nurture in the control of cancer. *European Journal of Cancer, 35,* 16-23.
35. Donahue, M. P. (1985). *Nursing: The finest art.* St. Louis: C. V. Mosby.
36. Duffy, J. (1979). *The healers: A history of American medicine.* Urbana: University of Illinois Press.
37. Ewing, J. (1940). A survey of cancer in children. In H. W. Dargeon (Ed.), *Cancer in childhood* (pp. 13-20). St. Louis: C. V. Mosby.
38. Farber, S. (1969). The control of cancer in children. In *Neoplasia in childhood* (pp. 321-327). Chicago: Year Book.
39. Fergusson, J. (1991). Pediatric oncology nursing: A historical perspective. Fifteenth Annual APON Conference: Keynote Address. Boston.
40. Foley, G. V. (1983). The role of the pediatric nurse clinician in pediatric oncology. In J. A. Beal (Ed.), *Issues and advanced practice in pediatric nursing* (pp. 155-174). Reston, VA: Reston Publishing.
41. Ford, L. (1979). A nurse for all settings: The nurse practitioner. *Nursing Outlook, 27,* 516-521.
42. Forte, K. (2001). Pediatric oncology nursing: Providing care through decades of change. *Journal of Pediatric Oncology Nursing, 18,* 154-163.
43. Freireich, E. J. (1997). The future of clinical cancer research into the next millennium. *Clinical Cancer Research, 3,* 2563-2570.
44. Freireich, E. J. (1997). Who took the clinical out of clinical research? Mouse versus man: 7th David A. Karnofsky Memorial Lecture 1976. *Clinical Cancer Research, 3,* 2711-2722.

45. Garrison, F. H. (1965). History of pediatrics. In F. Abt, & F. H. Garrison (Eds.), *Abt-Garrison history of pediatrics* (pp. 1-170). Philadelphia: W. B. Saunders.

46. Gehan, E. A. (1997). The scientific basis of clinical trials: Statistical aspects. *Clinical Cancer Research, 3,* 2587-2590.

47. Gleeson, R. M., McIlwain-Simpson, G., Boos, M. L., et al. (1990). Advanced practice nursing: a model of collaborative care, *MCN, 15,* 9-12.

48. Grant, M. M., & Padilla, G.V. (1990). *Cancer nursing research: A practical approach.* Norwalk, CT: Appleton & Lange.

49. Greene, P. (1983). The Association of Pediatric Oncology Nurses: The first ten years. *Oncology Nursing Forum, 10,* 59-63.

50. Greene, P. (1992). Personal communication. Atlanta.

51. Gutterman, J. U. (1997). Recreating an environment for clinical discovery. *Clinical Cancer Research, 3,* 2594-2597.

52. Hammond, G. D. (1986). The cure of childhood cancers, *Cancer, 58*(2 Suppl.), 407-413.

53. Hamric, A., & Spross, J. (1983). *The clinical nurse specialist in theory and practice.* New York: Grune & Stratton.

54. Harrison, H. E. (1990). The history of pediatrics in the United States. In F. A. Oski, C. D. De Angelis, R. D. Feigin, et al. (Eds.), *Principles and practice of pediatrics* (pp. 2-4). Philadelphia: J.B. Lippincott.

55. Heiney, S. P., & Wiley, F. M. (1996). Historical beginnings of a professional nursing organization dedicated to the care of children and adolescents with cancer and their families: The Association of Pediatric Oncology Nursing from 1974 to 1993. *Journal of Pediatric Oncology Nursing, 13,* 196-203.

56. Henke, C. (1980). Emerging roles of the nurse in oncology. *Seminars in Oncology, 7,* 4-8.

57. Hersh, E. M., & Stopeck, A. T. (1997). Advances in the biological therapy and gene therapy of malignant disease. *Clinical Cancer Research, 3,* 2623-2629.

58. Hilkemeyer, R. (1982). A historical perspective in cancer nursing. *Oncology Nursing Forum, 9,* 47.

59. Holland, J. F. (1997). Clinical trials in cancer. *Clinical Cancer Research, 3,* 2585-2586.

60. Jay, V. (1999). Legacy of Dr. Ewing. *Pediatric and Developmental Pathology, 2,* 597-598.

61. Kalisch, P. A., & Kalisch, B. J. (1978). *The advance of American nursing.* Boston: Little, Brown.

62. Kaplan, D. M., Grobstein, R., & Smith, A. (1976). Predicting the impact of severe illness on families. *Health and Social Work, 1,* 71-82.

63. Keil, H. (1950). The historical relationship between the concept of tumor and the ending—Oma. *Bulletin of the History of Medicine, 24,* 352-375.

64. Kids Count Data Book: State Profiles of Child Well-Being. (2000). Baltimore: The Annie E. Casey Foundation.

65. Kim, R. Y. (1996). Radiation oncology at the centennial. *Alabama Medicine, 65, (Feb-Apr)(8-10),* 6-8.

66. Komp, D. M. (1991). The medical care of young adults: The practice of ephebiatrics? *Journal of Adolescent Health, 12,* 291-293.

67. Koocher, G., & O'Malley, E. (1981). *The Damocles syndrome.* New York: McGraw-Hill.

68. Koten, J. W., Beukers, H., & DenOtter, W. (1999). History of cancer research in nosological perspective. *Anticancer Research, 19,* 4613-4626.

69. Kretchmer, N. (1991). Summary and conclusions. In B. L. Nichols, A. Ballabriga, & N. Kretchmer (Eds.), *Nestle nutrition workshop series* (Vol. 22, pp. 277-283). New York: Raven Press.

70. Lansky, S. B., Cairns, N. V., Hassanein, R., et al. (1978). Childhood cancer: Parental discord and divorce. *Pediatrics, 62,* 184-188.

71. Lee, S. J., Earle, C. C., & Weeks, J. C. (2000). Outcomes research in oncology: History, conceptual framework, and trends in the literature. *Journal of the National Cancer Institute, 92,* 195-204.

72. Mandni, J. A., & Orthner, D. K. (1988). The context and consequences of family change. *Family Relations, 37,* 363-366.

73. McGee, R. F. (1989). Oncology nursing: Five decades of growth. *Journal of Cancer Education, 4,* 167-173.

74. McGuire, D. B., & Ropka, M. E. (2000). Research and oncology nursing practice. *Seminars in Oncology Nursing, 16,* 35-46.

75. McManus, M. A., Newacheck, J. W., & Greaney, A. M. (1990). Young adults with special health needs: Prevalence, severity and access to health services. *Pediatrics, 86,* 674-682.

76. Micozzi, M. S. (1991). Disease in antiquity: The case of cancer. *Archives of Pathology Lab Medicine, 115,* 838-844.

77. Mihich, E. (2000). Historical overview of biologic response modifiers. *Cancer Investigation, 18,* 456-466.

78. Miller, R. W., & McKay, F. W. (1984). Decline in United States childhood cancer mortality 1950 through 1980. *Journal of the American Medical Association, 251,* 1567-1570.

79. Mott, S. R., James, S. R., & Sperhac, A. M. (1990). *Nursing care of children and families* (2nd ed.). New York: Addison Wesley Nursing.

80. Nichols, B. L. (1991). The European roots of American pediatrics. In B. L. Nichols, A. Ballabriga, & N. Kretchmer (Eds.), *Nestle nutrition workshop series* (Vol. 22, pp. 49-53). New York: Raven Press.

81. Nieswiadomy, R. M. (1987). *Foundations of nursing research.* Norwalk, CT: Appleton & Lange.

82. Nightingale, F. (1992). *Notes on nursing, commemorative edition.* Philadelphia: J. B. Lippincott.

83. Oppenheim, J. J., Murphy, W. J., Chertov, O., et al. (1997). Prospects for cytokine and chemokine biotherapy. *Clinical Cancer Research, 3,* 2682-2686.

84. Padilla, G. V., & Padilla, G. J. (1979). Nursing roles to improve patient care. In G. V. Padilla (ed.), *The clinical nurse specialist and improvement of nursing practice.* Wakefield, MA: Nursing Resources.

85. Patterson, J. T. (1987). *The dread disease: Cancer and modern American culture.* Cambridge, MA: Harvard University Press.

86. Pearson, H. A. (1990). Centennial history of the APS. *Pediatric Research, 27*(6 Suppl.), 54-57.

87. Pearson, H. A. (1991). Pediatrics in the United States. In B. L. Nichols, A. Ballabriga, & N. Kretchmer (Eds.), *Nestle nutrition workshop series* (Vol. 22, pp. 55-63). New York: Raven Press.

88. Pochedly, C. P. (1986). Biographical vignette: Dr. Lois Murphy. *American Journal of Pediatric Hematology Oncology, 8,* 58-62.

89. Rather, L. J. (1978). *The genesis of cancer: A study in the history of ideas.* Baltimore: Johns Hopkins University Press.

90. Raven, R. W. (1990). *The theory and practice of oncology: Historical evolution and present principles.* Park Ridge, NJ: Parthenon.

91. Ries, L. A. G. (1999). Childhood cancer mortality. In L. A. G. Ries, M. A. Smith, J. G. Gurney, et al. (Eds.), *Cancer incidence and survival among children and adolescents: United States SEER Program 1975-1995,* Na-

tional Cancer Institute, SEER Program. (NIH Pub. No. 99-4649, pp. 165-170). Bethesda, MD: National Cancer Institute.

92. Ries, L. A. G., Hankey, B. F., Miller, B. A., et al. (1991). *Cancer statistics reviewed 1973-1988.* (NIH Publication 91-2789). Bethesda, MD: National Cancer Institute.

93. Rodriguez, H. (1998). Cohabitation: a snapshot. (http://www.clasp.org/pubs/familyformation/cohab.html).

94. Ross, W. (1987). *Crusade: The official history of the American Cancer Society.* New York: Arbor House.

95. Ruccione, K., & Hinds, P. S. (1997). A living legend in pediatric oncology nursing: Genevieve Foley, RN, MSN. *Journal of Pediatric Oncology Nursing, 14,* 99-105.

96. Ruccione, K., & Kelly, K. P. (2000). State of the science: Pediatric oncology nursing in cooperative clinical trials groups comes of age. *Seminars in Oncology Nursing, 16,* 253-260.

97. Sattin, A. (Ed.). (1987). *Florence Nightingale: Letters from Egypt 1849-1850.* New York: Weidenfeld & Nicolson.

98. Schuyler, C. B. (1992). Florence Nightingale. In *Notes on Nursing* (Commemorative ed., pp. 3-17). Philadelphia: J. B. Lippincott.

99. Shimkin, M. B. (1977). *Contrary to nature.* Washington, DC: U. S. Department of Health, Education and Welfare.

100. Siegel, S. (1998). *Access to primary health care: Tracking the states.* Washington, DC: National Conference of State Legislatures.

101. Silver, H., & Ford, L. (1968). The pediatric nurse practitioner program. *Journal of the American Medical Association, 204,* 298-302.

102. Smith, M. A., Gurney, J. G., & Ries, L. A. G. (1999). Cancer among adolescents 15-19 years old. In L. A. G. Ries, M. A. Smith, J. G. Gurney, et al., (Eds.), *Cancer incidence and survival among children and adolescents: United States SEER Program 1975-1995,* National Cancer Institute, SEER Program. (NIH Pub. No. 99-4649, pp. 157-164). Bethesda, MD: National Cancer Institute.

103. Stagner, S. (1992). Personal communication. Memphis.

104. Stass, S. A., & Mixson, A.J. (1997). Oncogenes and tumors suppressor genes: Therapeutic implications. *Clinical Cancer Research, 3,* 2687-2695.

105. Still, G. F. (1931). *The history of paediatrics: The progress of the study of diseases of children up to the end of the XVIII century.* London: Oxford University Press.

106. Talbott, J. H. (1970). *A biographical history of medicine.* New York: Grune & Stratton.

107. Taylor, G., (Ed.). (1990). *Pioneers in pediatric oncology.* Houston: The University of Texas MD Anderson Cancer Center.

108. Truman, J. T., van Eys, J., & Pochedly, C. (1986). *Human values in pediatric hematology/oncology.* New York: Praeger.

109. van Eys, J. (1976). *The truly cured child.* Baltimore: University Park Press.

110. Ventura, S. J., & Bachrach, C. A. (October 18, 2000). Nonmarital childbearing in the United States, 1940-99. *National Vital Statistics Reports, 48,* 16 (revised).

111. Waechter, E. H., Phillips, J., & Holaday, B. (Eds.). (1985). *Nursing care of children* (10th ed.). Philadelphia: J. B. Lippincott.

112. Warshofsky, F. (1999). The Methuselah factor. Modern Maturity. (http://www.aarp.org/mmaturity/nov_dec99/methuselah.html).

113. Winchester, D. (1998). The Society of Surgical Oncology and the Commission on Cancer: Progress through synergism. *Annals of Surgical Oncology, 5,* 483-488.

114. Wolff, J. A. (1991). History of pediatric oncology. *Pediatric Hematology/Oncology, 8,* 89-91.

115. Zuelzer, W. W. (1987). Pediatric hematology in historical perspective. In D. G. Nathan, & F. A. Oski (Eds.), *Hematology of infancy and childhood* (3rd ed.). Philadelphia: W. B. Saunders.

2

Biologic Basis of Cancer in Children and Adolescents

Kathy Ruccione

Until the latter part of the twentieth century, many people were unaware that cancer ever occurred in children. This perception was reflected in the title of an article published in the Saturday Evening Post in the early 1950s: "Cancer Kills Children, Too."[97] Childhood cancer was not in the public eye. Today, even with greater public awareness of childhood cancer, cancer in children tends to be vastly overshadowed by the sheer numbers of adults diagnosed with cancer each year. In the United States approximately 12,400 children and adolescents younger than 20 years of age are diagnosed with cancer annually,[41] as compared with the approximately 1.2 million adults diagnosed with cancer each year.[2]

Yet in the United States and other developed countries where infectious disease is not the major cause of death due to illness in children, cancer in children and adolescents is a significant public health problem because it puts so many potential productive years of life at stake. For example, infant leukemia is a rare malignancy, but it has been projected that nearly 8000 potential person years of life are lost annually because of this disease, given its poor survival rates.[87] In addition, what we have learned about the etiologic mechanisms of pediatric cancers is one of the important "lessons from our children" enumerated by Donaldson.[25] These lessons have had impact far beyond pediatric oncology. The "children's lesson" in epidemiology grew out of observations of a childhood eye tumor (retinoblastoma), which prompted Knudson[57] to hypothesize a "two-hit theory" of oncogenesis, later confirmed when methods for laboratory study of the genetics of retinoblastoma became available.[10,16,17,95,96] This concept of cancer causation was then applied and extended to adult malignancies.

Childhood malignancies continue to be the focus of considerable investigation. The literature on molecular genetic alterations in cancer is dominated by work on childhood cancer, perhaps because the "fetal" or "embryonal" appearance of many childhood tumors suggests a more direct etiology in contrast to common carcinomas of adulthood. This work has been fruitful in developing a model of cancer etiology in general, with common pathways applicable to adult cancer as well. Similarly, epidemiologic studies in childhood cancer may be more productive than studies in adults, because the exposure experience of children is only a small window in comparison with that of an individual who develops a malignancy in middle or late age. Our growing understanding of the epidemiology and genetics of childhood cancer has important implications for cancer in general.

Over the past two decades numerous descriptive and analytic epidemiology studies have been conducted, largely under the auspices of the former Children's Cancer Group (CCG) Epidemiology Strategy Group. These studies have delineated risk factors worthy of more concentrated study and, just as importantly, have identified factors or exposures that do not seem to pose relevant risk. During this same period, profound changes brought about by discoveries in molecular biology enabled scientists to complete the first map of the human genome and begin to glimpse the genesis of cancer at the molecular level. Current studies are being conducted at the intersection of epidemiology and genetics, combining epidemiologic observations with clinical and biologic characteristics. Clearly, the better the biologic basis of pediatric cancers is understood, the more likely it is that we will be able to target treatment with greater efficacy and less toxicity; and if full understanding of their etiology can be translated into risk assessments and preventive health policies,[82] one day we may be able to prevent cancer from disrupting the life of any child.

EPIDEMIOLOGY OF CANCER IN CHILDREN AND ADOLESCENTS

More than 200 years ago an English physician named Percivall Pott proposed one of the first epidemiologic cause-and-effect linkages involving cancer in children. In 1775 Pott reported an excess incidence of squamous cell carcinoma of the scrotum among young chimney sweeps (Figure 2-1) in London.[84] He hypothesized that chemical agents in soot were responsible for the scrotal cancer in the "climbing boys." Later studies confirmed the association and demonstrated that the carcinogenic chemical agents in soot were polycyclic aromatic hydrocarbons. Dr. Pott's observation thus could be considered the world's first pediatric cancer epidemiology report.

Since that time we have learned that childhood cancer represents a number of different malignancies. Cancers in children and adolescents vary by type of histology, site of disease origin, race, sex, and age. These variations are evident when detailed incidence and survival data are compiled. At present, incidence is extrapolated from reports contributed by a set of geographically defined, population-based central cancer registries in several

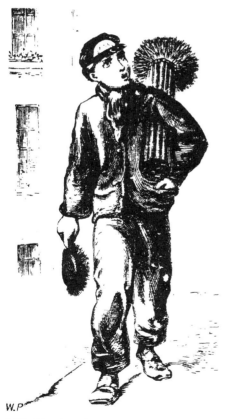

"Climbing boys," many younger than this lad, worked before child labor laws.

Figure 2-1

Chimney sweep.   (From Singer, N. [1995]. Chimney sweeps are plunging into their work again. *Smithsonian, 26*[6], 97-108.)

metropolitan areas and states participating in the Surveillance, Epidemiology and End Results (SEER) Program of the National Cancer Institute (NCI). Participants in the SEER Program were selected to represent urban and rural areas, as well as all ethnic groups. In 1999 the NCI published a landmark monograph that assembled the most detailed information available to date on the incidence of childhood cancer in the United States.[86] The monograph includes SEER Program data based on nearly 30,000 newly diagnosed cancers arising in children during the period from 1975 to 1995.

In the majority of states in the United States cancer is a reportable disease, and incidence data are compiled routinely by state and regional registries. In addition, the two major pediatric cooperative groups, CCG and the Pediatric Oncology Group (POG), which in the year 2000 merged into the Children's Oncology Group (C.O.G.), identify approximately 90% of children diagnosed with cancer under the age of 15 years in the United States.[88] Collaboration among C.O.G. and the regional and state registries is under way to establish a national population-based pediatric cancer research registry. The proposed Childhood Cancer Research Network will be an unexcelled centralized resource to facilitate studies addressing questions about etiology, health-related outcomes, cancer biology, and cancer control.[87]

INCIDENCE AND MORTALITY

In the United States each year approximately 150 out of every 1 million children younger than 20 years of age will be diagnosed with cancer.[86] That translates to 12,400 children or adolescents under age 20, of which 8,700 are under age 15. The recently published SEER pediatric monograph noted the following trends[41]:

- The overall incidence rate increased from the mid-1970s, but rates in the past decade have been relatively stable. In fact, there was an indication of a leveling off or a slight decline for the time period from 1990 to 1995 (Figure 2-2).
- Although there has been some disagreement,[53] most experts now attribute the small increases that were seen in the incidence of central nervous system (CNS) tumors, leukemias, and neuroblastoma in recent years to changes in diagnostic technology, reporting, and classification.[61]
- Overall, for all sites combined, cancer incidence was generally higher for males than for females.
- When divided into four groups by age, the highest incidence was among the youngest (younger than 5 years of age) and oldest (15 to 19 years of age), compared with the two intermediate age-groups.

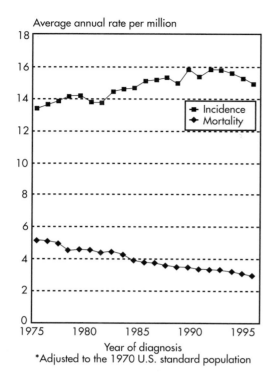

Average annual rate per million

Year of diagnosis
*Adjusted to the 1970 U.S. standard population

Figure 2-2

Trends in age-adjusted SEER incidence and U.S. mortality rates for all childhood cancers age <20, all races, both sexes. (From Reis, L.A.G., Smith, M.A., Gurney, J.G., et al. [1999]. *Cancer incidence and survival among children and adolescents: United States SEER Program 1975-1995* (p. 5). Bethesda, MD: National Cancer Institute, SEER Program. NIH Pub. No. 99-4649.)

- When examining a single year of age, the highest rates were in infants. Incidence rates declined as age increased to age 9, and then the incidence rates increased as age increased after age 9 (Figure 2-3).
- The majority of cancers (57%) among children less than 20 years of age were leukemia, tumors of the CNS, or lymphoma.
- Black children had lower incidence rates in 1990-1995 than white children overall and for many of the specific sites. Hispanic and Asian/Pacific children had cancer incidence rates intermediate to those for whites and blacks. American Indians had lower incidence rates than any other group.
- With newer, more effective treatment, death rates have declined dramatically for most childhood cancers, and survival rates have improved markedly since the 1970s (see Figure 2-2). Overall survival is now estimated at 80%, with the proportion varying with tumor type.[11] For a small but significant number, however, cancer is still fatal. Cancer remains the leading cause of death from disease in childhood.[2]

The caveat for anyone considering overall incidence and survival rates is to remember that there is considerable variation by sex, age, and race among the individual cancer types. When all are grouped together, these differences are masked. Specific information about the epidemiology of individual types of childhood cancer is presented within the chapter sections on those malignancies.

PATTERNS OF CHILDHOOD CANCER

In addition to its incidence, cancer in children and adolescents differs from cancers in adults in other ways. A major area of contrast is the tissue of ori-

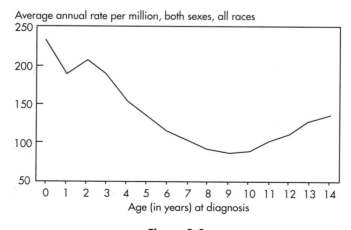

Average annual rate per million, both sexes, all races

Age (in years) at diagnosis

Figure 2-3

Age-specific cancer incidence among children under 15. (From Stat bite: Age-specific cancer incidence among children under 15. [1999] *Journal of the National Cancer Institute, 91,* 2076.)

gin. Most malignancies in adults are carcinomas, involving epithelial tissues, which occur very rarely in children. On the other hand, tumors in children often are composed of embryonal cell types (similar to fetal cells) that are uncommon among malignancies of adults.[18] The disparity between tissue types in pediatric versus adult cancers holds true for incidence until 15 years of age. Then, between 15 and 19 years of age, epithelial and nonepithelial cancers are equal in incidence. Thereafter, epithelial cancers predominate.[72]

Because childhood cancers most often arise from deep-seated tissue, they do not usually present obvious visual, palpable, or functional abnormalities until they are very large. They do not lend themselves to screening techniques that are useful for the more superficial or accessible adult cancers, such as Papanicolaou tests, skin biopsies, or mammograms. Thus almost 80% of children with cancer have distant metastases or systemic disease at the time of diagnosis. This challenge has led to the use of combined multimodal therapy, in turn requiring a multidisciplinary team approach to care, which has been highly successful and has served as a model for treatment of cancer in adults. Differences between adult and childhood cancers recently led to the enactment of the Federal Drug Administration Pediatric Rule.[36] The rule, which took effect in 2000, mandates that separate pediatric treatment studies must be performed because childhood cancers differ from the disease in adults in significant ways. Table 2-1 compares some of these differences.

Adult cancers usually are tabulated by primary site, but pediatric cancers are better grouped by their histologic type and primary site. The International Classification of Childhood Cancer (ICCC) recently was developed for this purpose. Using the ICCC groups, Figure 2-4 shows the incidence rates per million children. The highest rates are for groups I (leukemia), II (lymphoma), and III (CNS).

RISK FACTORS

Despite considerable epidemiologic effort, the specific etiologic pathway of any human malignancy, including childhood cancers, is unknown. Although it is known that genetic factors and certain prenatal and postnatal exposures can increase the risk of developing some childhood cancers, the process of finding the causes of disease is painstaking, and progress is usually slow. From clinical ob-

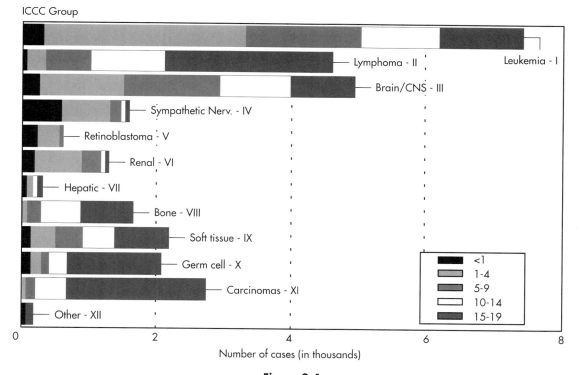

Figure 2-4

Number of cases of all childhood cancers by ICCC and age-group, all races, both sexes.   (From Reis, L. A. G., Smith, M. A., Gurney, J. G., et al. [1999]. *Cancer incidence and survival among children and adolescents: United States SEER Program 1975-1995* [p. 6]. Bethesda, MD: National Cancer Institute, SEER Program. NIH Pub. No. 99-4649.)

TABLE 2-1	CHARACTERISTICS OF CHILDHOOD CANCERS VERSUS CANCERS OF ADULTS	
Characteristic	**Childhood Cancers**	**Adult Cancers**
Frequency	Rare: <1% of all cancers	Common: >99% of all cancers
Primary sites	Involves tissues of reticuloendothelial system, central nervous system, muscle, bone	Involves organs such as breast, colon, lung, prostate
Histology	Most common type: nonepithelial (leukemia, lymphoma, central nervous system, sarcomas)	Most common type: epithelial (carcinomas)
Latency (from initiation to diagnosis)	Relatively brief latency	May be long (i.e., 20+ years); incidence increases with increasing age
Pathogenesis	Genetic alterations play a major role	Strong relationship to environmental and lifestyle factors; genetic factors have minor role
Preventable?	Minimal opportunity at present	80% estimated to be preventable
Opportunity for screening/early detection	Small percentage known to be at high risk can be monitored closely for early detection; screening tests generally not applicable	Many can be detected early by adherence to screening guidelines
Manifestations at diagnosis	Metastatic or systemic disease in ~80%	Local or regional disease
Pharmacokinetics (drug disposition), pharmacodynamics (tissue and organ sensitivity)	• Markedly different in children because of rapid developmental changes; many common tumor types have been responsive to chemotherapy • May tolerate higher doses and have less difficulty with acute toxicity • Vulnerable to long-term consequences (e.g., impaired growth and development, cognitive deficits, endocrine dysfunction, cardiotoxicity)	• Common tumor types have been less responsive to available chemotherapeutic agents • May have more difficulty with acute toxicity, but fewer long-term consequences
Presymptomatic genetic testing offered	Only under specific circumstances, following established guidelines for testing in children	Yes, for malignancies where genetic mutation has been identified (e.g., *BRCA1, BRCA2*)
Treatment per research protocols in cooperative groups as standard of care	Yes	No
Prognosis	70%-90% cure (depending on tumor type, stage)	<60% cure (depending on tumor type, stage)

Adapted from D. J. Fernbach & T. J. Vietti (Eds.). (1991). *Clinical pediatric oncology* (p. 2). St. Louis: Mosby–Year Book.

servations of patterns or associations, to descriptive studies of groups of individuals, to hypothesis-driven case-control studies, epidemiologists find clues and follow them up in subsequent studies. This is a brick-laying process in which some clues prove useful and others do not. Each current study is designed to assess whether or not previously identified clues are meaningful and play a role in the etiology of a particular cancer. No single study can prove that a certain exposure definitely causes a certain cancer, but each well-designed and well-executed study improves the understanding of the causes of these cancers.[41]

Epidemiologic studies do not give simple cause-and-effect answers to the question of why an individual child developed cancer. They can give information only on what exposures and characteristics increase risk and which do not. Risk factors vary with the different childhood cancers, and they range from known risk factors where there is strong scientific evidence for a causative association and exposures or characteristics with suggestive but not conclusive evidence to exposures or characteristics for which there is conflicting evidence and exposures or characteristics with limited evidence. Understanding these concepts of epidemiologic re-

TABLE 2-2	THE LANGUAGE OF EPIDEMIOLOGY
Terminology	**Meaning**
Relative risk	Whether or not an exposure increases the risk of cancer and how much it does is expressed in a measure called relative risk. The relative risk is the risk of disease in those with the exposure divided by the risk of disease in those without the exposure. Relative risk less than 1.0—the exposure appears to lower the risk of the disease. For example, a relative risk of 0.75 for taking vitamin X supplements indicates that those who took vitamin X had a risk that was 75% of that for individuals who did not take vitamin X. Or, taking vitamin X lowered one's risk by 25%. Relative risk of 1.0—the exposure does not affect the risk of the disease; the risk is the same in those with the exposure as in those without the exposure. Relative risk greater than 1.0—the exposure appears to increase the risk of the disease. For example, a relative risk of 3 for taking medication Y indicates that those taking medication had a risk that was three times that of those not taking the medication.
Risk factor	A characteristic or exposure that increases the risk of disease. A risk factor might be exposure to high levels of radon, having a diet low in vitamin A, having a family history of colon cancer, or smoking.
Case-control study	An epidemiologic study in which a group of individuals with a disease, the cases, are compared with a group of individuals without the disease, the controls. Exposures or characteristics that are more common in the cases than in the controls may be causes of the disease. Exposures or characteristics that are equally common in the cases and controls cannot be causes of the disease. Almost all studies of childhood cancer are case-control studies because this type of study is very useful in studying relatively uncommon diseases.
Cohort study	An epidemiologic study in which the incidence of disease is compared between a group of individuals with an exposure or characteristic and a group without that exposure or characteristic. For example, smokers and nonsmokers are followed, and the incidence of heart disease is compared in the two groups. Or, the incidence of breast cancer is compared in women with and without the *BRCA1* gene. This type of study is rarely feasible in investigating the etiology of childhood cancer. Since childhood cancer is rare, especially if we consider that each cancer should be studied separately, huge numbers of children (perhaps a million) would have to be followed to determine which children developed cancer.

From Bunin, G. (1998). *Children's Cancer Group nurses epidemiology notebook.*

search is essential to be able to read and critically evaluate study findings and to help patients and families interpret reported results. Table 2-2 summarizes definitions of key epidemiologic research terms. As defined in Table 2-2, risk factors are things that are known to increase the risk of disease. Exposures or characteristics that have been studied but are not yet known to be related to risk can be referred to as "potential risk factors," "possible risk factors," or just "factors being studied."

Various exposures have been investigated as risk factors for childhood cancer, including prenatal and postnatal exposures.

- *Prenatal exposures.* A modest increase in the risk of childhood leukemia has been associated with prenatal diagnostic irradiation.[18] Other *in utero* exposures associated with increased cancer risk in children include diethylstilbestrol (DES). Use of DES in pregnant women was associated with increased risk of clear-cell adenocarcinoma of the vagina in their daughters, with half of the cases occurring before age 20.[47] Very rarely, certain maternal cancers have been transmitted across the placenta to the fetus; these include melanoma, lymphoma, and bronchogenic carcinoma.[18]

- *Postnatal exposures.* Radiation can increase cancer risk in children. For example, children who survived atomic warfare in World War II had a higher risk of developing leukemia or solid tumors.[67] In the 1940s and 1950s children received therapeutic radiation for benign conditions such as thymus enlargement or ringworm of the scalp, and they had an increased risk of developing leukemia or solid tumors of the head and neck, beginning in older childhood or adulthood.[18] In addition, chemotherapy and radiation for treatment of childhood cancer increase the risk of subsequent cancers. Refer to Chapter 18 for additional information. A small proportion of childhood cancers has been linked with specific viruses; the best examples are nasopharyngeal carcinoma and some lymphomas associated with the Epstein-Barr virus.[67]

- Among the *possible* risk factors that have been studied, but with inconclusive or inconsistent findings, are certain *in utero* exposures (antinausea medications, barbiturates, antibiotics, marijuana, frequent alcohol use, and nitrosamine-containing substances). Other factors under investigation have included exposure to pesticides, electromagnetic fields, and motor vehicle exhaust. Potential associations between these exposures and certain childhood cancers have been found in some studies but not in others. The SEER Pediatric Monograph includes summaries of current knowledge on the causes of the various childhood cancers, categorized as known risk factors, factors for which evidence is suggestive but not conclusive, and factors for which evidence is inconsistent or limited.[86]

MULTIFACTORIAL ETIOLOGY

Epidemiologic studies to date suggest that not all children with a particular cancer developed it for the same reason. If they had, the causes would be simple, straightforward, and known by now. Instead, different individuals may develop the same cancer for different reasons. It is likely that no one factor, no single exposure or genetic trait, determines whether an individual will develop cancer. It appears that it is actually the interaction of many factors that produces cancer, a concept that is referred to as multiple causation or multifactorial etiology. Cancer may arise because of the predisposing characteristics of the individual interacting with the environment; with an interplay of genetic, immune, dietary, occupational, hormonal, viral, socioeconomic, lifestyle, and other factors related to the individual; and the biologic, social, or physical environment.

The concept of multiple causation is important in the interpretation of epidemiologic reports of risk factors for cancer. For example, a combination of laboratory and epidemiologic studies may show that exposure to a particular chemical can cause leukemia. Yet not all children who were exposed to this particular chemical develop leukemia, illustrating that there must be other factors that determine

TABLE 2-3	EVALUATING ASSOCIATIONS VS. CAUSES		
Epidemiologic Study Finds an Association	**Does Medication X Cause ALL?**	**Are There Other Explanations?**	
Imagine that a case-control study finds that more of the mothers of children with acute lymphoblastic leukemia (ALL) than mothers of controls used medication X during pregnancy.	Possibly	Yes: • Perhaps mothers of children with ALL were more accurate in their reporting of medication use than the control mothers were. Since mothers are asked in these studies to recall their use of medication and other substances during a pregnancy 5 or 10 years in the past, their reporting will not be completely accurate. However, mothers of children with cancer have probably thought about their exposures during the relevant pregnancies more intently than control mothers did in their search for an explanation of their children's illness. Case mothers may remember short episodes of medication use that control mothers may have forgotten about. A *recall bias* of this type would lead to an association between the medication and cancer, but the association would not be causal but spurious or false. • Another explanation of an association between the medication and cancer is that medication X is used to treat a medical condition and that the condition rather than the medication confers the risk. Epidemiologists would say that the condition is a *confounder* of the observed association between the medication and cancer.	

Adapted from L. A. G. Ries, M. A. Smith, J. G. Gurney, et al. (Eds.) (1999). *Cancer incidence and survival among children and adolescents: United States SEER Program 1975-1995* (p. 11). National Cancer Institute, SEER Program. NIH Pub. No. 99-4649. Bethesda, MD: National Cancer Institute.

which of the children exposed to the chemical will develop leukemia. Further studies would be needed to determine which factors interact with chemical exposure to cause leukemia.

ASSOCIATIONS VERSUS CAUSES

Anyone living in the information age with access to television, newspapers, or the Internet is exposed frequently—and confusingly—to reports of some chemical, dietary habit, or household product purported to increase or reduce the risk of cancer. Stories about the "carcinogen du jour" describe *associations* between an exposure and a cancer. In these reports usually people with cancer and people who did not have cancer were studied, and more of the people who developed cancer than those who did not develop cancer had the exposure. In epidemiology, though, an association link-

ing an exposure and cancer does not necessarily mean that the exposure *causes* cancer. Table 2-3 gives a hypothetical example of considerations that should be made in determining whether an association is a causal link.

Because an association does not necessarily denote a cause-and-effect relationship, epidemiologists need to be able to determine when an association does indicate disease causation. As noted previously, it is nearly impossible for a single study to prove that an exposure causes a disease, given the methods and processes of epidemiology and their limitations. Before an association between a disease and an exposure is considered a causal association, there must be a number of studies that epidemiologists can evaluate using the criteria shown in Table 2-4. All or most of these six criteria must be met (in no particular order of priority).

TABLE 2-4	CRITERIA FOR EVALUATING RISK FACTOR INFORMATION
Are there competing explanations?	*Other possible explanations* of the observed association must be ruled out, such as the medical condition rather than the medication. For example, if an association between eating hot dogs and developing a certain cancer is being studied, one must determine whether high dietary fat intake or infrequent fruit eating explains the association and rule out these factors before concluding that hot dog consumption is related to risk.
How strong is the association?	Epidemiologists consider the *strength* of the association, that is, the relative risk (see Table 2-2). An exposure associated with a ten-fold increase in risk is more likely to be a true cause than an exposure associated with a two-fold increase.
How consistent is the association?	The *consistency* of an association is considered. An association observed in many different studies in different populations using different methods is likely to be true.
Is there a dose-response relationship?	The observation of a *dose-response relationship* between the exposure and the disease increases confidence that the exposure is really a cause of the disease. In a dose-response relationship, the risk of disease increases with the dose of the exposure. For example, the relationship between cigarette smoking and lung cancer shows a dose-response in that heavy smokers have a higher risk than light smokers have.
Is the timing right?	The association must be *temporally correct,* meaning that we must be sure that the exposure actually preceded development of the disease. For example, a study might report that barbiturate use increased the risk of brain tumors. However, barbiturates are used to control seizures, which are often an early symptom of a brain tumor. Therefore it may not be clear if barbiturate use actually preceded the development of the brain tumor or if barbiturates were used to treat an early symptom before the brain tumor was diagnosed.
Is it plausible?	A *biologically plausible* association is more likely to be true than one without other supporting evidence. For example, we have more confidence that chemical X causes brain tumors in humans if it is known to cause brain tumors in animals.

Adapted from L. A. G. Ries, M. A. Smith, J. G. Gurney, et al. (Eds.) (1999). *Cancer incidence and survival among children and adolescents: United States SEER Program 1975-1995* (p. 11). National Cancer Institute, SEER Program. NIH Pub. No. 99-4649. Bethesda, MD: National Cancer Institute.

PARENTS' PERCEPTIONS ABOUT THE CAUSE OF CANCER

With few exceptions, our evolving understanding of the multifactorial origin of childhood cancer and the risk factor information emerging from epidemiologic studies do not provide definitive, clear, cause-and-effect answers for most parents who naturally want to know exactly what caused their child's cancer. In the absence of basic etiologic explanations, many parents of children with cancer form theories about the origins of their child's illness as they search for proximate cause and meaning in the experience. In a study of 175 sets of parents of children with acute lymphocytic leukemia (ALL), McWhirter and Kirk reported that the majority had formed theories as to why their children developed the disease; parents most often attributed the illness to environmental factors, radiation, chemicals, family history of cancer, and prior illness.[69] In another study, parents who volunteered their concerns about the cause of their child's cancer noted that environmental exposures and family health history were of prime importance to them.[89]

CANCER CLUSTERS

Sooner or later every pediatric oncology nurse will be asked about a suspected cancer cluster. A cancer cluster is a larger-than-expected number of people diagnosed with cancer during a limited time period in a specific geographic area. A well-known example is the cluster of leukemia reported in a parochial school in Niles, Illinois, between 1957 and 1960.[46] Study of this and other clusters began with high hopes that a single causative agent, probably a virus, would be discovered; however, no clear cause was found.[14] Individuals who suspect a cancer cluster should report it to their state or local health department or to the state cancer registry. When the suspected cancer cluster is reported, the state or local health officials will investigate it in a systematic way (Box 2-1). Early in the investigation, however, some putative clusters will be ruled out. Examples include:

- *"Clusters" of varied tumor types.* A concerned citizen may report 10 cancers that occurred in 2 years on two adjacent streets: three cases of lung cancer, three cases of cervical cancer, and four cases of breast cancer. These are common cancers, making it unlikely that there is a true cluster because it is not unexpected to see this many cancers in a small area. In addition, each of these cancers has been linked to different causes (e.g., smoking for lung cancer, patterns of sexual activity for cervical cancer, and hormonal and genetic factors for breast cancer). It is unlikely that some environmental toxin caused all three types of cancer. Generally, scientists believe that different

---

HOW STATE/LOCAL HEALTH OFFICIALS INVESTIGATE A CANCER CLUSTER

1. First, they obtain information from the informant about the number of cancers; the cancer sites; the age, race, and sex of each person with cancer; the location of the cluster; the time period; and the suspected cause, if any.
2. They confirm each reported cancer and obtain information on the specific diagnosis, site, and date of diagnosis.
3. The health officials use the number of confirmed cancers of each type and the population of the area of the suspected cluster to calculate cancer rates. The cancer rates for the area are compared with those for the state or county.
4. If the cancer rate in the area was higher (in a statistically significant way) than that in the county or state, it is considered a cancer cluster. At this point, the state or local health department would look further into possible causes of the cluster.

From Bunin, G. (1998). *Children's Cancer Group nurses epidemiology notebook.*

---

cancers have different causes. On the other hand, although different types of childhood cancers may indeed have different causes, we know very little about what causes cancer in children, and it is possible that exposures *in utero* or during infancy may affect many different organs and tissues. Therefore health officials investigating a suspected cluster of childhood cancer may include all types of childhood cancers in the investigation.

- *"Clusters" that include heterogenous tumors of the same anatomic site.* Consider a report of four brain tumors in a small community occurring in 1 year. Preliminary investigation by the health department determines that two were metastases from sites outside the brain and one was a recurrence of a tumor diagnosed 3 years earlier. Thus, actually only one resident of the community was diagnosed with a brain tumor in the year of interest and no cancer cluster existed.
- *Cancer "clusters" that actually reflect changing referral patterns rather than higher cancer rates.* For example, a hospital staff member may note an increase in cancer cases. It may be that the hospital is, in fact, seeing more cancer patients because other hospitals in the area are seeing fewer such patients. However, the number of cancers in the geographic area may not have changed at all.

Even when cancer clusters are sufficiently suspicious to be investigated, a cause is seldom discovered. There have been very few instances in the

United States in which a cause was found. Most of the latter involved an occupational group that was found to have a high incidence of a rare cancer, such as angiosarcoma of the liver in persons who work with vinyl chloride.[22] With thorough investigation, most suspected cancer clusters are found not to be true clusters. For example, in a report of the Missouri Department of Health, less than 20% of suspected clusters were actual clusters, that is, having more than the number of cancers that would be expected in the community.[24]

There are several issues that make "cluster busting" difficult. First, clusters can occur by chance; a high rate of cancer in an area may be unrelated to anything about the area or the people who live there. This does not mean that the cancers occurred by chance, but that the cancers developed for the same reasons as those occurring in people living elsewhere. In what appears to be a cluster of three cancers, one individual may have a family history of that cancer, another may have worked with a substance that increased his risk, and another may have a diet that increased her risk. Similarly, a street may have a higher-than-usual number of households with redheaded individuals. This might be because the redheaded individuals are all related to one another, or it might be a coincidence that the redheaded families ended up living on the same street.

Other clusters may not be chance occurrences and may indeed be related to some characteristic of the place or the people living there. However, we cannot distinguish clusters that are unrelated to the cause from those that are related to the cause. If a cluster is related to the cause of a particular cancer, the cause could be something about the location of the cluster or something about the people who live there. A natural exposure, such as high radon level, or a man-made exposure, such as a polluting industry, are possible explanations. Or the cause may be a characteristic of the people who live in the area. Perhaps the area's population includes many people of a specific ethnic group in which there is a genetic or dietary characteristic more common in this ethnic group than in other groups.

Over the years, thousands of possible cancer clusters have been reported to health authorities, including a few hundred that occurred in children. An explanation has been found for only a few cancer clusters in adults and for one cluster in children.[39] Yet public concern about industrial, air, or water pollution is magnified when a cancer cluster is suspected.[14] Whether or not a connection can be established, the perception of risk is as powerful as any demonstrated risk.[94] Thus, when individuals perceive a risk and are concerned about their well-being and the health of their children, demands for "cluster busting" are often made in outrage and

---

BOX 2-2

STUDIES OF DISEASE CLUSTERS: REASONS FOR THEIR LIMITED SCIENTIFIC VALUE

Individual clusters of disease are usually too small to constitute a useful epidemiologic study with adequate control of confounding factors.

Reported clusters often have vague definitions of disease, with cases that may be too heterogeneous for useful study.

The cluster is often defined by a community group (a sociologic not a scientific process), tending to produce clusters of causally unrelated cases.

The exposure or exposures under investigation are often poorly characterized, heterogeneous, and low in concentration.

The cluster often generates a torrent of publicity, making unbiased collection of data difficult or impossible.

From Rothman, K. J. (1990). Keynote presentation: A sobering start for the cluster busters' conference. *American Journal of Epidemiology, 132* (Suppl 1), S6-S13.

---

anger. The public expects that each cluster be investigated and the cause found.[14] This is a formidable problem for public health officials.

Although studies of clusters may be useful for reassuring the community or identifying sources of an environmental contamination that can then be cleaned up, clusters have given us very little information about the causes of cancer. Some of the reasons why the study of individual clusters does not offer bright prospects for advancing the science of epidemiology are listed in Box 2-2. More has been learned about cancer etiology from epidemiologic and laboratory research than from studying suspected clusters. Even more will be learned as epidemiologic studies focus on collecting direct evidence of exposure, such as the molecular changes that occur when carcinogens attach to deoxyribonucleic acid (DNA) (rather than relying on parents' memories of foods or chemicals they or their children were exposed to), and on looking for inherited variations in genes that may predispose children to cancer (e.g., by poorly metabolizing carcinogens in foods).[53] In this way, many current and proposed C.O.G. studies are most appropriately categorized as molecular genetic epidemiology studies. These studies are an attempt to zero in on environmental factors that trigger genetic damage at the molecular level.

MOLECULAR GENETICS

Molecular biology is the study of biologic processes at the level of the molecule. A major aspect of molecular biology is molecular genetics—the science

TABLE 2-5	DISCOVERIES IN MOLECULAR BIOLOGY	
Recent Medical Applications	**Future Medical Applications**
Testing for genetic predisposition to some childhood and adult cancer syndromes	Gene replacement therapy for selected diseases
Using amniotic fluid and chorionic villi sampling to examine fetal genes for disease	Organ replacement and repair using stem cell technology
Manufacturing drugs and vaccines by genetic engineering and protein expression	Antimicrobial agents that suppress resistance acquisition
Identifying specific genetic mutations and their roles in carcinogenesis	Interception of aberrant chemical signals in the signal transduction of cancer formation

From American Society of Clinical Oncology, B. L. Weber (Ed.). (2000). *ONCOSEP: Genetics, an oncology self-education program curriculum text* (p. 1). Dubuque, IA: Kendall.

that deals with DNA and ribonucleic acid (RNA). Most of the progress in molecular biology has been made since the middle of the twentieth century. Some of the discoveries that have already been translated into new medical applications and new items that will be added to the list in the foreseeable future are shown in Table 2-5. Each discovery or technologic innovation has built on previous discoveries and paved the way for the next, culminating in the current effort to map, sequence, and understand the functions of the entire human genome.

GENES AND THE HUMAN GENOME

All living organisms are made up of cells. Some are single celled, such as bacteria or yeast. Humans are made of approximately 1 trillion cells, and the cells are of many different types with different functions. Human cells are eukaryotic, meaning that the nucleus of each cell stores genetic instructions for making and organizing the cell (Figure 2-5). These instructions, the tightly packed DNA and structural proteins, are bundled in the chromosomes (named from root words meaning "colored bodies" [*chrom* = "color," *some* = "body"] because they show up in color when stained with special dyes). The chromosome is the largest unit of inheritance. The smallest unit of inherited information is a gene, a subunit of the chromosome. There are thousands of genes in each chromosome. Each gene carries the essential information for synthesizing a protein or part of a protein.

Chromosomes. Each type of chromosome has a different shape and pattern of staining and is numbered. In a cell or in a species, the number and structure of chromosomes is called its karyotype. A human karyotype normally has 23 pairs of chromosomes: 22 autosomes (nonsex chromosomes) and one pair of sex chromosomes (Figure 2-6). Each individual inherits two copies of each chromosome: one copy from the mother and one copy from the father. The two chromosomes in each pair are

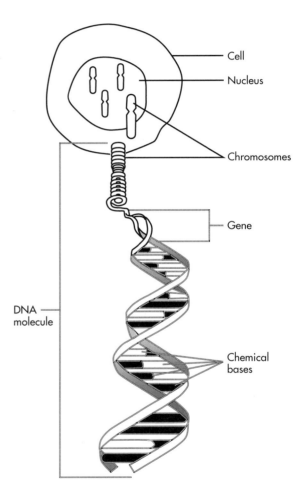

Figure 2-5

Double-helix: DNA molecule. (Artwork originally created for the National Cancer Institute. Reprinted with permission of the artist, Jeanne Kelly. Copyright 1996.)

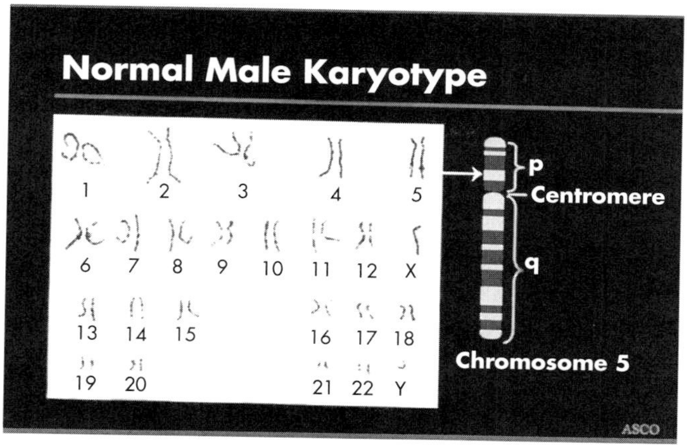

Figure 2-6

Normal male human karyotype.   (From American Society of Clinical Oncology, B.L. Weber [Ed.]. [2000]. *ONCOSEP: Genetics, an oncology self-education program curriculum text* [p. 2]. Dubuque, IA: Kendall.)

called homologous chromosomes. In girls, the sex chromosomes are composed of two X chromosomes. In boys, the sex chromosome pair consists of one X chromosome from their mother and one Y chromosome from their father. Thus the karyotypes are referred to as 46,XX for females and 46,XY for males. The nuclei of human cells are termed *diploid* (abbreviated *2N*) because their chromosomes are paired.

The study of chromosomes is known as cytogenetics. Karyotyping is a cytogenetic laboratory procedure for identifying chromosomal variation. This is done with lymphocytes or skin fibroblasts that are grown in tissue culture; single cells are isolated in metaphase when chromosomes are tightly condensed and prepared for microscopic study. In the dividing state, a chromosome looks like two U shapes, one inverted under the other, and joined together at their curved bases. The two sides of each U are called chromatids and are attached at a structure called the centromere. Generally the U's are different lengths; each is called an arm. The shorter arm is designated by the notation *p* for *petit,* and the longer arm is referred to as the *q*-arm. Thus a specific chromosome site, gene location, or abnormality is described by referring to the number and arm, p or q, of the chromosome; for example, the short arm of chromosome 1 is 1p or the long arm of chromosome 13 is 13q. Large chromosomal abnormalities are detectable at the level of resolution attainable by standard banding techniques, but smaller single-gene changes cannot be detected.

The DNA molecule.   All chromosomes contain a very long molecule (termed a *macromolecule*) called deoxyribonucleic acid (DNA). A molecule is

the smallest unit of a chemical and is composed of a combination of atoms; millions of different molecules can be made from the more than 100 types of atoms that exist. DNA molecules are among the largest molecules now known. DNA is an acid found in the nucleus; thus it is called a nucleic acid. DNA is similar to another nucleic acid—ribonucleic acid (RNA)—but it has one less atom of oxygen, hence the prefix in the term, *deoxy*-ribonucleic acid.[48]

The macromolecule DNA contains many molecules of sugar. Sugars have a certain arrangement of carbon atoms. The sugar molecule in DNA is called deoxyribose. In this molecule the atoms join together to form a ring. Phosphate molecules link the sugar molecules together into a very long chain. Each human chromosome has a single molecule of DNA that contains about 280 million sugars and 280 million phosphates.[48] The sugar-phosphate chain is the backbone of the DNA molecule. In DNA, each sugar molecule is attached to another kind of molecule called a nitrogenous base. The nitrogenous bases in DNA are of two types: the purines (double carbon-nitrogen rings) adenine and guanine, or the pyrimidines (single carbon-nitrogen rings) cytosine and thymine—known by their initials as A, G, C, T (Figure 2-7).

The arrangement of a base attached to a sugar attached to a phosphate molecule is called a nucleotide. There are rules for joining these bases by hydrogen bonds (pairing): C can pair only with G; T can pair only with A. Each of these linkages is known as a base pair. The complete set of instructions for the creation of an organism, that is, the number and structure of genes in a cell or species, is called its genome. The human genome contains approximately 3 billion base pairs. About 30% of

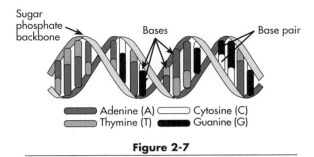

Sugar phosphate backbone — Bases — Base pair

☐ Adenine (A)   ☐ Cytosine (C)
☐ Thymine (T)   ☐ Guanine (G)

Figure 2-7

The DNA double helix. (From American Society of Clinical Oncology, B.L. Weber [Ed.] [2000]. *ONCOSEP: Genetics, an oncology self-education program curriculum text* [p. 2]. Dubuque, IA: Kendall.)

the base pairs are associated with the estimated 30,000 genes expressed in human cells. The remainder is termed *extragenic DNA;* the function of most extragenic DNA is not understood. Some parts are involved in regulating gene expression, and some may serve as spacers between genes or parts of genes.[4]

Watson and Crick[109,110] discerned that the DNA molecule is a gently twisted spiral staircase that carries the genes for each individual and is capable of endlessly copying itself. They showed the three-dimensional shape of DNA by making x-rays of crystallized DNA. They found that DNA contains not just one but two nucleotide chains of sugars and phosphates. Each base on one of the chains shares hydrogen atoms with one of the bases on the opposite chain to join the two chains together. This sharing is called a hydrogen bond. The complementary pairing of these chains causes the double-stranded DNA to form the shape of a twisting, turning staircase in which each step is a little higher than the last and a little to the left, so that the staircase moves upward in a spiral. This spiral shape is called a helix. Because DNA has two chains, it is called a double helix.[48] If a strand of DNA could be unwound, it would be 5 to 8 feet long, but only 50 trillionths of an inch wide.

The structure of DNA with its two chains is elegant, because it allows both replication of daughter DNA molecules and synthesis of the proteins that govern life. The complementary nucleotide chains ensure the accurate storage, retrieval, and transfer of genetic information.[4] Because of the complementary bonding, one strand of the double helix determines the nucleotide sequence of the other strand. This is the mechanism that is the basis for the faithful transmission of the instructions encoded in the base pairs during the process of copying or reading DNA.

Cell division. New cells are made by mitosis, the division of existing cells. During mitosis the cell doubles in size and then divides into two cells of equal size. For these new cells to work properly, each one must end up with exactly 46 molecules of DNA, each packaged into a chromosome. A cell that is preparing to divide first makes a copy of each of its 46 chromosomes and then gives each new cell a copy. To do this, the hydrogen bonds break between the bases in the two chains of the double helix, that is, they "unzip." Unzipping the double helix allows the bases in each chain to make a template for the new daughter molecules. Each base in an existing DNA chain pairs with a previously unattached partner by following the base pairing rules, and these newly attached bases join together to form a chain that builds alongside the original one. From one helix, two are produced with the same sequence of base pairs. The cells are then ready to divide (Figure 2-8).

There is another type of cell division, meiosis, which occurs in the only cells that do not have paired chromosomes: the haploid (abbreviated *N*) germ cells. When sperm or ova are being produced, diploid cells produce haploid gametes through meiosis. In meiosis, each chromosome first replicates, and each chromatid pairs with its homologue. Next, the homologues separate and migrate to opposite ends of the cells. The replicated chromatids remain attached at the centromere. Then a typical mitosis occurs, in which the 23 chromosomes separate at the centromere, producing haploid gametes that each have 22 unpaired chromosomes and one sex chromosome. Once fertilized, the sperm and ovum fuse to form a diploid (2N) cell, the zygote (see Figure 2-8).

When the zygote undergoes mitotic cell division, a complete set of chromosomes is replicated in every cell. If either of the gametes that formed the zygote contains a mutated gene, the mutation will be replicated in every cell of the offspring, producing a germ-line mutation. This phenomenon is of utmost importance, because germ-line mutation is the basis on which heritable disease, including familial cancer susceptibility, is transmitted.

Protein synthesis. One way of thinking of DNA is as a vast chemical information database that carries the complete set of instructions for making all the proteins a cell will ever need.[103] All proteins are made from chemicals called amino acids. Almost all living organisms use the same 20 amino acids as the building blocks of their proteins. It is the proteins that make the structure of cells and tissues, the antibodies of the immune system, and the enzymes for all the essential biochemical functions. The

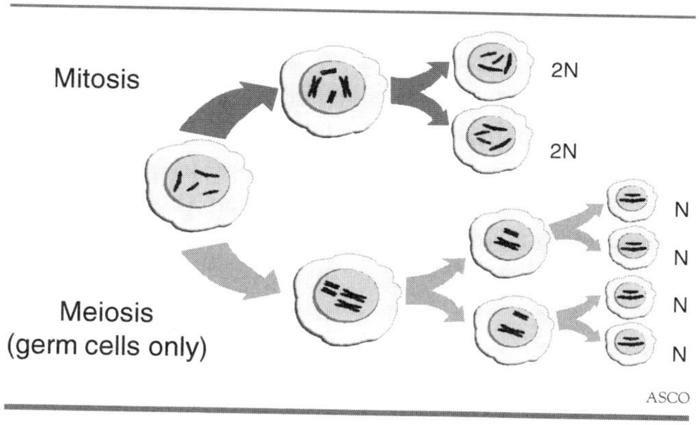

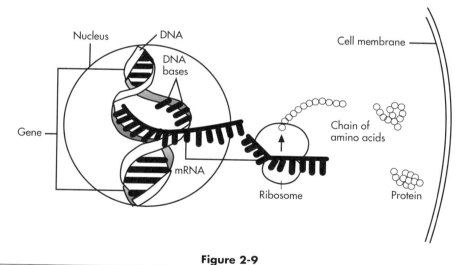

Figure 2-8

Mitosis and meiosis.   (From American Society of Clinical Oncology, B.L. Weber [Ed.] [2000]. *ONCOSEP: Genetics, an oncology self-education program curriculum text* [p. 3]. Dubuque, IA: Kendall.)

Figure 2-9

Transcription and translation.   (Artwork originally created for the National Cancer Institute. Reprinted with permission of the artist, Jeanne Kelly. Copyright 1996.)

DNA in each chromosome contains segments that carry the instructions for making a specific protein. Each of these segments is a gene, and each gene has a particular sequence of the four base pairs (nucleotides). The order of the nucleotides determines the amino acid sequence of the protein. Each triplet of nucleotides is termed a *codon;* a codon holds the code for a single amino acid. Most amino acids are encoded by more than one codon, but each codon can encode for only one amino acid.[4] A single gene can be made of thousands—or hundreds of thousands—of nucleotides, and with a few exceptions, there is a single corresponding protein for each gene. A large proportion, estimated to be about 95%, of DNA is made of repeated sequences that do not code proteins (these regions are called introns); protein-coding regions are called exons.

A gene works its magic by creating a template of itself made of messenger RNA, with one difference: it substitutes uracil for thymine, which in turn contains the code needed to manufacture a single protein molecule. This process is called transcription (Figure 2-9). The completed copy strand then travels out of the cell nucleus and into the cytoplasm to find a ribosome. The ribosome is like a microscopic workbench that holds the copy strand, reads its instructions, and joins amino acids together like beads of a necklace. The necklace of amino acids then folds up tightly in a shape that is unique to each protein. This process is called translation (see Figure 2-9). Cells are using gene recipes to make the proteins they need every second of every minute of every hour.[8] These very processes are the foundation of the biotechnology industry.

Cells use genes selectively. Within the entire complement of genes in each cell, some enable the production of proteins that are needed for basic cellular functions (called "housekeeping genes"), while others are inactive most of the time. Certain genes are active in the early development of the embryo and then shut down forever. Many genes carry the instructions for making proteins that enable cells to differentiate into various types (e.g., brain, bone, and muscle cells). When working normally, a cell activates only the genes it needs at the moment and suppresses all others.[103]

GENETIC MUTATION AND DISEASE

As noted previously, individuals inherit two copies of each chromosome pair, designated homologous chromosomes. In the population, genes may have variant sequences, called alleles. Because one copy of each homologous chromosome pair is inherited from each parent, an individual has two alleles for each gene. Each parent has a fifty-fifty chance of passing either allele to a child. In the case where both alleles have the same sequence, the child is considered to be homozygous for that allele. If the two alleles are different, the child is said to be heterozygous. Alleles are sometimes called "wild type" alleles if they have no known disease associations.

The strict definition of a mutation is any change in the normal base pair sequence of DNA, whether or not protein structure or function is altered.[4] That would mean that any allelic variation is a mutation. Yet there may be no pathophysiologic consequences to the mutation if the mutation is "silent" because it occurs in a noncoding region or if it is in a coding area that has redundancy for encoding an amino acid. Less formally, mutation usually refers to a DNA sequence change that does affect protein function, predisposing to disease. Depending on its location, a mutation can result in nonfunctional protein, over- or underexpression of the protein, or complete absence of the protein.

Mutations associated with cancer. Both germline and somatic mutations can contribute to cancer. Germ-line mutations are inherited from parental germ cells (ova or sperm). They are replicated in all the individual's cells. Individuals who inherit a germ-line mutation associated with a familial cancer syndrome have a tendency toward early onset of cancer and the occurrence of multi-

ple cancers because the mutation-damaged allele is present in every cell and there is only one normal allele to withstand exposure to carcinogens or additional errors during DNA replication. It is also possible to inherit a *de novo* germ-line mutation, which was not present in the parent's germ cells because it occurred at gametogenesis. Such a mutation becomes heritable by the next generation. Somatic mutations, occurring in nongerm cells, are not heritable. They may result from environmental exposures or errors that occur during DNA replication. It is thought that multiple mutations are needed to make a cell malignant, but it takes only one malignant cell to begin a tumor clone.[4] Mutations can produce various kinds of protein sequence changes, highlighted in Table 2-6.

Inherited cancer syndromes. Strictly speaking, cancer is not inherited; however, an increased susceptibility to cancer can be inherited. Familial cancer susceptibility occurs when a parent transmits a cancer-associated gene mutation.[4] Inherited cancer susceptibility syndromes account for only about 5% of newly diagnosed childhood cancer cases in the United States annually.[13,73] Genotype is an individual's genetic composition. Phenotype is a characteristic of an organism produced by interaction between the genotype and its environment.[4] Clinically, a phenotype can describe the manifestations of a trait or disease. For example, the DNA sequence of a *TP53* gene mutation (also known as *p53*) is a genotype; Li-Fraumeni malignancy is a phenotype. More than one phenotype can be produced by a single gene; indeed, Li-Fraumeni syndrome is characterized by various tumors.

The term *penetrance* is used to describe the proportion of individuals of the same genotype manifesting the correlated phenotype. If every individual with the same disease-predisposing genotype had the associated disease, penetrance would be 100%. When penetrance is incomplete, it is impossible even with genetic testing to predict which carriers of a particular disease-predisposing allele actually will be affected by the disease. Various mutations in the same gene may have varying degrees of penetrance.[4] Factors that can increase or decrease the penetrance of an altered cancer susceptibility allele include altered activity of DNA damage-response gene products (see next section), which enable mutations to accumulate in other genes, increasing the likelihood that a cell will undergo malignant transformation. Other factors affecting penetrance include exposure to carcinogens or to hormones and other reproductive factors. Penetrance is also affected by aging, so that the probability of developing a disease increases as a mutation carrier ages.

TABLE 2-6	PROTEIN SEQUENCE CHANGES RELATED TO MUTATIONS
Type of Change	**Description**
Point mutation	Change in a single base pair that can have an effect on the resulting protein. Types include missense mutations and nonsense mutations.
Small insertions and deletions	Involve one to a few (usually less than 100) base pairs. Types include frameshift mutations and in-frame mutations.
Splice-site mutations	Occur in the noncoding regions. May have profound effects on resulting protein, leading to disease.
Mutations in regulatory regions	Can result in reduced production or uncontrolled overproduction of an encoded protein. Can lead to disease.
Chromosomal disorders	Involve changes in large pieces of a chromosome. Many are associated with disease. Changes in germ line are often associated with abnormal development and/or mental retardation. May include large deletions or insertions of DNA, or translocations (segment of one chromosome breaks off and fuses with a nonhomologous chromosome with or without loss of genetic material). Translocations are often found in malignant tumor cells.
Polymorphisms	Changes in DNA sequence that have no effect or only a minor effect on protein function/production. Often used by geneticists to track inheritance patterns. They use linkage analysis to identify chromosomal regions that contain disease-associated genes and thereby to identify the specific genes themselves.

From American Society of Clinical Oncology, B. L. Weber (Ed.). (2000). *ONCOSEP: Genetics, an oncology self-education program curriculum text* (pp. 5-6). Dubuque, IA: Kendall.

TABLE 2-7	SOME AUTOSOMAL DOMINANTLY INHERITED CANCER SYNDROMES
Syndrome	**Associated Gene(s)**
Familial retinoblastoma	*RB1*
Li-Fraumeni	*TP53*
Familial adenomatous polyposis	*APC*
Hereditary nonpolyposis colorectal cancer	*MLH1, MSH2, MSH6, PMS1, PMS2*
Wilms tumor	*WT1*
Breast and ovarian cancer	*BRCA1, BRCA2*
Von Hippel-Landau	*VHL*
Cowden	*PTEN*

From American Society of Clinical Oncology, B. L. Weber (Ed.). (2000). *ONCOSEP: Genetics, an oncology self-education program curriculum text* (p. 8). Dubuque, IA: Kendall.

TABLE 2-8	SOME RECESSIVELY INHERITED CANCER SYNDROMES	
Syndrome	**Primary Tumor**	**Associated Gene(s)**
Ataxia telangiectasia	Lymphoma	*ATM*
Bloom syndrome	Solid tumors	*HLM*
Xeroderma pigmentosum	Skin cancer	*XPB, XPD, XPA*
Fanconi anemia	AML	*FACC, FACA*

From American Society of Clinical Oncology, B. L. Weber (Ed.). (2000). *ONCOSEP: Genetics, an oncology self-education program curriculum text* (p. 9). Dubuque, IA: Kendall.

Inherited disease susceptibility is transmitted on an autosome (chromosome in a somatic cell), and may be an autosomal dominant, autosomal recessive, or X-linked trait. In dominant susceptibility, an individual is heterozygous for the disease-related mutation; i.e., the individual inherited the mutated allele from one parent and the wild type allele from the other. In recessive inheritance, the individual will express the phenotype (disease) only if two copies of the mutated allele were inherited, one from each parent; the individual is homozygous for the disease-related mutation. The majority of cancer susceptibility syndromes are transmitted as autosomal dominant traits with incomplete penetrance. Tables 2-7 and 2-8 list examples of autosomal dominantly inherited and recessively inherited cancer syndromes. X-linked transmission occurs via an X chromosome rather than an autosome. If the disease is recessive, females would need to inherit two copies of the mutated allele to express the disease phenotype, because females have two X chromosomes; if only one allele is affected, the female would be an unaffected carrier. In contrast, a male would be affected if the abnormal X chromosome is inherited, and the mutation has 100% penetrance.

CANCER AS A GENETIC DISEASE

Progress in understanding cancer points to a fundamental concept: all cancer is a genetic disease, and perhaps, in a sense, all disease is genetic at the molecular level. That does not mean that all cancer is hereditary, but rather that for cancer to develop something must go awry in the genes. Recent discoveries in molecular biology are helping to solve the puzzle of cancer, showing how the normal cellular control mechanisms go awry to cause cancer and setting the stage for genetic testing and disease treatment. These new discoveries bring both promise and peril. To provide comprehensive care, health care providers must now be familiar with the concepts and language of molecular biology, understand its applications to cancer care, and be fully informed about its implications for clinical practice, research, and education.

GENES ASSOCIATED WITH
CANCER SUSCEPTIBILITY

Three classes of genes play major roles in triggering cancer. They are oncogenes, tumor-suppressor genes, and DNA damage response (repair) genes. When they are working normally, they choreograph the life cycle of the cell and the intricate steps by which the cell enlarges and divides.

Oncogenes. Proto-oncogenes encourage normal cell division and growth through a signaling process described later in this chapter (see Hallmarks of Cancer). When mutated, proto-oncogenes become carcinogenic oncogenes. Specific oncogenes may affect different parts of the signaling system or the amount of growth factors secreted, or they may interfere with the receptors. The changes cause the cell cycle to go out of control. Different tumors may show different abnormalities in the cell cycle. Examples of oncogenes involved in human cancer are N-*myc*, involved in neuroblastoma and glioblastoma, and *Bcl*-1, involved in breast and head and neck cancer.[112]

Tumor-suppressor genes. Although a damaged oncogene has been likened to a car having the accelerator pedal stuck to the floor, a damaged tumor-suppressor gene is like losing your brakes. Tumor-suppressor genes normally are the brakes that keep cell growth in check. If these genes are damaged or missing, the cell ignores inhibitory signals and grows out of control. Different parts of the signaling system are affected when different tumor-suppressor genes are lost or disrupted.

As discussed in the previous section ("Molecular Genetics"), cells have two copies of every gene, called alleles. The alleles provide a built-in safety

mechanism in case a normal tumor-suppressor gene is lost or inactivated. The loss of a functioning copy of a gene is called loss of heterozygosity (LOH). It has been proposed that two or more mutations must occur for tumors to arise. This concept, known as the "two-hit hypothesis," was first postulated by Knudson[57] to explain the etiology of retinoblastoma (Figure 2-10). In the hereditary form of a tumor, such as in retinoblastoma, the first "hit" occurs in a germ cell. That hit predisposes the individual's cells, in this case the retinal cells, to develop a malignancy after another mutation occurs. In the case of nonhereditary disease, both hits occur later in the development of the retina, and there is no constitutional predisposition to malignancy that could be passed on. This model, which may have many more than two steps in various forms of cancer, is true of all malignancies that have both heritable and nonheritable forms. The two-hit hypothesis was confirmed with a series of studies of retinoblastoma, which found a deletion of a specific band in the long q-arm of chromosome 13 in hereditary retinoblastoma.[10,16,17,95,96] When the retinoblastoma *(RB)* gene was cloned, it was shown to be a tumor-suppressor gene.[35] Deletion of an *RB* gene results in LOH, which predisposes the cell to tumor development.

Several other tumor-suppressor genes have been found in the past few years, of which the most significant is *p53,* because it is the most frequently mutated gene in human cancer. The *p53* gene helps to monitor the health of the cell and the integrity of its DNA. It is so important when functioning normally that it has been called the "guardian of the genome." Mutant inherited versions of the *p53* tumor-suppressor gene yield tumors at multiple sites, and possibly in different age-groups, a condition known as the Li-Fraumeni syndrome.[65] Other examples of tumor-suppressor genes involved in

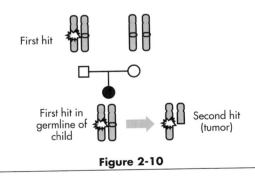

Figure 2-10

The two-hit hypothesis. (From American Society of Clinical Oncology, B. L. Weber [Ed.] [2000]. *ONCOSEP: Genetics, an oncology self-education program curriculum text* [p. 9]. Dubuque, IA: Kendall.)

human cancer include *WT1* (involved in some forms of Wilms tumor) and *BRCA1* and *BRCA2* (involved in breast cancer).[112]

A current area of research is focused on a cellular process called methylation,[52] altered in cancer, which may inactivate tumor suppressor genes. Although the prevailing view (the two-hit hypothesis), validated by many studies, is that tumor-suppressor genes are inactivated in cancer cells as a result of mutations in both alleles, there is evidence that so-called epigenetic mechanisms, such as alterations in DNA methylation in regulatory regions of the gene, may be another way that tumor-suppressor genes are inactivated.[52] There is some debate as to whether alterations in DNA methylation cause gene inactivation or are simply associated with it.[30] As more research is completed, it may be that methylation is part of the larger puzzle of carcinogenesis that may have potential as a useful marker for monitoring tumor presence and prognosis.[9] Another possibility is the development of demethylating agents to be used as a part of chemotherapy or chemoprevention.[99]

DNA repair (or damage response) genes. These are the genes that make sure that each strand of genetic information is correctly copied during cell division. When DNA repair genes are faulty, other mutations occur. Examples of disorders associated with faulty DNA repair genes and an increased risk of cancer include Bloom syndrome, ataxia-telangiectasia, Fanconi anemia, and hereditary nonpolyposis colon cancer. If these caretaker genes are mutated, cancer can arise from accumulation of mutations in critical growth-regulating genes, including proto-oncogenes and tumor-suppressor genes.[4]

NONTRADITIONAL INHERITANCE AND MITOCHONDRIAL MUTATIONS

As additional discoveries regarding the molecular biology of cancer are made, concepts of genetics are being challenged and revised. Newer concepts of nontraditional inheritance are emerging that may apply to Wilms tumor and perhaps to other types of cancer. These concepts include uniparental disomy, which means that under some circumstances both chromosomes of a pair can derive from the same parent. Genomic imprinting[31] means that the expression of a gene may be modified depending on whether the gene came from the mother or the father. In an example of genomic imprinting, studies of the *WT1* gene have shown that the copy of the gene inherited from the mother is lost more often than the copy from the father. This finding suggests that the mother's copy of the gene may have a role

in tumor suppression for which the father's copy cannot compensate.

Another line of research focuses on the genes in mitochondria, the tiny, energy-generating organs inside cells. Mitochondria seem to be ancient and entrenched parasites, descendants of bacteria that adapted and became part of cells. Mitochondria are inherited only from our mothers. Some types of blindness and degenerative disorders have been linked to mitochondrial DNA mutations, and testing is available for some of these mitochondrial disorders.[101] Discoveries about mitochondrial DNA, uniparental disomy, and genomic imprinting have opened new ways of thinking about genetic transmission of disease.

CONNECTING THE BIOLOGIC DOTS

From Mendel to the map. Although the term *gene* was not used until the 1900s,[108] we now understand that DNA was the invisible genetic blueprint for cellular activities since life began 4.6 billion years ago. Even in early agriculture-based societies, people knew that there was a force at work that determined the characteristics of living things, because they bred crops and animals for desired features. They were the first "genetic engineers." In the century between Gregor Mendel's experiments with plant genetics and the beginning of the Human Genome Project, numerous discoveries were made in various fields of study (Table 2-9), opening the door to twenty-first-century medicine and changing the definition of genetic disease (Box 2-3). The modern discipline of molecular genetics has come from the melding of several different areas of study, including biochemistry, biology, genetics, information sciences, and pathology.

The new millennium and the human genome. In June 2000 two rival teams of scientists jointly announced that their computers had identified virtually all 3 billion base pairs on the 23 chromosomes in the human genome, the blueprint for a human being.[100] The publicly funded consortium, the Human Genome Project (HGP), and Celera Genomics, a private commercial venture, had raced each other to complete a "working draft" of the human genome. Their methods differ, and they do not agree on the genome's exact size; neither side's version of the genome is complete, and neither has fully sequenced the DNA. But both versions will allow scientists to search for genes of interest. The genetic code has been cracked, and as Dr. Francis Collins, head of the Human Genome Project, said at the White House ceremony where the announcement was made, ". . . We have caught the first glimpses of our own instruction book, previously

TABLE 2-9	MILESTONES IN MOLECULAR BIOLOGY
Era	**Prominent Discoveries**
Nineteenth century	In the latter half of the nineteenth century an Austrian monk named Gregor Mendel did work that led to the discovery of gene function. Mendel crossbred pea plants and kept very careful records to analyze his results. He theorized that *hereditary factors* existed that were passed to offspring. These factors were indeed the genes, but his work went unnoticed until early in the 1900s.[55] By the 1870s scientists had the necessary microscopes to study chromosomes, which could be seen as cells divided.
Dawning of the twentieth century	Early in the twentieth century Mendelian genetics was rediscovered, and many of the details of how hereditary works were filled in as scientists observed similarities in the theoretical behavior of Mendel's units of heredity and the visible behavior of chromosomes. The first gene mapping was done in fruit flies. The *fruit fly geneticists* pioneered linkage analysis studies. They realized that when two types of traits tend to be inherited together, such as eye color and wing type, their genes are apt to lie on the same chromosome, and they are said to be linked. Genes that lie close to each other will tend to be inherited together. Linkage analysis could be done with fruit flies because they have only four pairs of chromosomes, making them manageable to study. Early in the 1900s Garrod first showed transmission of a characteristic in humans. He connected Mendelian heredity with his observations of metabolic disorders in individuals, which he called *inborn errors of metabolism.*[108]
The decades of the 1920s, 1930s, and 1940s	In the 1920s scientists began to focus attention on *gene mutations* and their effects. Muller hypothesized about possible types of mutations and showed that x-rays caused mutations in fruit flies.[55] In the 1930s the term *molecular biology* began to be used. The shape of the field, the focus of study, and the tools and methods that were developed were greatly influenced by the Rockefeller Foundation because of the projects it chose to fund. The foundation dedicated approximately $25 million for U.S. molecular biology research during the next 20 years.[54] In fact, it was the head of the Rockefeller Foundation's natural science division, Warren Weaver, who first used the term *molecular biology.*[111] In the 1940s a growing understanding of what genes do was articulated by Beadle and Tatum in their *one-gene-one-enzyme hypothesis,* now more generally phrased as the "one-gene-one-protein" concept.[101] They said that what the gene does is to specify production of an enzyme/protein.[55] The first direct evidence that human mutations alter the structure of proteins came through the study of the hemoglobin molecule.[80]
The 1950s	The chief breakthrough in the 1950s was Watson and Crick's discovery of the *structure of DNA*[109,110] and the beginning understanding of how genes express themselves and turn on or off. In work that was largely ignored at the time, Barbara McClintock discovered what she called *controlling elements,* that is, genetic factors that controlled the rate of gene expression.[55] During the 1950s the steps in protein synthesis were worked out. By the late 1950s scientists had the tools to better study chromosomes under the microscope, to count chromosomes, and to define abnormalities of chromosome number. The chromosome abnormalities in Down syndrome, Klinefelter syndrome, and Turner syndrome were first described at this time. The era of *karyotyping* had begun. The new field of *genetic counseling* developed. Discoveries of defective genes and the disorders they caused led Dr. Victor McKusick to compile them in a single book in 1966 entitled *Mendelian Inheritance in Man.*[68]
The 1960s and 1970s	In the 1960s scientists took another step forward with *somatic cell hybridization.* In this laboratory work, human cells and rodent cells were fused together into hybrid cells. When these cells were grown in culture, scientists could observe chromosomal defects and begin to map them to particular chromosomes. A staining method called *banding* made it possible to see the physical anatomy of the chromosome and advanced the ability to do human gene mapping.

From Ruccione, K. (1999). Cancer and genetics: What we need to know now. *Journal of Pediatric Oncology Nursing, 16,* 156-171.

TABLE 2-9	MILESTONES IN MOLECULAR BIOLOGY—cont'd
Era	**Prominent Discoveries**
	In the early 1970s a new set of techniques called *recombinant DNA* or genetic engineering was developed. This development meant that a fragment of DNA could be snipped out of one genome and spliced into (i.e., *recombined with*) another. The "Edward Scissorhands" of this scenario are proteins called restriction enzymes that can bind to and cut DNA at specific sites, depending on the sequence of base pairs. Another recombinant DNA technique known as molecular *cloning*—the ability to make multiple identical descendants of a gene transplanted into bacteria or yeast—made it possible to transcribe, translate, and make the gene's protein product in quantity. These recombinant techniques opened a new range of possibilities, including tracing a particular gene to a specific chromosome.
	Gene mapping catapulted further ahead with the discovery of restriction fragment length polymorphisms (*RFLPs*, pronounced "riflips"). The restriction enzymes generate DNA fragments of different lengths that form patterns of lines in a special gel. These patterns can be read in the same way that a scanning device at a supermarket can read a barcode on the bottom of a cereal box. The differences in the lengths of DNA fragments emerge because of a process called electrophoresis, which separates them. The heavier or longer ones end up on one side and the lighter or shorter ones on the other in a process called a *Southern blot.* In this way, "a baffling mystery was reduced to a graphic chart."[55]
The 1980s and 1990s	In the 1980s a new technique called *fluorescent in situ hybridization (FISH)* was developed as an improved method to map genes by using a "molecular probe." Chromosomes are isolated from cells and heated until each DNA double helix unzips into two complementary strands, then they are mixed with previously prepared, tagged DNA fragments. The fragments cling to their opposite partners (pair bonding rules apply), closing the zipper once more. Because the fragments glow under fluorescent light, scientists can more easily find abnormalities, such as when chunks of DNA break away from their home chromosomes and reattach to others.
	By the mid-1980s and 1990s discoveries about the *role of genes in disease* were coming along at a very fast pace, changing the definition of genetic disease. Equally important were the inventions that laid the technological foundation for the next wave of discoveries. Chief among these revolutionary new techniques was *gene amplification.* Just as the amplifier on a stereo system allows radio signals to be heard, gene amplification allows the genetic language of the cell to be deciphered. Amplification increases the total copies of a region of DNA to be studied. The most well known amplification technique, the *polymerase chain reaction (PCR),* earned its inventor, Kary Mullis, a Nobel Prize.
	In the 1990s more revolutionary innovations in biotechnology have included the *cloning of organisms from a single cell* (e.g., Dolly the sheep),[115] the creation of *artificial chromosomes,*[45] and the successful cultivation of human embryonic *stem cells* into immortal cell lines.[102] It was in this decade that some scientists began to believe that we needed to mobilize for a "genome sweepstakes," mapping and sequencing the complete human genome. What happened next, after considerable debate, was the launching of the *Human Genome Project,* designed to (a) find all the genes that humans possess, (b) determine their chromosomal location and structure, and (c) learn what regulates them. With this project, the most influential mapmakers of the twentieth century were charting the geography of genes. When the first catalog of human genetic disorders was compiled by Victor McKusick in 1966, it had approximately 1500 entries. By the late 1990s there was a continuously updated online version with thousands of entries. The technologies spinning off the Human Genome Project speeded up the rate of discovery of human disease genes so rapidly that a medically significant gene was being discovered almost every week.

known only to God."[100] Now the real work can begin.

In February 2001 the HGP and Celera published the first detailed sequence of the human genome, deciphering the order of the bases that make up DNA like the order of words in a sentence.[50,105] Scientists still need to produce a complete finished sequence, but already the map is yielding unexpected information. For example, the human genome is smaller than had been estimated, containing some 30,000 to 40,000 genes rather than the expected 100,000. Another surprising finding is that the highly complex human organism has only twice the genes of a fly or a worm. The next genomic step is to understand the function of genes and their proteins. Already, biologists are tracking down changes in DNA that underlie illness[20] and are mapping the precise chromosome location where the changes occur. This mapping is facilitated because more than 99% of all human DNA is identical. It is in the remaining fraction of a percent where the little changes lie that make one person different from another in characteristics such as hair color or cancer susceptibility. These differences represent a single change in the 3 billion letters that make up the human genome. Called single nucleotide polymorphisms (SNPs, pronounced "snips"), the differences can be used as landmarks on chromosomes. When these gene variants are tracked in a population, geneticists can determine the part they play in disease and learn why one person develops health problems such as cancer or heart disease and another does not. Both the Human Genome Project (in collaboration with a public/private SNP consortium which includes major pharmaceutical companies) and Celera Genomics have announced finding 2.8 million SNPs.

Finding out whether a gene has a counterpart in another organism, a field of study called comparative genomics, will assist in determining gene function. The mouse genome, already sequenced, will be extremely helpful in interpreting the human genome. One of the most daunting tasks ahead will be to study proteins' role in health and disease. Biologists have estimated that the functional set of human proteins, the proteome, could outnumber human genes by a factor of 10.[20] Really understanding what any protein or gene does will be the major challenge in biology for the twenty-first century.

CANCER AS A DISEASE OF THE MICROENVIRONMENT

Viewing cancer as a disease of the microenvironment reflects a deepening understanding of the role of the dynamic interactions between tumor cells and other cells and substances in their vicinity, and how they modulate each other in a highly choreographed ballet of malignancy. Recent reconceptualizations of cancer cell biology have proposed that cancer development depends on changes in the signals exchanged between malignant cells and nonmalignant cells present within tumor tissue, and between malignant cells and extracellular matrix proteins that form the connective tissue. Research is under way to map out the cells' signaling pathways, and their circuitry has been likened to an electronic integrated circuit in its complexity and finesse.[44]

IMMUNE REGULATION

The immune system is the body's intricate defense system against "foreign" molecules. When it is functioning well, it fights off infections by a variety of microorganisms such as bacteria, viruses, fungi, and parasites. When it malfunctions, diseases and disorders ranging from allergies to AIDS can result. The immune system functions through an elaborate and dynamic regulatory-communications network.[92] Millions of cells in the immune system exchange information continuously in a sensitive system of checks and balances to respond to threats promptly, appropriately, and effectively. The key element in this surveillance system is the ability to distinguish between self and non-self. The majority of cells carry molecular self-identification. Under normal conditions, the immune system does not attack cells marked as self, but when "foreign invaders" are encountered, the immune system mobilizes to eliminate them. Substances capable of triggering this immune response are termed *antigens*. Antigens provoke response by means of protrusions, called *epitopes*, on their surface (Figure 2-11). In some cases of mistaken identity, the im-

---

BOX 2-3

A CHANGING DEFINITION OF GENETIC DISEASE

- Single-gene or Mendelian genetic conditions, e.g., sickle cell disease and hemophilia.
- Multifactorial conditions, such as heart disease and cancer, which share a combination of genetic and environmental influences. These may be polygenic conditions, i.e., involving more than one gene.
- Acquired genetic conditions, such as AIDS or hepatitis C, in which a viral infection carries new genetic information into the host.

From Pollock, R. (1994). *Signs of life: The language and meanings of DNA.* Boston: Houghton-Mifflin.

mune system wrongly identifies self as non-self and initiates an attack, which can result in autoimmune diseases such as rheumatoid arthritis.

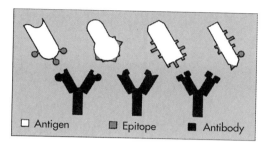

☐ Antigen   ▨ Epitope   ■ Antibody

Figure 2-11

Antigens and antibodies.   (From Schindler, L. W. [1993]. *Understanding the immune system* [p. 2]. Bethesda, MD: NIH Publication No: 93-529. U.S. Department of Health and Human Services. Public Health Service. National Institutes of Health. National Cancer Institute.)

Anatomy of the immune system.   The immune system has three primary functions: (1) defense against the entry of foreign microorganisms; (2) maintenance of homeostasis through the orderly removal of dead or damaged cells; and (3) surveillance to identify and destroy abnormal cells. These functions are carried out through the synchronized efforts of various organs, generally referred to as lymphoid organs because their chief role is in the growth, development, and deployment of lymphocytes, the white blood cells that are the foot soldiers of the immune system (Figure 2-12).

- *Bone marrow and thymus.* Cells that will become immune cells originate from progenitor stem cells in the bone marrow (Figure 2-13). Some stem cell descendents become *lymphocytes,* and others develop into *phagocytes*. Phagocytes are large immune cells capable of devouring cells and particles. Lymphocytes are grouped as B cells and T cells. B cells complete their maturation in the bone marrow, whereas T cells migrate

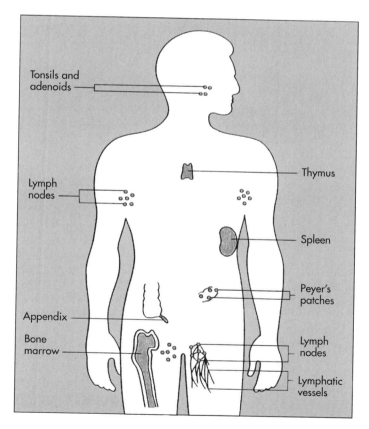

Figure 2-12

Organs of the immune system.   (From Schindler, L. W. [1993]. *Understanding the immune system* [p. 3]. Bethesda, MD: NIH Publication No: 93-529. U.S. Department of Health and Human Services. Public Health Service. National Institutes of Health. National Cancer Institute.)

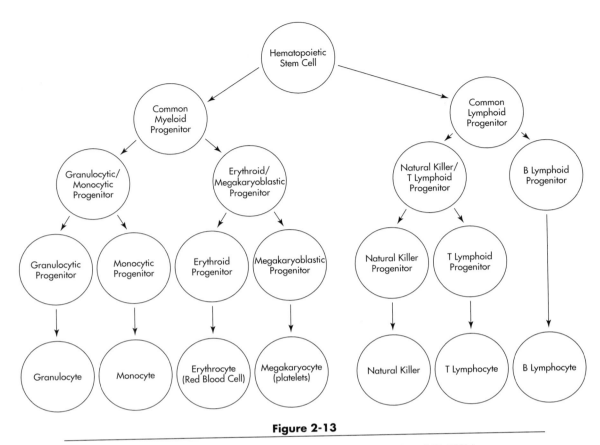

Figure 2-13

Cells of the immune system.   (Courtesy Kenneth A. Weinberg, MD, 2001.)

to the thymus, where they mature and learn to distinguish self from non-self.

- *Lymphatic vessels and lymph nodes.* B and T cells, after leaving the bone marrow and thymus, circulate freely throughout the body via a network of lymphatic vessels similar to blood vessels (except that, unlike the blood circulation which is pumped by the heart, this circulation is passive). Along the network of lymphatic vessels are small, bean-shaped lymph nodes that contain compartments housing B lymphocytes, T lymphocytes, and other cells that can enmesh antigens and present them to T cells for destruction.[92] The lymphatic vessels carry lymph, a clear fluid that continuously bathes body cells and carries immune cells. As the lymph drains out of tissues, it transports antigens through lymphatic vessels to lymph nodes where they can be filtered out and presented to immune cells to destroy. Blood vessels also supply lymph nodes and can transport lymphocytes to the nodes. Lymphatic vessels exiting the lymph nodes merge into the thoracic duct, which empties its contents

into the bloodstream.[92] Lymphocytes and other immune cells travel through the body in the blood to patrol tissues for foreign antigens, repeating the cycle of seeping into the lymphatic vessels and back to the lymph nodes.

- *Spleen.* The spleen has two main types of tissue: the red pulp, a disposal site for worn-out blood cells, and the white pulp containing lymphoid tissue. The lymphoid tissue stores various kinds of immune cells. Microorganisms carried into the red pulp are trapped by macrophages.
- *Other lymphoid tissue.* Many parts of the body contain clusters of lymphoid tissue, particularly around areas that serve as gateways to the body, such as the respiratory and gastrointestinal tracts. These include the tonsils and adenoids, the appendix, and Peyer's patches.

Cells of the immune system. The immune system includes cells that handle general defenses and cells that are trained to recognize specific targets. Only a limited number of specialized cells are stored, and when an antigen is encountered, the matched immune cells are signaled to multiply. When they are no longer needed in large supply, other signals suppress their growth. The major workhorses of the immune system are the lymphocytes, categorized as B cells and T cells. B cells, T cells, and natural killer cells (non-T, non-B cells) arise from a common lymphoid progenitor cell (see Figure 2-13).

B cells and antibodies. B cells make antibodies that are secreted into the body's fluids (also called humors, hence this type of immunity is termed *humoral immunity*). Each B cell can produce one specific antibody. When a B cell encounters its triggering antigen, it produces plasma cells that function as antibody factories. The plasma cells from the single B cell, because they are from the same family or clone, produce the same specific antibody (this is the basis for the concept of monoclonal antibody production by the biotechnology industry). Antibodies are large protein molecules with a typical structure that identifies them as immunoglobulins (Ig). Human immunoglobulins can be classified on the basis of that structure as IgM, IgD, IgG, IgA, and IgE (listed in the order that they are generated by B cells). Antibodies can work in various ways: by interlocking with toxins produced by some bacteria, forming antitoxins that disable directly; by opsonizing bacteria (coating them and making them vulnerable to scavenger cells that engulf and digest them); by forming antigen-antibody complexes that unleash serum enzymes known as complement; by blocking viruses from entering cells; and through antibody-dependent cell-mediated cytotoxicity, a phenomenon that makes cells coated with antibody vulnerable to attack by several types of white blood cells.[92]

T cells and lymphokines. T cells help the immune system in two ways: as regulatory cells orchestrating the system, and as cytotoxic cells that attack body cells that are infected or damaged. The regulatory T cells include "helper/inducer" cells (which carry the T_4 cell marker) that activate B cells, other T cells, natural killer cells, and macrophages. Cytotoxic T cells (usually carrying the T_4 marker) kill cells that have been infected by viruses or transformed by cancer, and reject tissue and organ grafts. T cells work primarily by secreting cytokines (specifically, lymphocytes secrete lymphokines; monocytes and macrophages secrete monokines). Cytokines are chemical messengers that can encourage cell growth, promote cell activation, direct cellular traffic, destroy target cells, and incite macrophages.[92] They are biologic response modifiers. Among the first cytokines to be identified

were the interferons (which activate macrophages and have antiviral properties), lymphotoxin (from lymphocytes), and tumor necrosis factor (from macrophages). The latter two kill tumor cells. As cytokines are identified and their structure is determined, they are named and numbered as interleukins (so-named because they serve as messengers *between* white cells). Examples include:

Interleukin-1 or IL-1: helps activate B cells and T cells

IL-2: promotes rapid growth or differentiation of mature T cells and B cells

IL-3: T cell–derived member of the family of colony-stimulating factors (CSF) that includes among its functions nurturing immature precursor cells into a variety of mature blood cells

IL-4, IL-5, IL-6: help various lymphoid and myeloid cells grow and differentiate

Natural killer (NK) cells. Like cytotoxic T cells, NK cells kill on contact. They kill by delivering chemicals that make a hole in the target cell's membrane, allowing fluids to seep in until the target cell bursts. In contrast to cytotoxic T cells, however, NK cells do not need to recognize a specific antigen before aiming their lethal weapons.

Phagocytes and granulocytes. Phagocytes are large white cells that can engulf and digest microorganisms and antigenic particles. Among the important phagocytes are monocytes and macrophages. After circulating in the blood, monocytes migrate into tissues and develop into macrophages (a name meaning "big eaters"). Macrophages have a role as scavengers, as initiators of immune response by presenting antigen to T cells, by secreting powerful chemicals, and by carrying receptors for lymphokines that allow them to be turned into "smart weapons" aimed at microorganisms and tumor cells. Another important phagocyte is the neutrophil, which is a granulocyte. The family of granulocytes (also known as polymorphonuclear leukocytes) also includes eosinophils and basophils. Chemicals in granulocytes help destroy microorganisms and play a role in acute inflammatory reactions.

Mounting an immune response. The body's first line of defense against invaders is the skin and mucous membranes, both because they are a physical barrier and because the immune system provides them with scavenger cells and IgA antibodies. The next level of defense is nonspecific, relying on immune system activities that don't require specifically matched weapons. Microorganisms that survive nonspecific defenses are met by specific responses of T cells and their lymphokines or by humoral responses of B cells secreting antibodies into body fluids. Although there is a traditional distinction between humoral (B cell) and cell-mediated (T cell) immunity, these activities are closely intertwined.

Cell-mediated immune response begins with a macrophage or other cell, which takes in an antigen, digests it, and then displays antigen fragments on its surface. This by itself is not sufficient to evoke the T cell's response, however. The antigen fragment must also have an MHC (major histocompatibility complex) molecule bound to it. MHC is a group of genes contained in a section of a specific chromosome that encode molecules that mark a cell as self and play a key role in immune defense. MHC markers determine which antigens an individual can respond to and how strongly, and they allow immune cells such as B cells, T cells, and macrophages to recognize and communicate with one another.[92] MHC genes and the molecules they encode vary widely among individuals (polymorphism), an important consideration in tissue transplants. One group of MHC proteins (class I MHC antigens) alert killer T cells to the presence of body cells that are infected or transformed into malignant cells and that need to be eliminated. Another group of MHC proteins (class II MHC antigens) help to focus T cell antigen recognition by binding to particles of foreign antigen.

T cells recognize antigens through a protein, a T cell receptor (TCR) for the antigen, on the cell surface. A T cell that fits the antigen-MHC complex binds to it, stimulating the antigen-presenting cell to secrete interleukins for T cell activation. A second go-ahead signal, called co-stimulation, is required. In co-stimulation, the antigen-presenting cell displays a special molecule that engages specific receptor molecules on the T cell, including one known as CD28.[92] Then a variety of T cells secrete lymphokines to stimulate growth of more T cells, and to bring other immune cells to the scene, direct activities at the site, activate cytotoxic cells, locate other affected body cells, and shut down the immune response when the invasion has been brought under control.

Immunity and cancer. When normal cells are transformed into cancer cells, it is thought that they form new or altered antigens on their surface that alert immune cells. A theory of immune surveillance holds that immune cells patrol the body and eliminate cells that have undergone malignant transformation. If the surveillance system breaks down or is overwhelmed, tumors develop. Evasive mechanisms could include the ability of the tumor cells to elude the immune system by altering or disguising their antigens, or to interfere with the immune system by stimulating production of suppressor T cells that block the cytotoxic T cells.

Although blood tests show that people can develop antibodies to various tumor antigens, there is no evidence to show that these antibodies are clinically effective in fighting tumors. A fundamental question in tumor immunology is whether tumor cells express antigens that T cells can recognize as foreign. Over the past 15 years various therapeutic strategies have been under investigation to try to increase the ability of T cells to kill tumor cells. These strategies include engineering T cells to recognize specific tumor-associated antigens, administration of growth factors (cytokines) to increase killing of tumor cells by T cells, and attempts to make engineered tumor cells that function as vaccines that would "teach" T cells to kill all the tumor cells in a patient.

Tumor-associated antigens are used for monitoring the course of disease and the effectiveness of treatment. Antigen markers are measured in the serum after being shed by tumor cells. T cell and B cell antigens are useful in differentiating between the various forms of leukemia and lymphoma, a distinction that is important in staging the disease and determining the intensity of treatment.

Other tumor markers (biomarkers). Cell-surface and cytoplasmic abnormalities foster or produce substances that are found on tumor cells or in blood, spinal fluid, or urine and are therefore identified as markers of specific tumors. Ideally these biomarkers can be detected and measured to aid in cancer surveillance, provide estimates of tumor burden, and indicate tumor regression or progression.[107] There are practical limitations to the use of biomarkers, however, which include inaccuracy in measurement and interpretation of findings. For example, nonmalignant disease can be associated with the presence of a tumor marker, or a tumor marker may only become detectable relatively late in the disease. Often tumor marker levels are not proportionate to actual tumor burden. Clinical application of tumor markers is more common in adult cancers such as prostate and ovarian cancer.

Tumor marker types relevant to childhood cancers include hormones, enzymes, and antigens (described above). Hormones inappropriately produced by tumor tissue include increased urinary catecholamines and their metabolites associated with neuroblastoma, α-fetoprotein in a variety of hepatic and germ cell tumors, and β-human chorionic gonadotropin in trophoblastic and other germ cell tumors. Enzymes may be expressed as an immature, fetal form of an enzyme or as the ectopic (produced by nonendocrine tissue) production of a normal enzyme; isoenzymes that have a variable form but function similarly to normal enzymes also are potential pediatric tumor markers. Neuron-specific enolase (NSE) is markedly elevated in children, particularly infants, with extensive neuroblastoma. Terminal deoxynucleotidyl transferase (TdT) is elevated with T-cell and B-cell leukemias and in some children with acute myeloblastic leukemia. TdT usefulness has been limited to measuring tumor responsiveness; it also may be elevated during febrile episodes or viral infection. Lactate dehydrogenase (LDH) may be elevated with a number of pediatric cancers, including ALL, non-Hodgkin's lymphoma, osteosarcoma, Ewing sarcoma, and neuroblastoma.

As research continues to characterize molecules shed by various kinds of tumor cells, more specific and sensitive markers may become available for earlier diagnosis, and accurate monitoring of disease progression. That is the goal of a coalition of National Cancer Institute-funded researchers, the Early Detection Research Network (EDRN).[104] EDRN investigators are analyzing blood, urine, saliva, and other tissue samples for abnormal proteins and genetic additions and deletions. If promising biomarkers are found, they will be validated in large-scale clinical trials. Ultimately, the best tests may not be single biomarkers, but rather patterns of markers for malignant and precancerous lesions.

HALLMARKS OF CANCER

During the past 20 years—a time that has been called the golden age of biology—a central mystery of cancer has already been solved. The main types of genes involved and the basic molecular steps toward cancer are known. Cancer arises because of genetic mutations in a cell. These mutations, in turn, can change the amount or activity of proteins involved in regulating cell life. The transformation from normal cell to malignant cell is a progressive multistep process, involving a succession of genetic changes. A cancer acquires the ability to circumvent normal control mechanisms and manipulate its local environment.[64] Important clues about how mutated genes contribute to cancer have come from studying what their counterparts do in normal cells, i.e., in their microenvironment. Hanahan and Weinberg have suggested that there are six essential alterations in normal cell physiology that collectively dictate malignant growth (Figure 2-14): self-sufficiency in growth signals, insensitivity to growth-inhibitory (antigrowth) signals, evasion

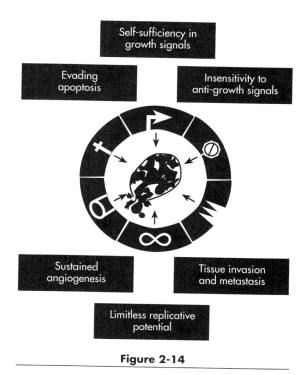

Figure 2-14

Acquired capabilities of cancer. (From Hanahan, D., Weinberg, R. A. [2000]. The hallmarks of cancer. *Cell, 100,* 57-70.)

of programmed cell death (apoptosis), limitless replicative potential, sustained angiogenesis, and tissue invasion and metastasis.[44] These mechanisms may represent an anticancer defense mechanism hardwired into cells and tissues, and their multiplicity may explain why cancer does not occur more often.[44]

1. *Self-sufficiency in growth signals.* Normal cells are dependent upon their tissue microenvironment for signals before they can move from a quiescent state into an active proliferative state. One scientist's description is that there are molecular "bucket brigades"[112] that relay growth-stimulating signals from outside the cell to deep into its interior (Figure 2-15). Cell-to-cell signaling for growth begins when one cell secretes proteins known as growth factors that move through spaces between cells and bind to specific receptors. The signal is passed to a succession of other proteins and finally to the nucleus, which alerts the cell to go through its growth cycle. A major area of cancer research has been focused on cancer cells and the genes within them, such as oncogenes that mimic normal growth signaling. Now an emerging view is that tumors are complex tissues in which mutant cancer cells have conscripted and subverted normal cell types to serve

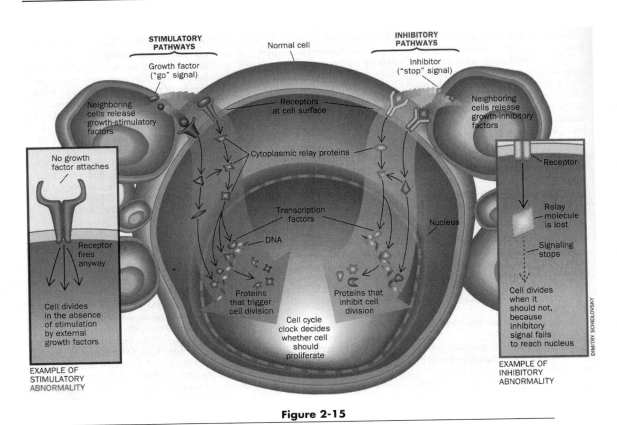

Figure 2-15

Molecular bucket brigades. (From Weinberg, R. A. [1996]. How cancer arises. *Scientific American, 275,* 62-70.)

as active collaborators.[44] In this concept of heterotypic cell biology, fibroblasts and endothelial cells may be induced to release growth-stimulating signals, and immune cells attracted to sites of malignant cells may promote rather than eliminate the cancer. This more dynamic view considers the interaction between cancer cells and their microenvironment.

2. *Insensitivity to antigrowth signals.* A cell may become malignant through overstimulation of the growth-promoting machinery in combination with evading or ignoring normal braking systems. The braking system, like the growth signal system, works with molecular "bucket brigades," in this case signaling that growth should stop. Another important discovery is the *cell clock,* that is, the destination point in the nucleus that promotes or inhibits growth. Normally the cell clock programs the events of the cell cycle through a variety of molecules. Of these molecules, two critical ones are cyclins and cyclin-dependent kinases (CDKs). It is now known that in almost every case of cancer, the cell clock is malfunctioning.[112]

3. *Evading apoptosis.* A recently described and important cellular defense against runaway cell division is apoptosis, which is a backup system that tells the cell to destroy itself if something essential is damaged or if controls are deregulated. Cancer cells may succeed in growing because they acquire the ability to evade apoptosis. Scientists have proposed that this ability to escape apoptosis may not only allow tumors to grow, but also make them more resistant to treatment.[112] Defects in the eradication of cells that accumulate genetic lesions lead to genomic instability, resistance to immune attack, and chemoresistance. With identification and cloning of the 11 enzymes (caspases) that are thought to play a major role in apoptosis, the search for useful interventions is headed for exponential growth.[71]

4. *Limitless replicative potential.* Another defense against runaway growth is a "counter" within the cells that keeps track of how many times cells reproduce themselves. The counters are molecular devices called telomeres and are located in DNA segments at the end of chromosomes. Usually, telomeres shorten a bit every time chromosomes

are replicated. Once they shrink below a certain threshold length, an alarm signals the cell to enter senescence and to stop reproducing. But cancer cells activate a gene for an enzyme called telomerase, which replaces telomeric segments and lets the cell replicate endlessly.

   5. *Sustained angiogenesis.* Another normal cell function is angiogenesis, i.e., the proliferation of new capillaries, which is normally activated during menstruation, placental nourishment of the fetus, and wound healing. Scientists have found that tumors can also switch on angiogenesis, which increases their blood supply and enables the tumor to expand.[33,34] Cells need close proximity to capillaries to survive, and tumors cannot expand beyond 1 to 2 mm^3 unless new blood vessel growth occurs. It appears that the ability to induce and sustain angiogenesis is acquired at some step during tumor development before formation of macroscopic tumor.[44] In tumor angiogenesis, the tumor produces proteins, growth factors such as VEGF (vascular endothelial growth factor) and bFGF (basic fibroblast growth factor) that activate endothelial cell growth and movement.[83] The action of these factors is counterbalanced by inhibitors of angiogenesis such as angiostatin or endostatin. Signals carried by regulatory molecules moving between cells and their microenvironment change the balance of angiogenesis inducers and inhibitors, thereby activating an "angiogenic switch." Angiogenesis is a very active area of research not only in cancer but also in developmental biology, cardiovascular disease, diabetes, and rheumatology because of the potential clinical application in increasing angiogenesis in patients with occlusive vascular disease and decreasing angiogenesis in patients with tumors.[29]

   6. *Tissue invasion and metastasis.* Most types of human cancer can produce cells that escape the primary tumor mass and move out, invade adjacent tissues, and then travel to distant sites to establish new tumors known as metastases. The new outposts provide an environment, at least initially, where nutrients and space are not limited. Not all cells in a tumor have the capability to travel to distant sites. The genetic instability of cancer cells, meaning their high mutation rate, enables the development of differentiated clones of cells within a tumor that have the characteristics for successful metastasis.

   Cancer cells with the capacity for invasion and metastasis disregard the normal tissue barrier of the extracellular matrix (ECM). The ECM is the structure that provides support for the development and organization of tissues. It consists of compartments separated by membranes, including the basement membrane that covers the blood vessels, muscle

cells, and nerves. Cells with invasive or metastatic capability have alterations in the proteins that are involved in tethering cells to their surroundings in tissue. These proteins include cell-cell adhesion molecules, which mediate cell-to-cell interactions, and integrins, which link cells to the extracellular matrix structure. Invasive and metastatic capability also involves extracellular enzymes called proteases. These substances play a role in degrading the extracellular matrix, allowing cancer cells to untether from the tumor and to establish themselves in other tissue.

   During invasion (1) tumor cells attach to the basement membrane when their cell-surface receptors bind to elements of the membrane; (2) enzymes are secreted that destroy basement membrane molecules and create an opening; and (3) tumor cells move through the opening into the tissue.[62,63] Without these changes in the regulation of the cell and its relationship to the ECM, a cancer would remain in situ. An active area of research is directed at understanding the precise role and mechanisms of various types of enzymes that have been implicated in the invasive process. These include plasminogen activators and matrix metalloproteinases (MMPs).[23] Cytokines and growth factors may play an important role in modulating secretion of proteolytic enzymes.

   Local invasion begins the multistep process of metastasis, referred to as the sequential metastatic cascade (Figure 2-16). Every step of the cascade must be completed for the development of clinically significant metastases.[64] For tumor cells to travel beyond local invasion, new blood vessel growth (neovascularization by angiogenesis) is essential.[33,34] Angiogenesis is an invasive process that requires: (1) degradation of the basement membrane and ECM surrounding blood vessels, (2) migration of endothelial cells toward an angiogenic stimulus, (3) proliferation of endothelial cells, and (4) alteration of the basement membrane as the new blood vessel forms. It is thought that plasminogen activators and MMPs are involved in various parts of this process. Recent studies have shown that tumor masses not only can induce new blood vessel growth by recruiting endothelial cells in angiogenesis, they also can develop a blood supply by other means, such as co-opting existing host vessels[49] or by forming tumor channels (called vascular mimicry).[66]

   Cancer cells are transported to distant sites via the general circulation or the lymphatics as individual cells or as emboli made up of tumor cells or tumor and host cells.[116] Tumor cells in the lymphatics are transported to regional lymph nodes.

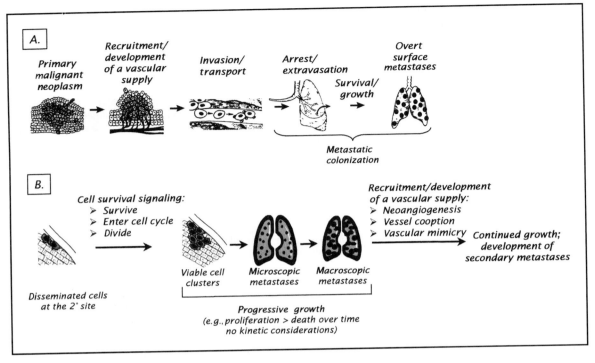

Figure 2-16

The metastatic cascade. (From Yoshida, B. A., Sokoloff, M. M., Welch, D. R., et al. [2000]. Metastasis-suppressor genes: A review and perspective on an emerging field. *JNCI, 92,* 1717-1730.)

Initially these regional nodes can serve as a barrier delaying the continued spread of the cancer cells, but eventually this protection becomes ineffective. At the secondary site, tumor cells arrest in the capillary beds because of their physical size or by binding to specific molecules in organs or tissues.[78,113] To escape the capillary circulation and create a metastatic site in tissue, tumor cells must first penetrate the layer of endothelial cells lining the inside of the capillary (extravasation). Tumor cells attach preferentially to endothelial surfaces, stimulating the endothelial layer to retract, exposing underlying tissue (the extracellular matrix). If the new microenvironment is suitable, a metastatic site is established. Additional new metastases can be initiated from both the secondary site and the primary tumor.

Individual primary tumors metastasize to particular anatomic sites preferentially. In 1873 Paget suggested a "seed and soil" theory to explain site-specific metastasis. This theory underscored the importance of conducive characteristics of the metastatic site (the soil) for the particular tumor cells (the seed) to grow. Specific factors thought to contribute to the preferential selection of the even-

tual site of metastasis for particular tumors include hormones, ECM proteins, growth-promoting factors, genetics, age, tumor angiogenesis at the metastatic site, immune status, and blood flow.[27] Table 2-10 shows common metastatic sites of childhood cancers.

Metastatic disease is responsible for most deaths due to cancer,[98] but the lethality of metastatic disease belies how inefficient it actually is. It is estimated that less than 0.01% of cancer cells that separate and spread from the primary tumor ever become a metastatic colony.[32,113] Tumor cells arriving at a secondary site have the potential to colonize, and they cannot be ignored in cancer treatment; however, an important emerging concept is that the mere presence of cells at a secondary site does not mean that metastatic colonization will occur.[116] Recent work has shown that a subset of metastasis-suppressor genes, distinct from oncogenes and tumor-suppressor genes, inhibits early steps in metastatic colonization.[116]

Invasion and metastasis are similar processes, both complex and incompletely understood. Both use similar strategies involving changes in the physical tethering of cells to their microenviron-

TABLE 2-10	METASTASIS IN SELECTED CHILDHOOD CANCERS	
Primary Tumor	**Incidence at Diagnosis**	**Metastatic Sites**
Neuroblastoma	60%	Lymph nodes, bone marrow, liver, bone
Rhabdomyosarcoma	10-30%	Lymph nodes, lung, bone, bone marrow, liver
Ewing sarcoma	14-50%	Bone, brain
Osteosarcoma	10-20%	Lung, bone
Wilms tumor	16%	Lung, liver
Retinoblastoma	5%	Bone, brain, bone marrow
Brain	Very rare	Spine

Courtesy Yves DeClerck, MD, 2001.

ment and activation of extracellular enzymes, called proteases, that can facilitate invasion of cancer cells into nearby tissue, across blood vessel walls, and through normal epithelial cell layers.[44] Elucidating the mechanisms of tumor invasion and metastasis has been described as the last great frontier for exploratory cancer research.[44] Discoveries in this field will have important implications for novel therapeutic approaches to controlling the growth and spread of malignant cells, discussed in the next section.

MOLECULAR MEDICINE

Considerable translational research is under way to bring molecular biology from bench to bedside. Some examples of current and predicted clinical applications of molecular biology include the following:

Genome-based diagnosis and disease management. Researchers are forecasting that within the next 20 years an individual's medical record will include his or her complete genome, as well as identification of specific alleles (SNPs) that increase the risk of disease.[26] The technology that will make this possible is DNA microarray, or "chip," analysis.[56,85,93] A microarray is a display of individual DNA sequences on a thin slice of glass or other solid support about the size of a postage stamp. On the surface of the "chip" in a grid pattern are strings of DNA representing thousands of gene variants. When a patient's DNA is added to the

chip, pieces stick to the matching strings because of complementary base pair binding, and the rest are washed away. Electronic scanners read the matches, and computer software analyzes the information. Recent advances in both molecular biology and high speed, high volume computer data analysis systems were prerequisites for the development of this innovation. In oncology, studies using gene expression profiling are under way to characterize genetic changes in neuroblastoma, CNS primitive neuroectodermal tumor or medulloblastoma, and childhood leukemias.[12]

Even more intriguing, perhaps, are the newer methods that will develop in the field of proteomics.[75] These techniques will allow researchers to analyze the proteins in a cell, which reflect the cell's responses to disease, diet, exercise, or other stimuli. Knowing what causes the changes that make a normal cell malignant or what causes disease progression in a cancer cell may make it possible to interfere with the disease process or reverse the effect. New technology that greatly speeds up the rate of protein analysis is under development. This will make it feasible to analyze samples from people with different types of cancer to try to identify better tumor markers for disease detection and monitoring response to treatment. In addition, researchers will try to identify key proteins that may make good targets for antibodies developed for use as cancer vaccines.

The day will come when doctors, reading a patient's individual proteomic, microarray gene expression, and polymorphism analyses, will be able to determine his or her susceptibility to a particular cancer, recommend preventive measures if applicable, and know simultaneously what the best genetically tailored treatment will be. The new hybrid of genomics and molecular pharmacology, *pharmacogenomics,* is evolving with a focus on profiling the expression of genes related to toxicity and response.[75] Microarray technology will be used to individually customize the most effective, least toxic therapy for individual patients and—by profiling tumor cell lines used for new drug development—will have clear application to clinical trials and developmental therapeutics. In addition, a likely outcome of the new genomic discoveries is that classification systems based on cellular genetic abnormalities will replace current classifications based on site of origin or histology.

Cytokines and other biologicals. Cytokines are molecules that coordinate and regulate cell life, growth, and death.[51] A number of cytokines are already in clinical use or in research protocols, including interferon, interleukin, tumor necrosis factor, and the hematopoietic cytokines (granulocyte-colony-stimulating factor, granulocyte macrophage-colony-stimulating factor, erythropoietin, thrombopoietin). Other biologicals include mediators of differentiation such as retinoic acid, which is being used for patients with promyelocytic leukemia and neuroblastoma.

Monoclonal antibodies. As described earlier in this chapter, many different antibodies are made by B lymphocytes. A population of identical cells that has arisen from the same ancestor cells is known as a clone, and the single kind of antibody produced by such a clone is a monoclonal antibody (MoAb). Methods for producing large quantities of MoAbs were discovered 25 years ago.[58] Since that time MoAbs have been used to treat cancer in the following ways: (1) as mediators of immune cytotoxicity through activation of complement or by action of lymphocytes and macrophages; (2) as inhibitors of specific functions mediated by the targeted antigen; and (3) as carriers of cytotoxic molecules or radionuclides to cells carrying the relevant antigen.[70,74] Despite early hope, and hype, MoAbs were mostly a therapeutic failure until some of their clinical problems could be overcome; side effects were serious, and efficacy was low.[38]

Now that there are better ways of using recombinant DNA technology to link antibodies to toxins, MoAb size has been reduced to better penetrate tumors, and fully human antibodies have been developed.[38] In adult oncology, two MoAbs have been approved by the FDA: Herceptin and Rituxan. Other MoAb-based drugs approved or in development include Mytolarg, an anti-CD33 antibody for treating relapsed acute myelogenous leukemia (AML), and radio-labeled antibodies for non-Hodgkin's lymphoma. Additional MoAb variations are in advanced development, including bispecific antibodies that attach both to tumor and to an effector or toxic molecule; antibody dimers, which deliver apoptotic signals to the targeted tumor cell; new drug-MoAb conjugates (similar to Mytolarg); and antibody mimetics, synthetic peptides that more easily penetrate tumors.[38]

Gene therapy. In gene therapy, functional copies of genes are transferred into somatic or germ cells (e.g., sperm, ova, or early embryo). Only somatic gene-directed therapy is currently approved for use in clinical trials. Germ-line therapy to eliminate inherited disease in future generations and enhancement gene therapy, or eugenics, are subjects of intense ethical debate. There are a number of somatic gene therapy trials in progress, although none have proved curative. Recently a storm of controversy unleashed by the publicity surrounding a young man's death in a gene therapy trial has focused attention on reporting of adverse events, government oversight of clinical trials, and human toxicity of gene therapy. Technical limitations still to be overcome include the difficulty of getting genes into the majority of target cells.

Some novel gene therapy strategies include designing tumor vaccines to rouse an immune response. Among the prime targets for vaccines are cancers caused by viruses (e.g., some cervical cancers). Recently, antigen-specific vaccines for melanoma have been studied. This work relies on activating an immune response against a tumor-associated antigen whose protein and DNA sequences are known. Using this information, investigators designed a synthetic peptide; the resulting peptide vaccines are given with cytokine.[28] Other tumor vaccines under investigation include recombinant vector-based vaccines using smallpox and avipoxvirus, and autologous dendritic cell peptide vaccines. Dendritic cells are a rare type of immune system cell, believed to be efficient at processing foreign antigens and starting the antigen-antibody response; dendritic vaccines would be made by attaching specific tumor antigens (e.g., from a pediatric sarcoma) to a patient's own dendritic cells and then reinfusing them into the patient to elicit an immune response.[28] In the future, constructing vaccines that combine a variety of antigens (e.g., polyvalent vaccines), testing how well antibody and vaccine-based approaches work together, and combining nonspecific and specific immunotherapies with other cancer therapies will be investigated. Other gene therapy strategies may include replacing damaged tumor-suppressor genes, restoring normal DNA repair gene function, and increasing an individual's tolerance for dose-intensified chemotherapy by transferring drug-resistance genes to normal, dose-sensitive tissues.[51]

Triplex and antisense agents. Two new approaches that can potentially attack viruses and cancers without harming normal tissues are being studied. Called triplex and antisense agents, they are synthetic short strands of nucleic acids. These nucleic acids (called oligomers or oligonucleotides) bind to selected sites on DNA or RNA that direct protein production. In triplex agents, the oligomer wraps around the double helix, making it a triple-stranded helix. The antisense agents are so named because the sequence on the RNA makes "sense" by serving as the code for the production of a protein. The sequence of the oligonucleotide designed to bind with it is "antisense."

These agents interfere with transcription and translation.[19]

Angiogenesis inhibitors.   Another group of drugs under study are the antiangiogenesis agents designed to block the generation of new blood vessels needed for tumor progression. There are four major methods of inhibiting angiogenesis currently under study: (1) inhibiting or neutralizing factors that stimulate angiogenesis; (2) inhibiting activated endothelial cells directly; (3) inhibiting proteolytic enzymes from breaking down the ECM; and (4) inhibiting the endothelial-specific adhesion molecule integrin.[81] Among the agents under study are angiogenic growth factor blockers such as interferon and anti-VEGF antibody; endothelial cell inhibitors such as thalidomide, endostatin, and angiostatin; MMP inhibitors such as Marimastat; and adhesion molecule inhibitors such as Vitaxin.[83] With identification of genes that are "turned on" in tumor angiogenesis, there is new potential for finding other drugs capable of switching off these genes.

Other novel anticancer agents.   Novel therapeutic strategies currently in development include agents to modulate the cell-to-cell signaling system that allows cell growth to work normally and stop cancer cells before they start, and to block telomerase in cancer cells and push them toward destruction.[112] Drugs like these that are target-specific rather than tumor-specific represent the new paradigm of cancer therapies. Other examples include ST1571, which targets a protein produced by abnormal genes in CML, and arsenic trioxide,[21,59] which targets mitochondrial membrane permeability to induce normal apoptosis.

Chemoprevention.   Chemoprevention is a strategy that uses natural and synthetic compounds to intervene in the early precancerous stages of cancer development.[43] Investigators are studying compounds in food, vitamin and mineral supplements, and drugs (e.g., tamoxifen and retinoids) to determine their ability to lower cancer risk. Ultimately, each individual could have a tailored chemoprevention strategy to stall carcinogenesis based on his or her personalized DNA "chip."

Genetic testing.   Genetic testing has already found application in paternity suits, in criminology (DNA "fingerprints"), and in solving historical mysteries. Carrier testing lets couples learn if they carry, and thus risk passing to their children, an allele for an inherited condition such as cystic fibrosis. Gene testing is being used to look for telltale DNA changes in tumor cells or precancerous cells.

Genetic testing that identifies people who are at increased risk of getting a disease is called predictive and presymptomatic testing.

There are two approaches in identifying a genetic risk of predisposing cancer mutation: direct testing and linkage analysis. Both involve examining DNA. In direct testing, the sequence of a susceptibility gene must be known in its normal and mutant forms. A mutation can then be sought directly in the DNA taken from lymphocytes in the blood. Direct testing is available for a number of genes; those relevant for pediatrics include *RB1* in retinoblastoma, *WT1* in Wilms tumor, and *p53* in Li-Fraumeni syndrome. Predictive tests for other pediatric cancers are on the horizon. In the foreseeable future, direct testing will become more readily available, less expensive, and less time-consuming than linkage analysis. Linkage analysis is used when there is a large family of affected members. In this situation, an individual's RFLP, the "barcode" DNA pattern (see Table 2-9), is compared with those of both affected and unaffected family members. If a marker for a known condition is present on a chromosome in those individuals with cancer, it is assumed that they have inherited the mutation as well. The presence of a mutation is not directly observed. It is inferred by the patterns of chromosome segregation.

The availability of presymptomatic genetic testing has intensified research into the psychologic effects of testing.[79,80,106,114] Further research about predisposition testing and follow-up care is needed, particularly in relation to the difficult choices when the decision involves testing children.[1,37] Guidelines have been established that mandate that testing be done on children only when: (1) a condition has childhood manifestations, (2) risk assessment indicates a high probability that genetic testing will be informative, (3) a test is available that will yield interpretable, nonambiguous results, and (4) effective surveillance measures exist for preventive care.[5] Hereditary cancer syndromes that meet these criteria include multiple endocrine neoplasia types 2A and B, familial retinoblastoma, and familial adenomatous polyposis.[4]

NURSING ASSESSMENT AND INTERVENTION

PATIENT AND FAMILY PERSPECTIVES ON CANCER

A fundamental nursing responsibility is assessment of the patient's and family's understanding of, and prior experience with, cancer. If, for example, their perspective on cancer is based on what they have seen in adult friends and relatives, it may be helpful to discuss important differences between cancer in children and adults. Most parents of children with cancer want to know what caused the illness. Often they are told that, as far as we know, nothing they did or did not do caused their child's cancer. Yet clinical experience has shown that many parents form their own theories about the origins of their child's illness. Because the biologic cause of most childhood cancers is not known, and because parents' etiologic explanations serve a purpose in defining the meaning of cancer in their lives, health care providers can support parents by acknowledging and validating the search for meaning, skillfully exploring parents' beliefs about their child's illness, and providing practical guidance about the nature and focus of current epidemiologic and genetic research.

Epidemiology and Genetic Studies

When parents ask whether environmental and genetic factors are being studied, nurses can let them know that epidemiologic studies have been or are being conducted to examine parental occupational exposure, radon, pesticides, electromagnetic fields, and other environmental exposures; these studies may prove informative for some childhood cancer cases. Nurses can explain that current epidemiologic studies often include genetic analyses to better understand how cancer may develop in cells in response to environmental exposures. It is important to emphasize that very little conclusive information is available yet and that the findings that have been reported need to be confirmed, to ask for parents' continued help in epidemiologic and genetic research, and to follow through on the ethical obligation to carefully and thoughtfully transmit results of the research back to parents as they are reported.[89] Nurses can use the SEER Pediatric Monograph tabulations of risk factor results of epidemiologic studies as a reliable resource for this teaching.[86] Nurses can help implement epidemiologic and genetic studies by virtue of being in a pivotal position to make sure all eligible patients are entered on study and by troubleshooting these protocols in their treatment centers. There is nursing representation in epidemiologic research through the C.O.G. Epidemiology Committee, and this committee also includes representation by a parent advocate. Opportunities for nurses to partner with parent advocates to improve understanding about the biology of childhood cancer are expected to grow as this area of research expands.

Need for Nursing Education

All families need reliable information in understandable terms to bridge the gap between what

they hear in the media and what is real and available in clinical practice. Nurses are experts at educating patients and families, in physical and psychosocial assessment, in communication and interpretation, in viewing the family as the focus of care, and in other areas essential to clinical situations engendered by the new advances in biology, particularly in genetics.[60] Nursing has been slow, however, to integrate new genetic information into clinical practice, research, and education. Most nurses practicing today do not have a strong knowledge base in genetics. A national survey of 1000 nurses conducted by the American Nurses Association found that the majority of respondents had no formal course in genetics during their initial professional preparation, and genetics content was not adequately addressed through other course offerings. Respondents expressed a decreasing sense of competence and confidence in their ability to discuss genetic issues with clients and recognized a need for continuing education in genetics.[91]

Efforts are under way to disseminate genetic knowledge so that nurses can better prepare for changes in practice, education, and research based on the new paradigm of genetic health care. In the past 5 years several planning meetings have been held[90] with the sponsorship of the Human Genome Project's Ethical, Legal, and Social Implications branch, leading to the formation of the National Coalition for Health Professional Education in Genetics (NCHPEG). NCHPEG's goal is to develop core curricula for all health care professionals, curricula for basic and advanced practice in specialty areas, and patterns of continuing education. The need is immediate, the stakes are high, and the only question is how rapidly and effectively the essential information can be communicated to nurses so that they can absorb this new information before discussing it with anxious patients and families. Nurses practicing in pediatric oncology must be committed to lifelong learning, and nowhere is this more evident or essential than in the dynamic areas of epidemiology and genetics. A number of educational programs are already available.[117] A variety of resources for use in patient and family education also are available (Table 2-11).

Updating Family Medical Histories

For nurses who practice in ambulatory settings, especially in posttreatment clinics, an important task is to update the family's medical history, with special attention to cancers that may have developed in any first-degree relatives (i.e., mother, father, brothers, sisters, children), second-degree relatives (i.e.,

TABLE 2-11	INFORMATION RESOURCES	
Print Media	**Video**	**Internet**
		GENETICS
• American Society of Clinical Oncology, B. L. Weber (Ed.). (2000). *ONCOSEP: Genetics, an oncology self-education program curriculum text*. Dubuque, IA: Kendall.	• University of California San Francisco (1996). *Winding your way through DNA—Promise and perils of biotechnology: Genetic testing*. San Francisco: The Regents of the University of California. Available from Pyramid Media, P.O. Box 1048, Santa Monica, CA 90406.	• American Medical Association Family History Tools (http://www.ama-assn.org/ama/pub/printcat/2380.html)
• Balkwill, F. (1993). *Cells are us*. Minneapolis: Carolrhoda Books. Available from Cold Spring Harbor Laboratory Press, 10 Skyline Drive, Plainview, NY 11803.	• National Center for Human Genome Research (1997) Office of Communications, National Center for Human Genome Research, 31 Center Drive, msc 2152, Building 31, Room 4B09, Bethesda, MD 20892-0911.	• Cancer Genetics Network (http://www.dccps.ims.nci.nih.gov/CGN/)
• Balkwill, F. (1993). *DNA is here to stay*. Minneapolis: Carolrhoda Books. Available from Cold Spring Harbor Laboratory Press, 10 Skyline Drive, Plainview, NY 11803.		• Cancer Genetics Web (http://www.cancer-genetics.org)
• Balkwill, F. (1993). *Amazing schemes within your genes*. London: Collins. Available from Cold Spring Harbor Laboratory Press, 10 Skyline Drive, Plainview, NY 11803.		• DNA Learning Center (Cold Spring Harbor Laboratory) (http://vector.cshl.org)
• Davies, S. M., & Ross, J. A. *C3 causes of childhood cancer newsletter*. Division of Pediatric Epidemiology-Clinical Research, University of Minnesota, 420 Delaware St. SE, Mayo Mail Code 422, Minneapolis, MN 55455.		• Genentech, Inc. *Biology education*. (http://www.gene.com)
• Gould, R. L. (1997). *Cancer and genetics: Answering your patients' questions, a manual for clinicians and their patients*. New York: PRR and the American Cancer Society. Available from PRR, Inc., 17 Prospect Street, Huntington, NY 11743.		• Genetics Science Learning Center (http://gslc.genetics.utah.basic)
• Herskowitz, J. (1993). *Double talking helix blues*. New York: Cold Spring Harbor Laboratory Press. Available from Cold Spring Harbor Laboratory Press, 10 Skyline Drive, Plainview, NY 11803.		• Human Genome Project Publications (http://www.ornl.gov)
• Scanlon, C., and Fibison, W. (1995). *Managing genetic information: Implications for nursing practice*. Washington, DC: American Nurses Publishing. Available from American Nurses Publishing, 600 Maryland Avenue, SW, Suite 100 West, Washington, DC 20024-2571.		• Howard Hughes Medical Institute (1997). *Blazing a genetic trail* (http://www.hhmi.org/GeneticTrail)
		• National Center for Biotechnology Information (gene maps). (http://www.ncbi.nlm.nih.gov)
		• National Center for Human Genome Research (http://www.nhgri.nih.gov)
		• Online Mendelian Inheritance in Man. (http://www.ncbi.nlm.nih.gov/omim)
		• Robert H. Lurie Cancer Center, Northwestern University Medical School, *The Genetics of Cancer web page*. (http://www.cancergenetics.org)
		• U.S. Department of Energy and The Human Genome Project (1996). *To know ourselves*. (http://www.ornl.gov)
		• U.S. Department of Energy, DOE Human Genome Program (1992). *Primer on molecular genetics*. (http://www.ornl.gov)

Continued

Adapted from Ruccione, K. (1999). Cancer and genetics: What we need to know now. *Journal of Pediatric Oncology Nursing, 16*, 156-171.

TABLE 2-11 INFORMATION RESOURCES—cont'd

Print Media	Video	Internet
• Schindler, L. W. (1993). *Understanding the immune system* (NIH Publication No: 93-529). Bethesda, MD: U.S. Department of Health and Human Services. Public Health Service. National Institutes of Health. National Cancer Institute. • U.S. Department of Health and Human Services, Public Health Service, National Institutes of Health (1997). *Understanding gene testing*. Bethesda, MD: National Cancer Institute (NIH Publication #97-3905). Available from National Cancer Institute, Office of Cancer Communications, Building 31, Room 10A28, Bethesda, MD 20892.		**DISPELLING MYTHS ABOUT CANCER CAUSES** • http://www.cdc.gov/hoax%5frumors.htm • http://www.mayohealth.org/mayo/0007/htm/myths/mht • http://www.urbanlegends.com • http://www.snopes.com • http://nonprofit.net/hoax/default.htm **ORGANIZATIONS** • American Society of Human Genetics (http://www.faseb.org) • International Society of Nurses in Genetics, Inc. (http://www.nursing.creighton.edu/isong) • National Human Genome Research Institute (http://www.nhgri.nih.gov) • Oncology Nursing Society Genetics SIG (http://www.ons.org)

Adapted from Ruccione, K. (1999). Cancer and genetics: What we need to know now. *Journal of Pediatric Oncology Nursing, 16*, 156-171.

grandparents, aunts, uncles, nieces, nephews, and grandchildren), and third-degree relatives (i.e., cousins). One reason to do this is that the individual patient may be part of a family not previously recognized as having a hereditary cancer syndrome. As the child matures over the years, other family members may be diagnosed with cancer, and a more complete portrait of the family's pattern of hereditary cancer will emerge. This valuable information will be missed if the family medical history is not updated at regular intervals.

Excellent family history forms are available[3,42] that can be photocopied and given to patients before the visit so that they can talk with other family members to get the most complete information possible. An important teaching point is to reassure patients and families that most cancers are not hereditary. However, in the rare cases in which multiple family members develop childhood cancer, screening other children in the family may be beneficial to improve the chance of early detection of a malignancy. A second teaching consideration is that estimating the risk of additional cases of cancer, either a second malignant neoplasm or new cancers in family members, is an inexact science. What matters to patients is their *perceived* risk, which is subjective and varies with individuals even with the same objective risk.

When the updated family history is reviewed, several cardinal features raise the index of suspicion for hereditary cancer syndromes. These include (1) cancer in two or more close relatives, (2) bilateral cancer in paired organs, (3) multiple primary tumors in the same individual, (4) atypical age of cancer occurrence, and (5) a specific constellation of tumors that comprise a known cancer syndrome.[42] A higher risk family should be encouraged to gather medical documentation of family members' cancers so they can be confirmed. Updating family medical histories is a shared responsibility of nurse, physician, and family.

REFERRALS FOR GENETIC COUNSELING AND TESTING

Individuals at increased risk can be referred for genetic counseling and possible genetic predisposition testing. Resources for genetic risk assessment and counseling are an increasingly important service for cancer treatment centers. Accessing these resources may require forging stronger (or making new) links between oncology and genetics services in the area. Additional resources include the lists of genetic counselors available in print[42] or on the National Cancer Institute's website (http://www.cancernet.nci.nih.gov/genesrch.shtml). Genetic coun-

selors can work collaboratively with the treatment or posttreatment team to coordinate the patient's care before and after testing if the patient and family decide to have testing performed.

Genetic testing has no medical parallel, and nurses must have a very enlightened view of the perils and promise of testing. Some have called genetic predisposition testing a "future diary" because it contains information about an individual's risk of disease that may—or may not—occur in the future.[7] Peering into someone's future diary is a previously unheard-of capability that carries substantial risk of genetic discrimination and raises major psychosocial, ethical, legal, and financial issues. Currently, recommended indications for genetic testing include (1) a confirmed, strong family history of cancer or a very early-onset disease exists, (2) the genetic test can be interpreted once performed, and (3) the results will influence medical management.[15] A number of uncertainties about predisposition testing exist because of unanswered questions about (1) the best methods for risk assessment and notification, (2) the actual cancer risks associated with mutations in cancer susceptibility genes, (3) medical management for those found to harbor a mutation, and (4) the psychosocial sequelae of this information.[15] For these reasons, most genetic testing is done within the context of clinical protocols, but it is expanding rapidly and moving into oncology and primary care settings. Establishing a liaison with genetic counseling experts will help health care providers know which genetic tests are available and where they can be performed.

A number of position statements related to genetics and genetic testing have been published, including statements about cancer predisposition genetic testing and risk assessment counseling,[76] informed consent,[40] genetic testing of children,[5] the disclosure of genetic information,[6] and the role of the oncology nurse in cancer genetic counseling.[77] Nurses must be familiar with these position statements and actively engage in continuous learning, because genetic testing is such a rapidly changing field.

Epidemiology and molecular biology are bringing us great discoveries and great problems, new prospects and new dilemmas. The implications are stunning and far-reaching. As genetics becomes central to the delivery of health care and preventive services, nurses will care for patients and families who have genetic concerns, whether these concerns are related to disorders or to screening, testing, and counseling options.[91] Clearly the rapidly moving stream of biologic discoveries is pushing us to think about genetics in new ways. Basic definitions of normality and disease are shifting. If all diseases have a genetic component and all humans carry approximately five recessive genes for lethal disorders, we need to change our idea about what is abnormal. As we educate ourselves in translating the story of science to our patients and families, we should be taking a leading role in researching the meaning and human impact of these discoveries, as well as exercising a voice in public policy to advocate patients' privacy and to encourage a greater acceptance of variation and vulnerability instead of stigmatization of people, especially children, who live with genetic injustices such as cancer. Understanding the biologic basis of cancer in all its ramifications for young people and their families is a critical challenge for pediatric oncology nurses in the twenty-first century.

ACKNOWLEDGMENT

The author is indebted to Greta Bunin, PhD, Yves DeClerck, MD, Julie Ross, PhD, and Kenneth Weinberg, MD, for their helpful comments on this chapter. NOTE: Portions of this chapter were previously published in Ruccione, K. (1999). Cancer and genetics: What we need to know now. *Journal of Pediatric Oncology Nursing, 16,* 156-171. Material about cancer clusters is largely drawn from Bunin, G. (1998). *Children's Cancer Group Nurses Epidemiology Notebook,* unpublished document.

REFERENCES

1. Ackerman, T. F. (1996). Genetic testing of children for cancer susceptibility. *Journal of Pediatric Oncology Nursing, 13,* 46-49.
2. American Cancer Society. (2000). *Cancer Facts and Figures.* (http://www.cancer.org).
3. American Medical Association. (2000). Family history tools. (http://www.ama-assn.org).
4. American Society of Clinical Oncology, Weber, B. L. (Ed.). (2000). *ONCOSEP: Genetics, an oncology self-education program curriculum text.* Dubuque, IA: Kendall.
5. American Society of Human Genetics. (1995). Points to consider: Ethical, legal, and psychosocial implications of genetic testing in children and adolescents. *American Journal of Human Genetics, 57,* 1233-1241.
6. American Society of Human Genetics. (1998). Statement of professional disclosure of familial genetic information. *American Journal of Human Genetics, 62,* 474-483.
7. Annas, G. J. (1993). Privacy rules for DNA databanks: Protecting coded "future diaries." *Journal of the American Medical Association, 270,* 2346-2350.
8. Balkwill, F. (1993). *Amazing schemes within your genes.* London: Collins.
9. Baylin, S. B., Belinsky, S. A., & Herman, J. G. (2000). Aberrant methylation of gene promoters in cancer: Concepts, misconcepts, and promise. *Journal of the National Cancer Institute, 92,* 1460-1461.
10. Benedict, W. F., Murphree, A. L., Banerjee, A., et al. (1983). Patient with chromosome 13 deletion: Evidence that the retinoblastoma gene is a recessive cancer gene. *Science, 219,* 973-975.
11. Bleyer, W. A. (1997). The U.S. pediatric clinical trials programmes: International implications and the way forward. *European Journal of Cancer, 33,* 1439-1447.
12. Bruggers, C., Carroll, W., Olson, J. (1999). The use of DNA chips to understand the clinical biology of pediatric tumors. *CCG Quarterly, 7(1),* 6-8.
13. Buckley, J. D., Buckley, C. M., Breslow, N. E., et al. (1996). Concordance for childhood cancer in twins. *Medical and Pediatric Oncology, 26,* 223-229.
14. Caldwell, G. G. (1990). Twenty-two years of cancer cluster investigations at the Centers for Disease Control. *American Journal of Epidemiology, 132* (Suppl. 1), S43-S47.
15. Calzone, K. A. (1997). Genetic predisposition testing: Clinical implications for oncology nurses. *Oncology Nursing Forum, 24,* 712-718.
16. Cavenee, W. K., Dryja, T. P., Phillips, R. A., et al. (1983). Expression of recessive alleles by chromosomal mechanisms in retinoblastoma. *Nature, 305,* 779-784.
17. Cavenee, W. K., Hansen, M. F., Nordenskjold, M., et al. (1985). Genetic origin of mutations predisposing to retinoblastoma. *Science, 228,* 501-503.
18. Chow, W., Linet, M. S., Liff, J. M., et al. (1996). Cancers in children. In D. Shottenfeld & J. F. Fraumeni, Jr., (Eds.). *Cancer epidemiology and prevention* (2nd ed., pp. 1331-1369). Oxford, MA: Oxford University Press.
19. Cohen, J. S., & Hogan, M. E. (1994). The new genetic medicines. *Scientific American, 271,* 74-82.
20. Cohen, P. (May 20, 2000). News. Now for the real challenge: Finding out how the players in this bio-drama strut their stuff. *New Scientist.* (http://www.newscientist.com).
21. Costantini, P., Jacotot, E., Decaudin, D., et al. (2000). Mitochondrion as a novel target of anticancer chemotherapy. *Journal of the National Cancer Institute, 92,* 1042-1053.
22. Creech, J. L., Johnson, M. N. (1974). Angiosarcoma of the liver in the manufacture of polyvinyl chloride. *Journal of Occupational Medicine, 16,* 150-151.
23. DeClerck, Y. A. (2000). Interactions between tumour cells and stromal cells and proteolytic modification of the extracellular matrix by metalloproteinases in cancer. *European Journal of Cancer, 36,* 1258-1268.
24. Devier, J. R., Brownson, R. C., Bagby, J. R., et al. (1990). A public health response to cancer clusters in Missouri. *American Journal of Epidemiology, 132* (Suppl. 1), S23-S31.
25. Donaldson, S. S. (1993). Lessons from our children. *International Journal of Radiation Oncology Biology Physics, 26,* 739-749.
26. Drell, D., & Adamson, A. (2000). Fast forward to 2020: What to expect in molecular medicine. (http://www.ornl.gov).
27. Dudjak, L. A. (1992). Cancer metastasis. *Seminars in Oncology Nursing, 8,* 40-50.28. Eastman, P. (2000). Molecular biology advances transforming tumor vaccine development. *Oncology Times, 22,* 24, 29.
29. Ellis, L. M., & Gallick, G. E. (2000). Promiscuous transcription of vascular endothelial growth factor and survival of tumors. *Journal of the National Cancer Institute, 92,* 1030-1031.
30. Fearon, E. R. (2000). BRCA1 and E-cadherin promoter hypermethylation and gene inactivation in cancer: Association or mechanism? *Journal of the National Cancer Institute, 92,* 515-517.

31. Feinberg, A. P. (1998). Genomic imprinting and cancer. In B. Vogelstein & K. W. Kinzler (Eds.), *The genetic basis of human cancer* (pp. 95-107). New York: McGraw-Hill.

32. Fidler, I. J. (1990). Critical factors in the biology of human cancer metastasis: Twenty-eighth G. H. A. Clowes memorial award lecture. *Cancer Research, 50,* 6130-6138.

33. Folkman, J. (1992). The role of angiogenesis in tumor growth. *Seminars in Cancer Biology, 3,* 65-71.

34. Folkman, J. (1997). Angiogenesis and angiogenesis inhibition: An overview. *EXS, 79,* 1-8.

35. Friend, S. H., Bernards, R., Rogelj, S., et al. (1986). A human DNA segment with properties of the gene that predisposes to retinoblastoma and osteosarcoma. *Nature, 323,* 643-646.

36. Fromer, M. J. (2000). ODAC subcommittee, FDA discuss differences between adult and childhood cancers. *Oncology Times, 22* (12), 24-25, 28.

37. Garber, J. E., & Diller, L. (1993). Screening children at genetic risk of cancer. *Current Opinion Pediatrics, 5,* 712-715.

38. Garber, K. (2000). New discoveries still abundant in monoclonal antibody research. *Journal of the National Cancer Institute, 92,* 1462-1464.

39. Gardner, M. J., Snee, M.P., Hall, A. J., et al. (1990). Results of a case control study of leukemia and lymphoma among young people near Sellafield Nuclear Plant in West Lumbria. *British Medical Journal, 300,* 423-429.

40. Geller, G., Botkin, J., Green, M., et al. (1997). Genetic testing for susceptibility to adult-onset cancer: The process and content of informed consent. *Journal of the American Medical Association, 277,* 1467-1474.

41. Gloeckler Ries, L. A., Percy, C. L., & Bunin, G. R. (1999). Introduction. In L. A. Gloeckler Ries, M. A. Smith, J. G. Gurney, et al. (Eds.), *Cancer Incidence and Survival among Children and Adolescents: United States SEER Program 1975-1995,* National Cancer Institute, SEER Program. (NIH Pub. No. 99-4649). Bethesda, MD: National Cancer Institute.

42. Gould, R. L. (1997). Cancer and genetics: *Answering your patients' questions. A manual for clinicians and their patients.* New York: PRR, Inc. and the American Cancer Society.

43. Greenwald, P. (1996). Chemoprevention of cancer. *Scientific American, 275,* 96-99.

44. Hanahan, D., & Weinberg, R. A. (2000). The hallmarks of cancer. *Cell, 100,* 57-70.

45. Harrington, J. J., Van Bokkelen, G., Mays, R. W., et al. (1997). Formation of *de novo* centromeres and construction of first-generation human artificial chromosomes. *Nature Genetics, 15,* 345-355.

46. Heath, C. W., Jr., & Hasterlik, R. J. (1963). Leukemia among children in a suburban community. *American Journal of Medicine, 34,* 796-812.

47. Herbst, A. L., Ulfelder, H., & Poskanzer, D.C. (1971). Adenocarcinoma of the vagina: Association of maternal stilbestrol therapy with tumor appearance in young women. *New England Journal of Medicine, 284,* 878-881.

48. Herskowitz, J. (1993). *Double talking helix blues.* New York: Cold Spring Harbor Laboratory Press.

49. Holash, J., Maisonpierre, P. C., Compton, D., et al. (1999). Vessel cooption, regression, and growth in tumors mediated by angiopoietins and VEGF. *Science, 284,* 1994-1998.

50. International Human Genome Sequencing Consortium. (2001). Initial sequencing and analysis of the human genome. *Nature, 409,* 860-921.

51. Israel, M. A. (1996). Molecular genetics in the management of patients with cancer. In J. M. Bishop & R. A. Weinberg (Eds.), *Molecular Oncology* (pp. 205-237). New York: Scientific American, Inc.

52. Jones, P. A., & Laird, P. W. (1999). Cancer epigenetics comes of age. *Nature Genetics, 21,* 163-167.

53. Kaiser, J. (1999). No meeting of minds on childhood cancer. *Journal of the National Cancer Institute, 286,* 1832-1834.

54. Kay, L. E. (1993). *The molecular vision of life: Caltech, the Rockefeller Foundation, and the rise of the new biology.* New York: Oxford University Press.

55. Kevles, D. J., & Hood, L. (Eds.). (1992). *The code of codes: Scientific and social issues in the human genome project.* Cambridge, MA: Harvard University Press.

56. Khan, J., Simon, R., Bittner, M., et al. (1998). Gene expression profiling of alveolar rhabdomyosarcoma with cDNA microarrays. *Cancer Research, 58,* 5009-5013.

57. Knudson, A. G., Jr. (1971). Mutation and cancer: Statistical study of retinoblastoma. *Proceedings of the National Academy of Sciences of the United States of America, 68,* 820.

58. Kohler, G., & Milstein, C. (1975). Continuous cultures of fused cells secreting antibody of predefined specificity. Nature, 256, 495-497.

59. Kroemer, G., & de Thé, H. (2000). Arsenic trioxide, a novel mitochondriotoxic anticancer agent? *Journal of the National Cancer Institute, 91,* 743-745.

60. Lashley, F. R. (1997). Thinking about genetics in new ways. *Image: Journal of Nursing Scholarship, 29,* 202.

61. Linet, M. S., Ries, L. A. G., Smith, M. A., et al. (1999). Trends in childhood cancer incidence and mortality in the United States. *Journal of the National Cancer Institute, 91,* 1051-1058.

62. Liotta, L. A., Steeg, P. S., & Stetler-Stevenson, W. G. (1991). Cancer metastasis and angiogenesis: An imbalance of positive and negative regulation. *Cell, 64,* 327-336.

63. Liotta, L. A. (1992). Cancer cell invasion and metastasis. *Scientific American, 226,* 63-65.

64. MacDonald, N. J., Steeg, P. S. (1993). Molecular basis of tumour metastasis. *Cancer Surveillance, 16,* 179-199.

65. Malkin, D. (1998). The Li-Fraumeni syndrome. In B. Vogelstein & K. W. Kinzler (Eds.), *The genetic basis of human cancer* (pp. 393-407). New York: McGraw-Hill.

66. Maniotis, A. J., Folberg, R., Hess, A., et al. (1999). Vascular channel formation by human melanoma cells in vivo and in vitro: Vasculogenic mimicry. *American Journal of Pathology, 155,* 739-752.

67. Marina, N. M., Bowman, L. C., Pui, C., et al. (1995). Pediatric solid tumors. In G.P. Murphy, W.L. Lawrence, & R. E. Lenhard, Jr. (Eds.), *American Cancer Society textbook of clinical oncology* (pp. 524-551). Atlanta: American Cancer Society.

68. McKusick, V. A. (1992). *Mendelian inheritance in man: Catalogs of autosomal dominant, autosomal recessive, and X-linked phenotypes.* Baltimore: Johns Hopkins University Press.

69. McWhirter, W. R., & Kirk, D. (1986). What causes childhood leukaemia? Some beliefs of parents of affected children. *Medical Journal of Australia, 145,* 314-316.

70. Mendelsohn, J. (2000). Use of an antibody to target geldanamycin. *Journal of the National Cancer Institute, 92,* 1549-1551.

71. Miller, M. (2000). Telling cells to die: Apoptosis research takes off. *Journal of the National Cancer Institute, 92,* 793.

72. Miller, R. W., Myers, M. H. (1983). Age distribution of epithelial cancers. *Lancet, 2,* 1250.

73. Narod, S. A., Siller, C., & Lenoir, G. M. (1991). An estimate of the heritable fraction of childhood cancer. *British Journal of Cancer, 63,* 993-999.

74. Old, L. J. (1996). Immunotherapy for cancer. *Scientific American, 275,* 136-143.

75. Oldendorf, B. (2000). Applying genomics and proteomics to cancer: DNA sequencing and microarray make it possible to measure expression of thousands of genes simultaneously, providing snapshot of cell's genome. *Oncology Times, 22, 20,* 23-24.

76. Oncology Nursing Society. (2000). Cancer predisposition genetic testing and risk assessment counseling. *Oncology Nursing Forum, 27,* 1349.

77. Oncology Nursing Society. (2000). The role of the oncology nurse in cancer genetic counseling. *Oncology Nursing Forum, 27,* 1348.

78. Pasqualini, R., & Ruoslahti, E. (1996). Organ targeting *in vivo* using phage display peptide libraries. *Nature, 380,* 364-366.

79. Patenaude, A. F., Basili, L., & Fairclough, D. L. (1996). Attitudes of 47 mothers of pediatric oncology patients toward genetic testing for cancer predisposition. *Journal of Clinical Oncology, 14,* 415-421.

80. Patenaude, A. F. (1996). The genetic testing of children for cancer susceptibility: Ethical, legal, and social issues. *Behavior Science Law, 14,* 393-410.

81. Pauling, L., Itano, H. A., Singer, S. J., et al. (1949). Sickle cell anemia: A molecular disease. *Science, 110,* 543-548.

82. Perera, F. P. (2000). Molecular epidemiology: On the path to prevention? *Journal of the National Cancer Institute, 92,* 602-612.

83. Philip, S. (2000). Angiogenesis inhibitors in oncology: The research continues. *Cancer Practice, 8,* 148-150.

84. Pott, P. (1775). *Chirurgical observations relative to the cataract, the polypus of the nose, the cancer of the scrotum, the different kinds of ruptures, and mortification of the toes and feet.* London: Hawes, Clarke, and Collins.

85. Ramsay, G. (1998). DNA chips: State-of-the art. *National Biotechnology, 16,* 40-44.

86. Ries, L. A. G., Smith, M. A., Gurney, J. G., et al. (Eds.). (1999). Cancer incidence and survival among children and adolescents: United States SEER Program 1975-1995, National Cancer Institute, SEER Program. (NIH Pub. No. 99-4649). Bethesda, MD: National Cancer Institute.

87. Ross, J. (2000). Personal communication.

88. Ross, J. A., Severson, R. K., Pollock, B. H., et al. (1996). Childhood cancer in the United States: A geographical analysis of cases from the Pediatric Cooperative Clinical Trials Groups. *Cancer, 77,* 201-207.

89. Ruccione, K. S., Waskerwitz, M., Buckley J., et al. (1994). What caused my child's cancer? Parents' responses to an epidemiology study of childhood cancer. *Journal of Pediatric Oncology Nursing, 11,* 71-84.

90. Ruccione, K. (1996). Genetics education in nursing takes a giant leap forward: A personal account. *APON Counts, 10,* 5-7.

91. Scanlon, C., & Fibison, W. (1995). *Managing genetic information: Implications for nursing practice.* Washington, DC: American Nurses Publishing.

92. Schindler, L. W. (1993). *Understanding the immune system* (NIH Publication No: 93-529). Bethesda, MD: U.S. Department of Health and Human Services. Public Health Service. National Institutes of Health. National Cancer Institute.

93. Shi, L. (2000). DNA microarray (genome chip): Monitoring the genome on a chip. (http://www.genechips.com).

94. Slovik, P. (1987). Perception of risk. *Science, 236,* 280-285.

95. Sparkes, R. S., Sparkes, M. C., Wilson, M. G., et al. (1980). Regional assignment of genes for human esterase D and retinoblastoma to chromosome band 13p14. *Science, 208,* 1042-1044.

96. Sparkes, R. S., Murphree, A. L., Lingua, R. W., et al. (1983). Gene for hereditary retinoblastoma assigned to human chromosome 13 by linkage to esterase D. *Science, 219,* 971-973.

97. Spencer, S. M. (1951). Cancer kills children too. *Saturday Evening Post, 233, 32,* 104-105.

98. Sporn, M. B. (1996). The war on cancer. *Lancet, 347,* 1377-1381.

99. Sporn, M. B. (2000). Retinoids and demethylating agents: Looking for partners. *Journal of the National Cancer Institute, 92,* 780-781.

100. The White House, Office of the Press Secretary. (2000). Remarks by the President, Prime Minister Tony Blair of England, Dr. Francis Collins, Director of the National Human Genome Research Institute, and Dr. Craig Venter, President and Chief Scientific Officer, Celera Genomics Corporation, on the completion of the first survey of the entire human genome project. (http://www.pub.whitehouse.gov).

101. Thompson, M. W., McInnes, R. R., & Willard, H. F. (1991). *Genetics in medicine.* Philadelphia: Saunders.

102. Thomson, J. A., Iskovitz-Eldor, J., Shapiro, S. S., et al. (1998). Embryonic stem cell lines derived from human blastocysts. *Science, 282,* 1145-1147.

103. U.S. Department of Health and Human Services. Public Health Service. National Institutes of Health. (1997). *Understanding gene testing.* (NIH Publication No: 97-3905). Bethesda, MD: National Cancer Institute.

104. Vastag, B. (2000). Detection network gives early cancer tests a push. *Journal of the National Cancer Institute, 92,* 786-788.

105. Venter, J. C., Adams, M. D., Myers, E. W., et al. (2001). The sequence of the human genome. *Science, 291,* 1304-1351.

106. Vernon, S. W., Gritz, E. R., Peterson, S. K., et al. (1999). Intention to learn results of genetic testing for hereditary colon cancer. *Cancer Epidemiology Biomarkers Prevention, 8,* 353-360.

107. Virji, M. A., Mercer, D. W., & Herberman, R. B. (1988). Tumor markers in cancer diagnosis and prognosis. *CA: A Journal for Clinicians, 38,* 104-126.

108. Vogelstein, B., & Kinzler, K. W. (1998). *The genetic basis of human cancer.* New York: McGraw-Hill.

109. Watson, J. D., & Crick, F. H. C. (1953). Molecular structure of nucleic acids: A structure of deoxyribose nucleic acid. *Nature, 171,* 737-738.

110. Watson, J. D., & Crick, F. H. C. (1953). Genetical implications of the structure of deoxyribonucleic acid. Nature, 171, 964-967. Reprinted in *Journal of the American Medical Association, 269,* 1967-1969.

111. Weaver, W. (1970). Molecular biology: Origins of the term. *Science, 170,* 591-592.

112. Weinberg, R. A. (1996). How cancer arises. *Scientific American, 275,* 62-70.

113. Welch, D. R., & Rinker-Schaeffer, C. W. (1999). What defines a useful marker of metastasis in human cancer? *Journal of the National Cancer Institute, 91,* 1351-1353.

114. Williams, J. K., Schutte, D. L., Evers, C. A., et al. (1999). Adults seeking presymptomatic gene testing for Huntington disease. *Image: Journal of Nursing Scholarship, 31,* 109-114.

115. Wilmut, I. (1997). Viable offspring derived from fetal and adult mammalian cells. *Nature, 385,* 810-813.

116. Yoshida, B. A., Sokoloff, M. M., Welch, D. R., et al. (2000). Metastasis-suppressor genes: A review and perspective on an emerging field. *Journal of the National Cancer Institute, 92,* 1717-1730.

117. Zawacki, K. L. (2000). Information sources: Cancer genetics and genetic testing. *Cancer Practice, 8,* 197-200.

II

Treatment

3

Diagnostic Evaluations and Staging Procedures

Marcia Leonard

Most families who have children with cancer agree that the period of diagnosis is one of the most difficult times of their cancer journey. The nurse caring for the child suspected of having a malignancy is in a unique position to offer support and guidance at this stressful time. To do this, however, the nurse needs a thorough understanding of the various measures used to diagnose pediatric malignancies and their usual sequence. Preparing the child and family for tests and procedures and facilitating patient safety are key nursing responsibilities.

ESTABLISHING THE DIAGNOSIS

Although cancer is the leading cause of death from disease in children 1 to 19 years of age in the United States, it is still uncommon.[29] The initial symptoms of childhood cancer can imitate other more benign problems such as infection or injury. Many children may be treated with several courses of antibiotics for persistent infectious symptoms or visit subspecialists for assessment of a specific pain or organ dysfunction. As a result of these factors the diagnosis of childhood cancer is often delayed, despite a family's persistence in repeatedly bringing their child to the family doctor or pediatrician.

The greatest aid in diagnosing malignant disease in children is a high index of suspicion, for there is no classic, universal symptom or symptom complex for cancer in children. The signs and symptoms are related to the age of the patient, the type of tumor, and the extent of the disease. Rather than focusing on any particular symptom or group of symptoms, the practitioner must be alert to children with persistence of symptoms.

The goals of the diagnostic and staging phase of treatment are to determine the presence of a cancer, to identify the type of cancer, and to determine its location throughout the body. Additionally, a thorough evaluation of baseline organ function is undertaken for the child who will undergo intensive chemotherapy. These procedures are carried out ex-

peditiously to allow appropriate therapy to begin as quickly as possible.

New and sophisticated tests that provide detailed information and prognostic data are available only at established pediatric cancer centers. As the science of pediatric oncology develops, classification of tumors and leukemia have become more precise and complex. Treatment is often stratified by these classifications, resulting in therapy that is more tailored to the individual. Treatment may be more aggressive for some but less intensive for others. Every child deserves state-of-the-art therapy and the psychosocial support provided by a team of professionals experienced in the care of children with cancer. Childhood cancer survival rate is positively influenced by the place of treatment and the use of cancer protocols.[21] Further studies have demonstrated the importance and the significant survival advantage to children and adolescents when treated on well-defined protocols in specialized children's cancer centers.[22]

Basic noninvasive imaging procedures confirming the presence of a mass and/or basic laboratory work suggesting organ dysfunction are often performed by the primary health care provider. In light of the results, a prompt referral must be made to a pediatric oncologist. Community-based diagnostic testing should be prompt and limited in scope. Many of the precise diagnostic tools required to identify pediatric malignancies correctly are unavailable in the community. An inconclusive diagnostic evaluation subjects the child and family to unnecessary expense and trauma and leads to treatment delays.

PATIENT HISTORY

Diagnosis begins by obtaining a detailed medical history. Special attention is given to factors that suggest the possibility of malignancy. The interview is best conducted in private, without interruptions, with consideration for the comfort of both the parents and child. The parents will be more relaxed if adequate provision has been made for the child's needs. An ill child is assigned to the care of an extended family member or a staff member. A more active child may be provided with toys or other activities. The parent may prefer to hold an infant or an older child, or the child may be placed on the examination table close to the parent.

The examiner begins the interview process by greeting both parent and child. Including a friendly comment to young children about appearance, clothing, or toy may help engage them. During the interview frequent eye contact is made with the child. Every attempt is made to engage the child verbally during anxiety-producing moments.

The older child and adolescent should actively participate in the initial history taking, since this sets the expectation of their involvement throughout their course of care. The adolescent is given the opportunity to provide information without parents in the room, usually after the initial interview with the parents and before the physical examination. The parents can be reassured that the pertinent findings of the physical examination will be shared with them. Respecting the teen's independence and establishing a sense of confidentiality are best achieved if begun at the onset of treatment.[10,24] Of course, if the adolescent is frightened and prefers to have the parents present, that wish is respected.

To collect relevant information, the examiner phrases questions in language that the parent and adolescent understand, listens carefully to the responses, and encourages the family to express ideas and concerns freely. If the parents are not fluent in English, an interpreter with some degree of medical knowledge is obtained.

Examiners elicit the information by following a specific pattern. First, they determine the chief complaint. Many health care professionals ask the parents, "Why did you come to see us today?" The duration of the illness or complaint that brought the child to the attention of a physician is recorded. The examiner then develops the sequence of the present illness by inquiring about the date symptoms first appeared, the order of occurrence, the diagnoses made by the referring health care provider who examined the patient, and response to any treatment prescribed. The health care professional must listen intently to the parent's description of the child's illness or complaint. Parents describe a child's problem as they perceive it, and their story frequently includes a theory regarding the cause of the problem. Understanding such theories may be helpful later in counseling parents.[1]

The examiner next reviews the child's history. The child's prenatal, neonatal, and subsequent growth and development are essential information. Genetic factors have an important role in pediatric cancers. Any history of immunodeficient or metabolic diseases or genetic disorders such as autoimmune diseases, neurofibromatosis, and Down syndrome is documented.[31] The examiner records all immunizations and past illnesses and obtains a thorough social history. A routine pediatric social history includes age, marital status, and occupation of the parents, including stepparents or those with whom the child lives, and the ages of siblings. The parent or the older child is asked to discuss school performance and adjustment. Information about the family's financial status, including insurance coverage, is obtained. The examiner inquires about the family's housing situation and available social and community resources.

Pertinent family medical history is also documented. Any history of cancer in family members, including the health status of grandparents, parents, and siblings, is noted, with special attention given to any pediatric cancers or indication of familial cancer syndromes (see Chapter 2). A family pedigree is constructed and documented on the medical record if there are several family members with cancer histories.

Finally, the patient history concludes with a review of body systems. The examiner attempts to elicit any symptoms that the parent has not recognized or considered relevant. Questions are asked about each body system. Before concluding the interview, the examiner asks the parent if all questions and concerns have been discussed. No concern is minimized or automatically dismissed.

PHYSICAL EXAMINATION

Physical examination begins as the examiner observes the child while obtaining the medical history. Initial impressions about the child-parent interaction, the child's general appearance, and whether the child behaves in an age-appropriate manner are made. A developmental assessment is an integral part of a pediatric physical examination. During the physical examination there must be regard for privacy and comfort (Figure 3-1). The child is treated with respect and consideration. An infant or toddler can be examined almost completely while on the parent's lap.

During the physical examination adolescents may raise concerns about their health or their bodies that were not mentioned in the initial interview. Many teens have misguided ideas about the cause of their illness, the extent of their symptoms, and the prognosis of childhood cancer. The skilled practitioner conveys to the adolescent that he or she is the primary concern of the medical team. The teen needs to be the primary source of information and is encouraged to be active and involved throughout treatment and decision making.[24]

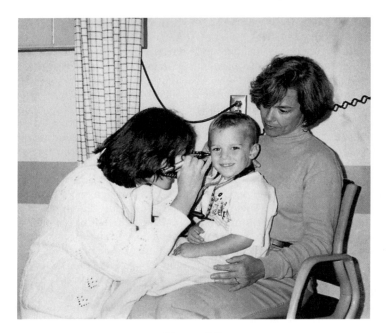

Figure 3-1

Young children may prefer to sit on their parent's lap during examination.

Vital signs are obtained and recorded during the initial examination. Height without shoes and weight are measured and plotted on the appropriate growth chart. Metric measurements are taken in order to calculate the patient's body surface area (BSA). The BSA is commonly used to calculate future chemotherapy doses, except for infants. Infant doses are typically calculated based on weight in kilograms, since infants have a proportionally greater BSA than older children who are larger than 10 km. Care must be taken to ensure that the height and weight measurements are accurate. Metric units are not the standard in the United States, and because of this unfamiliarity, incorrect values may be easily overlooked. Converting the metric height and weight into inches and pounds can provide a valuable double-check mechanism. The BSA is measured in square meters, m^2, and is computed with the use of a slide rule nomogram or chart or by using the following formula:

$$\sqrt{\frac{\text{Height (cm)} \times \text{weight (kg)}}{3600}}$$

The growth chart is an important tool for evaluating growth failure or dysfunction secondary to cancer treatment. Such dysfunction may be recognized sooner if baseline and incremental height and weight measurements are obtained and recorded regularly. The head circumference of infants and young children is also measured and recorded. The head circumference is considered the best assessment of brain growth and development in infants. Baseline and serial measurements may provide early clues to treatment toxicity or hydrocephalus.

The four methods of examination are incorporated: inspection, auscultation, palpation, and percussion. Each body system is assessed for abnormality. Careful physical examination may indicate the site of a primary tumor, spread to lymph nodes or other organs, or both. In addition, a detailed thorough documentation of physical findings is made.

Enlarged or abnormal areas discovered during the physical examination are recorded in concise, descriptive, and quantitative terms whenever possible. For example, "shotty" or "pea-sized" lymph nodes may have entirely different meanings to different examiners, whereas "1.5 cm × 1 cm" can mean only one size. Likewise, organ span, testicular size, abdominal girth, lymphadenopathy, and tumors, if present, are measured and their actual dimensions recorded.

After the initial history and physical examination, the health care provider orders a battery of tests to aid in confirming the diagnosis of a malignancy. These tests help define the source and the extent of the tumor and its effect on other organ systems in the body. The required tests fall into three broad categories: (1) blood or laboratory work; (2) imaging studies; and (3) direct examination of tumor for pathologic confirmation of diagnosis.

The nurse expedites the child's initial diagnostic phase by knowing and ensuring that the proper preparative regimens are maintained. She educates the family as to why "nothing by mouth" (NPO) status is necessary before some scans and makes sure that meals are not inadvertently delivered at those times. The nurse facilitates the sequencing of various tests, making sure that certain preparative procedures do not conflict with each other and that enough time is allowed to travel from one department to another. Timely scheduling of tests and scans permits more judicious use of sedation for the young child.

Parents often become frustrated by the length of time needed to establish the diagnosis and the deliberate pace of the workup. Children with cancer often have histories of numerous doctor or emergency room visits before arrival at the cancer center, and most parents are anxious for a definitive diagnosis. It is not unusual for parents to be eager to begin treatment and finally "do something." The nurse can help the family by emphasizing the vital importance of making an accurate diagnosis and fully defining the extent and histology of the malignancy before beginning treatment. The nurse who can sit patiently with the family, acknowledge their frustration, and provide information and support will do much to help them through a very anxious, difficult time.

BLOOD WORK AND LABORATORY STUDIES

In most medical centers the child routinely has a complete blood count (CBC), serum blood chemistries, and urinalysis at the time of admission. Depending on the location of the tumor, additional blood and urine studies are required.

COMPLETE BLOOD COUNT

The CBC is obtained from the peripheral blood. It is a measure of the formed elements that are suspended in plasma: erythrocytes (red blood cells—RBCs), leukocytes (white blood cells—WBCs), and platelets. Hemoglobin, the main physiologic component of RBCs, and hematocrit, the percentage of RBCs per volume of whole blood, are included. The CBC also includes qualitative and quantitative information about the RBCs, called the RBC indices. The RBC indices reflect the size, weight, and hemoglobin content of an individual RBC. The red cell indices include (1) MCV, the mean corpuscular volume; (2) MCHC, mean corpuscular hemoglobin concentration; and (3) MCH, the mean corpuscular hemoglobin. The MCV is the

mean volume of each RBC. MCH is a measure of the weight of hemoglobin in each RBC, and MCHC is the average amount of hemoglobin in each RBC but expressed as a percentage of the volume of the RBC.[11,23,28]

The CBC provides the total number of WBCs in the peripheral blood. The WBC differential is necessary to learn the percentage of each type of WBC present in the same specimen. Unlike the red blood cell, there is more than one type of white blood cell circulating at any one time. The differential identifies the relative proportions of the various types of WBCs that comprise the total white count. Five types of WBCs are normally present in blood: (1) basophils, (2) eosinophils, (3) monocytes, (4) lymphocytes, and (5) neutrophils. There are two stages of neutrophils: segmented neutrophils, referred to as *segs* or *polys,* and banded neutrophils, commonly called *bands* or *stabs.* All of these cells originate in the bone marrow from the same "pluripotent" stem cell; however, each cell line differentiates separately and has a unique function. To determine what percentage of each type of WBC is present, 100 WBCs are counted and each cell is identified and counted individually. The total of each type is reported as a percentage of the total number of WBCs (Table 3-1).[11,23,28]

Children with leukemia invariably have some degree of abnormality of the CBC at diagnosis. Typically the normal bone marrow is replaced by malignant cells, reflected by the abnormal CBC. However, a normal CBC does not guarantee that the bone marrow is free of tumor. A child with a solid tumor may also have malignant cells that have metastasized to the bone marrow but have not replaced the normal cells completely, thus expressing no significant alteration of the CBC.

SERUM CHEMISTRY

Biochemical evaluation of the blood serum is a routine screening procedure performed on admission. The biochemical studies of the child suspected of having cancer will measure and reflect ongoing metabolic processes and the status of specific organs.[5] Most laboratories have panels or combinations of serum chemistry tests that allow multiple assays from a single blood sample. These panels typically include "routine" electrolytes: sodium, potassium, chloride, and carbon dioxide. Tests that measure renal function (blood urea nitrogen, or BUN, and creatinine) and liver function (alanine aminotransferase, or ALT, asparate aminotransferase, or AST, and bilirubin) are also included. Some panels may measure various proteins such as the total protein and albumin, enzymes (amylase, lipase), and additional electrolytes (calcium, phosphorus, and magnesium).

TABLE 3-1	COMPLETE BLOOD COUNT	
Test	**Normal Values**	**Implications of Abnormal Values**
Hemoglobin (Hgb)	Infant, first day: 14-20 g/dL Child 1-5 yr: 10-14 g/dL Child 6-10 yr: 11-15 g/dL Adult female: 12-16 g/dL Adult male: 13.5-17.5 g/dL	Levels decreased with reduced RBC production, blood loss, and hemolysis; the hemoglobin level is usually approximately one third of the hematocrit.
Hematocrit (Hct)	Infant, first day: 42%-60% Child 1 yr: 34%-41% Child 6-10 yr: 33%-43% Adult female: 35%-48% Adult male: 39%-52%	Decreased with reduced RBC production, blood loss, and hemolysis; levels are easily influenced by fluid volume status; hypervolemia leads to lower hematocrit without actual decreased RBCs, and hypovolemia and hemoconcentration reflect a higher hematocrit than actually exists.
Mean corpuscular volume (MCV)	87-103 nm^3	Measures the average size of each RBC and reflects the maturity level and degree of hemoglobin content; low hemoglobin content results in a low MCV.
Mean corpuscular hemoglobin (MCH)	26-34 pg/cell	Measures the average amount of hemoglobin in each RBC; it reflects the amount of functional hemoglobin and will be lower in disorders of Hgb production.
Mean corpuscular hemoglobin concentration (MCHC)	31-37 g/dL	Measures the average amount of hemoglobin in an individual RBC.
Platelets	150,000-400,000 cells/mm^3	Production is affected by bone marrow disease and exposure to chemotherapy and radiation therapy; peripheral destruction may also reduce circulating levels.
White blood count	1 yr: 5,000-19,500 6 yr: 5,000-14,000 10 yr: 4,500-13,500 16 yr: 4,500-10,000	Increased values occur in infection and leukemia; elevated levels can occur with growth factor usage; decreased levels can occur with leukemia and chemotherapy.
Differential	Percentage of the total white blood count	Quantification of WBC types in blood.
Neutrophils Segs (polys)	1 yr: 23% 6 yr: 43% 10 yr: 46% 16 yr: 49%	Primary defense in bacterial and fungal infections; can phagocytize and kill bacteria.
Bands (stabs)	8%	Immature neutrophil, increased in number during infections, can also phagocytize and kill bacteria.
Lymphocytes	1 yr: 61% 6 yr: 42% 10 yr: 38% 16 yr: 35%	Involved in development of antibody and delayed hypersensitivity reactions; elevated in viral infections.
Monocytes	4%-5%	Large phagocytic cells involved in early phase of inflammatory response.
Eosinophils	3%	Increased in allergic disorders, parasitic diseases, and some rare forms of leukemia.
Basophils	0.5%	Contain histamine; function unknown.

Data from Henze, R. L., & Bullock, B. L. (2000). *Focus on pathophysiology*. Philadelphia: Lippincott; Nathan, D. G., & Orkin, S. H. (1998). *Nathan & Oski's hematology of infancy and childhood*. (5th ed., Vol 2). Philadelphia: W. B. Saunders; Parsons, L., & Patterson, K. L. (1993). Nursing assessment and diagnosis of hematologic function. In D. B. Jackson & R. B. Saunders (Eds.), *Child health nursing*. Philadelphia: JB Lippincott.

Serum lactate dehydrogenase (LDH) is not typically part of the panel. LDH is a cellular enzyme that contributes to carbohydrate metabolism. Specifically it catalyzes the conversion of lactic acid to pyruvic acid within cells. It is present in many cells of the body, including the liver, heart, kidney, and skeletal muscles. LDH is often elevated at the time of diagnosis in children with several types of malignancies, particularly lymphomas, leukemias, and bone tumors. LDH may be elevated for reasons other than malignancy; thus it cannot be considered a specific tumor marker. However, levels are obtained at diagnosis, and elevations that occur after remission is induced may be a sign of relapse.[18]

Alkaline phosphatase is an isoenzyme associated with bone, liver, and gastrointestinal (GI) metabolism. Levels are increased when cells such as osteoblasts, the cells that make bone, are active. Children with bone tumors usually have very high levels of this enzyme at diagnosis. Serial measurements may be indicative of response to therapy.[6] Normal bone growth in healthy children can also cause elevated values.[26]

Uric acid is routinely measured at diagnosis. It is one of the by-products of cell destruction and is released as cells lyse. Malignant cells, particularly in children with leukemia and non-Hodgkin's lymphoma, have a rapid doubling time and turnover rate. Consequently, uric acid levels may be elevated at diagnosis. Uric acid levels are monitored closely in children with cancer after therapy is initiated because levels can rise precipitously as the malignant cells are killed in response to chemotherapy, enhancing the possibility of tumor lysis syndrome, as described in detail in Chapter 13.

URINALYSIS

A urinalysis is obtained routinely on most children as a general renal screening test. The kidneys provide a semipermeable membrane that reabsorbs some substances from plasma and excretes others via urine. Urine is a complex, yellowish fluid consisting of approximately 95% water and 5% dissolved solids.[19] Urinalysis results reflect plasma homeostasis in a normally functioning kidney, or they may indicate pathology directly related to the genitourinary tract. The microscopic urinalysis measures the presence of WBCs, RBCs, casts, and epithelial cells. The macroscopic urinalysis measures specific gravity, pH, protein, glucose, and ketones. Children with renal or bladder tumors occasionally have hematuria as an initial presenting sign.[17]

TUMOR MARKERS

A tumor marker is any characteristic of a tumor cell, or product of such a cell, that serves to indicate, or "mark," the presence of that specific tumor cell.[8] Tumor-associated substances or tumor markers detected in body tissues, blood, urine, or cerebrospinal fluid (CSF) would ideally enable the clinician to screen patients for neoplastic development. Markers would also enable the physician to stage patients with malignant disease more effectively and predict the response to certain treatment modalities. Low concentration or levels of tumor markers could help identify minimal residual disease or signify an early recurrence ahead of clinical symptoms.[7] Unfortunately, in the pediatric population, there are only a few reliable tumor markers used for screening and detection purposes. Elevations of LDH and alkaline phosphatase are thought to have prognostic significance in certain childhood cancers such as lymphoma and osteosarcoma, but, in general, the results are too variable and lack sufficient sensitivity and specificity.

The best-documented and most sensitive markers are those associated with neuroblastoma, hepatoblastoma, and germ cell tumors. Tumor markers can help the physician differentiate among neuroblastoma, Wilms tumor, and hepatoblastoma, each of which may present similarly as a large abdominal tumor. Specific markers often clarify the diagnosis, but most importantly, their presence becomes a significant component for follow-up during therapy. Elevated marker values may also have a role in determining prognosis. Elevated levels of serum ferritin and neuron-specific enolase (NSE), a neuronal glycolytic enzyme, occur frequently with neuroblastoma. Abnormal levels of α-fetoprotein (AFP), normally occurring only in fetal cells, are found in patients with primary liver tumors. AFP can be of great value not only at diagnosis but also in screening for residual and/or recurrent liver tumors. β subunit of human chorionic gonadotropin (β-hCG) is produced by trophoblastic cells, and thus these levels, as well as AFP levels, are elevated in germ cell tumors of both gonadal and central nervous system (CNS) origin.

Vanillylmandelic acid (VMA), the main metabolite of epinephrine and norepinephrine, and homovanillic acid (HVA), the main metabolite of dopamine, metanephrine, and normetanephrine, are the catecholamines secreted by the adrenal medulla and sympathetic nervous tissue. Elevated catecholamine levels are found at diagnosis in 90% to 95% of patients with neuroblastoma either because of overproduction by individual cells or because of rapid release caused by defective storage within tumor cells.[2] VMA and HVA levels are considered elevated when values are more than 3.0 standard deviations above the mean for age.[4] Urine catecholamine collection is ordered if the child has an abdominal tumor that is suspicious for neuroblastoma. This may be obtained from one aliquot of urine, but a 24-hour collection may be requested. VMA and HVA excretion must be normalized to the milligrams of creatinine if single sample collection is ordered.[2]

Timed urine collections pose particular difficulties for the pediatric population. Babies and children still in diapers or with only daytime bladder control usually require an indwelling catheter to obtain acceptable collections. Older children need frequent reminders to save all urine and to use only one commode or urinal during the collection period. The stress and anxiety of hospitalization, combined with intravenous hydration, may cause enuresis in previously toilet-trained children. Diurnal variations occur in the excretion of catecholamines, and the loss of even one aliquot of urine may be crucial.[20] The physician is notified if urine loss occurs to determine whether to restart the 24-hour sample or continue with the present collection. The container for urinary catecholamine studies contains concentrated hydrochloric acid to maintain a pH of 2 to 3 throughout the collection period. Boys are instructed not to urinate directly into the jug.

In a percentage of patients with Hodgkin's disease, serum copper, a trace mineral found in plasma, is elevated at diagnosis. The level returns to normal with remission, and may be used to assess disease activity. Carcinoembryonic antigen (CEA), normally produced during rapid multiplication of epithelial cells, may be elevated with a number of malignancies, including retinoblastoma, neuroblastoma, and germ cell tumors.[26] Unfortunately, these tests have low specificity and poor reliability as tumor markers. Table 3-2 lists normal ranges of the various tumor-associated markers.

NURSING IMPLICATIONS

During the initial workup numerous other blood and laboratory tests may be ordered. It is crucial to evaluate organ systems other than those of tumor origin for any dysfunction caused by the disease and to evaluate baseline organ function before the initiation of therapy. The natural history of the cancer, its known pattern of spread, and proposed treatment influence the selection of tests.

The child with cancer will be subjected to hundreds of blood tests during the course of therapy. All newly diagnosed children will be assessed for the need of a venous access device. Venous access devices can eliminate much of the pain and trauma involved with repeated venipunctures; however, these devices do carry an additional risk for complica-

TABLE 3-2	**TUMOR-ASSOCIATED LABORATORY STUDIES**	
Laboratory Test	**Normal Range**	**Associated Malignancies**
Alkaline phosphatase	20-150 U/l	Bone tumors; NOTE: nonspecific elevations can occur in normal settings.
α-fetoprotein (AFP)	<20 ng/ml	Hepatomas Germ cell tumors (teratocarcinomas) Retinoblastoma
β human chorionic gonadotropin (β-hCG)	5 mIu/ml	Hepatoblastoma Germ cell tumors
Carcinoembryonic antigen (CEA)	2.5 ng/ml	Gastrointestinal cancers Neuroblastoma (elevations may occur in one or all)
Catecholamines (urine):		
Epinephrine	0-5 g/24 hr	
Homovanillic acid (HVA)	0-10 mg/24 hr	
Metanephrine	0-300 g/24 hr	
Norepinephrine	0-20 g/24 hr	
Normetanephrine	50-800 g/24 hr	
Vanillylmandelic acid (VMA)	2-10 mg/24 hr	
Copper	80-160 g/dl	Hodgkin's disease
Ferritin	7-150 g/l	Neuroblastoma
Lactate dehydrogenase (LDH)	60-170 U/l	Nonspecific Non-Hodgkin's lymphomas, acute lymphocytic leukemia (ALL), osteosarcoma, neuroblastoma, germ cell tumors, Ewing's sarcoma
Neuron-specific enolase (NSE)	15 ng/ml	Neuroblastoma

Data from Malarkey, L. M., & McMorrow, M. (1996). *Nurse's manual of laboratory tests and diagnostic procedures.* Philadelphia: W. B. Saunders; McFarland, M. B. (1995). *Nursing implications of laboratory tests.* Albany, NY: Delmar.

tions. For those children without a venous access device and for some specialized tests, venipuncture is frequently required. Every attempt is made to coordinate aspects of the child's care and obtain all daily blood specimens from a single venipuncture. The child must not be subjected to more than one or two venipunctures per day during acute phases of illness, with decreasing frequency as the child's condition improves. The nurse serves as the child's advocate, coordinating tests and intervening if excessive invasive procedures are requested.

Family and hospital personnel must be honest and open with the child from the beginning. The child's initial experience with painful procedures will be a learning experience for the entire family. An unpleasant experience may well determine behavior throughout the remainder of therapy. Sufficient time and energy is devoted to working with the child and family to promote a positive experience. Venipunctures are performed in the treatment room, which makes the child's bed and room a "safe place." The parents are allowed to stay with the child, if they wish, to provide support. At least initially, consider placing the child on the examination table with his or her arm or hand firmly held in place by someone other than the parents before performing venipuncture. It may be advisable to allow the child to sit up for the procedure once it has been determined that he or she can truly hold still. A second person is necessary to maintain proper positioning of the arm or hand, even with older children. Simple age-appropriate explanations for the blood work are given, reminding the child that the venipuncture is not a consequence of or punishment for bad behavior. Praise is given once the "poke" is over, and a small reward in the form of a special bandage, sticker, or small toy may be given.

DIAGNOSTIC IMAGING STUDIES

Diagnostic imaging helps define and delineate the primary tumor and examines regional and distant sites for spread. These studies are also crucial for follow-up to determine response to therapy. Once again, tests are ordered in a logical sequence, with the biology and known metastatic pattern in mind. Imaging falls into four general categories: (1) plain film radiography, (2) magnetic resonance studies, (3) nuclear medicine studies, and (4) ultrasonography.

PLAIN FILM RADIOGRAPHY

Radiology imaging studies include x-ray examinations, which use small amounts of electromagnetic energy to visualize organs and structures within the body. The four densities in the human body (air, water, fat, and bone) absorb radiation in varying degrees. The radio waves that pass through the patient's body are captured by photographic film and produce a corresponding image.[17] In passing through a patient, the x-ray beam is decreased according to the density of the various tissues through which it passes. X-rays turn the film black; therefore the less dense a material, the more x-rays get through and the blacker the film.[16] Air has the least density, causing dark images on film, and bone has the highest density, resulting in light images. The varying degrees of radiation absorption cause darker or lighter structures to appear on the film.

A chest x-ray study is obtained on almost every patient, either as a baseline or for diagnosis. A chest x-ray will provide information about the lungs, trachea, bronchi, diaphragm, mediastinum, heart, bony thorax, and pulmonary vasculature. To provide a three-dimensional image, x-ray studies are ordered as posterior-anterior (PA), indicating that the beam will be directed from the patient's back to front; and from side to side, called lateral images. X-ray studies of affected areas may also be ordered (e.g., leg studies if the child has a limp). These x-ray studies or "plain films" of specific areas are usually used for screening purposes and are followed by more extensive tests if indicated.

A skeletal survey is a collection of plain x-ray films of the entire skeletal system. This study is useful in detecting bony lesions in diseases that metastasize to the bone. Further corroborating studies may be ordered if the skeletal survey results are positive.

No pain is involved in obtaining x-ray films. However, the child must hold very still, and parents are not routinely allowed in the room. The nurse can help the child cooperate and minimize radiation exposure through patient education. Even young children understand the basic concept of a camera, film, and the taking of a picture. Simple statements explaining that the x-ray camera takes a picture of "your insides" may help a child to be less fearful and hold still. Reassurance that parents are waiting outside the door will also provide comfort. Very young children and babies may require assistive devices to maintain optimal positioning.[13] These are explained in a simple factual manner to the child and the parents before the test begins to avoid the impression that their use is punishment for noncompliance. Use of assistive devices must be time limited, applied gently with respect and consideration for the child, and employed only after other methods to gain the child's cooperation have been explored.

ULTRASOUND

Ultrasonography is a noninvasive procedure used to visualize body structures. The ultrasound probe is called a transducer and contains a crystal that vibrates when subjected to a small electric current. The vibrations produce sound waves. The transducer is held against the patient's skin, and the sound waves are intermittently transmitted to the tissues; this step is followed by periods of time during which the transducer "listens" for sound waves or echoes reflected back from the body tissues. These waves are then recorded on film, videotape, oscilloscope, or recorder and read by the ultrasonographer. No radiation is involved.

An ultrasound is most often ordered as an initial screening test for the child with a palpable mass. It is a fast and relatively inexpensive test with no known side effects. The ultrasound beam cannot penetrate air, so its usefulness is limited in the lung or in the GI tract if it is filled with gas.

The parent can stay with the child during the ultrasound examination. The child must hold still, but often a skilled technician, along with the parent's presence, can get even the younger child to cooperate. A jelly substance is applied to the skin to allow the transducer to move freely. Many children feel that the transducer tickles and may have a harder time holding still because of sensitive skin rather than fear. It is essential to keep excessive gas or air from the abdomen. When a baby cries, air is swallowed, and the ultrasound quality may suffer. Giving the baby a bottle with juice may help alleviate crying during the scan. Occasionally a full bladder is required to help differentiate various organs. Achieving this is very difficult for some children. Compliance may be improved with abundant verbal encouragement and praise, but children are not scolded if they urinate before the scan.

COMPUTED TOMOGRAPHY

Extensive computed tomography (CT) scans may be obtained in children with a known or suspected solid tumor. CT was developed in 1972 and has greatly diminished the need for many previously routine scans and tests. CT scan may also be referred to as computerized axial tomography (CAT) scan. The terms are interchangeable. CT scanning has rendered many older scans obsolete. Intravenous pyelogram (IVP), barium GI series, and lymphangiogram are rarely used today because superior imaging can be achieved with CT scans.

The conventional x-ray image is formed by the casting of shadows of internal structures when a large x-ray beam is projected through the area. The CT image, however, is formed in a two-step process. In the first step the CT scanner produces a narrow x-ray beam, which examines only one layer or slice of the body as the energy source rotates around the patient. Multiple slices are obtained as the patient is slowly moved through the tube. As previously stated, this x-ray beam is absorbed differently by body structures of different densities. Receptors, which are located directly across from the x-ray beam source, detect the number of x-rays remaining after the beams have passed through the body. This information is relayed to a computer and stored there. The x-ray beam source rotates 360 degrees around the body, imaging the body in slices, much like the slices in a loaf of bread. Thousands of readings are taken by the receptors and are recorded in the computer. The computer analyzes the receptor's readings and calculations at thousands of different points. In the second step the calculations are converted into an image on a video screen, which may be photographed or stored on videotape.

Radioiodinated contrast material highlights blood vessels and can be used to enhance the image of particular organs. Intravenous (IV) contrast is always used during brain CT scans if a tumor is present or suspected, and may be used to enhance other organs as well. The major characteristic of any contrast medium is its ability to alter the density of an organ in relation to the surrounding tissues.[34] The IV contrast may cause a temporary flush and a sensation of warmth, waves of nausea, and a metallic, salty, or bitter taste. The duration of these symptoms is usually only 1 to 3 minutes, but can be very frightening. The child must be told of this possibility before the scan and again just before the injection. Most radiology departments prefer that the child be NPO for 3 to 6 hours before the test to decrease the risk of aspiration should vomiting occur. IV contrast can be safely administered through central venous catheters, including implanted venous ports.

CT scanning of the abdomen and pelvis can be enhanced by oral contrast material. The family is instructed in the proper mixing, timing, and administration of the oral contrast medium if the child is an outpatient. For the medium to work effectively, the child must drink the entire volume before the scan. The parents may mix the material in a palatable drink such as fruit juice, Hawaiian Punch, or 7-Up. Several varieties of oral contrast are available. Specific instructions vary slightly with each brand. Some brands require oral ingestion 10 to 12 hours before the scan and again 2 hours before the scan to allow peristalsis to move the contrast material to all aspects of the GI tract. Other varieties may require only a single dose 1 to 2 hours before the scan. The volume of contrast depends on the child's age. Most children can be coaxed into drinking the contrast orally; however, some children refuse to drink the solution or may vomit the entire volume shortly after ingestion. In these cases the oral contrast may require administration through a nasogastric tube.

Today's modern scanners are much faster than those in the past, but the child undergoing a CT scan must remain very still for approximately 20 to 30 minutes. In addition, IV access is usually needed for contrast injection. Very young children typically require some form of sedation for motion control. Most children respond well to chloral hydrate (25 to 100 mg/kg; maximum total dose = 2 g or 100 mg/kg, whichever is less) administered by mouth 20 to 30 minutes before the scan.[14] Chloral hydrate is also available in rectal suppository form. In general, rectal medications are not used for the pediatric oncology patient because of the potential to cause trauma or infection in the rectal mucosa; however, chloral hydrate can be judiciously administered per rectum to patients who require sedation and cannot or will not swallow the drug. Most newly diagnosed patients with solid tumors do not have compromised bone marrow function. The nurse must ascertain, however, that the child is neither thrombocytopenic nor neutropenic before administering the drug by this route. If either condition is present, the nurse alerts the physician to recommend another drug.

For the occasional child who does not respond to chloral hydrate, stronger sedation is needed. Most pediatric radiology departments have protocols in place for pharmacologic sedation of children. Nurses must become familiar with their own institution's preferences. Commonly used sedative-hypnotic agents include midazolam, pentobarbital, methohexital, and thiopental.[14,37] Care must be taken not to overmedicate the child and depress respiration. A heavily sedated child must be continuously and closely monitored by a nurse or physician throughout the entire length of the scan. Patients are at high risk of complications immediately following the end of their scans, when procedural stimuli are discontinued.[14] The child cannot be transported while deeply sedated unless properly monitored.

Certain situations may demand that a child receive general anesthesia for diagnostic imaging. This may occur if multiple scans are needed, if the child is extremely anxious and fearful, or if the child is refractory to sedative agents such as chloral hydrate. Coordination and cooperation among the nursing staff, radiology department, and anesthesia staff are needed to promote a smooth and timely delivery of services.

Older children can cooperate during the CT scan if they have been adequately prepared ahead of time (Figure 3-2). Adolescents should likewise receive preparation and education before their first scan to diminish any fear of the unknown. The nurse can show the child or adolescent pictures of the CT scanner and explain positions expected during the scan. CT suites are usually somewhat chilly, and radiology tables are hard and uncomfortable. Children should practice holding their breath because this is sometimes required during the scan. Reassure children that the loud noises the machine makes will not hurt in any way. Let them know where their parents will be waiting during the scan. It is helpful if parents are on hand immediately after the completion of the study to praise and hug their children.

MAGNETIC RESONANCE IMAGING

The use of magnetic resonance imaging (MRI) has expanded greatly over the last decade, rendering obsolete many studies that were previously routinely ordered. MRI has become the scan of choice for certain malignancies, most notably brain and bone tumors. MRI scans use strong, steady magnetic fields created by a large round magnet. MR imaging is based on the fact that some nuclei—those with unpaired electrons—behave like tiny magnets.[32] Under normal conditions the protons inside the atoms that comprise the human body spin in random directions. The magnetic field produced by the MRI machine causes the protons to align and spin in the same direction. Throughout the scan a radio-frequency signal is intermittently beamed into the magnetic field, causing the protons to move out of their normal alignment. When the signal is stopped, the protons move back to their aligned positions and release energy. A receiver coil measures the energy released by the disturbed protons and the time it takes for the protons to return to the aligned positions. These measurements provide information about the type of tissue in which the protons lie and its condition. A computer then uses this information to create an image on a television monitor. A permanent copy of this image can be recorded on film or magnetic tape.

The MRI scan can last 60 minutes or more, and for most of that time the child must lie very still. Children, who are frightened by the loud noises made by the machine or become claustrophobic in the enclosed gantry, are sedated before the scan. The guidelines for motion control and sedation for MRI are the same as for CT scanning.

Because no x-rays are used during the scan, many MRI departments allow a parent to stay with the child during the entire procedure. There have been no short-term deleterious effects of magnetic field exposure described. Long-term side effects are as yet unknown but are probably negligible.[13] People with particular types of implanted metal objects

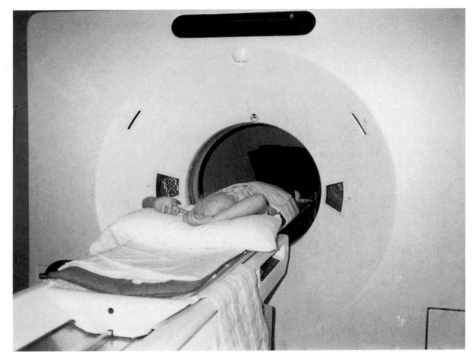

Figure 3-2

Child in place for a chest CT scan.

cannot enter the MRI scanner because of the strong magnetic field. Ferromagnetic metals are the major concern because these types of metals become very hot and can twist and torque in response to the strong magnetic field. Inner ear implants, intracranial aneurysm clips, intrauterine devices, and certain implanted venous ports may contain these metals.[3] Nonmagnetic metal is currently used in orthopedic devices, surgical clips, and suture material. Although these metals pose no danger, their presence may impair the quality and distort the MR image.[27] Pacemakers and prosthetic heart valves may be affected by the strong magnetic field of the MR signal. The radiologist must be informed of all pertinent metal and/or implant history and make the final decision regarding the safety of the MRI scan. Jewelry and other metallic objects must be removed before entering the area. Medical equipment such as IV poles, infusion controllers, and cardiac monitors may not be permitted in the MRI suite. Personnel working in MRI are familiar with the restrictions and can help the nurse prepare the patient appropriately.

MRI pictures are extremely precise, and often as much information can be obtained from MRI as from direct visualization of the tissue. MRI can tar-

get specific atoms, so it "sees" right through bone and clearly defines soft tissue and marrow space. MRI is able to visualize organs and to produce images in any plane. This is particularly useful for brain and spinal cord visualization[17] (Figure 3-3).

Gadolinium IV contrast is used as an enhancing agent during MRI at the discretion of the radiologist or oncologist. When assessing the spinal canal for metastatic brain tumors or paraspinal masses, gadolinium agents are commonly used.

MRI scanning time is slow, and patient movement affects scan quality. Patients who are having their upper body scanned must be enclosed deeply within the machine and are difficult to see or evaluate during the scan. The scanning machine produces a variety of very loud thumping noises. This can be a source of considerable anxiety and fear for children or adolescents. The guidelines for motion control and sedation are similar to those for CT scanning; however, children undergoing MRI may require deep sedation provided by anesthesia personnel.

NUCLEAR MEDICINE SCANS

Nuclear medicine scans use radioactive material, called isotopes, for diagnostic and therapeutic purposes. In comparison with other radiologic proce-

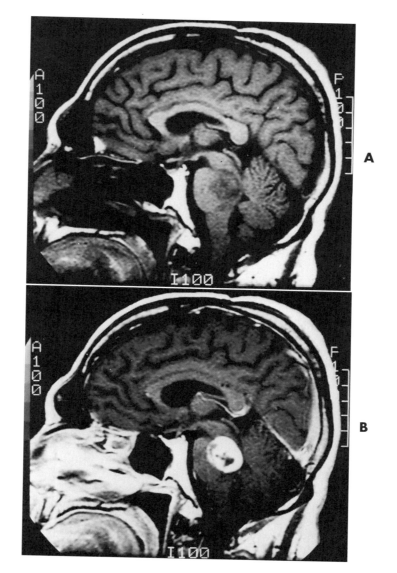

Figure 3-3

MRI scan. **A,** Without and, **B,** with gadolinium enhancement of patient with a brainstem glioma.

dures, nuclear imaging is less precise in providing anatomic information, but it is helpful in demonstrating physiologic activity.[17] Various radioisotopes or radionuclides such as technetium, xenon, gallium, and iodine can be used for nuclear medicine scans. A mandatory precaution before all nuclear medicine procedures, as is the case with x-ray studies and CT scans, is to ensure that the patient is not pregnant since pregnancy will affect how and whether the study is performed.

The radioisotope selected is a simple salt compound that cannot enter the targeted tissue until it is chemically linked to another element. A radioisotope bound to another compound is called a radiopharmaceutical. Once the radiopharmaceutical enters the body, it functions like the chemical the organ normally metabolizes so that the organ tissue "takes up" the radionuclide. For example, radioactive iodine concentrates in the thyroid just as stable iodine does. Radioisotopes delineate cancer in one of two ways: (1) the tumor concentrates the radionuclide from the rest of the organ in a "hot" spot or (2) the rest of the organ concentrates the radionuclide, and the tumor shows up as a "cold" spot.

Newly diagnosed patients may undergo multiple nuclear medicine scans before beginning therapy. Care must be taken to perform the tests in the proper sequence, since the various radiopharmaceuticals may interfere with each other and subsequent tests. For example, the radioisotope used for a bone scan can sometimes linger in the knee area and make the metaiodobenzylguanidine (MIBG) scan difficult to interpret. The glomerular filtration rate (GFR) is obtained after the MIBG scan, and there must be at least 1 day between the GFR and a bone scan. Coordination of tests with the nuclear medicine personnel will prevent scheduling conflicts and potential delays.

The gamma scintillation camera is the most common imaging device. The camera detects the gamma rays emitted after the IV administration of radionuclide, similar to a Geiger counter, and projects the image on a screen. The results can be transferred to x-ray film or paper.[35] Timing of the scan after administration of the radionuclide is dependent on its uptake in the targeted organ.

Various organs can be studied by means of nuclear medicine scans. Bone scans are the most commonly ordered nuclear medicine study in pediatric oncology. Thyroid scans are used to detect masses or tumors in the thyroid gland; however, this is a rare site of pediatric cancer. Kidney, liver or spleen, and brain scans are no longer routinely obtained because these organs can be more easily and better assessed by CT or MRI scan. Gallium scans are standardly ordered at diagnosis and for follow-up for patients with lymphoma. Gallium is also used to detect occult infections and inflammation in the immunocompromised cancer patient. It is particularly useful in detecting pelvic and abdominal abscesses. MIBG, positron emission tomography (PET), and single photon emission computed tomography (SPECT) scans are new and exciting applications of nuclear medicine and are described in further detail.

Bone Scan (Figure 3-4)

Technetium 99m (Tc 99m) labeled compounds, the radiopharmaceuticals used for bone scan, have a relatively low radiation exposure. The uptake of bone-seeking agents by the skeleton is nearly complete within 30 minutes after the IV injection. In practice, images are generally obtained after a 2- to 4-hour delay to permit additional renal clearance of the radiopharmaceutical from extracellular fluid. The bone scan is a highly sensitive method for detecting malignant lesions. However, increased focal accumulation of tracer may indicate a number of abnormalities in addition to malignant lesions. Bone scanning is based on the uptake of tracers by the crystal lattice of bone. The degree of uptake by a particular bone is related to bone blood flow and metabolism. Primary skeletal disease (e.g., osteosarcoma), secondary skeletal disease (e.g., metastases), inflammatory bone disease (e.g., osteomyelitis), and bone trauma are all associated with increased bone blood flow. Therefore the existence of any of these disease processes will be seen on a bone scan as increased uptake. Because of the nonspecificity of the bone scan, scan results are correlated with clinical findings and conventional radiographs such as a skeletal survey. The actual scan takes 30 to 60 minutes. No pain is involved with the scanning procedures, but the child must lie still during the procedure (Figure 3-5). Sedatives such as chloral hydrate are often used for young children.

The amount of radiation from radionuclide imaging is usually less than the amount of radiation received from diagnostic x-ray studies. The injected tracer is excreted in the urine and can be safely disposed of in the commode. The low dose of radiation will not affect parents or hospital staff. Urine produced immediately after the injection or scan should not be used for diagnostic purposes or samples for 24 hours.

Gallium Scan

Gallium is a radionuclide that is taken up or concentrated in areas of infection or inflammation and some malignancies. Lymphomas are particularly gallium avid tumors. Gallium is used at the time of diagnosis and staging in patients with lymphoma, but it is especially useful in follow-up to monitor the disease. Lymphomas can be detected via gallium scan, when CT scans are negative. Gallium is thought to be the best noninvasive way to determine if the tumor has completely disappeared after treatment. Gallium is injected intravenously, and imaging is performed 3 to 5 days later. The radionuclide must be injected before lymphoma therapy begins, but following injection therapy can begin if necessary without waiting for the images to be taken. Patients may require a bowel prep since gallium is normally excreted in the bowel and the presence of stool can interfere with evaluation of the abdomen.

MIBG Scan (Figure 3-6)

The radioisotope marker 1-metaiodobenzylguanidine (MIBG) was synthesized for the detection of pheochromocytoma, a benign tumor of the adrenal gland. MIBG is taken up and stored in tissues in a manner similar to norepinephrine; thus it accumulates in adrenergic tissues. MIBG is extremely useful in the diagnosis and follow-up of neuroblastoma, a tumor of the sympathetic nervous system.[2]

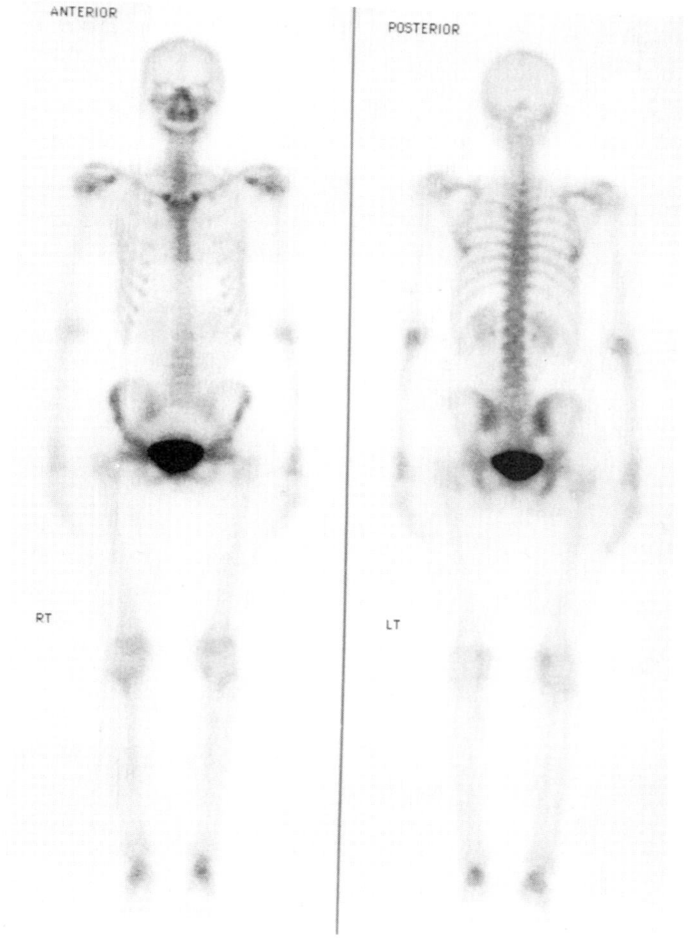

Figure 3-4

Anterior and posterior views of a normal bone scan.

MIBG is superior to bone scan in detecting metastatic neuroblastoma, particularly during therapy.[15] In clinical practice the two nuclear studies are often used in a corroborative fashion. As previously stated, bone scan uptake occurs in areas with any bone activity, including bone growth or repair. Bone scans may continue to read an area as positive with presumed malignancy when in fact the lesions have responded to therapy and active bone repair is occurring. MIBG, on the other hand, is picked up only by active tumor; therefore an area of bone regrowth would not take up the radioisotope. The major disadvantage of MIBG is that a small but significant percentage of biopsy-proven neuroblastomas do not take up MIBG.

The MIBG study requires imaging on 2 or 3 consecutive days after the tracer dose is given.

After injection of MIBG on day 1 the patient is seen 24, 48, and 72 hours later for imaging. Drugs such as phenothiazines, and sympathomimetics (e.g., pseudoephedrine), block the uptake of norepinephrine and thus MIBG. They should generally be avoided for 2 to 4 weeks before the scan.

MIBG is bound to radioactive iodide. Without adequate prophylaxis, the thyroid can take up the radioactive iodine that comes off MIBG, with damaging consequences. Administration of saturated solution of potassium iodide (SSKI) drops or Lugol's solution will block the uptake. It must begin 1 day before the scan and continue for 5 days if I-123 was used, and 10 days if I-131 was used as the radiopharmaceutical. Parents must be aware of the need for strict compliance with SSKI administration and the

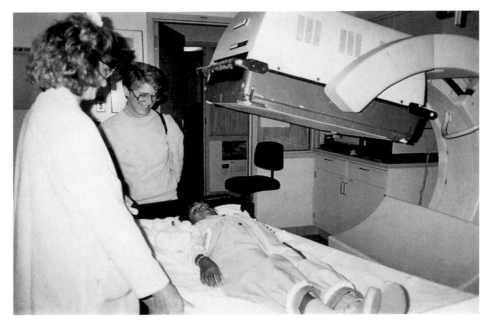

Figure 3-5

Child in proper position to begin bone scan.

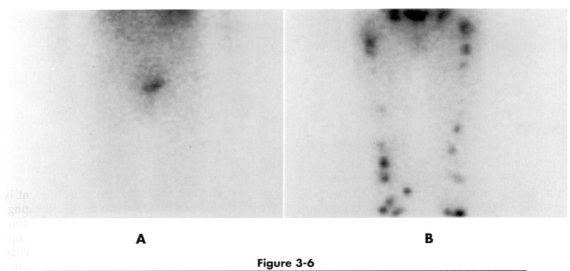

A   **B**

Figure 3-6

MIBG scans. **A,** Normal scan. **B,** Abnormal scan showing multiple areas of metastatic neuroblastoma.

potential for damage to the thyroid if radioactive iodine is absorbed.

As with most imaging studies, the child must
hold very still during the nuclear medicine scans.
Young children may require sedation. Older children should be informed about the scan and be
allowed to see the machine before the test. The
radioisotopes are usually injected through a
small-gauge butterfly needle. Some institutions
may not permit the use of central venous
catheters for radioisotope injection because of
the radioisotope's propensity to adhere to the
catheter lining and thus obscure the image in the
area of the catheter.

Positron Emission Tomography

PET is one of the newer scans added to the nuclear medicine arsenal. PET combines conventional nuclear medicine techniques with transaxial tomography (e.g., CT scans) to study blood flow and volume and protein metabolism of specific regions or organs. Substances normally used by the body, such as glucose, oxygen, nitrogen, carbon, or fatty acids, are made radioactive and administered intravenously before the PET scan. Once the isotope is injected, it emits subatomic particles called positrons (positively charged electrons). When a positron encounters an electron, which it does just after emission, both are destroyed and two gamma rays are released. These rays are recorded on a computer to be reconstructed as an image on a cathode ray screen.[33]

The most commonly used PET radiopharmaceutical is fluorine 18 (F-18-FDG), a labeled glucose analogue. It is one of the few known molecules with the ability to pass through the normal blood-brain barrier. Glucose is the only source of energy used by brain cells. By measuring the location and quantity of F-18-FDG, detailed information about the biochemical activity within cells and precise organ function can be determined. Brain metabolism is a reliable indicator of brain tissue viability and helps determine the degree of malignancy present. PET scan can also help distinguish recurrent or residual (i.e., active) tumor from necrotic tissues in other areas.

In general, there are no food or fluid restrictions before PET scanning; however, caffeine, nicotine, and alcohol should be avoided for 24 hours before the test. Sedative and tranquilizing drugs can also interfere with the test.

The positron-emitting radioisotopes used in PET typically have a very short half-life; thus local production of the radioisotopes in an in-house or regional cyclotron is required. Use of PET scanners has been limited to major centers with a cyclotron available, but this pattern is changing. To date, PET is used mainly for evaluation of tumors found in adults. Use in the pediatric population has been limited, but the next decade will no doubt bring additional clinical applications for the pediatric population.

Single Photon Emission Computed Tomography

SPECT is another new computer-aided nuclear medicine scan that is similar in concept to PET scan and combines the technique of conventional nuclear medicine imaging with that of CT. Rather than using x-rays, as in CT, the SPECT relies on gamma-emitting radioactive isotopes. Unlike PET scan, conventional isotopes such as technetium 99m and iodine 123 are used, greatly reducing cost and increasing accessibility. The image produced in SPECT is not merely in one plane; instead the gamma camera rotates 360 degrees around the patient. Therefore the targeted organ is reconstructed and displayed in axial, parasagittal, and coronal sections.[33] SPECT scan looks at only one photon (or gamma ray) instead of the double photons generated in PET and provides approximately half the information that a PET scan provides. The SPECT process is analogous to drawing the floor plan of a house by looking through the windows of the house. The viewer is confined to the outside of the house, but by walking around the house and looking into each window, one can see the details of the house.

Glomerular Filtration Rate

Precise kidney function can be assessed through measurement of the GFR. Two methods are used to calculate this rate, the plasma method and the Gates method.[33] Both methods employ the injection of a radiopharmaceutical agent such as technetium. The plasma method uses timed blood sampling to measure the level of the radiopharmaceutical. Following IV administration of the radiopharmaceutical, a blood sample is drawn 1 and 3 hours later. The agent is eliminated from the body by glomerular filtration; thus the level of radiotracer remaining in the blood at selected intervals can determine precise renal function. The volume of the technetium administered is very small, so any soft tissue extravasation will result in an inaccurate measurement. Films of the injection site may be taken to identify any such leakage.

The Gates method uses a scanning technique to determine the activity of the radiopharmaceutical measured over the kidneys. The technetium dose, as calculated by patient size or age, is counted by the camera before injection. The child is scanned for a period of time after injection. After the procedure is completed, the amount of radiopharmaceutical remaining in the syringe and IV catheter after removal is counted. The computer then calculates the filtration rate based on activity measured over the kidneys. Each kidney can be evaluated separately with this method. A peripheral IV must be inserted for this method since the minute volumes of the technetium must be carefully measured to ensure an accurate GFR.

Thallium Scans

Nuclear imaging using thallium-201 as the radioisotope is used for evaluating myocardial function, primarily in adults. Thallium-201 is being investigated for use in imaging osteosarcoma and some lymphomas in the pediatric setting. There have been reports that thallium may also work well in detecting residual tumor in Hodgkin's disease.[9]

Miscellaneous Studies

Several other tests or procedures are performed on the child with cancer once the diagnosis is suspected or confirmed but before initiating therapy. Baseline evaluations of certain organs are performed to ascertain normal function and as a means of evaluating treatment toxicity during the course of therapy. For children with a solid tumor, it is not unusual for some of these tests to be ordered even before the definitive surgical procedure. There is often a strong suspicion of the tumor type, and using free time to evaluate normal organs during the metastatic workup allows therapy to begin promptly after surgical recovery. Additionally, tests that require the child's full cooperation and participation are best obtained before surgery, when postoperative pain and discomfort will not interfere with performance.

A hearing evaluation is indicated before and during therapy with cisplatin. The older, cooperative child can be monitored with an audiogram. Skilled audiologists can perform an audiogram on children as young as 1 to 2 years of age; however, babies and some older children who are unable to cooperate will require brainstem auditory evoked response (BAER) testing. Auditory neural activity is recorded as it passes from the peripheral or cochlear end organ through the brainstem to the cortex. Both acoustic nerve response and upper brainstem response are measured.[26]

Normal cardiac function must be documented before anthracycline use. This is most commonly done with an echocardiogram and an electrocardiogram (ECG). An echocardiogram examines the sizes, shape, and motion of cardiac structures with high frequency sound waves, and ECG records the electric current generated by the heart. Some centers routinely perform a multigated angiography (MUGA) scan, a nuclear medicine study that evaluates cardiac function. The MUGA scan is more precise in evaluating cardiac function than an echocardiogram but is also more expensive and time-consuming. A sample of blood is tagged with the radioactive isotope Tc 99m. A scintillation camera measures the radioactivity emitted by the isotope as it passes through the left ventricle. The percentage of isotope ejected during each heartbeat can then be calculated to determine the ejection fraction, a reliable measure of ventricular function. The choice of a MUGA scan versus echocardiogram is generally up to individual institutions or physicians.

However, the same study must be consistently used to monitor the child throughout therapy.

Pulmonary function tests are used to diagnose and quantify the degree of restrictive lung disease. They may be performed before, during, and after bleomycin therapy or pulmonary irradiation, which is known to cause severe restrictive lung disease. Pulmonary function tests require full cooperation of the patient. During the test patients must inhale and exhale and hold their breath on demand. Pulmonary function tests therefore cannot be administered to young children, generally less than age 5 years, or to an uncooperative older child. Currently there is no reliable substitute for these tests; however, transcutaneous oxygen saturation monitoring measures the oxygen tension (pO_2) of blood and provides general information about lung function. Table 3-3 lists the various diagnostic imaging studies used for specific tumors.

PATHOLOGIC CONFIRMATION OF DIAGNOSIS

Once the entire metastatic workup is complete and laboratory and imaging studies indicate the likelihood of cancer, direct examination of the tumor is performed. The safest and most reliable method of obtaining tissue samples is used.

BONE MARROW ASPIRATION AND BIOPSY

When a child presents with an abnormal CBC and a history suspicious for malignancy, an examination of the bone marrow is warranted. The bone marrow is a potential site of metastasis for some solid tumors and the primary site for the leukemias. If leukemia is suspected, a bone marrow aspiration will provide the primary pathologic specimens needed to confirm the diagnosis. Not infrequently, this will be performed in a somewhat urgent fashion so treatment can begin quickly. Children with solid tumors that have the potential to metastasize to the bone marrow will also need their marrow sampled, but in this circumstance the aspiration and biopsy of marrow contents can often be delayed for a few days, while the staging workup is under way. Care can be coordinated so that the marrow examination is obtained while the child is in the operating room under general anesthesia for biopsy, debulking, or insertion of a central venous catheter. The judicious use of such timing spares the child the pain of the procedure and will not hamper or delay making the diagnosis. Coordination is required among the oncology, anesthesia, and surgery staff.

Bone marrow is the soft, spongelike material contained in the medullary cavity of bone. The

TABLE 3-3	DIAGNOSTIC IMAGING STUDIES FOR VARIOUS MALIGNANCIES	
Disease	**Primary Tumor**	**Metastatic Search**
Leukemia	Bone marrow aspirate and biopsy*	Spinal tap* Chest x-ray examination
Neuroblastoma	Computed tomography (CT) scan (abdomen, chest, pelvis)	Bone marrow aspirate and biopsy* Magnetic resonance imaging (MRI) for paraspinal lesion Chest x-ray examination Bone scan Metaiodobenzylguanidine (MIBG) scan Skeletal survey PET scan SPECT scan
Wilms tumor	Abdominal CT scan Abdominal ultrasound	Chest x-ray examination Chest CT scan Bone scan (unfavorable histology) Head CT/MRI scan (unfavorable histology) Skeletal survey (unfavorable histology)
Non-Hodgkin's lymphoma	CT scan of primary tumor area (abdomen, chest, pelvis)	Bone marrow aspirate and biopsy and spinal tap* Chest x-ray examination Chest CT scan Bone scan Skeletal survey Gallium scan SPECT scan Head CT scan if indicated
Hodgkin's disease	CT scan (chest, abdomen, neck, pelvis)	Chest x-ray examination Chest CT scan Bone marrow aspirate and biopsy* Gallium scan SPECT scan
Rhabdomyosarcoma	CT scan or MRI of primary tumor	Chest x-ray examination Chest CT scan Retroperitoneal CT scan (abdomen/pelvic tumor) Bone scan SPECT scan Head MRI or CT scan and spinal tap (for parameningeal tumors) Bone marrow aspirate and biopsy*

Bone tumors
  Osteosarcoma
  Ewing's sarcoma
	Extremity or involved bone MRI
	Bone x-ray examination
		Chest CT scan
		Chest x-ray examination
		Bone scan
		Bone marrow aspirate or biopsy for Ewing's sarcoma*
		Thallium scans

Hepatoblastoma	Abdominal CT or MRI scan	Chest x-ray examination Chest CT scan
Germ cell tumors	CT scan or MRI of primary site	Chest x-ray examination Chest CT scan Bone scan
Brain tumors	Brain CT scan or MRI with or without enhancement	MRI of spine with gadolinium if indicated Spinal tap* Bone marrow aspirate or biopsy* (medulloblastoma) Chest x-ray examination

*Not an imaging study; included for completeness.

cells of the bone marrow are responsible for hematopoiesis, the formation of blood. At birth all of the bones contain active marrow, but as the bones grow, the space in the medullary cavity is replaced with fat or yellow marrow. By late childhood the hematopoietic red marrow is found only in the skull, vertebrae, sternum, ribs, shoulder, and proximal ends of the long bones and pelvis. The most common sites for bone marrow examination in children are the anterior or posterior iliac crests. The tibia is sometimes used in infants. The spinous processes are used by some clinicians when both bone marrow aspiration and lumbar puncture are performed at the same time.

Historically, bone marrow aspiration was performed with little or no effective sedation or anesthesia. Over the past decade many advances in pain and anxiety management have been achieved. The development of short-acting opioids and sedatives, as well as specific antagonists to them, have enabled clinicians in pediatric oncology to render obsolete the days of screaming, frantic children pinned down on treatment room tables in an attempt to obtain bone marrow. In 1990 the American Academy of Pediatrics Subcommittee on the Management of Pain in Childhood Cancer published age-specific recommendations and guidelines for managing pain associated with bone marrow and lumbar puncture.[39]

Many pediatric centers perform all painful procedures under general anesthesia. Short-acting, quick-onset methods of achieving general anesthesia are widely available, and many cancer centers use the anesthesiology department to anesthetize the child during these procedures.

Other centers are using various medications to achieve "conscious sedation" for children undergoing bone marrow examination. Conscious sedation is a state of depressed consciousness, which still allows protective reflexes and patent airway to be maintained and permits patient response to verbal commands such as "open your eyes."[14] Midazolam (Versed) has become increasingly popular because of its rapid onset, short duration, and potent sedative and amnesic effect. Midazolam has no analgesic effect, so it is often used in combination with an opioid. Morphine sulfate, fentanyl, and meperidine have been used. The addition of these drugs can potentiate respiratory depression. Studies have reported apnea as a frequent side effect, and respiratory arrest has been reported secondary to anoxia.[38] Newer studies, however, have documented the safety and effectiveness of midazolam, with or without opiate analgesia, with careful monitoring.[30] Profound slumber is rarely obtained with midazolam, however, and children may still require personnel to assist and restrain them during the procedure. Nursing personnel must continuously monitor them; in addition, a pulse and oxygen saturation monitor is used during the short procedure and recovery period.

Lidocaine infiltration is needed before performing a bone marrow aspiration or biopsy. To help decrease the discomfort and stinging of the lidocaine injection, a topical analgesic can be used over the site. EMLA Cream (a eutectic mixture of lidocaine and prilocaine) can be very effective in numbing the skin. It must be applied at least 60 minutes before the procedure to be effective. Ethyl chloride or fluormethane sprays that numb the skin for a short period of time by cooling it have been used. Systems that deliver lidocaine transdermally via electrical current (Numby Stuff) are also available.

Marrow is easily and safely obtained from the pelvic bone from either the anterior or posterior iliac crest in the child. The child is permitted to climb onto the procedure table with minimal assistance and instructed to lie in a prone position if the posterior iliac crest is selected or supine if the anterior aspect of the bone will be used. If the child is chubby, a pillow or folded blanket can be placed under the abdomen to elevate the hips and facilitate access to the posterior site. Parents are allowed to stay during the procedure if they wish. The supporting parent may sit on a stool adjacent to the child's head. In this position the parent is able to offer physical and verbal support by talking to the child and holding his hand.

Several studies have shown that parents would like to stay with their child during painful procedures but are unsure about their role and have received little communication from the hospital staff in this area.[12] The nurse who briefly informs the parents of the positive effects of their presence during painful procedures, in effect grants "permission" for the parent or parents to remain. The parent who chooses to stay should not be placed in the position of having to physically restrain the child. Not only do parents have very little experience in proper restraining techniques, but also the experience may cause considerable distress to both parent and child. Parents are not forced to stay during the procedure against their wishes, nor should they feel guilty if they decide to leave.

Age-appropriate descriptions of the procedure, guided imagery, and distraction can all enhance the child's coping skills. Older children need help to hold still, and young children may require firm restraint. The parent can be there to offer love and support. Chapter 12 has a more in-depth review of procedural pain management in children.

When the desired site for bone marrow aspiration is identified, the area is prepared with a povidone-iodine solution. Surface anesthetic is most commonly injected through a small-gauge needle and syringe. A deeper injection of anesthetic may be given once the skin is numb. If a biopsy is required, the anesthetic is delivered directly into the periosteum of the bone.

After anesthesia has been achieved, the aspiration needle with stylet in place is inserted through the cortex of the bone with a slight twisting motion. The stylet is then removed, and a syringe is attached to the needle hub. Manual suction is applied until marrow appears in the syringe. If awake, the child will feel pressure as the needle goes through the periosteum of the bone and a sharp transient pain as the marrow is withdrawn into the syringe. Both sensations last only a few seconds.

When marrow appears in the syringe, the syringe is removed and the bone marrow expressed onto a glass slide. Bone marrow spicules will appear as whitish, granular particles throughout the bloody aspirate. Their presence indicates that the specimen is satisfactory. The hematologist or pathologist examining the cells on the slide under a microscope determines bone marrow cell morphology. In addition, a child with newly diagnosed or suspected leukemia will require additional bone marrow samples for cytogenetic analysis, and flow cytometry (immunophenotyping). Individual institutional studies or national clinical trials may require additional specimens of marrow.

The initial bone marrow aspirate on a newly diagnosed leukemic patient may be extremely difficult to withdraw because the marrow is very hypercellular and packed with leukemic cells. Sometimes puncturing more than one site is needed to obtain the proper specimens. These diagnostic marrow specimens may not contain the characteristic spicules. Although not ideal, these specimens are usually adequate for diagnosis. At times no marrow can be obtained via aspirate. This is referred to as a "dry tap." In these cases a bone marrow biopsy alone is used for diagnosis.

Many oncologists require a bone marrow biopsy for diagnosis and evaluation of children with cancer, especially for evaluation of children with solid tumors. A bone marrow biopsy consists of a solid core of bone and marrow that are removed in entirety, in addition to the aspiration. Bone marrow biopsy is also referred to as a trephine biopsy. This indicates the removal of a circular core with a specialized instrument, as opposed to a wedge biopsy that would be removed in an open surgical procedure. A Jamshidi biopsy needle is used to obtain a trephine bone marrow biopsy. The needle is manufactured by various companies in infant, pediatric, and adult sizes. The usual bone marrow sites are customarily used, but deeper local anesthesic is administered if the patient has not received a general anesthetic

agent. Local anesthetic should be infiltrated into the tissue and bone periosteum, in addition to the skin surface. Once the needle is inserted just into the periosteum, the introducer is removed and the needle is advanced to obtain a core biopsy. While obtaining the specimen, the practitioner must grasp and advance the needle firmly with both a rotating and rocking motion to cut a sliver of bone. The bone sliver remains in the core of the needle as it is removed from the patient. The biopsy material is ejected from the bottom of the needle core toward the top with a metal probe to prevent crushing the specimen. The specimen is then placed on a glass slide for immediate examination (called "touch preps") and then placed in a tube containing formalin for later study. It is not uncommon for solid tumor protocols to require two separate sites for bone marrow aspiration and biopsy. Sampling marrow from more than one site helps increase the likelihood of detecting bone marrow metastasis.[2]

A pressure bandage customarily is applied at the site of a bone marrow aspiration or biopsy if the child's platelet count is 50,000 or less. If the platelet count is adequate, a simple adhesive bandage is the only dressing necessary. The child or parent is instructed to remove the original dressing no earlier than 8 hours and no later than 24 hours after the procedure. Leaving the bandage in place for longer periods predisposes the immunocompromised child to infection. Many children are reluctant to have the dressing removed, especially the larger pressure bandage. In such a case the parent is advised to remove the bandage during the child's next bath because a wet bandage can be removed more easily.

LUMBAR PUNCTURE

Children with leukemia, lymphoma, parameningeal rhabdomyosarcoma, and certain brain tumors require a spinal tap or lumbar puncture as part of the diagnostic or staging workup. A lumbar puncture is a sterile procedure that provides information about the pressure and dynamics of the CSF circulation and, more importantly, the composition of the fluid. The procedure is explained to the child and parents in advance. The importance of correct positioning must be emphasized. The nurse can demonstrate the improved access obtained with proper positioning by bending and permitting the child to palpate between the nurse's vertebrae. Before the procedure the child is requested to void to ensure an empty bladder. Parents are informed that they are welcome to accompany the child, observe the procedure, and assist and support the child (Figure 3-7).

One of the available topical numbing agents—EMLA, or ethyl chloride spray, is recommended to anesthetize the skin surface before the lumbar

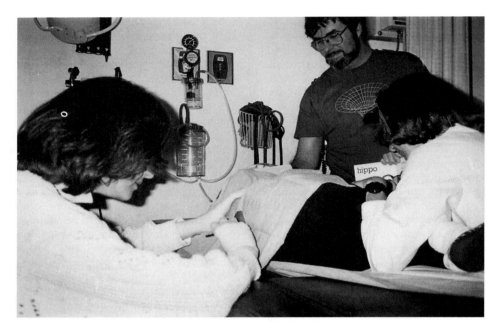

Figure 3-7

During a spinal tap both parent and nurse help comfort and distract a school-age child.

puncture. It will be necessary to have the child simulate the actual position to apply the EMLA cream appropriately. Care must be taken not to disrupt the occlusive dressing over the site with the child's clothes.

During the procedure the child is positioned on the table with knees drawn up under the chin and head bent over the chest. This position arches the lumbar section of the back, offers maximal widening of the interspinous spaces, and provides easy entry into the subarachnoid space. A nurse usually assists the child to maintain this position by using locked hands to provide support behind the child's knees and neck. The child's back must not rotate forward or backward, for this can make access to the lumbar spaces very difficult. The entire back in its curved position should be completely perpendicular to the table.

Occasionally, the child or adolescent may be unable to curl up adequately in the lying position. If this occurs, the child can be placed in a seated position. The child is seated on the table with legs dangling or supported on a stool. The child lays on top of an overbed tray table that is placed over the child's lap and supported with pillows. Care is taken to make sure the child is seated straight so that the spine will not be rotated. This position is not the treatment of choice since the distribution of the intrathecal chemotherapy may not be adequate.

However, ensuring a successful and atraumatic procedure is the priority.

The assisting nurse constantly provides verbal reassurance and continuously assesses the child's status. Physical support prevents sudden movements that could alter needle placement, causing tissue injury and bleeding, thus obscuring the correct diagnosis. Once the child's body is positioned correctly, the site is prepared with povidone-iodine, and intradermal and subcutaneous lidocaine is infiltrated. After skin preparation and the local anesthesia is administered, the child's position is rechecked and the spinal needle is inserted between the third and fourth or fourth and fifth lumbar vertebrae into the interspace. When the needle is in place, the nurse reassures the child that there will be no further pain. Children usually relax when they know the needle is in position.

The parent is encouraged to sit on a stool close to the child's head and to hold the child's hand. The parent is thus able to offer both physical and verbal support during the procedure. The child may be offered objects that will provide distraction once the needle is in place and the fluid is being collected. A helpful object for use with young children is "pop-up" storybooks. They seem to delight children and help them relax. The parent or restraining nurse can hold the book and read the story out loud while turning pages that pop out at the child.

The American Academy of Pediatrics Subcommittee on Cancer Pain in Children recommends some type of sedation during the initial lumbar puncture.[39] As is true for bone marrow procedures, many pediatric medical centers offer short-acting general anesthesia or sedation for lumbar punctures, as well. The administration and doses needed for spinal taps are similar to those necessary for bone marrow aspiration. At the completion of the lumbar puncture, the stylet is replaced (unless chemotherapy has been administered), the needle is withdrawn, and an adhesive bandage is placed over the site. The child and parents are informed that it may be helpful for the older child to remain flat or in Trendelenburg's position for 30 minutes to facilitate chemotherapy distribution throughout the CSF or to prevent a headache, although unlike in adults, this is not a common occurrence in children. The nurse may suggest that the child pass the time in quiet play.

The CSF is examined to determine if WBCs are present and to ascertain the numbers and differential of those cells. RBC levels are also noted. Biochemical evaluation of spinal fluid includes glucose and protein measurements. Abnormal amounts of glucose and protein obtained in the initial lumbar puncture may indicate disease. Specimens of fluid are sometimes sent for cell count, cytologic examination for cancer cells, and bacterial culture if indicated. It is important to ensure an atraumatic lumbar puncture for the initial determination of CNS spread of leukemia. The most experienced practitioner must perform the initial procedure because RBC contamination, especially in the child with a high circulating blast count, may be falsely positive for leukemia.

BIOPSY

With only a few exceptions, the child with a solid tumor must undergo a surgical biopsy to obtain tissue for direct examination. Pathologic confirmation is necessary and must precede any decision about choice and timing of treatment. As progress has been made in the treatment of childhood cancer, the approach to pathological analysis has become more complex. In the absence of curative therapy, each tumor was considered high risk and there was no need for risk classification. However, today many cancers are classified into risk categories based on pathological analysis, and treatment is applied accordingly. The modern diagnosis of childhood cancer requires a multimodal tumor analysis carefully planned ahead of biopsy by the pediatric oncologist, pathologist, and surgeon. Biopsy is best performed in the pediatric cancer center. Optimal use of the surgical specimen, including nonpreserved tumor samples needed for national cooperative group studies, can be performed only in specialized childhood cancer centers.

Precise biologic classification is performed by the pathologist using a variety of tests. The pathologist begins with light microscopy (standard microscopic evaluation) and electron microscopy to determine the morphology of the tumor. An electron microscope uses an electron beam rather than light for illumination and allows greater magnification and resolution. The tumor sections can be stained with various dyes to further define the cells' appearance. Light microscopic immunohistochemistry (IHC) is a nonmorphological method that detects a marker substance (antigen), within the tumor cell, that has reacted with an antibody specific for it.[36] Immunophenotyping uses monoclonal antibodies to further classify and describe tumor cells. Tumor cytogenetic analysis provides characteristic, sometimes diagnostic, identification of chromosomal abnormalities of many tumors. Molecular cytogenetic studies employing techniques of fluorescent in situ hybridization (FISH) and molecular genetic analysis (DNA amplification) can provide further, in-depth classification of tumors.

The surgeon, along with the oncologist, must decide if biopsy alone is sufficient for the child with a solid tumor or if complete surgical resection should be attempted. Needle biopsy, obtained with the help of CT or ultrasound, can be used to obtain diagnostic tissue. Performed by the interventional radiologist, CT guided biopsy makes lesions in the lung, liver, retroperitoneum, and abdomen readily accessible for examination. However, a fine (thin) needle is generally used, producing only a minimal amount of tissue, which is often inadequate for modern staging procedures. CT guided biopsy is often more valuable when used to identify isolated metastatic lesions.

Pediatric cancers encompass a diverse group of diseases, and there is no single surgical procedure with universal applications. Obviously, the primary goal is cure, which entails total eradication of all malignant cells. However, eradication may be achieved best with chemotherapy alone or chemotherapy and radiation combined rather than with surgery.

STAGING

Staging is defined as the extent of disease locally, regionally, and systemically at diagnosis or relapse and in most solid tumors is the cornerstone of appropriate, specific therapy. A system of staging has been designed for most pediatric tumors. Individual tumor staging systems will be described in the corresponding disease chapters.

Staging relates the extent of disease at diagnosis to the subsequent clinical course. It is based on the premise that cancers of similar histologic features and site of origin will extend and metastasize in a predictable manner.[25] Staging helps determine both prognosis and treatment.

The prognosis of most childhood cancers is dependent on the stage and/or the biology of the disease. Assessment of prognosis is therefore integral to determining appropriate therapy and improving the child's chance of achieving cure. Most large institutions discuss new patients with solid tumors at a multispecialty conference commonly called the tumor board. Pediatric cancer specialists, including medical oncologists and nurses, surgeons, radiation therapists, radiologists, and pathologists, convene to share their findings and to determine a strategy for treating the pediatric solid tumor patient. All of the data compiled during the staging and diagnostic workup are discussed and considered. Chemotherapy, radiation therapy, and surgery are all integral parts of a combined program of care, and each may play a role at a specific point. The timing of each is highly dependent on the effects of the other(s). During the tumor board meeting a plan of care is established, using the expertise of the various disciplines.

The diagnostic phase of cancer treatment is emotionally shattering to most families. Many parents are devastated, since the diagnosis will cause irrevocable changes in their lives. Nurses caring for a child at this time often become deeply involved in the child and family's life. This bond establishes the basis for intervention and support throughout therapy. A sound knowledge of the tests involved, the general sequence and timing of the diagnostic evaluation, and the disease itself permits nurses to respond realistically to the families. The diagnostic phase begins the long-term education, guidance, and support these families need and deserve.

REFERENCES

1. Barness, L. (1999). Pediatric history and physical exam. In J. A. McMillan, C. D. DeAngelis, R. D. Feigen, et al. (Eds.), *Oski's pediatric principles and practice* (pp. 39-52). Philadelphia: Lippincott.
2. Brodeur, G. M., & Castleberry, R. P. (1997). Neuroblastoma. In P. A. Pizzo & D. G. Poplack (Eds.), *Principles and practice of pediatric oncology* (3rd ed., pp. 761-797). Philadelphia: Lippincott-Raven.
3. Bushong, S. C. (1996). *MRI physical and biological principles.* (2nd ed.). St. Louis: Mosby.
4. Castleberry, R. P. (1997). Biology and treatment of neuroblastoma. *Pediatric Clinics of North America, 44,* 919-937.
5. Cavanaugh, B. (1999). *Nurse's manual of laboratory and diagnostic tests.* (3rd ed.). Philadelphia: F. A. Davis.
6. Dome, J. S., & Schwartz, C. L. (1997). Osteosarcoma. In D. O. Walterhouse & S. L. Cohn (Eds.), *Diagnostic and therapeutic advances in pediatric oncology* (pp. 215-253). Boston: Kluwer Academic.
7. Eissa, S. (1998). *Tumor markers.* London: Chapman & Hall.
8. Finlay, J. L., & Hann, H. W. (1992). Tumor markers. In G. J. D'Angio, D. Sinnian, A. T. Meadows, et al. (Eds.), *Practical pediatric oncology.* New York: Wiley-Liss.
9. Fletcher, B. D., Xiong, X., Kauffman, W. M., et al. (1998). Hodgkin disease: Use of T1-201 to monitor mediastinal involvement after treatment. *Radiology, 209,* 471-475.
10. Gundy, J. (1997). Pediatric physical examination. In R. A. Hoekelman, S. B. Friedman, & M. E. H. Wilson (Eds.), *Primary pediatric care* (3rd ed., pp. 55-98). St. Louis: Mosby.
11. Henze, R. L., & Bullock, B. L. (2000). *Focus on pathophysiology.* Philadelphia: Lippincott.
12. Kazak, A. E., Penati, B., Brophy, P., et al. (1998). Pharmacologic and psychologic interventions for procedural pain. *Pediatrics, 102,* 59-66.
13. Kirks, D. R. (1998). *Practical pediatric imaging: Diagnostic radiology of infants and children.* (3rd ed.). Philadelphia: Lippincott-Raven.
14. Krauss, B., & Green, S. M. (2000). Sedation and analgesia for procedures in children. *New England Journal of Medicine, 342,* 938-945.
15. Leung, A., Shapiro, B., Hattner, R., et al. (1997). Specificity of radioiodinated MIBG for neural crest tumors in childhood. *Journal of Nuclear Medicine, 38,* 1352-1357.
16. Lisle, D. (1996). *Imaging for students.* London: Oxford University.
17. Malarkey, L. M., & McMorrow, M. (1996). *Nurse's manual of laboratory tests and diagnostic procedures.* Philadelphia: W. B. Saunders.
18. Margolin, J. F., & Poplack, D. G. (1997). Acute lymphoblastic leukemia. In P. A. Pizzo & D. G. Poplack (Eds.), *Principles and practice of pediatric oncology* (3rd ed., pp. 409-462). Philadelphia: Lippincott-Raven.
19. McBride, L. J. (1998). *Textbook of urinalysis and body fluids.* Philadelphia: Lippincott-Raven.
20. McFarland, M. B. (1995). *Nursing implications of laboratory tests.* Albany, NY: Delmar.
21. Meadows, A. T., Kramer, S., Hopson, R., et al. (1983). Survival in childhood acute lymphocytic leukemia: Effect of protocol and place of treatment. *Cancer Investigation, 1,* 49-55.
22. Murphy, S. B. (1995). The national impact of clinical cooperative group trials for pediatric cancer. *Medical and Pediatric Oncology, 24,* 279-280.
23. Nathan, D. G., & Orkin, S. H. (1998). *Nathan & Oski's hematology of infancy and childhood.* (5th ed.). (Vol. 2). Philadelphia: W. B. Saunders.
24. Neinstein, L. S. (1996). *Adolescent health care: A practical guide.* (3rd ed.). Baltimore: Williams & Wilkins.
25. O'Mary, S. S. (1997). Diagnostic evaluation, classification and staging. In S. L. Groenwald, M. Goodman, M. H. Frogge, et al. (Eds.), *Cancer nursing: Principles and practice* (4th ed., pp. 175-201). Sudbury, MA: Jones & Bartlett.
26. Pagana, K. D., & Pagana, T. J. (1999). *Mosby's diagnostic and laboratory test reference.* St. Louis: Mosby.
27. Parker, B. (1997). Imaging studies in the diagnosis of pediatric malignancies. In P. A. Pizzo & D. G. Poplack (Eds.), *Principles and practice of pediatric oncology* (3rd ed., pp. 187-213). Philadelphia: Lippincott-Raven.
28. Parsons, L., & Patterson, K. L. (1993). Nursing assessment and diagnosis of hematologic function. In D. B. Jackson & R. B. Saunders (Eds.), *Child health nursing.* Philadelphia: J. B. Lippincott.

29. Ries, L. A. G., Smith, M. A., Gurney, J. G., et al. (1999). *Cancer incidence and survival among children and adolescents: United States SEER program 1975-1995.* Bethesda, MD: NIH Pub. No. 99-4649.

30. Rosen, D. A., & Rosen, K. R. (1998). Intravenous conscious sedation with midazolam in paediatric patients. *International Journal of Clinical Practice, 52,* 46-50.

31. Steuber, C. P., & Nesbitt, M. E. (1997). Clinical assessment and differential diagnosis of the child with suspected cancer. In P. A. Pizzo & D. G. Poplack (Eds.), *Principles and practice of pediatric oncology* (3rd ed., pp. 129-139). Philadelphia: Lippincott-Raven.

32. Sutton, D. (1994). *Radiology and imaging for medical students.* (6th ed.). Edinburgh: Churchill-Livingstone.

33. Torres, L. S. (1997). *Basic medical techniques and patient care in imaging technology.* (5th ed.). Philadelphia: Lippincott.

34. Tortorici, M., & Apfel, P. J. (1995). *Advanced radiographic and angiographic procedures.* Philadelphia: F. A. Davis.

35. Treseler, K. M. (1995). *Clinical laboratory and diagnostic tests: Significance and nursing implications.* (3rd ed.). Norwalk, CT: Appleton & Lange.

36. Triche, T. J. (1997). Pathology and molecular diagnosis of pediatric malignancies. In P. A. Pizzo & D. G. Poplack (Eds.), *Principles and practice of pediatric oncology* (3rd ed., pp. 141-185). Philadelphia: Lippincott-Raven.

37. Warner, T. M. (1997). Clinical applications for pediatric sedation. *CRNA—the Clinical Forum for Nurse Anesthetists, 8,* 144-151.

38. Yaster, M., Nichols, D. G., Deshpande, J. K., et al. (1990). Midazolam-fentanyl intravenous sedation in children: Case report of respiratory arrest. *Pediatrics, 86,* 463-467.

39. Zeltzer, L. K., Altman, A., Cohen, D., et al. (1990). American Academy of Pediatrics Report of the Subcommittee on the Management of Pain Associated with Procedures in Children with Cancer. *Pediatrics, 86,* 826-831.

4

Surgery

Holly Bagnall-Reeb
Shirley Perry

HISTORY

Long before the advent of chemotherapy and radiotherapy the specialists in the care of children with cancer were surgeons and pathologists. In the nineteenth century reports from European surgeons described the first successful nephrectomy for nephroblastoma and the first transperitoneal nephrectomy. In 1899 Max Wilms, a trained pathologist and surgeon, published a report of seven children with "mixed tumors."[41] Reported as embryonic mesodermal in origin, these tumors were undoubtedly nephroblastomas. Surgery remained the foundation of treatment for children with cancer for many years, with outcome dependent on the degree of surgical excision.

Pediatric surgery emerged as a distinct specialty in the 1930s. In the United States William Ladd, Chief of Surgery at Boston Children's Hospital, led the way. Concerned over the care and surgical management of children with cancer, he strongly believed that surgical intervention be performed by physicians who frequently operated on childhood tumors, not by general surgeons or urologists who infrequently encountered these cases. Ladd was one of the few surgeons at that time who advocated an aggressive approach in attempting to excise large abdominal tumors. In 1941 Ladd and colleagues reported 14 long-term survivors of Wilms tumor, 7 survivors with neuroblastoma, and 6 patients with ovarian tumors. Before that time there were only 16 such survivors reported in the English medical literature.[41]

The concept of a "team approach" for the treatment of pediatric oncology patients was pioneered by Boston Tumor Clinic pathologist Sydney Farber, who several years later initiated trials with chemotherapy as primary and adjuvant therapy.[41] Decisions regarding treatment were made following input from all relevant physician specialists. This multidisciplinary approach to the management of childhood cancer quickly spread to other pediatric centers nationwide.

In the period from 1946 to 1960 major developments in the surgical approach to pediatric cancers were made possible due to parallel advances in surgical techniques, anesthesia, and supportive care such as blood transfusions. C. Everett Koop, surgeon-in-chief at Children's Hospital of Philadelphia and subsequent Surgeon General, evaluated the impact of aggressive debulking surgery on unresectable neuroblastoma. He emphasized the importance of staging and monitoring the effects and clinical outcome of radiotherapy for this tumor type.[51,52] William Clatworthy from Children's Hospital in Columbus, Ohio, recognized the sensitivity of certain childhood tumors to chemotherapy and advocated a limited radical surgical approach to the management of rhabdomyosarcoma. Successful hepatic resections for primary malignant liver tumors were reported by Judson Randolph from Washington, D.C. Subsequently, Randolph became the first surgeon to become associated with a pediatric oncology cooperative group.[41]

The role of the pediatric surgeon affiliated with the pediatric oncology cooperative groups has developed over the past two decades, and surgical approaches to various tumors have been evaluated as part of group trials. The treatment of Wilms tumor exemplifies the effectiveness of a multidisciplinary team in the management of childhood cancer. Associated with a greater than 60% mortality rate in the 1950s, relapse-free survival rate at two years now exceeds 90%.[2] The diagnosis of pediatric cancers now relies on biologic staging, molecular techniques, or both, and surgery is required to obtain tissue samples for these evaluations.

Pediatric oncology nurses have been involved in the surgical committees within the cooperative groups for a number of years. They play an important role in group trials, assisting with study development, implementation, and data collection and interpretation. With the merger of the two pediatric cooperative groups that form the Children's Oncology Group (C.O.G.), nursing representation continues on the surgical committee. Refinements in the techniques of surgical intervention and innovations in instrumentation are expected to impact the approach to the management of pediatric tumors. Hence, the roles of the pediatric surgeon and pediatric surgical oncology nurse continue to evolve.

GENERAL PRINCIPLES

Surgery has been the foundation of cancer treatment for centuries. In some adult malignancies, it remains the essential modality. In pediatric cancer, however, the survival rate for children with cancer has improved over the past three decades largely due to multimodal treatment. Improvements in surgical techniques and intraoperative monitoring have contributed to the improved survival rate. While advances in chemotherapy and radiation therapy have reduced the need for radical surgical resections in children, few solid tumors are cured without surgical intervention. The role of surgery in the treatment of solid tumors is outlined in Table 4-1.

Surgeons play an important role in the initial diagnosis and treatment of the pediatric patient with a malignant disease. Clinical presentation and radiologic imaging give the oncologist a working differential. The tumor biopsy enables the pathologist to confirm the diagnosis.[6] Because of the increasing complexity of the pathologic analysis of pediatric cancers, which now includes molecular and other specialized tumor analyses, a multidisciplinary team consultation is necessary to plan the initial biopsy or surgery. Additionally, the surgeon is called upon to insert intravenous or enteral access devices. Common surgical techniques in the management of childhood tumors are outlined in Table 4-2.

PREOPERATIVE EVALUATION

The pediatric oncology patient undergoing surgery at any stage of treatment is often a challenge for the surgeon and the anesthesiologist.[82] Both the anatomic and physiologic alterations from the malignancy and the consequences of previous and concurrent therapy may have profound effects on the perioperative management of the patient; therefore a pediatric anesthesiologist should be consulted early.[63]

The surgeon uses diagnostic imaging to plan the surgical approach. Specialized scans and other x-rays may be necessary in addition to those done to evaluate tumor location or response to therapy. Collaboration between the primary pediatric oncologist and the surgeon is necessary to avoid duplication of studies. Close coordination between ser-

vices will also obviate the need for repeated sedation for procedures.

It is important to check the hemoglobin, white blood cell count, platelet count, and coagulation panel before surgery. Blood counts should be corrected as much as possible using packed red blood cell transfusions, granulocyte colony stimulating factor, and/or platelet transfusions if necessary. Generally, a platelet count above 30,000 to 50,000/mm^3 is preferable, although platelet transfusion at the time of surgical intervention can ensure that levels remain adequate for the procedure. A hemoglobin count of over 8.0 g/dl ensures that there will be adequate oxygenation during anesthesia.[7] Surgery may be delayed until blood counts stabilize, if clinically possible.

Before a splenectomy a child needs to be immunized, because the spleen contains macrophages, which provide defense against infections. Vaccines administered are to protect against *Haemophilus influenzae* type B (Hib); pneumococcal infections, with either the 23-valent pneumococcal polysaccharide (23PS) vaccine or a combination of the 23PS and the heptavalent pneumococcal conjugate vaccine (PCV7) depending on the child's age; and meningococcal infections. If the splenectomy is elective, the vaccines should be given at least 2 weeks in advance. The child who has had a splenectomy is routinely treated with penicillin and will require repeated pneumococcal vaccines.[83]

Electrolyte levels are checked before surgery, and any imbalances are corrected preoperatively. Most imbalances can be corrected preoperatively without impact on surgery; however, elective surgery should not be performed in the presence of severe hyperkalemia (potassium levels >5.5 mEq/L).[15] A bladder catheter may be placed intraoperatively for accurate assessment of urine output. Adequate perfusion is reflected in the maintenance of appropriate urinary output.

The anesthesiologist must be aware of the airway status of the child before surgery. A child with a mediastinal mass is at risk of respiratory collapse due to life-threatening airway compression, and therefore mild conscious sedation may be the only choice if tissue needs to be obtained for diagnosis.[82] Computed tomography (CT) is the reliable method of evaluating the extent of disease and tracheobronchial compression.[82] Chemotherapy, emergency radiation therapy, or steroids may be needed to shrink the tumor prior to anesthesia. A child who has had radiation to the lung or has received bleomycin should be identified to the anesthesiologist, because lung fibrosis can occur.

Any child who has received cardiotoxic drugs or mediastinal radiation is assessed preoperatively by

Text continued on p. 98

TABLE 4-1 TUMOR-SPECIFIC SURGICAL MANAGEMENT

Tumor	Characteristics	Surgical Management	Other Factors
WILMS TUMOR			
Mass in the kidney, either unilateral or bilateral **METASTASES** Contralateral kidney, lungs, liver, brain, mediastinum, abdomen	Abdominal mass with distortion of the kidney Large, soft, blotchy, and easy to rupture	The primary goal of surgery is complete resection. The incision is transabdominal-peritoneal (even if only biopsy is done). Surgery is important for staging with attention to local tumor extent, tumor rupture, and status of the regional periaortic, aortocaval, paracaval, and perirenal lymph nodes. The contralateral kidney is examined. Incorrect staging can lead to inappropriate therapy. Biopsy only is done in the case of unresectable or bilateral tumor. Chemotherapy and radiation are used to shrink the tumor, followed by second look surgery and resection. Partial nephrectomy is feasible in bilateral Wilms or in unilateral disease if tumor is large and chemotherapy has damaged the unaffected kidney.	Tumor spillage yields poorer prognosis. Intraoperative clips are placed if the tumor is unresectable. Renal transplant has been associated with high rate of tumor recurrence and hence is not recommended. Attempts at primary surgical excision of a large tumor with caval extension is a high-risk procedure. Cardiopulmonary bypass may be used if a large thrombus is suspected.
NEUROBLASTOMA			
Abdominal, pelvic (adrenal), thoracic, head and neck, and other **METASTASES** Bone marrow, bones, lungs, liver	Usually a fixed mass with metastases MIBG and urine catecholamines usually positive Biology studies used to stage disease (e.g., *nMYC*)	Surgery can be diagnostic, therapeutic, or palliative. Low stage/risk tumors need surgery alone with complete resection. High stage/risk tumors need biopsy only for staging and diagnosis. Treatment is chemotherapy, hematopoietic stem cell transplant, second look surgery, and radiation therapy. Biopsy is done of the closest and least invasive portion of the tumor. Fine needle aspirate (FNA) is a controversial issue, as biology studies require more tissue and complications have been reported. The incision for abdominal tumors is a large transverse incision based on the level of the tumor. Pelvic tumors may be very difficult to resect as they are usually attached to the sacral nerves. Thoracic tumors are approached through a posterolateral thoracotomy at the approximate level of the tumor.	Survival is not decreased by delayed surgery. The goal of large tumor surgery is complete resection, with or without microscopic residual. Resection and debulking help improve prognosis. Extensive surgery of unresectable tumor is associated with high rate of complications and should be avoided.

Data from Andrassy, R. J. (1998). General principles. In R. J. Andrassy (Ed.), *Pediatric surgical oncology* (pp. 13-34). Philadelphia: W. B. Saunders; Black, T. C. (1998). Neuroblastoma. In R. J. Andrassy (Ed.), *Pediatric surgical oncology* (pp 175-211.) Philadelphia: W. B. Saunders; Blandy, J. P., & Oliver, R. T. (2000). Genitourinary cancer. In N. J. Vogelzang, P. T. Scardino, W. U. Shipley, D. S. Coffey (Eds.), *Comprehensive textbook of genitourinary oncology* (pp. 462-500). Philadelphia: Lippincott Williams & Wilkins; Corpron, C. A., & Andrassy, R. J. (1998). Abdominal complications. In R. J. Andrassy (Ed.), *Pediatric surgical oncology* (pp. 477-479). Philadelphia: W. B. Saunders; Corpron, C. A., & Andrassy, R. J. (1997). Molecular and surgical advances in pediatric tumors. In R. E. Pollock (Ed.), *Surgical oncology* (pp. 51-69). Boston: Academic Publishers Norwell; DeCou, J. M., Bowan, L. C., Rao, B. N., et al. (1995). Infants with metastatic neuroblastoma have improved survival with resection of the primary tumor. *Journal of Pediatric Surgery, 30,* 937-940; Donaldson, S., Egbert, P. R., & Newsham, I. (1997). Retinoblastoma. In P. A. Pizzo & D. G. Poplack (Eds.), *Principles and practice of pediatric oncology* (3rd ed., pp. 699-716). Philadelphia: Lippincott-Raven; Dower, N. A., & Smith, L. J. (2000). Liver transplant for malignant liver tumor in children. *Medical and Pediatric Oncology, 34,* 136-140; Ehrenreich, B., & Miguel, L. S. (2000). Solid tumors. In B. V. Wise, C. McKenna, G. Garvin, et al. (Eds.), *Nursing care of the general pediatric surgical patient* (pp. 370-399). Gaithersburg, MD: Aspen; Herrera, J. M., Krebs, A., Harris, P., et al. (2000). Childhood tumors. *Surgical Clinics of North America, 80,* 747-760; Hudson, M. M., & Donaldson, S. S. (1997). Hodgkin's disease. In P. A. Pizzo & D. G. Poplack (Eds.), *Principles and practice of pediatric oncology* (3rd ed., pp. 523-543). Philadelphia: Lippincott-Raven; LaQuaglia, M. P. (1997). Childhood tumors. In L. I. Greenfield, M. W. Mulholland, & K. T. Oldham (Eds.), *Surgery: Scientific principles and practice* (pp. 2118-2140). Philadelphia: Lippincott-Raven; Palmer, J. S., Kletzel, M., Steinberg, G. D., et al. (1996). Testicular, sacrococcygeal, and other tumors. In J. C. Harvey & E. J. Beattie (Eds.), *Cancer surgery* (pp. 91-100). Philadelphia: W. B. Saunders; Woolley, M. M. (1993). Teratomas. In K. W. Ashcraft & T. M. Holder (Eds.), *Pediatric surgery* (2nd ed., pp. 847-862). Philadelphia: W. B. Saunders.

| TABLE 4-1 | **TUMOR-SPECIFIC SURGICAL MANAGEMENT—cont'd** |

Tumor	Characteristics	Surgical Management	Other Factors
RHABDOMYOSARCOMA			
Head and neck, genitourinary, extremities, other sites **METASTASES** Lung, lymph nodes	A mass, disturbing the affected organ(s) and nearby structures	The surgical procedure is site specific. Complete resection varies from site to site and is highest in the extremity tumors and lowest in head and neck. Complete resection of tumor is ideal if it can be performed with preservation of function and cosmetic form. Negative margins are essential. If the tumor is unresectable, an open biopsy is done, as several grams of tissue are needed for pathology. No tumor markers are known. Needle biopsy is appropriate in rare occasions. Debulking the tumor before chemotherapy and radiation is useful if it can be done safely. If the margins are positive and/or the tumor is unresectable, second look surgery is planned.	Lymph node dissection is important for staging and RT planning. The role of surgery in lung metastases is not clear. It is being performed in combination with chemotherapy and radiation therapy.
HEPATOBLASTOMA			
Liver tumor **METASTASES** Lungs	Massive tumor, which is a distinct, discrete mass in the liver Positive α-fetoprotein (AFP)	Primary resection of the entire tumor is ideal. A thoracoabdominal approach is recommended for all lobectomies (right and left partial, complete lobectomy, and trisegmentectomy). As much as 85% of the liver can be removed safely, and it will regenerate. FNA is often used in unresectable tumor. If the tumor is unresectable, chemotherapy is administered. The tumor shrinks and is less friable and easier to remove on second look surgery.	Liver transplants (living or cadaver) are done in extreme cases and are becoming more acceptable. Hemorrhage is a frequent and serious complication of liver dissection. Cardiopulmonary bypass may be needed and hypothermia induced before resection of the liver.

Continued

TABLE 4-1	**TUMOR-SPECIFIC SURGICAL MANAGEMENT—cont'd**		
Tumor	**Characteristics**	**Surgical Management**	**Other Factors**
GERM CELL			
GONADAL 36% Ovarian Testicular **EXTRAGONADAL 63%** Sacrococcygeal teratoma; mediastinal; abdominal	Large mass, visible or palpable at site Biochemical markers are present (β subunit of human chorionic gonadotropin [β-hCG], AFP)	**OVARIAN** Biopsy or oophorectomy is performed if most of the ovary is involved. If the tumor is benign, the ovary tissue is left in place. If the tumor is malignant, the ovary is removed and the other ovary biopsied. The uterus is left intact. **TESTICULAR** An orchiectomy is performed with no peritoneal lymph node dissection. The child is then treated with chemotherapy. **SACROCOCCYGEAL TERATOMA** The treatment of choice is complete surgical excision of the tumor including the coccyx bone. If the tumor is malignant, the child is treated with chemotherapy. If the tumor is benign, surgery alone is the treatment of choice.	Prosthesis of testes can be placed after recovery from surgery. Recurrence of benign teratoma is common. Close follow-up is needed after surgery.

Data from Andrassy, R. J. (1998). General principles. In R. J. Andrassy (Ed.), *Pediatric surgical oncology* (pp. 13-34). Philadelphia: W. B. Saunders; Black, T. C. (1998). Neuroblastoma. In R. J. Andrassy (Ed.), *Pediatric surgical oncology* (pp 175-211.) Philadelphia: W. B. Saunders; Blandy, J. P., & Oliver, R. T. (2000). Genitourinary cancer. In N. J. Vogelzang, P. T. Scardino, W. U. Shipley, D. S. Coffey (Eds.), *Comprehensive textbook of genitourinary oncology* (pp. 462-500). Philadelphia: Lippincott Williams & Wilkins; Corpron, C. A., & Andrassy, R. J. (1998). Abdominal complications. In R. J. Andrassy (Ed.), *Pediatric surgical oncology* (pp. 477-479). Philadelphia: W. B. Saunders; Corpron, C. A., & Andrassy, R. J. (1997). Molecular and surgical advances in pediatric tumors. In R. E. Pollock (Ed.), *Surgical oncology* (pp. 51-69). Boston: Academic Publishers Norwell; DeCou, J. M., Bowan, L. C., Rao, B. N., et al. (1995). Infants with metastatic neuroblastoma have improved survival with resection of the primary tumor. *Journal of Pediatric Surgery, 30,* 937-940; Donaldson, S., Egbert, P. R., & Newsham, I. (1997). Retinoblastoma. In P. A. Pizzo & D. G. Poplack (Eds.), *Principles and practice of pediatric oncology* (3rd ed., pp. 699-716). Philadelphia: Lippincott-Raven; Dower, N. A., & Smith, L. J. (2000). Liver transplant for malignant liver tumor in children. *Medical and Pediatric Oncology, 34,* 136-140; Ehrenreich, B., & Miguel, L. S. (2000). Solid tumors. In B. V. Wise, C. McKenna, G. Garvin, et al. (Eds.), *Nursing care of the general pediatric surgical patient* (pp. 370-399). Gaithersburg, MD: Aspen; Herrera, J. M., Krebs, A., Harris, P., et al. (2000). Childhood tumors. *Surgical Clinics of North America, 80,* 747-760; Hudson, M. M., & Donaldson, S. S. (1997). Hodgkin's disease. In P. A. Pizzo & D. G. Poplack (Eds.), *Principles and practice of pediatric oncology* (3rd ed., pp. 523-543). Philadelphia: Lippincott-Raven; LaQuaglia, M. P. (1997). Childhood tumors. In L. I. Greenfield, M. W. Mulholland, & K. T. Oldham (Eds.), *Surgery: Scientific principles and practice* (pp. 2118-2140). Philadelphia: Lippincott-Raven; Palmer, J. S., Kletzel, M., Steinberg, G. D., et al. (1996). Testicular, sacrococcygeal, and other tumors. In J. C. Harvey & E. J. Beattie (Eds.), *Cancer surgery* (pp. 91-100). Philadelphia: W. B. Saunders; Woolley, M. M. (1993). Teratomas. In K. W. Ashcraft & T. M. Holder (Eds.), *Pediatric surgery* (2nd ed., pp. 847-862). Philadelphia: W. B. Saunders.

TABLE 4-1	TUMOR-SPECIFIC SURGICAL MANAGEMENT—cont'd		
Tumor	**Characteristics**	**Surgical Management**	**Other Factors**
LYMPHOMA			
Lymphadenopathy or mass in abdomen, pelvis, mediastinum, bone **METASTASES** Bone marrow, mediastinal, pleural effusion, or bone	Palpable external lymph nodes in the groin, axilla, and cervical area Internal lymph nodes or mass (mediastinal, pelvic, bone) Tumor often gallium avid	The role of the surgeon is biopsy and staging. Usually a diagnosis can be made from peripheral lymph node dissection. In rare cases a thoracotomy or laparotomy may need to be performed to obtain tissue. If the biopsy is of the mediastinal mass, an attempt should be made to get a piece of tissue through the ribs. Bone marrow or thoracentesis can sometimes be diagnostic. A staging laparotomy is indicated only if the findings would alter therapy significantly.	These diseases are considered nonsurgical diseases. The treatment of choice is chemotherapy and radiation. If there is a mediastinal mass, there is a risk of respiratory collapse during anesthesia.
RETINOBLASTOMA			
METASTASES Bone marrow, other eye, and optic nerve	Leukokoria often present (cat's eye reflex)	Usually the spread of disease at diagnosis is so extensive that enucleation is the treatment of choice. An ophthalmologist usually performs enucleation. The orbit must be examined. If both eyes are affected, bilateral enucleation may be necessary.	Prosthesis will be placed after recovery from surgery. Follow-up is done of family members due to genetic link. Examination under general anesthesia is performed on a regular basis.

TABLE 4-2	COMMON SURGICAL TECHNIQUES IN PEDIATRIC ONCOLOGY
Surgical Techniques	**Comments**
FINE NEEDLE ASPIRATION (FNA) AND CORE BIOPSY	
A needle is placed in the tumor, and a portion is aspirated. A core needle (14 gauge or larger) is often used to keep the architecture of the tumor intact. Deep lesions may be biopsied with CT guidance.	Anesthesia—without sedation, with conscious sedation, or with general anesthesia. May be done with little planning in clinic, radiologic suite, or procedure room. May not provide a sufficient tissue sample. Negative results warrant an open biopsy if suspicion of malignancy still exists.
INCISIONAL BIOPSIES	
A portion of the tumor is taken out when a complete resection of the tumor is not feasible or thought to be necessary. Length of the incision and the location depend on the size and position of the tumor.	Anesthesia—general Often an initial incisional biopsy requires further surgery with wide excision of the entire biopsy tract at a later date.
TUMOR REMOVAL OR EXCISIONAL BIOPSY	
Complete resection of the tumor or residual metastatic disease is performed whenever possible. The type of incision and extent of surgery depends on the location and size of the tumor.	Anesthesia—general The goal is complete tumor resection, leaving negative margins, while retaining the patient's form and function.
SECOND LOOK SURGERY	
In large unresectable tumors, an initial biopsy is performed, and second look surgery is built into the future plan of care. The patient receives chemotherapy and radiation followed by radiologic imaging to determine the response to treatment.	Anesthesia—general Provides information on viability of removed tumor. Must be planned when the child is stable and has adequate neutrophils. Common in unresectable neuroblastoma, Wilms tumor, hepatoblastoma, rhabdomyosarcoma, and germ cell tumors.
DEBULKING	
Involves removing a portion of a tumor mass that cannot be completely resected. May be done as the first line of therapy or after several courses of chemotherapy or radiation.	Anesthesia—general May be done to relieve pressure on the spine, bowel, bladder, or other vital organs. Decrease in tumor load may give the chemotherapy a better chance of killing remaining tumor.
MANAGEMENT OF METASTASIS	
Operative removal undertaken if significant response in primary and improved prognosis is anticipated.	Anesthesia—general Biopsy at diagnosis if feasible and will impact treatment plan. If no response to therapy there is a greater chance that micrometastases will progress.

Data from Andrassy, R. J., & Hays, D. M. (1997). Pediatric surgical oncology. In P. A. Pizzo & D. G. Poplack (Eds.), *Principles and practice of pediatric oncology* (3rd ed., pp. 273-287). Philadelphia: Lippincott-Raven; Bowers, S. (2000). All about tubes: Your guide to enteral feeding devices. *Nursing 2000, 30*(12), 41-47; Eastridge, B. J., & Lefor, A. T. (1996). Chronic venous access in the cancer patient. In A. T. Lefor (Ed.), *Surgical problems affecting the patient with cancer: Interdisciplinary management* (pp. 183-209). Philadelphia: Lippincott-Raven; Herrera, J. M., Krebs, A., Harris, P., et al. (2000). Childhood tumors. *Surgical Clinics of North America, 80*, 747-760.

TABLE 4-2	COMMON SURGICAL TECHNIQUES IN PEDIATRIC ONCOLOGY—cont'd
Surgical Techniques	**Comments**

ENTEROSTOMAL TUBES

Inserted percutaneously through a stoma created on the abdomen. Used for nutritional support of malnourished patients or in patients intolerant of oral feeds. Placed by surgical, endoscopic, laparoscopic, or radiologic techniques.	Anesthesia—general Available devices: (1) Gastrostomy tube—short feeding tube placed into the stomach; (2) Percutaneous endoscopic gastrostomy (PEG) and dual access gastrostomy-jejunostomy (PEG/J) tube (gastrostomy lumen used for gastric decompressions, jejunostomy lumen used to deliver enteral feeds); (3) Low profile gastrostomy device (LPGD)—placed into a mature gastrostomy tract, protrudes just above the skin; (4) Jejunostomy tube—placed for postpyloric enteral feeding when bypassing the stomach is desired (gastric disease, GI obstruction, or aspiration risk).

CENTRAL VENOUS CATHETERS

Indwelling venous devices placed for long-term central venous access for administration of chemotherapy, TPN, antibiotic therapy, or administration of blood and blood products. Ideal position on operating table is with the patient flat and head pointing up. Trendelenburg position is not useful for subclavian access, as this vein does not dilate. Percutaneous access useful for subclavian or internal jugular veins. The internal and external jugular, cephalic, or saphenous veins can be accessed by cutdown. The device is passed either through an introducer (percutaneous approach) or through a venotomy (cutdown approach). The catheter is trimmed so that the tip is at the atriocaval junction (upper body) or at the confluence of the common iliac veins (saphenous vein approach). Intraoperative fluoroscopy is done to verify position of the catheter tip; chest radiograph is performed at the end of the procedure to evaluate for pneumothorax. PICC line placement is useful for intermediate-term therapy. It is inserted percutaneously via the basilic or cephalic veins.	Anesthesia—Usually general; conscious sedation may be possible for PICC placement. Decision regarding type of catheter depends on intensity of treatment, patient/family or clinician preference.

PALLIATIVE SURGERY

Operative procedure done to relieve pain, obstruction, or stop bleeding.	Anesthesia—general Decision to operate based on the child's comfort level and quality of life.

an echocardiogram and/or a multigaited angiography (MUGA) scan. A cardiologist may also be consulted. In tumors where imaging studies indicate that the disease has spread up the inferior vena cava, the anesthesiologist must be aware that the child may need bypass.

The anesthesiologist must also be aware of other physical anomalies. Intraoperative hypertension and tachycardia may occur with tumor manipulation in patients with neuroblastoma, and approximately 50% of these patients experience hypotension after removal of the tumor.[63]

Most oncologic surgeries are well planned, and there is time to obtain informed consent from the family and child. The benefits and risks of the surgery should be explained to the child and family,[30] who need to be prepared for potential complications and late effects of the surgical procedure.

The child and parent are prepared for the immediate pre- and postoperative period. Parents are involved as much as possible. Some institutions have developed programs to allow parental presence and involvement in the holding and recovery areas.[95] Operative preparation depends on the age of the child. Give the child as much choice as possible. Many institutions have child life staff who can work with the child (Figure 4-1). Physicians, nurses, and therapists explain procedures and answer questions. Preparation may include allowing the child to handle medical equipment, giving the child age-appropriate explanations of procedures, and arranging a tour of the operating room.

POSTOPERATIVE NURSING CARE

The pediatric oncology nurse is usually involved in the postoperative care of the child with cancer. The presence of immunosuppression secondary to cancer and cancer treatment makes the child with cancer a high-risk surgical patient. However, despite the complicated oncological problems these children face, pediatric oncology nurses must not forget the basic tenets of surgical nursing. A plan of care will include the following areas of concern.

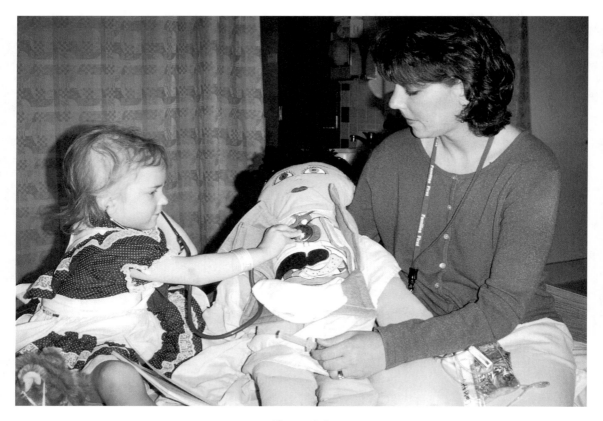

Figure 4-1

Child life specialist prepares child for surgical procedure.

AIRWAY

Report any concerns regarding air exchange or oxygen saturation. Incentive spirometer, early ambulation, position change, deep breathing and coughing, and chest physiotherapy can help to prevent postoperative atelectasis.

FLUID AND ELECTROLYTE BALANCE

Early in the postoperative period the child may be vulnerable to fluid and electrolyte imbalance. The operative record is checked to determine if fluid and electrolyte problems occurred during surgery. Aggressive hydration is usual with potassium added intravenously once the child has voided. Perfusion can be assessed by capillary refill, skin turgor, mucous membranes, accurate intake and output measurement, and measurement of electrolytes. Overhydration should be assessed once the initial postoperative period has passed or if significant imbalances in intake and output are observed.

PAIN CONTROL

Pain control is initiated intraoperatively or immediately postoperatively. Epidural and IV patient controlled analgesia (PCA) have become the standard in the early postoperative period. As the pain decreases, the analgesic may be tapered to the oral route. Incisional pain usually lasts for approximately 72 hours. Pain after 72 hours is considered to be primarily muscular pain.[30] Ambulation and use of the muscles generally provides better pain relief than using narcotics. Prudent use of opioid analgesics will minimize constipation from paralytic effects on the bowel. Use of medications before painful experiences, such as dressing change, initial ambulation, and suture or staple removal, will minimize the trauma of these procedures.

DIET

Postoperatively, the plan to resume a diet is dependent on the specific surgery performed. Most children who have had nonabdominal surgery are started on clear fluids the evening of surgery and advanced to a full diet as tolerated. Children who have had abdominal surgery must have normal peristalsis before beginning oral intake. Hyperalimentation or total parenteral nutrition (TPN) may be necessary if prolonged nothing-by-mouth (NPO) status is required.

WOUND CARE

Some types of incisions need extensive wound care. Wound drainage is monitored, the appearance of the wound is noted, and any signs of infection are reported. The family is taught how to do the dressing changes and advised when to return for a follow-up visit with their surgeon. Occasionally home health referral will be necessary to assist the family with complex wound care. The child and family are told when a bath or swimming is appropriate.

CARE OF DRAINS

The type of drain used and its purpose (e.g., chest tube, nasogastric tube, Hemovac drain) depend on the specific operation performed. It is very important to report the characteristics, amount, and texture of the drainage. The drain needs to be secured in place and irrigated as needed.

Preoperative and postoperative nursing care are essential components of the management of children with cancer. As treatment protocols become more intensive and surgical intervention more complex, knowledge and familiarity of the care of these patients is critical to successful outcomes.

AMBULATION

The importance of early ambulation in the postoperative recovery of a child who has undergone surgery cannot be overlooked. Ambulation prevents the development of atelectasis postoperatively, but it is also important to help maintain muscle tone after surgery.

SURGICAL PROBLEMS IN PEDIATRIC ONCOLOGY

Surgeons are regularly consulted to evaluate, assess, and treat complications of cancer and cancer treatment. Some of the most common abdominal complications are listed in Table 4-3. Others include wound healing, infection, and pneumothorax.

WOUND HEALING COMPLICATIONS

Wound healing complications can result following surgical intervention. Wound healing is divided into three phases. The inflammatory phase begins on the day of tissue injury and continues for approximately 5 days. This phase of wound healing is characterized by the interplay of platelets, acute inflammatory cells, growth factors, and cytokines. During the first few days the wound strength is less than 5% of normal strength.[79,93]

The proliferation phase is characterized by the formation of granulation tissue. This phase overlaps with the inflammatory phase, beginning on day three, and lasts for at least three weeks. During this time the tensile strength of the wound gains no more than 20% of the final strength.[79,93]

The remodeling phase continues from around the seventh day of tissue injury until at least one year. The tensile strength of the wound increases to about 50% of its original strength after 5 weeks. It

TABLE 4-3	ABDOMINAL COMPLICATIONS	
Complications	**Treatment**

NEUTROPENIC ENTEROCOLITIS (TYPHLITIS)

Inflammation of the cecum in a neutropenic patient, which can progress rapidly to gangrene, or perforation of the bowel. Symptoms are abdominal pain in the right lower quadrant, fever, distention, diarrhea, and vomiting. X-ray film shows bowel wall thickening and pneumatosis. CT scan confirms inflammation and extent.	Antibiotics, bowel rest (80% resolve) Laparotomy with removal of diseased bowel, with anastomosis or diversion if there is clinical deterioration, persistent gastrointestinal bleeding (despite resolution of neutropenia and thrombocytopenia), uncontrolled sepsis, evidence of perforation.

BOWEL OBSTRUCTION

Partial or complete obstruction caused by tumor, adhesions, constipation, ileus as a result of vincristine, or GVHD in HSCT. Perforation and necrosis are rare but possible.	Hydration, antibiotics, and laxatives are the first line of therapy. Nasogastric tube to relieve pressure. Surgery if does not resolve.

ULCERS

Single or multiple punctate, shallow, gastric or duodenal ulcers. Caused by chemotherapy, particularly steroids.	Antacids, H_2 blockers, bowel rest. Surgical intervention if bleeding continues.

RADIATION ENTERITIS

Radiation therapy directly affects rapidly dividing mucosal cells and may cause enteritis. Symptoms are nausea, vomiting, abdominal pain cramping, and intermittent diarrhea. In severe cases, obstruction, fistulization, and perforation.	Resolves once the therapy is completed. Bowel rest and antibiotics. Surgery to resect or remove affected intestinal segment if becomes severe.

PANCREATITIS

Inflammation of the pancreas. Symptoms are nausea, vomiting, and right-sided tenderness. The diagnosis is based on physical exam and elevated lipase and amylase. CT or ultrasound shows an enlarged and inflamed pancreas. The cause is tumor lysis and/or chemotherapy (asparaginase and possibly steroids).	Discontinuation of causative drug, diet restriction, antibiotics. Necrotizing pancreatitis may require surgical debridement or drainage of pseudocyst. Drainage may be done by CT guidance. NPO with TPN nutrition until symptoms resolve, then low-fat diet. May require NG tube.

Data from Alvarez, O. A., & Zimmerman, G. (2000). PEG-asparaginase-induced pancreatitis. *Medical and Pediatric Oncology, 34,* 200-205; Corpron, C. A., & Andrassy, R. J. (1998). Abdominal complications. In R. J. Andrassy (Ed.), *Pediatric surgical oncology* (pp. 477-479). Philadelphia: W. B. Saunders; Fisher, W. E., & Burak, W. E. (1996). Inflammatory lesions of the gastrointestinal tract. In A. T. Lefor (Ed.), *Surgical problems affecting the patient with cancer: Interdisciplinary management* (pp. 97-109). Philadelphia: Lippincott-Raven; Kun, L. E. (1997). General principles of radiation therapy. In P. A. Pizzo & D. G. Poplack (Eds.), *Principles and practice of pediatric oncology* (3rd ed., pp. 289-321). Philadelphia: Lippincott-Raven; Midis, G., & Skibber, J. (1996). Abdominal pain in the neutropenic cancer patient. In A. T. Lefor (Ed.), *Surgical problems affecting the patient with cancer: Interdisciplinary management* (pp. 3-23). Philadelphia: Lippincott-Raven; Shamberger, R. C. (1999). Preanesthetic evaluation of children with anterior mediastinal mass. *Seminars in Pediatric Surgery, 8,* 61-68.

is believed that the final recovery is only 80% of the tensile strength of normal skin.[79,93]

Antineoplastic agents may affect the outcome of surgical procedures by influencing wound healing. The majority of antineoplastic agents interfere with DNA or RNA replication, protein synthesis, and cell division. Chemotherapy directly affects the proliferative phase of wound healing by inhibition of fibroplasia, angiogenesis, and epithelialization. Only a few agents such as methotrexate and steroids affect wound strength during the remodeling phase.[79]

Neutropenia is normally seen 7 to 10 days after initiating chemotherapy. Chemotherapy administered preoperatively may interfere with the early phases of wound healing. The first wave of cells that migrate into the fresh wound include neutrophils.[93] However, it is believed that the presence of leukopenia has little or no effect on healing if the wound is uncontaminated. Surgical wounds heal without difficulty and do not have an increased risk of infection in children with a neutrophil count of 500/mm^3 or greater.[79] Typically, children's wounds heal very easily, and hence there is very little literature on wound healing in the child with cancer. One would anticipate problems with impaired wound healing in a malnourished or chronically anemic child.[79] It appears that the immediate preoperative and early postoperative time is when the child would be most vulnerable to impaired wound healing secondary to chemotherapy.

INFECTIONS

Surgeons are often asked to perform a biopsy on potential sites of infection to identify the causative agent. Fungal infections are a common cause of infection in the profoundly neutropenic patient. The usual fungal organisms are *Candida* species and *Aspergillus* species, and the most common sites of infection are the oral cavity, esophagus, gastrointestinal (GI) tract, and lungs. CT scan and/or ultrasound are used initially to evaluate possible sites of fungal infection. The characteristic bull's eye–shaped lesions appear when the granulocyte count begins to recover. A diagnosis is often difficult to confirm without biopsy, because positive blood cultures occur in less than 50% of patients with *Candida* species.[66] Open surgical biopsy may be necessary to accurately diagnose pulmonary or abdominal sites of fungal infection. Endoscopic examination is the most sensitive method to diagnose esophageal candidiasis. Biopsy is often necessary, since attempts to culture by bronchial washings or brushing may not provide a sufficient amount of tissue for diagnosis.[32]

Infections of the surgical wound or the central line site most often can be treated with appropriate antibiotics. If the infection is related to a foreign body, the device may need to be removed and the incision excised and drained. The signs of wound infections are tenderness, erythema, fever, and wound drainage. Wound infections usually do not occur until 5 to 7 days postoperatively. The treatment for a wound infection may involve excision and drainage of pus or serous fluid collection. If cellulitis is present, the wound infection is treated with appropriate antibiotics. Bruising at the incision site may occur, and expansion of the incision may represent the presence of an underlying hematoma. The surgeon may elect to debride a wound when infection inter-

feres with proper healing. A pseudocyst in any part of the body is first treated with antibiotics. Surgery may need to be performed and a temporary drain inserted to remove fluid.

PNEUMOTHORAX

Pneumothorax is defined as the collapse of a lung. Lung collapse can be spontaneous, a presenting symptom of metastatic lung disease, or a direct result of an invasive procedure (central line insertion or thoracotomy).[18] The common symptoms of pneumothorax are shortness of breath and severe chest pain. A chest x-ray demonstrating lung collapse confirms the diagnosis. Symptoms may not be apparent for up to 24 hours postoperatively. The treatment for pneumothorax is lung reexpansion with a chest tube. The chest tube is left in place until the daily chest x-rays and the patient's clinical condition show that the lung has reexpanded. If the pneumothorax is caused by metastatic disease, surgery may be planned to remove the metastatic disease, followed by resumption of chemotherapy.

VASCULAR ACCESS

Vascular access devices (VADs) play an integral role in the management of childhood cancer. Complex and intensive treatment regimens require multiple venous access and quickly deplete peripheral veins, causing significant stress for the child and family. Long-term, centrally placed venous catheters facilitate the delivery of prolonged and repetitive courses of chemotherapy as well as nutritional support, blood products, intravenous fluids, antimicrobials, pain medications, and other drugs. They are also useful for frequent blood sampling. Central venous catheter placement is one of the most frequently performed operations in cancer patients by pediatric surgeons.[91] The three types of centrally placed venous catheters commonly used in clinical practice are the peripherally inserted central venous catheter (PICC), tunneled external central venous catheter (CVC), and the implanted vascular access device, or "port." These catheters are made of Silastic, silicone, or polyurethane materials that are less thrombogenic and chemically inert than the more rigid polyvinyl catheters.[46]

PERIPHERALLY INSERTED CENTRAL VENOUS CATHETERS

Peripherally inserted central venous catheters (PICCs) have been used successfully in pediatric oncology patients requiring long-term and intermediate duration therapies. Both single- and double-lumen PICCs are available. Single-lumen pediatric sizes range from 1.9 French (F) to 3F. These catheters are placed percutaneously in the cephalic or basilic vein in the antecubital region and advanced to the central circulation through the subclavian vein to the superior vena cava. In many institutions they are placed by specially trained nurses on the unit or in the clinic, thus eliminating the need for a surgical procedure. This may be especially useful in situations where the patient is not a candidate for general anesthesia. Although indications for insertion of a PICC are consistent with those for tunneled external CVCs and implanted ports, they are not recommended for high volume or rapid bolus infusions, pressurized injections, or apheresis.[23] Additionally, these catheters are not indicated in patients with poor antecubital access as a result of prior repetitive venipunctures for chemotherapy and blood sampling or due to morbid obesity. Recently, implantable peripheral access ports have been developed for placement in the patient's forearm. These devices have limited application in the pediatric population due to the large (6F) size of the catheter.

TUNNELED EXTERNAL CATHETERS

Tunneled external CVCs are available as single-, double-, or triple-lumen devices, made of silicone or polyurethane material. Sizes range from 2.7F for infants to 14F for older children. The intravascular segment of the catheter is most commonly inserted percutaneously into an internal or external jugular vein. If the internal or external jugular veins cannot be accessed percutaneously, the catheter can be inserted by a cutdown approach. The extravascular segment of the catheter is tunneled subcutaneously from the vein insertion site to an area on the anterior chest wall. The Dacron cuff is positioned greater than 2 cm proximal to the catheter exit site to prevent dislodgement.[92] The purpose of this cuff is to promote tissue ingrowth, thereby stabilizing the catheter from inadvertent dislodgment and restricting migration of skin flora along the catheter tract.[46]

Tunneled external CVCs are the most commonly placed vascular access devices in children. Single-lumen catheters are indicated for frequent administration of chemotherapy, antibiotics, parenteral nutrition, and blood sampling; double-lumen catheters have the same indications but also allow for simultaneous administration of incompatible or continuous infusions of medications and fluids. Triple-lumen catheters have been reported in the pediatric oncology population and are used when multiple drugs are to be administered concur-

rently. However, these catheters are associated with a significantly higher complication rate compared with double- or single-lumen catheters.[28,46] Central venous catheters suitable for apheresis are also available. The tips of these catheters are staggered to minimize recirculation of blood, thereby maximizing stem cell collection. They are also more rigid to withstand the flow rates during the apheresis procedure.

External tunneled catheters allow for administration of therapy and blood sampling, thereby minimizing the need for peripheral venipuncture. Disadvantages include periodic dressing changes over the exposed catheter exit site, frequent irrigation of each lumen to maintain patency, altered body image, and restriction of physical activity (e.g., swimming).

IMPLANTED VASCULAR ACCESS DEVICES

Implanted vascular access devices consist of a subcutaneous reservoir or port with a silicone rubber septum attached to a silicone or polyurethane catheter. Implanted ports are available with single or double reservoirs and are made of stainless steel, titanium, or plastic. The plastic type is magnetic resonance imaging (MRI) compatible, lighter in weight, and does not interfere with radiation therapy or CT scans. The ports come in a variety of sizes and shapes (Figure 4-2). Silicone or polyurethane catheters are either pre-attached or are connected to the port with a locking device to prevent separation. The catheters range in size from 4F for the infant to 13F for the older child or young adult.

Following catheter insertion, the reservoir is placed in a subcutaneous pocket usually in the upper chest wall and secured with two or more nonabsorbable sutures to prevent movement. The port should not be placed directly under the incision line because of the potential for skin breakdown and infection with access through the incision. Because the port septum must be readily palpated before access, the implanted port must not be placed deep in the subcutaneous tissue, in the breast tissue of mature females, or in the breast tissue of prepubertal females who will develop breasts and obscure the port. Accessing these devices requires a percutaneous puncture over the port using a noncoring (Huber) needle. The port septum is designed for up to 2000 needle punctures. Discomfort associated with port access is reduced with the use of a topical anesthetic cream.[40]

Once the implanted port is placed and the catheter tip position is confirmed by x-ray, the port may be accessed for immediate use. Implanted ports are ideally indicated for the administration of intermittent chemotherapy, antibiotics, and other parenteral

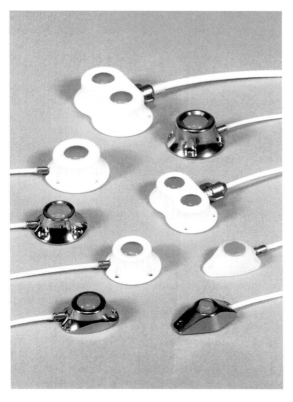

Figure 4-2

Examples of implanted ports. (Courtesy Sims Deltec, Inc., St. Paul, MN.)

therapies. Currently under investigation is a port suitable for apheresis.[64] Advantages of the implanted ports include fewer restrictions on patient activity, low catheter maintenance, and improved body image. Disadvantages include risk of extravasation with needle dislodgement, discomfort associated with port access, and an operative procedure for removal.

COMPLICATIONS OF LONG-TERM VENOUS ACCESS DEVICES

Although central venous access devices have greatly facilitated delivery of therapy to pediatric oncology patients, their insertion and frequent maintenance are not without complications. Potential complications during catheter placement include pneumothorax, hemothorax, arterial perforation, air embolism, nerve injury, and catheter malposition. In the hands of experienced pediatric surgeons, these complications are minimized.[91,92]

Infection and occlusion are the two major complications associated with the use and maintenance of central lines. Infection can be a potentially seri-

ous complication, leading to loss of access or causing significant morbidity and mortality.

Infection
Catheter-related bacteremia
The incidence of catheter-related infection and definitions used for clinical diagnosis are variable, and therefore it is difficult to compare results from existing studies. Catheter-related infections have been defined as: (1) any septic event in a patient with a central venous catheter, (2) sepsis that resolves following removal of the catheter, (3) the same organism isolated from both the peripheral blood and catheter tip, and (4) a greater number of organisms found in a sample of blood taken from the catheter than from a peripheral sample.[33] Catheter-related infection is typically based on the isolation of the same organism from a sample drawn from the catheter and peripheral blood.[50,88] A four- to five-fold difference in bacterial concentration between cultures taken from the catheter and peripheral blood is recommended to distinguish catheter-related and non–catheter-related bacteremia.[20,34] The introduction of semiquantitative and quantitative culture methods has greatly enhanced the ability to diagnose catheter-related infections. These culture techniques have greater specificity in classifying a catheter-related infection than do broth cultures, where a clinically insignificant amount of microorganisms may result in a positive culture.[62]

The pathogenesis of catheter-related infections is multifactorial. Data show that the majority of catheter-related infections result from migration of skin organisms at the exit site through the subcutaneous tissue, with eventual colonization of the catheter tip.[88] Silver ion-impregnated catheter cuffs were postulated to reduce the incidence of bloodstream infections by inhibiting the migration of bacteria. However, results from a large prospective randomized study of over 200 tunneled CVCs did not reveal a statistically significant difference in the reduction of tunnel infections or catheter-related bacteremia.[38]

Catheter hub contamination is also an important contributor to intraluminal colonization of the catheter.[77,84] Minimizing catheter entry and improving staff compliance with catheter care procedures have shown to reduce the incidence of catheter infection.[84,85] The recent introduction of needleless systems has gained widespread acceptance among health care professionals. Little data presently exists about these devices' impact on the risk of catheter-related infections.[33] Studies are needed to fully evaluate the impact of these innovative caps on infection risk.

Hematogenous seeding of the catheter from a distant focus of infection and infusion of contaminated solutions have also been postulated as causes of catheter infections.[60] Additional pathogenic determinants of catheter-related infections are catheter material and the adherence properties of certain microorganisms. Silicone or polyurethane catheters are more resistant to the adherence of microorganisms than polyvinyl chloride or polyethylene catheters. Coagulase-negative staphylococci adhere to the surface of polymer catheters. Certain strains produce an extracellular polysaccharide or "slime" that potentiates the pathogenicity of coagulase-negative staphylococci by acting as a barrier to host defenses (leukocytes) and inhibiting the effects of antimicrobial agents. *S. aureus,* a frequent pathogen in catheter-related infections, readily adheres to fibrin commonly present on the surfaces of catheters. In vitro studies of antimicrobial or antiseptic-impregnated catheters have shown a reduction in bacterial and biofilm formation on catheters.[87] Studies using antimicrobial-coated long-term tunneled catheters are needed to determine efficacy, risk of toxicity, and emergence of resistant organisms.

Infection risk and type of catheter

Several studies have compared the incidence of catheter-related infection in totally implanted devices and external tunneled catheters. The occurrence of catheter infection would be expected to be lower in ports, as these devices require less manipulation for flushing and site care. Various studies have reported a lower catheter infection rate in pediatric oncology patients with implanted ports versus external CVCs,[67,81] but these results have been contested by studies showing no statistical difference between types of catheters.[67] Comparison of data is difficult, as definitions of catheter-related infection are inconsistent and catheter maintenance techniques vary between institutions. Large, prospective studies are needed to make a valid comparison of these VADs.

Multilumen catheters have been associated with a higher infection rate. One study[90] found that multilumen catheters had twice the infection rate compared with single-lumen devices. Yet other investigators have found no difference in infection rates between single- and double-lumen catheters despite an increase in the number of manipulations in the double-lumen catheter group.[81,92] Decisions regarding the number of catheter lumens must be based on type and duration of therapies. Patients requiring intermittent infusions may benefit from single-lumen devices, whereas double-lumen cath-

eters can be used for patients requiring intensive therapy or simultaneous infusions of two or more solutions.

Catheter site care

Insertion site care is considered to be an important factor in preventing catheter-related infection, as studies have shown that lapses in technique may increase exit site colonization.[70] Most of the studies have reported on the antibacterial effect on the hands of hospital personnel, with few discussing the effect on skin surrounding the catheter. However, one comparative trial of cutaneous antiseptic regimens showed that 2% aqueous chlorhexidine was superior to 10% povidone-iodine or 70% alcohol in preventing catheter-related infections.[61] At present the 2% chlorhexidine used in this trial is not available for use in the United States. A sustained-release chlorhexidine gluconate patch has been used as an antiseptic dressing, with initial studies showing a reduction in the incidence of bacterial colonization at the catheter exit site.[88] Studies investigating the use of antimicrobial ointments at the catheter exit site to reduce catheter-related infections have yielded conflicting results. Moreover, the application of polyantibiotic ointments that are not fungicidal may significantly increase the incidence of catheter colonization with *Candida* species.[88]

One of the most controversial areas in catheter site care is the use of transparent, semipermeable, polyurethane dressings. These dressings permit visual inspection of the exit site and require less frequent changes than do gauze and tape dressings. A meta-analysis of infection risk with two types of catheter dressings revealed a higher incidence of catheter sepsis in catheters with transparent dressings than in those with gauze dressings.[88,91] Randomized, controlled studies are needed to determine optimal CVC site care.

Treatment and prevention of catheter infections

Because patients requiring long-term access have a limited number of sites for catheter placement, efforts to treat catheter infections and preserve access have been extensively investigated. Management of catheter-related infections while leaving the device intact has been reported with success rates ranging from 57% to 93%.[92] Successful treatment is based on the type of causative organism. Gram-positive organisms are usually the cause of catheter-related infections, the most common being *Staphylococcus epidermidis.* Gram-negative organisms may also seed the bloodstream from gastrointestinal sources, especially in neutropenic patients.[86] Hence, in the setting of suspected catheter-related bacteremia, initial treatment may include vancomycin with or without an aminoglycoside, with therapy subsequently changed, if necessary, based on organism sensitivity.[48] Antibiotics must be alternated between each catheter lumen, because the infection may be limited to a single lumen. Rotating antibiotics through each lumen also prevents a reservoir of infection.[37]

Antibiotic "locks" have been evaluated for the treatment of catheter-related infections as an alternative to systemic antimicrobial therapy.[34,72] Results from studies using a dilute vancomycin flush for the prevention of catheter infections have not been uniformly successful.[71,80]

VAD infections due to fungal colonization have a much lower catheter salvage rate. The incidence of *Candida*-related catheter infections is higher in infants and children as compared with adults (3.8% and 1.2%), with complications from fungal infections more severe in the younger patient.[3] Successful treatment in most cases requires removal of the catheter and amphotericin B therapy.[24]

The current recommended approach for the treatment of catheter-related bacteremia is to administer antibiotics through the catheter, alternating lumens if multiple lumens present, and to repeat both peripheral and catheter blood cultures within 24 to 48 hours. Therapy is continued for 14 to 21 days. Catheter removal is warranted if fever, bacteremia, or clinical signs of sepsis persist.[49]

Exit site or port pocket infections are defined as the presence of tenderness, induration, erythema, or purulent drainage within 2 cm of the catheter exit site or subcutaneous port.[33] These infections may be cured with oral antibiotics; however, parenteral antibiotics should be instituted for neutropenic patients. Pseudomonas-positive cultures from the subcutaneous site may warrant catheter removal.[37] Catheter tunnel or port-pocket infections may be difficult to treat and usually result in removal of the device.[37]

A number of studies have reported an association of device-related infection with catheter thrombosis. This finding is predicated on the concept of fibrin sheath and glycocalyx biofilm formation on the catheter surface, which has been shown to occur within three months of catheter insertion.[8] Organisms such as *Staphylococcus aureus* and *Candida albicans* adhere to the fibrin matrix, forming biofilm, which provides a sanctuary against antibiotic penetration. This may result in persistent catheter bacteremia or recurrence of catheter infection following treatment. Thrombolytics, in conjunction with antibiotic therapy, have been evaluated in the treatment of catheter infections.[50]

Two small studies demonstrated the benefit of using a thrombolytic prophylactically in decreasing the incidence of catheter infection.[12,35] However, another study failed to show any clinical benefit to adding urokinase to the antibiotic regimen.[55] Further studies are needed to establish the efficacy of thrombolytic therapy in the treatment of catheter-related infection.

Occlusions

Intermittent, sluggish, partial withdrawal occlusion (PWO) or total occlusion of catheter function may result from several mechanisms. Patency may be affected by anatomical obstruction, usually due to compression of the catheter between the first rib and clavicle or improper catheter tip placement. Less commonly, occlusion may result from precipitation of poorly soluble solutions caused by administration of incompatible drug-to-drug or drug-to-solution infusates.

The most common cause of catheter occlusion is thrombus formation within the lumen of the device, in the portal reservoir, or around the catheter tip. Figure 4-3 depicts the types of thromboses affecting catheter function. Venous stasis, hypercoagulability, and local trauma to the intima of the vein wall (caused by the catheter or infusate) are contributing factors to the development of catheter thrombosis. Improper catheter tip placement has also been associated with a higher incidence of catheter thrombosis.[45] The catheter tip should be at the junction of the superior vena cava/right atrial junction, below the level of the carina. Suboptimal catheter care also influences the rate of catheter occlusion. Despite routine flushing with heparin or saline, the incidence of catheter thrombosis has been reported as high as 31%.[10] Restoration of patency is paramount in the pediatric oncology patient because of limited peripheral sites and frequent need for blood draws.

Treatment of thrombotic occlusions

Catheter occlusions resulting from thrombus formation are treated with the instillation of a thrombolytic agent. Following reports of success rates of up to 98%,[57] urokinase was the standard of care for almost two decades in restoring patency to obstructed central venous catheters. Recently, however, urokinase has not been available because of the Food and Drug Administration's (FDA) concern for potential transmission of viral illnesses based on the production of urokinase from fetal kidney cells.[89]

Recombinant tissue plasminogen activator (rt-PA) has been used to restore patency to occluded

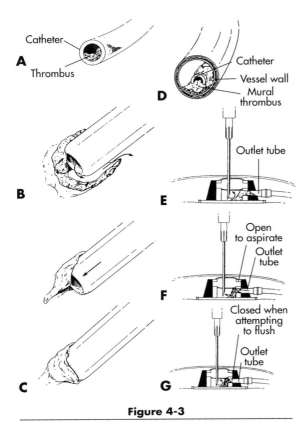

Figure 4-3

Examples of catheter-related occlusions. **A,** Intraluminal thrombus or clot. **B,** Fibrin sleeve. **C,** Fibrin tail. **D,** Mural thrombus. **E,** Portal reservoir obstruction. **F and G,** "Reverse ball-value" effect. (From Bagnall-Reeb, H. A. [1998]. Diagnosis of central venous access device occlusion. *Journal of Intravenous Nursing, 21,* S115-S121.)

central venous catheters. A fibrin specific thrombolytic agent, rt-PA, may pose less risk of hemorrhage. Because the product is produced through recombinant DNA technology, the relative risk of viral transmission is avoided. The instillation of 2 mg (1 mg/ml concentration) rt-PA was shown to be effective in restoring patency to obstructed central venous catheters.[9,39] A recombinant formulation of urokinase for catheter clearance is currently under study. Recommendations for the evaluation and treatment of catheter occlusions are listed in Figure 4-4.

Catheter-related venous thrombosis

Indwelling central venous catheters account for as much as 40% of deep vein thromboses in the upper extremities.[11] Thrombosis of the subclavian vein may be asymptomatic due to the development of collateral circulation. Prominent superficial veins over the chest wall and clavicle may be seen. In ad-

dition to the factors listed previously for the formation of thromboses, the duration of line placement, size of catheter in relation to vessel size, underlying disease (lymphoma, neuroblastoma, germ cell tumors), and use of medications known to affect coagulation (i.e., asparaginase) have been postulated as causing venous thrombosis.[69]

Treatment of venous thrombus

Catheter removal, followed by systemic anticoagulation with heparin and/or warfarin (Coumadin), has been one approach to the management of venous thrombosis.[3] A less aggressive approach has been taken with a local infusion of urokinase either directly through the existing line or through the placement of a separate line distal to the affected vein.[36] Studies to determine dose, efficacy, infusion time, and drug safety are under way using current investigational thrombolytic agents such as rt-PA (alteplase, reteplase) and recombinant urokinase.

Prophylaxis

In an effort to reduce the incidence of thrombus formation associated with central venous catheters, low-dose heparin has been added to total parenteral nutrition admixtures. One study reported a reduction to one third that observed in patients without heparin.[31] Daily low-dose prophylactic warfarin (1 mg/day) has been successfully used to reduce the incidence of venous thrombosis in adult cancer patients.[13] Further studies are warranted to determine the safety and efficacy of prophylactic anticoagulant treatment in children with cancer who have central venous catheters.

PATIENT AND FAMILY EDUCATION

Compliance with catheter care regimens in the home setting is key to the prevention of catheter-related complications. With same-day surgical placement of a catheter and shortened hospital stays becoming common medical practice, the importance of early family education about line care maintenance is paramount. Compliance and standardization of line care between the treating institution and home health care agency is important to reduce confusion and anxiety in the child and family. Teaching is performed based on the parent and child's education level and preferred methods of learning.

Strict adherence to hand washing, aseptic technique, and catheter irrigation is crucial for the prevention of catheter-related complications, yet studies examining compliance with such protocols reveal that many patients fail to comply with line care instruction.[17] Studies examining the effect of education and reinforcement of line care in the

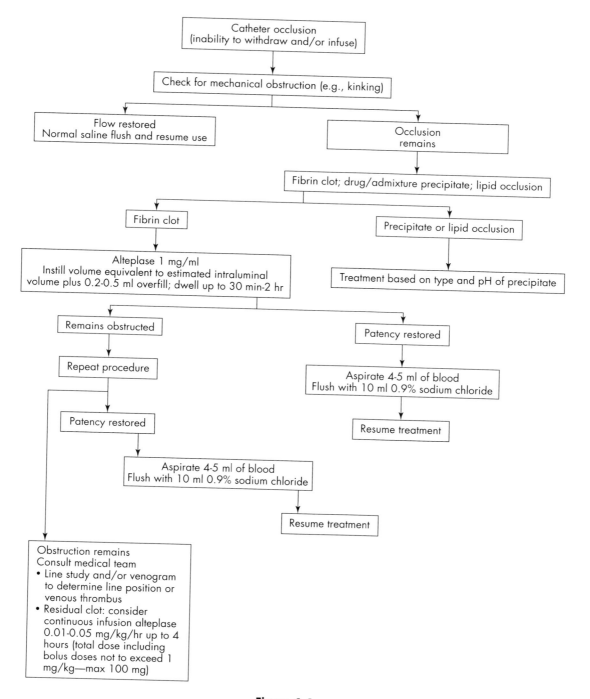

Figure 4-4

Guidelines for the treatment of obstructed catheters.   (Data from Michelson, A. D., Bovill, E., Monagle, P., et al. [1998]. Antithrombotic therapy in children. *Chest, 114,* 748S-769S; Bagnall, H. A., Gomperts, E., & Atkinson, J. B. [1989]. Continuous infusion low-dose urokinase in the treatment of central venous catheter thrombosis in infants and children. *Pediatrics, 83,* 963-966; Haire, W. D., Atkinson, J. B., Stephens, L. C., et al. [1994]. Urokinase versus recombinant tissue plasminogen activator in thrombosed central venous catheters: A double-blinded, randomized trial. *Thrombosis and Haemostasis, 72,* 543-547.)

home setting are needed to enhance nursing practice and improve patient outcomes.

Central venous catheters have improved the delivery of parenteral therapies in patients requiring long-term access and intensive drug regimens. Catheter selection depends on intended use, patient population, and family/clinician preference. Two common complications associated with the use of these devices, infection and occlusion, can be minimized by adherence to institutional protocols for catheter insertion, dressing changes, and drug and fluid administration.

ENTERAL ACCESS

Cancer therapy frequently alters the nutritional status of the pediatric oncology patient. The effects of these therapies—loss of appetite, lethargy, nausea, and vomiting—impact the patient's ability to sustain adequate nutritional stores and weight. Studies have shown that poor nutritional status correlates with decreased activity, lethargy, irritability, and delays in therapy.[6] Nutritional support using the intestinal tract is preferred, as absorption of nutrients throughout the intestinal tract improves visceral protein synthesis compared with nutrients given intravenously. Enteral feeding maintains the functional integrity of the gastrointestinal tract by preventing atrophic changes. Additionally, the risk of cholestasis is decreased through the stimulation of bile flow. Compared with parenteral feeding, using the gut for enteral formulas decreases infection risk.[16]

A variety of techniques are available for administering enteral nutrition. The patient must have a functioning gastrointestinal tract and the ability to tolerate feedings with management of nausea, vomiting, and diarrhea. The access route chosen depends on the portion of the gastrointestinal tract to be accessed and used for feeding, the planned duration of feeding, and the risks of an operative procedure. Access can be achieved nonoperatively, or it may require a surgical procedure for placement. Delivery of formula into the stomach (intragastric feeding) ensures the best exposure and absorption in the small bowel. This is an important factor for patients with a limited amount of small bowel. Additionally, directing the diet into the stomach allows the formula to be physiologically adjusted before it goes into the small bowel and allows for a greater selection of diet formulas. This versatility of intragastric feedings must be balanced against the increased risk of gastric overload, reflux, vomiting, or aspiration.[7]

Nasogastric feeding tubes can easily be placed, and their smaller size compared with nasogastric suction tubes allows for more comfortable insertion and maintenance. Newer, less viscous formulas can be administered through smaller-caliber tubes. These smaller catheters also decrease the risk of reflux and aspiration. Nasogastric feeding has been successfully used for both short-term and long-term patient nutrition.[7]

Gastrostomy tubes may be placed endoscopically or surgically. After removal of the tube, the stoma closes spontaneously. This method of intragastric feeding has the same advantages as using nasogastric tubes.[7]

Delivery of the formula directly into the small bowel (intrajejunal feeding) eliminates the problems of reflux, vomiting, and gastric overload associated with intragastric feeding. This is an important factor in anorexic or vomiting patients receiving chemotherapy. Mechanical or inflammatory processes that can affect gastric emptying do not affect intrajejunal feeds. Another advantage of intrajejunal feeding is that it can be initiated concurrently with nasogastric decompression in the early postoperative period.[7] Additionally, intrajejunal feeding is not affected by oral intake. This form of nutrition is indicated for both long-term and short-term feeding.

Nursing assessment of the patient receiving enteral feeding includes close attention to weight, fluid intake and output, and gastrointestinal function. Calcium, phosphorus, and magnesium are monitored regularly. Delayed gastric emptying can cause a high gastric residual of formula. The use of prokinetic medications such as metoclopramide hydrochloride may help alleviate this problem. Nasogastric tubes should be taped securely without pressure on the nares. Skin irritation or excoriation can develop around gastrostomy or jejunostomy tubes, increasing the risk of infection, especially in neutropenic patients. Diligent site care, including the use of topical or oral antibiotics, may be warranted. The risk of obstruction is minimized by routinely flushing the tube before and after administering feedings, medications, and boluses. No fluid has been found to be superior to water for maintaining patency. The tube is flushed every 4 to 6 hours in patients receiving continuous feedings. Large syringes are used (30 to 60 ml) to prevent rupturing the tube. Patency can be restored in clogged tubes by using enzymatic solutions such as pancrelipase (Viokase) or by instilling cola.[76] Enteral tubes may be left in place for 4 to 6 weeks before replacing. Nursing care of enteral tubes is outlined in Table 4-4.

Substantial evidence exists that enteral feeding provides gut mucosal protection and reduces the risk for local and systemic sepsis.[6] Clinicians

TABLE 4-4	**ENTERAL ACCESS CARE**
Assessment	**Interventions**
Device position	Nasogastric: • Mark tube or record incremental measurements • Nasal bridle/umbilical tape to secure G-tube/J-tube: • Dry dressing or abdominal binder Monitoring tip location: • Auscultation • Aspiration • pH paper testing pH $>$ 6 intestinal; pH $<$ 6 gastric • Radiographic evaluation
Site care	Nasogastric: • Secure tube without pressure on nostril • Change tape/location every other day G-tube/J-tube: • Remove dressing 24 hr after placement; leave open to air • Daily cleansing with soap and water followed by a water rinse • Crusty drainage: ½ strength peroxide solution • Granulation tissue: silver nitrate 2-3 $\times$ per week • Purulent drainage: antibiotic or antifungal treatment
Maintaining tube patency	Routine flush with water every 4 hr for continuous feeds and before and after intermittent feeds or medications
Declogging tubes	Flush with water Pancrealipase and sodium bicarbonate (½ tsp Viokase mixed with ⅛ tsp baking soda in 5 ml water)

Data from Lord, L. M. (1997). Enteral access devices. *Nursing Clinics of North America, 32,* 685-702.

should be aware of the benefits of enteral feeding and consider this method of nutrition for the pediatric oncology patient requiring nutrition support.

INNOVATIVE SURGICAL TECHNIQUES

Over the past decade the treatment and surgical management of the child with cancer has significantly improved. Present-day pediatric oncology surgery has become extremely complex, with newer procedures requiring greater technical skills with advanced equipment. The aim of surgery is to remove the tumor while preserving as much anatomical and physiologic function as possible. The nurse must be knowledgeable about these recent advancements in order to effectively plan and implement preoperative and postoperative care.

MINIMALLY INVASIVE SURGERY

During the past decade minimally invasive surgical techniques have been documented for a variety of abdominal and thoracic procedures. *Minimally invasive surgery* (MIS) is a term used to describe surgical procedures accomplished with instruments directed through cannulas. Also known as minimal access surgery and video-assisted surgery, this approach has been reported in the pediatric surgical literature for laparoscopic cholecystectomy, appendectomy, fundoplication, splenectomy, and pull-through procedures. In addition, thoracoscopic procedures have been described using this technique.[19,43,44] Advantages of MIS over an open surgical approach for a specific operation include smaller wound size, less tissue exposure, and minimal tissue and organ manipulation.

The advantages of MIS in the pediatric setting include less discomfort, shorter hospital stay, improved cosmesis, earlier return to routine activities, and potential earlier resumption of adjuvant therapy.[43] The addition of a video camera allows the surgeon to stand upright rather than bent over, and the entire surgical team can observe the operation in progress. Disadvantages of this technique include the possibility of intra-abdominal hemorrhage, organ injury, or gas embolism with trocar insertion; tumor spillage; and sampling error. Additional expense and inability to perform the MIS operation are other limitations to this technique.[19,59] Technically, MIS is more challenging to the surgeon, because the distance between the surgeon's eyes and hands is lengthened, which potentially makes hand-eye coordination more difficult. The procedure is more complex and may lengthen operative time compared with the equivalent "open" procedures.

Not all patients are candidates for MIS.[6] Because most children undergoing MIS require general anesthesia, the patient must be able to tolerate a pneumoperitoneum or one-lung ventilation for thoracoscopic procedures. Computed tomography (CT) or magnetic resonance imaging (MRI) are helpful in identifying specific areas within the tumor for biopsy or within the lymph nodes for resection. The child and family must be prepared for the possibility of conversion to an open technique, especially if the tumor lies deep within the lung or liver or if excessive or uncontrolled bleeding occurs.[43]

For pediatric oncologic procedures, laparoscopy has been successfully used for staging; for biopsies of lymph nodes, liver, or abdominal masses; and for evaluation of residual, recurrent, or metastatic tumor.[44] Advances in MIS over the past 2 decades have led to extensive use of thoracoscopy for biopsy or resection of mediastinal or hilar masses, biopsy of pulmonary infiltrates, and irrigation and debridement of empyema.[43] Metastatic lung lesions have been successfully resected using this approach, thus improving long-term survival. The surgeon's inability to directly palpate lesions not visualized is a limitation to this technique.[43]

The body's response to MIS differs from traditional open procedures. Because there is less stress imposed on the body, postoperative pain, fluid, and respiratory management and activity restrictions are much less. Since the patient may be discharged from the hospital earlier, it is important that family education begins early.

ORGAN TRANSPLANTATION

Organ transplant has limited application as treatment for pediatric solid tumors, due in part to the metastatic nature of most tumor types as well as local invasion of adjacent tissues. Reports of successful organ transplant have been described for bilateral Wilms tumor, hepatoblastoma, and hepatocellular carcinoma.

Bilateral Wilms tumor

The recommended surgical approach to patients with bilateral Wilms tumor involves initial biopsy of both kidneys followed by preoperative chemotherapy. Radical excision of the tumor is not recommended initially because of the sensitivity of this tumor to systemic chemotherapy. Partial nephrectomy or wedge resection may be performed as long as at least two thirds or more of renal parenchyma remains bilaterally. Definitive resection is delayed until there is a reduction in tumor burden.[73] For patients unresponsive to chemotherapy and radiation therapy, bilateral nephrectomy may be indicated. If renal transplant is considered, a waiting period of approximately 2 years is recommended to rule out the presence of or subsequent development of metastatic disease.[74,75]

Liver transplantation in hepatic cancer

Hepatic tumors include hepatoblastoma and hepatocellular carcinoma. Liver transplantation is an uncommon treatment modality in hepatoblastoma due to the success of multimodal therapy.[4] Patients who are not cured by conventional therapy may be eligible for a liver transplant. Eligibility for transplant is based on the extent of tumor, absence of extrahepatic metastases, and angiography that confirms patency of the portal venous system. Isolated intrahepatic disease is a prerequisite for transplantation. Survival rates of 63% to 100% have been reported in patients transplanted for unresectable hepatoblastoma.[4,54]

Hepatocellular carcinoma (HCC) in children can occur secondary to viral or metabolic liver disease such as hepatitis B or tyrosinemia. In general, HCC is not as chemosensitive as hepatoblastoma, and liver transplantation has been investigated in tumors not responsive to systemic chemotherapy. Survival after liver transplantation has dramatically improved with the advent of new immunosuppressive regimens and refinement of surgical procedures and postoperative management.

Future directions

The pace of technological development in the field of surgery continues to accelerate. The scope has expanded beyond physicians and nurses to include scientists, computer specialists, and bioengineers. Surgery has entered the digital era with several surgical procedures and devices presently directed by computer technology. Patient care is being performed through computer-assisted techniques, and soon physicians will be able to diagnose and perform surgical treatment in remote and distant areas without actually being physically present. The gateway into this new paradigm will be the physician's computer workstation, where medical information, data, and devices can be manipulated. The future era of surgery involves robotics, telepresence, and virtual reality.

Robotics

Several types of surgical robotic systems have been developed. These machines are supervised and manipulated by specially trained surgical teams (Figure 4-5). Current systems are in operation for renal, orthopedic, cardiac, ophthalmologic, and neurosurgical procedures. These systems are able to perform surgery with a higher degree of accuracy than is capable by human hands. Some systems feature voice-activated equipment so surgeons can adjust lighting, change camera angles, and maneuver robotic arms without the assistance of technicians or nurses. One such robot named Zeus compensates for the motion of a beating heart, enabling surgeons to perform bypass surgery without stopping a patient's heart.[78]

Telepresence

Telepresence is the ability to perform a task or procedure from a distance using a remote manipulator and video image. A surgery workstation is equipped with dexterous manipulator and stereoscopic camera. Next to the surgical suite is a workstation with a three-dimensional monitor and instrument handle controllers that have the dexterity and sensory feedback similar to devices used in open procedures. This remote-controlled system was developed to solve the three deficiencies of MIS: (1) the absence of three-dimensional imaging, (2) poor dexterity, and (3) loss of sensory feedback. Currently under trial through the U.S. military, this system provides the surgeon, who may be physically distant from the actual operative site, with the sense of touch and monitors that display "real-time" updates on the patient's condition.[78]

Virtual reality

Similar to telepresence, which performs actual procedures, virtual reality permits surgical intervention

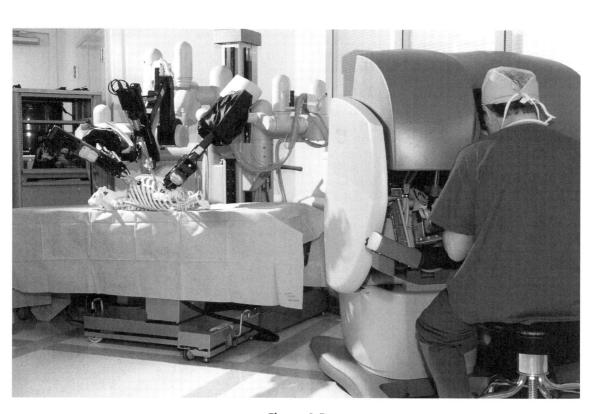

Figure 4-5

Robotic surgery: The da Vinci Surgical System (Intuitive Surgical, Mountain View, CA). (Courtesy St. Vincent Medical Center, Department of Cardiac Surgery, Portland, OR.)

on imaginary bodies. Imaginary three-dimensional computer images of human anatomy are reconstructed, allowing a person to enter the program through the use of a helmet-mounted display and Dataglove. The person is dissociated from the real world and immersed in a "virtual" world—able to pick up, move, and interact with objects as if they really existed. One medical application of virtual reality is the "Visible Human Project." Designed as a three-dimensional recreation of a human cadaver, the surgeon in training can navigate around and behind organs, providing perspectives of the interrelationship of organs that are not possible with cadavers. Use of this technology will allow surgical teams to practice their technique on a simulator, comparable to pilots' using a flight simulator for take-offs and landings.[19,78]

The clinical application of this technology has immense possibilities in the field of pediatric surgical oncology. Tumors once deemed inoperable may be totally excised through the use of robotic technology. Likewise, distant surgeons who are specialists in the particular tumor type may perform difficult or complex surgical procedures. Physicians and nurses will be able to network and consult with an international array of experts through digital information and three-dimensional video imaging. Family and patient education will be facilitated through the use of a three-dimensional patient image depicting tumor location and extent of disease.

The pediatric oncology nurse, in this era of digital information, has a vast array of tools available for education and family teaching. Knowledge of available resources and how to use these novel products and devices will be paramount and must be integrated into curricula. The future of nursing practice is rapidly evolving in this digital era; our challenge is to develop understanding of and expertise in caring for children undergoing these techniques.

Advances in surgical devices and techniques in pediatric oncology are occurring at an unprecedented rate. Nursing roles are changing with these advancements, and pediatric oncology nurses now take an active part in the complex management of these patients. Nurses serve as members of the health care team as clinicians, educators, and surgical assistants. Over the past two decades pediatric oncology nurses have developed a strong collaborative relationship with pediatric surgeons, specializing as surgical nurse practitioners and coordinators. With the advent of robotic surgical technology, new programs are being developed to prepare nurses as surgical robotic specialists. This is an era of rapid change and opportunity for pediatric nurses in the field of surgical oncology.

REFERENCES

1. Abbott Laboratories, Data on file.
2. Adzick, N. S., & Nance, M. L. (2000). Pediatric surgery. *New England Journal of Medicine, 342,* 1726-1732.
3. Alexander, H. R. (1994). Infectious complications associated with long-term venous access devices. In H. R. Alexander (Ed.), Vascular access in the cancer patient (pp. 113-127). Philadelphia: J. B. Lippincott.
4. Al-Qabandi, W., Jenkinson, J. A., Buckels, A. D., et al. (1999). Orthotopic liver transplantation for unresectable hepatoblastoma: A single center's experience. *Journal of Pediatric Surgery, 34,* 1261-1264.
5. Alvarez, O. A., & Zimmerman, G. (2000). PEG-asparaginase-induced pancreatitis. *Medical and Pediatric Oncology, 34,* 200-205.
6. Andrassy, R. J. (1998). General principles. In R. J. Andrassy (Ed.), *Pediatric surgical oncology* (pp. 13-34). Philadelphia: W. B. Saunders.
7. Andrassy, R. J., & Hays, D. M. (1997). Pediatric surgical oncology. In P. A. Pizzo & D. G. Poplack (Eds.), *Principles and practice of pediatric oncology* (3rd ed., pp. 273-287). Philadelphia: Lippincott-Raven.
8. Andremount, A., Paulet, R., Nitenberg, G., et al. (1988). Value of semiquantitative cultures of blood draws through catheter hubs for estimating the risk of catheter tip colonization in cancer patients. *Journal of Clinical Microbiology, 26,* 2297-2299.
9. Atkinson, J. B., & Bagnall, H. A. (1990). Investigational use of tissue plasminogen activator (t-PA) for occluded central venous catheters. *Journal of Parenteral and Enteral Nutrition, 14,* 310-311.
10. Bagnall, H. A., Gomperts, E., & Atkinson, J. B. (1989). Continuous infusion low-dose urokinase in the treatment of central venous catheter thrombosis in infants and children. *Pediatrics, 83,* 963-966.
11. Bagnall-Reeb, H. A. (1998). Diagnosis of central venous access device occlusion. *Journal of Intravenous Nursing, 21,* S115-S121.
12. Bagnall-Reeb, H. A., Saltzman, D. A., Smith, C. M, et al. (1993). Prophylactic scheduled urokinase for the prevention of right atrial catheter infection. *Oncology Nursing Forum, 20,* 315.
13. Bern, M. M., Lokich, J. J., Wallach, S. R., et al. (1990). Very low doses of warfarin can prevent thrombosis in central venous catheters. *Annals of Internal Medicine, 112,* 423-428.
14. Black, T. C. (1998). Neuroblastoma. In R. J. Andrassy (Ed.), *Pediatric surgical oncology* (pp. 175-211). Philadelphia: W. B. Saunders.
15. Blandy, J. P., & Oliver, R. T. (2000). Genitourinary cancer. In N. J. Vogelzang, P. T. Scardino, W. U. Shipley, et al. (Eds.), *Comprehensive textbook of genitourinary oncology* (pp. 462-500). Philadelphia: Lippincott Williams & Wilkins.
16. Bowers, S. (2000). All about tubes: Your guide to enteral feeding devices. *Nursing 2000, 30(12),* 41-47.
17. Boyer, C. L., & Wade, D. C. (1998). The impact of compliance on quality outcomes in the home infusion population. *Journal of Intravenous Nursing, 21(5S),* S161-S165.
18. Briassoulis, G., Hatzis, T., Paphitis, C., et al. (1999). Acute spontaneous pneumomediastinum in a child with Hodgkin's disease and pulmonary fibrosis. *Pediatric Hematology Oncology, 16,* 175-180.
19. Browne, A. F., & Tkacz, N. J. (2000). Minimally invasive surgery. In B. V. Wise, C. McKenna, G. Garvin, et al. (Eds.), *Nursing care of the general pediatric surgical patient* (pp. 110-120). Gaithersburg, MD: Aspen.

20. Capdevila, J. A., Planes, A. M., Palomar, M., et al. (1992). Value of differential quantitative blood cultures in the diagnosis of catheter-related sepsis. *European Journal of Clinical Microbiology and Infectious Diseases, 11,* 403-407.

21. Corpron, C. A., & Andrassy, R. J. (1997). Molecular and surgical advances in pediatric tumors. In R. E. Pollock (Ed.), *Surgical oncology* (pp. 51-69). Boston: Academic Publishers Norwell.

22. Corpron, C. A., & Andrassy, R. J. (1998). Abdominal complications. In R. J. Andrassy (Ed.), *Pediatric surgical oncology* (pp. 477-479). Philadelphia: W. B. Saunders.

23. Cunningham, R.S., & Ravikumar, T.S. (1995). A review of peripherally inserted central venous catheters in oncology patients. *Surgical Oncology Clinics of North America, 4,* 429-441.

24. Dato, V. M., & Dajani, A. S. (1990). Candidemia in children with central venous catheters: Role of catheter removal and amphotericin B. *Pediatric Infectious Disease Journal, 9,* 309-314.

25. DeCou, J. M., Bowan, L. C., Rao, B. N., et al. (1995). Infants with metastatic neuroblastoma have improved survival with resection of the primary tumor. *Journal of Pediatric Surgery, 30,* 937-940.

26. Donaldson, S., Egbert, P. R., & Newsham, I. (1997). Retinoblastoma. In P. A. Pizzo & D. G. Poplack (Eds.), *Principles and practice of pediatric oncology* (3rd ed., pp. 699-716). Philadelphia: J. B. Lippincott.

27. Dower, N. A., & Smith, L. J. (2000). Liver transplant for malignant liver tumor in children. *Medical and Pediatric Oncology, 34,* 136-140.

28. Eastridge, B. J., & Lefor, A. T. (1995). Complications of indwelling venous access devices in cancer patients. *Journal of Clinical Oncology, 13,* 233-238.

29. Eastridge, B. J., & Lefor, A. T. (1996). Chronic venous access in the cancer patient. In A. T. Lefor (Ed.), *Surgical problems affecting the patient with cancer: Interdisciplinary management* (pp. 183-209). Philadelphia: Lippincott-Raven.

30. Ehrenreich, B., & Miguel, L. S. (2000). Solid tumors. In B. V. Wise, C. McKenna, G. Garvin, et al. (Eds.), *Nursing care of the general pediatric surgical patient* (pp. 370-399). Gaithersburg, MD: Aspen.

31. Fabri, P. J., Mirtallo, J. M., Ruberg, R. L., et al. (1982). Incidence and prevention of thrombosis of the subclavian vein during total parenteral nutrition. *Surgical Gynecology and Obstetrics, 155,* 238-240.

32. Fisher, W. E., & Burak, W. E. (1996). Inflammatory lesions of the gastrointestinal tract. In A. T. Lefor (Ed.), *Surgical problems affecting the patient with cancer: Interdisciplinary management* (pp. 97-109). Philadelphia: Lippincott-Raven.

33. Flynn, P.M. (2000). Diagnosis, management, and prevention of catheter-related infections. *Seminars in Pediatric Infectious Diseases, 11,* 113-121.

34. Flynn, P. M., Shenep, J. L., Stokes, D. C., et al. (1987). In situ management of confirmed central venous catheter-related bacteremia. *Pediatric Infectious Disease Journal, 6,* 729-734.

35. Fraschini, G., Becker, M., Bruso, P., et al. (1991). Comparative trial of urokinase vs heparin as prophylaxis for central venous ports. *Proceedings of the American Society of Clinical Oncology, 10,* 337.

36. Fraschini, G., Jadeja, J., Lawson, M., et al. (1987). Local infusion of urokinase for the lysis of thrombosis associated with permanent central venous catheters in cancer patients. *Journal of Clinical Oncology, 5,* 672-678.

37. Greene, J. N. (1996). Catheter-related complications in cancer therapy. *Infectious Disease Clinics of North America, 10,* 255-295.

38. Groeger, J. S., Lucas, A. B., Coit, D., et al. (1993). A prospective, randomized evaluation of the effect of the silver impregnated subcutaneous cuffs for preventing tunneled chronic venous access catheter infections in cancer patients. *Annals of Surgery, 218,* 206-210.

39. Haire, W. D., Atkinson, J. B., Stephens, L. C., et al. (1994). Urokinase versus recombinant tissue plasminogen activator in thrombosed central venous catheters: A double-blinded, randomized trial. *Thrombosis and Haemostasis, 72,* 543-547.

40. Halperin, D. L., Koren, G., Attias, D., et al. (1989). Topical skin anesthesia for venous, subcutaneous drug reservoir and lumbar punctures in children. *Pediatrics, 84,* 281-284.

41. Hays, D. M. (1998). Pediatric surgical oncology: The background. In R. J. Andrassy (Ed.), *Pediatric surgical oncology* (pp. 1-11). Philadelphia: W. B. Saunders.

42. Herrera, J. M., Krebs, A., Harris, P., et al. (2000). Childhood tumors. *Surgical Clinics of North America, 80,* 747-760.

43. Holcomb, G.W. (1998). Minimally invasive surgery. In R. J. Andrassy (Ed.), *Pediatric surgical oncology* (pp. 123-135). Philadelphia: W. B. Saunders.

44. Holcomb, G. W., Tomita, S. S., Haase, G. M., et al. (1995). Minimally invasive surgery in children with cancer. *Cancer, 76,* 121-128.

45. Horne, M. K., & Mayo, D. J. (1997). Low-dose urokinase infusions to treat fibrinous obstruction of venous access devices in cancer patients. *Journal of Clinical Oncology, 15,* 2709-2714.

46. Horwitz, J. R., & Lally, K. P. (1998). Vascular access. In R. J. Andrassey (Ed.), *Pediatric surgical oncology* (pp. 137-153). Philadelphia: W. B. Saunders.

47. Hudson, M. M., & Donaldson, S. S. (1997). Hodgkin's disease. In P. A. Pizzo & D. G. Poplack (Eds.), *Principles and practice of pediatric oncology* (3rd ed., pp. 523-543). Philadelphia: Lippincott-Raven.

48. Hughes, W. T., Armstrong, D., Bodey, G. P., et al. (1997). Guidelines for the use of antimicrobial agents in neutropenic patients with unexplained fever. *Clinical Infectious Disease, 25,* 551-573.

49. Jones, G. R. (1998). A practical guide to evaluation and treatment of infections in patients with central venous catheters. *Journal of Intravenous Nursing, 21,* 5134-5142.

50. Jones, G. R., Konsler, G. K., Dunaway, R. P., et al. (1993). Prospective analysis of urokinase in the treatment of catheter sepsis in pediatric hematology-oncology patients. *Journal of Pediatric Surgery, 28,* 350-355.

51. Koop, C. E. (1968). Neuroblastoma: Two years' survival and treatment correlations. *Journal of Pediatric Surgery, 3,* 178-179.

52. Koop, C. E., Kiesewetter, W. B., & Horn, R. C. (1955). Neuroblastoma in childhood: Survival after major surgical insult to tumor. *Surgery, 38,* 272-278.

53. Kun, L. E. (1997). General principles of radiation therapy. In P. A. Pizzo & D. G. Poplack (Eds.), *Principles and practice of pediatric oncology* (3rd ed., pp. 289-321). Philadelphia: Lippincott-Raven.

54. Laine, J., Jalanko, H., Saarinen-Pihkala, U. M., et al. (1999). Successful liver transplantation after induction chemotherapy in children with inoperable, multifocal primary hepatic malignancy. *Transplantation, 67,* 1369-1372.

55. La Quaglia, M. P. (1997). Childhood tumors. In L. I. Greenfield, M. W. Mulholland & K. T. Oldham (Eds.), *Surgery: Scientific principles and practice* (pp. 2118-2140). Philadelphia: Lippincott-Raven.

56. La Quaglia, M. P., Caldwell, C., Lucas, A., et al. (1994). A prospective randomized double-blind trial of bolus urokinase in the treatment of established Hickman catheter sepsis in children. *Journal of Pediatric Surgery, 29,* 742-745.

57. Lawson, M., Bottino, J. C., Hurtubise, M. R., McCredie, K. B. (1982). The use of urokinase to restore the patency of occluded central venous catheters. *American Journal of Intravenous Therapy and Clinical Nutrition, 5,* 29-32.

58. Lord, L. M. (1997). Enteral access devices. *Nursing Clinics of North America, 32,* 685-702.

59. Mailbach, C. B. (1996). The future of minimally invasive surgery. *Nursing Management, 10,* 32V-32AA.

60. Maki, D. G., & Martin, W. T. (1975). Nationwide epidemic of septicemia caused by contaminated infusion products: Growth of microbial pathogens in fluids for intravenous infection. *Journal of Infectious Disease, 131,* 267-672.

61. Maki, D. G., Ringer, M., & Alvarado, C. J. (1991). Prospective randomized trial of povidone-iodine, alcohol, and chlorhexidine for prevention of infection associated with central venous and arterial catheters. *Lancet, 338,* 339-343.

62. Maki, D. G., Weise, C. E., & Sarafin, H. W. (1977). A semiquantitative culture method for identifying intravenous catheter-related infection. *New England Journal of Medicine, 296,* 1305-1309.

63. Mathes, D. D., & Bogdonoff, D. L. (1996). Preoperative evaluation of the cancer patient. In A. T. Lefor (Ed.), *Surgical problems affecting the patient with cancer: Interdisciplinary management* (pp. 273-304). Philadelphia: Lippincott-Raven.

64. Megerman, J., Levin, N. W., Ing, T. S., et al. (1999). Development of a new approach to vascular access. *Artificial Organ, 23,* 10-14.

65. Michelson, A. D., Bovill, E., Monagle, P., et al. (1998). Antithrombotic therapy in children. *Chest, 114,* 748S-769S.

66. Midis, G., & Skibber, J. (1996). Abdominal pain in the neutropenic cancer patient. In A. T. Lefor (Ed.), *Surgical problems affecting the patient with cancer: Interdisciplinary management* (pp. 3-23). Philadelphia: Lippincott-Raven.

67. Mueller, B. U., Skelton, J., Callender, D. P. E., et al. (1992). A prospective randomized trial comparing the infectious and non-infectious complications of an externalized catheter versus a subcutaneously implanted device in cancer patients. *Journal of Clinical Oncology, 10,* 1943-1948.

68. Palmer, J. S., Kletzel, M., Steinberg, G. D., et al. (1996). Testicular, sacrococcygeal, and other tumors. In J. C. Harvey & E. J. Beattie (Eds.), *Cancer surgery* (pp. 91-100). Philadelphia: W. B. Saunders.

69. Priest, J. R., Ramsay, N. K., Bennett, A. J., et al. (1982). The effect of L-asparaginase on antithrombin, plasminogen and plasma coagulation during therapy for acute lymphoblastic leukemia. *Journal of Pediatrics, 100,* 990-995.

70. Puntis, J. W. L., Holden, C. E., Smallman, S., et al. (1991). Staff training: A key factor in reducing intravascular catheter sepsis. *Archives of Diseases in Children, 66,* 335-337.

71. Rackoff, W. R., Weiman, M., Jakobowski, D., et al. (1995). A randomized, controlled trial of the efficacy of a heparin and vancomycin solution in preventing central venous catheter infections in children. *Journal of Pediatrics, 127,* 147-151.

72. Rao, J. S., O'Meara, A., Harvey, T., et al. (1992). A new approach to the management of Broviac catheter infection. *Journal of Hospital Infection, 22,* 109-116.

73. Ritchey, M. L. (1998). Wilms tumor. In R. J. Andrassy (Ed.), *Pediatric surgical oncology* (pp. 155-174). Philadelphia: W. B. Saunders.

74. Ritchey, M. L., Green, D. M., Thomas, P., et al. (1996). Renal failure in Wilms' tumor patients: A report from the National Wilms' Tumor Study Group. *Medical and Pediatric Oncology, 26,* 75-80.

75. Rudin, C., Pritchard, J., Fernando, O.N., et al. (1998). Renal transplantation in the management of bilateral Wilms' tumour (BWT) and of Denys-Drash syndrome (DDS). *Nephrology, Dialysis Transplantation, 13,* 1506-1510.

76. Saks, N., & Meeks, R. S. (1998). Nutrition support in children with cancer. In M. J. Hockenberry-Eaton (Ed.), *Essentials of pediatric oncology nursing: A core curriculum* (pp. 164-169). Glenview, IL: Association of Pediatric Oncology Nurses.

77. Salzman, M. B., Isenberg, H. D., Shapiro, J. F., et al. (1993). A prospective study of the catheter hub as the portal of entry for micro-organisms causing catheter-related sepsis in neonates. *Journal of Infectious Diseases, 167,* 487-490.

78. Satava, R. M. (1996). Future directions. In B. V. McFadden, Jr., & J. L. Ponsky (Eds.), *Operative laparoscopy and thoracoscopy* (pp. 929-939). Philadelphia: Lippincott-Raven.

79. Schaffer, M., & Barbul, A. (1996). Chemotherapy and wound healing. In A. T. Lefor (Ed.), *Surgical problems affecting the patient with cancer: Interdisciplinary management* (pp. 305-319). Philadelphia: Lippincott-Raven.

80. Schwartz, C., Henrickson, K. J., Roghmann, K., et al. (1990). Prevention of bacteria attributed to lumenal colonization of tunneled central venous catheters with vancomycin-susceptible organisms. *Journal of Clinical Oncology, 8,* 1591-1597.

81. Severien, C., & Nelson, J. D. (1991). Frequency of infections associated with implanted systems versus cuffed, tunneled Silastic venous catheters in patients with acute leukemia. *American Journal of Diseases in Children, 145,* 1433-1438.

82. Shamberger, R. C. (1999). Preanesthetic evaluation of children with anterior mediastinal mass. *Seminars in Pediatric Surgery, 8,* 61-68.

83. Shanholtz, C. (1996). Infections in the immunocompromised patient. In A. T. Lefor (Ed.), *Surgical problems affecting the patient with cancer: Interdisciplinary management* (pp. 343-372). Philadelphia: Lippincott-Raven.

84. Sitges-Serra, A., Linases, J., Perez, J.L., et al. (1985). Catheter sepsis: The clue is the hub. *Surgery, 97,* 355-357.

85. Stotter, A. T., Ward, H., Waterfield, A. H., et al. (1987). The key to prevention of catheter sepsis in intravenous feeding. *Journal of Parenteral and Enteral Nutrition, 11,* 159-162.

86. Tancrede, C. H., & Andremont, A. O. (1985). Bacterial translocation and gram-negative bacteremia in patients with hematological malignancies. *Journal of Infectious Disease, 152,* 99-103.

87. Trooskin, S. Z., Donetz, A. P., Harvey, R. A., et al. (1985). Prevention of catheter sepsis by antibiotic bonding. *Surgery, 97,* 547-551.

88. U.S. Department of Health and Human Services, Public Health Service, Centers for Disease Control and Prevention. (1996). Guidelines for the prevention of intravascular device-related infections. *American Journal of Infection Control, 24,* 262-93.

89. U.S. Food and Drug Administration Letter, January, 1999.

90. Vane, D. W., Ong, B., Rescorla, F. J., et al. (1990). Complications of central venous access in children: A review of 2281 catheter insertions. *Pediatric Surgery International, 5,* 174-178.

91. Wiener, E. S., & Albanese, C. T. (1998). Venous access in pediatric patients. *Journal of Intravenous Nursing, 21,* 5122-5133.

92. Wiener, E. S., McGuire, P., Stolar, C., et al. (1992). The CCSG prospective study of venous access devices: An analysis of insertions and causes for removal. *Journal of Pediatric Surgery, 27,* 155-164.

93. Witte, M. B., & Barbul, A. (1997). General principles of wound healing. *Surgical Clinics of North America, 77,* 509-525.

94. Woolley, M. M. (1993). Teratomas. In K. W. Ashcraft & T. M. Holder (Eds.), *Pediatric surgery* (2nd ed., pp. 847-862). Philadelphia: W. B. Saunders.

95. Ziegler, D. B., & Prior, M. M. (1994). Preparation for surgery and adjustment to hospitalization. *Nursing Clinics of North America, 29,* 655-669.

5

Radiation Therapy

Patsy McGuire Cullen
Joyce D. Derrickson
Jennifer A. Potter

Radiation as a therapeutic modality originated with the discovery of x-rays by Roentgen, a German physicist, in 1895. The element radium was isolated by Marie and Pierre Curie in 1898. Shortly thereafter, both Henri Becquerel, a French physician, and Pierre Curie observed radiodermatitis firsthand, on the chest, after carrying radium in their coat pockets. Interest in the area of radiation quickly sparked many experiments. Emil Grubbe, a medical student in Chicago, reproduced Becquerel and Curie's experience by exposing his hand to an x-ray cathode tube and observing a similar skin reaction. Therapeutic uses of radiation for malignancy developed rapidly for conditions with superficial lesions, such as basal cell carcinoma.[26,31] In the early part of the twentieth century radiation was also used in the treatment of many nonmalignant conditions, including thyrotoxicosis, rheumatism, herpes, and gout.[27,59]

Initially, the therapeutic benefit of radiation was hindered by many scientific and technical factors. For several decades treatment was administered with insufficient understanding of radiation biology and no concept of dosage. The treatment rationale was to deliver radiation sufficient to produce skin erythema.[33] Superficial tumors such as skin lesions responded to this treatment. The technology of the day, however, limited therapeutic usefulness in the treatment of deep-seated tumors because of unacceptable dose depth characteristics, resulting in severe and often irreversible toxicity.

In 1922 Regaud developed the practice of administering radiation over a period of days or weeks. Fractionation, the process of dividing the total radiation dose into small equal portions in a set schedule, was developed approximately 10 years later by Coutard.[5,31] However, the application of the modality to a broad spectrum of malignancies was hampered until increasingly sophisticated equipment became available. Following the development of the atomic bomb in World War II,

technology became available that led to the production of more sophisticated teletherapy equipment using high-energy gamma radiation from cobalt 60. Subsequently, the development of the linear accelerator, which produced high-energy photon beams, further advanced and refined treatment capabilities.[27,65] Increased electronic sophistication and the advent of computer-assisted equipment have further facilitated the administration of radiation therapy in a more precise fashion, with minimal "scatter" or diffusion of radiation away from the planned treatment field to surrounding normal tissues.

Although radiation therapy has been used for almost a century, understanding the most effective use of this modality in the treatment of children with cancer continues to evolve (Table 5-1). Equipment is regularly upgraded and refined to ensure accuracy. Both acute and late effects are now better managed as research findings are integrated into clinical practice. This has become particularly important in the radiation of the pediatric patient, as children and adolescents who have not yet completed growth and development are susceptible to the long-term effects of radiation.

As the radiation experience may be a frightening one for the child and family, proper preparation and instruction are necessary. The pediatric oncology nurse must have a basic understanding of the physical and biological principles underlying radiation therapy in order to educate children and families and to provide effective symptom management.

BIOLOGY AND PHYSICS OF RADIATION

The goal of radiation therapy in cancer treatment is delivery of a therapeutic dose of radiation to tumor cells while sparing healthy tissue. Radiation causes single-strand or double-strand breaks in the DNA molecule, which results in the inability of tumor cells to divide, the inability to repair DNA damage,

TABLE 5-1	ROLE OF RADIATION THERAPY IN THE TREATMENT OF CHILDHOOD CANCER
Type of Cancer	**Role of Radiation**
Acute lymphocytic leukemia	Historically used for CNS prophylaxis.
	Currently reserved for CNS or testicular relapse.
Brain tumors	Primary therapy for many CNS tumors.
Neuroblastoma	Part of multimodality therapy. Treatment of residual, bulky, unresectable, or disseminated disease.
Non-Hodgkin's lymphoma	Used exclusively in emergency situations when tumor mass is causing spinal cord compression, respiratory distress, superior vena cava syndrome, orbital proptosis, or cranial nerve palsy.
Wilms tumor	Reserved for local control in stage III disease and whole lung radiation in stage IV disease with pulmonary metastases.
Hodgkin's disease	Radiosensitive tumor, multimodal treatment, radiation generally limited to low dose, involved field. Adolescents receive higher doses on rare occasions.
Acute myelocytic leukemia	Historically used for CNS prophylaxis.
Rhabdomyosarcoma	Used for local control when complete resection is not possible, in emergency situations, or for management of metastatic disease.
Osteosarcoma	Radioresistant tumor, radiation rarely used; can be seen as a radiation induced second malignancy.
Ewing's sarcoma	Radiosensitive, used for local control in bones that are considered indispensible or inoperable, or management of metastic disease. Use limited by risk of secondary malignancies.

From Ruble, K., & Kelly, K. P. (1999). Radiation therapy in childhood cancer. *Seminars in Oncology Nursing, 15,* 292-302.

or death during cellular division. The specific process that causes this cellular damage is ionization, a complex process whereby a source of radiation emits energy sufficient to cause cellular atoms the radiation encounters to lose electrons orbiting around the nucleus. Liberated electrons attach themselves to other nearby atoms, converting these atomic fragments to a negatively charged state. A chain reaction is set up as electrons continue to displace other orbiting electrons, generating a release of energy. This energy has the capacity to cause both physical and chemical changes in living cells, which further results in modifications in cell structure and function.[26,35,92]

Therapeutic radiation is classified as either electromagnetic (x-rays, gamma rays) or particulate (alpha particles, beta particles, neutrons). Electromagnetic radiation is characterized by high energy and absence of mass[27,92] and may be machine generated (x-rays) or produced spontaneously through emission by radioactive substances undergoing decay (gamma rays). Examples of these radioactive substances include cobalt (frequently used in the past), and iridium, cesium, and iodine, which are more commonly used today. Both x-rays and gamma rays emit photons, discrete packets of energy. They have no electromagnetic charge, but their energy is transferred to the absorbing medium when they collide with the orbiting electrons of an atom. Three differ-

ent types of electromagnetic radiation are currently used in clinical practice. Superficial radiation covers the keV (kilo electron volt) range. Orthovoltage radiation spans the midrange of 125 to 500 keV. Megavoltage radiation involves the range above 500 keV. The level of penetration increases as the voltage level increases. Megavoltage radiation, unlike orthovoltage and superficial radiation, achieves its maximal dose deep in the tissues rather than on the skin surface. When superficial or orthovoltage therapy is used, skin reactions are often the dose-limiting toxicity. With the more commonly used skin-sparing machines of today, severe skin problems are rare. These physical properties of the different types of radiation are key concepts employed in planning radiation treatment.

Electromagnetic radiation undergoes ionization by three methods.[26,92] In the photoelectric effect, photon interaction results in the ejection of a tightly bound electron. The empty space created is subsequently filled by another electron from the atom's outer shell or from outside in a domino-like fashion. All, or at least a majority, of the photon's energy is lost in this process. The photoelectric effect varies with the cube of the atomic number (Z^3); thus, the higher the atomic number, the less the absorption. This explains why lead, which has a high atomic number, is such an effective shielding agent. It also means that at lower photon energies, bones will absorb more radiation than muscle or soft tissues, a concept also important to the field of diagnostic radiology. The Compton effect is the name given to this process of ionization where the photon gives up part, but not all, of its energy in a single interaction. A portion is reformulated as a secondary photon capable of causing subsequent ionization processes (Figure 5-1). Finally, high-energy photons are also capable of interacting with the atom's nucleus; when this occurs, the resultant energy is converted to matter. Two charged particles (positive and negative electrons) result from this interchange. Ionization that occurs in this manner is referred to as the pair production process and is possible only at energies higher than 1.02 MeV (mega or 1,000,000 electron volts). Electrons produced by the pair production process are also capable of further ionization reactions.

Radiation is not dependent upon the cell cycle for its effect. It causes lysis of the cell membrane or a break in both strands of DNA and prompts cellular death. DNA and RNA may be damaged by ionizing radiation in at least three ways, including base damage to pyrimidines (cytosine, thymine, and uracil), single strand breaks, and double helical breaks in DNA. These processes are responsible for the immediate tumoricidal effects and the acute toxicities. Cellular death is delayed when only a single DNA strand has been damaged. Such cells may not die until they attempt to divide, when the cellular defect in base RNA or DNA may become apparent. This helps to explain the variance in rapidity of tumor response to radiation treatment. Cell kinetics will help determine the speed of cell death following radiation. Whereas a rapidly dividing tumor will "melt away" with radiation treatment, a slowly dividing tumor will respond to radiation over weeks or months.

Normal and malignant cells that divide frequently are most susceptible to the effects of radiation. Highly mitotic normal cells, such as those of the skin, gastrointestinal mucosa, hair follicles, and bone marrow, are particularly susceptible to radiation effects. Tumors with rapid proliferation, such as leukemia and lymphoma, often respond quickly to radiation therapy. Conversely, tumors that divide more slowly are affected more slowly and respond over a more prolonged period of time. They often require a higher total dose of radiation for adequate treatment effect.

Molecular oxygen is considered the most important modifier of the biologic effect of radiation because the oxygen in the cell leads to the formation of free radicals that increase the damage to the cell's DNA.[35,92] Studies have consistently shown that higher doses of radiation are required under hypoxic conditions to achieve optimal cell destruc-

tion.[26] Thus tumors with necrotic or poorly oxygenated regions may respond less well to radiation. Conversely, well-oxygenated tissues and tumors have enhanced response to radiation. Red blood cell transfusions are given to maintain the hemoglobin above 10 g/dl during radiation therapy to enhance this oxygen effect.

Malignant cells have less ability to recover from the acute effects of radiation therapy than do normal cells. Both normal and malignant cells, however, attempt to repair themselves within three to four hours after exposure to radiation. Some of the late nontumor tissue effects arising in the irradiated treatment field may be related to failure of repair.[68,70] Repair may be inhibited by a variety of related factors, such as hypothermia; certain chemotherapeutic agents including dactinomycin, anthracyclines, bleomycin, cisplatin, and methotrexate; and tissue hypoxia. Each of these have been shown to inhibit cellular self-repair.*

RADIATION TREATMENT PLANNING

Before implementing a plan for radiation therapy, the overall goal of treatment must be defined. For most children, radiation therapy is used with curative intent; for some children with recurrent or metastatic disease, radiation therapy provides excellent palliation of troublesome symptoms (see Table 5-1). The following data must be assembled before initiating therapy: (1) the goal of therapy; (2) pertinent facts about the tumor such as size, location, and histologic grade; (3) relative volume of necrotic or poorly vascularized tissue within the

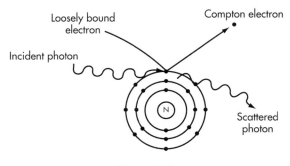

Figure 5-1

The Compton effect is the dominant reaction of the photon energies commonly used in radiation therapy. *N*, nucleus. (From Mieszkalski, G. B., Brady, L. W., Yaeger, T. E., et al. [2000]. Radiotherapy. In R. E. Lenhard, R. T. Osteen, & T. Gausler (Eds.), *Clinical oncology* (pp. 165-174). New York: American Cancer Society.)

*References 1, 35, 44, 55, 69, 76.

treatment field as assessed by imaging studies; (4) coexisting medical conditions; and (5) the age, physiologic, and psychologic condition of the child. The radiation oncologist then determines the total dose, volume, and number of radiation treatments to deliver as well as the frequency of treatment. The entire planning process may take hours to several days to complete.[26,35,65]

The therapeutic ratio, the relationship between the dose of radiation required to kill the tumor and the dose of radiation that normal adjacent tissue can safely tolerate, is established before the initiation of therapy. The radiation field is designed to exclude as much surrounding normal tissue as possible. Under most circumstances, the volume to be treated is prescribed as a dose that controls the tumor while not exceeding the tolerance of the tissue to be irradiated, and includes the volume of the tumor plus areas of potential local spread.[10,65]

Radiation therapy is fractionated, divided into separate small treatments or fractions, and delivered over a specified period of days or weeks. The usual range of time for radiation therapy is dependent on the total dose to be delivered. For example, radiation to the central nervous system (CNS) to prevent or treat CNS leukemia may be accomplished in approximately two weeks, whereas partial brain radiation for a malignant brain tumor may take six to seven weeks due to the higher total dose required to control the tumor.[22]

As a rule, the majority of radiation treatment plans used today require sophisticated analyses and equipment to establish an appropriate treatment field.[65] This may be accomplished by interfacing a treatment-planning computer with a computed tomography (CT) or magnetic resonance imaging (MRI) scan. The radiation absorbed dose (rad) defines the interaction between radiation and matter. In 1984 the term *gray* was officially designated as the unit of absorbed dose, measured in joules per kilogram. One gray (Gy) equals 100 rads or 100 cGy. Both terms (*rad* and *cGy*) have been used interchangeably in the past; however, Gy is now the preferred nomenclature and will be used throughout this text.

Once the specific treatment plan for a given patient has been established, an x-ray film of the designated treatment area is obtained. A simulator machine uses a diagnostic rather than a therapeutic-ranged dose of radiation to simulate the treatment field in terms of size, shape, angle, and volume. The radiographs obtained during this procedure are used to demonstrate adequate coverage of the tumor volume and the reproducibility of the treatment field. These films are kept as a permanent part of the patient's treatment record and are also used for quality-control purposes.

Today many children undergo three-dimensional conformal radiation therapy.[22] Conformal techniques focus the radiation beam, thereby avoiding unnecessary radiation exposure to surrounding normal tissue. Simulation for this type of radiation therapy is more complex than for traditional simulation.[35a]

The treatment field is defined in a variety of ways using skin marks or tattoos. Inked lines are sometimes replaced during treatment by tiny permanent tattoos that assist with reconstruction of the treatment field.[27,65] Although not painful, the procedure may be viewed by children as intrusive, and careful attention to patient and family preparation is essential. Today external marks are applied more often to an immobilization device such as a mask or cradle to avoid applying marks to the child's skin. A variety of external devices and molds are useful to immobilize the pediatric patient for purposes of treatment reproducibility (Figure 5-2).

Shielding devices constructed of lead are individually designed for each patient and used to protect healthy surrounding tissues and organs from unnecessary radiation exposure. Newer equipment allows the physician to "shape" the radiation beam. Using multileaf collimation, individual or multiple "leaves" open or close in such a way that cumbersome lead blocks used for shielding are not necessary.[51,64]

Conscious sedation or general anesthesia may be required to ensure adequate immobilization and accuracy for very young children.[22] Additionally, in certain situations the need for a surgical procedure such as ovarian transposition (oophoropexy) may be identified during the planning phase.

The accurate planning, organization, and implementation of the radiation program is a true team

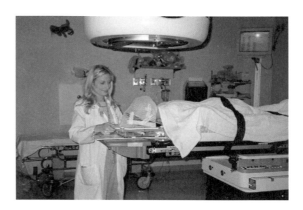

Figure 5-2

Plastic mesh head immobilization device.

effort that requires the input, involvement, and expertise of a variety of involved professionals. Most children treated for cancer in the United States and Canada are treated on carefully constructed treatment protocols reviewed and approved by the National Cancer Institute and developed and supervised by the Children's Oncology Group, a federally funded pediatric cancer research consortium. Experts in the field develop radiation guidelines for each protocol, and radiation performance is closely monitored by the Quality Assurance Review Center (QARC).

The radiation oncologist is a physician who clinically supervises and directs the therapy, manages the patient's care during treatment, delineates the area for treatment, and prescribes the appropriate radiation dose and plan of care. The radiation physicist and dosimetrist are instrumental in planning the specific treatment field. Trained radiation therapists deliver the prescribed therapy. Registered nurses and advanced practice nurses specializing in radiation oncology provide physical assessment, psychologic support, education, symptom management, and longitudinal follow-up.[80] Child life specialists may be involved in age-specific preparation and support for individual patients.

Once the radiation planning has been accomplished, the actual treatment sessions begin. Radiation treatments are generally scheduled daily on a Monday to Friday schedule. In an emergency situation, such as airway compromise or spinal cord compression, after-hours or weekend treatment may be necessary. For certain tumors, hyperfractionated schedules that employ multiple treatments at specific intervals during the same day are being investigated. Total body irradiation for bone marrow transplantation is also typically given according to a hyperfractionated schedule. Theoretically, such schedules allow an increase in the total delivered dose without an associated increase in late toxicity.[10,14,17,25]

Treatment verification films are obtained at various points during therapy to assess the reproducibility of the treatment fields. These portal films can be used to compare the proper positioning of the patient and the appropriate shielding of sensitive organs.

PSYCHOSOCIAL AND DEVELOPMENTAL CONSIDERATIONS

Adults undergoing radiation therapy have linked the distress surrounding this treatment to issues such as misconceptions or lack of knowledge about the treatment and its effects as well as their concern for their family's distress.[42,89] Children experience

distress as a result of the physical and psychologic ramifications of cancer and the necessary treatment. The child's developmental level may affect the manifestations of this response, with younger children tending to display more overt behavioral coping strategies.[94] Although study of specific radiation therapy–associated distress in children is limited, like adult studies the cancer distress experience for children has been linked to factors such as fear of the unknown and concern for their family.[94] In addition, the patient's developmental level, history of previous encounters with health care professionals, comorbid conditions, and the parental anxiety level significantly impact the child's ability to cooperate with radiation therapy procedures.[2,22,71,75,94] Meticulous nursing care entails attention to the multidimensional distress experience of the pediatric radiation-oncology patient.

Radiation treatment requires considerable cooperation on the part of the patient. Simulation procedures at the beginning of therapy often take an hour or more to complete. Thereafter, total treatment time may be as little as 5 to 10 minutes. However, since treatment demands complete cooperation to ensure accuracy, developmental level and distress response can significantly affect the treatment routine.

Developmentally, children younger than 3 years of age are unable to remain still without assistance. Young children (less than 3 years) have little ability to understand complex explanations of the anticipated procedure. They require pharmaceutical assistance in order to assure accurate delivery of therapy. A mild sedative such as lorazepam (Ativan) or diazepam (Valium) administered 1 hour before the scheduled treatment time, conscious sedation, or a short-acting general anesthetic such as propofol is indicated.[39] In addition to this pharmaceutical intervention the separation anxiety experienced by this age group should be addressed through consistent caregivers and parental presence.[71]

Unlike the young child, a preschool child (4 to 6 years of age) may benefit from behavioral intervention strategies and explanations that focus on sensory information. Explanations need to be simple and concrete and are best given within a few minutes of the actual procedure. Preschool children's magical thinking and developmental tendency toward fears of bodily intrusion and separation from their parents can be addressed through the employment of play therapy, exploration, and rewards.[2,71,75] For example, rewards may come in the form of a trip to the "treasure box." Allowing children to wear their own clothes into the treatment suite may be helpful, especially with preschool-age children who have fears about body integrity.[39]

These interventions take time and planning and require a team commitment to this approach.

Behavioral intervention strategies may also be more formal. Some programs have been shown effective in eliminating the need for pharmaceutical intervention in this age-group. For example, the Starbright Hospital Pals Program[79] is specifically directed to the preschool-age child undergoing radiation therapy. (For more information please refer to http://www.starbright.org or call 310-479-1212.) Other behavioral modification methods have also been successfully employed to desensitize preschool children to the new environment, thereby allowing them to achieve success in motion control without pharmaceutical intervention.[2,75]

Barring other conditions, school-age children (7 to 12 years) generally tolerate radiation treatments without pharmaceutical intervention. They are able to process sophisticated information. Because they are task-oriented and eager to please, school-age children are often interested in the actual workings of the equipment and should be encouraged to ask questions.[2,39,71] Appropriate preparation for the procedure includes explanations, tours, and teaching mediums (e.g., videos, coloring books) to alleviate the fear of the unknown.[22] Parents can help their child learn to cope with the required immobilization by having their child practice lying still on a flat surface at home, making a game out of this, and rewarding positive behavior.[2]

Like the school-age child, the adolescent can generally cope well with the radiation procedure itself. Adolescents are able to formally process information and plan for the future.[71] Sensitivity to concerns about body image is warranted. Education and explanation of the treatment are important in decreasing the distress they experience as a result of uncertainty.[56,71] With body image being a main concern, adolescents may be particularly resistant to the idea of the permanent skin tattoos applied to reconstruct the treatment field accurately.[39,71]

Side effects of treatment, treatment outcomes, safety, and equipment are areas of concern for patients and families.[2,42,71,89] Distress may be enhanced by fear of the unknown and misinformation.[34,89] Parents may mistakenly believe that their child will be "radioactive" after leaving the radiation department and worry that their child's skin, clothing, urine, and stool will be contaminated and dangerous to others. This is not the case, and no radiation safety precautions are required for those undergoing external beam radiation therapy. Since many children receiving radiation treatment also attend school or day care centers, school personnel and other students may need to be provided with this basic information.[24]

Children experience many sources of distress during their cancer treatment, including concern for their families' distress levels.[94] Because patient and family distress levels are intimately related, supporting the family is integral to the support of the child.[2,71,94] Anticipatory guidance throughout treatment and assistance in managing side effects helps to alleviate patient and family distress.[42,71,89] Concrete explanations of the mechanisms of radiation and printed information about the procedure are useful. The child and family should be informed that even though radiation is a brief and silent treatment, the machinery involved in the delivery of the therapy might make noise. In addition, close collaboration between radiation department personnel and pediatric oncology nursing staff provides a smooth transition when this modality is part of the comprehensive treatment plan.[39]

Immobilization Devices

Reproducibility in positioning is essential to delivering safe and effective treatment. In addition to a cooperative child, immobilization devices are essential. The devices themselves, however, may increase a child's anxiety level and make pharmaceutical intervention necessary. In general, individualized molds and devices allow the most accurate delivery. The use of head holders, bite blocks, chin supports, mesh casts fit to the individual patient, customized vacuum fixation bags, or individualized casts may be employed to ensure reproducibility of treatment positioning each day[22,35,58] (see Figure 5-2). Each center will employ an immobilization device that works for them.

SIDE EFFECTS OF RADIATION THERAPY

The majority of side effects of radiation develop within the first 2 to 3 weeks from the initiation of treatment.[80] The acute effects of radiation therapy are generally the result of damage to tissues with rapidly dividing cells and are location and dose dependent[35] (Table 5-2). These acute effects usually appear within days to weeks from the beginning of treatment, continue throughout the course of treatment, and last for several weeks to months following completion.[35] Since most children receiving radiation therapy are treated on an outpatient basis, it is important that parents and caregivers receive adequate information about anticipated side effects and management.[80]

Skin

As a tissue with rapid renewal properties, the skin is particularly susceptible to radiation effects. These range from mild to severe. Hyperpigmenta-

TABLE 5-2	ACUTE RESPONSES TO RADIATION THERAPY
Site	**Response**
Skin	Loss of epidermal layer
	Erythema, dryness
	Wet desquamation
	Hyperpigmentation
GI tract	Mucositis
	Proctitis
	Dysphagia
	Ulceration
	Nausea, vomiting
	Diarrhea
	Anorexia/malnutrition
Salivary glands	Decreased formation of saliva
	Dry mucous membranes
	Taste distortion
	Dysphagia
Kidneys/bladder	Cystitis
Bone marrow	Myelosuppression
	Anemia
	Thrombocytopenia
Hair follicle	Hair loss
Lungs	Pneumonitis
Heart	Myocarditis/pericarditis
Brain/spinal cord	Edema
Ovary/testes	Amenorrhea
	Decrease in sperm production

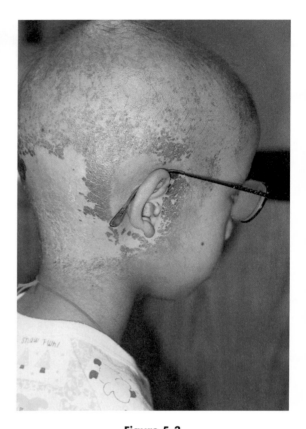

Figure 5-3

Dry desquamation after cranial irradiation.

tion results from stimulation of melanocytes in the radiation field.[34,35,88] The function of sweat and sebaceous glands may lessen or cease.[32,88] In addition, erythema may occur, progressing to dry desquamation (Figure 5-3), moist desquamation, and, rarely, ulceration and necrosis.[32,34,35] Only skin located within the radiation field, including the exit site, will develop a reaction.

A typical skin reaction may appear at the irradiated site 2 to 3 weeks into therapy and increase until 1 to 2 weeks after the treatments have ended.[34,35] The skin may be pruritic with concomitant inflammation, erythema, hyperpigmentation, dryness (e.g., flaking), and irritation (Table 5-3). This dry desquamation can progress to moist desquamation with areas of denudation as the epidermis loses its renewal cells.[34,35,88] A subacute cutaneous reaction may be experienced 2 to 4 months after completion of therapy that includes late phase erythema.[88]

It is advisable to instruct parents to observe the skin regularly for areas of breakdown and to avoid friction, scrubbing, and the use of abrasive skin products. Children will be most comfortable if clothing is loose rather than constrictive. Curved

TABLE 5-3	SKIN REACTIONS TO EXTERNAL BEAM RADIATION
Stage I	Inflammation
	Erythema
	Mild edema
Stage II	Dry desquamation
Stage III	Moist desquamation
Stage IV	Ulceration
	Fibrosis
	Atrophy

body areas and skin folds, such as in the axilla or groin, may be sites of excoriation and may require special attention[32,34,88] (Box 5-1).

Certain creams, deodorants, and lotions can enhance skin reactions by causing radiation particles to pause as they enter the surface. These should be avoided.[32] Patients should use only skin products recommended by the radiation staff on the area receiving radiation. For best results, these should be applied several times per day as both a prophylactic and treatment measure. Any product should be completely removed and the skin should be clean and dry immediately before daily treatments. Pruritus can be treated with a corticosteroid cream such as 1% triamcinolone acetonide.[34,84] If a reaction progresses to a moist desquamation, cleansing with normal saline and leaving the area open to air or dressing with moisture- and vapor-permeable dressings is advisable. Topical application of antibiotic creams such as 1% silver sulfadiazine can also be considered. Heat or very hot water should be avoided, and the irradiated area should be protected. After bathing, pat the skin dry with a soft towel and avoid rubbing or excessive abrasion. Parents are instructed to avoid removing the radiation marks or applying coverlets or tape to the skin in the radiated field.[32,34,88] Care must be taken when the central venous line dressing is in the field of radiation, with removal of the dressing before the treatment each day and close monitoring and treatment for local skin reaction (see Box 5-1). The radiation oncology nurse will assess the skin on an ongoing basis for evidence of reaction and provide guidance.

Recommended moisturizing products must be free of alcohol or perfumes because of their drying effect and must not be water resistant (e.g., petroleum jelly). These agents leave a residue in the radiation field that may enhance the reaction. Specific cleansing agents include mild soaps such as Dove or warm water rinses without soap. Moisturizing products should be water soluble, such as those that are aloe vera or lanolin based. Specific mois-

turizers include Lubriderm and Eucerin.[34,35,84,88] Studies are ongoing in an effort to find products for radiation-induced skin reactions.

Most skin reactions resolve within several weeks of onset. Following resolution, the skin will usually feel and appear normal except for a temporary slightly hyperpigmented appearance. Depending on the dose of radiation, the healed epidermal layer may be somewhat atrophic and more fragile due to damage to vascular and connective tissue. Exposure of irradiated skin to the sun should be minimized to avoid later skin damage.[34,35,88]

ALOPECIA

Radiation produces local alopecia in the radiation field, including the scalp if it was involved. Following the radiation effect on scalp hair, and in descending order, is the effect of radiation on facial hair, eyebrows, eyelashes, axillary hair, pubic hair, and body hair.[88] Loss usually begins around the third week of treatment.[35] In general, radiation doses of 25 to 30 Gy will lead to temporary thinning of hair, and doses of 45 to 55 Gy will cause complete alopecia. These are generally temporary and reversible. Doses greater than 55 Gy generally result in permanent thinning or loss.[88] Children and their families need factual information about the nature of hair loss and should be encouraged to obtain appropriate head coverings suitable to the child's age, gender, and developmental level.

GASTROINTESTINAL

Oral

Radiation to the head and neck, as in facial or cranial parameningeal tumors near the base of the skull, may cause side effects that significantly impact the child's quality of life.[2] In addition, normal developmental events such as tooth exfoliation and eruption may lead to more complications.[38] Children who receive head and neck radiation may develop abnormal or blunted tooth roots and may be candidates for early permanent tooth loss if ongoing, consistent dental care is not given.[52,53]

Oral mucositis or radioepithelitis and the related pain, infection, and nutritional problems may occur. The sensitivity response of the oral epithelial barrier may develop within a week from the start of treatment and can progress to an ulcerative state.[12,35] Concurrent administration of certain chemotherapeutic agents can significantly increase the severity of this response to treatment.[2,82] Some studies have shown that the prophylactic use of antimicrobial lozenges in radiation-induced mucositis may reduce the severity.[12] Refer to Chapter 11 for more information on the care of the child with mucositis.

Another radiation-induced complication may be xerostomia (dry mouth). This results from damage to the salivary glands leading to hyposalivation. This then may lead to dental caries, altered taste sensation, difficulty with mastication, dysphagia, and infection.[23,52] Studies have shown that radiation-induced xerostomia actually changes the microflora of the oral cavity, including increased incidence of colonization by *Candida albicans*.[11,12,38] Comfort measures for xerostomia include the use of extra oral lubricants, moist foods, and rinsing with half-strength hydrogen peroxide preparations to clear thick mucous.[2,23,29] A sialagogue (medication for increasing the flow of saliva) should be considered if age-appropriate. In addition, antifungal preparations such as nystatin are considered for prophylactic measures. However, care must be taken to continue meticulous monitoring, as the patient may still develop candidiasis.[12]

Anticipatory guidance and appropriate education throughout treatment is necessary. Care must be taken to maintain moisture of the mucous membranes by frequent intake of fluids. A mouth care regimen is employed from the outset. A complete baseline dental evaluation by a pedodontist with knowledge in the area of pediatric oncology is recommended before the initiation of head and neck radiation therapy. Fluoride carriers (appliances similar to orthodontic retainers that are filled with topical fluoride solution) and fluoride mouth washes are indicated to minimize risk of radiation caries. The rinses are better tolerated by children.[2]

ESOPHAGITIS/DYSPHAGIA

Radiation to the chest or upper back, including craniospinal radiation, can cause esophagitis, leading to odynophagia, and dysphagia with its related complications. Milk and milk products can help ease discomfort. Sucralfate (Carafate), an agent commonly used in ulcer regimens, often helps relieve symptoms and may decrease the severity of the esophagitis induced by radiation.[12] Esophagitis may also be exacerbated by gastrointestinal reflux. This can be addressed through pharmaceutical intervention.[2] Again, anticipatory guidance and ongoing assessment of these common radiation effects must continue throughout treatment. Refer to Chapter 11 for further management recommendations.

Nausea and Vomiting

Nausea and vomiting, generally seen only with radiation to the abdomen or the brain, can be alleviated by the use of antiemetic agents. Phenothiazine agents, such as chlorpromazine and prochlorperazine, are discouraged, as these agents can cause excessive sedation and extrapyramidal side effects.

The serotonin-antagonist antiemetic agents, such as ondansetron (Zofran) and granisetron (Kytril) have been found to be very effective in controlling these symptoms. Nutritional ramifications of nausea and vomiting must also be promptly addressed. Refer to Chapter 11 for additional information about the treatment of nausea and vomiting.

Nutrition

In addition to the nutritional issues that arise with nausea, vomiting, and altered oral mucosal integrity, the problems of dehydration and weight loss must be promptly addressed, especially in the young child who must be NPO for daily general anesthesia or sedation. Malnutrition and weight loss are common in the pediatric oncology patient due to a number of factors including a combination of increased metabolic demands and the necessary treatment approaches.[9,46] Radiation treatment requiring daily or twice daily restriction of oral intake can have an additive effect, leading to malnutrition. A child may quickly lose greater than 5% of preillness weight, which is a recommended cutoff for nutritional intervention in children.[46] One strategy that may be employed to ameliorate this loss includes the scheduling of treatment of young children in the early morning to facilitate oral intake throughout the remainder of the day. For additional information on nutritional intervention, refer to Chapter 11.

Diarrhea

Radiation therapy delivered to the pelvis or lower back may cause diarrhea. A low-residue diet, elimination or restriction of milk and milk products, and optimal fluid intake may be used to relieve gastrointestinal symptoms. The anal mucosa is inspected regularly for evidence of ulceration, especially if neutropenia has developed. Meticulous skin care is mandatory when radiation is delivered to the groin and perianal areas. Daily sitz baths may provide comfort and hygiene. Antidiarrheal agents may be indicated but used only under the close supervision of the oncology team. Parents are instructed not to take the child's temperature via the rectal route. Likewise, rectal suppositories and enemas are contraindicated.

Pneumonitis

Patients who receive high doses of radiation to a large volume of the lungs can develop pneumonitis. Pneumonitis is a complication in up to 20% of patients who receive radiation to the chest.[74] Symptoms of acute radiation pneumonitis usually develop within 2 to 12 weeks after completion of treatment, and a subacute fibrosis may develop 3 to

6 months after the completion of therapy.[74] Pneumonitis is generally a self-limited pulmonary inflammation resulting from damage to the alveolar cells and endothelial layer that may present with cough, dyspnea, or low-grade fever. It may be asymptomatic, with only radiographic findings.[35,74] Prompt attention should be sought for respiratory symptoms such as tachypnea, orthopnea, dyspnea, nonproductive cough, increased respiratory effort, or diminished oxygen saturation. Supportive therapy includes the administration of oxygen, systemic corticosteroids, and cough suppressants. Coughing and deep breathing exercises should be encouraged to help prevent pneumonia.[74] Tapering of steroids must be very slow and conservative following lung irradiation. Prophylaxis for Pneumocystis carinii pneumonia is indicated for children undergoing radiation therapy and particularly for those maintained on steroids or concomitant chemotherapy regimens.[2,15] Subacute or chronic radiation pneumonitis can be a life-threatening condition, necessitating hospitalization and occasionally mechanical ventilation.

Cystitis

Cystitis can occur after radiation to the pelvis or lower back. Inadequate fluid intake and an alkaline urinary pH accelerate the development of cystitis. Encouraging a high fluid intake and maintaining an acidic (<7.0) urinary pH by increasing the child's intake of citrus juices, for example, is helpful in this regard. If symptoms persist or worsen, a urinalysis and urine culture should be obtained, urinary tract analgesics prescribed, and appropriate antibiotic therapy instituted if bacterial infection is demonstrated.[80]

Fatigue

Many patients receiving radiation therapy report vague symptoms of fatigue and malaise that develop after the initiation of treatment. Headache may be a complaint of children receiving cranial radiation. Children feel energetic during the early hours of the day and may want to attend school in the morning. They often, however, display decreased energy reserve and require more sleep and a daily nap.[28]

Over the past decade fatigue has been recognized as a significant complication of cancer and its treatment, which can affect a patient's quality of life.[4,30,63,93] One adult study investigating radiation-induced fatigue found that it usually improved 3 to 6 months after the completion of treatment.[30] However, many adult cancer survivors report persistent fatigue.[45,93] The recognition of fatigue in adult cancer patients and survivors has led to re-

search in pediatric patients, and recently a conceptual model for cancer-related fatigue in children and adolescents was developed.[28] A study of adult childhood cancer survivors found that fatigue significantly impacted their daily lives,[37] and research in pediatrics is ongoing. Nursing interventions directed toward assessment of potential causes of fatigue during radiation include medications and other conditions or psychologic factors. The nurse can offer education and anticipatory guidance to the patient and family in ameliorating this symptom.[30,45,63,93]

Postradiation somnolence syndrome is related specifically to neurologic changes following cranial irradiation and is probably the result of temporary demyelinization.[35] It usually occurs 3 to 12 weeks after completion of cranial irradiation and may last a few days to a few weeks.[22,72] Symptoms may include varying degrees of lethargy, nausea and vomiting, anorexia, headache, ataxia, dysarthria, and dysphagia.[2,35]

Somnolence syndrome is worrisome for staff and families alike, as the symptoms may suggest worsening of CNS symptoms related to the child's underlying disease. After confirmation that tumor progression or regrowth has not occurred, care revolves primarily around supporting the patient and family until symptoms abate.

Bone Marrow Suppression

The effect of radiation therapy on the hematopoietic system must not be overlooked. Areas of bone marrow in the radiation field are affected in a manner similar to the effects of chemotherapy. Neutropenia, anemia, and thrombocytopenia may all result and contribute to the cumulative toxicities the child experiences. Radiation to major sites of active bone marrow including the pelvis and sternum often results in myelosuppression.[2] For example, the child receiving radiation to the spinal axis may sustain prolonged thrombocytopenia and anemia. Because the effectiveness of radiation is related to the availability of oxygen, maintenance of the hemoglobin level of at least 10 g/dl is recommended. Hemoglobin values below this level may limit tumor cell kill and compromise the efficacy of therapy.[35,83] Children receiving radiation to large areas of bone marrow will have weekly complete blood counts (CBCs) performed, with results communicated to the radiation oncology department. Packed red blood cell and platelet transfusions are indicated in the event of persistently low blood counts.

Combined Modality Therapy

Plateaus in cure rates of pediatric cancers led to the use of combined modality treatment strategies.

These were designed to overcome obstacles to established therapies and provide synergistic effect on tumor cell kill. Ideally, treatment strategies will not have similar toxicity patterns and therefore can be used to the fullest extent possible. The use of chemotherapy, surgery, and radiation therapy has significantly improved the survival rates in many childhood malignancies.[20,44] Combined treatment plans may include concurrent or alternative sequencing of chemotherapy and radiation therapy. Specifically, the chemotherapy and radiation treatments may be remote, sequential, alternating, or simultaneous treatment.[85] The strategy will depend to a large extent on the interaction of the toxicity profiles, the synergistic properties of combined modalities, and the specific intent of the treatment (e.g., chemotherapy as a debulking strategy before radiation therapy versus chemotherapy as a radiosensitizer).[20,44] To improve the treatment of pediatric malignancies the feasibility of employing different treatment modalities instead of standard treatment is under ongoing review.[81]

The effects of multimodal treatment require close monitoring, because the toxicities may be exacerbated.[44] One example of this is the recall phenomenon that may be observed when chemoradiotherapy is employed. Recall is an inflammatory reaction of affected tissues. Radiation recall may be seen when the administration of certain chemotherapeutic agents follows radiation therapy. Reverse recall may be seen when radiation follows chemotherapy treatment.[44] This phenomenon is thought to be an exacerbation of subclinical DNA damage caused by one modality when the second modality is employed. Often radiation recall is seen as a cutaneous reaction; however, it can involve deeper tissues such as the lung, mucous membranes, esophagus, and gastrointestinal tract. Cutaneous manifestations include painless erythema, desquamation, and necrosis.[44,82] It may occur even when chemotherapy and radiation therapy are administered remotely from one another (days to years).[44,48,82] Box 5-2 lists the drugs that cause radiation recall.

Specific precautions with combined modality therapy should be recognized. For example, dactinomycin followed by radiation can lead to pneumonitis.[44] The heart damage caused by doxorubicin can be increased when the chest is irradiated.[69] Methotrexate followed by cranial radiation leads to an increased incidence of acute encephalopathy.[44] Methotrexate and craniospinal radiation can also lead to a chronic neurotoxicity known as leukoencephalopathy. The incidence is increased when radiation precedes intrathecal or intravenous methotrexate. It may result in de-

---

BOX 5-2

CHEMOTHERAPEUTIC AGENTS ASSOCIATED WITH RADIATION RECALL

Bleomycin
Cyclophosphamide
Cytarabine
Dactinomycin
Daunorubicin
Docetaxel
Doxorubicin
Etoposide
Fluorouracil
Hydroxyurea
Idarubicin
Lomustine
Melphalan
Methotrexate
Paclitaxel
Tamoxifen
Trimetrexate
Vinblastine

From Susser, W. S., Whitaker-Worth, D. L., & Grant-Kels, J. M. (1999). Continuing medical education: Mucocutaneous reactions to chemotherapy. *Journal of the Academy of Dermatology, 40,* 367-398.

---

creased cognitive function and focal neurologic signs or seizures. In severe cases, the neuronal injury can lead to coma or death.[49]

Certain chemotherapeutic agents are being employed as radiosensitizers. Drugs such as cisplatin, carboplatin, doxorubicin, mitomycin-C, hydroxyurea, paclitaxel, and the camptothecins are used as or are being investigated for their potentiating effects.[36,69,90] Similar to but separate from the recall phenomenon is the radiation enhancement phenomenon, seen when chemotherapy and radiation are administered for their synergistic effect. They must be administered together or within 7 days of each other. Enhancement may occur in any organ and synergises the damage caused by each modality separately. The process is generally self-limited, but some additional supportive care measures may be needed.[82]

The acute effects of radiation are summarized in Table 5-2. The long-term effects of this treatment modality are varied and depend on site of radiation therapy, dose of therapy delivered, use of other treatment modalities, and age at the time of therapy. Radiation therapy can lead to a number of chronic postradiation syndromes that may result in, among other things, chronic pain.[3] Recent research has also shown that chest irradiation can lead to subclinical myocardial damage, increasing the risk of congestive heart failure and coronary artery disease.[61] Radiation including the long bones has

TABLE 5-4	DELAYED AND LATE RESPONSES TO RADIATION THERAPY
Site	**Response**
Skin	Fibrosis/atrophy
	Telangiectasis, ulceration
GI tract	Fibrosis
	Loss of taste sensation
	Enteritis
	Bowel obstruction
Salivary glands	Xerostomia
	Dental caries
Kidneys/bladder	Renal insufficiency
	Bladder fibrosis
Bone marrow	Chronic anemia
	Aplasia (rare)
Hair	Permanent epilation (hair loss)
Lungs	Fibrosis
Heart	Pericarditis
	Valvular disorders
	Vascular compromise
	Cardiomyopathy
Brain	Loss of cognitive ability
	Attentional difficulties
	Leukoencephalopathy
Neuronal	Peripheral neuropathy
Neck	Thyroid dysfunction
Eyes	Cataracts
	Decreased tear production
	Radiation retinopathy
	Scleral melting
Bone	Alteration in bone growth
	Fractures
Neuroendocrine	Hypothalamic/pituitary dysfunction
Ovary/testis	Sterility
Other	Second malignancy

been linked to an increased incidence of fractures.[86] The neuropsychologic effect of cranial radiation on the developing brain significantly impacts survivors' quality of life.[54] Problems with attention, memory, mental processing speed, and behavior have been identified and present ongoing challenges for patients and families.[47,54,57,71] Issues such as growth retardation, body asymmetry, endocrine dysfunction, cataracts, and cognitive problems are summarized in Table 5-4 and are discussed in detail in Chapter 18.

INNOVATIVE TREATMENT APPROACHES

HYPERFRACTIONATION

Hyperfractionation refers to the delivery of more than one radiation treatment per day, without altering the duration of the overall treatment course. In the pediatric arena, hyperfractionated radiation therapy is used for bone marrow conditioning regimens before transplantation. It has been studied in the treatment of aggressive CNS tumors (specifically those in the brainstem) and nonresected soft tissue and bone sarcomas, such as rhabdomyosarcoma and Ewing's sarcoma.[14,22,25,35] The rationale underlying this approach is that treating tumors with a high proliferation rate more than once a day may increase tumor cell kill and decrease repair between fractions. Although each individual fraction delivers a lower dose, the total dose over the entire treatment period is higher. Preliminary data in brain tumor patients do not indicate a higher incidence of toxicity with this approach, although the need for longitudinal analysis is indicated.[14] There is the potential for serious or possibly irreversible toxicity, and pilot studies with meticulous attention and assessment must be undertaken before this treatment approach is routine. Scheduling multiple treatments a day may be problematic for patients and families, especially if sedation is required. Coordination between family schedules and radiation department is essential.

INTRAOPERATIVE RADIATION THERAPY

Intraoperative radiation therapy (IORT) involves delivery of radiation treatment in the operating room directly to the tumor or tumor bed during surgery. Theoretic advantages are the area to be treated is directly visualized, the treatment field is precisely defined, and normal adjacent structures can be protected from the radiation beam.[7,18,19,21,67]

A commonly administered pediatric intraoperative radiation dose for a solid tumor is 10 Gy, although higher doses are possible. The tumor bed is measured to accommodate introduction of a Lucite cone, which in turn is attached to the radiation machine. After resection of as much of the tumor as possible, the radiation dose is delivered, and then the operative procedure is completed. The highest theoretic benefit of intraoperative radiation is for microscopic or minimal residual disease. In the pediatric setting, intraoperative radiation therapy has been used in patients with rhabdomyosarcoma, neuroblastoma, Wilms tumor, and Ewing's sarcoma, as well as primitive neuroepithelioma. Studies of small numbers of children suggest that local control is improved with the addition of this method of therapy.[7,19,21]

Initial concerns regarding increased infection rates and delayed wound healing have not been borne out.[7,67] In unresectable tumors treated with IORT possible metabolic and renal abnormalities from tumor lysis have not been reported. A primary limiting factor of this modality is the logistic dilemma of orchestrating a multidisciplinary, and often multiinstitutional, effort. Many institutions do not have the facilities for IORT, and transportation to a new facility can cause stress for both patient and family. If IORT is planned, a preoperative tour is advisable so that staff, patient, and family will feel more comfortable. Although indications for IORT are limited in pediatrics, this modality provides an innovative treatment for specific difficult clinical situations.

INTERSTITIAL RADIATION THERAPY

Interstitial radiation therapy, also known as implant therapy or brachytherapy, has limited use in children. In contrast to external beam radiation therapy, the radioactive material is implanted directly into the tumor bed. The radiation sources used (iridium, radioactive iodine, and cesium) have limited penetration, so large local doses of radiation can be administered with minimal delivery to adjacent tissues. Such implants provide an additional "boost" for specific tumors without inflicting significant damage to normal tissues.[22,62,91]

Interstitial implants may provide improved local control for recurrent retinoblastoma, soft tissue tumors, and certain malignant brain tumors. Although experience in children is limited, interstitial implants have been used in adults with malignant brain tumors who had received prior radiation therapy.[13,60] In such situations the interstitial afterloading catheters are placed with CT guidance and are then loaded with the radioactive isotope. The catheters are left in place for a specific time and deliver a specific dose. Research in this area is ongoing.

The use of interstitial radiation therapy in children requires organized multispecialty care. Nurses and allied health personnel who care for these children must stringently follow safety precautions. Sources of radiation are cesium, iridium, and gold or iodine 125 seeds, and the radiation is delivered in enclosed or sealed sources. The radiation from these sources is not absorbed systemically by the body, nor is it excreted like unsealed sources of radiation such as iodine 131, which is used for treatment of thyroid cancer.

General guidelines for care of a child receiving brachytherapy using sealed sources include assigning the child to a private room with a private bath, placing a caution sign on the door, and ensuring appropriate shielding to avoid contact with other patients. Health care personnel must wear a dosimeter badge at all times while caring for their patients. Pregnant health care workers must not care for these patients, and pregnant women, or children under 18 years of age, must not visit. The amount

of time per visit is determined by the amount of radiation emitted, but generally it is limited to 30 minutes per visitor per day. In the unlikely event that the radioactive source becomes dislodged, it is retrieved only by the responsible radiation oncologist using long-handled forceps and deposited in a lead container. The necessary isolation practice may prove stressful to the pediatric patient, and appropriate education and orientation of the child, family, and involved health care workers must be conducted before the initiation of this therapy.[10,22]

CHEMICAL MODIFIERS

Two categories of compounds are being evaluated as adjuvants to radiation therapy at the present time: (1) radiosensitizers and (2) radioprotectors. Radiosensitizers theoretically increase oxygenation to hypoxic cells and thereby render them more sensitive to the effects of radiation, or they may work through interference with the cell cycle of rapidly dividing cells.[83] To date, radiosensitizers have failed to prove useful or tolerable, but research in adults is ongoing.[73,83] As discussed previously, certain chemotherapeutic agents are also being employed and investigated for their radiosensitization properties.[22]

Radioprotectors theoretically shield normal cells from radiation damage by using substances absorbed by healthy cells but not by tumor cells. Amifostine is a drug that has recently been shown to provide radioprotective effects for adults undergoing radiation therapy and multimodal therapy.[6,8,50,87] It is also being studied in the pediatric population as a chemoprotectant and will likely be trialed soon as a radioprotectant.

THREE-DIMENSIONAL CONFORMAL RADIATION

Three-dimensional (3-D) conformal radiation therapy delivers high-dose radiation tailored to the target volume while delivering a low dose to the patient's nontarget tissues. This innovative delivery system was made possible by a variety of technological advances. Refinements in CT and MRI imaging capabilities now provide accurate three-dimensional representations of the patient's anatomy and tumor volume. Additionally, the computer industry has recently produced equipment to support this technology. Radiation accelerator manufacturers have used this advanced microcircuitry and computer technology to produce equipment that more precisely shapes the delivered radiation so it "conforms" to the anatomy of the patient and the tumor to be treated. This method is particularly appealing in radiation treatments designed to achieve local tumor control while preserving normal function and minimizing long-term morbidity.

Three-dimensional conformal radiation therapy requires proper patient immobilization for precise reproducibility of the radiation field on a daily basis. Sophisticated new immobilization systems are required to achieve this end[51,58,64] (Figure 5-4). The target volume and organs at risk must be carefully identified. The dose prescription, design of the beam shape, and orientation of the beam in 3-D requires careful calculation and subsequent evaluation prior to implementation. While 3-D conformal radiation is not yet available at all treatment centers, it is available in most pediatric cancer centers and is expected to replace the conventional simulator and two-dimensional dose planning systems within the next 10 years.

RADIOSURGERY

Radiosurgery is a highly sophisticated 3-D technique that employs stereotactic localization to direct radiation to a small, precisely defined target.[40,41,43,66] Stereotaxis refers to a precise positioning in space and most often applies to specific areas of the brain. Such focused radiation is delivered by multiple independent sources directed to a single target by a gamma knife or linear accelerator. Immobilization is paramount in this type of treatment. This is now possible because of newer, more effective immobilization devices and sedation techniques.[40,66,80]

The ablative dose can be delivered either in a single session or in multiple sessions. Fractionated radiosurgery or stereotactic radiotherapy combines precision volume delivery with the biologic advantages of fractionating the total dose.[40,66,80] This method is ideal for certain inoperable lesions that are small and well defined. It is used in the treatment of some low-grade gliomas and is undergoing investigation in recurrent lesions or those resistant to standard radiation.[40] Stereotactic radiosurgery in the pediatric population has been trialed in various intracranial tumor types, including low-grade and high-grade gliomas and recurrent ependymomas.[16,77,78]

Generally, the acute side effects of stereotactic procedures in the treatment of intracranial lesions in children are minimal. They include discomfort from the pressure of the frame and a mild headache.[80] Occasionally, edema will occur months later, which may lead to some neurologic deficit depending on the site. The effect of this treatment modality on long-term sequelae of cranial radiation in children has yet to be determined.[39]

NURSING IMPLICATIONS

As stated throughout this chapter, nurses have a large role to play in caring for the pediatric patient undergoing radiation therapy. The ramifications of this type of treatment are both acute and chronic. While the use of this method with other modalities has lead to increased survival rates in many types of childhood cancer, the effects of treatment on normal growing tissues can be immense. The impact can lead to lifelong challenges.

Nurses working with the radiation-oncology pediatric patient have the opportunity to help to provide multidimensional care for the patient and family. In addition, they may provide coordination of care among various disciplines working with the patient, including child life, psychology, medical oncology, and surgery. The child's needs range from the psychosocial concerns surrounding the treatment itself to acute toxicity issues to anticipatory guidance in managing long-term effects. In the context of a therapeutic relationship, the nurse can help guide the family through symptom management strategies and setting realistic long-term goals.

With an understanding of the treatment rationale and its effects on the tumor and normal tissue, the nurse can be an excellent educator for the entire family. As stated previously, uncertainty is intimately related to patient distress. Nurses who are sensitive to the developmental needs of the patient and to the informational needs of the family are in an excellent position to significantly impact the quality of life during the radiation experience. Thorough nursing assessment, planning, and intervention can significantly alter a child's experience.

FUTURE DIRECTIONS

Research efforts are ongoing in the field of radiation therapy in an effort to provide sophisticated treatment that results in effective tumor cell kill

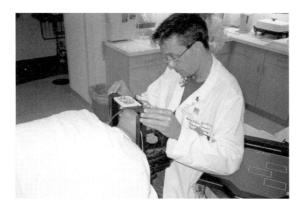

Figure 5-4

Head immobilization device.

while sparing normal tissue. These efforts are critical in the field of pediatric oncology, where survival rates for most tumors are good and the need to prevent long-term morbidity is paramount. Research focusing on developing ever more sophisticated equipment is ongoing. The enrollment of the majority of eligible children on nationally supported clinical trials enables data to be accumulated in a systematic and timely fashion. National monitoring centers also help ensure consistent quality of delivered treatment. While radiation therapy is a complicated modality, pediatric oncology nurses can assist in the education of patients and families by providing ongoing information and clarification.

ACKNOWLEDGMENT

The authors express sincere appreciation to Sarah Donaldson, MD, for her careful review of this chapter.

REFERENCES

1. Begg, A. C. (1998). Prediction of radiation response. In S. A. Leibel & T. L. Philips (Eds.), *Textbook of radiation oncology* (pp. 55-68). Philadelphia: W. B. Saunders.
2. Bucholtz, J. D. (1994). Comforting children during radiotherapy. *Oncology Nursing Forum, 21,* 987-994.
3. Caraceni, A. (1996). Pain and palliative care: Clinicopathologic correlates of common cancer pain syndromes. *Hematology Oncology Clinics of North America, 10,* 58-78.
4. Clarke, P. M., & Lacasse, C. (1998). Cancer-related fatigue: Clinical practice issues. *Clinical Journal of Oncology Nursing, 2,* 45-53.
5. Coutard, H. (1934). Principles of x-ray therapy of malignant disease. *Lancet, 2,* 1-8.
6. Curran, W. J. (1998). Radiation-induced toxicities: The role of radioprotectants. *Seminars in Radiation Oncology, 8*(4, Suppl. 1), 2-4.
7. Doebelbower, R. R., & Abe, M. (1990). *Intraoperative radiation therapy.* Boca Raton, FL: CRC Press.
8. Dorr, R. T. (1998). Radioprotectants: Pharmacology and clinical applications of amifostine. *Seminars in Radiation Oncology, 8* (4, Suppl. 1), 10-13.
9. Dragone, M. A. (1996). Cancer. In P. L. Jackson & J. A. Vessey (Eds.), *Primary care of the child with a chronic condition* (pp. 193-231). St. Louis, Mo.: Mosby–Year Book.
10. Dunne-Daly, C. F. (1999). Principles of radiotherapy and radiobiology. *Seminars in Oncology Nursing, 15,* 250-259.
11. Epstein, J. B., Chin, E. A., Jacobson, J. J., et al. (1998). The relationships among fluoride, cariogenic oral flora and salivary flora rate during radiation therapy. *Oral Surgery, Oral Medicine, Oral Pathology, Oral Radiology and Endodontics, 86,* 286-292.
12. Epstein, J. B., & Chow, A. W. (1999). Oral infection, oral complications associated with immuno-suppression and cancer therapies. *Infectious Disease Clinics of North America, 13,* 901-923.
13. Fontanesi, J., Rao, B. N., Fleming, I. D., et al. (1994). Pediatric brachytherapy. *Cancer, 74,* 733-739.

14. Freeman, C. R., Bourgouin, P. M., Sanford, P. A., et al. (1996). Long-term survivors of childhood brain stem gliomas treated with hyperfractionated radiotherapy: Clinical characteristics and treatment-related toxicities. *Cancer, 77,* 555-562.
15. Freifield, A. G., Walch, T. J., & Pizzo, P. A. (1997). Infectious complications in the pediatric cancer patient. In P. A. Pizzo & D. G. Poplack (Eds.), *Principles and practice of pediatric oncology* (3rd ed., pp. 1069-1114). Philadelphia: Lippincott-Raven.
16. Grabb, P. A. (1996). Stereotactic radiosurgery for glial neoplasms of childhood. *Neurosurgery, 38,* 696-701.
17. Griebel, M., Friedman, H. S., Halperin, E. C., et al. (1991). Reversible neurotoxicity following hyperfractionated radiation therapy for brain stem glioma. *Medical and Pediatric Oncology, 19,* 182-186.
18. Gunderson, L. L. (1994). Rationale for and results of intraoperative radiation therapy (Editorial). *Cancer, 74,* 537-541.
19. Haase, G. M., Meagher, D. P., McNeely, L. K., et al. (1994). Electron beam intraoperative radiation therapy for pediatric neoplasms. *Cancer, 74,* 740-747.
20. Habrand, J. L. (1998). Combined chemoradiotherapy of tumors in the child. *Cancer Radiotherapy, 2,* 752-759.
21. Halberg, F. E., Harrison, M. R., Salvatierra, O., et al. (1991). Intraoperative radiation therapy for Wilms' tumor in situ and ex vivo. *Cancer, 67,* 2839-2843.
22. Halperin, E. C., Constine, L. S., Tarbell, N. J., et al. (1999). *Pediatric radiation oncology* (3rd ed.). Philadelphia: Lippincott Williams & Wilkins.
23. Hamlet, S., Faull, I., Klein, B., et al. (1997). Mastication and swallowing in patients with postirradiation xerostomia. *International Journal of Radiation Oncology, Biology and Physics, 37,* 789-796.
24. Hassey, K. M. (1987). Principles of radiation safety and protection. *Seminars in Oncology Nursing, 3,* 23-29.
25. Hebert, M. E., Halperin, E. C., Oakes, W. J., et al. (1993). Multiple-fraction-per-day radiotherapy for patients with brain stem tumors. *Journal of Neurosurgery, 17,* 131-138.
26. Hellman, S. (1991). Principles of radiation therapy. In V. T. DeVita, S. Hellman, & S. A. Rosenberg (Eds.), *Cancer: Principles and practice of oncology* (3rd ed., pp. 227-255). Philadelphia: J. B. Lippincott.
27. Hilderley, L. J. (1992). Radiation oncology: Historical background and principles of teletherapy. In K. Hassey-Dow & L. J. Hilderley (Eds.), *Nursing care in radiation oncology* (pp. 3-15). Philadelphia: W. B. Saunders.
28. Hockenberry-Eaton, M., Hinds, P. S., Alcoser, P., et al. (1998). Fatigue in children and adolescents with cancer. *Journal of Pediatric Oncology Nursing, 15,* 172-182.
29. Hockenberry-Eaton, M., & Kline, N. E. (1997). Nursing support of the child with cancer. In P. A. Pizzo & D. G. Poplack (Eds.), *Principles and practice of pediatric oncology* (3rd ed., pp. 1209-1228). Philadelphia: Lippincott-Raven.
30. Irvine, D. M., Vincent, L., Graydon, J. E., et al. (1998). Fatigue in women with breast cancer receiving radiation therapy. *Cancer Nursing, 21,* 127-135.
31. Kaplan, H. (1979). Historic milestones in radiobiology and radiation therapy. *Seminars in Oncology, 4,* 479-490.
32. Kelly, L. D. (1999). Nursing assessment and patient management. *Seminars in Oncology Nursing, 15,* 282-291.
33. Kim, R. Y. (1996). Radiation oncology at the centennial. *Alabama Medicine, 65 (8,9,10),* 6-8.
34. Korinko, A., & Yurick, A. (1997). Maintaining skin integrity during radiation therapy. *American Journal of Nursing, 97*(2), 40-44.

35. Kun, L. E. (1997). General principles of radiation therapy. In P. A. Pizzo & D. G. Poplack (Eds.), *Principles and practice of pediatric oncology* (3rd ed., pp. 289-321). Philadelphia: Lippincott-Raven.

35a. Kutcher, G. J., Mageras, G. S., Burman, C. M. (1998). Three-dimensional radiation therapy. In S. A. Leibel & T. L. Phillips (Eds.), *Textbook of radiation oncology* (pp. 138-149). Philadelphia: W. B. Saunders.

36. Lamond, J. P., Mehta, M. P., & Boothman, D. A. (1996). The potential of topoisomerase I inhibitors in the treatment of CNS malignancies: Report of a synergistic effect between topotecan and radiation. *Journal of Neuro-oncology, 30,* 1-6.

37. Langveld, N., Ubbink, M., & Smets, E. (2000). I don't have any energy: The experience of fatigue in young adult survivors of childhood cancer. *European Journal of Oncology Nursing, 4,* 20-28.

38. Lawson, L. (1989). Oral-dental concerns of the pediatric oncology patient. *Issues in Comprehensive Pediatric Nursing, 12,* 199-206.

39. Lew, C. C. (1992). Special needs of children. In K. Hassey-Dow & L. J. Hilderley (Eds.), *Nursing care in radiation oncology* (pp. 177-202). Philadelphia: W. B. Saunders.

40. Lew, C., & LaVally, B. (1995). The role of stereotactic radiation therapy in the management of children with brain tumors. *Journal of Pediatric Oncology Nursing, 12,* 212-222.

41. Loeffler, J., Alexander, E., Shea, M., et al. (1992). Radiosurgery as part of the initial management of patients with malignant gliomas. *Journal of Clinical Oncology, 10,* 1379-1385.

42. Louise, I., & Jodrell, N. (1999). The distress associated with cranial irradiation: A comparison of patient-nurse perceptions. *Cancer Nursing, 22,* 126-133.

43. Lundquist, C. (1995). Gamma knife radiosurgery. *Seminars in Radiation Oncology, 5,* 197-204.

44. Madhu, J. J. (1998). Radiotherapy and chemotherapy. In S. A. Leibel & T. L. Phillips (Eds.), *Textbook of radiation oncology* (pp. 69-89). Philadelphia: W. B. Saunders.

45. Mast, M. E. (1998). Correlates of fatigue in survivors of breast cancer. *Cancer Nursing, 21,* 136-142.

46. Mauer, A. M., Burgers, J. B., Donaldson, S. S., et al. (1990). Special nutritional needs of children with malignancies: A review. *Journal of Parenteral and Enteral Nutrition, 14,* 315-324.

47. McCabe, M. A., Getson, P., Brasseux, C., et al. (1995). Survivors of medulloblastoma: Implications for program planning. *Cancer Practice, 3,* 47-53.

48. McDonald, C. J., Muglia, J. J., & Vittorio, C. C. (2000). Alopecia and cutaneous complications. In M. D. Abeloff, J. O. Armitage, A. S. Litcher, et al. (Eds.), *Clinical oncology* (2nd ed., pp. 980-999). Philadelphia: Churchill-Livingstone.

49. McDonald, S., Garrow, G. C., & Rubin, P. (2000). Neurologic complications. In M. D. Abelhoff, J. O. Armitage, A. S. Litcher, et al. (Eds.), *Clinical oncology* (2nd ed., pp. 1000-1022). Philadelphia: Churchill-Livingstone.

50. Mehta, M. (1999). Amifostine and combined-modality therapeutic approaches. *Seminars in Oncology, 26* (2, Suppl. 7), 95-101.

51. Mohan, R. (1995). Field shaping for three-dimensional conformal radiation therapy and multileaf collimation. *Seminars in Radiation Oncology, 5,* 86-93.

52. Mueller, W. A., Cullen, J. W., Abrams, R. B., et al. (1990). Late effects of cancer therapy on developing dentition. *Journal of Dental Research, 69,* 250.

53. Mueller, W. A., Cullen, J. W., Abrams, R. B., et al. (1991). Effect of cranial radiation on tooth abnormalities in ALL patients. *Journal of Dental Research, 70,* 424.

54. Mulhern, R. K., Kepner, J. L., Thomas, P. R., et al. (1998). Neuropsychological functions of survivors of childhood medulloblastoma randomized to receive conventional or reduced craniospinal irradiation: A Pediatric Oncology Group study. *Journal of Clinical Oncology, 16,* 1723-1728.

55. Myerson, R. J., Moros, E., & Roti-Roti, J. C. (1998). Hyperthermia. In C. A. Perez & L. W. Brady (Eds.), *Principles and practice of radiation oncology* (3rd ed., pp. 637-683). Philadelphia: Lippincott-Raven.

56. Neville, K. (1998). The relationships among uncertainty, social support, and psychological distress in adolescents recently diagnosed with cancer. *Journal of Pediatric Oncology Nursing, 15,* 37-46.

57. Nicholaou, N. (1999). Radiation treatment plan and delivery. *Seminars in Oncology Nursing, 15,* 260-269.

58. Olch, A. J., & Lavey, R. S. (2000). Evaluation of a new relocatable head fixation system. In W. Schlegel & T. Bortfeld (Eds.), *Proceedings of the 13th International Conference on the Use of Computers* (pp. 594-596). New York: Springer.

59. Perez, C. A., Brady, L. W., & Roti-Roti, J. L. (1998). Biologic basis of radiation therapy. In C. A. Perez & L. W. Brady (Eds.), *Principles and practice of radiation oncology* (3rd ed., pp. 1-78). Philadelphia: Lippincott-Raven.

60. Perez, C. A., Grigsby, P. W., & Williamson, J. F. (1998). Clinical applications of brachytherapy I: Low dose rate. In C. A. Perez & L. W. Brady (Eds.), *Principles and practice of radiation oncology* (3rd ed., pp. 487-560). Philadelphia: Lippincott-Raven.

61. Pihkala, J., Happonen, J. M., Virtanen, K., et al. (1995). Cardiopulmonary evaluation of exercise tolerance after chest irradiation and anticancer chemotherapy in children and adolescents. *Pediatrics, 95,* 722-726.

62. Pisters, P. W. T., Harrison, L. B., Woodruff, J. M., et al. (1994). A prospective randomized trial of adjuvant brachytherapy in the management of completely resected soft tissue sarcoma of the extremity and superficial trunk. *Journal of Clinical Oncology, 6,* 1150-1155.

63. Portenoy, R. K., & Itri, L. M. (1999). Cancer-related fatigue: Guidelines for evaluation and management. *Oncologist, 4*(1), 1-10.

64. Purdy, J. A. (1996). 3-D radiation treatment planning: A new era. In J. L. Meyer & J. A. Purdy (Eds.), *Frontiers in radiation therapy and oncology* (pp. 2-15). Basel, Switzerland: Karger.

65. Purdy, J. A. (1998). Principles of radiologic physics, dosimetry and treatment planning. In C. A. Perez & L. W. Brady (Eds.), *Principles and practice of radiation oncology* (3rd ed., pp. 243-280). Philadelphia: Lippincott-Raven.

66. Rafferty-Mitchell C., Scalon, J. P., Laskoroski-Joris, L. (1999). Gamma knife radiosurgery. *American Journal of Nursing, 99*(10), 52-59.

67. Rich, T. A. (1998). Intraoperative radiation therapy. In C. A. Perez & L. W. Brady (Eds.), *Principles and practice of radiation oncology* (3rd ed., pp. 629-636). Philadelphia: Lippincott-Raven.

68. Robison, L. L. (1997). General principles of the epidemiology of childhood cancer. In P. A. Pizzo & D. G. Poplack (Eds.), *Principles and practice of pediatric oncology* (3rd ed., pp. 1-10). Philadelphia: Lippincott-Raven.

69. Rotman, M., Aziz, H., & Wasserman, T. H. (1998). Chemotherapy and irradiation. In C. A. Perez & L. W. Brady (Eds.), *Principles and practice of radiation oncology* (3rd ed., pp. 705-722). Philadelphia: Lippincott-Raven.

70. Rubin, P., Constine, L. S., & Williams, J. P. (1998). Late effects of cancer treatment: Radiation and drug toxicity. In C. A. Perez & L. W. Brady (Eds.), *Principles and practice of radiation oncology* (3rd ed., pp. 155-211). Philadelphia: Lippincott.

71. Ruble, K., & Kelly, K. P. (1999). Radiation therapy in childhood cancer. *Seminars in Oncology Nursing, 15,* 292-302.

72. Ryan, J. (2000). Clinical issues: Radiation somnolence syndrome. *Journal of Pediatric Oncology Nursing, 17,* 50-53.

73. Shibotamoto, Y. (1997). A phase I/II study of a hypoxic cell radiosensitizer KO-2285 in combination with intraoperative radiotherapy. *British Journal of Cancer, 76,* 1474-1479.

74. Shuey, K. M. (1994). Heart lung and endocrine complications. *Seminars in Oncology Nursing, 10,* 177-188.

75. Slifer, K .J., Bucholtz, J. D., & Cataldo, M. D. (1994). Behavioral training of motor control in young children undergoing radiation treatment without sedation. *Journal of Pediatric Oncology Nursing, 11,* 55-63.

76. Sneed, P. K., Stauffer, P. R., Li, G. C., et al. (1998). Hyperthermia. In S. A. Leibel & T. L. Phillips (Eds.), *Textbook of radiation oncology* (pp. 1241-1262). Philadelphia: W. B. Saunders.

77. Somaza, S. C. (1996). Early outcomes after stereotactic radiosurgery for growing pilocytic astrocytomas in children. *Pediatric Neurosurgery, 25,* 109-115.

78. Stafford, S. L., Pollack, B. E., Foote, R. L., et al. (2000). Stereotactic radiosurgery for recurrent ependymoma. *Cancer, 88,* 870-875.

79. Starbright Hospital Pals. (2001). (http://www.starbright.org).

80. Strohl, R. A. (1990). Radiation therapy: Recent advances and nursing implications. *Nursing Clinics of North America, 25,* 309-329.

81. Strother, D., Bowman, L., Fraga, A., et al. (2001). High-dose chemotherapy and peripheral blood stem cell rescue following craniospinal irradiation is feasible for patients with medulloblastoma, *Journal of Clinical Oncology, 19,* 2696-2704.

82. Susser, W. S., Whitaker-Worth, D. L., & Grant-Kels, J. M. (1999). Continuing medical education: Mucocutaneous reactions to chemotherapy. *Journal of the Academy of Dermatology, 40,* 367-398.

83. Urtasun, R. C. (1997). Chemical modifiers of radiation. In S. A. Leibel & T. L. Phillips (Eds.), *Textbook of radiation oncology* (pp. 42-53). Philadelphia: W. B. Saunders.

84. Vanna, D. (2000). Helping patients cope with skin problems caused by radiation. *RN, 63*(2), 73.

85. Vokes, E. E., & Weichselbaum, R. R. (1990). Concomitant chemoradiotherapy: Rationale and clinical experience in patients with solid tumors. *Journal of Clinical Oncology, 8,* 911-934.

86. Wall, J. E., Kaste, S. C., Greenwald, C. A., et al. (1996). Fractures in children treated with radiotherapy for soft tissue sarcoma. *Orthopedics, 19,* 647-664.

87. Wasserman, T. (1999). Radioprotective effects of amifostine. *Seminars in Oncology, 26*(2 Suppl. 7), 78-84.

88. Weiss, P. A., & O'Rourke, M. E. (1999). Cutaneous manifestations of cancer and cancer treatment. *American Journal of Nursing, 99*(4 Suppl.), 13-16.

89. Wengstrom, Y., & Forsberg, C. (1999). Justifying radiation in oncology nursing: A literature review. *Oncology Nursing Forum, 26,* 741-750.

90. Wilkins, D. E. (1996). Cisplatin and low dose irradiation in cisplatin resistant and sensitive human glioma cells. *International Journal of Radiation Oncology, Biology and Physics, 36,* 105-111.

91. Williamson, J. F. (1998). Physics of brachytherapy. In C. A. Perez & L. W. Brady (Eds.), *Principles and practice of radiation oncology* (3rd ed., pp. 405-468). Philadelphia: Lippincott-Raven.

92. Withers, H. R., & McBride, W. H. (1998). Biologic basis of radiation therapy. In C. A. Perez & L. W. Brady (Eds.), *Principles and practice of radiation oncology* (3rd ed., pp. 79-118). Philadelphia: Lippincott-Raven.

93. Woo, B., Dibble, S. L., Piper, B. F., et al. (1998). Differences in fatigue by treatment methods in women with breast cancer. *Oncology Nursing Forum, 25,* 915-920.

94. Woodgate, R., & McClement, S. (1998). Symptom distress in children with cancer: The need to adopt a meaning-centered approach. *Journal of Pediatric Oncology Nursing, 15,* 3-12.

6

Chemotherapy

Alice G. Ettinger
Dana M. Bond
Theresa D. Sievers

Every day researchers are looking for the "magic bullet"—the one drug that will eliminate cancer. Perhaps someday an immunization will prevent the development of cancer. Until that day, we rely heavily on agents that are primarily cytotoxic to cancer cells. These agents are known as chemotherapy. The word chemotherapy actually refers to drug or chemical treatment of all diseases. However, commonplace use of this word is limited to the antineoplastic agents used to treat malignancies.

Chemotherapy agents have been identified in various ways. During World War I it was discovered that soldiers exposed to nitrogen gas developed low white blood cell (WBC) counts. In the 1940s nitrogen mustard, a derivative of the nitrogen gas, was developed as an anticancer agent. Interestingly, the second antibiotic discovered after penicillin was dactinomycin, an agent now used for cancer treatment.[40] The development of other chemotherapeutic agents to treat cancers of all types followed.

Numerous anticancer agents have been discovered incidentally while developing drugs for other purposes. These drugs were ultimately found to have excessive toxicity when used for their original purpose. An example is daunorubicin. This antibiotic was originally isolated from a colony of *Streptomyces* and was subsequently found to have significant antileukemic activity.[88]

Other drugs were specifically developed for cancer treatment, such as methotrexate, a folic acid antagonist that interferes with metabolic pathways, or thioguanine and mercaptopurine, antimetabolites that inhibit enzyme production for DNA synthesis. Researchers continue to look for new highly effective agents that will help in the battle against cancer.

PRINCIPLES OF ANTICANCER CHEMOTHERAPY

Chemotherapeutic agents take advantage of the difference between normal cells and cancer cells. Cancer cells have a rapid rate of cellular division compared with most other normal body tissues. Antineoplastic agents are designed to kill rapidly dividing cells. To understand how chemotherapy works, it is essential to review normal cellular proliferation, consisting of DNA replication and cell division.

CELL CYCLE

There are five phases in the growth cycle that ultimately lead to replication or death of the cell. Figure 6-1 depicts these phases. Mitosis (M) represents the phase of cell division. Between mitotic events, the cell is in an interphase period distinguished by two gaps, G_1 and G_2, occurring before and after DNA synthesis (S). After mitosis, some cells enter G_0, a period that is considered out of cycle, or resting. During G_0, cells are not actively dividing. In any body tissue, there are cells present in each of the phases of growth.[43]

G_1, the first gap, is the postmitotic phase in which synthesis of ribonucleic acid (RNA) and protein occurs. G_1 has the most variable time span (8 to 48 hours) and is the phase in which cells spend the greatest portion of their active lives. The length of time that a cell spends in this phase influences the rate of cell proliferation. Rapidly growing cell populations have very few cells in this phase, whereas slow-growing populations have many cells in this phase.

The S phase is the synthesis phase in which the cell replicates its DNA in preparation for cellular division. This phase lasts 10 to 20 hours. After the S phase is a resting period called G_2 in which a second gap occurs. This premitotic phase lasts 2 to 10 hours and is the phase in which RNA synthesis is completed.

Mitosis, actual cell division, takes approximately 1 hour to complete and is accomplished in a four-step sequence shown in Figure 6-1. During the prophase, the nuclear membrane breaks down and disintegrates, and the chromosomes begin to clump. During metaphase, the chromosomes align

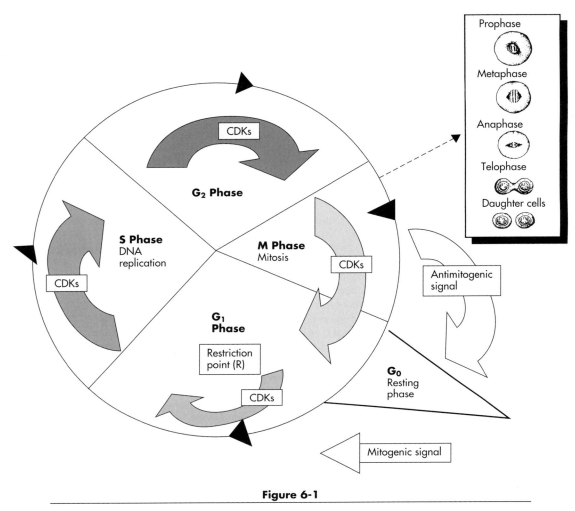

Figure 6-1

Cell cycle and cell division.

in the middle of the cell, in preparation for cell division. Then the chromosomes separate and move to the centrioles during anaphase. The final step is telophase, in which cell division results in the production of two identical daughter cells.

G_0 represents a resting phase when cells are not dividing. Normal cells are in this phase for the majority of the time. Cancer cells in this phase are extremely difficult to treat, because they are resistant to the cytotoxic effects of chemotherapy.[84]

The cell cycle is regulated by extracellular factors, such as mitogens and growth factors, which ensure that the cell cycle proceeds in the usual sequence[55] (see Figure 6-1). DNA that has mutated or cells that become damaged are prevented from replicating by intracellular control mechanisms, or enzymes known as cyclin-dependent kinases (CDKs).[52] Normal cells and cancer cells proceed

through the cell cycle in a similar fashion. However, normal cells reproduce in response to feedback mechanisms, whereas cancer cells are unresponsive and replicate uncontrollably.

Age and developmental status influence cellular proliferation. In adults many cell populations are inactive, such as muscle cells and neurons that do not replicate because they are irreversibly differentiated. Some cells replicate only under special circumstances, such as the normally quiescent hepatocytes of children and adults that proliferate only after hepatic injury. Hematopoietic cells and the mucosal cells lining the gastrointestinal tract replicate constantly in adults and children to repair normal daily wear and tear. Because these cells are replicating more frequently than other cells, they are more likely to be affected by chemotherapy. Hence, chemotherapy commonly causes bone mar-

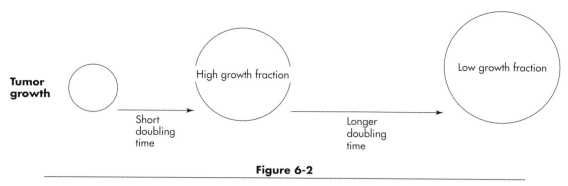

Figure 6-2

Gompertzian tumor growth model.

row and gastrointestinal side effects, most notably myelosuppression resulting in immunosuppression and mucositis that is secondary to both epithelial cell destruction and to a lesser extent bone marrow suppression. In addition, children and adolescents have more body tissues with dividing cell populations because of growth and are therefore susceptible to acute and long-term adverse effects on cerebral and somatic growth and development.

TUMOR CELL KINETICS

The development of a therapeutic plan, referred to as a protocol, for the treatment of malignancies incorporates cellular dynamics and the tenets of the Gompertzian model (Figure 6-2). Originally derived by the eighteenth-century mathematician Gompertz, this mathematical model theorizes that tumors grow exponentially at first, with a high growth fraction and a very short doubling time. The growth fraction is the percentage of cells undergoing division at any one time. The doubling time is the time for any given number of cells to double. The growth fraction decreases and the doubling time slows as the tumor size increases.[89]

As cells accumulate, a small mass is formed, and as the mass grows, the oxygen supply becomes inadequate to supply the cells in the center of the mass. The mass outgrows the blood supply, leading to anoxia of the tumor cells and a subsequent slowing of the cell cycle. Some of the cells will enter the G_0 phase and will eventually die or become temporarily resistant to most chemotherapeutic agents. These resting cells may have time to repair damaged DNA and thus reenter the proliferating pool.

Basic science research has elucidated the differences between cancer cells and normal cells by defining how growth pathways are activated and inactivated by oncogenes and cancer suppressor genes (see Chapter 2). The myriad biologic factors that influence cancer cell growth continues to be an area of interest in the development of anticancer agents.

Normal cells have a defined number of cell divisions and are programmed for cell death as they age or are seriously damaged. This concept of preprogrammed cell death, or apoptosis, is essential to the life cycle of normal cells.[89] Studies are under way to understand apoptosis more clearly and to identify how the process of apoptosis influences cellular resistance to chemotherapy. Genetic factors appear to play a role. Overexpression of *bcl-2* has been tied to chemotherapy resistance. Interactions between *bcl-2* and *p53* may also be important in cellular response and lack of response to chemotherapy.[46]

RESISTANCE

Often, malignant cells are sensitive to chemotherapy, and remission and cure are achieved. However, some cancer cells demonstrate either an intrinsic or acquired resistance to chemotherapeutic agents.[11] The mechanisms of drug resistance in cancer cells include the following: (1) decreased drug uptake by the cell, (2) increased efflux of drug out of the cell as a result of changes in the cell membrane, (3) detoxification of drugs in the cell as a result of metabolic changes, (4) increased DNA repair, (5) alterations in the structure of drug receptor sites or targets, or (6) decreased sensitivity to apoptosis. Any one of these drug resistance mechanisms can occur alone or in combination in cancer cells.[11]

Multidrug resistance gene.   Resistant malignant cells contain the gene known as the multidrug resistance (MDR) gene. In intrinsic cases, the MDR gene is present from the onset of the disease, even before exposure to any chemotherapeutic agents. In the acquired form, the presence of the MDR gene is the result of genetic mutation following exposure to antineoplastic drugs. One of the best-understood mechanisms of resistance as a result of the MDR gene involves the presence of a protein on the cell surface called P-glycoprotein. This protein acts as an efflux pump to eliminate certain chemotherapeutic agents rapidly from the cell, particularly anthracyclines, vinca alkaloids, epipodophyllotoxins, taxanes, and several miscellaneous agents such as dactinomycin and topotecan. Alkylating agents, antimetabolites, cisplatin, carboplatin, and hydroxyurea are not associated with MDR.

Basic science research and clinical trials are investigating the causes of and prevention strategies for MDR. Some classes of drugs such as calcium channel blockers, cyclosporines, antibiotics, and steroids have shown the ability to modulate MDR by inhibiting P-glycoprotein.[11]

Dose intensity. In an effort to reduce the development of resistance, chemotherapeutic agents should be administered at maximum dose intensity, defined as the maximum tolerated dose and the shortest possible interval between doses.[5] Improved supportive care of patients, including colony stimulating factors, aggressive antibiotic regimens, and safer transfusion practices allow dose-intensive chemotherapeutic regimens to be administered. Treatment regimens are typically developed with multiple, alternating agents in an attempt to prevent the development of resistance.[44]

COMBINATION CHEMOTHERAPY

Therapeutic protocols use a combination of drugs that individually are active against a specific disease. Drugs used in combination may have synergistic or enhanced effect against malignant cells. It is not completely understood how agents work synergistically to provide maximum cell kill, but it is known that certain agents display a greater antitumor effect when used together than when used alone. Because tumor cells do not progress through the cell cycle at the same time, it is important to use agents that exert effects at different stages of the cell cycle.

To minimize the risk of severe toxicity, the use of chemotherapeutic drugs with different side effect profiles is an essential strategy used to combine agents.[42] Myelosuppression is usually the most serious dose-limiting toxicity for many chemotherapeutic agents, thus the scheduling and dose of drugs is important to consider. Higher doses of all agents can be administered if the nadir, or low point of blood counts, occurs at different times. Optimal scheduling requires that drugs are administered at the highest possible dose and given as frequently as possible to prevent the develop-

ment of resistance. However, there must be adequate time between cycles to allow for healthy tissues to recover. The principles for selecting antineoplastic agents for combination chemotherapy regimens include the use of agents with the following characteristics:

1. They are individually active against a specific disease entity.
2. They show synergy—display a greater antitumor effect when used together rather than as single agents.
3. They exert effects at different phases of the cell cycle.
4. They have toxicities that do not overlap by organ system or timing, which minimizes the risk of severe or lethal effects.
5. They are given at regular intervals (cycles), minimizing the time between cycles.
6. They are given at the highest possible dose and as frequently as possible.

PHARMACOKINETICS

Pharmacokinetics is the study of drug absorption, distribution, metabolism, and excretion—or how the body processes the drug. Pharmacodynamics is the study of the relationships between drug concentration and drug effect—or how the drug affects the body.[26,73] Principles of pharmacokinetics and pharmacodynamics are used in the development of therapeutic protocols to optimize drug dose and schedule to achieve the greatest cell kill while minimizing toxicity.[26]

The following definitions are helpful in understanding the principles of pharmacokinetics:

Bioavailability is the rate and extent of absorption of a drug.

Biotransformation is the enzymatic metabolism of a drug.

Clearance is the rate of drug elimination calculated in terms of volume of plasma containing a drug, cleared per unit of time.

The half-life of a drug is the time needed to reduce the concentration of the drug by 50% within the body.

The area under the concentration time curve (AUC) is the exposure to drug over time.

Although these principles help determine the optimal route, schedule, and dose of a drug, both physiologic and cellular factors are involved in the failure of chemotherapy to induce the expected response (Table 6-1).

PHARMACODYNAMICS

The study of pharmacodynamics is concerned with the concentration of drug available at receptor sites

TABLE 6-1	**INDIVIDUAL FACTORS THAT ALTER PHARMACOKINETICS OF ANTICANCER AGENTS**
Abnormality	**Cause**
Absorption (bioavailability)	Surgery
	Radiotherapy
	Chemotherapy
	Concomitant agents affecting gastrointestinal motility (e.g., opiates, antiemetics)
	Nausea/vomiting
	Chronic medications (e.g., phenytoin, verapamil)
Distribution	Weight loss
	Obesity
	Decreased body fat
	Pleural effusions or ascites (methotrexate)
Metabolism	Genetically determined variability in drug-metabolizing enzymes
	Hepatic dysfunction
	Renal dysfunction
	Nutritional status (malnutrition)
	Concomitant medication, including chemotherapeutic agents
Excretion	Hepatic dysfunction
	Renal dysfunction
	Reabsorption in the small intestine

Data from Ratain, M. J. (2001). Section 1—Pharmacokinetics and pharmacodynamics: Pharmacology of cancer chemotherapy. In V. T. DeVita, Jr., S. Hellman, & S. A. Rosenberg (Eds.), *Cancer Principles and practice of oncology* (6th ed., pp. 335-344). Philadelphia: Lippincott Williams & Wilkins.

or targets in the body and how the drug concentration produces a response or clinical effect. Clinical effects can be intended and unintended. Intended effects are the goals of the prescribed therapy. Unintended effects are side effects or adverse effects. Rarely, an unintended effect of a drug will sometimes be determined to be beneficial.

The method of drug administration influences the bioavailability of the drug, and thus the ultimate effect on the patient. The same total dose of an agent administered by rapid versus prolonged intravenous (IV) infusion may result in significantly different efficacy and toxicity. The use of biochemical modulators, such as leucovorin for rescue of methotrexate, may allow the safe use of a potentially lethal dose and produce a higher cell kill.

Factors within each person, which can change over time, influence the pharmacodynamics and pharmacokinetics of chemotherapeutic drugs[68] (see Table 6-1). Such variables include age, gender, organ function, genetic factors, and exposure to other chemicals including cigarette smoking and alcohol use. Therefore it is essential to evaluate patients before each course of chemotherapy and make dose adjustments if necessary. For instance, many agents produce increasing amounts of myelosuppression after each subsequent dose. Al-though this may represent the continuous exposure of the bone marrow to the drug, thus slowing the production of new cells, it may also represent decreased clearance of the drug, resulting in increased drug exposure.[73]

Some definitions may help in understanding how chemotherapy is used in the treatment of patients with malignancies.

Multimodel therapy is the use of chemotherapeutic agents with other forms of treatment such as surgery and/or radiation.

Adjuvant chemotherapy is the use of chemotherapy in addition to surgery or radiation to treat residual disease or undetected metastasis.

Combination chemotherapy is the use of several chemotherapeutic agents to treat a specific type of tumor in a multidrug regimen.

Neoadjuvant chemotherapy is used preoperatively in an effort to reduce bulk disease before a definitive surgical procedure is performed.

Sanctuary therapy is chemotherapy administered to an area where malignant cells may be sequestered and concentrations of systemic chemotherapy may not be sufficient to eradicate them. The central nervous system (CNS), which is protected by the blood-brain barrier, is an example. Chemotherapy is administered intrathecally, through lumbar puncture or through an Ommaya reservoir, directly into the spinal fluid that bathes the brain and spinal cord to eliminate malignant cells (Figure 6-3).

CLASSIFICATION OF CHEMOTHERAPEUTIC AGENTS

Chemotherapeutic agents are classified according to their chemical structure, biologic source, or effect on the cell cycle. Effects on the cell cycle are categorized as cell cycle (phase) specific or cell cycle (phase) nonspecific. Table 6-2 describes the various categories of chemotherapy agents. Classification is determined by one or more of the following properties:

1. Cell cycle specific agents exert an effect during a specific phase of the cell cycle, with the maximal effect on rapidly dividing cells.
2. Cell cycle nonspecific agents act on cells regardless of their phase. These agents are dose dependent—the degree of cell kill is directly proportional to the dose administered. They are effective on cancer cells that grow slowly because they are cytotoxic even to resting cells.
3. Biologic agents are naturally occurring substances, such as growth factors and hormones.

Alkylating agents. Alkylating and alkylating-like agents were among the first drugs to be used for the treatment of malignancies. They can be used as single agents or in combination with other drugs and are considered cell cycle phase nonspecific. These agents are most active against cancer cells in the G_0 (resting) phase. Their action is exerted when they contribute their alkyl group to sites on macromolecules such as DNA. This may cause DNA strand breaks, nucleotide base deletions, and/or ring openings, thereby resulting in interference with replication and transcription. This ultimately causes cytotoxicity and mutagenicity in the cancer cells, and also potentially in normal cells. This class varies considerably in the onset and duration of action. For example, nitrogen mustard acts directly and almost instantly, but cyclophosphamide, which must be metabolically activated, is slower and has relatively longer lasting effects.

Antimetabolites. Antimetabolites are agents that are structurally similar (analogs) to the normal cellular metabolites that are required for cell function and replication. They interfere with normal cell metabolism, interacting directly with specific enzymes, either inhibiting production of the enzyme or producing a nonfunctional end product. Cell processes dependent on the enzyme or the end product are thus blocked, causing interruption in

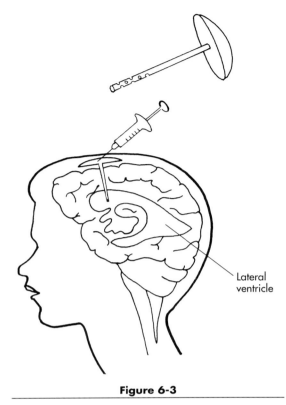

Figure 6-3

Ommaya reservoir. (From Cornwell, C. M. [1990]. The Ommaya reservoir: Implications for pediatric oncology. *Pediatric Nursing, 16*, 249.)

the synthesis of protein, RNA, or DNA within the cell. For example, methotrexate competes with folic acid to bind the enzyme dihydrofolate reductase. When methotrexate binds with this enzyme, folic acid cannot be metabolized further, interfering with DNA synthesis. For this reason, folic acid is administered as a rescue medication following high doses of methotrexate.

Antitumor antibiotics. Antineoplastic antibiotics are natural agents synthesized by a variety of species of bacteria and fungi. These agents interfere with cellular metabolism via numerous mechanisms. Generally they form relatively stable complexes with DNA, inhibiting synthesis of DNA or RNA or both.

Anthracyclines. The anthracyclines are a group of highly colored compounds (known as rhodomycins) which include daunorubicin, doxorubicin, and idarubicin, and the similar drug, mitoxantrone. Their mechanism of action includes intercalation or covalent DNA binding and subse-

TABLE 6-2	CLASSIFICATION OF CHEMOTHERAPEUTIC AGENTS	
Classification	**Agents**	**Mechanism of Action**
AGENTS THAT DAMAGE DNA		
Alkylating agents		Cross-link DNA strands; most active in G_0 phase; react with electrons in cells to form covalent bonds causing lethal results to DNA
Mustard derivatives	Chlorambucil	
	Cyclophosphamide	
	Ifosfamide	
	Mechlorethamine	
	Melphalan	
Nitrosoureas	Carmustine (BCNU)	
	Lomustine (CCNU)	
Aziridines	Thiotepa	
	Mitomycin C	
Alkyl sulfonates	Busulfan	
Triazenes	Dacarbazine	
	Temozolomide	
Hydrozines	Procarbazine	(MAO inhibitor)
Platinum complexes	Carboplatin	Inhibit DNA synthesis
	Cisplatin	
	Oxaliplatin	
Topoisomerase I inhibitors	Topotecan	Unlink coiled DNA resulting in single-strand cleavage
	Camptothecin	
	Irinotecan	
Topoisomerase II inhibitors		Unlink coiled DNA resulting in double-strand cleavage
Anthracyclines	Daunorubicin	
	Doxorubicin	
	Idarubicin	
	Mitoxantrone	
Antimetabolites		Structural analogues of nucleotide bases (building blocks of DNA and RNA); inhibit nucleic acid synthesis; falsely incorporate into DNA double helix
Folic acid antagonists	Methotrexate	Inhibit dihydrofolate reductase, a necessary enzyme in folate metabolism; interrupt normal cellular metabolism; S phase specific
	Trimetrexate	
Pyrimidine antagonists	5-Azacytidine	
	5-Fluorouracil	
	Cytosine arabinoside	
	Gemcitabine	
Purine antagonists	6-Mercaptopurine	
	6-Thioguanine	
	Fazarabine	
	Fludarabine	
	Cladribine	
	Pentostatin	

Adapted from Renick-Ettinger, A. (1993). Chemotherapy. In G. V. Foley, D. Fochtman, & K. H. Mooney (Eds.), *Nursing care of the child with cancer* (2nd ed., pp. 81-116). Philadelphia: W. B. Saunders; Minter, B., & Ryan, J. (Eds.). (1998). *Pharmacological agents in pediatric oncology nursing* (4th ed.). Glenview, IL: Association of Pediatric Oncology Nurses.

Continued

TABLE 6-2	CLASSIFICATION OF CHEMOTHERAPEUTIC AGENTS—cont'd	
Classification	Agents	Mechanism of Action
Plant alkaloids		Bind to microtubules in cell, causing metaphase arrest
Vinca alkaloids	Vinorelbine	M phase specific
	Vinblastine	
	Vincristine	
	Vindesine	
Epipodophyllotoxins	Etoposide	Late S or early G phase; inhibit microtubulin formation (also topoisomerase II inhibitors)
	Teniposide	
Taxanes	Paclitaxel	M phase specific; bind to microtubules and inhibit their disassembly
	Docetaxel	
Anticancer antibiotics		Inhibit DNA replication and/or RNA transcription; active in all phases
Anthracyclines	Daunorubicin	
	Doxorubicin	
	Idarubicin	
	Mitoxantrone	
Chromomycins	Dactinomycin	
Miscellaneous	Bleomycin	Most active in G_2 or M phase
	Mitomycin	
Hormonal agents	Corticosteroids	Interfere with protein synthesis and cellular metabolism
Miscellaneous agents		
Ribonucleotide reductase inhibitor	Hydroxyurea	Interferes with ribonucleotide reductase enzyme system, which inhibits DNA synthesis
Enzymes	Asparaginase	Inhibit DNA, RNA, and protein synthesis by hydrolyzing serum asparagine to nonfunctional aspartic acid and ammonia
	Pegaspargase	

Adapted from Renick-Ettinger, A. (1993). Chemotherapy. In G. V. Foley, D. Fochtman, & K. H. Mooney (Eds.), *Nursing care of the child with cancer* (2nd ed., pp. 81-116). Philadelphia: W. B. Saunders; Minter, B., & Ryan, J. (Eds). (1998). *Pharmacological agents in pediatric oncology nursing* (4th ed.). Glenview, IL: Association of Pediatric Oncology Nurses.

quent formation of free radicals. In addition, they cause inhibition of topoisomerase II, an enzyme that allows long strands of DNA to pass through each other as they untangle.[84] Anthracyclines interfere with this activity by blocking the rejoining of the cleaved DNA strands.[89]

Free radical formation and inhibition of topoisomerase II are responsible for most of the cytotoxicity of these agents. Oxygen radicals are generated by anthracyclines as superoxides, produced when an electron is donated to an oxygen molecule, and then converted to hydrogen peroxide and finally a hydroxyl radical.[84] The hydroxyl radical attacks both DNA and cell membrane lipids. Although most normal tissues and tumor cells possess enzymes to detoxify hydrogen peroxide, heart muscle cells lack this enzyme, resulting in selective damage by anthracyclines to cardiac tissue. Cardioprotective agents are now undergoing evaluation with the administration of anthracyclines.

Other antitumor antibiotics include bleomycin and dactinomycin. Bleomycin is a polypeptide iso-lated from the fungus *Streptomyces verticullus*. It causes single- and double-strand DNA breaks, most commonly in the G_2 or M phase. Dactinomycin is used in the treatment of solid tumors and binds to DNA, causing single-strand DNA breaks.

Plant derivatives. Plant derivatives are drugs from naturally occurring plant material or manufactured from compounds originally extracted from plants. The vinca alkaloids, vincristine, vinblastine, vinorelbine, and vindesine, are plant derivatives. These agents are known as tubulin interactive agents because they interfere with normal microtubule formation and function, causing arrest during mitosis. This results in a lack of a mitotic spindle that causes chromosomes to be dispersed throughout the cytoplasm. The vinca alkaloids may have some effect on cells in the G_1, and S phase, but predominantly the effect is in the M phase.

The taxanes are plant derivatives that have shown antitumor effect in recent clinical trials.

Paclitaxel is extracted from the bark of the Pacific yew tree, *Taxus brevifolia,* and docetaxel is a semi-synthetic compound similar in structure and action. These agents bind to microtubules and inhibit microtubular disassembly, which is necessary for completion of mitosis and normal cellular functioning.

The epipodophyllotoxins, etoposide and teniposide, are plant derivatives thought to inhibit topoisomerase II and produce DNA strand breaks. They appear to exert their effects in the late S and early G phases of the cell cycle, rather than the M phase as originally thought.[84]

The camptothecin plant derivatives, topotecan and irinotecan, are semisynthetic agents believed to inhibit topoisomerase I, an enzyme responsible for maintaining the structure of DNA. These agents bind with the DNA-enzyme complex causing DNA strand breaks and cell death.

Corticosteroids.   Steroids appear to enter the cell passively and bind with macromolecules in the cytoplasm of the cell. This complex then enters the cell nucleus, binds with DNA, and modifies the transcription process. The use of steroids in the treatment of pediatric cancer is limited primarily to prednisone and dexamethasone.

Antiangiogenic agents.   Angiogenesis is the growth of new microvessels, particularly from capillary endothelial cells. Under normal conditions the vascular endothelium is a tissue with a very low cell division rate—turnover times are measured in hundreds of days. In contrast, the average turnover time for bone marrow is 5 days, sustained by approximately 6 billion cell divisions per hour. Furthermore, it is known that benign neoplasms are sparsely vascularized and tend to grow slowly, whereas malignant neoplasms are highly vascular and fast growing, increasing the probability that tumor cells will enter the circulation and produce metastases.[37]

During angiogenesis, endothelial cells can proliferate as rapidly as bone marrow cells. Pathologic angiogenesis rarely stops spontaneously and has until recently been difficult to suppress. Therefore the goal of antiangiogenic therapy is to return proliferating microvessels to their normal resting state and to prevent their regrowth.[41]

Antiangiogenic agents are a new classification of drug developed for this purpose. These agents are not directly cytotoxic but rather can be used to limit further tumor growth and development of metastases. Some inhibitors of angiogenesis currently in clinical trials include angiostatin, endostatin, and thalidomide.[38]

Miscellaneous agents.   Chemotherapeutic agents that do not fit a particular classification are referred to as miscellaneous agents. They include the enzymes asparaginase and pegaspargase, as well as hydroxyurea and procarbazine.

Asparaginase is an enzyme produced from the bacteria *Escherichia coli* or *Erwinia,* which functions to inhibit DNA, RNA, and protein synthesis by hydrolyzing serum asparagine to the nonfunctional products aspartic acid and ammonia. It is cell cycle nonspecific. Pegaspargase is also produced from the bacteria but is coated with a compound called polyethylene glycol that decreases the immunogenicity of the natural enzyme.[31] Hydroxyurea inhibits DNA synthesis and causes cell death in the S phase.

CLINICAL TRIALS

A clinical trial is a scientific experiment designed to evaluate the use of drugs and other therapies to prevent, diagnose, and manage disease in human subjects.[15] Once an investigational drug or treatment is approved for study in humans, a series of clinical trials progresses sequentially through three phases before approval for general use by the U.S. Food and Drug Administration (FDA). Each phase of study explores a different research question. Phase I trials investigate toxicity, phase II trials investigate efficacy, and phase III trials determine the effectiveness of a drug or treatment in comparison with another. Phase IV studies may be conducted after the FDA has approved the drug for marketing (Box 6-1).

DRUG APPROVAL

Before a drug is approved for widespread use in the United States, it must be approved by the FDA. The approval process is time consuming and complex. After a compound is identified or synthesized in the laboratory, it is screened for pharmacologic activity and tested in laboratory animals in a phase called preclinical testing. If animal testing proves successful, the agent moves on to clinical testing, beginning with the application to the federal government for an investigational new drug (IND). The application must include specific reasons and scientific evidence that support the hypothesis that the agent will be effective in humans with specific diseases or conditions. Once the application is approved, the clinical trials process in humans can begin.[65]

PHASES OF CLINICAL TRIALS

Phase I.   Phase I clinical trials are the initial safety trials in human subjects. An increasing dose of drug is administered to a small number of pa-

PHASES OF CLINICAL TRIALS

PHASE I
Initial safety trial in humans. Increasing dosages of a drug are given to a small number of patients to determine the maximum tolerated dose (MTD). Patients are carefully monitored for side effects to identify dose-limiting toxicities (DLTs). Typically performed in patients with refractory disease.

PHASE II
Determines the efficacy of a drug, measured by antitumor activity for a specific disease or group of diseases and estimates tumor response rate. Patients are carefully monitored for side effects to further define the safety and toxicity profile of the drug.

PHASE III
Compares the efficacy of at least two treatments, typically the experimental treatment versus the current standard therapy. Treatment may consist of one drug or a combination of drugs or treatments such as chemotherapy, radiation therapy, and surgery. Comparisons are generally done in prospective randomized trials. Patients are carefully monitored for side effects, as additional safety and efficacy data is obtained for larger numbers of patients.

PHASE IV
May be conducted after the U.S. Food and Drug Administration has approved the drug for marketing. Postmarketing surveillence and other studies continue to evaluate the drug's mechanism of action, further investigating toxicity and safety profiles, side effects, adverse drug reactions, and quality of life and cost issues that are discovered during phases I through III trials.

tients with the single goal of determining the maximum tolerated dose (MTD). The MTD is based on the emerging side effect profile and toxicity as a result of drug administration.

Dose escalation studies typically begin with a very low dose in adult patients and may require as many as 10 to 20 dose escalations before the dose-limiting toxicity (DLT) is obtained. Typically three patients are entered on a dose level before increasing to the next level. Dose escalations occur if no significant (grade IV) toxicity is reported. If a patient experiences a grade IV toxicity, the next patient is entered at the previous dose level. Escalations continue until the MTD is established. Because of the limited number of children available to participate in phase I trials, a lengthy dose escalation trial that requires many patients is not feasible. Phase I trials sponsored by the National

Cancer Institute (NCI) usually wait for completion of adult phase I trials. Pediatric trials are then begun at 80% of the MTD reached in the adult studies, reducing the number of dose escalations to fewer than 5, thereby reducing the number of children needed to complete the study.[80]

It is important to note that children appear to tolerate some drugs differently than adults.[80] Significant differences between children and adults have been found in drug disposition (pharmacokinetics) and drug action (pharmacodynamics). Physiologic differences between children and adults, such as body composition, renal function, and hepatic metabolism, cause differences in drug disposition. In addition, children appear to differ from adults regarding susceptibility to the toxic effects of drugs.[80] These differences may cause a greater or lesser degree of toxic effects. For example, pediatric trials of all-*trans*-retinoic acid[80] produced a higher degree of central nervous system toxicity than adult phase I trials. Conversely, pediatric patients appeared to tolerate higher doses of paclitaxel with less toxicity in phase I dose escalation trial than adults.[80]

Nursing care of the patient on a phase I trial includes a comprehensive assessment and careful monitoring for side effects. Documentation is crucial to the ultimate success of the clinical trial and determination of the side effect profile of a particular drug. The medication side effects are tracked to determine the dose-limiting toxicities (DLTs).[67,74,81] The Common Toxicity Criteria (CTC) is the National Cancer Institute's scoring system used to grade toxicities on clinical trials.[27] Documentation must be clear and accurate to allow for accurate coding of toxicities.

It is important to note that the goal of a phase I trial is to establish the MTD of a new agent and not to treat the patient's cancer, although it is hoped that ultimately the drug will prove efficacious. Nurses can provide clarification of the clinical trial goals for patients and their families. It is important to make clear the goal of the trial without eliminating the patients' and families' hope for improvement in their child's condition.[67,74,81]

Phase II. The goal of phase II trials is to determine a treatment's efficacy. In a clinical trial for cancer patients, this is measured by antitumor activity against a specific disease or select group of diseases.[15,53,67,74,81] Ultimate goals of the phase II trial are to determine the tumor response rate and further define the drug (or treatment) safety and toxicity profile.[53,67,74,81]

Patients who enter onto phase II trials have often been heavily pretreated with chemotherapy, and therefore their disease may have developed resistance and in some cases multiple drug resistance. In an effort to identify new agents for very high-risk (often stage IV) disease, scientists may introduce a "phase II window" before the initiation of protocol treatment. This method of evaluation helps to provide a more accurate test of new agents in chemotherapy-naïve patients and is limited to trials for these difficult-to-treat diseases. These studies are monitored very carefully to ensure the child is not subjected to undue risk, either because of drug toxicity or delay in initiation of therapy known to be active against the child's disease.[19]

Nursing care of the patient on a phase II trial also requires a comprehensive assessment, careful monitoring for side effects, and detailed documentation. It is imperative that the nurse be aware of the information gained in phase I trials about the side effect profile of the drug and toxicities and can categorize toxicities as common or rare in terms of frequency. The nurse must also understand the goal of the trial and ensure that the patient and family understand.[67,74,81] Compliance with both treatment and diagnostic studies that measure tumor response is critical to the success of the clinical trial.

Phase III.   Phase III clinical trials compare the efficacy of two or more treatments. Treatment may consist of a single drug or a combination of drugs or treatments such as chemotherapy with radiation therapy. The experimental treatment is compared with what is considered standard therapy or the best results of the previous phase III trial. Comparisons are typically performed in a prospective randomized fashion.[74,81]

A randomized clinical trial (RCT) refers to the study design for comparing two or more treatments. Patients are randomly assigned to receive one of the therapies being studied. The study design is important because it must control for factors that could bias or influence the outcomes of a study and therefore any conclusions about which treatment is better.[74,81]

Nursing care for patients on phase III trials also requires a comprehensive assessment, careful monitoring for side effects, and detailed documentation. Patient compliance with treatment evaluations and diagnostic studies that measure tumor response is critical. Nurses provide patient and family education regarding the clinical trial, randomization, and the preparation for diagnostic tests and laboratory studies. The concept of randomization in cancer treatment is difficult to accept.[74,81] Nurses need to acknowledge the family's ambivalence and concern regarding this issue, reinforce explanations regarding study objectives, and support patients and families in the decision-making process.

Most phase III clinical trials in pediatric oncology compare regimens that are all considered to be effective treatment for the child's particular cancer. Study objectives determine the specific goals for the trial such as increased survival, decreased toxicity, or improved quality of life.

Phase IV.   Phase IV studies are conducted after a drug or treatment has gained FDA approval. These postmarketing surveillance and pharmacoepidemiologic studies continue to evaluate the drug's mechanism of action, toxicity, and safety profiles. In addition, evaluation of quality of life, cost, and other issues that arose during the phases I through III trials are done.[81]

PROTOCOL DOCUMENTS

A well-designed clinical trial has a clearly defined set of objectives, logical and feasible methodology, and a clearly written protocol. The protocol document provides a detailed plan for conducting the research (Box 6-2). Strict adherence to the specifications in the plan is critical to the successful completion of the study and accurate interpretation of the data. Protocol documents often serve as the only reference material available to providers caring for patients enrolled on clinical trials. Information about investigational agents and treatments cannot be found in commonly used drug reference texts such as the *Physician's Desk Reference* (PDR) or even the hospital formulary. Therefore the accuracy, clarity, completeness, and internal consistency of the protocol document are essential.[79]

BOX 6-2

COMMON ELEMENTS OF THE PROTOCOL DOCUMENT

1. Abstract
2. Overview/schema/roadmap
3. Objectives/purpose
4. Background and significance
5. Patient eligibility criteria
6. Data to be accessioned
7. Response criteria
8. Agent/pharmaceutical information
9. Treatment plan
10. Dose modifications
11. Patient follow-up
12. Off-study criteria/patient, trial discontinuation
13. Statistical analysis/considerations
14. Informed consent
15. References/appendices

The agent or pharmaceutical information section provides a detailed review of all drugs and treatments in the proposed study. Drug preparation guidelines may be included. If drug administration information is included, it should match the drug information in the treatment section of the protocol.[79]

The treatment section contains specific instructions for administration of therapy. Some protocols contain instructions for supportive care as well. It is important to note that although protocols contain detailed instructions for administration of therapy, information to guide the provision of nursing care generally is not included.[48] Individualized, compassionate nursing care is not only essential to the patient and family, it is essential to the success of the protocol.[48]

PROTOCOL EVALUATION

Nurses must correctly interpret the specifications in the protocol document regarding drug administration, patient monitoring, and data collection. Nursing review of the protocol focuses on evaluation of patient safety, patient care requirements, ethical considerations, treatment feasibility, and compliance with obtaining the informed consent. Ideally nurses are involved in the development of preprinted order sets and other aspects of protocol implementation.

Notification of nursing staff and initiation of education regarding the protocol are best done before activation of the study. Prior notification ensures that nurses have sufficient knowledge about a protocol to safely and effectively care for the patient enrolled on the study. Information about investigational drugs includes the drug's therapeutic indication, dose range, side effect profile, and administration and monitoring requirements.

Nurses must fully understand the clinical trial process and important issues in conducting clinical trials to effectively provide patient and family education. In addition to ensuring that informed consent is obtained before patient enrollment on a clinical trial, the nurse participates in the ongoing education of patients and families throughout the clinical trial. Some patients require additional support at the time a clinical trial ends. Nurses must be aware of this during times of transition for the patient and family.

Successful completion of the protocol demands that patients be compliant with the prescribed treatment, diagnostic testing, and monitoring requirements. Nurses can enlist patients and families to partner with the health care team in providing safe and effective care. Box 6-3 lists information patients and families need to know about clinical trials.

BOX 6-3

WHAT PATIENTS AND FAMILIES NEED TO KNOW ABOUT CLINICAL TRIALS

1. Overall treatment plan and treatment goals
2. Purpose/objective(s) of the study
3. Specific treatment proposed (e.g., chemotherapy, radiation therapy, surgery)
4. Response expected from treatment on the study if known
5. Advantages and disadvantages (risks and benefits) of proposed treatment
6. Alternative treatment(s) available
7. Response of others receiving same treatment to date, if available
8. Expected and possible short-term and long-term side effects
9. Preventing, managing, and reporting side effects
10. Diagnostic tests required (e.g., magnetic resonance imaging [MRI], computed tomography [CT] scan, diagnostic and laboratory tests)
11. Impact of proposed treatment on daily life (e.g., define activity restrictions, time off from work/school, frequency of anticipated hospitalizations and length of stay, frequency of outpatient examinations, therapies, diagnostic tests, laboratory tests, need for nursing care in the home); will need to explain how the clinical trial may be different from regular treatment
12. Impact of proposed treatment on family members in terms of added burden of care

---

PEDIATRIC CANCER CLINICAL TRIALS

Well-designed and carefully conducted clinical trials are essential to the evaluation process for new drugs and treatments in children with cancer.[53,67,80] Access to clinical trials is critical for all children and adolescents with cancer because enrolling in a clinical trial and treatment at a pediatric tertiary care center have been shown to confer a significant survival advantage.[15,66,70,83,87]

A relatively small number of children are diagnosed with cancer annually; therefore pediatric clinical trials are typically conducted as multiinstitutional trials within a cooperative group. Most single institutions do not have enough eligible patients to yield significant findings and to complete studies in a timely manner.[74,80] In an effort to reduce duplication of effort, expedite evaluation of new agents, and improve access to clinical trials, four national pediatric oncology clinical trial groups (Children's Cancer Group [CCG], Intergroup Rhabdomyosarcoma Study Group [IRSG], National Wilms Tumor

Study Group [NWTSG], and Pediatric Oncology Group [POG]) recently merged to form a single cooperative group. The new group is the Children's Oncology Group (C.O.G.), dedicated to improving outcomes for children and adolescents diagnosed with cancer.

Although more than 70% of children diagnosed with cancer in the United States are entered into at least one clinical trial, this number is far lower for adolescents between 15 and 19 years of age.[15,74] In contrast to adult cancer clinical trials, minority children diagnosed with cancer are enrolled on clinical trials at the same rate as nonminority children.[14] Therefore efforts should be focused on improving access and increasing enrollment of adolescents and young adults.

A successful clinical trial depends on careful planning and preparation of the study protocol and protocol documents, in addition to detailed attention to compliance with protocol specifications.[53,67,80] Pediatric oncology nurses are integral members of the study development team and the health care team involved in the care of children enrolled on clinical trials. Nurses play key roles in the many stages of clinical trial development and implementation including the following: (1) developing the study and drafting protocol documents; (2) participating as institutional review board (IRB) members; (3) providing direct patient care; (4) providing patient, family, and staff education; (5) managing the study, including collection of data and specimens; and (6) participating in the auditing process.[74,81] Treatment toxicities are assigned a code as developed by the National Cancer Institute.[27] Accurate and complete documentation of all patient responses to chemotherapy will ensure the most accurate assessment and analysis of protocol-related complications and will improve care for children in the future.

NURSING IMPLICATIONS IN CHEMOTHERAPY ADMINISTRATION

ROLE OF THE PEDIATRIC ONCOLOGY NURSE

The role of the nurse in chemotherapy administration has changed in the past decade as scope and practice standards,[3] responsibilities, methods, and treatment settings have changed. Today's nursing education, pediatric oncology certification, and the health care environment have afforded the opportunity for nurses to assume a more active lead in the team of professionals who prescribe and administer chemotherapy for children with cancer. This team consists of the physician, pharmacist, advanced practice nurse, and staff nurse responsible for chemotherapy administration and/or

postchemotherapy monitoring of the patient. Each has the responsibility for the safe and effective administration of chemotherapeutic agents.[69]

Nurses administer chemotherapeutic agents in a variety of settings such as inpatient hospital units, ambulatory care units, and in the home. Chemotherapy may be administered orally, parenterally, intrathecally, and even topically. Nurses in each type of setting must be well versed in the proper administration and disposal techniques. In addition, family members should also understand the indication for the medication, expected and potential side effects, and how to administer the drug correctly.

Nurses administering chemotherapy should have achieved established competencies and knowledge of basic pediatric oncology and chemotherapy.[3,40] According to institutional standards and guidelines, nurses receive instruction about chemotherapy administration and demonstrate their skills through examination and a clinical practicum or skills demonstration.

In addition to a formal credentialling process, standardized chemotherapy education programs are offered by organizations such as the Oncology Nursing Society. Pediatric content in these programs is being enhanced. Additionally, many nurses value the credentialing process offered by the Oncology Nursing Credentialing Corporation (ONCC) to provide the credentials CPON (certified pediatric oncology nurse).[25,50] Certification ensures standard knowledge about pediatric oncology practice. Some institutions offer employment incentives to nurses who achieve certification.[25] Studies of nurses' self-reported value of certification find that nurses report increased confidence, competence, credibility, and control in their practice after achieving certification.[18] To date studies have yet to link specialty-nursing certification to improved patient outcomes.[18,50]

PRETREATMENT PHASE

Assessment.   The nurse is cognizant of any intervening issues that have occurred such as surgery, radiation, or other treatments. The history includes allergies and experience with prior illnesses, hospitalizations, and medications. If prior chemotherapy has been given, document how the patient tolerated it, what antiemetics were used, when they were given, and how they worked. Also, determine what other medications the patient is taking, including vitamins, chemotherapeutic agents, allergy medications, cold preparations, and any other over-the-counter preparations, including complementary or alternative medications such as nutritional supplements and herbs.

Treatment plan review. Before the initiation of treatment, the nurse reviews the child's treatment protocol to verify the phase and day of treatment, drug, dose, and pretreatment studies required before administration, as well as antiemetic therapy orders. Also, it is important to recheck the height and weight of the patient and compare with the last recorded values and then calculate the body surface area (BSA) based on this information. Review the pretreatment laboratory values, including imaging studies, tests, and special evaluations that may have been performed.

Dose calculation. Chemotherapy doses are computed according to the child's weight in kilograms or BSA. BSA is calculated using the child's height (in centimeters) and weight (in kilograms). This calculation determines the child's BSA in meters squared (m^2). Most chemotherapy doses are calculated using a milligrams-per-square-meter formula. Several different methods may be used to determine the BSA. The most commonly used method employs a mathematical formula. Alternatively, a nomogram or special graph may be used to plot the BSA according to the patient's height in centimeters and weight in kilograms.

The equation used to calculate body surface area is as follows:

$$\sqrt{\frac{\text{Height (cm)} \times \text{Weight (kg)}}{3600}} = \text{BSA}$$

Children who weigh less than 10 kg or who are under the age of 12 months require a milligrams-per-kilogram formula rather than a BSA formula. Some treatment regimens decrease chemotherapy doses for these infants by 50%. The rationale for this approach stems from the fact that virtually every aspect of the distribution, excretion, and metabolism of chemotherapeutic agents is quantitatively and qualitatively altered in newborns and young infants. Unique to this age-group is the rapid change in the relative volume of fluid compartments that occurs during the first 9 months of life. The use of BSA does not account for the changes in the distribution of body water compartments that occur with age. Therefore the BSA method is not appropriate for the child less than 10 kg.[56]

Dosage for intrathecal and intra-Ommaya therapy is based on age because the volume of cerebral spinal fluid (CSF) is a known quantity according to the age of the person. Spinal fluid volume is proportionally much greater in infants and young children, reaching adult volume by the age of 3 years. Therefore a chemotherapy dose based on BSA might underdose a young child and overdose an adolescent.[13]

Dose adjustment. Dose reductions are made if there has been severe toxicity from prior treatment. Alternatively, dose escalations may be made if the full dose is tolerated without the usual anticipated toxicity. Many treatment regimens specify the percentage of dose adjustment and dose adjustment criteria. Some chemotherapeutic agents such as dactinomycin and doxorubicin are radiosensitizers, requiring dose reductions during concomitant radiotherapy. These agents also cause radiation recall, a skin reaction in an area where radiation was previously given. This reaction can occur after administration of radiosensitizing drugs and may necessitate a dose adjustment. Agents that have cumulative toxicities, such as bleomycin and doxorubicin, have maximal lifetime dose restrictions.

Informed consent. Ensure that informed consent for treatment has been obtained and is available on the patient's chart. The pediatric oncology nurse does not have responsibility for obtaining informed consent for treatment or clinical trial participation. However, the nurse shares the ethical responsibility with the physician investigator to ensure that children and adolescents and their families understand the treatment protocol, associated toxicities, and any other issues related to clinical trials. Chapter 33 reviews ethical issues surrounding informed consent.

CHEMOTHERAPY ERROR PREVENTION AND MANAGEMENT

Pediatric oncology nurses have a key role in preventing and reducing medication errors in children with cancer. Clinical trial protocols and cancer treatment regimens are becoming increasingly complex and intensive.[39,57] The chemotherapy medication process is also complex and involves staff nurses, nurse practitioners, physicians, and pharmacists who must work together in complex health care systems.

Chemotherapeutic agents are considered "high-risk" agents because of the narrow therapeutic index (difference between treatment and toxic or lethal dose) and need for careful patient monitoring.[23,24] Errors prescribing, compounding, dispensing, and administering chemotherapeutic agents have resulted in significant morbidity and mortality.[39,85] The consequences of medical errors in terms of harm to all patients and added health care costs have been well documented over the past several years. In the United States alone, it is estimated that 100,000 deaths, 1 million injuries, and over $10 billion in added health care costs are attributed to preventable medical errors annually.[9,20] Medication errors are the most common cause of injury to hospitalized patients. Medication errors resulting in injury are the most preventable.[10,17,62,76,82]

Errors may occur anywhere in the medication-use process: from the decision to treat the patient, to writing the medication order, to transcription of the order, to admixing or compounding the drug, to administration of the drug, and finally to proper monitoring of the patient for side effects and toxicity.[7,36,61] Medical error is defined by the Institute of Medicine (IOM) as the "failure to complete a planned action as intended or the use of a wrong plan to achieve an aim."[51] An adverse event is defined as "an injury caused by medical management rather than by the underlying disease or condition of the patient."[51]

Prescribing error is the most common cause of medication error, occurring in up to 5% of all inpatient orders written.[6] These prescribing errors are attributed to choice of the wrong drug, wrong dosage, wrong form or concentration of the drug, wrong route of administration, and wrong time or frequency of administration.[6,62-64] Prescribing errors are more likely to occur when the prescriber lacks immediate knowledge about the drug such as the correct dosage, indications, contraindications, interactions, or side effect profile or lacks current information about the patient such as allergies, comorbidities, weight, and up-to-date laboratory results.[63,64]

Illegible prescriptions and improper transcription contribute to a significant number of medication errors.[75] Misinterpretation of medication prescriptions or orders is attributed to many factors such as illegible writing, use of abbreviations, improper placement of zeros and decimals, obscured decimals on lined paper, drugs with similar names, and use of the apothecary system to dose medications rather than the standard metric system.[22]

Use of computerized order entry or prescription systems has clearly demonstrated success in reducing prescribing error, particularly when the computer systems are encoded with rules to prevent incomplete and inaccurate orders and wrong drug choices.* Significant error prevention has also been attributed to the development of preprinted (legible) orders, facilitating accurate interpretation by pharmacists and nurses.[7,61] These computer order entry systems were designed to support, not control, clinical decision making and therefore achieved acceptance by the prescribing clinical staff.

Although computerized order entry systems are ideal, they are not available in all clinical settings. Recommendations made by the Institute for Safe Medication Practices (ISMP) and others to standardize the prescribing vocabulary can significantly improve prescription legibility and clarity and ensure correct interpretation of chemotherapy orders.[22,39] Kohler et al.[57] provide detailed recommendations about the use of specific nomenclature for prescribing cancer treatment regimens to decrease misinterpretation of chemotherapy orders.

In addition to prescribing errors, other factors such as improper pharmacy compounding, dispensing, and labeling; drug administration errors; inadequate patient monitoring; inadequate patient education; and manufacturers' using similar names or labels for different drugs can predispose to medication errors.[21] The most common medication errors in infants are incorrect dose due to incorrect patient weight or misplaced decimal points. Infants were significantly more likely to suffer from tenfold overdoses due to decimal point misplacement than were other types of patients.[1,58]

Most medication errors have multiple causes and multiple opportunities for prevention. Dr. Lucian Leape, one of the authors of the IOM report released in November 1999, stated: "Errors are caused by faulty systems, processes and conditions that lead people to make mistakes."[51] Error prevention and reduction strategies are based on designing and implementing error-resistant systems capable of preventing, detecting, and correcting errors.

Nurses should participate in the multidisciplinary review of clinically significant errors that occur in their practice setting. The investigation into errors focuses on and evaluates what caused the error, not who caused the error. Identification of "organizational precursors" such as unsafe systems and faulty mechanical devices or medical equipment is key to making care delivery systems safer.[51] Patterns of error must be identified and a standard medication error index used for categorizing the severity of error.[28] Information about patterns of error that occur in a particular setting is valuable and should be shared with staff in an ongoing forum.[30] Specific error reduction strategies for chemotherapy include the following:
1. Elimination of verbal orders for chemotherapy
2. Use of delivery systems for oral, intravenous, intrathecal, and gastric solutions that are not compatible with one another
3. Use of a controlled delivery system for intravenous chemotherapy that is not given by intravenous bolus
4. Avoiding labels that truncate the name of the patient or medication

---

*References 8, 32, 33, 54, 71, 72, 78.

5. Using labels that include full patient name, drug, total dose calculated in milligrams and milliliters, and route of administration
6. Developing guidelines for ordering, admixing, compounding, and administering chemotherapy
7. Use of preprinted order forms or order templates
8. Development of a verification process for prescribing, dispensing, and administering chemotherapy[24,28,58,60,82]
9. Emphasizing importance of positive patient identification

Multidisciplinary independent dose calculation when prescribing, dispensing, and administering chemotherapy is a key to preventing errors due to dosing.[23,39] Box 6-4 lists steps in the verification process for prescribing and administering chemotherapeutic agents.

Access to current pediatric drug references and easily accessible patient-specific data is essential. The treatment plan for pediatric oncology patients may include clinical trial protocol documents. These protocol documents serve as reference material for providers who prescribe, dispense, and administer chemotherapy on a clinical trial.[39,79]

Paper or electronic access to the current protocol version is critical. Amendments or revisions made to the protocol documents after activation of the study may include significant changes in drug dosages, schedules, and patient monitoring. Providers must be able to verify the patient's correct treatment regimen, cycle, week, and day for each chemotherapy order written, dispensed, and administered.

Pediatric oncology providers must receive ongoing education about new drugs and clinical trial protocols. This education includes information about the drug's therapeutic indication, dose range, side effect profile, administration, and monitoring requirements. All health care providers should receive some training and education about error reporting, error reduction strategies, and the importance of communication and teamwork.[77] New employees should demonstrate competency before prescribing, dispensing, or administering chemotherapy.[23,39]

It is estimated that 20% of patients in the United States are not literate enough to understand and follow directions on prescriptions.[29] Patients who understand their treatment plan and medication schedule comply with the plan and medications at a higher rate.[34] The value of patient and family education should not be underestimated. The patient and family are partners in providing safe care. Remind patients that they must let their caregivers know of drug and food allergies and all prescription and over-the-counter medications they are tak-

---

BOX 6-4

VERIFICATION PROCESS FOR PRESCRIBING AND ADMINISTERING CHEMOTHERAPY

1. Patient name, diagnosis, allergies
2. Signed, informed consent for treatment obtained before initiation of therapy
3. Treatment plan/protocol, regimen, cycle, week, day
4. Current weight/height (<5% change)
5. Dose according to treatment plan/protocol (calculate dose independently, write out dose calculations if prescribing, have another licensed person review the order set)
6. Dose adjustments or modifications consistent with specifications in the treatment plan/protocol (calculate dose adjustments independently, and write out dose calculations if prescribing)
7. Current laboratory values
8. Results of diagnostic testing
9. Order includes generic name of drug, dose, dose calculation, dose modification and calculation, route, frequency, administration guidelines, required monitoring and, if needed, admixture fluid type, volume, and rate

---

ing, including nutritional supplements, vitamins, and herbal remedies. Provide patients and families with written information as a follow-up to verbal instructions. Written information should include the drug name, indication, contraindications, usual and actual doses, expected and possible adverse effects, and methods for preventing or managing side effects.[34] Visual learning aids such as videos should be available for those whose preferred learning style is not the written word. Listen carefully to the expressed concerns of patients about their medications to establish and maintain an open dialogue. Box 6-5 lists information patients should know about their medications.

TREATMENT PHASE

Typically only specially trained registered nurses give chemotherapy.[40] All procedures must be explained to the child and family. Prehydration requirements as indicated by the protocol must be met before chemotherapy administration. A plan for antiemetic management must be in place for each patient. This plan is based on the emetogenic potential of the agent[2,47] (see Chapter 11) and the patient's previous experience with the treatment. Verify chemotherapy against the order and protocol with another licensed person as described in the previous sections. Protective devices such as gloves, gowns, and Luer-Lok syringes must be used to protect the child and nurse from accidental

<table>
<tr><td>

BOX 6-5

WHAT PATIENTS NEED TO KNOW ABOUT THEIR MEDICATIONS

1. Overall treatment plan and treatment goals
2. Name of medication (brand name and generic name)
3. Indication for the medication/purpose for taking it
4. Dose of medication, including strength (mg/cc or mg/tab)
5. How and when to take the medication and for how long
6. How to measure the medication, especially if liquid
7. What food or drink the medication can be taken or mixed with
8. What food, drink, or other medications should be avoided
9. Contraindications to taking the medication
10. Expected and possible side effects
11. Methods for preventing or managing side effects
12. If side effects occur, when to report symptoms
13. If side effects or problems occur, whom to call (regular and off hours)

</td><td>

BOX 6-6

SURVIVAL SKILLS: CHEMOTHERAPY ADMINISTRATION

Double check dose before administration
  With the protocol and the order
  With another RN or licensed professional
Wear gloves while preparing chemotherapy for infusions and during administration
Know/review these pertinent drug facts
  Baseline lab/other studies within normal limits?
  Common side effects?
  Vesicant?
  Emetogenic?
  Prehydration required?
  Light sensitive?
  Postadministration monitoring needs?
Have emergency equipment available
Prepare patient and family
  Side effects of drugs
  Schedule of events
  What to expect without overemphasizing side effects such as nausea and vomiting
  Does the child have any rituals that assist coping?
Keep emesis basin, trash can within reach but out of sight
Know who and where your resources are
Remember, it is not as important to memorize facts about each chemotherapy drug that you give. More importantly, you should know what you need to know about the agent, where to find this information and how to apply the information to the clinical situation.

From Kathy Patterson Kelly, RN, MN, *Pediatric Oncology Program.* Staff development program used to train pediatric nurses for chemotherapy administration. Children's Hospital, University of Missouri Health Care, Columbia, MO.

</td></tr>
</table>

exposure to the toxic antineoplastic agents. If the agent is a potential vesicant, proper precautions are implemented to avoid extravasation. Certain chemotherapy agents require "rescue" medications such as mesna or leucovorin. Ensure these medications are given precisely as prescribed. Box 6-6 describes the "survival steps" necessary to follow every time the nurse administers a chemotherapy agent.

Safe handling. Because chemotherapy is currently administered in many settings, health care personnel, support personnel, and families continue to be at risk of exposure to antineoplastic drugs. Because the risks from the prolonged exposure are unknown and no safe level of exposure has been identified, meticulous attention must be given to handling and disposal of these agents.[86]

The Occupational Safety and Health Administration (OSHA) has developed guidelines to protect workers from undue exposures to cytotoxic agents.[49] OSHA has issued guidelines for safe handling and disposal, which focus on minimizing exposure through absorption and inhalation. According to these guidelines, all persons at risk for contact must be educated in the safe handling of these agents.[45]

All drugs are prepared aseptically in a class II biologic safety cabinet, which is cleaned, serviced,

and maintained at specified intervals. The environment is clean and free of interruptions; no food or drink should be present. Personnel preparing chemotherapy wear disposable surgical gowns, which tie in the back and have cuffs. Unpowdered latex gloves should be worn at all times. Alternative gloves are provided for the employee with a latex allergy. Drugs are transported to the patient in a sealed, zip-closed bag and labeled as chemotherapy so that proper handling and disposal will be followed.

Individuals who administer the drugs should wear gloves. If tubing is not primed within the biologic safety cabinet, the end of the tubing is placed in a sealable plastic bag with sterile gauze to catch any fluid. The end of the tube is wiped with alcohol to remove any drug. All tubing and syringes must have Luer-Lok connections to prevent accidental disconnection.

All wastes associated with chemotherapy are treated as hazardous waste, including containers, tubing, needles, syringes, bag, gloves, and protective pads. Body excretions from the individual receiving the drug may contain active metabolites up to 48 hours after administration and are handled according to universal precautions. Linens and clothing contaminated with chemotherapy or body excreta from a patient who has received chemotherapy are handled with gloves and disposed of as hazardous waste. In addition, wearing a disposable gown during handling of contaminated linens is recommended to protect staff. If the linens are wet, they are placed in impenetrable, waterproof bags to protect all other personnel who come in contact with them. Gloves should be worn when changing diapers or assisting with urinals, bedpans, and emesis basins for up to 48 hours after the patient has received chemotherapy.

Patients receiving therapy at home must also be educated in proper handling and disposal of chemotherapy waste. This information is incorporated into family teaching to avoid unnecessary cytotoxic exposures. The Environmental Protection Agency has made available patient fact cards, entitled "Disposal Tips for Home Health Care," which explain how to handle needles and syringes. Patients and/or their families can contact their state or community environmental programs or local sanitation departments for specific details for their area.

In cases of accidental exposure to the drug, contaminated clothing is removed promptly and the affected skin washed thoroughly with soap and water. If the eye is involved, immediately flood the eye for at least 5 minutes with water or isotonic eyewash. Prompt medical follow-up is recommended for all exposures.

A spill kit should be maintained in all dispensing and treatment areas in the event of an accidental drug spill. Spills must be cleaned up immediately. Traffic through the area is restricted until cleanup is completed. For a large spill, absorbent sheets or pads are placed on the spill to cover and contain it completely. Powder spills are covered with moist towels. Personnel handling the spill must wear protective apparel. The area must be thoroughly cleaned and all contaminated materials disposed of as hazardous waste.

Physicians and oncology nurses have a responsibility to protect themselves and the environment from the potential hazards of chemotherapeutic agents through safe practice techniques. This information must also be incorporated into family teaching to avoid unnecessary cytotoxic exposures. Each institution will have specific policies and procedures regarding the safe handling of chemotherapeutic agents and cytotoxic spills. Often the question arises whether it is safe for nurses to give antineoplastic agents if they are trying to conceive or are pregnant. Historically studies indicated potential risk. However, recent studies that incorporated the use of safe handling techniques indicate minimal risk to the pregnancy or unborn child. The decision about whether a nurse will administer chemotherapy during pregnancy should be made on an individual basis between the nurse and employer.[16]

Drug administration techniques. Chemotherapy administration occurs after the physiologic and psychoeducational parameters have been met. Medications are inspected for any discoloration, particulate matter, or other sign of contamination. Because any medication may cause an allergic or adverse reaction, the nurse must be prepared to treat any potential outcome. The patient who is to receive medications known to cause allergic reactions, such as asparaginase or etoposide, is monitored closely. Emergency drugs and equipment must be readily available.[69] Chapter 13 reviews the nursing care of the child who develops anaphylaxis.

Oral. Many chemotherapeutic agents are available only for oral administration. Most chemotherapy medications are given on an empty stomach (1 hour before or 2 hours after meals) to facilitate absorption. It may be necessary for the nurse and family to find creative methods to give oral medications to children. Principles of pediatric drug administration apply to chemotherapeutic agents. The following interventions are recommended for the child who has difficulty taking oral medications.

- Teach children to swallow tablets by starting with small candies, such as Tic Tacs or M&M's. Consult with Child Life staff as needed.
- Do not crush unpleasant tasting medications, such as prednisone. Try to administer the pill whole (if it is small enough) to avoid the taste or place pill in a gelatin capsule. Place the dose in a food that might disguise the taste of the drug, such as ice cream, flavored gelatin, peanut butter, syrup, fruit roll, or jelly. Be sure to use only a small amount of food, so the drug can be more easily given. Avoid using the child's favorite foods to disguise medications.
- Educate parents to administer antiemetics as ordered to avoid vomiting of oral medication. (For additional information, see Chapter 11.)

- Repeat oral dose if vomiting occurs immediately after administration and the tablet or capsule can be visualized in the vomitus.[45] Some protocols recommend repeating the dose if vomiting occurs within 30 minutes; check with physician regarding need for repeat dose.
- It may be necessary to watch older children take their oral medications.

Nonadherence to treatment among older children and adolescents is a complex issue.[59] During adolescence, teenagers develop independence and are motivated to be like their peers. They may find the side effects so unpleasant that they do not take their medications. Open discussion with the teen and family may allow the adolescent to express feelings and frustrations, thus leading to improved compliance.

Subcutaneous/intramuscular.   Use the smallest gauge needle available to decrease injection pain. In addition, ice or a topical anesthetic or other needleless method of applying local anesthesia such as EMLA or Numby Stuff may be applied to the site before injection to decrease needle pain; unfortunately, these agents will not reduce the pain associated with injection of the drug into the tissue. Be aware of the platelet count; additional pressure will be needed if the platelet count is below 50,000/mm^3.[69]

Intrathecal.   Extreme care must be taken to ensure sterile technique during drug preparation and administration to prevent introduction of infection into the central nervous system. Typically the volume of drug administered should be equal to the cerebrospinal fluid removed. Most children will lie flat 30 minutes to 1 hour after intrathecal administration to facilitate drug distribution and to prevent headache.[69] Do not bring other medications into the procedure room to be given via other routes. Accidental administration of the wrong drug into the CNS can be fatal.[4,35,90]

Intravenous.   Recommendations for venipuncture sites (forearm preferred) for adults with cancer are often not possible in children. Typically the best available vein is used and venipuncture performed by the most skilled nurse available. Avoid antecubital sites and sites distal to recent venipunctures. Consider replacing any peripheral intravenous lines that are over 24 hours old before giving vesicant chemotherapy. Before administration of any intravenous agent, vein patency must be ensured. Although many children will have a central venous catheter (CVC) placed, the nurse must still estab-lish patency of a CVC in a similar fashion to peripheral IVs, because CVCs can become displaced. Vein patency will need to be assessed regularly during continuous infusion chemotherapy.

There are many controversial issues surrounding the administration of vesicant chemotherapy via peripheral veins. Issues such as sequencing of vesicant medication with nonvesicant medications, use of the antecubital fossa, gauge of intravenous catheter, and side arm versus direct push methods for administration are examples. Excellent resources for the many issues surrounding the intravenous administration of chemotherapy are detailed in the Oncology Nursing Society's cancer chemotherapy guidelines[40] and the Association of Pediatric Oncology Nurses' pharmacological agents books.[69] Nurses are also directed to their institution's individual policies and procedures for recommendations for intravenous administration of chemotherapy agents.

Extravasation.   Some chemotherapeutic agents are vesicants and can cause tissue damage if not administered directly into the vein. The degree of tissue damage is related to the vesicant potential of the drug and the concentration and quantity of drug extravasated.[45] The appearance of an area where a vesicant or irritant extravasated can range from erythema and hyperpigmentation to blister formation, ulceration, and tissue sloughing and necrosis. Symptoms may range from tingling, burning, and pain to complete loss of mobility. Infectious complications may also result, especially if the patient is neutropenic. Appearance and symptoms may not be present at first and may develop later.

Agents that have the potential to irritate tissue if an extravasation occurs are referred to as irritants. Although they may not cause serious damage, they can produce a reaction ranging from erythema and burning to pain and inflammation at the injection site. Table 6-3 summarizes some of the antidotes and methods used for local tissue reaction after extravasation (Figure 6-4).

Guidelines for the treatment of extravasation:
1. Prevention is the best way to avoid the sequelae of extravasation. Careful administration by persons skilled in IV therapy prevents serious complications. However, extravasation has occurred even in the most skilled nursing hands.
2. Some chemotherapeutic agents have an antidote identified for infusion through the needle and infiltration into the surrounding tissues. If an extravasation antidote is given, first aspirate any residual drug from the needle and tubing before administering the antidote.

TABLE 6-3	VESICANT AND IRRITANT CHEMOTHERAPEUTIC AGENTS AND EXTRAVASATION ANTIDOTE			
Chemotherapeutic Agents	**Antidote**	**Local Care**		**Comments**
VESICANT AGENTS				
Dactinomycin (Actinomycin D)	None	Ice as comfort measure Elevate extremity and do not use for several days		More pronounced if receiving or previously received radiotherapy May need surgical consult
Daunorubicin (Daunomycin) Doxorubicin (Adriamycin) Epirubicin Idarubicin (Idamycin) Mitomycin C (Mutamycin)	None	Apply ice for 15 min every 3-4 hr as tolerated for 24-48 hr Elevate extremity and do not use for several days Infuse hydrocortisone 1 ml intradermally surrounding extravasation site Topical dimethyl sulfoxide (DMSO) 99% applied to site every 6 hr for 14 days		May need surgical consult Can be used for small amount of extravasation Apply DMSO to large area surrounding extravasation site
Mechlorethamine (Nitrogen Mustard)	Isotonic sodium thiosulfate	Mix 4 ml 10% sodium thiosulfate with 8.4 ml sterile H_2O Inject 1-4 ml through existing IV line or subcutaneously (SQ) at extravasation site		
Vinblastine (Velban) Vincristine (Oncovin) Vindesine (Eldisine) Vinorelbine (Navelbine)	Hyaluronidase	Mix 150 units/ml hyaluronidase with 1 ml of normal saline (NS) Inject 1.4 ml through existing IV line or SQ at extravasation site		
IRRITANT AGENTS				
Irritant agents cause pain, venous irritation, and/or chemical phlebitis Carboplatin Carmustine (BCNU) Dacarbazine (DTIC) Etoposide (VP-16) Ifosfamide Teniposide (VM-26)		Apply cold pack to IV site and along vein		Slowing infusion rate and/or increasing diluent may decrease pain associated with administration of irritant agents

Data from Goodman, M. (2000). Chemotherapy: Principles of administration. In C. H. Yarbro, M. G. Frogge, M. Goodman, et al. (Eds.), *Cancer nursing: Principles and practice* (5th ed., pp. 385-443). Sudbury, MA: Jones & Bartlett; Tortorice, P. V. (2000). Chemotherapy: Principles of therapy. In C. H. Yarbro, M. G. Frogge, M. Goodman, et al. (Eds.), *Cancer nursing: Principles and practice* (5th ed., pp. 352-384). Sudbury, MA: Jones & Bartlett.

3. Notify the physician immediately if there is a definite or suspected extravasation. It may be necessary for a plastic surgeon to be consulted for a serious extravasation.

4. An extravasation kit containing agents used as antidotes must be available on the unit where chemotherapeutic agents are administered.

5. The extravasation site should be kept clean and dry. If a blister occurs, it should not be lanced. Protect the area with a light, nonocclusive dressing, and evaluate the area at 24 hours, 48 hours, and 7 days, then PRN if pain is present. Increase monitoring frequency if the skin changes progress.

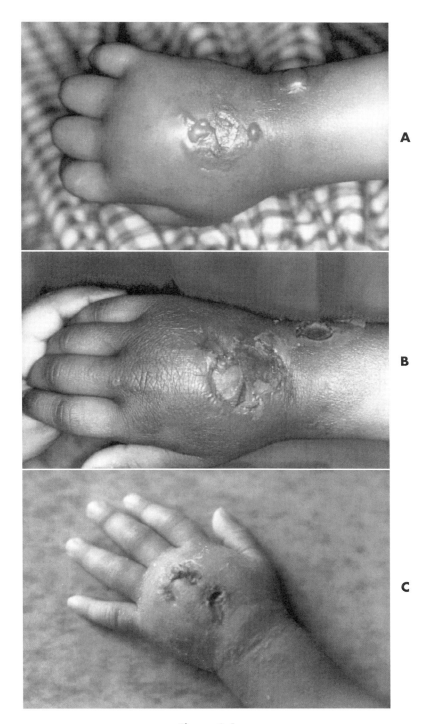

Figure 6-4

Examples of vesicant extravasations. **A,** Extravasation 1 week after infiltration of vesicant chemotherapy. **B,** Same extravasation 7 to 10 days later. **C,** Extravasation nearing completion of the healing process.   (Courtesy Peter F. Coccia, MD, University of Nebraska Medical Center, Omaha.)

6. Document the incident according to policy. Describe the date, time, needle type and gauge used, site and size of infiltrate, approximate amount of drug infiltrated, nursing management, physician notification, and patient instruction regarding follow-up care. In some institutions, photographs are taken of the site at the time of the incident and then at each follow-up visit.

The use of CVCs has made it easier and safer to administer vesicant agents. However, a CVC that does not demonstrate a blood return should not be used for administration of a vesicant agent unless a dye study (an x-ray examination in which a radiopaque dye is injected and then followed by x-ray through the CVC) is performed. When a continuous infusion vesicant agent is being administered, frequent observation of the exit site and the surrounding area, as well as periodic checks for blood return, is necessary. Know the institutional policy regarding administration of chemotherapeutic agents.

Documentation. Documentation of chemotherapy administration can be accomplished by carefully constructed checklists or via a detailed narrative note. The essential elements of documentation include the following: (1) patient name, date, time; (2) vein selection, gauge and length of needle inserted or type of central line; (3) site assessment before and after infusion; (4) establishment of blood return before, during, and after administration; (5) amount and type of flushing solution; (6) drug name, route, dose (including volume in milliliters), and infusion duration; (7) patient tolerance; (8) patient education related to drugs received, toxicities, and management; and (9) follow-up care.[40]

Legal issues in chemotherapy administration. Chemotherapy medication errors are the most significant legal issue related to chemotherapy administration. Because these agents have a very small margin of safety, errors can be fatal. The previous section described recommendations for the prevention of chemotherapy errors. In addition, adverse outcomes related to vesicant extravasations or hypersensitivity reactions are potential litigation risks. Nurses can best defend themselves from litigation involving chemotherapy administration by knowing national standards and adhering to institutional practices for safe chemotherapy administration and administration of vesicants and carefully documenting chemotherapy administration practices, including patient and family education.[40]

POSTTREATMENT PHASE

Monitoring of the child and adolescent after chemotherapy administration is as critical as the administration of the actual agents. Adverse reactions or toxicities will often present during this time. Each agent has a specific toxicity profile and recommendations for monitoring parameters after administration. Table 6-4 covers the most commonly administered chemotherapy agents, administration recommendations, side effects, and associated nursing implications. The plan of care is derived from the nurse's knowledge of the child's disease and the expected treatment-related side effects, all placed within the context of the child's developmental maturation. Part III of this book reviews pertinent nursing management issues related to the supportive care of children and adolescents with cancer after chemotherapy administration.

PATIENT/FAMILY EDUCATION

The diagnosis of cancer is devastating to the child and family. The initial days are filled with fear, shock, and "information overload." When chemotherapy is first being administered, parents may feel that something unusual will take place. They may believe that side effects will occur immediately, and they must be vigilant to wait for the occurrence.

Parents and families rely on the nurse to provide ongoing education about chemotherapy administration procedures and anticipated side effects. Reinforce the name and expected side effects for each drug administered. Remind patients and families that rapidly growing cells, including blood cells, hair, and the gastrointestinal (GI) mucosa are affected by most chemotherapeutic agents[12] (refer to Part III). Assure them that antiemetic therapy will be administered before chemotherapeutic agents known to cause nausea and/or vomiting. Give them explicit information about the time frame for the expected side effects. Providing written information is often reassuring. The consent form may be used as a reference point, because it includes expected side effects for each agent. Box 6-7, on p. 171, illustrates a typical checklist that can be used for newly diagnosed patient and family education.

When administering chemotherapy, explain the procedures, the agents being used, and the expected or potential side effects. Present all of the information to the child at an age-appropriate level and repeat as necessary. Children cooperate more fully if they are included in the discussions about their care. It may be necessary to improvise a strategy involving rewards for appropriate behaviors.

Many people are involved in the care of the child with cancer in addition to parents. These include

Text continued on p. 171

TABLE 6-4	CHEMOTHERAPEUTIC AGENTS			
Drug	**Classification**	**Route**	**Side Effects**	**Special Considerations**
Asparaginase (Elspar) Erwinia asparaginase PEG-asparaginase (pegaspargase, Oncaspar)	Enzyme from *Escherichia coli* or *Erwinia carotovora* PEG-asparaginase is *E. coli* asparaginase conjugated with polyethelyne glycol Inhibits protein synthesis by hydrolyzing serum asparagine to nonfunctional aspartic acid and ammonia Cell cycle nonspecific	Intramuscular (IM), IV	Common: local allergic reaction, hyperammonemia, low fibrinogen Occasional: rash, hyperglycemia, abnormal liver function tests, coagulation abnormalities Rare: hypersensitivity with anaphylaxis, nausea, vomiting, anorexia, somnolence, lethargy, pancreatitis, convulsions, thrombosis, edema, CNS ischemic attack, renal compromise	IV administration is associated with increased risk of anaphylaxis. Have emergency equipment and drugs available. Observe patient for at least ½ hr after dose. Coagulation abnormalities place child at risk for thrombus formation or bleeding.
Bleomycin sulfate (Blenoxane)	Antibiotic	IV, IM, subcutaneous (SQ)	Common: none Occasional: hyperpigmentation, pneumonitis, high fever 2-6 hr after administration Rare: anaphylaxis, fever, hypotension, nausea, vomiting, anorexia, skin rash, mucositis, pulmonary fibrosis, renal failure	High fevers may occur without anaphylaxis; give earlier in the day so does not occur at night. Rare, lethal anaphylactoid reactions with severe fever and hypotension—have emergency equipment available. If test dose required, administer 1-2 Units IM; wait 1 hr and give remaining dose. Lower dose may need to be given when pulmonary radiotherapy is used. *Continued*

Data from Almuete, V., Brisby, J., Delman, B., et al. (2000). 2000 Guide for the administration and use of cancer chemotherapeutic agents. *Oncology Special Edition, 3,* 51-55; Balis, F., Hocenberg, J., & Poplack, D. G. General principles of chemotherapy. In P. A. Pizzo & D. G. Poplack (Eds.). *Principles and practice of pediatric oncology* (3rd ed., pp. 215-272). Philadelphia: Lippincott-Raven; Henry, D., Cartwright, J., & Sinsabaugh, D. (2000). *Children's Oncology Group pharmacology manual.* Arcadia, CA: Children's Oncology Group Operations Center; Renick-Ettinger, A. (1993). Chemotherapy: In G. V. Foley, D. Fochtman, & K. H. Mooney (Eds.), *Nursing care of the child with cancer* (2nd ed., pp. 81-116). Philadelphia: W. B. Saunders.

TABLE 6-4	CHEMOTHERAPEUTIC AGENTS—cont'd			
Drug	**Classification**	**Route**	**Side Effects**	**Special Considerations**
Bleomycin sulfate (Blenoxane) —cont'd				Pulmonary function tests are done as baseline, throughout course of therapy, and for a period of time after therapy; patients can develop fibrosis with decreased diffusion capacity. Monitor cumulative dose.
Busulfan (Myleran)	Alkylating agent	By mouth (PO) 2 mg tablets	Common: myelosuppression, mild nausea, vomiting, "bronzing" of the skin	Prophylactic anticonvulsant therapy may be useful in patients receiving high doses of the drug.
			Occasional: seizures with high dose, oral mucositis, skin breakdown, decreased adrenal function	
			Rare: skin rashes, veno-occlusive disease (VOD), amenorrhea, testicular atrophy, gynecomastia, myasthenia symptoms, cataract, atrophic bronchitis	
Carboplatin (Paraplatin)	Heavy metal alkylating agent	IV infusion	Common: nausea, vomiting, myelosuppression	IV infusion over 15 min or longer.
			Occasional: electrolyte disturbances	Aluminum reacts with carboplatin, causing precipitate formation and loss of potency; therefore do not allow needles or IV sets containing aluminum parts to come in contact with the drug.
			Rare: metallic taste, peripheral neuropathy, hepatotoxicity, renal toxicity, ototoxicity, secondary leukemia	Elimination dependent on glomerular filtration rate (GFR) and may be prescribed based on GFR and area under the curve (AUC) desired.

Agent	Classification/Action	Administration	Side Effects	Nursing Considerations
Carmustine (BCNU, BiCNU)	Nitrosourea Lipid-soluble alkylating agent that crosses blood-brain barrier Cell cycle nonspecific	IV infusion	Common: burning with peripheral administration, nausea, vomiting, myelosuppression, alopecia, late pulmonary dysfunction Occasional: marked facial flushing, liver dysfunction, thrombophlebitis at injection site Rare: brownish discoloration of skin, renal dysfunction, pulmonary fibrosis, secondary malignancy	Avoid extravasation of local contact with skin or conjunctiva. Avoid rapid infusion, which is associated with burning and/or hypotension. Use glass containers and polyethylene-lined administration sets for stability.
Cisplatin (Platinol)	Heavy metal alkylating agent Inhibition of DNA synthesis	IV infusion	Common: nausea, vomiting, anorexia, myelosuppression, hypomagnesemia, high-frequency hearing loss, nephrotoxicity Occasional: metallic taste, electrolyte disturbances, hearing loss in the normal hearing range Rare: anaphylactic reaction, peripheral neuropathy, tinnitus, seizure, liver toxicity, secondary malignancy	Synergistic with radiation therapy. Aluminum reacts with cisplatin, causing precipitate formation and loss of potency; therefore do not allow needles or IV sets containing aluminum parts to come in contact with drug. Premedicate with antiemetics; continue throughout and beyond course of therapy, causes delayed nausea and vomiting. During course of therapy carefully monitor input and output (I&O). Maintain urinary output at least at 2 ml/kg/hr. Administer furosemide (Lasix) or mannitol as ordered to ensure adequate urinary output. Intensifies aminoglycoside toxicity and should be used with caution when administered concurrently. To decrease risk of hypomagnesemia, supplement with magnesium.

Continued

Data from Almuete, V., Brisby, J., Delman, B., et al. (2000). 2000 Guide for the administration and use of cancer chemotherapeutic agents. *Oncology Special Edition, 3*, 51-55: Balis, F., Hocenberg, J., & Poplack, D. G. (2000). General principles of chemotherapy. In P. A. Pizzo & D. G. Poplack (Eds.). *Principles and practice of pediatric oncology* (3rd ed.. pp. 215-272). Philadelphia: Lippincott-Raven: Henry, D. Cartwright, J., & Sinsabaugh. D. (2000). *Children's Oncology Group pharmacology manual.* Arcadia, CA: Children's Oncology Group Operations Center; Renick-Ettinger, A. (1993). Chemotherapy. In G. V. Foley, D. Fochtman, & K. H. Mooney (Eds.). *Nursing care of the child with cancer* (2nd ed., pp. 81-116). Philadelphia: W. B. Saunders.

TABLE 6-4	CHEMOTHERAPEUTIC AGENTS—cont'd			
Drug	**Classification**	**Route**	**Side Effects**	**Special Considerations**
Corticosteroids (prednisone, dexamethasone, hydrocortisone, methylprednisolone)	Lympholytic Decreases edema produced by tumor or caused by tumor necrosis	PO IV Intrathecal (IT) Equivalent potency: • Cortisone 5 • Hydrocortisone 4 • Prednisone 1 • Methylprednisolone 0.8 • Dexamethasone 0.15	Common: hyperphagia, immunosuppression, personality changes, Cushing's syndrome, pituitary-adrenal axis suppression, acne Occasional: poor wound healing, stomach upset, hyperglycemia, gastritis, muscle weakness, osteonecrosis Rare: pancreatitis, electrolyte imbalance, gastrointestinal (GI) bleeding, increased intraocular pressure, hypertension, aseptic necrosis of femoral head, growth retardation, striae, osteopenia, peptic ulcer, cataracts	Decrease salt intake; protect from infection; observe for hyperglycemia. To decrease or prevent GI upset, take with meals or snacks; may need to take with histamine H_2-receptor antagonist such as cimetidine, ranitidine. May mask fever or infection.
Cyclophosphamide (Cytoxan)	Alkylating agent	IV push or infusion PO tablets	Common: anorexia, nausea, vomiting, myelosuppression, alopecia, gonadal dysfunction/sterility Occasional: metallic taste, hemorrhagic cystitis, syndrome of inappropriate antidiuretic hormone (SIADH) Rare: transient blurred vision, cardiac toxicity with arrhythmias (in higher doses), myocardial necrosis, pulmonary fibrosis, secondary malignancy, bladder fibrosis	Maintain adequate hydration, urinary output. Check urine for blood frequently. Outpatient therapy should be given early in the day when possible so that toxic metabolites do not accumulate in bladder overnight. Encourage patient to urinate before going to bed at night to empty bladder completely. Administration of high doses of cyclophosphamide should be preceded and followed by IV fluids and mesna.
Cytarabine (ara-C, cytosine arabinoside, Cytosar-U)	Antimetabolite	IV, SQ, IM, IT	Common: nausea, vomiting, anorexia, conjunctivitis with higher doses, myelosuppression, stomatitis,	Administer steroid eyedrops to prevent conjunctivitis with high dose.

Drug	Classification	Administration	Side Effects	Nursing Considerations
			Occasional: flulike symptoms with fever, diarrhea Rare: encephalopathy, cerebellar dysfunction, or pulmonary capillary leak with higher doses; rash, hepatotoxicity, VOD, pneumonitis, gonadal dysfunction With intrathecal administration: Nausea, vomiting, headache, pleocytosis, fever, learning disability, rash, somnolence, meningismus, convulsions, paresis, myelosuppression, ataxia	
Dactinomycin (actinomycin D, Cosmegen)	Antineoplastic antibiotic	IV push Gold color	Common: nausea, vomiting, local ulceration if extravasated, myelosuppression, alopecia, skin photosensitivity or hyperpigmentation Occasional: diarrhea, mucositis, immune thrombocytopenia, radiation recall Rare: hepatotoxicity	Vesicant—severe tissue damage if extravasation occurs. Protect from light. Avoid preservatives. Do not filter. Radiation recall may occur in an area of previous radiotherapy.
Daunorubicin (daunomycin, Cerubidine) and Doxorubicin (Adriamycin)	Anthracycline antibiotic	IV push or infusion Red color	Common: subclinical cardiac arrhythmias, nausea, local ulceration if extravasated, pink or red color to urine, myelosuppression, alopecia Occasional: stomatitis, hepatotoxicity, mucositis, cardiomyopathy (cumulative and dose dependent) Rare: anaphylaxis, allergic reaction, rash, secondary malignancy	Vesicant—severe tissue damage if extravasation occurs. Warn patient and family about urine discoloration. Cardiac studies with echocardiogram or multigated angiography (MUGA) scan should be done periodically to monitor cardiac function—must have acceptable cardiac ejection fraction. Monitor cumulative dose.

Continued

Data from Almuete, V., Brisby, J., Delman, B., et al. (2000). 2000 Guide for the administration and use of cancer chemotherapeutic agents. *Oncology Special Edition, 3,* 51–55; Balis, F., Hocenberg, J., & Poplack, D. G. General principles of chemotherapy. In P. A. Pizzo & D. G. Poplack (Eds.), *Principles and practice of pediatric oncology* (3rd ed., pp. 215–272). Philadelphia: Lippincott-Raven; Henry, D., Cartwright, J., & Sinsabaugh, D. (2000). *Children's Oncology Group pharmacology manual.* Arcadia, CA: Children's Oncology Group Operations Center; Renick-Ettinger, A. (1993). Chemotherapy. In G. V. Foley, D. Fochtman, & K. H. Mooney (Eds.), *Nursing care of the child with cancer* (2nd ed., pp. 81–116). Philadelphia: W. B. Saunders.

TABLE 6-4	CHEMOTHERAPEUTIC AGENTS—cont'd			
Drug	**Classification**	**Route**	**Side Effects**	**Special Considerations**
Etoposide (VP-16, VePesid)	Plant alkaloid Epipodophyllotoxin	IV infusion over 60 min; severe hypotension if given in less than 30 min PO—50 mg capsules Capsules must be refrigerated	Common: nausea, vomiting, myelosuppression Occasional: alopecia, enhanced damage due to radiation, diarrhea Rare: hypotension, anaphylaxis, skin rash, peripheral neuropathy, stomatitis, secondary malignancy	Severe hypotension can occur with rapid infusion. Concentrations above 0.4 mg/ml have unpredictable stability in solution. Do not refrigerate intravenous solution, PO capsules must be refrigerated.
5-Fluorouracil (5-FU, fluorouracil, Adrucil)	Antimetabolite	IV push, IV infusion, PO (parenteral form may be given orally but is absorbed poorly) Intrahepatic artery	Common: nausea, vomiting, metallic taste, immunosuppression, myelosuppression Occasional: diarrhea, stomatitis, sun sensitivity, hyperpigmentation, dry skin, palmar-plantar erythrodysesthesia (red painful skin irritation) Rare: hypotension, angina, electrocardiogram (ECG) changes, tearing, conjunctivitis and blurred vision, partial loss of nails, headache, visual disturbances, cerebellar ataxia, proctitis	Take on empty stomach (at least 1 hr before or 2 hr after food). For oral administration mix parenteral solution of 5-FU with flavored water or carbonated beverage; avoid acidic fruit juice.
Hydroxyurea (Hydrea)	Antimetabolite	PO	Common: myelosuppression with rapid drop in WBC count Occasional: nausea, vomiting, stomatitis, anemia Rare: rash, facial erythema, dysuria, renal tubular damage, headache, dizziness, jaundice, radiation recall, hallucination, convulsions, nail changes	Take on empty stomach (1 hr before or 2 hr after meals). Dose often titrated to WBC count. Do not add to solutions that are acidic or carbonated, alkaline solutions preferred.
Idarubicin (Idamycin)	Anthracycline	IV slow push or infusion	Analogue of daunorubicin with similar activity and side effects	Vesicant—severe tissue damage if extravasation occurs. Protect from light. See daunomycin. Perhaps less cardiotoxicity than doxorubicin and daunorubicin.

Medication	Administration	Description	Toxicity	Comments
(isophosphamide, Ifex)	min		Common: nausea, vomiting, anorexia, myelosuppression, alopecia Occasional: somnolence, confusion, weakness, seizure, SIADH, hemorrhagic cystitis, cardiac toxicities with arrhythmias at high dosages, myocardial necrosis, Fanconi's renal failure Rare: encephalopathy, peripheral neuropathy, acute renal failure, pulmonary fibrosis, secondary malignancy, bladder fibrosis	cystitis if given without uroprotection from mesna. Can be mixed with mesna. More severe symptoms may occur at higher doses and after rapid injection. Must receive PO or IV hydration beginning 3-6 hr before and 24 hr after dose. Must monitor I&O and urinary specific gravity. Fanconi's renal failure more common with history of cisplatin, prior kidney damage, and greater than 70-100 g/m² cumulative dose. May require electrolyte supplementation with magnesium (Mg), potassium (K^+), and phosphorus (PO_4).
Interferon (Intron A, Roferon-A)	IV over 15-30 min, SQ, IM	Protein produced by recombinant DNA technology	Common: none Occasional: fever, headache, fatigue, anorexia, nausea, myalgia, arthralgia, diarrhea, depression, confusion Rare: vomiting, chills, stomatitis, somnolence, psychosis, elevated transaminases, myelosuppression, peripheral neuropathy, sinus tachyarrhythmias, hypocalcemia, hyperkalemia, anaphylaxis, dyspnea, hypotension, rash, dizziness, impotence, alopecia, menstrual disorder	Premedication with magnesium choline salicylate, acetaminophen, or if not contraindicated, nonsteroidal antiinflammatory drugs (NSAIDs), may reduce fever and myalgias.

Data from Almuete, V., Brisby, J., Delman, B., et al. (2000). 2000 Guide for the administration and use of cancer chemotherapeutic agents. *Oncology Special Edition, 3,* 51-55; Balis, F., Hocenberg, J., & Poplack, D. G. (2000). General principles of chemotherapy. In P. A. Pizzo & D. G. Poplack (Eds.), *Principles and practice of pediatric oncology* (3rd ed., pp. 215-272). Philadelphia: Lippincott-Raven; Henry, D., Cartwright, J., & Sinsabaugh, D. (2000). *Children's Oncology Group pharmacology manual.* Arcadia, CA: Children's Oncology Group Operations Center; Renick-Ettinger, A. (1993). Chemotherapy. In G. V. Foley, D. Fochtman, & K. H. Mooney (Eds.). *Nursing care of the child with cancer* (2nd ed., pp. 81-116). Philadelphia: W. B. Saunders.

Continued

TABLE 6-4	CHEMOTHERAPEUTIC AGENTS—cont'd			
Drug	**Classification**	**Route**	**Side Effects**	**Special Considerations**
Irinotecan (CPT-11, Camptosar)	Topoisomerase I inhibitor	IV over 60 min	Common: transient early diarrhea, nausea, vomiting, abdominal pain, anorexia, fever, dehydration, alopecia, asthenia, myelosuppression, later diarrhea, alopecia Occasional: elevation in transaminases, alkaline phosphatase, bilirubin, creatinine, constipation, pain at infusion site Rare: dermatitis, tremor, hematuria, hypoproteinemia, glucosuria, mucositis, headache, dizziness, disorientation/confusion, facial hot flushes, colitis, pulmonary infiltrates, pneumonitis	May require antidiarrheal for control of diarrhea: atropine for early diarrhea, loperamide for delayed diarrhea.
Lomustine (CCNU, CeeNU)	Nitrosourea	PO	Common: nausea, vomiting, myelosuppression Occasional: anorexia Rare: elevation of liver enzymes, pulmonary toxicity, renal toxicity, cumulative myelosuppression	PO in one dose on an empty stomach, 1 hr before meals or 2 hr after meals.
Mechlorethamine (nitrogen mustard, Mustargen, HN2)	Alkylating agent	IV over 5 to 10 min	Common: nausea, vomiting, anorexia, metallic taste, phlebitis, alopecia, diarrhea, myelosuppression, gonadal dysfunction/sterility, necrosis if extravasated Occasional: weakness, lethargy Rare: anaphylaxis, rash, fever, headache, tinnitus, secondary malignancy	Vesicant—can also cause skin irritation with local contact (use sodium thiosulfate and ice). Use within 1 hr after reconstitution. May cause thrombosis, phlebitis, and discoloration of vein.
Melphalan (Alkeran, L-PAM, L-sarcolysin)	Alkylating agent	PO—2 mg tablets IV (investigational)	Common: anorexia, ulceration if extravasated, nausea, vomiting, myelosuppression, mucositis, diarrhea, alopecia Occasional: lethargy	Infusion over 15-30 min. Good hydration for 24 hr after IV dose. Furosemide may be given to maintain urinary output after IV

Drug	Classification	Route/Dose	Side effects	Nursing considerations
			fibrosis, sterility, secondary malignancy	Take on empty stomach.
Mercaptopurine (Purinethol, 6-MP)	Antimetabolite	PO—50 mg tablets IT (investigational)	Common: myelosuppression Occasional: anorexia, nausea, vomiting, diarrhea, mucositis Rare: anaphylactic reaction, urticaria, hepatic fibrosis, hyperbilirubinemia	Reduce oral dose 75% if given with allopurinol. Take daily dose at one time, preferably at bedtime on an empty stomach.
Methotrexate (amethopterin, MTX)	Antimetabolite	PO—2.5 mg tablets IV push or infusion IM IT	Common: transaminase and bilirubin elevations Occasional: nausea, vomiting, anorexia, diarrhea, myelosuppression, stomatitis, photosensitivity, learning disability Rare: dizziness, malaise, blurred vision, allergic reaction, peeling, redness and tenderness of skin—especially soles and palms, alopecia, folliculitis, renal toxicity, leukoencephalopathy, seizures, acute neurotoxicity, lung damage, liver damage, hyperpigmentation, osteoporosis, osteonecrosis and soft tissue necrosis, progressive CNS deterioration Intrathecal administration: nausea, vomiting, headache, pleocytosis, fever, convulsions, learning disability, rash, somnolence, meningismus, convulsions, paresis, myelosuppression, somnolence, ataxia, leukoencephalopathy, progressive CNS deterioration	Renal impairment will enhance toxicity. Advise patients to use sunscreen; severe sunburn can occur even with low weekly doses. When intermediate or high-dose methotrexate is given, leucovorin is administered as a rescue agent. Avoid vitamins containing folic acid to avoid the metabolic block caused by methotrexate. Hydration and urine alkalinization are used with higher dose infusions. Methotrexate readily enters body fluids; patients with effusions may have delayed clearance. Do not give concomitant trimethoprim and sulfamethaxozole, NSAIDs, aspirin because delayed clearance and increased toxicities may occur.

Data from Almuete, V., Brisby, J., Delman, B., et al. (2000). 2000 Guide for the administration and use of cancer chemotherapeutic agents. *Oncology Special Edition, 3*, 51-55; Balis, F., Hocenberg, J., & Poplack, D. G. (2000). General principles of chemotherapy. In P. A. Pizzo & D. G. Poplack (Eds.). *Principles and practice of pediatric oncology* (3rd ed., pp. 215-272). Philadelphia: Lippincott-Raven; Henry, D., Cartwright, J., & Sinsabaugh, D. (2000). *Children's Oncology Group pharmacology manual*. Arcadia, CA: Children's Oncology Group Operations Center; Renick-Ettinger, A. (1993). Chemotherapy. In G. V. Foley, D. Fochtman, & K. H. Mooney (Eds.), *Nursing care of the child with cancer* (2nd ed., pp. 81-116). Philadelphia: W. B. Saunders.

Continued

TABLE 6-4	**CHEMOTHERAPEUTIC AGENTS—cont'd**			
Drug	**Classification**	**Route**	**Side Effects**	**Special Considerations**
Mitoxantrone (Novantrone, DHAD)	Topoisomerase II inhibitor	IV infusion Dark blue solution	Common: cardiac arrhythmias, nausea, vomiting, worsening side effects due to radiation, local ulceration if extravasated, bluish-green color to urine, myelosuppression, immunosuppression, alopecia Occasional: stomatitis, hepatotoxicity, mucositis, cardiomyopathy (dose dependent) Rare: anaphylaxis, allergic reactions, rash, secondary malignancy	Vesicant—severe tissue damage if extravasation occurs. Not recommended for patients who have received full doses of anthracycline. Do not give IV push.
Paclitaxel (Taxol)	Plant product isolated from the stem bark of the western yew *Taxus brevifolia* or the needles of related plants Plant alkaloid	IV infusion	Common: pain, swelling, erythema if extravasated, myelosuppression, diminished or absent deep tendon reflexes, alopecia, fatigue Occasional: acute anaphylactic reaction, nausea, vomiting, headache, skin rash, mucositis, diarrhea, fever, glove and stocking numbness, hyperesthesia with burning sensation, mild to severe myalgias, increased triglyceride levels Rare: fever, bradycardia, seizures, swelling, erythema, coma, pulmonary toxicity, diplopia, blurred vision, flashing lights, confusion and disorientation, taste changes, pancreatitis, abdominal pain, hemorrhagic cystitis	Irritant—avoid extravasation. Premedicate with diphenhydramine, dexamethasone, and an H_2 receptor blocker. Do not administer in any bag or tubing containing polyvinyl chloride (PVC). Use filters because small fibers can appear after dilution.
Procarbazine (Matulane)	Alkylating agent	PO—50 mg capsules IV (investigational)	Common: nausea, vomiting, diarrhea, anorexia, inhibits monoamine oxidase (MAO) activity, myelosuppression, alopecia Occasional: headache, flulike syndrome,	Hypotension and/or CNS depression may occur in the presence of alcohol, narcotics, antihistamines, phenothiazines, phenytoin (Dilantin), tricyclic

			Side effects	Nursing considerations
Retinoic acids (13-*cis*-retinoic acid, isotretinoin [Accutane is investigational in cancer]) All-*trans* retinoic acid (tretinoin [Vesanoid])	Differentiating agents Vitamin A and its derivatives stimulates clonal proliferation of erythroid and myeloid progenitor cells and play a role in growth, reproduction, epithelial cell differentiation, and immune function	PO	hemolytic anemia, pruritis, rash, depression, insomnia, convulsions, coma, stomatitis, pulmonary reaction, hypertension, secondary malignancy Common: dry skin, dry mucosa, inflammation of the lips Occasional: nausea, vomiting, rash, conjunctivitis, musculoskeletal pains, fatigue, headache, triglyceride elevation, cholesterol elevations, transaminase elevations, retinoic acid syndrome with hyperleukocytosis Rare: changes in skin pigmentation, nonspecific GI complaints, dizziness, pseudotumor cerebri, RBC count decreases, WBC count decreases, respiratory distress, fever, hypotension, skeletal hyperostosis	tyramine-rich foods such as aged cheese, wine, bananas, yogurt. Take ½ hr before or 2 hr after meals. Take with food or milk to enhance absorption. Monitor lipid levels. Avoid sun exposure, use good lubricant for skin. Monitor nutritional status.
Teniposide (VM-26, Vumon)	Plant alkaloid Epipodophyllotoxin	IV infusion over 60 min	Common: nausea, vomiting, myelosuppression Occasional: alopecia, enhanced damage due to radiation, diarrhea Rare: hypotension, anaphylaxis, skin rash, peripheral neuropathy, stomatitis, secondary malignancy	Irritant—avoid extravasation. Do not use PVC-containing bags or tubing to administer. Do not refrigerate diluted solutions. Heparin can precipitate; must be flushed from lines. Anaphylaxis or hypotensive reaction with rapid infusion. Flush vein before and after administration.

Data from Almuete, V., Brisby, J., Delman, B., et al. (2000). 2000 Guide for the administration and use of cancer chemotherapeutic agents. *Oncology Special Edition, 3,* 51-55; Balis, F., Hocenberg, J., & Poplack, D. G. General principles of chemotherapy. In P. A. Pizzo & D. G. Poplack (Eds.), *Principles and practice of pediatric oncology* (3rd ed., pp. 215-272). Philadelphia: Lippincott-Raven; Henry, D., Cartwright, J., & Sinsabaugh, D. (2000). *Children's Oncology Group pharmacology manual.* Arcadia, CA: Children's Oncology Group Operations Center; Renick-Ettinger, A. (1993). Chemotherapy. In G. V. Foley, D. Fochtman, & K. H. Mooney (Eds.), *Nursing care of the child with cancer* (2nd ed., pp. 81-116). Philadelphia: W. B. Saunders.

Continued

TABLE 6-4	CHEMOTHERAPEUTIC AGENTS—cont'd			
Drug	Classification	Route	Side Effects	Special Considerations
Thioguanine (6-thioguanine, 6-TG)	Antimetabolite	PO 40-mg tab	Common: myelosuppression Occasional: anorexia, nausea, vomiting, diarrhea, mucositis Rare: anaphylactic reaction, urticaria, hematuria, crystalluria, hepatic fibrosis, hyperbilirubinemia	Take oral dose at one time, preferably at bedtime on empty stomach.
Thiotepa (Triethylenethio-phosphoramide, Thioplex)	Alkylating agent	IV infusion IT IM SQ Intracavitary Intratumor	Common: nausea, vomiting, anorexia, myelosuppression, mucositis and esophagitis at higher doses in conditioning regimens for bone marrow transplant (BMT), gonadal dysfunction/infertility Occasional: pain at injection site, dizziness, headache; inappropriate behavior, confusion, somnolence, increased liver transaminase, increased bilirubin, hyperpigmentation of the skin at higher dose in conditioning regimens for BMT Rare: hives, skin rash, febrile reaction	Use 0.22-micron filter to eliminate haze with IV infusions; solutions that are grossly opaque or contain obvious precipitation should not be used. Dilute reconstituted solutions with NS before use. Should be used within 8 hr.
Topotecan (Hycamtin)	Plant alkaloid Topoisomerase I inhibitor	IV IT	Common: myelosuppression, alopecia Occasional: nausea, vomiting, diarrhea, mucositis, flulike symptoms, headache, rash, elevated transaminases, elevated alkaline phosphatase, elevated bilirubin, asthenia Rare: abdominal pain, rigors, microscopic hematuria Intrathecal: Nausea, vomiting, headache, fever, back pain, possible leukoencephalopathy, seizures, or	Administer IT doses over 5 min to avoid potential adverse reactions.

Drug	Classification	Route	Side effects	Comments
(VLB, vincaleukoblastine, Velban)	Plant alkaloid	IV push	Common: myelosuppression, alopecia Occasional: constipation, loss of deep tendon reflexes, paresthesias Rare: nausea, vomiting, anorexia, bone pain, allergic reaction, stomatitis, peripheral neuropathy, hoarseness, ptosis, double vision	Vesicant—severe tissue damage if extravasation occurs. Administer stool softeners; increase bulk and fiber in diet.
Vincristine (VCR, Oncovin)	Plant alkaloid	IV push	Common: local ulceration if extravasated, hair loss, loss of deep tendon reflexes Occasional: jaw pain, weakness, constipation, numbness, tingling, clumsiness Rare: paralytic ileus, ptosis, vocal cord paralysis, myelosuppression, CNS depression, seizures, SIADH	Vesicant—severe tissue damage if extravasation occurs. Refrigerate and protect from light. Stool softeners may be given prophylactically or for constipation. Liver dysfunction or concomitant radiation therapy to the liver may enhance toxicity. Must have special overwrap label that bears the statement, "Do not remove covering until moment of injection. Fatal if given intrathecally. For intravenous injection only." Infants may have difficulty sucking because of jaw pain. Maximal single dose: 2 mg regardless of BSA. A few Hodgkin's disease protocols do not cap the dose at 2 mg. Always check.

Data from Almuete, V., Brisby, J., Delman, B., et al. (2000). 2000 Guide for the administration and use of cancer chemotherapeutic agents. *Oncology Special Edition, 3,* 51-55; Balis, F., Hocenberg, J., & Poplack, D. G. General principles of chemotherapy. In P. A. Pizzo & D. G. Poplack (Eds.), *Principles and practice of pediatric oncology* (3rd ed., pp. 215-272). Philadelphia: Lippincott-Raven; Henry, D., Cartwright, J., & Sinsabaugh, D. (2000). *Children's Oncology Group pharmacology manual.* Arcadia, CA: Children's Oncology Group Operations Center; Renick-Ettinger, A. (1993). Chemotherapy. In G. V. Foley, D. Fochtman, & K. H. Mooney (Eds.), *Nursing care of the child with cancer* (2nd ed., pp. 81-116). Philadelphia: W. B. Saunders.

Continued

TABLE 6-4	CHEMOTHERAPEUTIC AGENTS—cont'd			
Drug	**Classification**	**Route**	**Side Effects**	**Special Considerations**
MISCELLANEOUS DRUGS				
Allopurinol (Zyloprim)	Enzyme inhibitor; blocks uric acid production by inhibiting xanthine oxidase	PO IV	Common: rash, fever Occasional: granulomatous hepatitis, ocular lesions, alopecia, slight bone marrow suppression, drowsiness, peripheral neuropathy, GI complaints Rare: agranulocytosis, toxic epidermal necrolysis, severe systemic vasculitis, exfoliative dermatitis	Dose reduction is required in moderate to severe renal impairment. Increased toxicities may occur when used with 6-MP or azathioprine—use with great caution. With cyclophosphamide, warfarin, oral antidiabetic drugs, ampicillin, amoxicillin, or thiazide diuretics, use with caution. Maintain adequate hydration. Physically incompatible with methotrexate—do not give in same IV fluid.
Amifostine (Ethyol)	Organic thiophosphate cytoprotective agent	IV	Common: nausea, vomiting, flushing, hypotension, hypocalcemia (with multiple daily or multiple day dosing) Occasional: sleepiness, dizziness, sneezing Rare: hiccups, chills	If multiple doses are administered within a 24-hr period, monitor serum calcium levels and supplement as needed. Administer with patient lying down. Have normal saline bolus at bedside. Monitor blood pressure frequently during infusion (every 3-5 min). Hypotension often occurs toward the end of the infusion. If hypotension develops, place patient in Trendelenberg's position and administer NS bolus (20 ml/kg over 20 min). If blood pressure normalizes, resume infusion. Doses are given immediately before radiation therapy or chemotherapy. Inspect parenteral solutions for particulate matter or discoloration. Do not use if cloudiness or precipitate is observed.

Drug	Action	Route	Side Effects	Comments
Dexrazoxane (Zinecard)	Iron chelator that interferes with iron-mediated free radical generation	IV Slow push or rapid infusion	Common: Pain on injection, phlebitis, myelosuppression Occasional: transient increases in triglycerides, amylase, and alanine transaminase (ALT), mild nausea, vomiting, and diarrhea Rare: neurotoxicity (headache, constipation)	Use with NS solutions only. Compatibility with other solutions has not been examined. Recommended dose ratio of dexrazoxane:doxorubicin is 10:1. After completing infusion of dexrazoxane, doxorubicin must be given before elapsed time of 30 min from beginning of dexrazoxane infusion.
Leucovorin calcium (Wellcovorin, citrovorum factor, folinic acid)	Antidote Bypasses the inhibitor action of folic acid antagonist (methotrexate)	PO IV IM	Rare: allergic sensitization, rash	Used as cellular rescue when intermediate- or high-dose methotrexate is given. May be given as a single dose after IT methotrexate. Must be given exactly at the times ordered.
Mesna (Mesnex)	Uroprotective agent	IV push IV infusion IV form may be given PO	Common: bad taste with oral use Occasional: nausea, vomiting, stomach pain Rare: headache; pain in arms, legs, and joints; fatigue; rash; transient hypotension; allergy; diarrhea	False positive test for urinary ketones. Not compatible with cisplatin. May be mixed with cyclophosphamide or ifosfamide. Must be give exactly at the times ordered. IV dose may be given orally at a higher dose, orally has a foul taste. Do not use the multidose vial in young infants or neonates because preservative benzyl alcohol is used.

Data from Almuete, V., Brisby, J., Delman, B., et al. (2000). 2000 Guide for the administration and use of cancer chemotherapeutic agents. *Oncology Special Edition, 3,* 51-55; Balis, F., Hocenberg, J., & Poplack, D. G. General principles of chemotherapy. In P. A. Pizzo & D. G. Poplack (Eds.), *Principles and practice of pediatric oncology* (3rd ed., pp. 215-272). Philadelphia: Lippincott-Raven; Henry, D., Cartwright, J., & Sinsabaugh, D. (2000). *Children's Oncology Group pharmacology manual.* Arcadia, CA: Children's Oncology Group Operations Center; Renick-Ettinger, A. (1993). Chemotherapy. In G. V. Foley, D. Fochtman, & K. H. Mooney (Eds.), *Nursing care of the child with cancer* (2nd ed., pp. 81-116). Philadelphia: W. B. Saunders.

Continued

TABLE 6-4	CHEMOTHERAPEUTIC AGENTS—cont'd			
Drug	**Classification**	**Route**	**Side Effects**	**Special Considerations**
Trimethoprim and sulfamethoxazole (Bactrim, Septrax, Co-Trimoxizole)	Antibiotic used prophylactically to prevent *Pneumocystis carinii* pneumonia	PO IV	Occasional: neutropenia, anorexia, nausea, vomiting, diarrhea, GI upset, hepatic dysfunction, rash Rare: Stevens-Johnson syndrome, toxic epidermal necrolysis	May be given as prophylaxis for *P. carinii* on a schedule of 3 consecutive days weekly. If allergic to Bactrim, may use aerosolized pentamidine or PO dapsone. Must be diluted in 5% dextrose in water (D5W) solution for IV administration; infuse parenteral solution over 60-90 min; monitor for hyponatremia. Not compatible with other drugs in IV solution. Avoid use during methotrexate infusion: delays methotrexate clearance and increases risk of toxicities. Use sunscreen during use because Trimethoprim increases sensitivity to sun.

Data from Almuete, V., Brisby, J., Delman, B., et al. (2000). 2000 Guide for the administration and use of cancer chemotherapeutic agents. *Oncology Special Edition, 3,* 51-55; Balis, F., Hocenberg, J., & Poplack. D. G. General principles of chemotherapy. In P. A. Pizzo & D. G. Poplack (Eds.), *Principles and practice of pediatric oncology* (3rd ed., pp. 215-272). Philadelphia: Lippincott-Raven; Henry, D., Cartwright, J., & Sinsabaugh, D. (2000). *Children's Oncology Group pharmacology manual.* Arcadia, CA: Children's Oncology Group Operations Center; Renick-Ettinger, A. (1993). Chemotherapy. In G. V. Foley, D. Fochtman, & K. H. Mooney (Eds.), *Nursing care of the child with cancer* (2nd ed., pp. 81-116). Philadelphia: W. B. Saunders.

BOX 6-7

FAMILY EDUCATION CHECKLIST: WHAT THE FAMILY SHOULD KNOW

TREATMENT PLAN

The type of chemotherapy the child is receiving and its side effects

The date, time, and location of the next appointment

Important telephone numbers

The days on which blood counts should be done

IMPORTANT SIGNS TO REPORT

Signs of infection

- Fever (temperatures of 101° F/38.3° C and above)
- Cough or rapid breathing
- Earache
- Sore throat
- The child's inability to bend his or her neck
- Stomach pain
- Red or irritated skin around the child's bottom
- Blisters, rashes, ulcers on the skin
- Redness, swelling, pus around the central line

Change in behavior or level of consciousness

Break in the central line

Bleeding, increased bruising, or petechiae

Difficulty or pain when eating, drinking, or swallowing

Changes in bowel habits (e.g., constipation, diarrhea)

Paleness, increased fatigue

Inability to drink or eat

Exposure to chicken pox

IMPORTANT PRECAUTIONS

Do not give the patient aspirin (Ecotrin) or products containing aspirin.

Do not take the child's temperatures rectally or otherwise manipulate that area, and do not give the patient suppositories.

HEALTHCARE HABITS AND INFECTION PRECAUTIONS

Good handwashing

Proper nutrition

Proper mouth care

Avoidance of crowds and contagious persons

Daily bath or shower

Sufficient rest

Knowing the proper way to take a temperature

SUPPORTIVE MEDICATIONS (INCLUDING THE REASON FOR THEIR USE AND INFORMATION ABOUT DOSAGE AND ADMINISTRATION)

Pneumocystis carinii prophylaxis (e.g., Bactrim)

Colony-stimulating factor therapy (e.g., G-CSF)

Supplemental or adjuvant medications (e.g., allopurinol, magnesium, calcium)

MISCELLANEOUS

Nutritional support (e.g., total parenteral nutrition, lipids, supplements)

Care of a central line

From Hando, S. (1998). Family education. In M. Hockenberry-Eaton (Ed.), *Essentials of pediatric oncology nursing: A core curriculum* (p. 217). Glenview, IL: Association of Pediatric Oncology Nurses.

grandparents, siblings, extended family members, teachers, school nurses, and babysitters, to name a few. Each person is vital to the child's care, and each should be comfortable with the treatment being given. These other caregivers need education about the treatment and associated side effects. With the parents' permission, offer other caregivers written materials—available from the NCI, American Cancer Society (ACS), Association of Pediatric Oncology Nurses (APON), the Internet, and many other sources, or give information that has been developed by you or your institution. Provide explanations, review the written information, and schedule time for "teaching" sessions with all caregivers.

Caution is necessary with all medications, supplies, and equipment at home. Remind parents that siblings may be curious about the medications in the household. Therefore it is imperative that they understand the disease and treatment or medications necessary for the care of the child with can-

cer. Medications, needles, and syringes must be stored in a locked box and kept out of reach. Children must never be told that their medication is candy.

In this fast-paced world where patients and families have access to information at the same time as health care professionals, it is important that the nurse be cognizant of new developments. Often the media reports on new agents that have been tested and marketed only for adults. Parents will come to you asking about these agents. If you are familiar with the agent, carefully explain it to the parents, noting the similarities and differences in adults and children. If you are unfamiliar with a treatment, tell them that you will seek the information and then share it with them.

There are many new agents being tested in pediatric oncology (Table 6-5). These agents may be fast-tracked to be marketed. The concept of using a new agent must be carefully explained to families and patients. They should not be made to feel like

TABLE 6-5	PHASE I/II AGENTS: NEW CANCER MEDICINES IN DEVELOPMENT FOR CHILDREN	

Agent	Tumor Types	Phase
O6-benzylguanine (with BCNU)	Brain tumors	Phase I
506U78 (Ara-G prodrug)	Refractory or recurrent T cell malignancies	Phase II
6-Mercaptopurine-IV	ALL, refractory leukemia or lymphoma	Phase II/III
6-Thioguinine-IV	Acute leukemia	Phase I
Aastrom Cell Production System stem and progenitor cells	Pediatric leukemia	Phase I/II
Aptosyn exisulind	Precancerous colon polyps in children with familial adenomatous polyposis	Phase II (ages 9-18)
Arsenic trioxide	Leukemia	Phase I
Gemcitabine (Gemzar)	Refractory leukemia, lymphoma, solid tumors	Phase I/II
Trastuzumab (Herceptin)	Osteosarcoma	Phase II
Homoharringtonine	Leukemia	Phase II (ages 12 and older)
Topotecan (Hycamtin)	Brain cancer, leukemia, neuroblastoma, sarcoma, solid tumors	Phase I/II
ImmTher	Ewing's sarcoma	Phase II (ages 6-18)
Interleukin-4	Refractory acute leukemia	Phase I
Irofulven (MGI-114)	Solid tumors	Phase I
Liposomal all-*trans* retinoic acid (IV) (Atragen)	Acute promyelocytic leukemia	Phase II
BNP1350 (Karenitecin)	Solid tumors	Phase I (ages 1-20)
Bryostatin I	Solid tumors	Phase I
Busulfex Busulfan (Orphan drug)	Combined with cyclophosphamide as conditioning regimen for HSCT in CML	Phase II (newborn-16)
Buthionine sulfoximine with BCNU	Melanoma, neuroblastoma	Phase I
Irinotecan (Camptosar)	Refractory solid tumors	Phase I
Cereport/RMP-7	Brain tumors	Phase II (ages 6-18)
Cytarabine liposome injection (DepoCyt) (orphan drug)	Lymphomatous meningitis, neoplastic meningitis	Phase I (newborn-18)
Dolastatin 10	Refractory solid tumors	Phase I
Ewing's sarcoma and alveolar rhabdomyosarcoma peptide vaccine	Sarcoma	Phase II

Adapted from New cancer medicines in development for children. (2000). *Oncology Times, 22*(10), 34-35.

"guinea pigs" but should understand that every chemotherapeutic agent that is presently marketed and used as standard therapy was once a new, investigational agent.

It is possible to intensify chemotherapy regimens because of the care that can be afforded patients today. Growth factors, transfusion therapy, and improved antibiotic therapy are a few of the supportive care methods available to improve the outcome for children and adolescents undergoing chemotherapy. (See Part III for further information.)

The importance of cooperative clinical trials cannot be overemphasized. It is through this method of research that children and adolescents with cancer are being cured today. With the merger of the pediatric cooperative groups and the forma-

TABLE 6-5	PHASE I/II AGENTS
	NEW CANCER MEDICINES IN DEVELOPMENT FOR CHILDREN—cont'd

Agent	Tumor Types	Phase
Fenretinide	Solid tumors	Phase I
G3139	Leukemia	Phase I (ages 16 and older)
Leridistim	Chemotherapy induced neutropenia	Phase III (ages 2-21)
MTP-PE	Osteogenic sarcoma	Phase III
Multiple-drug-resistance inhibitor	Enhance potency of anticancer drugs	Phase II
Gemtuzumab ozogamicin (Mylotarg)	AML	Phase I (ages 18 and younger)
Oprelvekin (Neumega)	Chemotherapy induced thrombocytopenia	Phase I/II (ages 1-18)
Sandostatin LAR (OncoLAR)	Osteosarcoma	Phase I
Prednisolone sodium phosphate oral solution (Orapred)	ALL	Application limited (infants-adults)
Phenylacetate	Brain tumors	Phase II
Aldesleukin (interleukin-2) (Proleukin)	Leukemia, myelodysplastic syndromes	Phase III
PSC-833 (MDR reversing agent)	Refractory leukemia	Phase I
R115777	Brain tumors, refractory solid tumors	Phase III (ages 2-18)
Rebeccamycin analogue	Neuroblastoma, solid tumors	Phase II
SR 29142 (urate oxidase)	Prevention and treatment of hyperuricemia in association with treatment of malignancies	Application submitted
STI 571	Philadelphia chromosome positive leukemia	Phase I (newborn-16)
Paclitaxel (Taxol)	Leukemia, solid tumors	Phase I
Docetaxel (Taxotere)	Recurrent solid tumors	Phase II
Thrombopoietin	Chemotherapy related thrombocytopenia	Phase III
Tirapazamine	Solid tumors	Phase I
Tomudex	Leukemia, solid tumors	Phase I/II
All-*trans*-retinoic acid (Vesanoid)	Recurrent neuroblastoma, Wilms tumor	Phase II
Xcytrin	Gliomas	Phase I (ages 2-15)
ICRF-187, dexrazoxane (Zinecard) (cardioprotectant)	Leukemia, lymphoma	Phase III

tion of the Children's Oncology Group, clinical trials can be opened and completed rapidly, thereby ensuring that results will be available more quickly.

Finally, the nurse makes the ordeal of a cancer diagnosis more bearable for the patient and family. Caregiver, support giver, and teacher are only a few of the roles the nurse fulfills. Families always appreciate the importance of a competent, knowledgeable, friendly, kind nurse as the most important force that gets them through the process.

ACKNOWLEDGMENT

The authors would like to thank Kim Eberson, RN, from the Children's Hospital at University of Missouri Health Care for her careful review of the chapter.

REFERENCES

1. Anderson, B. J., & Ellis, J. F. (1999). Common errors of drug administration in infants: Causes and avoidance. *Pediatric Drugs, 1,* 93-107.
2. ASHP Therapeutic guidelines on the pharmacologic management of nausea and vomiting in adult and pediatric patients receiving chemotherapy or radiation therapy or undergoing surgery. (1999). *American Journal of Health-System Pharmacists, 56,* 729-764.
3. Association of Pediatric Oncology Nurses. (2000). *Scope and standards of pediatric oncology nursing practice.* Washington, DC: American Nurses Publishing.
4. Bain, P. G., Lantos, P. L., Djurovic, V., et al. (1991). Intrathecal vincristine: A fatal chemotherapeutic error with devastating central nervous system effects. *Journal of Neurology, 238,* 230-234.
5. Balis, F. M., Holcenberg, J. S., & Poplack, D. G. (1997). General principles of chemotherapy. In P. A. Pizzo & D. G. Poplack (Eds.), *Principles and practice of pediatric oncology* (3rd ed., pp. 215-272). Philadelphia: Lippincott-Raven.
6. Bates, D. W., Boyle, D. L., Vander Vliet, M., et al. (1995). Relationship between medication errors and adverse drug events. *Journal of General Internal Medicine, 10,* 199-205.
7. Bates, D. W., Cullen, D., Laird, N., et al. (1995). ADE Prevention Study Group. Incidence of adverse drug events and potential adverse drug events: Implications for prevention. *Journal of the American Medical Association, 274,* 29-34.
8. Bates, D. W., Leape, L. L., Cullen, D. J., et al. (1998). Effect of computerized physician order entry and a team intervention on prevention of serious medication errors. *Journal of the American Medical Association, 280,* 1311-1316.
9. Bates, D. W., Spell, N., Cullen, D. J., et al. (1997). The cost of adverse drug events in hospitalized patients. *Journal of the American Medical Association, 277,* 307-311.
10. Bedell, W. E., Deitz, D. C., & Leeman, D. (1991). Incidence and characteristics of preventable iatrogenic cardiac arrests. *Journal of the American Medical Association, 265,* 2815-2820.
11. Berg, D., Centrilla, L., Halsey, J., et al. (1999). Overcoming multidrug resistance: Valspodar as a paradigm for nursing care. *Oncology Nursing Forum, 26,* 711-720.
12. Berger, A. M., & Clark-Snow, R. A. (2001). Adverse effects of treatment. In V. T. DeVita, Jr., S. Hellman, & S. A. Rosenberg (Eds.), *Cancer: Principles and practice of oncology* (6th ed., pp. 335-344). Philadelphia: Lippincott Williams & Wilkins.
13. Bleyer, W. A., & Dedrick, R. L. (1977). The clinical pharmacology of intrathecal methotrexate. 1. Distribution kinetics in nontoxic patients after lumbar injection. *Cancer Treatment Reports, 61,* 703-708.
14. Bleyer, W. A., Tejeda, H., Murphy, S., et al. (1997). Equal participation of minority patients in U.S. national pediatric cancer clinical trials. *Journal of Pediatric Hematology/Oncology, 19,* 473-477.
15. Bleyer, W. A., Tejeda, H., Murphy, S., et al. (1997). National cancer clinical trials: Children have equal access; Adolescents do not. *Journal of Adolescent Health, 21,* 366-373.
16. Brant, J. (1995). Is it safe for pregnant nurses to be exposed to chemotherapy agents? *ONS News, 10*(3), 5.
17. Brennan, T. A., Leape, L. L., Laird, N. M., et al. (1991). Incidence of adverse events and negligence in hospitalized patients. *New England Journal of Medicine, 324,* 37-36.

18. Cary, A. H. (2001). Certified registered nurses: Results of the Study of the Certified Workforce. *American Journal of Nursing, 101* (1), 44-52.
19. Castleberry, R. P., Cantor, A. B., Green, A. A., et al. (1994). Phase II investigational window using carboplatin, iproplatin, ifosfamide, and epirubicin in children with untreated disseminated neuroblastoma: A Pediatric Oncology Group study. *Journal of Clinical Oncology, 12,* 1616-1620.
20. Classen, D. C., Pestonik, S. L., Evans, R. S., et al. (1997). Adverse drug events in hospitalized patients: Excess length of stay, extra costs, and attributable mortality. *Journal of the American Medical Association, 277,* 301-306.
21. Cohen, M. R. (1999). Causes of medication errors. In M. R. Cohen (Ed.), *Medication errors* (pp. 1-8). Washington, DC: American Pharmaceutical Association.
22. Cohen, M. R. (1999). Preventing medication errors related to prescribing. In M. R. Cohen (Ed.), *Medication errors* (pp. 8.1-8.23). Washington, DC: American Pharmaceutical Association.
23. Cohen, M. R., Anderson, R. W., Attilo, R. M., et al. (1996). Preventing medication errors in cancer chemotherapy. *American Journal of Health-System Pharmacists, 53,* 737-746.
24. Cohen, M. R., & Kilo, C. M. (1999). High-alert medications: Safeguarding against errors. In M. R. Cohen (Ed.), *Medication errors* (pp. 5.1-5.40). Washington, DC: American Pharmaceutical Association.
25. Coleman, E. A., Frank-Stromborg, M., Hughes, L. C., et al. (1999). A national survey of certified, recertified, and noncertified oncology nurses: Comparisons and contrasts. *Oncology Nursing Forum, 26,* 839-849.
26. Collins, J. M. (1996). Pharmacokinetics and clinical monitoring. In B. A. Chabner, & D. L. Longo (Eds.), *Cancer chemotherapy and biotherapy: Principles and practice* (2nd ed., pp. 17-30). Philadelphia: Lippincott-Raven.
27. *Common toxicity criteria.* (1999). Bethesda, MD: National Cancer Institute.
28. Cousins, D. D., & Calnan, R. (1999). Medication error reporting systems. In M. R. Cohen (Ed.), *Medication errors* (pp. 18.1-18.20). Washington, DC: American Pharmaceutical Association.
29. Doak, C. C., Doak, L. G., & Root, J. H. (1996). *Teaching patients with low literacy skills.* Philadelphia: J. B. Lippincott.
30. Espinosa, J. A., & Nolan, T. W. (2000). Reducing errors made by emergency physicians in interpreting radiographs: Longitudinal study. *British Journal of Medicine, 320,* 737-740.
31. Ettinger, L. J., Ettinger, A. G., Avramis, V. I., et al. (1997). Acute lymphoblastic leukaemia: A guide to asparaginase and pegaspargase therapy. A review from the Children's Cancer Group Asparaginase Task Force. *BioDrugs, 7,* 30-39.
32. Evans, R. S., Classen, D. C., Pestotnic, S. L., et al. (1994). Improving empiric antibiotic selection using computer decision support. *Archives in Internal Medicine, 154,* 878-884.
33. Evans, R. S., Pestonik, S. L., Classen, D. C., et al. (1998). A computer assisted management program for antibiotics and other anti-infective agents. *New England Journal of Medicine, 338,* 232-238.
34. Falvo, D. R. (1994). *Effective patient education: A guide to increased compliance* (2nd ed.). Gaithersburg, MD: Aspen.
35. Fernandez, C. V., Esau, R., Hamilton, D., et al. (1998). Intrathecal vincristine: An analysis of reasons for recurrent fatal chemotherapeutic error with recommendations for prevention. *Journal of Pediatric Hematology/Oncology, 20,* 587-590.

36. Ferner, R. E. (1992). Errors in prescribing and giving drugs. *Journal of the Medical Defense Union, 8,* 60-63.

37. Fidler, I. J., Kerbel, R. S., & Lee, M. E. (2001). Biology of cancer: Angiogenesis. In V. T. DeVita, Jr., S. Hellman, & S. A. Rosenberg (Eds.), *Cancer: Principles and practice of oncology* (6th ed., pp. 137-147). Philadelphia: Lippincott Williams & Wilkins.

38. Finley, R. S. (2000). Overview of promising new anticancer agents. *Oncology nursing updates, 7*(4), 1-15.

39. Fischer, D. S., Alfano, S., Knobf, M. T., et al. (1996). Improving the cancer chemotherapy use process. *Journal of Clinical Oncology, 14,* 3148-3155.

40. Fishman, M., & Mrozek-Orlowski, M. (Eds.). (1999). *Cancer chemotherapy: Guidelines and recommendations for practice* (2nd ed.). Pittsburgh: Oncology Nursing Press.

41. Folkman, J. (2001). Antiangiogenic therapy. In V. T. DeVita, Jr., S. Hellman, & S. A. Rosenberg (Eds.), *Cancer: Principles and practice of oncology* (6th ed., pp. 509-519). Philadelphia: Lippincott Williams & Wilkins.

42. Friedland, M. L. (1996). Combination chemotherapy. In M. C. Perry (Ed.), *The chemotherapy source book* (2nd ed., pp. 101-107). Baltimore: Williams & Wilkins.

43. Gilewski, T., & Bitran, J. D. (1996). Adjuvant chemotherapy. In M. C. Perry, (Ed.), *The chemotherapy source book* (2nd ed., pp. 79-100). Baltimore: Williams & Wilkins.

44. Goldie, J. H. (1996). Drug resistance. In M. C. Perry (Ed.), *The chemotherapy source book* (2nd ed., pp. 63-78). Baltimore: Williams & Wilkins.

45. Goodman, M. (2000). Chemotherapy: Principles of administration. In C. H. Yarbro, M. G. Frogge, M. Goodman, et al. (Eds.), *Cancer nursing: Principles and practice* (5th ed., pp. 385-443). Sudbury, MA: Jones & Bartlett.

46. Gribbon, J., & Loescher, L. J. (2000). Biology of cancer. In C. H. Yarbro, M. H. Frogge, M. Goodman, et al. (Eds.), *Cancer nursing: Principles and practice* (5th ed., pp. 17-34). Sudbury, MA: Jones & Bartlett.

47. Hesketh, P., Dris M., Greensberg, S. M., et al. (1997). Proposal for classifying the acute emetogenicity of cancer chemotherapy. *Journal of Clinical Oncology, 15,* 103-109.

48. Hinds, P. S., & Herring, P. L. (1998). The guidance not given by clinical trial protocols. *Journal of Pediatric Oncology Nursing, 15,* 1-2.

49. Hockenberry-Eaton, M., & Kline, N. (1997). Nursing support of the child with cancer. In P. A. Pizzo & D. G. Poplack (Eds.), *Principle and practice of pediatric oncology,* (3rd ed., pp. 1209-1228). Philadelphia: J. B. Lippincott.

50. Hughes, L. C., Ward, S., Grindel, C. G., et al. (2001). Relationships between certification and job perceptions of oncology nurses. *Oncology Nursing Forum, 28,* 99-106.

51. Institute of Medicine. (1999). *To err is human: Building a safer health system.* Washington, D.C.: National Academy Press.

52. Israels, E. D., & Israels, L. G. (2000). The cell cycle. *The Oncologist, 4,* 510-513.

53. Jenkins, J., & Hubbard, S. (1991). History of clinical trials. *Seminars in Oncology Nursing, 7,* 228-234.

54. Johnston, M. E., Langton, K. B., Haynes, R. B., et al. (1994). Effects of computer-based clinical decision support systems on clinician performance and patient outcome: A critical appraisal of research. *Annals of Internal Medicine, 120,* 135-142.

55. Kastan, M. B., & Skapek, S. X. (2001). Molecular biology of cancer: The cell cycle. In V. T. DeVita, Jr., S. Hellman, S. A. Rosenberg (Eds.), *Cancer: Principles and practice of oncology* (6th ed., pp. 91-110). Philadelphia: Lippincott Williams & Wilkins.

56. Kenney, L. B., & Reaman, G. H. (1997). Special considerations for the infant with cancer. In P. A. Pizzo, & D. G. Poplack. (Eds.), *Principles and practices of pediatric oncology* (3rd ed., 343-356). Philadelphia: Lippincott-Raven.

57. Kohler, D. R., Montello, M. J., Green, L., et al. (1998). Standardizing the expression and nomenclature of cancer treatment regimens. *American Journal of Health-System Pharmacists, 55,* 137-144.

58. Koren, G., Barzilay, Z., & Greenwald, M. (1986). Tenfold errors in administration of drug doses: A neglected iatrogenic disease in pediatrics. *Pediatrics, 77,* 848-849.

59. Kyngäs, H. A., Kroll, T., & Duffy, M. E. (2000). Compliance in adolescents with chronic diseases: A review. *Journal of Adolescent Health, 26,* 379-388.

60. Leape, L. L. (1994). Error in medicine. *Journal of the American Medical Association, 272,* 1851-1857.

61. Leape, L. L., Bates, D. W., Cullen, D. J., et al. (1995). ADE Prevention Study Group. Systems analysis of adverse drug events. *Journal of the American Medical Association, 274,* 35-43.

62. Leape, L. L., Brennan, T. A., Laird, N., et al. (1991). The nature of adverse events in hospitalized patients: Results of the Harvard medical practice study II. *New England Journal of Medicine, 324,* 377-384.

63. Lesar, T. S., Briceland, L. L., Delcoure, K., et al. (1990). Medication prescribing errors in a teaching hospital. *Journal of the American Medical Association, 263,* 2329-2334.

64. Lesar, T. S., Briceland, L. L., & Stein, D. S. (1997). Factors related to errors in medication prescribing. *Journal of the American Medical Association, 277,* 312-317.

65. Lunik, M. C. (1994). Managing oncology research protocols. *Topics in Hospital Pharmacy Management, 14,* 11-21.

66. Meadows, A. T., Kramer, S., Hopson, R., et al. (1983). Survival in childhood acute lymphocytic leukemia: Effect of protocol and place of treatment. *Cancer Investigation, 1,* 49-55.

67. Melink, T. K., & Whitacre, M. Y. (1991). Planning and implementing clinical trials. *Seminars in Oncology Nursing, 7,* 243-251.

68. Miller, A. A., Ratain, M. J., & Schilsky, R. L. (1996). Principles of pharmacology. In M. C. Perry (Ed.), *The chemotherapy source book* (2nd ed., pp. 27-41). Baltimore: Williams & Wilkins.

69. Minter, B., & Ryan, J. (Eds.). (1998). *Pharmacological agents in pediatric oncology nursing* (4th ed.). Glenview, IL: Association of Pediatric Oncology Nurses.

70. Murphy, S. B. (1995). The national impact of clinical cooperative group trials for pediatric cancer. *Medical and Pediatric Oncology, 24,* 279-280.

71. Pestonik, S. L., Classen, D. C., Evans, R. S., et al. (1996). Implementing antibiotics practice guidelines through computer-assisted decision-support: Clinical and financial outcomes. *Annals of Internal Medicine, 124,* 884-890.

72. Raschke, R. A., Gollihare, B., Wunderlich, T. A., et al. (1998). A computer alert system to prevent injury from adverse drug events: Development and evaluation in a community teaching hospital. *Journal of the American Medical Association, 280,* 1317-1320.

73. Ratain, M. J. (2001). Section 1—pharmacokinetics and pharmacodynamics: Pharmacology of cancer chemotherapy. In V. T. DeVita, Jr., S. Hellman, & S. A. Rosenberg (Eds.), *Cancer: Principles and practice of oncology* (6th ed., pp. 335-344). Philadelphia: Lippincott Williams & Wilkins.

74. Sadler, G. R., Lantz, J. M., Fullerton, J. T., et al. (1999). Nurses' unique roles in randomized clinical trials. *Journal of Professional Nursing, 15,* 106-115.

75. Schiff, G. D., & Rucker, T. D. (1998). Computerized prescribing: Building the electronic infrastructure for better medication usage. *Journal of the American Medical Association, 279,* 1024-1029.

76. Schimmel, E. M. (1994). The hazards of hospitalization. *Annals of Internal Medicine, 60,* 100-110.

77. Sexton, J. B., Thomas, E. J., & Helmreich, R. L. (2000). Error, stress, and teamwork in medicine and aviation: Cross sectional surveys. *British Medical Journal, 320,* 745-749.

78. Shojania, K. G., Yokoe, D., Platt, R., et al. (1998). Reducing vancomycin use utilizing a computer guideline: Results of a randomized controlled trial. *Journal of American Medical Informatics Association, 5,* 554-562.

79. Sievers, T. D., Lagan, M. A., Bartel, S. B., et al. (2001). Variation in administration of cyclophosphamide and mesna in the treatment of childhood malignancies. *Journal of Pediatric Oncology Nursing, 18,* 37-45.

80. Smith, M., & Ho, P. T. (1996). Pediatric drug development: A perspective from the Cancer Therapy Evaluation Program (CTEP) of the National Cancer Institute (NCI). *Investigational New Drugs, 14,* 11-22.

81. Spilker, B. (1996). *Guide to clinical trials.* Philadelphia: Lippincott-Raven.

82. Steel, K. I., Gertman, P. M., & Crescenzi, C. (1981). Iatrogenic illness on a general medicine service at a university hospital. *New England Journal of Medicine, 304,* 638-642.

83. Stock, W., Sather, H., Dodge, R. K., et al. (2000). Outcome of adolescents and young adults with ALL: A comparison of Children Cancer Group (CCG) and Cancer and Leukemia Group B (CALGB) regimens, *Blood, 96,* 467a (abstract 2009).

84. Tortorice, P. V. (2000). Chemotherapy: Principles of therapy. In C. H. Yarbro, M. G. Frogge, M. Goodman, et al. (Eds.), *Cancer nursing: Principles and practice* (5th ed., pp. 352-384). Sudbury, MA: Jones & Bartlett.

85. Trinkle, R., & Wu, J. K. (1996). Errors involving pediatric patients receiving chemotherapy: A literature review. *Medical and Pediatric Oncology, 26,* 344-351.

86. U.S. Department of Labor, Office of Occupational Medicine: Occupational Safety and Health Administration. (1986). *OSHA work practice guidelines for personnel dealing with cytotoxic (antineoplastic) drugs.* Publication No. 8-1.1. Washington, D.C.: U.S. Government Printing Office.

87. Wagner, H. P., Dingeldein-Bettler, L., & Berchthold, W. (1995). Swiss Pediatric Oncology Group (SPOG). Childhood NHL in Switzerland: Incidence and survival of 120 study and 42 non-study patients. *Medical and Pediatric Oncology, 24,* 281-286.

88. Weiss, R. B., Sarosy, G., Clagett-Carr, K., et al. (1986). Anthracycline analogs: The past, present, and future. *Cancer Chemotherapy and Pharmacology, 18,* 185-197.

89. Yarbro, J. W. (1996). The scientific basis of cancer chemotherapy. In M. C. Perry (Ed.), *The chemotherapy source book* (2nd ed., pp. 3-18). Baltimore: Williams & Wilkins.

90. Zaragoza, M. R., Ritche, M. L., & Walter, A. (1995). Neurologic consequences of accidental intrathecal vincristine: A case report. *Medical and Pediatric Oncology, 24,* 61-62.

Biotherapy

Myra Woolery-Antill

For more than a century scientists and researchers have been intrigued by the intricate and complex functions of the body's immune system, especially the role it plays in disease development and disease prevention. Early scientific manipulation of the immune system was referred to as immunotherapy. Clinical reports concerning the use of immunotherapy date back to the late 1800s; however, research and extensive exploration were hindered by unsophisticated scientific technology, limited quantities and crude preparations of immune substances, and inconsistent, often disappointing clinical results. Researchers' interest in immunotherapy has been influenced directly by technologic advances, and the scientific developments are often compared to a roller coaster ride.[76,91]

Many cancer researchers have postulated that progress in the understanding of the immune system will assist in the identification of risk factors for the prevention and treatment of many cancers. Researchers have known for decades about the existence of substances occurring in minute quantities in the body that influence immune system functioning. These substances, now referred to as biologic response modifiers (BRMs) or biologics, encompass a diverse group of agents (e.g., hematopoietic growth factors, interleukins, monoclonal antibodies, tumor necrosis factor, and interferons). They were initially named according to cellular origin and function. Several BRMs are interdependent and belong to the cytokine network (Figure 7-1). Cytokines are naturally occurring glycoproteins produced by a variety of cells. They are responsible for the regulation and function of other cells in the body.[6,108]

The term *biologic response modifiers* includes not only agents but also therapeutic approaches capable of modifying physiologic and/or immune responses. The terms *biologics, BRM, immunotherapy,* and *biotherapy* are often used interchangeably; however, they are not necessarily synonymous. Since the activities and clinical responses elicited in patients receiving BRMs are not neces-

sarily confined to the immune system, as once speculated, many researchers no longer consider the term *immunotherapy* reflective of the diverse activities and responses elicited. Therefore many now refer to this body of knowledge and technology as biotherapy.

Scientific advances of the late 1970s and early 1980s, particularly in molecular biology, genetic engineering, and immunology, led to the reemergence of the concept of immunotherapy. Renewed enthusiasm emerged for conducting research using BRMs to modulate or alter the individual's immune system for the treatment of various diseases and their side effects.

One example of an important scientific advance in the field of biotherapy is hybridization technology, which spawned the development of first generation monoclonal antibodies (MoAbs). This technology is based on the immune system's response to a foreign antigen. The antibodies produced from this process are MoAbs. Once the technology was refined in vitro, hybridization technology and MoAb production were used in many clinical trials in the diagnosis and treatment of cancer. In fact, MoAbs can be produced to screen proteins made by recombinant deoxyribonucleic acid (DNA) molecules, demonstrating the interrelatedness of the many advances in biotechnology.[97,98]

Further examples of scientific advances are the techniques developed through genetic engineering. These opened an exciting field involving recombinant DNA technology (Figure 7-2). This technology involves identifying the genes on a particular area of a DNA strand that codes for a specific cell function, such as protein synthesis. Using an enzyme preparation, the DNA can be broken at the ends of the area of interest and removed from the strand. This portion of DNA is inserted into a plasmid, a spliced ring of DNA, and introduced into a chosen host organism such as *Escherichia coli*. After subsequent cloning procedures, multiple copies of the DNA fragment are produced within the vector, unaffected by the host cell's chromo-

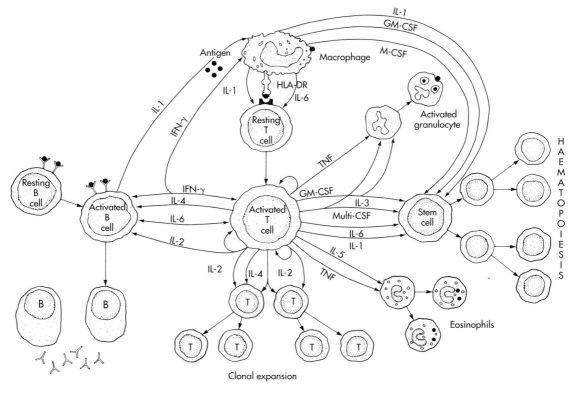

Figure 7-1

Positive interactions in the cytokine network when antigen is encountered. (From Balkwill, F. R. [1989]. *Cytokines in cancer therapy.* Oxford: Oxford University Press.)

somes. The molecules constructed by this method are called recombinant DNA. Researchers can further manipulate these molecules for use in laboratory and clinical settings, including drug production (e.g., interferon), study of genetic diseases, and cancer research.[97,98]

The increased availability of recombinant preparations sparked rapid progress in this field of study. The phase I, II, and III clinical trials of BRMs increased dramatically in the 1980s and 1990s. Over the last several years biotherapy has been incorporated as adjuvant therapy. As new medical advances occur, clinical trials continue to assist in defining the role this treatment modality will have in children with cancer. It is clear that children do not necessarily experience the same therapeutic effects and/or side effects with BRMs as adults. The pediatric oncology nurse caring for patients receiving BRMs or biologic agents must have a basic understanding of the concepts of immunology, hematopoiesis, and biotherapy. Unlike chemotherapy, radiation, and hematopoietic stem cell transplantation, which have direct cytotoxicity,

BRMs possess a variety of biologic actions and may or may not be directly cytotoxic. Biotherapy has emerged and is recognized as the fourth modality of cancer treatment.[87]

HEMATOPOIETIC GROWTH FACTORS

HEMATOPOIETIC CASCADE

Hematopoiesis is a dynamic process involving the proliferation, differentiation, and maturation of stem cells found in the bone marrow into circulating blood cells (red blood cells [RBCs], white blood cells [WBCs], and platelets) (Figure 7-3). The complex set of hierarchical events responsible for this process is known as the hematopoietic cascade. All hematopoietic lineages are derived from a small pool of pluripotent stem cells that are uncommitted to any blood cell lineage. These cells have the ability to self-replicate (reproduce stem cells), proliferate, and differentiate (develop into any blood cell lineage). As differentiation proceeds, cells take on specific cell lineage characteristics and no longer have the capacity for self-renewal.

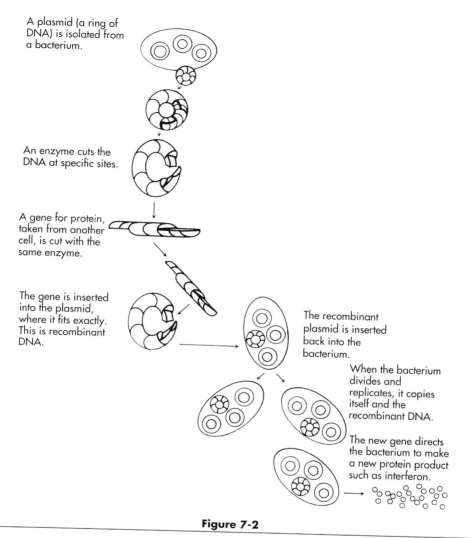

Figure 7-2

Genetic engineering.   (From Schindler, L. W. *Understanding the immune system.* NIH Publication 90-529. Bethesda, MD: U.S. Department of Health and Human Services, National Institutes of Health, March 1990, p. 32.)

Pluripotent stem cells (the most primitive cells of the bone marrow) can become multipotent progenitors of myeloid or lymphoid lineage. The myeloid progenitor gives rise to the colony forming unit (CFU) of granulocytes, erythroid, monocyte, and megakaryocytes (CFU-GEMM). The CFU-GEMM leads to the development of various cell lineages and eventually to precursors. Precursors are the earliest recognizable cell of various blood cell lineages. For example, the proerythroblast is the earliest recognizable cell in erythrocyte or RBC lineage. Through the process of differentiation, precursors develop into the functional components of circulating blood, which have a limited time span and must be continually replaced. Alterations

in production of blood cells can occur as a result of a crisis (e.g., infection, bleeding), certain disease processes, and specific medical treatments.[101]

OVERVIEW OF HUMAN HEMATOPOIETIC GROWTH FACTORS

Human hematopoietic growth factors (HGFs), historically referred to as colony stimulating factors (CSFs) because of their ability to stimulate the formation of blood colonies of various lineage, are naturally occurring cytokines and are responsible for stimulating and regulating the complex process of hematopoiesis. Each cytokine exerts its influence at a different point in the hematopoietic cascade (see Figure 7-3). HGFs can exhibit either mul-

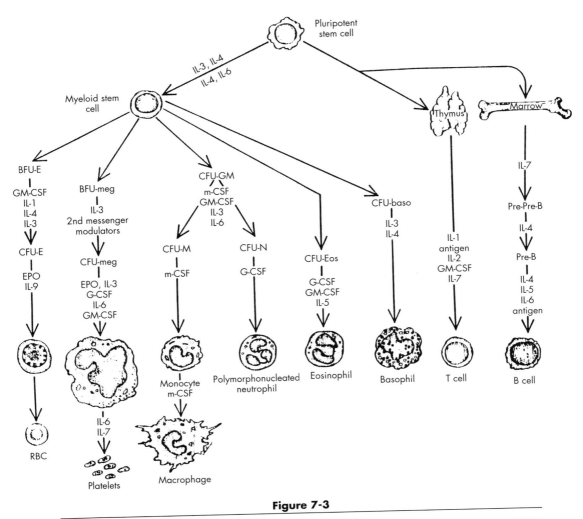

Figure 7-3

Interactions of colony stimulating factors with hematopoietic precursors. (From Delmonte, L. [1990]. Demystifying blood growth factors. *Oncology Times, 12,* 11.)

tilineage (affecting uncommitted precursors) or single-lineage (affecting committed precursors) effects. Examples of HGFs having multilineage effects are Interleukin-3 (IL-3) and granulocyte macrophage colony stimulating factor (GM-CSF). Examples of single-lineage HGFs are erythropoietin (EPO), granulocyte colony stimulating factor (G-CSF), and macrophage colony stimulating factor (M-CSF). In addition, many HGFs augment the various functions of mature blood cells. Examples of clinical application of HGFs for pediatrics include the following: (1) hematopoietic reconstitution acceleration; (2) amelioration of the side effect of myelosuppression; (3) decrease in transfusion requirements with decreased exposure to blood products; (4) reduction in the length of hospitalization secondary to fever and neutropenia; (5) facilitation of the design and successful implementation of more aggressive dose-intensive regimens without the need for bone marrow reinfusion; and (6) mobilization of stem cells for peripheral blood stem cell transplants.[42,51,57,79]

Hematopoietic growth factors (HGFs) play a primary therapeutic role in alleviating the severity of myelosuppression associated with the disease process and/or treatment. This is important because the longer patients are neutropenic, with absolute neutrophil counts below 500, the greater the risk for the development of infection and/or septicemia. HGFs alleviate the severity of neutropenia by shortening the period of myelosuppression and decreasing the depth of the nadir (the point of the lowest neutrophil count). As a result, patients are less susceptible to opportunistic infections. The HGF dose is titrated (increased, decreased, or discontinued) to maintain the WBC count and differential or hemoglobin level within a specified range. Children receiving HGFs require frequent monitoring of their blood counts to evaluate the response to HGF therapy. The optimal timing and duration of therapy for the different HGFs to produce the desired effects and the interactions between HGFs vary based on the clinical application. Patients receiving HGFs that affect the production of WBCs usually experience a rapid increase in their WBCs over the first few days after beginning HGF therapy. Once the effects of the antineoplastic agent are evident, they experience a decrease of their blood counts. When the child's bone marrow recovers from the effect of chemotherapy, the WBCs begin to rise rapidly. After cessation of HGF therapy, the WBCs begin to decrease within the first 24 hours with return to the patient's normal values in 4 to 7 days. Often the platelets will remain low until the HGF is discontinued as the bone marrow is preferentially stimulated to produce WBCs rather than platelets. Once the HGF is stopped, the platelet count will recover within a few days.

With the change in how new biologic agents are classified and named, many of the newer HGFs are also known as interleukins. Those interleukins that act as HGFs and are currently being studied will be discussed in this section.

Erythropoietin

Erythropoietin (EPO) was the first hematopoietic growth factor (HGF) identified more than 40 years ago as an important regulatory factor in erythropoiesis (the development of erythrocytes). The gene for EPO is located on chromosome 7q11-22 (Table 7-1). This factor is produced primarily by the kidneys in response to the amount of oxygen available to the tissues and renal cells. EPO production is increased in the presence of anemia or tissue hypoxia. EPO induces RBC production by stimulating proliferation, differentiation, and maturation of erythroid progenitors. However, the proliferation of immature progenitors into mature erythrocytes requires the presence of EPO, IL-3, and GM-CSF. EPO is the most lineage restricted of the hematopoietic growth factors identified to date.[1,70]

Successful cloning and expression have resulted in adequate supplies for clinical trials. EPO was the first HGF to be used clinically. Initial trials with recombinant EPO were conducted in patients with end stage renal disease who required hemodialysis and frequent blood transfusions. Results of these studies demonstrated that erythropoiesis was stimulated by EPO and transfusion requirements were minimized or eliminated as soon as 1 week after starting EPO therapy.[45,101]

Clinical trials have been conducted in children with human immunodeficiency virus (HIV) who were anemic secondary to treatment with zidovudine (AZT). EPO alleviated the distressing side effects related to anemia, thus increasing tolerance to therapy with zidovudine. EPO administration has also been studied in cancer patients with anemia secondary to chemotherapy or disease process. Patients with low endogenous EPO levels achieved the best responses. In the cancer patient it may take 2 to 6 weeks before the hematocrit begins to respond and 6 to 8 weeks before a significant rise is observed. For cancer patients the cost of EPO therapy as well as the risk/benefit ratio must be considered. The side effects and risk of exposure to blood borne diseases are less.[9,11,16,41,50,64]

When EPO was administered to patients after hematopoietic stem cell transplantation (HSCT), allogeneic recipients experienced acceleration of erythropoiesis, whereas autologous recipients experienced no acceleration.[63] EPO is well tolerated, with injection site pain being the most common side effect (Table 7-2). Doses of EPO are adjusted to achieve the targeted hemoglobin or hematocrit. A common dose is 150 units/kg administered 3 times per week. EPO appears to have a role for patients who object to blood transfusions on religious grounds, such as Jehovah's Witnesses, by potentially eliminating the need for red blood cell transfusions.[2,31]

Granulocyte Macrophage Colony Stimulating Factor

Granulocyte macrophage colony stimulating factor (GM-CSF) is the cytokine responsible for regulating the production of granulocytes, monocytes, and eosinophils. This glycoprotein is produced by T cells, endothelial cells, and fibroblasts. The gene for this cytokine is localized to chromosome 5q21-32 (see Table 7-1).[39] GM-CSF has multilineage effects, stimulating the proliferation, differentiation, and maturation of granulocytes, monocytes, and eosinophils. Other biologic activities include inducing mature neutrophils and monocytes to increase phagocytosis, augmenting antibody-dependent cellular cytotoxicity, increasing tumoricidal killing, stimulating cytokine production, and enhancing monocyte tumor necrosis factor.

Text continued on p. 190

TABLE 7-1	BIOTHERAPY: FDA APPROVED BIOLOGIC AGENTS			
Biologic Agent	Chromosome Location	FDA Approved Indications	Commercial Product	Administration
HEMATOPOIETIC GROWTH FACTORS				
EPO (erythropoietin alpha)	7q11-22	Anemia related to: • Chronic renal failure (CRF) • Zidovudine treated HIV infection • Cancer chemotherapy • Allogeneic blood transfusion in surgery patients	Epoetin-alpha (Epogen) Manufacturer: Amgen Epoetin-alpha (Procrit) Manufacturer: Ortho Biotech	Can be administered IV Titrate dosage as needed to achieve and maintain desired hemoglobin value **DOSAGE** **Cancer Chemotherapy** 150 units/kg subcutaneously (SQ) 3 times per week until targeted hemoglobin reached **Zidovudine Treated HIV Infection** 100 units/kg SQ 3 times per week until targeted hemoglobin reached **CRF (Initial Dosing)** 50 units/kg 3 times per week IV or SQ **VIAL SIZE** 2,000, 3,000, 4,000, or 10,000 units/ml **STORAGE** Refrigerate until use **LABS** CBC and reticulocyte count at least weekly; usually takes 2-6 weeks for effects to be evident; check iron level, baseline endogenous serum erythropoeitin levels
GM-CSF (granulocyte macrophage colony stimulating factor)	5q21-32	**Neutropenia** Accelerate bone marrow recovery **BMT** Mobilize stem cells for peripheral blood stem cell transplant Myeloid reconstitution Graft delay or failure	Sargramostim (Leukine) Manufacturer: Immunex	Can be administered IV bolus or continuous infusion; if concentration less than 10 mg/ml, albumin should be added **DOSAGE** **Neutropenia** 250 mcg/m²/day for 3 weeks or until post nadir (absolute neutrophil count) ANC ≥1500 cells/mm³ for 3 consecutive days Administer SQ daily or IV infusion over 2-4 hours First dose administered 24 hours after last dose of

250 mcg/m²/day IV over 24 hours or SQ daily

Graft Delay or Failure
250 mcg/m²/day IV over 2 hours for 14 days

VIAL SIZE
Liquid preparation available in 500 mcg/vial
Lyophilized preparation available in 250 mcg vials; reconstitute with 1 ml of sterile water; gently swirl and avoid shaking

STORAGE
Refrigerate until use

LABS
CBC 2-3 times per week

G-CSF (granulocyte colony stimulating factor)	Filgrastim (Neupogen) Manufacturer: Amgen	17q11.2-21	**Neutropenia** Accelerate bone marrow recovery **HSCT** Graft delay or failure Mobilize stem cells for PBSC transplant Myeloid reconstitution **Severe Chronic Neutropenia**	SQ is the most common route of administration; can be administered IV bolus or continuous infusion **DOSAGE** **Neutropenia** 5-10 mcg/kg/day SQ until post nadir ANC ≥10,000 cells/mm³ First dose administered 24 hours after last dose of cytotoxic chemotherapy or after bone marrow infusion **PBSC Mobilization** 10 mcg/kg/day for at least 4 days before first leukopheresis **VIAL SIZE** 300 mcg (1 ml), 480 mcg (1.6 ml) **PREFILLED SYRINGE** 300 mcg (0.5 ml), 480 mcg (0.8 ml) **STORAGE** Refrigerate until use **LABS** CBC 2-3 times per week

Continued

TABLE 7-1	BIOTHERAPY: FDA APPROVED BIOLOGIC AGENTS—cont'd		
Biologic Agent	**Chromosome Location**	**FDA Approved Indications**	**Commercial Product**	**Administration**

HEMATOPOIETIC GROWTH FACTORS—cont'd

Biologic Agent	Chromosome Location	FDA Approved Indications	Commercial Product	Administration
IL-11 (interleukin-11)	19q13.3-13.4	Severe thrombocytopenia	Oprelvekin (Neumega) Manufacturer: Genetics Institute	**DOSAGE** 50 mcg/kg in adults; 75-100 mcg/kg in peds SQ: first dose 6-14 hours after last dose of chemotherapy; continue until post nadir platelet count is ≥50,000 mm^3 or maximum 21 days **VIAL SIZE** 5 mg/vial; reconstitute with 1 ml of sterile water; gently swirl and avoid shaking **STORAGE** Refrigerate until use **LABS** CBC with platelet count

INTERFERONS

Biologic Agent	Chromosome Location	FDA Approved Indications	Commercial Product	Administration
Alpha interferon	9p21	Hairy cell leukemia Melanoma AIDS related Kaposi's sarcoma Hepatitis C Hemangioma Chronic myelogenous leukemia (Roche) Hepatitis B (Schering)	IFN alpha-2A (Roferon-a) Manufacturer: Roche IFN alpha-2b (Intron-a) Manufacturer: Schering	**DOSAGE** See manufacturer insert; varies according to indication; administered SQ or IM **Roche** *Single Use Vial Size:* 3, 6, or 36 million international units (MIU)/ml, 9 MIU/.09 ml *Multidose Vials:* 9 MIU/0.9 ml or 18 MIU/3 ml *Prefilled Syringe (SQ Route Only):* 3, 6, or 9 MIU/0.5 ml **Schering** *Single Use Vial Size:* 3, 5, or 10 MIU/0.5 ml *Multidose Vials:* 18 or 25 MIU *Multidose Pen Size (6 Doses):* 3, 5, or 10 MIU/0.2 ml *Storage:* Refrigerate until use

Agent	Location	Indications	Product/Manufacturer	Details
Gamma interferon	12q24	Chronic granulomatous disease (CGD); Chronic neutropenia	Manufacturer: Berlex/Chiron Labs IFN Gamma-1b (Actimmune) Manufacturer: Genentech	0.25 mg (8 MIU) SQ every other day **VIAL SIZE** 0.3 mg (9.6 MIU) lyophilized powder; reconstitute with 1.2 ml of diluent; gently swirl and avoid shaking **STORAGE** Refrigerate until use **LABS** CBC and chemistries including liver function tests **DOSAGE** *Body Surface Area (BSA) >0.5 m²:* 50 mcg/m² (1.5 MIU/m²) *BSA <0.5 m²:* 1.5 mcg/m²/dose Administer 3 times per week **VIAL SIZE** 100 mcg (3 MIU) **STORAGE** Refrigerate until use **LABS** CBC and chemistries, including renal and liver function tests, every 3 months
INTERLEUKINS				
IL-2 (interleukin-2)	22q11.2-12	Metastatic renal cell carcinoma Metastatic melanoma Investigational for other indications	Aldesleukin (Proleukin) Manufacturer: Chiron Therapeutics	**DOSAGE** 5-20 MIU SQ 3×/week (600,000 or 720,000 IU/kg IV over 15 minutes every 8 hours for 15 doses) **VIAL SIZE** 22×10^6 IU; reconstitute with 1.2 ml sterile water; yields 18 MIU/ml; gently swirl and avoid shaking **STORAGE** Refrigerate until use

Continued

TABLE 7-1	BIOTHERAPY: FDA APPROVED BIOLOGIC AGENTS—cont'd			
Biologic Agent	**Chromosome Location**	**FDA Approved Indications**	**Commercial Product**	**Administration**
MONOCLONAL ANTIBODIES				
Chimeric human/murine monoclonal antibody (MoAb) (targets CD20+ antigen found on pre-B and B cells)		B cell non-Hodgkin's lymphoma (NHL)	Rituximab (Rituxan) Manufacturer: Genentech	**DOSAGE** 375 mg/m²/week IV infusion for 4 doses (day 1, 8, 15, 22) *Initial Infusion:* Start at 50 mg/hr; increase rate by 50 mg/hr every 30 minutes to a maximum rate of 400 mg/hr as tolerated by patient *Subsequent Infusions:* Start at 100 mg/hr; increase rate by 100 mg/hr every 30 minutes to a maximum rate of 400 mg/hr as tolerated by patient **VIAL SIZE** 100 mg/10 ml or 500 mg/50 ml; maximum infusion concentration is 4 mg/ml **STORAGE** Refrigerate until use; avoid shaking
Humanized MoAb		Organ rejection prophylaxis Investigational for pediatric leukemia	Daclizumab (Zenapax) Manufacturer: Roche	**DOSAGE** 1 mg/kg IV bolus over 15 minutes; first dose 24 hours before transplant and subsequent doses every 14 days × 4 doses **VIAL SIZE** 25 mg/ml; dilute for infusion **STORAGE** Refrigerate until use
Murine monoclonal antibody		Organ rejection Investigational for management of graft-	Muromonab-CD3 (OKT3 or Orthoclone) Manufacturer: Ortho	**DOSAGE** 5 mg/day IV bolus over <1 minute for 14 days; begin when graft rejection identified

Humanized MoAb	Metastatic breast cancer that overexpresses human epidermal growth factor receptor 2 (HER2) Investigational for osteosarcoma	Trastuzumab (Herceptin) Manufacturer: Genentech	**VIAL SIZE** 5 mg/ml; use 0.22 micron filter to withdraw solution from vial; avoid shaking **STORAGE** Refrigerate until use **DOSAGE** Initial dose 4 mg/kg IV over 90 minutes; subsequent doses 2 mg/kg IV weekly over 30 minutes **VIAL SIZE** 400 mg as lyophilized preparation **STORAGE** Refrigerate until use

RETINOIDS

All-trans retinoic acid (tRA)	Acute promyelocytic leukemia (APL)	Tretinoin (Vesanoid) Manufacturer: Roche	**DOSAGE** Induction therapy—45 mg/m²/day orally divided into two doses until remission confirmed; discontinue 30 days after remission or 90 days after treatment initiation, whichever comes first Take with food **SIZE** Available in 10 mg capsules **LABS** CBC, coagulation profile, liver function tests, cholesterol and triglyceride levels
13-cis-retinoic acid	Investigational for neuroblastoma	Isotretinoin	

TABLE 7-2	SIDE EFFECTS ASSOCIATED WITH BIOLOGIC AGENTS			
Biologic Agent	**Flulike Syndrome**	**Cardiopulmonary**	**Gastrointestinal**	**Integumentary**
HGFs				
• G-CSF	Fever (rare) • None or low grade	Hypotension (rare)	Anorexia	Rash (rare)
• GM-CSF	Fever (common) • Low grade HA (transient or mild) Chills Myalgias	Hypotension (occasional) First dose syndrome (rare)	N/V (occasional) Diarrhea (occasional)	Erythema • At injection site Rash (rare)
• EPO	HA (rare)	Hypotension (rare)	Diarrhea (rare)	Rash (rare)
• IL-11	Fever (occasional) Chills (occasional) HA (mild)	Common • Peripheral edema Occasional • Tachycardia • Dyspnea	Anorexia (occasional) Diarrhea (occasional)	Rash (rare)
Interleukin-2	Fever (common) • Dose related • Duration up to 18 hours • T_{max} in 10-12 hours Malaise Fatigue	Common • Capillary leak (dose related • Hypotension • Fluid retention • Dyspnea	N/V (common) Diarrhea (common) Anorexia (common) Mucositis (occasional)	Erythema (common) Pruritus (common) Rash (common) Sun sensitivity Injection site reactions
Monoclonal antibodies	Fever (common) • Various patterns Chills/rigors (common) HA (rare) Malaise	Common • Capillary leak • Fluid retention Occasional • Hypotension • Hypertension • Dyspnea, wheezing • Anaphylaxis (rare)	N/V (occasional) Diarrhea (rare) Abdominal cramps	Urticaria (common) Pruritus (common) Erythema (occasional)
Interferons				
• Alpha	Fever and chills (common) HA (common) Myalgias (common) Fatigue (chronic)	Hypotension	Taste changes Anorexia (common) N/V (occasional) Diarrhea (occasional)	Rash Dry skin Pruritus Injection site reactions
• Beta	Fever and chills HA (common) • Mild to moderate Fatigue (chronic)	Hypotension • Dose related	Abdominal pain Diarrhea (occasional) Dry mouth	Urticaria Injection site reactions
• Gamma	HA (common) • May be severe Fatigue (chronic)	Hypotension • Dose related	Anorexia (common) N/V (occasional) Diarrhea (occasional) Abdominal pain	Injection site erythema and/or tenderness
Retinoids	Fever (common) HA (common) Malaise Fatigue	Occasional • Hypotension • Hypertension • Flushing • Dyspnea	N/V (common) Diarrhea (occasional)	Dry skin and mucous membranes (common) Pruritus (occasional) Sun sensitivity

N/V, Nausea/vomiting; *HA*, headache.
NOTE: Most side effects are dose related and reversible.

Renal/Hepatic	Musculoskeletal	CNS
Elevated liver enzymes Elevated uric acid	Bone pain (common)	
Elevated liver enzymes Elevated creatinine and BUN	Bone pain (common)	Insomnia Anxiety
BUN and creatinine	Injection site pain Trunk pain (rare)	
Decreased serum albumin and transferrin Decreased serum protein Electrolyte changes	Bone pain	Papilledema Insomnia
Oliguria (common) Increase in creatinine and BUN (common) Elevated liver enzymes	Myalgias (common) Arthralgias	Lethargy (occasional) Confusion (occasional) Cognitive changes Agitation Psychoses Sleep disturbances
Elevated liver enzymes Electrolyte changes	Arthralgias Generalized pain Neuropathic pain	Anxiety Agitation Insomnia
Elevated liver enzymes, creatinine, and BUN Proteinuria	Myalgias (common) Arthralgias (common)	Lethargy (common) Confusion (occasional) Mental status changes (rare) Depression
Elevated liver enzymes Proteinuria Elevated BUN	Myalgias (common) Arthralgias (common) Pain	Depression Psychosis
Elevated triglycerides and liver enzymes	Myalgias (common) Arthralgias (common) Back pain	Depression
Elevated triglycerides, cholesterol, liver enzymes	Bone pain (common) Myalgias (common) Arthralgias (common)	Visual disturbances Irritability Conjunctivitis Pseudotumor cerebri

CNS, Central nervous system.

Since 1987, when recombinant GM-CSF first became available, multiple studies have been conducted in a variety of disease processes. Initial human trials validated observations from animal trials that the use of GM-CSF results in an increase in neutrophils, monocytes, and eosinophils, which return to baseline on discontinuation of therapy. GM-CSF has been shown to decrease the duration of myelosuppression following chemotherapy and to accelerate hematopoietic reconstitution following HSCT.

GM-CSF has been administered by a variety of routes (subcutaneously [SQ] and intravenously [IV] by continuous infusion or bolus) and in various dosages. The maximum tolerated dose (MTD) varies slightly according to the recombinant preparation used. SQ doses as low as 5 mcg/kg/day stimulate bone marrow reconstitution. The side effects observed clinically with low dose administration include a flulike syndrome (or constitutional symptoms), low grade fever, chills, fatigue, myalgia, bone pain, nausea, anorexia, rash, and occasional thrombocytopenia. Bone pain usually begins 2 to 3 days after initiation of GM-CSF in areas of high bone marrow concentration. Severity of this side effect generally ranges from mild to moderate. Erythema at the injection site of patients receiving SQ administration has been noted. Serious side effects observed with high doses of GM-CSF include fluid retention, pleural effusion, and capillary leak syndrome (i.e., a fluid shift caused by increased vascular permeability) (see Table 7-2). Eosinophilia has been observed. The potential long-term effects warrant further exploration.[3,39]

An event associated with GM-CSF known as the first dose phenomenon has been identified. It is characterized by facial flushing, the urge to defecate, changes in blood pressure, and transient oxygen desaturation. This reaction generally appears on the first day of administration, but it can occur on subsequent cycles on day 1, even if the patient has not had a previous reaction. This phenomenon has been observed in adults and to a lesser extent in the pediatric population. It demonstrates the importance of nursing assessment and careful, thorough documentation of side effects and interventions. Vital signs are generally taken at baseline and 15 minutes, 1 hour, and 2 hours after SQ administration. Patients should be monitored for approximately 2 hours after administration. With Food and Drug Administration (FDA) approval in 1991, GM-CSF has become more widely available in the clinical setting and is marketed in the United States as sargramostim (Leukine). The most common dosage is 250 mcg/m^2/day, and it is administered daily until the absolute neutrophil count (ANC) is greater than or equal to 1500 for 3 consecutive days.[61]

Granulocyte Colony Stimulating Factor (G-CSF)

This cytokine is responsible for regulating the production of granulocytes. The granulocyte colony stimulating factor (G-CSF) gene is located on chromosome 17q11.2-21 (see Table 7-1). G-CSF is considered to be lineage specific because it stimulates the late proliferation and differentiation of progenitor cells committed to granulocyte lineage. In addition, it increases neutrophil phagocytosis and enhances the activity of erythropoietin. The first clinical trials were designed to evaluate the ability of G-CSF to accelerate neutrophil recovery after chemotherapy.[116] Results of clinical trials revealed G-CSF was better tolerated than GM-CSF, with medullary bone pain (a dull, transient ache) the only consistent side effect. This side effect most often begins 2 to 3 days after initiation of therapy in response to neutrophil proliferation and is relieved once the neutrophils begin appearing in the circulating blood. Unlike GM-CSF, a dose limiting toxicity was not reached with G-CSF. G-CSF has been administered by a variety of routes (SQ, and IV by infusion and bolus) in doses ranging from 3 to 20 mcg/kg/day. The most common dose and route of administration are 5 mcg/kg/day SQ. The timing of administration after myelosuppressive chemotherapy is 24 hours after the last dose of chemotherapy.

G-CSF received FDA approval for the treatment of myelosuppression in 1991 and is marketed in the United States as filgrastim (Neupogen). Since then, the use of G-CSF in the pediatric setting has increased. To date no long-term side effects have been associated with G-CSF, but continual monitoring for potential long-term side effects is necessary. A long-acting pegylated G-CSF preparation (SD/01 filgrastim) is under clinical investigation. This preparation is being evaluated in the pediatric sarcoma patient population. Early study results were encouraging and suggested that the long-acting preparation administered once, 24 hours after the last dose of chemotherapy, is as effective as daily doses of G-CSF in accelerating bone marrow recovery. If the long-acting preparation is found to be as effective in phase III clinical trials, it has the potential to change current administration practices.[26,100] For the pediatric patient population this is expected to have a positive effect on quality of life.

Interleukin-11

The interleukin-11 (IL-11) gene is located on chromosome 19q13.3-13.4 (see Table 7-1). This cytokine is responsible for regulating the production of megakaryocytes and was first isolated in 1990. IL-11 is considered to be lineage specific because it stimulates the late proliferation and differentiation of progenitor cells committed to megakaryocyte lineage. Clinical trials revealed IL-11 was effective in inducing platelet recovery and decreasing the number of platelet transfusions needed.[19,30] It received FDA approval in 1997 and is marketed under the name oprelvekin (Neumega). It is administered SQ beginning 6 to 24 hours after the last dose of chemotherapy and continuing daily until the post nadir platelet count is greater than or equal to 50,000 cells/mm³. The most common side effects include edema of the arms or legs, dyspnea, tachycardia, and conjunctival redness. IL-11 is used in situations where severe thrombocytopenia is anticipated. The goal is to prevent or minimize thrombocytopenia and decrease the number of platelet transfusions. The cost/benefit ratio of IL-11 therapy must be considered. Its use is usually reserved for potentially severe thrombocytopenia or patients resistant to platelet transfusions.[15,90,93,104,107]

CLINICAL APPLICATIONS OF HEMATOPOIETIC GROWTH FACTORS

Hematopoietic growth factors (HGFs) are being used in a variety of clinical settings and increasingly as an adjunct to cancer and HIV treatments. It is anticipated that the use of HGFs alone and in combination is likely to continue to increase. Optimal timing of administration to produce desired outcomes will be further refined as a result of ongoing clinical investigations. Currently no long-term side effects have been identified, but continued monitoring is needed.[18,36,77,84,86]

The American Society of Clinical Oncology (ASCO) released its first evidence-based practice guideline recommendations for the use of HGFs in 1994. Continued revisions of these practice guidelines based on findings from clinical application are needed to refine the practice of HGF administration. The recommendations were last updated in 2000. Each section of the guidelines addresses an issue related to HGF administration and includes clinical outcomes, alternative approaches, highlights of last revision, update from clinical studies since the last revision, and a recommendation. Highlights of the 2000 recommendations can be found in Table 7-3. According to the guidelines, the recommended dosing of filgrastim for peripheral blood stem cell (PBSC) mobilization is 10 mcg/kg/day. For all other situations the recommended filgrastim dosing is 5 mcg/kg/day, and the sargramostim dosing is 250 mcg/kg/day. The preferred route of administration is SQ.[77]

A 1998 survey of pediatric oncologists revealed a greater use of hematopoietic growth factors (HGFs) for primary and secondary management of neutropenia than their adult oncology counterparts and the current ASCO recommendations for HGF use. Pediatric oncologists used HGFs more often for delayed neutrophil recovery rather than making a chemotherapy dose reduction. Unlike adult patients, most pediatric patients actively participate in a clinical trial in which the HGF use is delineated. The more dose-intensive treatments and increased toxicities associated with pediatric protocols may explain the differences in practice. Further investigation is needed.[80]

Adjunct to Intensive and/or Myelosuppressive Chemotherapy

Clinical trials have examined the role of hematopoietic growth factors (HGFs) in accelerating bone marrow recovery. A number of comparison studies have been conducted to examine the efficacy of different HGFs.* Most of the HGFs administered to children are used in conjunction with chemotherapy. For example, one of the most challenging problems of treating aggressive cancers, such as Burkitt's lymphoma, is the need to give chemotherapy in rapid pulses. The intensive regimens often result in prolonged neutropenia leading to delays in chemotherapy cycles. With the addition of HGFs such as GM-CSF or G-CSF to decrease the period of aplasia, the time between cycles is maintained as designed.[94,116] This advancement has led to more effective therapy and increased the long-term survival of children diagnosed with aggressive lymphomas. As a result, fewer patients experience delays in therapy or reduction in chemotherapy doses secondary to inadequate bone marrow recovery at the time the next cycle is due. In a study of children diagnosed with acute lymphoblastic leukemia, investigators demonstrated G-CSF was effective in ameliorating the toxicities associated with the administration of a dose-intensive chemotherapy regimen.[25] Although the administration of GM-CSF or G-CSF to patients with leukemia to increase dose intensity and facilitate the adherence to therapy schedule is effective in decreasing therapy toxicities, it has not increased disease-free survival.[69] IL-11 has been used to minimize treatment modifications because of prolonged platelet recovery.[15] Large collaborative research studies are needed to explore the benefits of dose-intensive regimens and the use of HGFs. Results of cost analysis studies have been variable, warranting further exploration. When examining the cost of the administration of HGFs, the clinician needs to consider the impact on quality of life.[3,10]

*References 25, 36, 37, 60, 96, 117.

TABLE 7-3	HIGHLIGHTS OF ASCO 2000 RECOMMENDATIONS FOR THE USE OF HEMATOPOIETIC COLONY STIMULATING FACTORS (CSFs)
Guidelines	**Recommendations**
Primary prophylaxis	Routine use of CSFs not recommended
	CSFs should be reserved for patients at high risk of experiencing prolonged fever and neutropenia and for special populations such as those with AIDS-related lymphoma or elderly
Secondary prophylaxis	Dose reduction should be considered as primary option for patients who have experienced delays in therapy
	Lack of published data demonstrating improved disease free survival when treatment scheduled maintained
CSF therapy	**AFEBRILE NEUTROPENIC PATIENTS**
	Routine initiation of CSF not recommended
	FEBRILE NEUTROPENIC PATIENTS
	Not recommended for uncomplicated fever and neutropenic episodes ($\leq$10 days)
	High-risk patients may receive CSFs; however, the benefits are unproven
	Pediatric patients: studies have demonstrated some clinical benefit
Increase chemotherapy dose intensity	Recommend dose modifications of chemotherapy for neutropenia and treatment related toxicities
	More clinical trials needed to define impact or overall survival and quality of life
Adjuncts to progenitor cell transplantation	Recommend for mobilization of peripheral blood stem cells (PBSCs) and after PBSC infusion
	Optimal dose of CSF still investigational
Patients with acute leukemia	Consider if shortening of hospitalization outweighs costs of CSF administration
	No evidence of improvement in clinical response to therapy
	Small benefits observed in children with acute lymphocytic leukemia (ALL)
	Further investigation needed
Patients receiving concurrent chemotherapy and irradiation	Not recommended, especially for patients receiving mediastinal radiation
	May be considered for prolonged delays caused by neutropenia in patients receiving large field irradiation
Pediatric patients	Guidelines for adults generally applicable unless pediatric data available
	Pediatric oncologists use CSFs more often than ASCO guidelines recommend and rarely choose reduction in chemotherapy as an option. Most CSFs given in conjunction with clinical trial.
CSF dosing and route	**DOSAGE**
	Filgrastim 5 mcg/kg/day
	Sargramostim 250 mcg/kg/day
	PBSC mobilization: filgrastim 10 mcg/kg/day
	Subcutaneous route is preferred
Initiation and duration of CSF administration	Optimal timing and duration remain investigational

Adjunct to Hematopoietic Stem Cell Transplantation

Peripheral blood stem cell (PBSC) mobilization. One of the difficulties encountered in HSCT is obtaining adequate stem cells. Historically, the only way to obtain stem cells was through bone marrow harvesting (multiple bone marrow aspira-

tions under general anesthesia). Children with aggressive hematologic malignancies often relapsed before harvesting or during the time between the harvesting procedure and the beginning of the pretransplant conditioning regimen. With PBSC mobilization, these children can often maintain a remission during the collection procedure. PBSC mobilization involves the administration of a hematopoietic growth factor (HGF), such as G-CSF, approximately 4 days before stem cell collection. Once the peripheral WBC count is greater than 1000/mm^3, the stem cells can be harvested via apheresis. On the day of stem cell collection(s) the dose of G-CSF is administered approximately 2 hours before apheresis. Stem cells are collected over the next 2 to 3 days, depending on the number of progenitor cells obtained. PBSC mobilization has proven effective in obtaining adequate stem cells from autologous and allogeneic sources. This procedure appears to be better tolerated by donors and eliminates the risks associated with general anesthesia. Refer to Chapter 8 for details on peripheral stem cell harvesting.[26,99,116]

Post bone marrow reinfusion.   Hematopoietic growth factors (HGFs) are administered to accelerate hematopoietic reconstitution and decrease the period of aplasia. This has led to reduced hospital stays for HSCT recipients. Clinical trials evaluated GM-CSF, G-CSF, and M-CSF after high-dose cytotoxic therapy with autologous rescue. Reports of reduced incidence of bacteremia encouraged investigators to explore the use of these HGFs in a variety of transplant settings.[83,115,116] HGFs such as G-CSF are standard therapy after bone marrow or PBSC infusion to accelerate bone marrow recovery. Clinical studies are still needed to determine the optimal timing of administration after stem cell reinfusion. A prospective randomized study of filgrastim administered at different time points after unrelated HSCT demonstrated no differences in hematologic recovery, bacteremia, or transfusion requirements between early versus delayed initiation of G-CSF. This study suggests that delaying G-CSF administration can safely decrease the costs. The results indicate that G-CSF is most effective with mature progenitor cells committed to neutrophil differentiation.[43] Further clinical investigation is needed to validate these findings and to determine the optimal start time for G-CSF.

Adjunct to HIV management.   Many children with HIV infection experience myelosuppression at some point during their disease. The administration of antiretroviral therapies such as zidovudine (AZT) often results in neutropenia and anemia, requiring a decrease in dose or discontinuation of therapy. EPO and/or G-CSF have been used to treat myelosuppression associated with therapy and/or secondary to the disease process itself. In general the administration schedule is 3 times per week to achieve the desired outcome.[116]

Investigational Hematopoietic Growth Factors (HGFs)

Several other HGFs have been identified and are presently investigational. They include IL-1, or hematopoietin, which is involved in the early differentiation of hematopoietic pluripotent stem cells; IL-5, which plays a role in eosinophil differentiation; and IL-6, or thrombopoietin (TPO), which is involved in the production of platelets. The role, if any, these factors can play in conjunction with cancer therapy continues to be investigated.

Stem Cell Factor

Stem cell factor (SCF), also known as steel factor or c-kit ligand, is a multilineage HGF found on chromosomes 12q22-24. It affects the earliest undifferentiated multipotential progenitor cells responsible for myeloid and lymphoid lineage development. By itself it has little colony stimulating effect. However, in concert with other HGFs, it orchestrates the complex process of hematopoiesis. Clinical studies have administered SCF in doses beginning as low as 5 mcg/kg SQ and up to 30 mcg/kg. In several randomized clinical studies SCF combined with G-CSF significantly increased the number of progenitor cells obtained through leukopheresis. Although the increased side effects may not be warranted for every patient, the addition of SCF may be beneficial for patients in whom G-CSF alone is not effective in mobilizing enough progenitor cells for transplant. Early studies of the effects of SCF on acute myeloid leukemia blasts demonstrated that SCF may induce apoptosis in these cells.[24,111,113] Ongoing investigation is needed to determine other roles of SCF. The FDA, after reviewing results of clinical investigations, has recommended approval of Stemgen, manufactured by Amgen; however, details of the availability and license indications have not been released.

The most common side effects are injection related (i.e., erythema or edema) and mild to severe hypersensitivity reaction. Urticaria with respiratory distress has been reported in approximately 3% to 12% of patients who received doses greater than 15 mcg/kg. Mast cell stimulation by SCF may be a contributing factor. Premedication with an antihistamine and decreasing the dose of stem cell factor (SCF) have been effective interventions. Although it affects cells earlier in the hematopoietic cascade, the benefits do not outweigh the side effects at this time.[24,113]

Interleukin-3

Naturally occurring interleukin-3 (IL-3) is produced primarily by T lymphocytes. The gene for this complex glycoprotein is located on chromosomes 5q21-31. IL-3 has multilineage effects and can support the formation of various types of single and multilineage colonies. It has often been called multi-CSF because it is capable of stimulating multipotential hematopoietic stem cells to differentiate. Initially it was thought to be more effective in counteracting the myelosuppressive effects of irradiation and chemotherapy than GM-CSF or G-CSF.[113]

The focus of early IL-3 clinical trials has been in adult patients with bone marrow failure (e.g., aplastic anemia) and malignancies, although there have been attempts to stimulate hematopoiesis in children with aplastic anemia and myelodysplastic syndrome. Although IL-3 is multilineage, it does not appear to be superior to G-CSF and is less well tolerated. Its role in pediatric oncology has yet to be defined.[65]

Side effects of IL-3 include fever, flulike symptoms, including malaise, and myalgias, swelling of the face and extremities, mild splenomegaly, a pruritic papular rash, and injection site inflammation. Headaches have been a dose limiting toxicity. Eosinophilia and basophilia can also occur, which may lead to a rise in plasma histamine.[65,113]

Thrombopoietin

This hematopoietic growth factor (HGF) is lineage specific because it affects the later steps of platelet formation. It stimulates the proliferation, differentiation, and maturation of megakaryoblasts to megakaryocytes that produce platelets. The discovery and cloning of this HGF in 1994 enhanced the understanding of megakaryocytopoiesis, and investigations continue to determine the role thrombopoietin (TPO) might play in the management of cancer and its treatment related side effects. Two recombinant forms of thrombopoietin have been developed. Thrombopoietin (rhTPO), manufactured by Genentech, Inc., is a full-length glycolated version.[54] In clinical studies thrombopoietin has been administered IV and SQ and has demonstrated an increase in platelet count leading to a decrease in the duration of thrombocytopenia. A mild transient headache was associated with the administration of TPO. Otherwise it is well tolerated. Clinical studies are needed to determine the optimal dosing and schedule.[55,73,88,109]

Megakaryocyte growth development factor (MGDF) is a truncated pegylated derivative of thrombopoietin developed by Amgen that is administered SQ and has been shown to increase platelet counts, decreasing the severity and duration of thrombocytopenia.[7,110,113] Phase III clinical studies investigating the role of MGDF revealed the development of neutralizing antibodies. Further investigations have been suspended.[85]

Macrophage Colony Stimulating Factor

The cytokine that regulates the production of macrophages is known as macrophage colony stimulating factor (M-CSF). The gene for this glycoprotein is located on chromosome 5q33.1. M-CSF is lineage specific because it stimulates the proliferation and differentiation of progenitor cells committed to the macrophage lineage. In addition, M-CSF activates mature macrophages and augments host defenses by enhancing the antimicrobial and tumoricidal properties of macrophages. After treatment with chemotherapy, it may be able to induce hematopoietic progenitor cells to enter the cell cycle, resulting in an increased number of progenitor cells in the marrow and the spleen. In an animal study a continuous infusion of M-CSF for 14 days resulted in an increase in monocytes.[14]

Enhanced tumor infiltration by macrophages stimulated with M-CSF and possible usefulness in treatment of refractory fungal infections are a few of the roles being investigated. Animal studies have been most promising, but the benefits of M-CSF in humans have not been established and this agent remains investigational. Thrombocytopenia is a dose limiting toxicity.[14,42,74]

THE INTERLEUKINS

The class of cytokines called interleukins includes protein molecules that send messages between leukocytes. The many types of interleukins are grouped according to their biologic activities. The nomenclature system devised by participants at the Sixth International Congress of Immunology in 1986 assigns a number to each interleukin.[6] The group decided to name newly discovered substances according to their biologic actions. After establishing the human amino acid sequence, the molecule is to be given an interleukin number corresponding to the order in which it was identified. Often researchers in different laboratories "discover" the same substance performing different functions in separate experiments at the same time, explaining why many of the interleukins have more than one name. When the amino acid sequence is unveiled, the researchers can then determine if the substance truly is a newly identified cytokine. If the unique properties of a substance are confirmed, another numbered interleukin is added to the list.[8]

Although all of the substances assigned to the growing list of interleukins may not directly affect cancer cells, their activities as cytokines may indirectly assist in cancer therapy. The interleukins are produced by and regulate many cell types. Each has a specific function within the immune system. The goal of administration of interleukins is the enhancement of the body's natural immune system.

There have been a total of 18 interleukins identified to date. Two have received regulatory approval, and several others are in clinical trials. The remaining interleukins are in various stages of exploration. As we continue to explore and learn more, additional interleukins will be identified and classified. With each discovery, our understanding of the complex interactions of the immune system become clearer. The significance of the various interleukins identified and their place in pediatric cancer therapy will become more evident as reports of research results become available.

INTERLEUKIN-2

When identified in 1976, the cytokine now known as interleukin-2 (IL-2) was originally known as T-cell growth factor. Researchers have validated its potential as a potent immunotherapeutic agent. Since 1983, when the DNA sequence of the gene coding for IL-2 was established, researchers have had access to a large supply of IL-2 produced by recombinant gene technology. Studies have shown that the presence of IL-2 stimulates cells known as lymphokine-activated killer (LAK) cells to lyse fresh tumor cells while sparing normal cells. LAK cells may proliferate in the lungs, liver, spleen, kidneys, and mesenteric lymph nodes. Controlling tumor cell proliferation is the goal of incorporating IL-2 into cancer therapy.[91,92]

The regression of certain experimental tumors in animals in the presence of IL-2 paved the way for use of this substance in clinical trials. The first human studies involved metastatic malignant melanoma and renal cell carcinoma. Treatment with IL-2 depends on its potential to promote direct cell-mediated destruction of tumor cells and to mobilize cells capable of destroying neoplasms. These cells include LAK cells, activated natural killer (NK) cells, tumor-infiltrating lymphocytes (TILs), and certain T and B cells. TILs and LAK cells have been used in the technique of adoptive cellular therapy, which relies on IL-2 to stimulate certain immune system cells in the laboratory; then the cells are readministered to cause tumor regression in the host organism. The process of obtaining LAK or TIL cells is difficult, lengthy, and costly.[4,21]

After extensive clinical trials, IL-2 was FDA approved in 1992 for the treatment of metastatic renal cell cancer and subsequently for metastatic malignant melanoma in 1998. It is marketed in the United States as aldesleukin (Proleukin). The recommended dose and schedule are 600,000 or 720,000 international units/kg IV every 8 hours for a total of 15 doses as tolerated by the patient (see Table 7-1). The majority of patients receiving high dose IL-2 on this schedule are not able to tolerate all 15 doses. Although the side effects are reversible, patients often require intensive care unit (ICU) support because of the toxic multisystem side effects. Most of the side effects are the direct result of capillary leak and/or renal insufficiency. The predictable need for ICU support and the low percentage of responders have limited the use of high dose IL-2.[118]

Since receiving FDA approval, a variety of administration routes (bolus, SQ, continuous infusion), dosages (low, intermediate, high) and schedules have been studied for IL-2 in an attempt to define the optimal conditions needed to achieve the desired outcome. Better tolerance was observed with the continuous infusion route rather than bolus administration. Additionally, IL-2 has been incorporated into therapeutic regimens with chemotherapeutic agents such as cyclophosphamide, dacarbazine, and fluorouracil. Studies have used IL-2 with other biologic agents including interferon (IFN), monoclonal antibodies (MoAbs), tumor necrosis factor (TNF), and adoptive cells such as lymphokine-activated killer (LAK) cells and tumor-infiltrating lymphocytes (TILs). Clinical trials to date have not demonstrated improved efficacy of IL-2 with LAK or TIL cells compared with IL-2 alone. Further research with these combinations is necessary to identify the clinical use in anticancer therapy.[33,91,92]

IL-2 in the laboratory setting has been shown to enhance the cytotoxic activity of natural killer (NK) cells against solid tumors such as neuroblastoma and rhabdomyosarcoma in children. IL-2 has been administered to children with a variety of cancers (e.g., neuroblastoma, osteosarcoma, Ewing's sarcoma, leukemia, rhabdomyosarcoma, hepatoblastoma) via a number of different administration routes (IV bolus, continuous infusion, SQ) and schedules. Studies of the cytotoxic activity of IL-2 have been disappointing in the pediatric population.[21]

The results of pediatric clinical trials suggest that IL-2 may have the lowest response rate in children who have been heavily pretreated with intensive high dose chemotherapy. However, children who have not been affected by the toxicities of multiple antineoplastic agents may be able to tolerate a more aggressive dose schedule of IL-2 and receive the full benefit of this biologic response modifier without eliciting early multisystem toxicities. When administered to children with a small tumor burden, IL-2 elicits the best response. This is because a desirable effector-to-target ratio is established with a large amount of IL-2–activated cells (effectors) compared with a small number of tumor cells (targets).[21]

A number of clinical investigations have evaluated the potential role of IL-2 in the HSCT setting.[68,72,81,112] Two studies demonstrated improved disease free survival for the control of minimal residual disease after autologous HSCT or peripheral blood stem cell transplantation (PBSCT). Patients with neuroblastoma received low dose IL-2 by continuous infusion, and the other study patients received IL-2 and alpha interferon.[81,112] Different administration schedules have also been investigated. IL-2 was administered after autologous HSCT to pediatric patients diagnosed with acute leukemia who were at high risk for relapse. One group received a continuous infusion of IL-2 over 2 weeks as an induction dose after HSCT followed by a 3-week rest. Then a six-cycle maintenance schedule consisting of a monthly 72-hour infusion was initiated. The other group received IL-2 before harvesting, and some patients received IL-2 after HSCT as above.[68] These studies demonstrate that IL-2 can safely be incorporated into regimens using HSCT. IL-2 was well tolerated, with fever, chills, anorexia, rash, and gastrointestinal (GI) symptoms being the most common side effects observed. Larger clinical studies are needed to validate the findings and to determine the most effective dosage, route of administration, and schedule.

Currently there is interest in exploring the immunomodulating role that IL-2 may play in augmenting the immune system. According to the National Cancer Institute's Physician Data Query Base, clinical trials are investigating the role of IL-2 on the ability to maintain or restore immune function in HIV infected children. Low dose IL-2 is administered SQ. IL-2 is also being studied in the cancer population to determine if it is able to boost the immune system.

Most toxicities of IL-2 are dose related and reversible (see Table 7-2). The child receiving IL-2 must have a thorough pretreatment examination, since IL-2 is known to affect many body organs, especially at the high dose level. Documented toxicities in children receiving low dose IL-2 therapy (1×10^6 units/m^2 3 times weekly for 3 weeks) include fever, nausea, vomiting, and mild hypotension. Toxicity with higher dose therapy (3×10^6 units/m^2 3 times weekly for 3 weeks) was more severe, including fluid retention, significant hypotension, increased creatinine, oliguria, and elevated liver enzymes. Diuretics are administered to treat peripheral edema. Acetaminophen and indomethacin are administered before and after to treat fever. Although the classic flulike syndrome usually resolves after the IL-2 is discontinued, associated myalgias, malaise, and anorexia may last for several weeks. Fatigue develops over time and has a cumulative effect.[21,47]

INVESTIGATIONAL INTERLEUKINS

Interleukin-1

Researchers originally discovered the cytokine known as interleukin-1 (IL-1) in the 1940s, when it was named "endogenous pyrogen." Since that time, numerous sources and functions of the IL-1 molecule have been identified. It is also known as lymphocyte-activating factor (LAF), hemopoietin-1, and mononuclear cell factor (MCF). Although nearly all cell types can produce it, monocytes and macrophages are generally considered to be the most important sources of IL-1.

Interleukin-1 is involved in the majority of regulatory aspects of the immune response. It activates T-cells, directly stimulating the events of the cytokine cascade. This chain reaction begins with the stimulation of the immune system by a foreign antigen and concludes with the intricate network of activities known as the humoral and cellular immune responses (see Figure 7-1).

Laboratory studies in animals have revealed several therapeutic uses for IL-1. It can protect normal cells against the effects of radiation. It can also stimulate recovery of bone marrow after myelosuppression from chemotherapy and radiation. The ability to stimulate platelet production and differentiation in thrombocytopenic patients has been demonstrated in the clinical setting, but further research is needed to determine the benefit in treatment schemas. Side effects reported in preliminary trials include fever with chills or rigors, tachycardia, hypertension, headache, and mild myalgias. These symptoms resolve shortly after completion of the infusion.

Interleukin-3

Interleukin-3 (IL-3) is considered a hematopoietic growth factor (HGF) and has been historically referred to as multi-CSF. Refer to the section on HGFs for further detail.

Interleukin-4

Interleukin-4 (IL-4) was first named B cell growth factor-1 (BCGF-1). It later emerged as T cell growth factor-2 (TCGF-2). The function of IL-4 is to enhance the cytotoxic activity of activated B and T cells. This capability enables it to play a role in the body's fight against mutated cells. IL-4 has the potential to initiate activity in any tumor-infiltrating lymphocyte (TIL), which can infiltrate tumor cells and cause cell lysis under the appropriate immunologic conditions.[6] Clinical trials continue and so far have not demonstrated the same positive antitumor results in humans as those seen in animal studies. Side effects include fever, nasal congestions, headache, GI side effects (nausea and vomiting, diarrhea), anorexia, fatigue, capillary leak, dyspnea, and weight loss.

Interleukin-5

Interleukin-5 (IL-5) primarily regulates the differentiation of eosinophils. As a cytokine, its importance as an adjuvant to chemotherapy has not been described. However, levels of IL-5 may be increased by certain tumors in which eosinophilia is often a clinical finding. In addition, IL-5 is associated with the presence of IL-2 receptors on activated B cells, but the significance of this association is still not clear.

Interleukin-6

The discovery of Interleukin-6 (IL-6) was made by several separate research teams investigating various immunologic functions. It has been named B cell differentiating factor (BCDF), beta-2 interferon (IFN-2), plasmacytoma growth factor, hybridoma growth factor, hepatocyte-stimulating factor (HSF), and T-activating factor (TAF). IL-6 is similar to IL-1 in its ability to regulate the immune response of nonimmune cells. The role in cancer therapy is to stimulate the pluripotent hematopoietic stem cell. It can also promote killer T cell production. Studies suggest that IL-6 will play an important role in the production of platelets. Clinical trials continue and have involved the use of IL-6 alone and in combination with G-CSF or GM-CSF. The most common route of administration is SQ. Side effects include flulike syndrome with fatigue, mild nausea and vomiting, cardiovascular (hypotension, dizziness, mild to moderate pedal edema, bradycardia) and pulmonary (dyspnea, cough, nasal congestion). Flulike symptoms were the most common. Erythema at the injection site has also been observed.[65]

Interleukin-7

Extensive investigation into the regulation and differentiation events governing hematopoiesis in bone marrow led to the identification of the factor supporting the proliferation of precursor B cells. The substance, now known as interleukin-7 (IL-7) and also called lymphopoietin-1, is secreted by cells in the spleen, thymus, and kidney. Subsequent studies indicate that IL-7 also regulates cytotoxic T

lymphocytes (CTL) and lymphokine-activated killer (LAK) cells. Much has yet to be learned about IL-7, its multiple interactions with other cytokines, and its potential therapeutic applications.

Interleukin-8

Interleukin-8 (IL-8) plays a role in the inflammatory process and is secreted by a variety of cells. The ability to stimulate capillary endothelial cell growth may play a role in angiogenesis.

Interleukin-9

Interleukin-9 (IL-9) is derived from T cells. It is responsible for induction of T-helper cells and IgE immunoglobulin production by B cells, and it acts as a growth factor for mast cells.

Interleukin-10

Interleukin-10 (IL-10) was first known as cytokine synthesis inhibitory factor (CSIF), B derived T cell growth factor, and mast cell growth factor III. It is produced by B cells, some T cells, monocytes, and macrophages. IL-10 has been associated with a variety of regulatory functions including: (1) enhancement of B lymphocyte proliferation leading to an increased production of immunoglobulins; (2) inhibition of T cell cytokine secretion; (3) suppression of T cell cytokine production; and (4) inhibition of inflammatory cytokine production. IL-10 is overexpressed in patients with HIV infection.

IL-10 may play a role in the treatment of several different conditions, such as HIV and graft-versus-host disease (GVHD). One laboratory study demonstrated the ability to inhibit juvenile myelomonocytic leukemia cells. Further investigation is needed, and clinical trials continue.[48] Side effects identified thus far include flulike syndrome with fever and headaches.

Interleukin-11

Interleukin-11 (IL-11) is considered a hematopoietic growth factor (HGF). Refer to the section on HGFs for further detail.

Interleukin-12

Interleukin-12 (IL-12) has also been referred to as natural killer (NK) cell stimulatory factor and is produced primarily by monocytes. It stimulates activated CD4+ and CD8+ T cells. The role in GVHD is being explored.

Clinical studies of IL-12 are ongoing. Side effects include flulike syndrome (chills, fatigue, headache, and myalgias were not influenced by dose), GI (nausea and vomiting were rare, stomatitis was dose related), and myelosuppression regardless of dose.

Interleukin-13 Through Interleukin-18

These interleukins are in the earliest stages of clinical development and study. Interleukin-13 (IL-13) plays a role in the chronic inflammation process by blocking the activation of monocyte and macrophage cytokines. It is also involved in B cell proliferation and stimulation. Interleukin-14 (IL-14) has an effect on B cells. Interleukin-15 (IL-15) has similar properties as IL-2 and is involved in stimulating T lymphocytes. It is capable of activating natural killer (NK) cells and stimulates lymphokine-activated killer (LAK) activity. Interleukin-16 (IL-16) is produced by CD8+ T cells and plays a role in T cell mediated inflammatory process. Interleukin-17 (IL-17) induces other cytokine production and induces protein tyrosine kinase mediated signaling. Interleukin-18 (IL-18) induces protein tyrosine kinase mediated signaling and stimulates T cells to produce gamma interferon.

MONOCLONAL ANTIBODIES

The Nobel Prize–winning introduction of hybridoma technology by Kohler and Milstein in 1975 resulted in the development of highly specific agents called monoclonal antibodies (MoAbs) (Figure 7-4).[58] This technique involves injecting a target antigen into a mouse, which then makes an antibody to the injected antigen. When stimulated, B cells can differentiate to plasma cells and secrete a specific antibody. The spleen is a reservoir for these antibody-secreting lymphocytes. Using a mouse that has been injected with tumor cells (acting as the antigen), researchers can induce antibody production. The foreign tumor cells initiate antibody production. Antibody-secreting B lymphocytes from the injected mouse's spleen are removed and placed in culture with a single strain of immortal cancer cells. The B lymphocytes and cancer cells, including their nuclei, fuse to form a hybridoma, which shares the genetic information of both the B lymphocytes and the cancer cell. The immortal hybridoma can produce a perpetual supply of cancer-specific antibody, the MoAb. The MoAb produced is specific for a target antigen, usually a glycoprotein, expressed on the surface of a particular type of cancer cell. Thus, researchers have mimicked the immune system's response to foreign substances with antigen-antibody complex formation, by applying this lock-and-key concept to cancer-targeted interventions with anticancer MoAbs.[53]

Target-specific MoAbs have been used to detect the presence of tumors. Using a sample of the patient's blood, an oncologist can more specifically test for the presence of tumors that have specific antigen markers or secrete identifiable antigens. Small amounts of tumor-associated antigen, such as carcinoembryonic antigen (CEA), can be identified using MoAbs in laboratory immunoassays.[89]

The first cancer-specific MoAbs were developed to detect certain lymphocytic leukemia, melanoma, and lymphoma cells. The production of human antimouse antibodies (HAMAs) in patients treated with murine (mouse) MoAbs appears responsible for most of the reported side effects of first generation MoAb administration and posed one of the early obstacles to administering MoAbs. These side effects include hypotension, dyspnea, fever, chills, diarrhea, bronchospasm, tachycardia, and pruritus. Serologically detectable HAMAs in children receiving MoAb therapy signals an increased risk for anaphylaxis in subsequent administrations. The development of HAMAs limited the ability to administer multiple cycles of murine MoAbs to children. Usually by the third administration the majority of patients developed HAMAs. Clinical trials with first generation MoAbs were disappointing.[114]

To bypass the interspecies reactions and reduce side effects caused by infusing mouse MoAbs, researchers have produced human MoAbs (primarily human protein) and human-mouse chimeric, or combination, MoAbs through genetic engineering. The advantages of using these hybridomas include a diminished risk of sensitization and an increased capability of activating a more appropriate and effective human immune response.

With the advances in genetic engineering and changes in how MoAbs are developed, there has been a renewed interest in treatment with MoAbs. The ability to combine a murine variable region with a human constant has decreased one of the most problematic aspects, the development of HAMA response. The reduction and improvement in clinical management of the hypersensitivity reaction enabled clinicians to use MoAbs for longer periods without the risk of anaphylactic shock. The efficacy of this therapy is beginning to be realized. Trials with this next generation of MoAbs have yielded fewer toxicities, better response rates, and longer remissions.[44,59]

MoAbs have been used in clinical studies to diagnosis cancers, to treat cancers, to purge autologous bone marrow of residual cancer cells, and to prevent or treat GVHD after HSCT. When using MoAbs to treat cancer, patients with minimal tumor burden responded better. The role of MoAbs continues to be investigated. Investigators are developing monoclonal antibodies to target specific receptors found on cancer cells but only minimally or not at all on normal cells. Of special interest in pediatrics is the G_{D2} receptor that is found on cer-

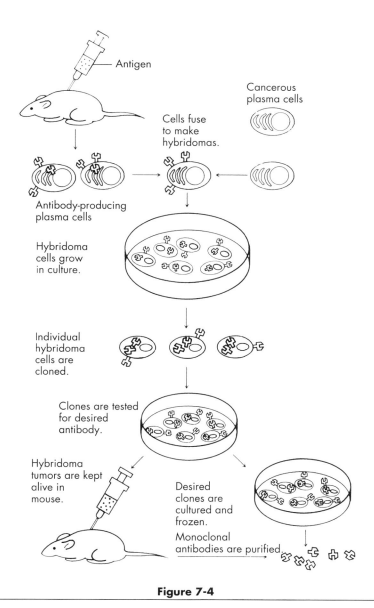

Figure 7-4

Hybridization technology. (From Schindler, L. W. *Understanding the immune system.* NIH Publication 90-529. Bethesda, MD: U.S. Department of Health and Human Services, National Institutes of Health, March 1990, p. 29.)

tain types of cancer cells and selectively on normal cells such as neurons and pain fibers. The G_{D2} antigen is highly expressed on neuroblastoma cells and selectively expressed on some brain tumors, melanoma, soft tissue sarcomas, and osteogenic sarcoma cells.[22,23,121]

RADIOIMMUNODETECTION (RAID)

Researchers have been able to couple MoAbs with radioisotopes, such as iodine-131 (I^{131}) and

indium-111 (In^{111}), and the lower energy radionuclides iodine-123 (I^{123}) and technetium-99 (TC^{99}).[52] Advances in chelation technology have led to the coupling and exploration of yttrium-90 (Y^{90}) for imaging. These radioimmunoconjugates, which combine a MoAb with a radioisotope, have greatly enhanced the diagnostic capabilities of MoAbs. Radioimaging techniques using total body gamma scan or single photon emission computed tomography (SPECT) can detect tumors in primary and metastatic sites, which may not be detected by other currently available means. The diagnostic workup is thus more thorough and allows monitoring of disease sites more accurately during and after therapy. Two MoAbs have received FDA approval for diagnostic purposes in adult cancers. OncoScint CR/OV was approved for detection of colorectal and ovarian cancer. ProstaScint was approved for detection of prostate cancer.[5,114] The development of radiolabeled MoAbs for diagnostic imaging remains investigational in children.[21]

TREATMENT

The effectiveness of MoAbs as a single agent in treatment plans has not generally been impressive. Through the process of opsonization (making bacteria and tumor cells susceptible to phagocytosis), MoAbs are capable of activating complement and stimulating antibody-dependent cell-mediated cytotoxicity. Although some tumor regression may occur, this process does not significantly affect larger tumor burdens.

To overcome this limitation in treatment, researchers have linked MoAbs to chemotherapy (chemoimmunoconjugates); radioactive particles, including iodine preparations (radioimmunoconjugates); cytotoxic agents such as Ricin A-immunotoxin; or other biologic agents. Treatment with these immunoconjugates potentially allows the accurate administration of toxins, radiation, or antineoplastic agents to the sites of disease while limiting the destruction of surrounding tissue. This seek-and-destroy concept, whereby the target-specific antibody delivers a lethal agent to the cancer cell, brings to life Paul Ehrlich's image of MoAbs as "magic bullets."[46] Studies of these MoAbs were disappointing. The toxic effects encountered secondary to the administration of these MoAbs and the low percentage of responders limited clinical investigation and exploration.

Clinical trials using radiolabeled MoAb 3F8 in children with chemotherapy resistant and/or disseminated neuroblastoma are setting the stage for using radioactive or "hot" target-specific antibodies for other malignancies. Early clinical trials with radiolabeled MoAb 3F8 demonstrated that over 10 mg/m^2 of 3F8 antibody can be administered with over 12 mCi/kg of I^{131}. Although there were minimal acute radiation side effects, prolonged myelosuppression with marked thrombocytopenia was observed. Marrow toxicity necessitated the incorporation of stem cell rescue, with previously harvested marrow, into the design of protocols using treatment with multiple infusions of radiolabeled MoAbs.[20] The use of I^{131} and Y^{90} are being investigated. I^{131} is used in the treatment of thyroid cancers. Research is

being conducted using intrathecally administered radiolabeled MoAbs for leptomeningeal disease.

Safety issues must be considered when children receive MoAb preparations. The institution's radiation safety department must work with the medical and nursing teams to develop appropriate guidelines. Depending on the type and amount of radioisotope administered, patients may need to be isolated in a manner similar to those who are implanted with radioactive sources. The implications when the patient is very young are especially important, since parents may need to minimize close contact with their developing child. It is therefore important to establish a mechanism for the child to visualize and have interactions with the parent. Using an absorbing shield at the bedside and establishing organized sequences for interactions when the child's level of radioactivity is high will decrease the risks of radiation exposure to the family and health care team while still providing essential contact and support to the isolated child. The child life worker or recreation therapist can assist in identifying age-appropriate activities such as toys, games, and videos that may be helpful for the child during isolation.

The radiation safety department monitors the radioactivity levels daily and determines the contact restrictions. The expected amount of time necessitating isolation varies by treatment protocol and may range from several days to weeks, based on the dosage and administration sequence of the isotope. In some cases there may be a period just before administration of a scheduled dose of radioimmunoconjugate when a child's radioactivity is at a safe level; this time may be used to allow the child to "escape" isolation briefly. The nurse and family can determine if this would benefit the child and plan an appropriate activity outside of the isolation room.

Several MoAbs are being investigated in children. According to CancerNet, gemtuzumab ozogamicin (CMA-676) and trastuzumab (Herceptin) are both undergoing clinical trial investigation. In a phase II randomized study gemtuzumab is administered with or without high dose cytarabine to patients with recurrent or refractory leukemia that expresses CD33+ receptors (cancernet.nci.nih.gov). Trastuzumab is in phase II investigation for the treatment of patients with recurrent osteosarcoma. It is being infused intravenously over 30 to 90 minutes weekly (cancernet.nci.nih. gov). Clinical investigations of anti-ganglioside (G_{D2}) MoAbs alone and in combination regimens are ongoing and have yielded encouraging results in patients with minimal residual disease. Three anti-G_{D2} MoAbs (3F8, 14.G2, ch 14.18) are currently being investigated in pediatrics.[22,23,35,78,121] Two studies of 3F8 administered to children with stage 4 neuroblastoma have been conducted. The results of a phase II study of children refractory to treatment demonstrated a 19% response rate and support for the use in patients with minimal residual disease.[23] The other study, in which 3F8 was administered following completion of a chemotherapy regimen, again supports the benefits in patients with minimal residual disease.[22] Toxicities in both studies included fever, severe pain, urticaria, and anaphylactic reactions.

In a phase I study of ch 14.18 in patients with refractory neuroblastoma or osteosarcoma, the maximum tolerated dose was safely administered. Side effects included infusion-related pain, fever, urticaria, tachycardia, and hypertension.[121] In another phase I study investigators evaluated the effect of administering escalating doses of ch 14.18 with GM-CSF in children with neuroblastoma after HSCT. Ch 14.18 was administered intravenously over 5 hours for 4 consecutive days within 8 weeks of HSCT. The maximum tolerated dose for ch 14.18 with GM-CSF was determined.[78]

In a phase I-II trial 33 children with refractory neuroblastoma received 14.G2a alone and in combination with IL-2. In this study the maximum tolerated dose of 14.G2a administered with IL-2 was determined followed by an evaluation of the toxicity profile for 14.G2a when administered alone. Side effects included fever, pain, rash, and anaphylactic reactions.[35] Clinical trials of IL-2 and MoAbs continue.[105] The use of MoAbs to purge autologous bone marrow continues to be investigated. One study examined the use of two MoAbs to purge marrow and did not find any better results than standard purging methods.[49] Further investigation is needed.

Several MoAbs have been approved for treatment; some include (1) rituximab (Rituxan) for treatment of CD20+ non-Hodgkin's lymphoma (NHL) and recurrent or refractory low grade NHL (studies in pediatrics are ongoing[28]); (2) trastuzumab (Herceptin) for the treatment of metastatic breast cancer; (3) daclizumab (Zenapax) and (4) muromonab-Cd3 (Orthoclone OKT3) for organ rejection (see Table 7-1). Studies are investigating the use of daclizumab in treatment of refractory ALL,[71] rituximab after HSCT, trastuzumab in the treatment of recurrent osteosarcoma, and muromonab-Cd3 for treatment of GVHD.

MoAbs are usually administered intravenously. Less toxicity has been seen with the administration of MoAbs as compared with myeloablative chemotherapy. Side effects are generally transient and can be mild to moderate (see Table 7-2). Infusion related side effects are common. Premedications are given before administration; however, this has not completely eliminated the risk of reactions. Slowing the rate of infusion may also be helpful. The child needs to be monitored during infusion for signs of hypersensitivity and anaphylaxis. Management includes the administration of additional antihistamines and epinephrine. Flulike symptoms are common. The side effects are less of a problem with chimeric and humanized derived MoAbs. A rare but more serious and potentially life-threatening infusion-related event known as infusion-related complex has been identified. It is generally observed with the first infusion but can occur with subsequent doses. Clinical manifestations include hypoxia, pulmonary infiltrates, adult respiratory distress syndrome, myocardial infarction, ventricular fibrillation, or cardiogenic shock. Patients with preexisting cardiac and pulmonary conditions or those with a previous history of a cardiopulmonary adverse event appear to be at greater risk and must be monitored closely during infusions. Pain is another side effect that may be severe despite the administration of premedications such as morphine. For children receiving anti-G_{D2} MoAbs this is most likely the activation of G_{D2} receptors on pain fibers.

INTERFERONS

In 1957 Isaacs and Linderman first described interferon as a single soluble protein with antiviral activity. Since its initial discovery three major types of interferons (alpha, beta, and gamma) and a broad spectrum of properties have been identified. Interferons (IFNs), members of the cytokine network, are part of a complex family of proteins and glycoproteins capable of inhibiting viral replication, modulating immune responses, altering cellular proliferation, and inhibiting angiogenesis. However, the precise mechanism of action is still not clearly understood.[82]

In addition to its antiviral activity, which may play a role in HIV therapy, IFN antiproliferative, immunomodulatory, and vascular properties may play a role in cancer therapy. For instance, IFNs have been shown to prolong the cell cycle by delaying the entry of cells into the S phase, thereby increasing the number of cells in the G_1 phase. This is an important phenomenon when considering the combination of IFNs with other treatment modalities to achieve the maximum therapeutic effect. The majority of cells have been found to contain two different types of IFN cell receptors; however, the number varies from approximately 100 to 2000 receptors per cell. The role this variation in the number of IFN cell receptors plays has yet to be determined.[119]

Since only minute amounts of IFNs are synthesized in the body, extensive clinical trials could not be conducted until 1981, when recombinant forms of interferon (rIFN) became available. The goal of phase I, II, and III trials was to define the maximum tolerated dose, optimal schedule, route of administration, and maximum biologic response. Although studies in pediatrics have been limited, ongoing trials have incorporated IFN alone and in combination with other agents and/or treatment modalities. Currently IFN has received FDA approval for the treatment of 10 diseases (see Table 7-1). With increased understanding of the biologic properties of IFN, further exploration of potential clinical applications for this agent will occur.[89]

Administration and dosing vary with each type of IFN, manufacturer, and indication for use. It is important to consult the package insert when administering IFN. Anecdotal reports indicate that nighttime administration helps to decrease the side effects and is better tolerated by patients.

The side effects and their intensity differ with each type of IFN, the dose, route of administration, and patient factors (e.g., age, clinical condition). The majority of the side effects (see Table 7-2) are manageable and reversible. Based on findings from clinical trials, younger patients appear to tolerate IFN better than older patients. The acute side effects include a flulike syndrome, which mimics these flulike symptoms (also referred to as constitutional symptoms): fever, chills, fatigue, headache, malaise, nausea, and diarrhea. Fevers associated with IFN usually peak within 6 hours of administration and resolve within 4 to 8 hours. Although the symptoms may be severe initially, the patient's body adjusts to the IFN over time. This process is known as tachyphylaxis. Premedicating the patient with acetaminophen and then remedicating every 4 hours for the first 24 hours benefits many patients. Chronic side effects generally occur 3 to 4 weeks after initiation of therapy and include fatigue, anorexia, and mental status changes such as slowed thinking, forgetfulness, and depression. Fatigue, often a dose limiting side effect, can be minimized by administering IFN at bedtime.[*]

ALPHA INTERFERONS

Naturally occurring alpha interferon (IFN-α) is derived primarily from leukocytes and is often referred to as a type I interferon. More than 20 different subtypes of IFN-α have been identified. The genes encoding IFN-α are located on the short arm of chromosome 9. IFN-α was the first recombinant IFN available and is the most widely studied of all the IFNs. It has been used to treat a variety of cancers; however, the hematologic malignancies (e.g., hairy cell leukemia, chronic myelogenous leukemia) appear to be the most responsive. Results of clinical trials indicate that IFN-α may be more effective in patients with minimal tumor burden than in patients with extensive tumor burden; therefore it may play a more active role as adjuvant therapy after the tumor burden is reduced by another treatment modality (e.g., chemotherapy, radiation, surgery). A few studies have indicated a potential role for the administration of IL-2 and IFN-α after HSCT to reduce relapse rate.

In 1986 IFN-α became the first cytokine to receive FDA approval for the treatment of hairy cell leukemia, Kaposi's sarcoma, and condyloma acuminatum. Additionally, IFN-α has been approved for the treatment of hepatitis C and chronic hepatitis B. IFN-α has been administered by a variety of routes (subcutaneous, intramuscular, intraperitoneal, intravenous) and in different dosages. The MTD is $5\text{-}100 \times 10^6$ units/m^2 or 25-500 mcg/m^2. It may take 1 to 3 months to observe a response to IFN-α therapy.[21] Although the potential role IFN-α will play in pediatric oncology is not yet known, it is currently being studied in a variety of other settings. Clinical trials examining the potential role of IFN-α in the treatment of juvenile laryngeal papillomatosis (a benign tumor of the larynx) in the pediatric population were conducted, and results were encouraging. The role of IFN administered alone for neuroblastoma yielded disappointing results.[22] A phase II study of IFN-α and cytarabine for the treatment of pediatric HIV malignancy is ongoing.

BETA INTERFERONS

Interferon-beta (IFN-β), also referred to as a type I interferon, is derived primarily from fibroblasts and epithelial cells. It is similar to IFN-α genetically, structurally, and in activity, and also competes for the same cell surface receptor. It is FDA approved for use in multiple sclerosis. Clinical trials in cancer are limited and thus far have not demonstrated any superiority of IFN-β over IFN-α in efficacy. There are currently no known ongoing trials in pediatrics; therefore the unique functions of IFN-β and its role(s) in pediatric oncology and HIV treatment remain to be determined.[27]

GAMMA INTERFERON

Interferon-gamma (IFN-γ) is produced primarily by T cells and natural killer (NK) cells and is often referred to as a type II interferon. The genes responsible for encoding IFN-γ production are located on chromosome 12. The genes responsible for encoding IFN-γ receptors are located on chromosome 21. Although this cytokine has functions similar to that of the other IFNs, its immunomodulatory functions apparently are more prominent.[21] In vitro and in vivo studies have revealed synergy between IFN-γ and several other cytokines (e.g., IFN-α, IFN-β, IL-2) and with chemotherapy and/or radiation.[12]

The side effects associated with IFN-γ are similar to those observed with IFN-α. However, more frequent headaches, prolonged fevers, and an increase in liver enzymes and serum triglycerides have also been observed. The role of IFN-γ in cancer therapy will probably not be as a cytotoxic agent, but as an adjuvant to therapy by modulating host responses, altering cellular structure, and/or inhibiting cellular growth. A phase I-II study exploring the use of IFN-γ in the treatment of chronic granulomatous disease revealed significantly fewer bacterial and fungal infections. In 1990 IFN-γ received FDA approval for this indication. This result may indicate a potential role for IFN-γ in the management of fever and neutropenia associated with cancer therapy.[21]

RETINOIDS

Retinoids are derivatives of vitamin A, also known as retinol, which have received much publicity for their role in the treatment of acne and as antiaging creams. Vision, fertility, growth, immune function, and epithelial differentiation are influenced by these natural derivatives. Although the existence of retinoids has been known for more than 50 years, it was not until the 1990s that investigation of their potential role in the treatment of cancer began. Retinoids are classified as immunomodulators in cancer therapy because they facilitate differentiation and suppress proliferation of cells. The retinoid derivatives all-trans retinoic acid (ATRA), 13-cis-retinoic acid, and 9-cis-retinoic acid are under clinical investigations. Optimal dosing and scheduling need to be defined.[67]

Clinical studies with ATRA revealed dramatic results in remission induction for patients with acute promyelocytic leukemia (APL). ATRA received FDA approval in 1995. It is now considered standard therapy for induction of APL. However, clinical studies have shown that it is not effective for the maintenance phase. Following induction, consolidation with daunorubicin and cytarabine is initiated. Survival rates increased from 51% to 81%.[102,106,120]

Clinical trials continue to investigate other retinoic acid derivatives (i.e., 13-cis-retinoic acid, 9-cis-retinoic acid) and their potential role in the treatment of childhood cancers. The use of isotretinoin (13-cis-retinoic acid) in the treatment of neuroblastoma has been investigated. A double randomized study of high-risk patients with neuroblastoma demonstrated that autologous HSCT was superior to chemotherapy alone and the addition of isotretinoin after HSCT recovery or completion of chemotherapy increased long-term survival rates.[66] Isotretinoin has demonstrated activity in juvenile chronic myelogenous leukemia (JCML) and is being investigated. Results of a pilot study were encouraging, with children surviving beyond the mean survival achieved with conventional chemotherapy regimens. Isotretinoin was well tolerated, and minimal toxicity was observed. The mechanism of action and the role isotretinoin will play in the treatment of JCML is still under investigation. One thought is that it may be used to control JCML for those children preparing for HSCT.[17,62] Additionally clinical trials are being conducted to evaluate the combination of retinoids with other cancer treatment modalities.[8,89]

Retinoids are administered orally with food and are usually well tolerated by patients. The most common side effects include dermatologic changes (e.g., dry skin, lips, and mucous membranes; pruritus; increased pigmentation; desquamation), conjunctival redness or irritation, bone pain, arthralgias, anorexia, fatigue, and headache (see Table 7-2). Children appear to be less tolerant especially of the CNS side effects such as headache and pseudotumor cerebri. Tachyphylaxis develops over time.[40]

It is important to monitor patients carefully for any signs of toxicity. For example, patients can develop acute hypervitaminosis A, characterized by drowsiness, irritability, headache, and/or vomiting. Another potentially fatal syndrome occurring in approximately 25% of patients with APL, known as retinoic acid syndrome, requires early recognition and immediate treatment most often with high dose corticosteroids. The etiology of this syndrome is unknown; however, the symptoms are similar to those observed with capillary leak and may be the result of a cytokine release. Symptoms usually appear 2 to 21 days after initiation of therapy and do not appear to be reversed when the drug is stopped. Symptoms include fever, respiratory distress, interstitial pulmonary infiltrates, pleural and/or pericardial effusions, and weight gain.[34,40]

For postmenarchal females a pregnancy test should be obtained before initiation of therapy. Females are encouraged to use two forms of contraceptives during treatment with retinoids and for 1 month after completion of therapy because of the teratogenetic effects of this therapy.

SIDE EFFECTS OF BRMS

Biotherapy often results in significant toxicities that can occur acutely or chronically and are generally noncumulative. The side effects associated with each biologic agent are often influenced by the dose, route of administration, and schedule. As always, it is best to keep in mind that there are differences in the immune systems of adult and pediatric patients, and a thorough assessment of each individual will ensure the identification of expected and unexpected side effects. In general, the side effects related to biotherapy in children do not overlap those associated with chemotherapy and/or radiation and are generally reversible once administration of the agent is stopped. Prolonged, severe fatigue, widely observed as a significant side effect in adult patients treated with biologic agents, has not been universally reported or documented in the pediatric population. Recovery from the effect(s) may occur instantaneously or take several weeks. The most unique side effect associated with biotherapy, occurring almost universally, is known as the flu-like syndrome. It is characterized by fever, chills, rigors, myalgias, headache, and fatigue. The severity of this syndrome is variable. Edema, resulting from vascular leakage, combined with lymphocyte mobilization and infiltration, compounds the symptoms ascribed to this phenomenon (see Table 7-2).

Nursing Management

The management of the side effects associated with the administration of biologic agents presents a unique challenge for nurses. Knowledge of measures to treat side effects associated with chemotherapy and radiation is useful. These interventions can serve as a starting point in the management of side effects associated with biotherapy; however, they may prove ineffective for the unique manifestations of the interactions between biologic agents and the patient's immune system. Emphasis should be placed on comprehensive ongoing physical and psychosocial assessment, observation for subtle changes in physical status or behavior, and documentation of side effects. This will enable nurses to recognize trends and devise a plan of action for expected clinical situations.

Many of the interventions fall into one of three categories. The first is the implementation of preventative measures, such as patient teaching or administration of premedications to prevent allergic reactions or pain. The second is to reduce side effects as they occur. This includes correction of fluid or electrolyte imbalances, administering analgesics, antipyretics, or antihistamines, and adjusting therapy administration if possible. Third, individual strategies are devised to provide for patient comfort. Reducing side effects will usually improve patient comfort, but in addition there are many nonprescriptive ways to manipulate the environment to relax the patient and improve tolerance. These can range from providing quiet surroundings or an age-appropriate roommate to identifying distraction activities. Two important measures are continued explanations of nursing and medical activities related to the therapy and the emotional support before, during, and after treatment. Despite increasing knowledge about the acute side effects and their management, further research is needed to identify and refine effective symptom management interventions. In addition, studies are needed to determine long-term side effects associated with this therapy and its impact on quality of life.[32,38,95] Table 7-4 reviews recommended nursing interventions for the side effects associated with biotherapy. Refer to Chapter 11 for more information about treatment of disease and treatment-related complications.

As the excitement of new cancer therapies builds and research in the clinical setting becomes more aggressive, the pediatric oncology nurse's role takes on new dimensions and more responsibilities. Child and family safety, education, and support; data collection and documentation; and peer education are important elements. The pediatric oncology nurse must develop an understanding of the components of the immune system, the process of hematopoiesis, and the intimate interactions of biologic agents with each other and with other elements of the immune system. In addition, excellent assessment skills are necessary to recognize subtle changes that may occur. The nurse must be aware of the particular side effects most commonly associated with each biologic agent, as well as the general side effects experienced in varying degrees by any patient receiving anticancer therapy. As new combination therapies are developed, many unexpected side effects can occur.

In addition to the challenges of physical care, the nurse must also recognize the child and family's need for psychosocial support. Often, children receiving biologic agents are participating in experimental therapy or clinical trials, which adds another component to the child and family's physical and psychosocial care. Families may have experienced multiple unsuccessful treatment attempts before the use of biologic agents. They depend on the nurse to provide information and reassurance and look to the nurse for answers, guidance, support, and hope.

Clinical application of protocols using biother-

TABLE 7-4	NURSING INTERVENTIONS FOR MANAGEMENT OF BIOTHERAPY SIDE EFFECTS
Side Effect	**Interventions**
Flulike syndrome	Assess for signs and symptoms (S/S) associated with flulike syndrome.
	Monitor temperature, identify fever pattern in response to therapy, and report unusual fever spikes.
	Pharmacologic agents
	• Premedicate before administration if appropriate; acetaminophen is most commonly used.
	• Administer antipyretic such as acetaminophen, ibuprofen, and/or indomethacin every 4 hours as needed for fever; for high fevers consider alternating schedule.
	• Administer parenteral meperidine for rigors.
	Provide comfort measures such as warm blankets; for high fevers consider cooling blanket or tepid bath.
	Evaluate S/S of fatigue; teach ways to balance activities and conserve energy (e.g., naps, rest periods, prioritizing and delegating activities).
	Educate about S/S and when to notify health care team.
Cardiopulmonary	Assess baseline cardiopulmonary status and for S/S of cardiopulmonary side effects during therapy.
	Monitor vital signs (VS) and pulse oximetry as indicated; monitor for orthostatic changes as indicated.
	Administer oxygen if indicated.
	Capillary leak
	• Weigh patient and assess for edema; measure abdominal girth.
	• Assess intake and urinary output.
	• Monitor for tachycardia and hypotension; instruct patient to stand slowly and report any dizziness.
	• Administer albumin, diuretics, fluids, and low dose dopamine as needed.
	Infusion related (most often observed with monoclonals)
	• Premedicate with acetaminophen and diphenhydramine; premedicate with narcotic if ordered.
	• Start infusion slowly and escalate rate as tolerated; monitor VS every 15 to 30 minutes during infusion or as ordered.
	• Adverse reactions
	• Hypersensitivity: slow infusion rate if symptoms (e.g., hives, rash) noted; administer medications as ordered.
	• Anaphylaxis: stop infusion and administer emergency medications as needed.
	• Notify prescriber and report adverse drug reaction according to institutional guidelines.
	Educate about symptoms and when to notify health care team.
Renal/hepatic	Monitor laboratory values.
	Monitor intake and output; encourage oral intake.
	Assess for jaundice and/or hepatomegaly.
	If patient is receiving acetaminophen, monitor total 24 hour dose.
Gastrointestinal	Assess for S/S of gastrointestinal side effects.
	Assess dietary habits and elimination patterns.
	Encourage oral intake; encourage small frequent meals; use dietary supplements as needed.
	Obtain dietary consult.
	Monitor for S/S of fluid and electrolyte imbalances.
	Pharmacologic agents
	• Antiemetics (avoid steroids)
	• Antidiarrheals
	Educate about S/S and when to notify health care team.

Continued

TABLE 7-4	NURSING INTERVENTIONS FOR MANAGEMENT OF BIOTHERAPY SIDE EFFECTS—cont'd
Side Effect	**Interventions**
Integumentary	Obtain baseline skin assessment and skin history.
	Assess skin integrity for color and areas of irritation, redness, breakdown, scaling, and moisture.
	Skin care
	• Bathe daily using hypoallergenic soaps (e.g., Dove, Basis) or bath oils (e.g., Alpha Keri).
	• Apply hypoallergenic water based emollient lotions and creams frequently (e.g., Alpha Keri, aloe).
	• Sun protection: minimize sun exposure and use a sunscreen with SPF 15 or greater.
	Pruritis
	• Use colloidal oatmeal baths (e.g., Aveeno).
	• Administer anitpruritic medications as needed; diphenhydramine and hydroxyzine are common.
	• Instruct patient to wear loose fitting and cotton clothing.
	Injection sites
	• Monitor for erythema, induration, and/or inflammation.
	• Rotate injection sites.
	• Minimize volume of injection.
	Educate about S/S and when to notify health care team.
Musculoskeletal	Assess patient's history of pain: note onset, location, duration, and sensation.
	Administer acetaminophen, ibuprofen, and/or indomethacin for arthralgia, myalgia, headache, and bone pain as needed.
	Provide comfort measures (e.g., apply moist heat to affected areas).
	Use distraction and relaxation techniques.
	Educate about S/S and when to report to health care team.
Central nervous system	Assess baseline neurologic and mental status.
	Monitor neurologic and mental status frequently during therapy; note any changes (e.g., confusion, agitation, anxiety, lethargy), and evaluate impact on activities of daily living.
	Maintain safe environment; orient child to person, place, and time as indicated; provide memory prompts as needed.
	Instruct family about potential mental status changes; reassure them that changes are related to treatment, are agent and dose related, and generally subside after treatment.
	Educate about S/S and when to notify health care team.

apy facilitates nursing research. Pediatric oncology nurses are in a unique position to contribute to this body of knowledge. Thorough assessment and documentation before, during, and after the treatment period will provide important data necessary to develop policies, procedures, and standards of care for the child receiving biotherapy. Patient information (e.g., teaching booklets and videos) for the child and family must be developed for patients receiving biotherapy and for the various biologic agents. It is also the pediatric oncology nurse's responsibility to disseminate information regarding biotherapy to colleagues. The professional nurse who accepts this challenge welcomes the opportunity to contribute to the body of science and continue to advance this growing treatment modality.

RESEARCH ACTIVITIES AND FUTURE DIRECTIONS

The complex nature of biologic agents' interactions makes the determination of the most effective routes of administration, dose levels, and dose scheduling essential. Clinical trials of this decade will be designed to determine whether biologic agents in combination with each other or as adjuvant with other treatment modalities are efficacious in the treatment of pediatric oncologic diseases and their associated side effects. Many combination clinical trials to address these issues are currently being conducted in the pediatric population. Some of the more widely used combinations involve biologic agents with other biologic agents, biologic agents with chemotherapy, and biologic agents with radiotherapy. The physician data query

(PDQ), a computerized database of clinical trials funded by the National Cancer Institute and the website http://cancertrials.nci.nih.gov are excellent resources for ascertaining information concerning active clinical trials using biologics and/or biologic agents in cancer treatment. Information about clinical trials can also be accessed through the toll-free number 1-800-4-CANCER. Current and future research will help to clarify the many interrelated functions and activities of biologic agents.

Advances and new developments in biotechnology have a direct effect on the field of biotherapy and cause renewed enthusiasm for this therapeutic approach. Although the development and use of hematopoietic growth factors (HGFs) has yielded much success, the use of other BRMs as immunomodulators and/or for cytotoxicity have had only limited success with some specific cancers. The emergence of biotherapy as the fourth modality in cancer therapy poses a challenging new frontier that is still in its infancy in comparison with the other treatment modalities.

REFERENCES

1. Adamson, J. W. (1998). Epoetin alfa: Into the new millennium. *Seminars in Oncology, 25 (Suppl. 7)*, 76-79.
2. Akingbola, A., Custer, J. R., Bunchman, T. E., et al. (1994). Management of severe anemia without transfusion in a pediatric Jehovah's Witness patient. *Critical Care Medicine, 22,* 524-528.
3. Armitage, J. O. (1998). Emerging applications of recombinant human granulocyte-macrophage colony-stimulating factor, part I. *Blood, 92,* 4491-4508.
4. Atkins, M. (1997). Interleukin-2 in metastatic melanoma. Establishing a role. *Cancer Journal: from Scientific American, 3 (Suppl 1),* 57-58.
5. Bacquiran, D. C., Dantis, L., & McKerrow, J. (1996). Monoclonal antibodies: Innovations in diagnosis and therapy. *Seminars in Oncology Nursing, 12,* 130-141.
6. Balkwill, F. R. (1989). *Cytokines in Cancer Therapy.* Oxford: Oxford University Press.
7. Basser, R., Underhill, C., Davis, I., et al. (2000). Enhancement of platelet recovery after myelosuppressive chemotherapy by recombinant human megakaryocyte growth and development factor in patients with advanced cancer. *Journal of Clinical Oncology, 18,* 2852-2861.
8. Battiato, L., & Wheeler, V. (2000). Biotherapy. In S. L. Groenwald, H. Frogge, M. Goodman, et al. (Eds.), *Cancer nursing principles and practice* (5th ed., pp. 543-579). Boston: Jones & Bartlett.
9. Beck, M. J., & Beck, D. (1995). Recombinant erythropoietin in acute chemotherapy induced anemia of children with cancer. *Medical and Pediatric Oncology, 25,* 17-21.
10. Bennett, C., Stinson, T., Lane, D., et al. (2000). Cost analysis of filgrastim for prevention of neutropenia in pediatric T-cell leukemia and advanced lymphoblastic lymphoma: A case for prospective economic analysis in cooperative group trials. *Medical and Pediatric Oncology, 34,* 92-96.
11. Bolonaki, I., Stiakaki, E., Lydaki, E., et al. (1996). Treatment with recombinant human erythropoietin in children with malignancies. *Pediatric Hematology/Oncology, 13,* 111-121.
12. Bonnem, E. M., & Oldham, R. K. (1987). Gamma-interferon: Physiology and speculation on its role in medicine. *Journal of Biologic Response Modifiers, 6,* 275-301.
13. Borden, E., & Parkinson, E. (1998). Side effects of interferons alpha: Possible clinical causes and intervention strategies. *Seminars in Oncology, 25 (1 Suppl 1),* 1-78.
14. Bukowski, R. M., McLain, D., & Finke, J. (1996). Clinical pharmacokinetics of interleukin 1, interleukin 2, interleukin 4, tumor necrosis factor, and macrophage colony-stimulating factor. In B. A. Chabner & D. L. Longo (Eds.), *Cancer chemotherapy and biotherapy* (2nd ed., pp. 609-638). Philadelphia: Lippincott-Raven.
15. Cario, M. S. (2000). Dose reductions and delays: Limitations of myelosuppressive chemotherapy. *Oncology, 14(9 Suppl 8),* 21-31.
16. Casadevall, N. (1998). Update on the role of epoetin alfa in hematologic malignancies and myelodysplastic syndromes. *Seminars in Oncology, 25 (Suppl 7),* 12-18.
17. Castleberry, R. P., Emanuel, P. D., Zuckerman, K. S., et al. (1994). A pilot study of isotretinoin in the treatment of juvenile chronic myelogenous leukemia. *New England Journal of Medicine, 331,* 1680-1684.
18. Champlin, R. E., & Figlin, R. A. (Eds.) (1996) Evolving clinical applications of hematopoietic growth factors. *Seminars in Oncology, 23 (2 Suppl 4),* 1-30.
19. Chang, M., Suen, Y., Meng, G., et al. (1996). Differential mechanisms in the regulation of endogenous levels of thrombopoietin and interleukin-11 during thrombocytopenia: Insight into the regulation of platelet production. *Blood, 88,* 3354-3362.
20. Cheung, N. V. (1991). Immunotherapy: Pediatric neuroblastoma as a model. *Pediatric Clinics of North America, 38,* 425-441.
21. Cheung, N. V. (1997). Principles of immunotherapy. In P. A. Pizzo & D. G. Poplack (Eds.), *Principles and practice of pediatric oncology* (3rd ed., pp. 323-342). Philadelphia: Lippincott-Raven.
22. Cheung, N. V., Kushner, B. H., Cheung, I. Y., et al. (1998). Anti-G_{D2} antibody treatment of minimal residual stage 4 neuroblastoma diagnosed at more than 1 year of age. *Journal of Clinical Oncology, 16,* 3053-3060.
23. Cheung, N. V., Kushner, B. H., Yeh, S., et al. (1998). 3F8 monoclonal antibody treatment of patients with stage 4 neuroblastoma: A phase II study. *International Journal of Oncology, 12,* 1299-1306.
24. Chopra, R., & Scarffe, J. H. (2000). The biology and clinical use of stem cell factor. In J. O. Armitage & K. H. Antman (Eds.), *High dose cancer therapy: Pharmacology, hematopoietins, stem cells* (3rd ed., pp. 455-465). Philadelphia: Lippincott Williams & Wilkins.
25. Clarke, V., Dunstan, F. D. J., & Webb, D. K. H. (1999). Granulocyte colony-stimulating factor ameliorates toxicity of intensification chemotherapy for acute lymphoblastic leukemia. *Medical and Pediatric Oncology, 32,* 331-335.
26. Crawford, J., & Lee, M. E. (2000). Recombinant human granulocyte colony-stimulating factor support of the cancer patient. In J. O. Armitage & K. H. Antman (Eds.), *High dose cancer therapy: Pharmacology, hematopoietins, stem cells* (3rd ed., pp. 411-436). Philadelphia: Lippincott, Williams, & Wilkins.
27. Costello, K., & Conway, K. (1997). Nursing management of MS patients receiving interferon beta-1b therapy. *Rehabilitation Nursing, 22,* 62-66.

28. Davis, T., Grillo-Lopez, A. J., White, C. A., et al. (2000). Rituximab anti-DS20 monoclonal antibody therapy in non-Hodgkin's lymphoma: Safety and efficacy of re-treatment. *Journal of Clinical Oncology, 18*, 3135-3143.

29. Donnelly, S. (1998). Patient management strategies for interferon alfa-2b as adjuvant therapy of high-risk melanoma. *Oncology Nursing Forum, 25*, 921-927.

30. Du, X., & William, D. A. (1997). Interleukin-11: Review of molecular, cell biology and clinical use. *Blood, 89*, 3897-3908.

31. Estrin, J. T., Ford, P. A., Henry, D. H., et al. (1997). Ery-thropoietin permits high-dose chemotherapy with periph-eral blood stem-cell transplant for Jehovah's Witness. *American Journal of Hematology, 55*, 51-52.

32. Farrell, M. M. (1996). Biotherapy and the oncology nurse. *Seminars in Oncology Nursing, 12*, 82-88.

33. Fefer, A. (1997). Interleukin-2 in the treatment of hema-tologic malignancies. *Cancer Journal: from Scientific American, 3 (Suppl. 1)*, S35-S36.

34. Frankel, S., Eardley, A., & Lauwers, G. (1992). The "retinoic acid syndrome" in acute promyelocytic leukemia. *Annals of Internal Medicine, 117*, 292-296.

35. Frost, J. D., Hank, J. A., Reaman, G. H., et al. (1997). A phase I/IB trial of murine monoclonal anti-G_{D2} antibody 14.G2a plus interleukin-2 in children with refractory neuroblastoma. *Cancer, 80*, 317-333.

36. Furman, W. L. (1995). Cytokine support following chemotherapy in children. *International Journal of Pedi-atric Hematology/Oncology, 2*, 163-167.

37. Furman, W., Luo, X., Marina, N., et al. (1998). Compari-son of cytokines in children with recurrent solid tumors treated with intensive chemotherapy. *Journal of Pediatric Hematology/Oncology, 20*, 62-68.

38. Gale, D. M. (1997). Part II: Nursing management guide-lines. In *Biotherapy: Considerations for Oncology Nurses, (Vol 2, 3-5)*. Washington Crossing: Scientific Frontiers.

39. Ghalie, R. G., & Tallman, M. S. (2000). Granulocyte-macrophage colony-stimulating factor. In J. O. Armitage & K. H. Antman (Eds.), *High dose cancer therapy: Phar-macology, hematopoietins, stem cells* (3rd ed., pp. 393-410). Philadelphia: Lippincott Williams & Wilkins.

40. Gillis, J. C., & Goa, K. L. (1995). Tretinoin, *Drugs, 50*, 897-923.

41. Glaspy, J., Bukowski, R., Steinberg, D., et al. (1997). Im-pact of therapy with epoetin alfa on clinical outcomes in patients with non-myeloid malignancies during cancer chemotherapy in community oncology practice. *Journal of Clinical Oncology, 15*, 1218-1234.

42. Griffin, J. D. (1997). Hematopoietic growth factors. In V. T. DeVita, S. Hellman, & S. A. Rosenberg (Eds.), *Can-cer: Principles and practice of oncology* (5th ed., pp. 2639-2657). Philadelphia: Lippincott-Raven.

43. Hagglund, H., Ringden, O., Oman, S., et al. (1999). A prospective randomized trial of filgrastim (r-metHuG-CSF) given at different times after unrelated bone mar-row transplantation. *Bone Marrow Transplantation, 24*, 831-836.

44. Hall, S. S. (1995). Monoclonal antibodies at age 20: Promise at last? *Science, 270*, 915-916.

45. Henry, D. H. (1998). Epoetin Alfa and high-dose chemotherapy. *Seminars in Oncology, 25 (Suppl 7)*, 54-57.

46. Himmelweit, B. (Ed.) (1975). *The collected papers of Paul Ehrlich*. Oxford: Pergamon Press.

47. Hossan, E., & Rieger, P. (1997). Interleukin-2 therapy nursing management plus education equals success in the ambulatory setting. In *Biotherapy: Considerations for oncology nurses, (Vol 2, pp. 1-7)*. Washington Crossing: Scientific Frontiers.

48. Iverson, P. O., Hart, P. H., Claudine, S., et al. (1997). In-terleukin (IL)-10, but not IL-4 or IL-13, inhibits cytokine production and growth in juvenile myelomonocytic leukemia cells. *Cancer Research, 57*, 476-480.

49. Jabado, N., Le Deist, F., Cant, A., et al. (1996). Bone marrow transplantation from genetically HLA-nonidenti-cal donors in children with fatal inherited disorders ex-cluding severe combined immunodeficiencies: Use of two monoclonal antibodies to prevent graft rejection. *Pe-diatrics, 98*, 420-428.

50. Jilani, S. M., & Glaspy, J. A. (1998). Impact of epoetin alfa in chemotherapy-associated anemia. *Seminars in Oncology, 25*, 571-576.

51. Johnston, E. M., & Crawford, J. (1998). Hematopoietic growth factors: The reduction of chemotherapeutic toxic-ity. *Seminars in Oncology, 25*, 552-561.

52. Jurcic, J. G., Scheinber, D. A., & Houghton, A. N. (1997). Monoclonal antibody therapy of cancer. *Cancer Chemotherapy Biological Response Modifiers, 17*, 195-216.

53. Karius, D., & Marriott, M. A. (1997). Immunologic ad-vances in monoclonal antibody therapy: Implications for oncology nursing. *Oncology Nursing Forum, 24*, 483-496.

54. Kaushansky, K. (1997). Thrombopoietin: Platelets on de-mand? *Annals of Internal Medicine, 126*, 731-733.

55. Kaushansky, K. (1998). Thrombopoietin. *New England Journal of Medicine, 339*, 746-754.

56. Kiley, K. E., & Gale, D. M. (1998). Nursing management of patients with malignant melanoma receiving adjuvant alpha interferon-2b. *Clinical Journal of Oncology Nurs-ing, 2*, 11-16.

57. King, C. R. (1996). Colony-stimulating factors. In M. B. Burke, G. M. Wilkes, & K. Ingwerson (Eds.), *Cancer chemotherapy: A nursing approach* (2nd ed., pp. 85-88). Boston: Jones & Bartlett.

58. Kohler, G., and Milstein, C. (1975). Continuous cultures of fused cells secreting antibody of predefined speci-ficity. *Nature, 256*, 495-497.

59. Kostis, C., & Callaghan, M. (2000). Rituximab: A new monoclonal antibody therapy for non-Hodgkin's lym-phoma. *Oncology Nursing Forum, 27*, 51-59.

60. Lachance, D. H., Oette, D., Schold, S. C., et al. (1995). Dose escalation trial of cyclophosphamide with sar-gramostim in the treatment of central nervous system (CNS) neoplasms. *Medical and Pediatric Oncology, 24*, 241-247.

61. Lieschke, G. H., Ceban, J., & Morstyn, G. (1989). Char-acterization of the clinical effects after the first dose of bacterially synthesized recombinant human granulocyte-macrophage colony-stimulating factors. *Blood, 74*, 2634-2643.

62. Lippman, S. M., & Davies, P. (1997). Retinoids, neopla-sia and differentiation therapy. In H. M. Pinedo, D. L. Longo, & B. A. Chabner (Eds.), *Cancer chemotherapy and biological response modifiers annual* (pp. 349-362). New York: Elsevier.

63. Locatelli, F., Zecca, M., Pedrazzoli, P., et al. (1994). Use of recombinant human erythropoietin after bone marrow transplantation in pediatric patients with acute leukemia: Effect on erythroid repopulation in autologous versus al-logeneic transplants. *Bone Marrow Transplantation, 13*, 403-410.

64. MacMillian, M., & Freedman, M. (1998). Recombinant human erythropoietin in children with cancer. *Journal of Pediatric Hematology/Oncology, 20*, 187-189.

65. Maslak, P., & Nimer, S. D. (1998). The efficacy of IL-3, SCF, IL-6, and IL-11 in treating thrombocytopenia. *Sem-inars in Hematology, 35*, 253-260.

66. Matthay, K. K., Villablanca, J. G., Seeger, R. C., et al. (1999). Treatment of high-risk neuroblastoma with intensive chemotherapy, radiotherapy, autologous bone marrow transplantation and 13-cis-retinoic acid. *New England Journal of Medicine, 341,* 1165-1173.

67. Mayne, S. T., & Lippman, S. M. (1997). Retinoids and carotenoids. In V. T. DeVita, S. Hellman, & S. A. Rosenberg (Eds.), *Cancer: Principles and practice of oncology* (5th ed., pp. 585-599). Philadelphia: Lippincott-Raven.

68. Messina, C., Zambello, R., Rossetti, F., et al. (1996). Interleukin-2 before and/or after autologous bone marrow transplantation for pediatric acute leukemia patients. *Bone Marrow Transplantation, 17,* 729-735.

69. Michel, G., Landman-Parker, J., Auclerc, M. F., et al. (2000). Use of recombinant human granulocyte colony-stimulating factor to increase chemotherapy dose-intensity: A randomized trial in very high-risk childhood acute lymphoblastic leukemia. *Journal of Clinical Oncology, 18,* 1517-1524.

70. Miller, C. B. (2000). Erythropoietin. In J. O. Armitage & K. H. Antman (Eds.), *High dose cancer therapy: Pharmacology, hematopoietins, stem cells* (3rd ed., pp. 437-454). Philadelphia: Lippincott Williams & Wilkins.

71. Multani, P. S., & Grossband., M. L. (1998). Monoclonal antibody-based therapies for hematologic malignancies. *Journal of Clinical Oncology, 16,* 3691-3710.

72. Nagayama, H., Takahashi, S., Takahashi, T., et al. (1999). IL-2/LAK therapy for refractory acute monoblastic leukemia after unrelated allogeneic bone marrow transplantation. *Bone Marrow Transplantation, 23,* 183-185.

73. Nash, R., Kurzrock, R., DiPersio, J., et al. (1997). Safety and activity of recombinant human thrombopoietin (rhTPO) in patients with delayed platelet recovery (DPR). *Blood, 90 (Suppl. 1),* 262a.

74. Nemunaitis, J. (1997). A comparative review of colony-stimulating factors. *Drugs, 54,* 709-729.

75. O'Brien, S., Kantarjian, H., & Talpaz, M. (1996). Practical guidelines for the management of chronic myelogenous leukemia with interferon alpha. *Leukemia and Lymphoma, 23,* 247-252.

76. Oldham, R. K. (Ed.) (1998). *Principles of cancer biotherapy* (3rd ed.). Boston: Kluwer Academic.

77. Ozer, H., Armitage, J., Bennett, C., et al. (Eds.) (2000). 2000 update of recommendations for the use of hematopoietic colony-stimulating factors: Evidence-based clinical practice guidelines. *Journal of Clinical Oncology, 18,* 3558-3585.

78. Ozkaynak, M. F., Sondel, P. M., Krailo, M. D., et al. (2000). Phase I study of chimeric human/murine anti-ganglioside G_{D2} monoclonal antibody (ch 14.18) with granulocyte-macrophage colony stimulating factor in children with neuroblastoma immediately after hematopoietic stem-cell transplantation: A Children's Cancer Group study. *Journal of Clinical Oncology, 18,* 4077-4085.

79. Parkinson, D. R., & Grimm, E. A. (1997). Cytokines: Biology and applications in cancer medicine. In J. F. Holland, R. C. Bast, D.L. Morton, et al. (Eds.), *Cancer medicine* (4th ed., pp. 1213-1226). Baltimore: Williams & Wilkins.

80. Parsons, S. K., Mayer, D. K., Alexander, S. W., et al. (2000). Growth factor practice patterns among pediatric oncologists: Results of a 1998 Pediatric Oncology Group survey. *Journal of Pediatric Hematology/Oncology, 22,* 227-241.

81. Pessin, A., Prete, A., Locatelli, F., et al. (1998). Immunotherapy with low-dose recombinant interleukin 2 after high-dose chemotherapy and autologous stem cell transplantation in neuroblastoma. *British Journal of Cancer, 78,* 528-533.

82. Peska, S., & Trotta, P. P. (1997). Recombinant alfa-interferons from naturally occurring genes. *Seminars in Oncology , 24(3 Suppl. 9),* 1-104.

83. Petros, W. P., & Peters, W. P. (1996). Colony stimulating factors. In B. A. Chabner & D. L. Longo (Eds.), *Cancer chemotherapy and biotherapy* (2nd ed., pp. 639-654). Philadelphia: Lippincott-Raven.

84. Pitlet, L. R. (1996). Hematopoietic growth factors in clinical practice. *Seminars in Oncology Nursing, 12,* 115-129.

85. Prow, D., & Vadhan-Raj, S. (1998). Thrombopoietin: Biology and potential clinical applications. *Oncology, 12,* 1597-1608.

86. Rahiala, J., Perkkio, M., & Riikonen, R. (1999). Prospective and randomized comparison of early versus delayed prophylactic administration of granulocyte colony-stimulating factor (filgrastim) in children with cancer. *Medical and Pediatric Oncology, 32,* 326-330.

87. Reiger, P. T. (1996). Biotherapy: The fourth modality. In M. B. Burke, G. M. Wilkes, & K. Ingewersen (Eds.), *Cancer chemotherapy: A nursing process approach* (2nd ed., pp. 43-73). Boston: Jones & Bartlett.

88. Reiger, P. T. (Ed.) (1996). Biotherapy: Present accomplishments and future projections. *Seminars in Oncology Nursing, 12,* 81-171.

89. Reiger, P. T. (1999). *Clinical handbook for biotherapy.* Boston: Jones and Bartlett.

90. Reynolds, C. H. (2000). Clinical efficacy of rhIL-11. *Oncology, 14(9 Suppl. 8),* 32-40.

91. Rosenberg, S. A. (1997). Principles of cancer management. In V. T. DeVita, S. Hellman, & S. A. Rosenberg (Eds.), *Cancer: Principles and practice of oncology* (5th ed., pp. 349-373). Philadelphia: Lippincott-Raven.

92. Rosenberg, S. A. (1997). Keynote address: Perspectives on the use of interleukin-2 in cancer treatment. *Cancer Journal: From Scientific American, 3(Suppl. 1),* S2-S6.

93. Rust, D. M., Wood, L. S., & Battiato, L. (1999). Oprelvekin: An alternative treatment for thrombocytopenia. *Clinical Journal of Oncology Nursing, 3,* 57-62.

94. Saarinen-Pihkala, U. M., Lanning, M., Perkkio, M, et al. (2000). Granulocyte-macrophage colony-stimulating factor support in therapy of high risk acute lymphoblastic leukemia in children. *Medical and Pediatric Oncology, 34,* 319-327.

95. Sandstrom, S. K. (1996). Nursing management of patients receiving biological therapy. *Seminars in Oncology Nursing, 12,* 152-162.

96. Savarese, D. M. (1997). Clinical impact of chemotherapy dose escalation in patients with hematologic malignancies and solid tumors. *Journal of Clinical Oncology, 15,* 2765-2768.

97. Schindler, L. (1992). Understanding the immune system. *NIH Publication No. 92-3229.* Bethesda, MD: U.S. Department of Health and Human Services.

98. Schindler, L. (1996). The immune system and how it works. *NIH Publication No. 96-3229.* Bethesda, MD: U.S. Department of Health and Human Services.

99. Schmitz, N., Linch, D., Dreger, P., et al. (1996). Filgrastim-mobilised peripheral blood progenitor cell transplantation in comparison with autologous bone marrow transplantation: Results of a randomised phase III trial in lymphoma patients. *Lancet, 347,* 353-357.

100. Schwab, G., Roskos, L., Molineux, G., et al. (1998). A phase I study of SD/01 in normal volunteers. *Experimental Hematology, 26,* 709.

101. Seiff, C. A., Nathan, D. G., & Clark, S. C. (1998). The anatomy and physiology of hematopoiesis. In D. G. Nathan & S. H. Orkin (Eds.), *Nathan and Oski's hematology of infancy and childhood* (5th ed., pp. 162-223). Philadephia: W. B. Saunders.

102. Singh, D. K., & Lipmann, S. M. (1998). Cancer chemoprevention. Part 1: Retinoids and carotenoids and other classic antioxidants. *Oncology, 12,* 605-610.

103. Skalla, K. (1996). The interferons. *Seminars in Oncology Nursing, 12,* 97-105.

104. Smith, J. W. (2000). Tolerability and side-effect profile of rhIL-11. *Oncology, 14(9 Suppl 8),* 41-47.

105. Sondel, P. M., & Hank, J. A. (1997). Combination therapy with interleukin-2 and antitumor monoclonal antibodies. *The Cancer Journal: from Scientific American, (3 Suppl. 1),* S121-S127.

106. Taliman, M. S., Andersen, J. W., Schiffer, C. A., et al. (1997). All-trans-retinoic acid in acute promyelocytic leukemia. *New England Journal of Medicine, 337,* 1021-1028.

107. Tepler, I., Elias, L., Smith, J. W., et al. (1996). A randomized placebo-controlled trial of recombinant human interleukin-11 in cancer patients with severe thrombocytopenia due to chemotherapy. *Blood, 87,* 3607-3614.

108. Thompson, A. W. (Ed.) (1998). *The cytokine handbook* (3rd ed.). San Diego: Academic Press.

109. VadhanRaj, S. (1998). Recombinant human thrombopoietin: Clinical experience and in vivo biology. *Seminars in Hematology, 35,* 261-268.

110. Vadhan-Raj, S., Murray, L. J., Bueso-Ramos, C., et al. (1997). Stimulation of megakaryocyte and platelet production by a single dose of recombinant human thrombopoietin in patients with cancer. *Annals of Internal Medicine, 126,* 673-681.

111. Vik, T. A., Ryder, J. W., Melemed, A. S., et al. (1997). Soluble stem cell factor treatment of MAL blasts induces apoptosis as it modulates MAP kinase activity. *Blood, 90(Suppl 1),* 386a.

112. Vivancos, P., Granena, A., Sarra, J., et al. (1999). Treatment with interleukin-2 (IL-2) and interferon (INF alpha 2b) after autologous bone marrow or peripheral blood stem cell transplantation in onco-hematological malignancies with a high risk of relapse. *Bone Marrow Transplantation, 23,* 169-172.

113. Vose, J. M. (2000). Other cytokines (IL-11, thrombopoietin, flt-3 Ligand, and IL-3). In J. O. Armitage & K. H. Antman (Eds.), *High dose cancer therapy: Pharmacology, hematopoietins, stem cells* (3rd ed., pp. 467-475). Philadelphia: Lippincott Williams & Wilkins.

114. Weiner, L. M. (1999). An overview of monoclonal antibody therapy of cancer. *Seminars in Oncology, 26(4 Suppl. 12),* 41-50.

115. Weinthal, J. A. (1996). The role of cytokines following bone marrow transplantation: Indications and controversies. *Bone Marrow Transplantation, 18 (Suppl. 3),* S10-S14.

116. Welte, K., Gabrilove, J., Bronchud, M. H., et al. (1996). Filgrastim (r-metHuG-CSF): The first 10 years. *Blood, 88,* 1907-1929.

117. Wexler, L. H., Weaver-McClure, L., & Steinberg, S. M. (1996). Randomized trial of recombinant human granulocyte-macrophage colony-stimulating factor in pediatric patients receiving intensive myelosuppressive chemotherapy. *Journal of Clinical Oncology, 14,* 901-910.

118. Wheeler, V. (1996). Interleukins: The search for an anticancer therapy. *Seminars in Oncology Nursing, 12,* 106-114.

119. Witt, P. L. (1996). Pharmacology of interferons: Induced proteins, cell activation, and antitumor activity. In B. A. Chabner & D. L. Longo (Eds.), *Cancer chemotherapy and biotherapy* (2nd ed., pp. 585-607). Philadelphia: Lippincott-Raven.

120. Wujcik, D. (1996). Update on the diagnosis of and therapy of acute promyelocytic leukemia and chronic myelogenous leukemia. *Oncology Nursing Forum, 23,* 478-487.

121. Yu, A. L., Utterreuther-Fischer, M. M., Huang, C., et al. (1998). Phase I trial of a human-mouse chimeric antiganglioside monoclonal antibody ch14.18 in patients with refractory neuroblastoma and osteosarcoma. *Journal of Clinical Oncology, 16,* 2169-2180.

GLOSSARY

Adoptive Cellular Therapy - Technique of passive immunity whereby immune system cells possessing antitumor capabilities are manipulated in the laboratory and then transferred to the tumor-bearing organism to stimulate tumor regression; LAK cells and TILs are used in adoptive cellular therapy.

Antibody-Dependent Cell-Mediated Cytotoxicity (ADCC) - Process by which neutrophils, monocytes, macrophages, and lymphocytes recognize bound antibody on a target cell and kill that cell.

Biologic Response Modifiers (BRMs) - Naturally occurring or synthesized substances that can enhance, regulate, or restore functions of the immune system.

Biotechnology - Science that uses living specimens to create or modify a substance.

Capillary Leak Syndrome - Phenomenon of increased vascular permeability; vascular fluid leakage occurs most often in the lungs, liver, spleen, kidney, and thymus.

Cell Surface Receptor Site - Unique structure on the membrane of the cell body where binding can occur.

Colony-Forming Unit (CFU) - Hematopoietic progenitor cell that has the ability for self-renewal.

Colony Stimulating Factors (CSF) - Family of glycoproteins involved in stimulating and regulating the complex steps of hematopoiesis; used interchangeably with hematopoietic growth factors.

Commitment - Process by which a hematopoietic progenitor cell loses the ability for self-renewal and develops the characteristics of a specific blood cell lineage.

Cytokines - Glycoproteins that are produced by a variety of cells; they are responsible for regulation and function of other cells.

Erythropoiesis - Production of red blood cells (erythrocytes)

Erythropoietin (EPO) - Lineage-specific glycoprotein responsible for stimulating the proliferation, differentiation, and maturation of red blood cells (erythrocytes) from committed erythroid precursors.

Flulike Syndrome (FLS) - Collection of symptoms, including fever, myalgia, malaise, and anorexia, frequently observed in patients receiving biotherapy; also known as constitutional symptoms.

Genetic Engineering - Technology that enables scientists to combine gene segments from two separate organisms.

Granulocyte Colony Stimulating Factor (G-CSF) - Lineage-specific glycoprotein responsible for the production and maturation of white blood cells known as granulocytes or neutrophils from committed precursor cells.

Granulocyte Macrophage Colony Stimulating Factor (GM-CSF) - Multilineage glycoprotein responsible for the proliferation, differentiation, and maturation of granulocytes, monocytes, macrophages, and eosinophils.

Hematopoiesis - Dynamic process involving the proliferation, differentiation, and maturation of blood cells; steps involved in hematopoiesis are referred to as the hematopoietic cascade.

Hematopoietic Growth Factors (HGF) - Family of glycoproteins that stimulate and regulate the complex steps of hematopoiesis.

Hybridoma - Cell created by fusing a secretory cell with an immortal cancer cell that can indefinitely produce a desired immune system product.

Interleukins - Cytokines that relay information between leukocytes to modulate their activities.

Lymphokine-Activated Killer (LAK) Cells - Lymphocytes that have been cultured with IL-2 to produce cells with cytolytic capabilities.

Macrophage Colony Stimulating Factor - Lineage-specific glycoprotein responsible for the proliferation, differentiation, and maturation of monocytes and macrophages from committed precursor cells.

Myeloablative - Term that describes agents and treatment modalities that affect bone marrow production; patients receiving myeloablative therapy are profoundly neutropenic for several weeks, often requiring marrow reinfusion for blood cell counts to recover.

Myelosuppressive - Term to describe agents or treatment modalities that have a transient effect on the production of blood cells; a decrease in any or all of the blood cell lines can occur.

Natural Killer (NK) Cells - Large granular lymphocytes that are not antigen specific and attack cells that appear foreign, such as tumor cells and infected cells.

Opsonization - Process whereby foreign substances are coated by antibodies to enhance their recognition and destruction by phagocytic cells.

Pluripotent Stem Cell - Most primitive cell in bone marrow that has the potential to self-replicate or differentiate into myeloid or lymphoid cell lineages.

Precursor Cell - Most primitive and recognizable cell of a specific blood cell lineage; precursors are cells that are intermediate between pluripotent stem cells and mature blood cells; they are unable to self-replicate but produce mature blood cells through differentiation and maturation.

Stem Cell - Gives rise to various precursors of the different blood cell lineages and has the ability to self-replicate and differentiate.

Tumor-Infiltrating Lymphocytes (TILs) - Lymphoid cells produced in response to stimulation with IL-2 that are capable of infiltrating solid tumors and exerting lytic activity.

8

Hematopoietic Stem Cell Transplantation

Lydia Gonzalez Ryan
Karen Marie Kristovich
Maureen S. Haugen
Kelly D. Coyne
M. Maureen Hubbell

Significant advances have been achieved in the field of hematopoietic stem cell transplantation (HSCT) in the past decade.[15,116] A variety of sources of stem cells are now available for transplantation. Peripheral blood stem cells (PBSCs) have greatly reduced use of bone marrow to reconstitute hematopoiesis following myeloablative chemotherapy. Refined techniques for stem cell separation have facilitated successful engraftment with much smaller numbers of stem cells. Umbilical cord blood (UCB) has become an established source of allogeneic stem cells for transplantation.

Since only about 35% of patients have a genotypically human lymphocyte antigen (HLA) identical sibling donor, patients who do not have a matched related (family) donor are being transplanted with marrow grafts obtained from unrelated donors. With the dramatic evolution and refinement of HLA typing techniques and interpretation, it is now possible to find a compatible unrelated donor among the millions of volunteers registered. Although success has steadily improved in recent years, graft-versus-host disease (GVHD) and other immune dysfunction are still major causes of morbidity and mortality.[43]

Among the exciting changes in HSCT is the increasing use of autologous PBSCs to treat a select group of chemotherapy-responsive pediatric patients with high-risk solid tumors.[75] The patient's own stem cells are collected from the peripheral blood and are then reinfused at a later date following intensive chemotherapy. Advances in the understanding of the biology of peripheral hematopoietic stem cells have driven the design of treatment regimens that allow for dose intensification without unacceptable hematologic toxicity. The use of cluster designation (CD) 34+ selected PBSCs to limit the risk of tumor cell contamination has facilitated prompt hematologic recovery from these highly intensified treatments. Because autologous PBSC therapy is not a true "stem cell transplant" but rather the "return" of the patient's own stem cells, autologous PBSC transplants are now being referred to as stem cell reinfusions or stem cell rescues.

Progress in the treatment of infections and multiorgan dysfunction, in symptom management, and in the understanding of immunobiology has had an impact on stem cell transplantation.[93] Coincident with these advances has been the growing realization that the best clinical management involves a multidisciplinary approach. Stem cell transplant nursing has evolved as a highly specialized practice, incorporating hematologic, oncologic, immunobiologic, and critical care concepts.

PRINCIPLES OF HEMATOPOIETIC STEM CELL TRANSPLANTATION

BASIC CONCEPTS

The bone marrow is the soft tissue that fills the cavities of the bone. Its primary functions are to provide and maintain the body's source of blood cells through hematopoiesis and to maintain the integrity of the immune system through lymphopoiesis. The pluripotent stem cell, which is capable of self-replication, proliferation, and multilineage differentiation (both myeloid and lymphoid), is the key progenitor cell responsible for these functions. Stem cells needed for transplantation can be distinguished by their physical properties. These stem cells are found within the mononuclear fraction of the collected sample, or suspension. Appropriate cell populations are identified by staining cell surface molecules with a monoclonal antibody (MoAb) linked to fluorescent dyes. These cluster designation (CD) antigens and the MoAbs that attach to them are assigned CD numbers. The antibody assay associated with the identification of those stem cells necessary for engraftment is the CD34 assay. Although not all CD34+ cells are true stem cells, this assay represents one of the most accurate ways to determine stem cell purity.

A stem cell transplant is possible because these stem cells can be removed from one individual through a process called "harvesting" and transplanted or infused into a recipient. The transplanted stem cells migrate to the recipient's marrow spaces, engraft, and produce a new hematopoietic and immune system in the recipient.

Stem cell transplantation is performed for the treatment of cancer, diseases that affect the immune and hematopoietic systems, and certain metabolic diseases. Hematopoietic stem cells can be obtained from a related or unrelated donor (allogeneic) or from the patient (autologous). When the donor stem cell source is derived from a twin, the transplant is referred to as syngeneic. The stem cells can be harvested from the bone marrow, the peripheral blood, or the umbilical vein of the placenta.

In allogeneic HSCT, HLA typing is used to determine the most genetically compatible stem cell donor for a patient. HLA is a protein antigen tissue-type marker located on an individual's nucleated cells. The genes of the HLA system reside on the short arm of chromosome 6, clustered in three distinct regions designated class I, class II, and class III. Although class III genes play an important role in the immune system, they do not function as major transplantation agents. Both class I and II genes, on the other hand, control T-cell recognition and histocompatibility in transplantation. It is the HLA system that is responsible for recognizing foreign tissue and activating the immune system to fight it, thereby triggering graft-versus-host disease (GVHD).[49,54]

There are over 15 class I genes in the human genome. Most pertinent to transplantation are the HLA-A, HLA-B, and HLA-C antigens. Class II genes, also referred to as HLA-D region genes, are further divided into distinct subregions designated as DR (B1-5), DQ (A1, B1), DO, DN, and DP. Class I and II antigens are closely linked and inherited in blocks called haplotypes. The three HLA genes thought to be most important to match for allogeneic stem cell transplant are HLA-A, HLA-B, and HLA-DRB1[9] (Figure 8-1).

The HLA can be typed by either a blood test or more recently a buccal swab. Because all the HLA genes are located next to one another on a single

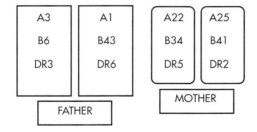

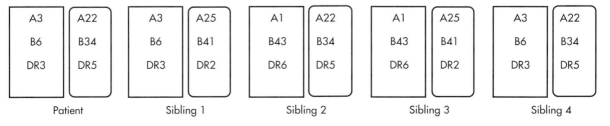

Figure 8-1

An example of HLA-DR typing.   (From Forte, K. [1997]. Alternative donor sources in pediatric bone marrow transplantation. *Journal of Pediatric Oncology Nursing, 14,* 214.)

The day a stem cell transplant is performed is universally known as "day zero." When a child is admitted to the hospital before transplant, minus numbers are assigned to the days leading up to and preparing for the procedure. After a transplant is performed, the count forward begins, with many milestones of recovery occurring within the first 100 days. From beginning to end a stem cell transplant can take up to one whole year to complete.

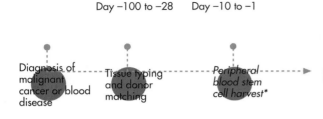
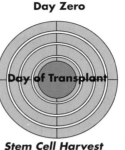
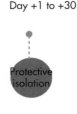

Day −100 to −28	Day −10 to −1	**Day Zero**	Day +1 to +30
Diagnosis of malignant cancer or blood disease	Tissue typing and donor matching	Peripheral blood stem cell harvest*	Day of Transplant	Protective isolation

Day −100 to −28 / Tissue typing and donor matching

A child requiring an external stem cell donor source must have his or her tissue type identified and matched with a suitable donor. Since tissue types are based on inherited genetic material, siblings are one likely donor source, with a 25 percent chance of a match.

Day −10 to −1 / Peripheral blood stem cell harvest*

Stem cells are gathered from the bloodstream through an intravenous line or special catheter, or from the bone marrow of the selected unrelated donor. This type of harvest is conducted before chemotherapy.

Day −10 to −6:
Admission to the Hospital.

Day −6 to −1:
Chemotherapy and/or radiation are given to eradicate the disease and to eliminate the immune system so that it will not figh the new cells when they are introduced.

Stem Cell Harvest From Bone Marrow*

Stem cells are gathered from the bloodstream or bone marrow of the selected unrelated donor or from the bloodstream of the patient. This type of harvest is conducted before chemotherapy.

Day of Transplant
The child receives the new stem cells as an intravenous infusion— no anesthetic is needed. Once the stem cells are infused, they migrate to the bone marrow, where they engraft, or "settle," and begin producing new and healthy blood cells.

Protective isolation

To avoid a potentially lethal infection in the weeks following a transplant, strict protective isolation precautions must be observed. Precautions include being confined to the hospital room and floor and having limited contact with visitors and items brought in from outside.

* Process dependent on stem cell source to be used.

Figure 8-2

Countdown to day zero: steps in an allogeneic stem cell transplant.   (Adapted from Simon, T. [2000, Spring]. The long road to day zero and beyond. *Carousel—The Magazine of Children's Memorial Hospital,* 1-3.)

chromosome, they are usually inherited as a package. Children receive one chromosome carrying the HLA genes from their mother (maternal haplotype) and one chromosome from their father (paternal haplotype). Any two children in a family have a one-in-four chance of receiving the same two chromosomes from their parents. Children receiving the same pair of chromosomes will be HLA identical and will express the same HLA antigens on their cells. Children receiving the same chromosome from one parent but a different one from the other

parent are haploidentical. Recent developments in deoxyribonucleic acid (DNA)-based techniques for HLA typing, replacing older less specific serologic techniques, have provided tools that more completely define the extent of HLA polymorphism within given populations and have improved matching of donor and recipient.[9,49,54,107,118]

With very few exceptions, all stem cell transplant patients must undergo ablative therapy before receiving their infusion of stem cells. The ablative therapy, also known as the conditioning regimen,

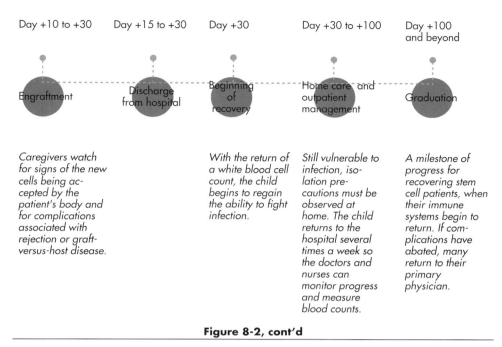

Day +10 to +30	Day +15 to +30	Day +30	Day +30 to +100	Day +100 and beyond
Engraftment	Discharge from hospital	Beginning of recovery	Home care and outpatient management	Graduation
Caregivers watch for signs of the new cells being accepted by the patient's body and for complications associated with rejection or graft-versus-host disease.		With the return of a white blood cell count, the child begins to regain the ability to fight infection.	Still vulnerable to infection, isolation precautions must be observed at home. The child returns to the hospital several times a week so the doctors and nurses can monitor progress and measure blood counts.	A milestone of progress for recovering stem cell patients, when their immune systems begin to return. If complications have abated, many return to their primary physician.

Figure 8-2, cont'd

Countdown to day zero: steps in an allogeneic stem cell transplant.

is an intensive, very high-dose combination chemotherapy with or without total body irradiation (TBI). It is designed to destroy any unwanted cell population (e.g., cancer cells) and suppress the body's immune system. Effective suppression of the immune system is essential to prevent rejection of the donor stem cells in patients receiving allogeneic transplants. The greater the incompatibility between the patient's HLA type and the donor stem cells, the higher the risk of GVHD.

Immediately after completion of the ablative therapy, the patient will receive the harvested stem cells. In autologous HSCT the stem cells are harvested from the patient weeks to months before the ablative therapy and are frozen (cryopreserved) until they are needed. Autologous stem cells can be obtained peripherally or from a bone marrow harvest. In allogeneic HSCT the stem cells are harvested from the selected donor. When the ablative therapy is complete, the stem cells are transfused directly into the patient. Stem cells can be obtained from the bone marrow itself, from the peripheral circulation, or from the placental blood via the umbilical vein. The process by which the transplanted stem cells successfully take root and grow in the patient's marrow cavities is known as engraftment and usually occurs 10 to 21 days after the infusion of the stem cell product.[44]

Although the precise mechanism by which the intravenously (IV) infused stem cells "home" or

migrate to the bone marrow cavities is unknown, it is speculated that the process involves molecules on the infused hematopoietic cells that have preferential binding sites on bone marrow stromal cells. After infusion, the cells probably circulate throughout the blood system until the hematopoietic cells come in contact with the bone marrow tissue in the empty cavities. Once in contact with the stromal tissue, the hematopoietic cells engraft and begin replication and differentiation.

Aggressive supportive care to manage the effects of pancytopenia and other toxicities resulting from the ablative therapy is the hallmark of posttransplant medical and nursing care. The success of any stem cell transplant depends on the quality and quantity of the stem cell source, the effectiveness of the pretransplant conditioning regimen, successful multilineage engraftment with effective immune reconstitution, and cure or stabilization of the disease state for which the transplant was performed.

ALLOGENEIC HEMATOPOIETIC STEM CELL TRANSPLANTATION

Allogeneic HSCT is used in many diseases (Figure 8-2). In some, transplants correct congenital or acquired defects in marrow production, immune function, or both. In others, they restore hematopoiesis after high-dose (myeloablative) cytotoxic therapy for malignancy.[52,68,113,123] There is increasing interest in using HSCT in several pediatric diseases for which transplants were not used or were rarely used in the past. These include thalassemia, sickle cell disease, inborn errors of metabolism, and autoimmune diseases, such as systemic lupus erythematosus and severe rheumatoid arthritis. These diseases currently account for fewer than 5% of HSCT; however, their combined incidence is high, and if ongoing trials confirm the efficacy of HSCT, the numbers should increase dramatically.

An understanding of immunology and immunogenetics is critical to comprehending transplant-related concepts such as engraftment, GVHD, development of tolerance, immune reconstitution, and control of malignancy. Whereas autologous transplantation immunology focuses primarily on the rate and quality of immune reconstitution and the control of malignancy, understanding allogeneic HSCT demands a mastery of how and if the above functions interface to achieve successful outcomes.[74]

Allogeneic HSCT differs fundamentally from solid organ transplantation. Solid organ grafts contain only limited numbers of cells with immunologic function, and the primary clinical concern is preventing rejection by the recipient's immune system. The conditioning regimen administered before a HSCT eliminates most, though not all, elements of the recipient's immune system. The transplanted stem cell collection contains larger numbers of precursors and mature cellular elements that replace those of the recipient's immune system. Thus, the immune system in the recipient (patient) is restored by the donor graft. The primary clinical concern in HSCT therefore is not only preventing rejection by recipient cells that survive the conditioning regimen, but also preventing donor cells from causing immune-mediated injury in the patient (recipient), GVHD, while allowing immune reconstitution. Immune reconstitution represents the establishment of humoral and cellular immunity, the ability of the patient to recognize and control pathogens.[96]

Immunosuppressive drugs are administered for a period of time after transplantation primarily to prevent GVHD. One of the goals of HSCT is to achieve tolerance between the donor and the recipient, and to have durable engraftment of donor lymphoid and hematopoietic cells in the absence of GVHD. Immunocompetence is achieved when the recipient's immune system can effectively respond to antigens such as viral and bacterial infections. Graft rejection after allogeneic HSCT is demonstrated by either the lack of engraftment or the development of pancytopenia and marrow aplasia after initial engraftment. The diagnosis of graft rejection can be difficult because lack of initial engraftment and pancytopenia can also be caused by drug toxicity and certain viral infections.[129]

With the exception of some transplants for immunodeficiencies, the infusion of stem cells is preceded by intensive immunosuppressive and/or cytotoxic therapy, referred to as the preparative or conditioning regimen. Conditioning regimens are designed to eliminate malignant or abnormal cells and, in allogeneic transplants, host recipient immune cells that mediate rejection.

UNRELATED/MISMATCHED ALLOGENEIC HSCT

HSCTs from HLA–phenotypically identical unrelated donors are an alternative for patients who lack a family donor. Unrelated HSCT has been made feasible by development or expansion of registries of HLA-typed individuals who are willing to serve as marrow donors. Selection of unrelated donors is currently based on matching for HLA-A, HLA-B, and HLA-DRB1. Ongoing studies are evaluating the necessity of and outcome associated with matching for HLA-C, HLA-DQ, and HLA-DP. With registries currently available in the United States and in other countries, it is possible to identify an HLA-A, HLA-B, phenotypically identical DRB1-matched unrelated donor for at least 50% of patients in need.[126] In the pediatric population the use of umbilical cord stem cells has made it possible to identify potential donors for many more patients. The immunogenetic relationship (level of HLA disparity) between the donor and recipient profoundly influences the outcome of HSCT.[36,43]

In the 1970s and early 1980s essentially all HSCTs used stem cells collected from the marrow of HLA-matched related donors. Clinical trials focused on bone marrow transplantation and its role in a variety of malignant and nonmalignant disorders. The limitations of HLA technology and lack of a donor pool made the likelihood of finding an alternative donor for an individual patient extremely low. The few transplants done with HLA-matched unrelated donors were associated with high risks of GVHD, graft failure, and poor outcome.

In the 1980s national and international groups organized marrow donor registries with HLA-typed volunteers who agreed to be donors for unrelated patients. These donors now total close to 4 million worldwide and are computerized due to the collaborative efforts of the National Marrow Donor Program (NMDP) and many other national registries (e.g., Bone Marrow Donors Worldwide [BMDW])[52] (Table 8-1).

Establishment of large donor pools dramatically increased the use of unrelated donor transplants,

TABLE 8-1	MAJOR NATIONAL UNRELATED DONOR REGISTRIES	
Organization	**Address**	**Number of Donors (As of February 2001)**
National Marrow Donor Program (NMDP): a coordinating center for national bone marrow and cord blood donor searches	3001 Broadway St. N.E., Suite 500 Minneapolis, MN 55413-1753 USA Tel: (612) 627-5801* Fax: (612) 627-5810* Tel: (800) MARROW2 or may use the NMDP contact form at the NMDP website**	Over 3 million marrow donors 8,895 cord units (some repetition with other smaller national cord banks)
Caitlin Raymond International Registry: a coordinating center for international bone marrow and cord blood donor searches	University of Massachusetts Medical Center 55 Lake Ave. N. Worcester, MA 01655 USA Tel: (508) 334-8969 Fax: (508) 334-8972 E-mail: info@crir.org http://www.crir.org	44,610 marrow donors 3,998 cord units
Gift of Life Bone Marrow Foundation: donor recruitment, patient advocacy, search correlation, family studies/genealogy; composed almost entirely of Jewish volunteer donors	P.O. Box 6429 Delray Beach, FL 33482 USA Tel: (561) 274-8200 Fax: (561) 274-8206 E-mail: info@HLAMatch.org http://www.hlamatch.org	41,411 marrow donors
New York Cord Blood Registry: national cord blood searches	The Fred H. Allen Laboratory of Immunogenetics The New York Blood Center 310 East 67th St. New York, NY 10021 USA Tel: (212) 570-3230 Fax: (212) 570-3393 E-mail: prubins@nybc.org stem@nybc.org	Over 10,000 cord units
American Red Cross Cord Blood Program: lists cord blood units from multiple Red Cross sites	55 Lake Ave. N. Worcester, MA 01655 USA Tel: (781) 461-2145 Fax: (781) 461-2269 E-mail: AloscoSh@USA.Red Cross.org	2,850 cord units
American Bone Marrow Donor Registry: marrow donor information, registration, and regional donor center locations; is coordinated via the Caitlin Raymond International Registry	P.O. Box 8841 Mandeville, LA 70470-8841 USA Tel: (985) 626-1749 Fax: (985) 626-7414 E-mail: jakabmdr@bellsouth.net	27,775 marrow donors
Bone Marrow Donors Worldwide (BMDW): lists HLA phenotypes of marrow donors and cord units across the world	Europdonor Foundation Building 1, E3-Q Leinden University Medical Center Albinusdreef 2 2333 ZA Leinden The Netherlands http://www.bmdw.org	Combined marrow/cord units totaling over 7 million

* For professionals only.
** Donors and prospective donors: http://www.marrow.org

Continued

TABLE 8-1	MAJOR NATIONAL UNRELATED DONOR REGISTRIES—cont'd	
Organization	Address	Number of Donors (As of February 2001)
University of Colorado Cord Blood Bank: national cord blood searches	University of Colorado Health Science Center Bone Marrow Transplant Program Cord Blood Bank 4200 E. Ninth Ave., B190 Denver, CO 80262 USA Tel: (303) 372-8398 Fax: (303) 372-7570 E-mail: Judith.King@UHColorado.edu	Unknown at the time of chapter publication

from 10% in 1985 to greater than 25% in 1998.[53] Although some settings report survival after such transplants as comparable to HLA-identical sibling transplants, risks of graft failure and GVHD are much greater. Unrelated donor transplants are still associated with longer delays caused by the lengthy and rigorous search and evaluation process, as well as the reluctance to enter into a difficult and more risky approach to transplant.[52]

Partially matched relatives may offer a greater possibility of finding a donor. About 10% of all allogeneic transplants are from relatives who share one HLA haplotype and are mismatched for one or more antigens on the unshared haplotype.[89] Although stem cell transplant results with more than one antigen disparity have been disappointing, recent studies suggest that aggressive pretransplant and posttransplant immunosuppression may improve outcomes.[51]

High resolution HLA matching capabilities, access to interpretive HLA consultants, and thorough international searches can maximize the potential matches found, and impact overall outcomes for patients undergoing unrelated HSCT.[107] Most pediatric allogeneic HSCTs are done with stem cells collected from marrow or umbilical cord blood. In the adult arena, however, stem cells are increasingly being collected from donors peripherally rather than via bone marrow harvest. Cells collected from peripheral blood contain large numbers of mature T lymphocytes, which may mediate a more intense GVHD reaction. Additionally, blood-derived stem cells require stimulation with granulocyte colony stimulating factor (GCSF), which may be placing healthy donors at an unnecessary theoretical risk for leukemic conversion. No data exist correlating this presumed risk to actual case reports. Early patient accounts have demonstrated

rapid hematopoietic recovery and acceptable acute GVHD after HLA-identical related peripheral blood allografts.[12] Concerns exist about the development of chronic GVHD.[11,66] Pediatric donors present yet another challenge to PBSC donation since these healthy individuals may have to be exposed to large bore cannulas or apheresis catheters, GCSF stimulation, and long hours of large volume leukapheresis.

UMBILICAL CORD TRANSPLANTATION

Umbilical cord blood, collected at birth, contains large numbers of stem cells. This occurs because fetuses normally generate generous quantities of CD34+ cells in their liver and bone marrow during development. These cells are present in the circulation and, therefore, in the umbilical cord. Because cord blood is richer in stem cells than adult peripheral blood or bone marrow, much less volume is required to reconstitute hematopoiesis.[42]

Umbilical cord blood also has reduced immunoreactivity, which lessens the risk of rejection by the recipient's immune system, as well as GVHD. It is believed that cord blood has a muted immune system and naive stem cells, not yet educated to attack specific antigens. Although the reason for their reduced immunoactivity is unknown, T cells (the white cells responsible for this targeted immune response) present in cord blood may be more tolerant or may be influenced by a suppressive effect of circulating maternal cells within the cord.[26,38]

Although results are still preliminary, umbilical cord blood has proved to be an exciting source of stem cells for gene therapy and tissue transplantation, as well. It appears that umbilical cord stem cells have a greater capacity for retroviral transduction (the mechanism by which the gene is transplanted into the body), making their use more advantageous than bone marrow.[38]

Another critical difference between umbilical cord blood and bone marrow is that cord blood is rarely contaminated by viruses such as cytomegalovirus (CMV) or Epstein-Barr virus (EBV). For the stem cell patient population, these viruses are associated with significant morbidity and mortality.

In 1988 Dr. Elaine Gluckman performed the first successful umbilical cord blood transplant in a patient with Fanconi's anemia.[114] Since that time, it has been demonstrated that umbilical cord blood contains sufficient numbers of hematopoietic stem and progenitor cells to engraft small patients (less than 50 kg). Engraftment is durable, and collection is safe. Umbilical cord blood, once collected, can be tested and available within several weeks.

Furthermore, because a greater percentage of the volunteer donors currently in the NMDP registry are Caucasian, patients from other ethnic and racial groups are underrepresented in the potential donor pool. Every year compatible donors cannot be found for approximately tens of thousands of people in the United States in need of HSCTs. With large scale umbilical cord blood collections across state, ethnic, and racial lines, the potential donor pool becomes enormous.

The speed and efficiency of umbilical cord blood procurement is especially important for diseases requiring immediate therapy. Because every step along the way is critical, the search for and procurement of bone marrow is time consuming and costly with limited donor availability. Clearly, cord blood is a far more advantageous and attractive alternative. By reducing complications, increasing the pool of suitable donors, and decreasing the time needed for potential donor searches, the use of umbilical cord blood has become an attractive alternative in pediatric transplantation.

Several reports have suggested that cord blood transplantation is associated with a lower incidence of acute and chronic GVHD.[121] The difference may be due to immunologic properties of umbilical cord T cells (relative immaturity) that reduce their capacity to induce GVHD. This, in turn, permits more HLA mismatching between donor and recipient than is usually acceptable with HSCTs.[72] However, because the incidence of GVHD correlates with age, and because most cord blood transplants are performed in children, it is not clear whether the degree or rate of GVHD differs in comparable allogeneic transplants. Comparison studies in the unrelated setting are also complicated by differences in donor-recipient histocompatibility and the specificity of the methods used to ascertain histocompatibility.[69]

Compared with hematopoietic stem cells from marrow, hematopoietic stem cells in cord blood have distinctive engraftment advantages: (1) the capacity to form more colonies in cultures; (2) a higher cell-cycle rate; and (3) increased production of growth factors. However, cord blood has a limited number of nucleated cells, the precursors of neutrophils and platelets. The number of nucleated cells infused per kilogram of recipient weight is thought to be a major factor in the recovery of neutrophil and platelet counts. As a rule, the smaller the total count of nucleated cells in any given cord blood collection, the more compromised the neutrophil and platelet recovery may be. Overall, recipients of cord blood transplants have delayed neutrophil and platelet recovery, which increases the risk of infection and bleeding.[120] In the absence of prospective studies, it has been difficult to recommend an optimal number of cells in a cord blood collection that is needed for long-term engraftment.

Overall survival for children with umbilical cord transplants does not differ significantly from those with marrow transplants. Variables associated with improved survival among recipients of cord blood transplants are age less than 6 years, weight less than 20 kg, CMV-negative serologic status in the recipient, and HLA compatibility with the donor.[40]

Research suggests that umbilical cord blood is as effective as bone marrow as a source of hematopoietic stem cells for children. Since few patients have umbilical cord blood from an HLA-identical sibling available, the real opportunities are in unrelated transplantation.

PERIPHERAL BLOOD STEM CELL TRANSPLANTATION

PBSCs can also be used as hematopoietic stem cells following high dose therapy for both malignant and nonmalignant disease. Their ease of collection and the faster engraftment kinetics make them ideal in both the pediatric and adult arenas. The suggested positive attributes of peripheral blood stem cell transplantation (PBSCT) or rescue (PBSCR) include (1) elimination of the hospital admission and general anesthesia for harvesting; (2) lower risk of tumor contamination; (3) the ability to offer dose intensive therapy to patients with unharvestable bone marrow; and (4) a possible economic advantage over marrow transplantation.[12,50]

Allogeneic Peripheral Blood Stem Cell Transplantation

Recently, allogeneic PBSCT has also been considered as an alternative to allogeneic bone marrow transplantation. The use of PBSCT has made it easier to obtain larger numbers of stem cells per harvest, which is necessary in the newer immunoablative and adoptive immunotherapy approaches to transplantation. Uncertainty about the impact and demands on healthy donors, as well as the fact that the donor is often a minor, has resulted in limited application of this technique in children. At this time this methodology is used when the donor is an adult, when a second transplant from a minor is required, or when large numbers of stem cells are required from a low weight donor.[70]

Autologous Peripheral Blood Stem Cell Rescue

In pediatrics the use of high dose therapy with autologous PBSCRs is indicated for metastatic and recurrent pediatric solid tumors and in some high-risk diseases at initial presentation (Figure 8-3). Solid tumors commonly treated with this approach include high-stage neuroblastoma and rhabdomyosarcoma, recurrent or refractory Wilms tumor, germ cell tumors, hepatoblastoma, bone sarcomas, Hodgkin's disease and non-Hodgkin's lymphoma, and certain high-risk brain tumors. To be eligible for a PBSCR, the child's tumor must show evidence of chemosensitivity, have a poor prognosis with conventional therapies, and exhibit a steep dose-response curve with traditional select chemotherapeutic agents such as alkylating agents.[48,67,71,108]

Stem cells are collected by leukopheresis weeks to months before admission for PBSCR. Following high-dose therapy, the newly infused stem cells give rise to both a new hematopoietic and immune system. Hematopoietic recovery with PBSCR is more rapid than from a bone marrow transplant, occurring approximately 7 to 10 days earlier. It may be that a larger number of progenitor cells are collected, or a higher percentage of peripheral progenitor cells are already committed to a line of differentiation, and/or the number of cells in cell cycle is greater in peripherally collected stem cells. Also the stem cells may be influenced by the priming procedure used to mobilize them. It is known that the reconstitution and durability of peripheral stem cell progenitor cells are the same or better than that of marrow progenitors.[50,64] Although the use of PBSCs is rapidly growing, many unanswered questions and challenges remain.

Whether purging autologous grafts of malignant tumor cells can improve outcome remains unknown. Gene marking studies show that contaminating tumor cells in bone marrow grafts can contribute to relapse. However, retrospective analyses have not demonstrated a significant reduction in the risk of relapse by purging, indicating that tumor control throughout the body is the major problem. Prospective studies with unpurged PBSC collec-

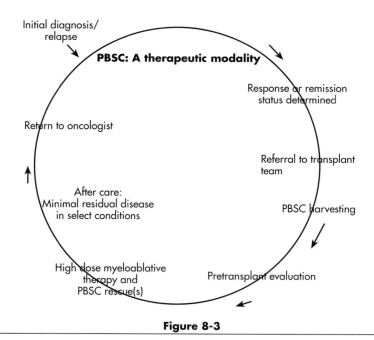

Figure 8-3

Autologous PBSC rescue: the therapeutic trajectory.

tions have yielded results similar to those with purged PBSC collections.[11] Nevertheless, frequent contamination in the mobilized PBSC collections demonstrates that the tumor cells survive in the patient's body. Therefore, there is a need for more effective cytoreductive regimens and nontoxic methods for tumor purging.[11,25,61]

Pharmacologic methods of purging have resulted in substantial delays in engraftment. Immunomagnetic purging, on the other hand, has had a minimal effect on the rate of engraftment and reduces the detectable tumor contamination by several log. A recent complementary approach is positive selection of hematopoietic stem cells based on CD34+ expression. This is a procedure where the stem cell collection is "purged" of tumor cells indirectly by selecting out the CD34+ cells, ideally creating a sample of true stem cells without tumor. This method is feasible and facilitates a 2 to 3 log depletion of tumor cells in the collected sample.[25,45]

Other challenges continue. Among them are the true prognostic efficacy of PBSCR in select diseases, the best techniques for mobilizing PBSCs, the feasibility of harvesting PBSCs from young children under 25 kg, and the management of minimal residual disease.[112]

PRETRANSPLANT PERIOD

REFERRAL AND CONSULTATION

Patients referred for HSCT require a comprehensive clinical evaluation and in-depth counseling by an experienced multidisciplinary team. Most transplant candidates are referred by hematologists or oncologists to a tertiary center where the transplant procedure will be performed. Patients are also referred by other providers such as immunologists and geneticists for nonmalignant childhood disorders.

The most critical factor for a smooth transition from the referring institution to the transplant center is the communication of information between the health care teams and the family. This will help to maintain consistency and foster the family's trust in the transplant program. Information about the stem cell transplant process and specific routines used by the transplant center must be accurate and detailed. Differences in technique or routines between the referring center and the transplant program must be presented in a way that does not prejudice the family or jeopardize the development of trust in the transplant center. Box 8-1 lists the responsibilities associated with the referral and consultation phase.

PRE–STEM CELL TRANSPLANT EVALUATION

Before the conditioning regimen or transplant admission, all prospective patients, donors, and their families participate in a comprehensive evaluation process (Box 8-2). The pretransplant evaluation includes a thorough clinical assessment of the child and donor (if relevant) and provides an introduction to the transplant center, transplant team, and the stem cell transplant process. The evaluation is performed a maximum of 28 days before the actual day of the transplant to obtain the most representative clinical, organ, and performance status. Appropriate baseline tests confirm the child's overall clinical condition and disease status. In allogeneic transplants the donor also undergoes a rigorous evaluation, including a physical examination, laboratory testing, and psychological/educational preparation to ensure that this is an appropriate candidate, willing and able to undergo the harvest process.

A psychosocial assessment of the family will identify areas of needed support or resource allocation (Box 8-3). The pre–stem cell transplant evaluation period is a time of anxiety and uncertainty for the child and family. Their fears are only heightened if the transplant is delayed or if evaluation tests indicate that the transplant is contraindicated (e.g., relapse or significant organ damage has occurred). Obtaining insurance coverage or raising necessary funds can sometimes delay the transplant procedure. This compounds the already existing anxiety and leads to tremendous frustration for all involved.

PATIENT AND FAMILY EDUCATION

The education and preparation of the patient and family before transplantation are critical to their subsequent adjustment and adaptation (Box 8-4). Many have already had initial discussions with their primary referring physicians, have received written materials, and/or have obtained information from the Internet even before they have met the transplant team. The initial meeting with the transplant team is important, therefore, to clarify the process of transplantation and possible existing misconceptions and to establish trust. Often the first meeting occurs close to the initial diagnosis, for example, in patients with stage IV neuroblastoma or high-risk leukemia, or in the first few weeks after relapse.

Visual pictures or figures (see Figures 8-2, 8-3) are extremely helpful to orient families to transplant for the first time. The first meeting focuses on information sharing and establishing the patient as a potential transplant candidate—not on decision making. The session is general, well organized, and individualized to the needs of the particular patient

---

BOX 8-1

REFERRAL AND CONSULTATION PROCESS

Referral is obtained. The following data are gathered:
• Basic demographic information
• Review of medical history and summary
• Reason for referral

Transplant and referral teams discuss disease and remission status, performance status, role of transplantation within the disease trajectory, and logistical variables.

Initial appointment is made with the patient and family to discuss rationale for transplant option, type and source of stem cell transplant, potential risks, toxicities and complications, proposed preparatory-conditioning regimen, timing of transplant, and expected outcomes.

Transplant team discusses patient's eligibility, appropriateness for transplantation, potential stem cell sources, and best curative intent. Patient is placed on an "Upcoming/New Patient List."

In the case of allogeneic transplantation:
HLA typing is ordered or obtained, and a search for a donor begins. If an unrelated donor search is expected, an international search is initiated based on the best available, highest resolution typing. Family, umbilical cord, and marrow options are discussed, and all results are compared to determine the best source for the individual patient's circumstances.

In the case of autologous peripheral or marrow transplantation:
Dates for marrow or peripheral harvest(s) are scheduled in conjunction with the planned date of the transplant. If PBSCT is planned, the appropriate catheter is also discussed and may be placed at this time.

A thorough psychosocial assessment of the patient and family is undertaken to evaluate financial resources, social supports, religious, cultural, and ethnic variables, and family dynamics. Additionally, issues surrounding compliance, follow-up, and aftercare demands are explored with the family.

Multiple visits and counseling sessions are scheduled in the weeks following referral to consolidate the preparation and evaluation of the patient and family. Extensive verbal and written information and education are provided to the family and referring physician/institution. Out-of-state referrals can be conducted via teleconferencing.

Search results and/or total stem cell doses (cord nucleated cell counts, yields from peripheral stem cell collections) are reviewed, and the best stem cell source and total targeted nucleated cell dose is obtained.

Financial coverage for the transplant is secured. Insurance benefits are reviewed and authorization for transplantation is obtained before the scheduled transplant. A letter of medical necessity is formulated, and information is communicated to the payor, referring physician, and family. When relevant, a global case rate or individual payment contract is negotiated at this time.

BOX 8-2

COMPREHENSIVE PRE-HSCT EVALUATION

STAGING–DISEASE RELATED TESTS (AS APPROPRIATE)
Bone marrow aspirate and biopsy
Spinal tap/cerebral spinal fluid assessment
Radiologic tests (computerized tomography scans, magnetic resonance imaging, bone scan, x-rays, gallium scans)
Tissue biopsy (liver, reevaluation/staging surgery)
Tumor markers

COMPREHENSIVE ASSESSMENT/ORGAN PERFORMANCE STATUS
Catheter/venous access issues
Psychosocial assessment
Nutritional evaluation
Occupational/physical therapy evaluation
Ancillary support evaluation (education/academic support, child life, clergy)
Transfusion history/transfusion support planning
Blood product donor screening and preparation
Significant drug intolerance/allergies

Genetic disease status evaluation (if applicable)
Dental evaluation
Hearing evaluation
Multiple gated angiography (MUGA), echocardiogram, ECG
Chest x-ray scans
Pulmonary function tests
Sinus films
Sperm/ova banking

LABORATORY TESTS
Complete blood count
Renal, hepatic, electrolyte, endocrine serum tests
Hepatitis screen (A, B, C)
HIV
CMV
Herpes simplex virus
Human T-cell lymphotrophic virus (HTLV)
Rapid plasma reagin (RPR) (syphilis screen)
Coagulation tests

Psychosocial Assessment of the Pediatric Transplant Candidate

- Assent/consent to undergo transplant
- Understanding of diagnosis, treatment plan, and prognosis
- History of sexual or physical abuse or neglect
- Past psychiatric history/substance abuse
- Developmental assessment
- Interests, hobbies, and coping strategies
- Behavioral/school problems
- Problems with peer/family relationships
- Compliance issues
- Problems with prior hospitalization experiences
- Previous methods of coping with treatment and hospitalizations
- Pain tolerance/experiences
- Understanding of advanced directives
- Awareness of aftercare/follow-up demands post-transplant

Adapted from Blume, K., & Amylon, M. (1999). The evaluation and counseling of candidates for hematopoietic cell transplantation. In E. D. Thomas, K. Blume, S. Forman (Eds.), *Hematopoietic and stem cell transplantation* (pp. 371-380). Malden, MA: Blackwell Science.

and family.[14] Families are then given time to absorb and validate the information, discuss it with trusted family members and/or consultants, and seek second or third opinions if desired. Subsequent meetings are used to share protocol and informed consent information, make the necessary decisions, and schedule the transplant and related tests. During this preparatory time patient and family coping strategies are identified, a psychosocial assessment is completed, and resources and support systems are activated.

ALLOGENEIC HEMATOPOIETIC STEM CELL TRANSPLANTATION

Donor Search

When a sibling or family donor is not suitable or available, an unrelated donor search is instituted. The goal is to provide a panel of suitable donors with histocompatibility at more than two loci. The ideal donor, of course, is one who is an identical match to the recipient at all HLA-A, HLA-B, and HLA-DRB1 antigens (see Figure 8-1).

National and international searches are conducted among donor registries through the NMDP, the American Bone Marrow Donor Registry, and

Patient and Family Education Plan

Extensive discussions with patients and families and provision of supportive educational materials: written, computer based, and/or audiovisual
Orientation to transplant team, unit, and processes
Role and rationale of stem cell transplant
Preparatory/conditioning regimen
Role of the pretransplant testing
Type of transplant
- Autologous versus allogeneic
- Myeloablative versus submyeloablative conditioning
- Single versus sequential autologous PBSC
- Related versus unrelated allogeneic
Donor preparation
- Peripheral versus marrow collection
- If peripheral, cannulas versus apheresis catheter (if applicable)
- Preoperative teaching (if applicable)
- Pre-SCT testing of donor
- Expected/scheduled appointments for donor
Peripheral stem cell harvest information
Transplant-related restrictions and routines
Discussion of stem cell infusion and its effects
Peritransplant complications/toxicities
Do not resuscitate, intensive care issues

Advanced directives
Graft-versus-host disease
- Acute and chronic disease
- Potential for "trading one disease for another"
- Immunosuppressive therapy
Discharge guidelines/planning process
Home care management
Potential posttransplant complications
Posttransplant aftercare demands, follow-up, expectations
Family/sibling issues
Financial counseling
Lodging and transportation resources
Community and hospital-based resources
Potential long-term effects of therapy
Written schedule given to family as to the process
Pre-SCT labs, diagnostics, appointments
Harvest/donor-related dates/appointments
Timing of conditioning/transplant
Admission date and time
Important traumatic events (e.g., urinary catheter placement, central venous access placement)
Day of stem cell infusion
Highlights of key periods/events (expected onset of GVHD, potential discharge dates)

smaller registries throughout the world. The search process for an unrelated donor through the NMDP is outlined in Figure 8-4. In pediatrics, umbilical cord blood collections are increasingly available as potential sources of unrelated stem cells. Some large registries routinely provide preliminary searches of affiliated cord banks, and other potential umbilical cord blood matches can be found by searching independent umbilical cord blood registries.

Since 1988 BMDW has provided a periodically updated list of each HLA phenotype from over 60 registries and cord banks and the number of donors expressing that phenotype. BMDW currently lists the HLA phenotypes for more than 6 million donors from around the world.[53]

A preliminary search of available donors can be done within 72 hours. The list may vary in level of detail and in the resolution of available HLA typing.

Some marrow donors typed in recent years may have very high level HLA typing performed, whereas others done in the early 1980s, for example, may have only serologic preliminary typing recorded. Cord blood banks generally carry out initial HLA-A, HLA-B, and HLA-DR typing using DNA based methods at an intermediate level of resolution, expediting the process of finding a compatible donor. The results of the preliminary search are then presented to the transplant team for evaluation.

An unrelated search is influenced by factors such as diagnosis, type of transplant planned, and the weight of the patient. The insurance source may direct when and where and by whom a search can be done, as well as how many potential donors can be considered at one time. If there are limited financial resources, the searcher may pursue donor sources with fees that are not incurred until the time

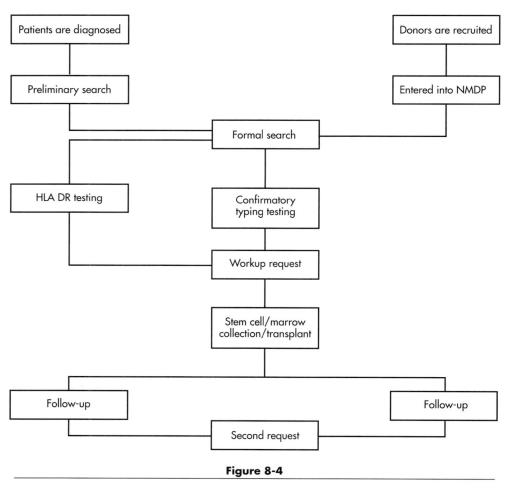

Figure 8-4

Steps involved in a search of the NMDP Registry. (Data from Howe, C., & Radde-Stepaniak, T. [1999]. Hematopoietic cell donor registries. In E. D. Thomas, K. Blume, & S. Forman [Eds.], *Hematopoietic and stem cell transplantation* [pp. 503-512]. Malden, MA: Blackwell Science.)

of collection or where fewer steps, and therefore costs, are necessary. The ethnicity of the patient may also guide the search, directing it to specific international registries or banks. Among the most critical variables influencing the selection process are the age and weight of the child—whether a cord unit can be used; the rate of disease progression—whether there is time to do an expanded search; and in the case of leukemia, the role that graft versus leukemia may play in curative intent—what degree of HLA disparity will be tolerated.

Ultimately, one or several donors believed to be the best potential candidates are selected and confirmatory typing is performed. Confirmatory typing involves repeating the HLA typing at the transplant center or a designated laboratory capable of doing high resolution HLA testing. It can be time-consuming and costly, especially if several donors are screened. Therefore it is done only when there is a reasonable likelihood that the patient will proceed to transplant.

The preliminary search results must be carefully reviewed and prioritized before continuing to the next stage. This is the formal search, where individual donors are investigated, ultimately leading to final donor selection. In the unrelated marrow donor setting, the priority is generally placed on DRB1 matching to eliminate those who will not match at that locus. However, preliminary donor typing is often incomplete and the search may require linking with other antigens, or reviewing common haplotypes, to select donors who may be a true match at higher resolution typing. Often the experience of an HLA expert is required, which is available through large registries such as the NMDP. If several donors with similar likelihood of histocompatibility are available, transplant center–specific preferences in donor characteristics such as age, sex, parity, and CMV status are considered. In the cord blood setting, where donor typing is often more complete, eliminating those who do not have a cell dose appropriate for the patient's weight will narrow the search. A greater level of mismatch may be acceptable in the cord blood setting, including a DRB1 mismatch. These factors often result in a shorter search time for cord blood donors.

NMDP donor recruitment and eligibility criteria. Marrow donation is a complex process, and the recruitment of donors relies on truly informed consent. The recruitment process involves a gradual presentation of information and a graded commitment from the donor. First the donor is presented with written information about marrow transplantation and marrow donation. All donors are screened for HIV risk initially. The donor is then asked to sign a consent for their HLA type to be listed in the program, although this does not mean they consent to donate their marrow. If they should match a recipient, each further step in the donor process provides more detailed information and asks for a greater commitment from the donor.

NMDP guidelines for interaction between donor and recipient. Throughout the recruitment and donation process, the donor's identity is known only to donor center staff. Confidentiality is maintained throughout the marrow donation. Recipients often wish to express their thanks by card, letter, or a small gift. These are conveyed through the transplant center coordinator. Any correspondence from the donor is passed from the donor center coordinator to the transplant center coordinator, who then forwards it to the recipient. After 1 year if the donor and recipient both desire contact, this can be arranged after obtaining written consent.

Donor Evaluation

Parental consent is required for a minor child to donate bone marrow for transplantation. Special consents may be required for a very young child or a child with developmental disabilities. Children 6 years of age and older assent to the procedure after reviewing developmentally appropriate information. Children can safely donate marrow,[97] and successful marrow collections can be done in infants as small as 6 to 9 kg, with one case reported in an infant as small as 3.95 kg.[117] In general, transplant physicians prefer to wait until an infant donor is at least 6 months of age. Usually, children are more likely to need a blood transfusion following marrow harvest. Autologous red cells can be recovered from the collected marrow and reinfused following the marrow harvest, thus avoiding allogeneic blood transfusion. This is the preferred practice. Otherwise, the pediatric donor is asked to donate an autologous unit 7 to 10 days before the harvest.

When donors for HSCT have been identified, they undergo a preharvest evaluation similar to that of the patient. The baseline information obtained is used to monitor the donor throughout the harvest process, to diagnose comorbidity that may preclude the use of a particular donor, and to obtain the necessary molecular (chromosomal) data to document engraftment in the recipient.

Bone Marrow Harvest

Emotional preparation and teaching are essential for the donor. Whether the donor is an allogeneic sibling or an autologous donor, the harvest experience is new and frightening. Age-appropriate information explaining how marrow is removed from the bone marrow spaces is given with emphasis on the fact the body will replace the marrow after the harvest. In the hematologically healthy donor, the marrow begins to replenish itself immediately.

Emotional support and encouragement are also provided to the parents during the bone marrow harvest. Many parents struggle with the ethical conflict of subjecting a healthy child to the risks of surgery and anesthesia to collect marrow that may or may not be curative therapy for their ill child.

Harvesting is performed in the operating room using sterile technique. A team of bone marrow harvesters (usually two or three individuals) prepare the posterior iliac crests under sterile conditions. The bone marrow aspiration needles are inserted numerous times, often 50 to 100 times, on each side to aspirate the appropriate amount of marrow. Although there are multiple needle sticks into the bone, for the most part only two "holes" are actually punctured through the skin. The same entry port is then used to insert the needles into the bone. The marrow is placed in heparinized culture medium to prevent clotting. It is filtered through several fine and coarse mesh screens to remove bone spicules, fat particles, and blood clots, which can cause emboli in the recipient.

After the harvest procedure the site is cleansed and covered with pressure dressings. The entry sites are monitored for bleeding. The donor and parents are instructed to keep the sites clean and dry to prevent infection. The donor is likely to experience mild to moderate muscle and bone pain in the hips, which is easily alleviated with nonopioid analgesics such as acetaminophen or ibuprofen. Typically the donor is released from the hospital the same day of the harvest. Supplemental iron is not usually needed.

Although the volume of marrow collected provides an estimate of an "adequate" harvest, the actual number of mononuclear cells obtained is the essential parameter. The requisite amount of harvested cells is based on the weight of the recipient. Typically a dose of 2 to 6 $\times$ 10^8 nucleated cells per kilogram of the recipient's weight is collected. The usual volume desired is approximately 10 to 20 ml per kilogram of the recipient's weight. This volume is most safely and easily obtained when the donor is larger than the recipient or is older than toddler age; however, successful bone marrow harvesting has been reported for donors less than 2 years of age. Once the fresh marrow is collected, it is given to the patient the same day.

The harvest procedure is nearly the same for the autologous stem cell transplant donor except that the amount of marrow collected is also contingent on the quality of marrow reserve (which may be depleted from previous chemotherapy and/or radiotherapy). It is often necessary to collect an additional amount of marrow to compensate for a potentially inadequate harvest. Autologous stem cell transplant donors are also more likely to have existing organ system disease (e.g., nephrotoxicity) that may place them at greater risk for complications from general anesthesia.

Unlike fresh allogeneic marrow, autologous marrow is cryopreserved, or frozen, until the patient has completed the preparative regimen. A cryopreservative protective agent such as dimethyl sulfoxide (DMSO) or hydroxyethyl starch is added to the marrow before freezing to protect the stem cells from lysis caused by the extreme temperature. Cryopreserved marrow can be thawed and infused several years after harvest without appreciable loss in stem cell viability, although there is little research to suggest how long marrow may be stored without damage to the cells. All samples, either autologous or allogeneic, are tested for cell counts and bacterial and fungal contamination.

Cord Blood Banking and Storage

Cord blood banks have been developed around the world, and considerable efforts are under way to standardize banking processes and procedures. These banks have facilitated the widespread availability of a stem cell source with a lower rate of viral infection and greater ethnic diversity.

As public awareness has increased, intrigue, concern, and even fear have surfaced over umbilical cord blood collection. Families must know the types, purpose, fees, and current pediatric recommendations for cord blood banking. The obstetrician or midwife collecting the unit must be familiar with cord blood collection. It is imperative that the health care professional receive instructions from the bank or institution receiving and banking the cord blood. At this point, each bank has its own procedure and equipment for collection (Figure 8-5).

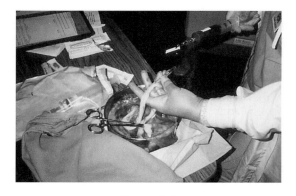

Figure 8-5

A cord blood harvest.

Expectant mothers with a child who may need an allogeneic stem cell transplant are urged to bank the umbilical cord blood from the new baby at delivery as a potential source of stem cells. It is important to address procurement of placental blood early in the pregnancy in order to: (1) facilitate the informed consent process; (2) assess the family's medical history; (3) examine factors potentially affecting cord blood collection; (4) educate the delivering obstetrician or midwife; and (5) arrange for collection, processing, transport, and storage of the unit.[30]

Informed consent is a crucial issue. Consumers must be educated to make informed decisions about cord blood collection and storage. Consent includes discussion of testing, collection, processing, storage, cost, and ultimate potential uses of the umbilical cord unit. Expectant families need to understand that extensive infectious disease testing will be performed on the mother, as well as the cord blood obtained. They must be prepared for full disclosure of results. Consent requires an explanation of the actual collection process at delivery and potential uses and limitations of the collection.

Familial and genetic history must be obtained. Genetic conditions affecting the hematopoietic system would preclude the cord blood donation. These conditions include hemoglobinopathies (e.g., sickle cell anemia, thalassemias), deficiencies of erythrocytic enzymes (e.g., glucose-6-phosphate dehydrogenase deficiency), congenital anemias (e.g., Fanconi's anemia), and congenital immunologic defects (e.g., severe combined immune deficiency, bare lymphocyte syndrome).[94] The Placental Blood Program in New York City, directed by Dr. Pablo Rubinstein, uses an interview before cord blood donation, which is intended to elicit a thorough family and infectious disease history. It is critical to obtain any prenatal history of high-risk behaviors and/or infectious exposures of the mother and fetus. Infectious organisms potentially passed from mother to child may also contaminate placental blood and be transmitted to the cord blood recipient. Individuals donating to cord blood banks must also provide ethnic background, since this will be important in donor selection criteria. The need to provide follow-up of the donor to detect for possible transmission of genetic or infectious diseases has become significant and may be problematic for cord bankers and transplanters alike.

AUTOLOGOUS PERIPHERAL BLOOD STEM CELL RESCUE

Mobilization

Hematopoietic progenitor and stem cells reside normally in the bone marrow and are detected in very small numbers in the circulation. In order to collect a sufficient number of PBSCs, a methodology has been devised to "move" them out of the marrow compartment. This process is referred to as mobilization and occurs (1) during the recovery phase following myelosuppressive chemotherapy; (2) with administration of growth factors such as granulocyte colony stimulating factor (G-CSF) or granulocyte macrophage colony stimulating factor (GM-CSF); and (3) after the combination of chemotherapy and growth factors.

Harvesting (Collection)

Although the exact identity of the cells needed for durable engraftment is not clear, it is theorized that they are part of the leukocyte group known as mononuclear cells, which includes lymphocytes and monocytes. These cells exhibit a narrow range of densities, which makes it possible to separate them from plasma, red cells, and platelets. Anticoagulated blood is centrifuged, causing cells to distribute according to their density in the centrifugal field. Cells in the specified density range for the mononuclear cell layer are then collected.[73] The COBE Spectra Auto PBSC System is an automated system used to collect PBSCs. This machine can function with a low extracorporeal volume and can operate at very low blood flow rates (10 ml/minute).

The collection (leukapheresis) refers to the actual day of the procedure and the volume collected. A harvest event refers to several collections after one mobilization. Depending on the disease or reason for collecting, there may be multiple harvest events in an attempt to collect sufficient targeted cells. The number of collections and harvest events increases if CD34+ selection or purging is required or in the case of sequential transplants. All of these situations require more stem cells.

The apheresis machine centrifuges blood drawn from the patient, draws the stem cell layer into a collection bag, and returns the rest (i.e., plasma, red cells, platelets) to the patient (Figure 8-6). The mechanics of this machine are similar to a dialysis machine and require two venous access lines—a line to draw from and one to act as the return. Several venous access devices can be used: a double lumen central venous catheter (CVC), an apheresis catheter, or two large bore IV cannulas. In children who have small vessels, especially those under 25 kg, larger bore IV cannulas may not be feasible. In these cases apheresis catheters or double lumen CVCs are used. Some centers use femoral arterial lines and a secondary IV line.[28]

Targeted cell dose. The cell dose for PBSC transplantation initially was a given number of mononuclear cells per kilogram of body weight. As more information about the identity of the cells de-

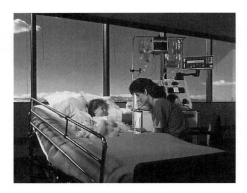

Figure 8-6

A child undergoing stem cell harvest (with machine).

veloped, other measures of stem cell content were introduced. Currently, CD34 counts are widely used. After a harvest event, cell collections are analyzed to determine if enough of the appropriate cells have been collected to engraft the patient. Although only a fraction of the CD34+ cells are truly stem cells, good correlations between CD34+ dose and engraftment time have created confidence in this assay.[99]

Although some institutional variation exists, the targeted PBSC dose ranges necessary for engraftment are approximately 2×10^8/kg of total mononuclear cells, with a presumed minimum CD34+ cell dose of 1-2 $\times 10^6$/kg. The correlation between CD34+ cell dose and engraftment has not been clearly proven, but it is presumed to increase the process of immune system reconstitution.[64]

Timing of collection. The timing of PBSC collection requires considerable organization, coordination, and proactive planning. The goal is an optimal harvest (the highest cell dose, mobilizing the largest numbers of progenitors) with the least amount of leukaphereses (harvest events).[45,73]

The white blood count, and sometimes the CD34+ cell count, is monitored to determine when to initiate the PBSC collection. If chemotherapy or hematopoietic growth factors are used for mobilization, the objective is to identify the point when the patient is recovering from the nadir, when the bone marrow is turning out many progenitor cells. Once patients recover their blood counts, it is too late to collect cells since they have presumably "differentiated" most of the mobilized progenitors. When growth factors are used for mobilization, collections are usually done on the fifth day after the start of growth factors—at the point when they

have the greatest effect. Additional days on growth factors do not improve yield.

Purging or CD34+ Selection

Debate still exists about the role of residual malignant cells, which may contaminate harvested PBSCs. The data suggest that the infusion of contaminated cells is not the major source of relapse, but transplanters would prefer to do more to purify the graft. Therefore investigation of purging methods continues. In pediatric transplantation the two most common purging methods used are immunologic purging with MoAbs and CD34+ selection techniques. Immunologic purging involves sedimentation, filtration, and tumor removal, usually with immunomagnetic beading (the MoAb attaches to the malignant cell, and both are subsequently removed by attachment to magnetic beading). Another purging technique is the positive selection of CD34+ cells with an immunoaffinity column. Selection of CD34+ cells does not reduce the number of progenitor and stem cells since the column preferentially selects them out. The process can result in a 2 to 5 log depletion of malignant cells since the column leaves behind unwanted cells.[99]

Processing, Testing, and Storage

Once the apheresis procedure is completed, a sample of the collection is removed for total cell count, CD34 count, bacterial and fungal cultures, colony assay, and immunophenotypic analysis. Testing for minimal residual disease in the collection by either immunocytology or molecular testing is an institutional or protocol specific practice. Dimethyl sulfoxide (DMSO) is added as a cryoprotectant, and collections are then frozen in a controlled-rate liquid nitrogen freezer. Collections are often spun to remove excess plasma and reduce the volume before freezing. This is important when there are multiple leukapheresis events and collections and many bags have to be given to equal the desired cell dose. Potentially the more bags needed to achieve the targeted cell dose, the more fluid infused on the day of transplant. In pediatric patients under 20 kg this could lead to fluid overload and/or excessive DMSO toxicity.

Clinical considerations for harvesting PBSCs in pediatrics are summarized in Box 8-5. Although institutional and/or protocol parameters may vary slightly, the stages in the process remain fairly constant. As experience in pediatric harvesting has increased, transplantation centers have refined the process to include very small children under 20 kg.* PBSC harvest and collection in these small children pose many challenges, but it is feasible, effective,

---

*References 1, 28, 45, 50, 59, 112.

BOX 8-5

PERIPHERAL BLOOD STEM CELL HARVEST: CLINICAL CONSIDERATIONS

I. PREHARVEST
Previous therapy: potential effects on stem cell yield
Central venous access device*
Mobilization techniques
• Chemotherapy + cytokine vs. cytokine alone
Desired cell dose†
Consideration of timely delivery of scheduled chemotherapy
Patient condition at time of harvest
• Anemia, thrombocytopenia
• Infectious status
• Malignancy status
Protocol markers: CD34+ selection, purging, and/or large volume leukapheresis*

II. AT HARVEST
Immediately before initiation of harvest:
• Obtain CBC and type/hold.
• Prime extracorporeal line with irradiated, leukopoor filtered PRBCs if child <25 kg.
• Obtain CD34+ count if required by protocol.
Anemia and thrombocytopenia *are not* contraindications to PBSC harvest.
Patient monitoring throughout harvest:
• Hypovolemia, sepsis, citrate toxicity

Process a *minimum* of two blood volumes per pheresis procedure (~4-6 hours).*

III. SPECIFIC ISSUES: <25-KILOGRAM CHILD
Citrate toxicity
Hypovolemia at initiation of leukapheresis
Adequate flow rates through small catheters
Ability to do large volume leukapheresis in 1 day (>3 blood volumes)
Behavioral considerations for long and/or repeated collections

IV. QUALITY CONTROL OF STEM CELL PRODUCT
Collection processed for volume reduction and stem cell purification by density gradient separation
Product evaluation:
• Total mononuclear and CD34+ cell counts
• Cell viability, colony assay formation
• Bacterial and fungal contamination
Minimal residual disease testing
• Immunocytology
• Molecular testing

*See catheter guidelines (Table 8-2) for criteria specifications in large leukapheresis or purging.
†Large volume leukapheresis, purged products, and/or CD34+ selected samples may require 4-6 blood volumes.

---

and safe. Technical challenges include obtaining adequate venous access, using alternative modes of anticoagulation, and obtaining extracorporeal volume balance. Psychosocial challenges include issues of assent and the ability to distract patients for the duration of a prolonged collection.[45,50]

Vascular Access

In pediatric patients, particularly those under 20 kg, apheresis procedures are performed using a subcutaneously (SQ) tunneled, double-lumen CVC. The apheresis (dialysis-style) catheter is one of the most feasible and effective because of its large lumens, stiff material, and minimal recirculation characteristics. It is capable of high flow rates and is associated with decreased collapse rates and flow occlusion under negative pressure.[45,73] However, when an apheresis catheter is required for leukapheresis, it has meant an additional surgical intervention with additional anesthesia and associated risks.

Both the benefits and risks of apheresis catheters must be considered. Apheresis catheters often crack at the junction where the catheter meets the caps. They are stiff, large, and uncomfortable. Whereas they may be most reasonable for a short

window during an apheresis event, they are not practical for long-term use. A traditional tunneled CVC is more appropriate.

Smaller lumen CVCs, however, have limitations in the apheresis setting. These CVCs are not as rigid, tend to collapse, occlude easily under negative pressure, and have proven to recirculate blood. These limitations will affect flow rates. Lower flow rates mean more time and therefore less numbers of cells collected, increased frustration for families and staff, and potentially additional harvest events. Many pediatric centers have found that tunneled CVCs in size 10 french (Fr) or greater significantly decrease these limitations. The larger the catheter, the fewer the flow problems. Although the procedure is reported feasible with an 8 Fr catheter, greater patience and expertise are required.

Controversies and institutional variance exist about which catheter to use for apheresis. At the start of therapy when a CVC is needed and there is a potential for leukaphresis harvesting, the following questions should be asked:
• Does the patient weigh less than 20 kg?
• Are prolonged chemotherapy, blood products, IV medication, and blood sampling required?

TABLE 8-2	PERIPHERAL BLOOD STEM CELL APHERESIS: PRINCIPLES OF CENTRAL VENOUS CATHETER SELECTION

Apheresis catheters are not required in pediatrics.

The larger the inner sheath of the catheter diameter, the greater and faster the flow.

Large volume leukapheresis, CD34+ selection, and other purging techniques require more stem cells, longer collection times, and/or greater number of apheresis events.

An appropriate double lumen CVC can be used through all phases of therapy: induction, harvesting, myeloablation, infusion, and supportive care.

Essential CVC characteristics:
- Provides a minimal outflow rate of 15-20 ml/min
- 8 Fr or greater double lumen catheter
- Durable sheath, stiff material to decrease collapse and flow occlusion under negative pressure
- Implanted port devices contraindicated

Patient Weight	Catheter Recommendation
<20 kg	10 Fr Hickman double lumen or 7-9 Fr single lumen draw line and 7 Fr double return
	8 Fr can be used in select situations but has significantly slower flow rates.
20-40 kg	8 Fr MedComp (Sl18P or SL24P)
	12 Fr Hickman
>40 kg	12.5 Fr MedComp (SL28)
	12 Fr Hickman

From Gorlin, J. B., Humphreys, D., Kent, P., et al. (1996). Pediatric large volume peripheral blood progenitor cell collections from patients under 25 kg: A primer. *Journal of Clinical Apheresis, 11,* 195-203; Marson, P., Petris, M. G., De Silvestro. G., et al. (1998). Collection of peripheral blood stem cells in pediatric patients: A concise review on technical aspects. *Bone Marrow Transplantation, 22* (Suppl. 5), S7-S11.
MedComp, 1499 Drive, Hasleysville, PA.
Hickman: Bard Access Systems, Davol Division, 5425 W. Amelia Earhart Drive, Salt Lake City, UT 84116.

- Is leukapheresis planned? How many harvesting events are planned? Are CD34+ selection and/or purging going to be required?
- What is the developmental stage of the child?
- Are the parents or guardians aware of all that is involved? If possible, can they be involved in decision making?

The principles of catheter selection are outlined in Table 8-2.

Volume of Extracorporeal Circulation

Leukapheresis for PBSC collection may induce volume shifts as fluid is withdrawn or infused, most significantly when the patient's blood is initially withdrawn into the machine. In the child who weighs less than 20 kg with smaller blood volumes, even a small shift can be significant. For this reason it is necessary to prime the tubing system of the apheresis machine with blood (usually about 150 ml of packed red blood cells [pRBCs] per apheresis procedure). The red cell units used for priming must be irradiated and leukocyte depleted.

Anticoagulation

Leukapheresis for PBSC collection requires temporary anticoagulation to prevent clotting and oc-

clusion of the tubing system. Anticoagulation in this procedure is traditionally ensured by adding acid-citrate dextrose (ACD) to the collection when the pRBCs are infused. Citrate can produce side effects, most significantly hypocalcemia and resulting hypotension. The risk of this rare and often preventable complication may be greater in small children (<20 kg).* To minimize this potential complication, some institutions administer oral calcium supplements before the harvest procedure. In smaller children the anticoagulation regimens may include extremely low dose ACD plus heparin, or heparin alone.

Social Challenges

Apheresis in small children challenges the skills of a pediatric nurse. It is difficult to convince a young child to sit still or within the limited geographic area of a recliner or bed, but it can be done. Children do not need to be sedated—they need to be distracted and entertained. Careful planning and preparation of activities and the use of creative play are helpful. Consultation with child life specialists, teachers, and family members will also help. Plans

---

*References 1, 28, 45, 50, 59, 112.

should include rotation of activities and audiovisual, manipulation and fine motor, and table play. Frequent snacks and behavioral rewards can be extremely effective.

PERITRANSPLANT PROCESS

ADMISSION PROCEDURES

Children are usually admitted to the transplant unit either the day of or the day before beginning the conditioning regimen. Some patients may be transferred from another hospital directly to the inpatient unit of the transplant center. The extent of isolation precautions varies with the child's clinical condition and institutional policies. Comprehensive HSCT isolation guidelines have recently been published by the Centers for Disease Control (CDC). This has been an invaluable tool in standardizing protective measures.[47]

On admission to the transplant unit, nurses provide the child and family with (1) a practical orientation to the patient care environment, including the type of isolation room used and isolation techniques; (2) a description of the roles and responsibilities of members of the multidisciplinary team; (3) a list of guidelines governing unit activities; and (4) a discussion of the routine nursing care provided in a usual patient day. Most HSCT units have nursing standards of care for patient education and orientation.

Knowledge of the child's medical history, developmental history, and experiences with hospitalization guide the assessment, development, and implementation of strategies designed to integrate the child and family into the HSCT environment. For example, from prior hospitalization experiences, a child with a malignancy will be somewhat familiar with the side effects of chemotherapy and radiation. In contrast, a child with a new diagnosis of severe aplastic anemia or severe combined immunodeficiency syndrome (SCIDS) will need a different, more intensive teaching approach.

A major risk for these patients is life-threatening infections that can occur during prolonged granulocytopenia after marrow infusion. The type of isolation used can prevent and/or minimize exposure to exogenous sources of infection. Gut decontamination and skin cleansing measures are used to suppress or eliminate the endogenous microbial flora of the patient. Many centers introduce a low-bacteria diet at or immediately following the preparative regimen in an attempt to decrease the risk of bacterial contamination from food products. Although standards vary from center to center, restricted diets are usually continued until mucositis is fully resolved (autologous transplants) and/or

there is evidence of initial immunoreconstitution (allogeneic transplants).

An important nursing goal is to minimize the impact of being in isolation on an already stressed child and family. Touring the unit before admission helps, as does reassuring the child and family that all types of personal belongings, from clothing and toys to stereos, televisions, videocassette recorders (VCRs), and computers, are commonly permitted. Special care is taken on admission to sterilize or thoroughly clean objects before bringing them into the isolation room. Personal items and reminders of home, family, friends, and pets are encouraged, particularly for children and families traveling a far distance. Parents of younger children are encouraged to create photo albums of important people, pets, places, and home that can be used for storytelling or in creative play therapy with the child. Home videos can be entertaining and therapeutic. Adolescents may prefer a video or photographs of special moments with their friends in addition to reminders of home. Classmates from school should be encouraged to write and send cards and other items of interest. Cassette recordings from family and friends are also important to have and help to ease feelings of isolation and separation. The active involvement of the child life therapy staff is paramount to assist children in coping with the necessary isolation during and after transplant.

Once the child is admitted, the parents and the child, if old enough, are encouraged to take an active role in the daily routine, assisting with bathing, central line and dressing care, and medication administration. Nurses work with the child and family to develop plans for managing care throughout the hospitalization. Children are encouraged to decorate their isolation room. To relieve the tedium and boredom that normally develop with a prolonged hospital stay, parents are encouraged to divide a child's toys into groups that are given back at different intervals. Most personal items brought by the child can be sterilized or cleaned effectively for use in the isolation room.

PREPARATIVE REGIMENS

Immediately before the bone marrow infusion, the child receives the chemotherapy conditioning regimen with or without total body irradiation (TBI). Regimen selection is influenced by the disease and the type of HSCT. For patients with malignant diseases, the regimen must provide tumor reduction, and ideally, disease eradication. The ideal properties of HSCT preparative regimens are outlined in Table 8-3. In allogeneic transplants the risk of graft rejection necessitates vary-

TABLE 8-3	IDEAL PROPERTIES OF HSCT PREPARATIVE REGIMENS		
	Allogeneic for Malignant Disease	**Allogeneic for Nonmalignant Disease**	**Autologous for Malignant Disease**
Immunosuppression (antigraft rejection)	Yes	Yes	No
Eradicate malignancy (antitumor)	Yes	No	Yes
Make space for new marrow (ablation)	Yes	Yes	Yes
Avoid/minimize overlapping toxicity	Yes	Yes	Yes

Adapted from Dix, S., & Yee, G. C. (1997). Pharmacologic and biologic agents. In M. B. Whedon & D. Wujick (Eds.), *Blood and marrow stem cell transplantation: Principles, practice, and nursing insights* (2nd ed., pp. 101). Sudbury, MA: Jones & Bartlett.

ing degrees of immunosuppression. In autologous transplants immunosuppression to prevent graft rejection is not necessary. TBI, total lymphoid irradiation (TLI), cyclophosphamide, and antithymocyte globulin (ATG) may be used to provide effective immunosuppression and prevent graft rejection.

Removal of unwanted cell populations requires agents with antineoplastic, and thus myeloablative, effects. Cyclophosphamide, busulfan, cytarabine, and the nitrosoureas (i.e., carmustine, lomustine) have antineoplastic or myeloablative effects and are used most often in conditioning regimens for hematologic malignancies and certain nonmalignant disorders. Combinations of known tumoricidal agents are used against malignant solid tumors. The majority of conditioning regimens use a combination of drugs that do not have overlapping toxicities, with or without radiation therapy. Rarely is only a single agent used. Chemotherapy is administered in myeloablative doses, resulting in a dramatic increase in side effects rarely seen outside of the HSCT setting. Astute assessment skills are critical to monitor and intervene effectively for both anticipated and unanticipated side effects and toxicities during the conditioning procedure (Table 8-4).

TOTAL BODY IRRADIATION

TBI remains the primary therapeutic modality for autologous and allogeneic HSCT for patients with hematologic malignancies. TBI has excellent immunosuppressive properties. It is active against a wide variety of malignancies, even those with proven chemotherapy resistance, and can penetrate the sanctuary sites of the central nervous system (CNS) and testicles.

There is extensive experience using 10 to 16 Gy TBI as a single or fractionated dose, preceding or following high doses of cyclophosphamide (alone or with other agents).[96] Experimental studies and clinical trials indicate that TBI given in fractions is more tolerable than single dose administration. Studies also suggest that antileukemia effects and normal tissue toxicity of TBI have a steep dose-response curve.[96]

The side effects associated with the administration of TBI are relatively well tolerated and include fatigue, nausea, and vomiting. Some transplant centers are administering TBI in the outpatient setting.[4] Post-TBI effects include nausea and vomiting, diarrhea, hypotension, capillary leak syndrome, and a respiratory distress syndrome. TBI may enhance the toxicities resulting from other agents used in the conditioning regimen. The late effects of TBI include cataracts, restrictive and obstructive lung disease, interstitial pneumonitis, leukoencephalopathy, cognitive impairment leading to poor school performance, and endocrinopathies such as gonadal failure, hypothyroidism, and growth hormone deficiency.[96,110] Extensive efforts have been made to develop non–TBI containing transplantation regimens. Many patients have already received dose-limiting radiotherapy before transplant. For other patients avoiding the long-term sequelae of TBI, particularly the associated growth and development problems in children, is desirable.

SEQUENTIAL REGIMENS WITH PBSC SUPPORT

Using less intensive or submyeloablative antineoplastic regimens given repeatedly as an alternative to single, high-dose marrow ablative therapy (tandem high-dose chemotherapy) has only recently been explored. The concept is to increase dose intensity with sequential regimens each followed by PBSC rescues, theoretically destroying minimal residual disease and disrupting the ability of malignant cells to "recover" from previous high dose chemotherapy. Phase I trials of this procedure in pediatric transplantation have focused on high risk neuroblastoma, high risk or recurrent CNS tumors, and other high risk solid tumors.[46,57,98,101]

TABLE 8-4	HIGH-DOSE CHEMOTHERAPY REGIMENS		
Agent	MTD	Dose-Limiting Toxicities	Clinical Monitors/Interventions

MARROW-ABLATIVE SINGLE AGENTS USED IN HIGH-DOSE REGIMENS WITH STEM CELL SUPPORT

Agent	MTD	Dose-Limiting Toxicities	Clinical Monitors/Interventions
Total body irradiation	10-16 Gy	GI, hepatic, pulmonary	*During TBI:* Effects include fatigue, nausea, vomiting. *Post-TBI:* Effects include significant skin and mucosal toxicity resulting in diarrhea, nausea, vomiting, hypotension, capillary leak syndrome, and respiratory distress syndrome. *Interventions:* Antiemetics provided around-the-clock may be required, aggressive skin care to affected areas, continuous opioid infusion to manage pain of skin and gut toxicity, and IV fluid/nutritional support.
Busulfan	20 mg/kg	GI, hepatic, pulmonary	Associated with variable pharmacokinetics (PK); children have lower mean plasma busulfan levels than adults given the same dose; PK levels are followed closely to facilitate adjustments and achieve targeted steady state plasma levels. *Interventions:* Close monitoring for tolerance/compliance with full oral dose administration; occasionally use of nasogastric tube may be necessary to ensure a patient receives and absorbs total dose; can affect seizure threshold, especially in adolescent patients—administration of prophylactic phenytoin (Dilantin) is given throughout conditioning regimen to prevent seizure activity; associated with occurrence of veno-occlusive disease (VOD)—signs and symptoms of VOD are monitored—institute daily weights, measurement of abdominal girths, fluid restrictions, pain management.
Melphalan	200 mg/kg	GI	No specific clinical monitors/interventions required outside of standard HSCT routines; can be administered as outpatient with no observable side effects.
Thiotepa	1135 mg/m^2	CNS, GI	Associated with significant skin and mucosal toxicity; mucositis is common and can be severe; dermatologic toxicity is manifested as acute erythoderma, which can be maculopapular and desquamating, or as a generalized rash consisting of total body hyperpigmentation or bronzing, which may persist for several months; effects begin several days following administration; no observable/reportable side effects during infusion; can be administered as outpatient, then patient is admitted for supportive care/isolation. *Interventions:* Aggressive skin care, pain management; multiple daily baths recommended during days of infusion in an attempt to minimize skin toxicity (drug is excreted primarily through sweat).

NON–MARROW ABLATIVE SINGLE AGENTS USED IN HIGH-DOSE REGIMENS WITH STEM CELL SUPPORT

Agent	MTD	Dose-Limiting Toxicities	Clinical Monitors/Interventions
Cyclophos-phamide	200 mg/kg	Cardiac	Associated with hemorrhagic cystitis, myocarditis, syndrome of inappropriate antidiuretic hormone (SIADH). *Interventions:* Aggressive IV fluid support during and after administration; monitoring for blood, "racking" of urine; mesna administration and/or bladder irrigation; cardiac monitoring during infusion; concomitant cardiac contractility agents may be used in the evidence of affected cardiac function; fluid adjustment and sodium level monitoring if suspicion of SIADH.

Data from Bensinger, W., & Buckner, D. (1999). Preparative regimens. In E. D. Thomas, K. Blume, & S. Forman (Eds.), *Hematopoietic cell transplantation* (p. 124). Malden, MA: Blackwell Science; Sanders, J. E. (1999). Stem-cell transplant preparative regimens. *Pediatric Transplantation, 3*(Suppl. 1), 23-34.

GI, Gastrointestinal; *CNS,* central nervous system; *MTD,* maximum tolerated dose.

Continued

TABLE 8-4	HIGH-DOSE CHEMOTHERAPY REGIMENS—cont'd		
Agent	MTD	Dose-Limiting Toxicities	Clinical Monitors/Interventions
NON–MARROW ABLATIVE SINGLE AGENTS USED IN HIGH-DOSE REGIMENS WITH STEM CELL SUPPORT—cont'd			
Etoposide	2400 mg/m²	GI	Associated with significant mucositis and diarrhea when administered in high doses.
			Interventions: Aggressive fluid/platelet support, pain management, oral hygiene.
AGENTS USED IN HIGH-DOSE REGIMENS WITHOUT DETERMINATION OF MTD WITH STEM CELL SUPPORT			
Carboplatin	2000 mg/m²	Hepatic, renal	Associated with hepatic and renal toxicities; Dose is usually determined by a formula based on renal function.
Cytarabine	36 g/m²	CNS	Associated with significant gastrointestinal, skin, and mucosal toxicity; radiation recall effects are often seen.
			Interventions: Aggressive skin care to affected areas, pain management, IV fluid, and nutritional support; eyedrops to prevent conjunctivitis.

Data from Bensinger, W., & Buckner, D. (1999). Preparative regimens. In E. D. Thomas, K. Blume, & S. Forman (Eds.), *Hematopoietic cell transplantation* (p. 124). Malden, MA: Blackwell Science; Sanders, J. E. (1999). Stem-cell transplant preparative regimens. *Pediatric Transplantation, 3*(Suppl. 1), 23-34.
GI, Gastrointestinal; *CNS,* central nervous system; *MTD,* maximum tolerated dose.

ALLOGENEIC TRANSPLANTATION WITH IMMUNOABLATIVE (SUBMYELOABLATIVE) REGIMENS

There is increasing evidence that stable chimerism can be achieved with submyeloablative doses of TBI and/or chemotherapeutic agents.[83,103] Partial but stable grafts would benefit patients with nonmalignant diseases such as thalassemia or sickle cell anemia. In these patients total elimination of the recipient graft is not necessary (complete graft) because a partial graft (mixed chimera) may bring about the needed correction of the underlying hematologic disorder.

The goal of this approach for patients with malignancies, particularly leukemia, is to develop nontoxic methods of achieving donor chimerism while maximizing posttransplantation immunotherapy. Sufficient immunosuppression is provided to achieve engraftment of an allogeneic hematopoietic graft and to also allow the subsequent development of a graft-versus-malignancy effect. Advantages of this method include the reduction of ablative and toxic chemotherapy and radiation given in the preparative regimen and potentially fewer inpatient hospitalizations. By eliminating or reducing radiation and certain chemotherapeutic drugs from the conditioning regimen, peritransplant organ toxicity and posttransplant long-term effects may be reduced. The risks of this approach are not well defined and are dependent on the donor source and the actual submyeloablative/immunoablative approach. Potential risks are the increased incidence of nonengraftment and GVHD.[22,103,104]

STEM CELL INFUSION

Infusion of the stem cells is similar to transfusion of a blood component. Allogeneic, unprocessed marrow may be transported directly from the surgical suite to the patient's room and infused to the recipient through a CVC. If the marrow is plasma depleted, purged, or otherwise processed, there may be a delay of hours or days before reinfusion. Autologous, cryopreserved marrow or PBSCs are removed from the liquid nitrogen tank and thawed in a warm water bath before infusion.

The stem cell infusion can be infused by gravity or given as an IV push infusion. In some institutions the physicians or transplant coordinators reinfuse the marrow; HSCT nurses are responsible for reinfusion in others. Generally the infusion lasts 30 to 90 minutes, depending on the stem cell volume and the patient's size. Frequently the patient receives antiemetics and/or diphenhydramine before the infusion to decrease the potential for an allergic reaction to the donor marrow (associated with ABO incompatibility). Procedures for correct identification of the patient must be followed carefully.

The stem cell infusion is usually anticlimactic for the patient and family. Although it signifies optimism and hope for cure, it is less eventful than the evaluation process and preparative regimen. At the time of transplant many patients and families have other fears and preoccupations, including fear of complications, fear of disease recurrence, and fear that the HSCT will not engraft. Patients may complain of nausea, particularly if DMSO was used as the cryopreservative. DMSO is metabolized and excreted in the lungs, which produces a characteristic strong garlic breath odor for 24 to 48 hours that may distress the patient and family. During the infusion measures are taken to keep the child comfortable and to provide emotional support to the entire family. Some families ask to carry out rituals or celebrations as a way to bring meaning and significance to the infusion procedure.

Side Effects and Complications of Allogeneic Stem Cell Infusion

Hemolytic transfusion reactions.   Acute reactions can occur when the donor's red blood cells and the recipient's plasma are incompatible. Undetected serologic incompatibilities can be a contributing cause, but most immediate reactions occur when clerical or other identification errors lead to an ABO mismatch. Symptoms include shock, chills, fever, dyspnea, chest pain, back pain, headache, abnormal bleeding, and disseminated intravascular coagulation (DIC). Other indicators include hemoglobinemia, hemoglobinuria, elevated bilirubin, and renal failure. Treatment includes management of shock and administration of fluids and diuretics.

Delayed reactions usually occur in patients with red blood cell antibodies undetected at the time of transplant. These reactions usually present within 4 to 14 days after transplantation. Symptoms include unexplained anemia, positive direct antiglobulin test (DAT), fever, hemoglobinuria, and elevated bilirubin.

Transmission of infectious disease.   (In spite of careful donor screening and blood testing before infusion) infectious diseases that can be transmitted include:
- Viral hepatitis, hepatitis B, and hepatitis C
- Human retrovirus HIV and Human T-lymphotrophic virus (HTLV)
- CMV
- EBV
- Others: malaria, toxoplasma, and parvovirus.

Febrile reactions.   These can occur when antibodies to white cell antigens react against foreign leukocytes.

Allergic reactions.   These are caused by the presence of donor plasma proteins or to processing reagents or processing antibiotics. Patients can be premedicated with antihistamines to prevent allergic reactions.

Side Effects and Complications of Autologous Peripheral Blood Stem Cell Infusion

Bacterial contamination.   This is commonly but not exclusively due to the normal skin flora.

DMSO reactions.   Symptoms include coughing/choking, sneezing/bronchial spasms/dyspnea, nausea/vomiting, hypertension, diarrhea, or abdominal cramping.

Allergic reactions.   These are caused by allergens to processing reagents or processing antibiotics. Patients can be premedicated or treated with antihistamines to prevent or treat allergic reactions.

Circulatory overload.   Pulmonary edema can result when excessive volume is infused. Thawed bone marrow infusions rarely exceed 200 ml total volume, so this is a concern primarily in the small patient or one with renal problems.

Depletion of coagulation proteins and platelets.   Citrate and heparin used in the collection and infusion procedures can deplete coagulation proteins and cause bleeding.

Microaggregates.   Particles of fibrin, bone, and cell clumps can cause emboli.

Metabolic complications.   These can include:
- Citrate toxicity: citrate anticoagulant can bind to ionized calcium in the body, and the depletion of calcium can cause muscle tremors and dysarrhythmias
- Acidosis
- Hyperkalemia/hypokalemia: alterations in potassium can occur because of excessive red cell lysis during cryopreservation.

Infusion of hemolyzed blood.   This can result in hemoglobinuria, chills, fever, or DIC.

Throughout the infusion the patient is assessed for fever, hypertension, tachycardia, and/or tachypnea, which may indicate a transfusion reaction or emboli, and other symptoms of side effects or complications. Transplant centers have established protocols for stem cell infusion and the management of infusion-related complications. Specific flow sheets are maintained to document and chronicle the marrow infusion.

ACUTE TOXICITIES

Acute toxicities related to HSCT occur within the first 100 days after transplant, with a mortality rate of 20% to 25% in recipients of allogeneic transplants and 5% to 15% in autologous and PBSCR patients combined.[5] Toxicities of transplantation vary according to the preparative regimen, level of immunosuppression, organ status before transplant, and the type of transplant itself. Single organ dysfunction in the posttransplant period predicts the subsequent development of multiple organ dysfunction.[43] Therefore it is postulated that it is not confined to one organ, but a manifestation of a more generalized abnormality.[43] One such abnormality suspected to have a relationship to organ dysfunction is the anticoagulant deficiencies observed in HSCT patients.

The greater morbidity and mortality associated with allogeneic HSCT is related to the host immunosuppression required to achieve donor engraftment and prevent GVHD. For allogeneic HSCT the leading causes of morbidity and mortality include acute GVHD, bacterial and fungal infections, CMV infections, idiopathic pneumonitis, and organ dysfunction caused by chemotherapy or radiotherapy or medications used during transplantation.[36] Acute GVHD contributes to organ dysfunction and also necessitates increased immunosuppression, which increases the risk of infection.

For autologous HSCT the most frequent causes of morbidity and mortality are opportunistic infections and organ dysfunction caused by chemotherapy or radiotherapy. Many complications are interrelated and can occur simultaneously. The management of one problem may exacerbate or cause another. Figure 8-7 illustrates onset and time interval of major complications.

The post-HSCT process is divided into three phases: early (Day 0 to engraftment), intermediate (engraftment to Day 100), and late (after Day 100). The early phase focuses on the management of acute life-threatening toxicities. The intermediate period begins with engraftment and extends to the start of immune reconstitution, usually around Day +100. In PBSCR therapy, this period can end as early as Day +60, whereas in unrelated transplants with significant immunosuppression, it can extend well past Day +180. Nursing and medical

care focuses on the resolution of acute toxicities, patient and family teaching, management of minimal residual disease, and control and management of GVHD and its associated complications. The late or long-term phase begins with the start of immune reconstitution and care focuses on posttransplant follow-up and rehabilitation.

Early Phase

Hematologic complications. All HSCT patients experience prolonged marrow aplasia following cytoreductive therapy. The hematologic recovery time is affected by stem cell source (marrow, peripheral blood, umbilical cord blood), manipulation of cells (purging, T-cell reduction), GVHD, and infection. Some HSCT protocols use growth factors (e.g., G-CSF, GM-CSF) to shorten the period of neutropenia and decrease the risk of infection. Cytokines can also be useful for delayed or failed engraftment.

Nursing care focuses on management of neutropenia, anemia, and thrombocytopenia. Patients will require supportive red blood cell and platelet transfusions. All blood products are irradiated to eliminate any remaining immunocompetent lymphocytes in the product. Patients who are profoundly immunocompromised can develop GVHD just from lymphocyte contamination of these products alone. Irradiation does not compromise the functional qualities of the cells.[20] Blood products are also leukocyte depleted to minimize viral contamination, particularly CMV. (Refer to Chapters 11 and 14 for additional information about blood product administration.)

Hemorrhage is always a risk for thrombocytopenic patients. During the early phase of HSCT tissue and organ damage can increase the risk for bleeding. Although these patients may hemorrhage from any site, bleeding from oral mucosa is most common. Spontaneous gingival bleeding can occur when platelets are below 15,000/mm³. Therefore most centers try to keep the platelet count above 20,000/mm³. A higher platelet count may be required to achieve hemostasis if severe oral bleeding or gastrointestinal bleeding occurs. (Refer to Chapters 11 and 14 for additional information about platelet transfusions.)

Hemorrhagic cystitis occurs in 10% of HSCT patients and is most likely due to irritation of the bladder mucosal cells by the drug metabolites of cyclophosphamide and ifosfamide.[100] Bladder toxicity may be minimized by forced diuresis with or without mesna, a bladder protectant agent used in many HSCT protocols that include these drugs as part of the conditioning regimen. Hemorrhagic cystitis can develop a few days after the stem cell infu-

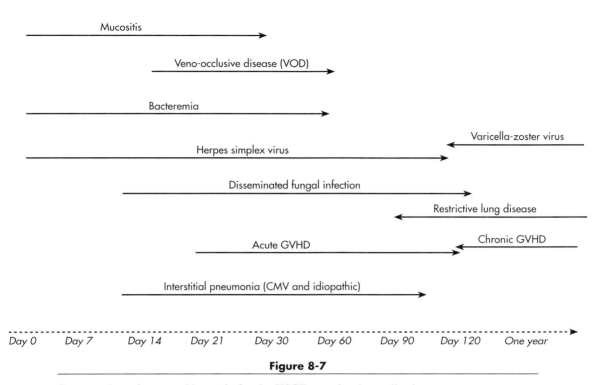

Figure 8-7

Common time of onset and interval of major HSCT–associated complications.   (Adapted from Press, O., Schaller, J.R., & Thomas, E.D. [1987]. Bone marrow transplant complications. In L.H. Toledo-Pereyra (Ed.), *Complications of organ transplantation.* New York: M. Dekker.)

sion but most commonly occurs around day 21 to 35[100] with variable severity. When hemorrhagic cystitis occurs much later, other causes should be explored. Both adenovirus and BK virus (a polyomavirus) have been identified as causes of delayed hemorrhagic cystitis (up to 100 days posttransplantation).[100] Severe cystitis can be extremely painful and debilitating, requiring prolonged hospitalization. Supportive care measures are instituted and may include a Foley catheter to decrease the risk of urinary obstruction from clots and bladder irrigation if necessary.

Thrombocytopenic patients are also at risk for CNS hemorrhage, particularly if hypertension occurs. Administration of cyclosporine or facrolimus (FK506) for GVHD prophylaxis and control may increase the risk of bleeding because of their effects on cerebral vasculature.[33]

Infections.   During the early phase of transplant, patients are neutropenic and immunosuppressed. With no functioning immune system and alterations in mucosal integrity, the patient is susceptible to bacterial, fungal, and viral infections. Gram-negative bacteria, mainly *E. coli, Klebsiella,* and *Pseudomonas,* have been the most frequent

cause of bacteremia in HSCT patients. However, in recent years gram-positive pathogens have become more prevalent, specifically coagulase-negative staphylococci and *Staphylococcus aureus.* The increase in staphylococcal infections may be related to the use of indwelling CVCs. *Candida* and *Aspergillus* are the most common fungal infections. Candidal infections usually arise from damaged mucosa, whereas *Aspergillus* is exogenous and airborne. Medical centers where construction is occurring have demonstrated a higher incidence of *Aspergillus* infections. High-energy particulate air (HEPA) filter systems have been shown to reduce this risk.[47] Prolonged neutropenia is the greatest risk factor for developing fungal infection. The most common viral infection in the early posttransplant phase is herpes simplex virus (HSV). Reactivation of HSV occurs in 80% of seropositive patients.[95] Acyclovir prophylaxis can decrease the risk of reactivation. Gingivostomatitis is the common manifestation, but disseminated disease may occur in the lungs, liver, or gastrointestinal (GI) tract. (Refer to Chapter 10 for additional information about infections complications.)

Most febrile episodes are related to infections, although persistent fevers without an identifiable etiology are commonly seen during the hematologic nadir.[95] All fevers should be regarded as infectious in origin until proven otherwise. Other signs and symptoms of infection may be obscured if the patient is neutropenic. Bacterial or fungal infections can rapidly become life threatening if untreated. Fungus should be considered a possible pathogen in patients with persistent fevers on broad spectrum antibiotics, in patients who have been heavily pretreated, and/or in those who have had prior episodes of prolonged neutropenia. (Refer to Chapter 10 for additional information about infections complications.)

Gastrointestinal. In the GI tract the mucous membranes separate the host from the external environment. The immune component of this defense consists of immunoglobulins, intraepithelial lymphocytes, and aggregates. The second component is created by an intact epithelial lining, mucous coat, and native microbial flora. Almost all HSCT patients have breakdown in the integrity of the mucosal defense system. It is impaired by chemotherapy and radiotherapy, allowing gut flora to invade the damaged epithelial lining and increasing the risk of bacteremia. Mucositis usually peaks 10 to 14 days after the stem cell infusion and causes swelling and pain. The severity can vary greatly. In severe cases sloughing of the epithelium can occur, and in extreme cases the sloughing can extend into the pharynx and the esophagus, causing gagging, inability to swallow, and airway compromise. Mucositis may be exacerbated by HSV infection and methotrexate treatment for GVHD prophylaxis. Patients with moderate to severe mucositis may need a continuous opioid infusion. Children 5 to 7 years of age and older can use patient-controlled analgesia. There is currently no preventative therapy for mucositis. To minimize discomfort and decrease the risk of infection, proper cleansing of the oral and perianal mucosa is important. To decrease the rate of gut-derived bacteremia, some transplant centers use oral, nonabsorbable antibiotics for gut decontamination until hematologic recovery. (Refer to Chapter 11 for additional information about mucositis.)

Hepatic. Veno-occlusive disease (VOD) of the liver is a major toxicity that can occur after cytoreductive therapy and is one of the leading causes of death during transplantation. It is a clinical syndrome characterized by hyperbilirubinemia, hepatomegaly, and fluid retention. The reported incidence varies greatly, from 2% to 54% of HSCT patients.[102] Presently there is no proven method of prevention or adequate treatment for

established VOD. Early detection of symptoms and institution of supportive care measures are critical. Often right upper quadrant pain or liver tenderness, caused by stretching of the liver capsule, is the initial symptom, which occurs 8 to 10 days after the start of cytoreductive therapy. Early weight gain and fluid retention may also be presenting signs.[79]

The exact sequence of events leading to VOD is only partially understood. It is believed that cytoreductive therapy damages liver endothelial cells in the venules and sinusoids, resulting in local activation of the clotting cascade.[79] Cytokines released by damaged cells may also contribute to ongoing local damage. The endothelial cells and fibrin deposition occlude sinusoidal pores, eventually causing intrahepatic obstruction to venous blood flow.[58] As a result, the sinusoids become dilated and engorged. There is leakage of protein-rich fluid from the sinusoids into the extravascular spaces, overwhelming the lymphatics and leaking through the capsule of the liver, causing ascites. The obstruction of blood flow leaving the liver eventually results in fibrosis and necrosis of the hepatocytes.

Diagnosis of VOD is made by clinical evaluation. Both the Seattle[102] and Baltimore[58] groups have developed diagnostic criteria. The Seattle definition requires two of three clinical manifestations by day 20: jaundice, painful hepatomegaly, or fluid retention. The Baltimore criteria include jaundice and two of the following: ascites, weight gain greater than 5%, or hepatomegaly (usually painful). The severity of VOD ranges from mild (requiring no treatment) to moderate (requiring treatment, usually supportive) to severe (irreversible even with treatment). Multiorgan failure follows the initial symptoms by several days, and the incidence depends on the severity of VOD.[79] Risk factors for the development of VOD include elevated transaminases before cytoreductive therapy, prior radiation therapy with fields including the liver, ongoing antiviral or antibacterial treatment at the start of cytoreductive therapy, and previous HSCT.[58]

Several agents to reduce the incidence or severity of VOD have been evaluated, including continuous low dose heparin infusion.[7,10,21] Due to inconclusive results or research study design flaws, the role of heparin remains unclear. Other drugs studied include prostaglandin E1,[10,39] ursodiol (Actigall),[32] and pentoxifylline.[13,19] Unfortunately there is still no proven prophylaxis or treatment for VOD.

Supportive management focuses on the conflicting and difficult tasks of maintaining intravascular volume to optimize intrahepatic and renal perfusion in patients with capillary leak syndrome. Renal insufficiency commonly complicates the management of VOD, and the use of diuretics remains controversial. Close attention to intake and output measures, monitoring abdominal girth, and daily weights are imperative.

Pulmonary. Pulmonary edema and pulmonary infection can be seen within the first 4 weeks following stem cell infusions. Pulmonary edema is caused by capillary leakage most often resulting from chemotherapy toxicity or radiotherapy toxicity. With careful use of diuretics and precise fluid management, the edema can resolve and the patient can recover. Infectious complications are either pneumonia (intraalveolar lobar consolidations) or pneumonitis (interalveolar wall thickening) and can be caused by bacteria (gram-negative or gram-positive), viruses (CMV, HSV), or fungus *(Aspergillus, Candida).*[17]

Renal. Renal insufficiency is a frequent complication following HSCT. Both cytoreductive therapy and nephrotoxic supportive medications (e.g., cyclosporine, amphotericin, vancomycin, gentamicin, acyclovir) can adversely affect renal blood flow and tubular function. In prerenal conditions glomerular filtration rate or blood flow is compromised by changes in the systemic circulation resulting in structural damage. Systemic circulatory disturbances can be caused by third spacing of fluid, VOD with capillary leak syndrome, dehydration, septic shock, and hemorrhage. In intrarenal conditions the structural components of the kidney are damaged, resulting in acute tubular necrosis (ATN). Damage to the renal tubules, often caused by renal tubular acidosis (RTA), produces obstruction within the tubules, impairing reabsorption and secretion, altering fluid, electrolyte, and acid-base balances, and affecting the elimination of waste products. The kidney can withstand a greater than 50% decrease in function before signs or symptoms are observed.[89] Younger children are more adversely affected by fluid shifts because of their larger body surface area relative to their total body weight. Attention must be paid to medication dosage adjustments in renal insufficiency.

Neurologic. Cyclosporine, FK506, and cytoreductive therapy can cause neurologic complications. Cyclosporine and FK506 are widely used to prevent and treat acute GVHD and cause complications varying from mild, reversible tremors to encephalopathy and CNS ischemia. Toxicity is indicated by elevated serum drug levels but can also occur at therapeutic levels.[27,33] Cytoreductive therapy induces pancytopenia, leaving the patient

at risk for infection and hemorrhage, both of which can be debilitating or even fatal when they occur in the CNS. Seizures can occur during the early phase and can be associated with infection, hemorrhage, hypertension, electrolyte abnormalities, or cyclosporine/FK506 toxicity. Seizures are also a side effect of some chemotherapeutic agents used in preparatory regimens, including busulfan and cytarabine.

Intermediate Phase

Infections. In allogeneic patients the intermediate phase is characterized by acute GVHD and its therapy and T-cells decreased in number and function. The highest risk is for viral infections, normally controlled by T cells and associated with high morbidity and mortality.[95] Viral infections during this phase are more frequent in allogeneic than autologous patients because of the added immunosuppression of allogeneic HSCT. Although T-cell defects can exist in autologous HSCT patients, severe viral infections are rare. All patients with an indwelling device in place, such as a CVC, will be at risk for bacteremia despite resolution of neutropenia. All allogeneic patients are at risk for persistent or repeated bacterial infections caused by the quantitative and qualitative disorders associated with profound immunosuppression.

CMV is one of the most dangerous infectious complications in allogeneic HSCT and most commonly occurs 45 to 60 days posttransplant.[92] Although recently there have been significant improvements in the detection and prevention of CMV infections, they remain a major complication in HSCT. CMV causes multiorgan disease, including pneumonia, gastroenteritis, hepatitis, retinitis, and encephalitis. CMV, like HSV, has the ability to establish lifelong and latent infections after primary exposure.[92] The outcome of therapy for disseminated CMV disease is poor; therefore preventive measures are very important. The three strategies of preventive therapy are as follows:

1. Prevention of primary infection
2. Prophylaxis—prevention of reactivation
3. Preemptive therapy—prevention of development of disseminated disease when reactivation has occurred

Most transplant centers have adopted one of the following options for prevention of CMV disease if the patient or donor is seropositive pretransplant[90]:

1. Universal prophylaxis—All patients at risk are given ganciclovir after engraftment through day 100.
2. Preemptive therapy—Patients are monitored for CMV infection. If the virus is detected,

treatment with ganciclovir is initiated. Monitoring is usually by weekly blood testing and includes cultures, CMV ribonucleic acid (RNA) by polymerase chain reaction (PCR), or measurement of CMV antigenemia. Day 35 bronchoalveolar lavage may also be performed.[81]

Intravenous immunoglobulin (IVIG) or hyperimmune globulin is sometimes used in addition to ganciclovir. Patients receiving ganciclovir are at risk for renal insufficiency and neutropenia. Dose adjustments are needed if either occur. The risk of CMV infection has been shown to increase with the occurrence and increasing severity of acute GVHD (aGVHD). Thus in the presence of aGVHD, CMV surveillance is often maximized.[76]

Pulmonary. Interstitial pneumonitis is the most common pulmonary complication. It occurs in about 40% of HSCT patients and is fatal in about 60% of the cases.[23] Few pulmonary complications appear during the first 4 weeks posttransplant except for the diffuse alveolar hemorrhage which usually occurs around the time of engraftment.[91]

Interstitial pneumonia. With or without evidence of infection, interstitial pneumonia is reportedly the leading cause of respiratory failure in HSCT patients. The toxicity of the conditioning regimen and the presence of CMV in the lung are major underlying factors that cause interstitial pneumonia. Due to improved prevention and treatment, the incidence induced by pathogens other than CMV, notably *Pneumocystis carinii,* herpes simplex, and varicella zoster, has diminished substantially over the past decade.[23] *Toxoplasma gondii* pneumonia is another rare cause of interstitial pneumonia that usually occurs only in association with CNS or cardiac manifestations.[17]

Idiopathic pneumonia syndrome. Idiopathic pneumonia syndrome is a noninfectious interstitial pneumonia that is not clearly understood. As with CMV pneumonia, the establishment of the marrow graft often seems to be a prerequisite.[91] This observation, and the association of idiopathic pneumonia syndrome with allogeneic grafting and GVHD, strongly suggests that immunologic reactions, as well as the toxicity from the conditioning regimen, are involved in the pathogenesis. Like CMV pneumonia, there is some evidence that T lymphocytes play a key role in the initial immunologic event.[91]

The basic clinical and histopathological features of idiopathic pneumonia syndrome are well defined and include dyspnea, nonproductive cough, hypoxemia, nonlobar radiographic infiltrates, diffuse alveolar damage, interstitial pneumonitis, and absence of lower respiratory tract infections. As molecular techniques for infection detection are further developed, the role of possible occult infection may be further defined.

Once it occurs, the overall mortality rate of idiopathic pneumonia syndrome exceeds 70%.[91] No promising therapeutic options have as yet emerged. The use of ventilatory support remains a matter of debate. Treatment failure in patients receiving ventilatory support may be due to irreversible lung damage at the time of intubation or the additional injuries caused by barotrauma and by pulmonary oxygen toxicity.[23]

ENGRAFTMENT AND RECOVERY

Approximately 10 to 21 days (depending on the type of transplant) following the stem cell infusion, the stem cells begin to find their home and produce normal blood cells. This process is called engraftment. The graft (stem cell infusion) contains a wide variety of cell types that differ in cell function and life span. Survival, distribution, and differentiation of engrafted donor cells are of central importance to the recovery of marrow function following HSCT. Some of the cells will contribute to short-term engraftment and then die off, whereas others are responsible for durable, long lasting immunoreconstitution and hematopoeisis.[16]

Informative genetic markers are used in allogeneic HSCT to confirm engraftment and distinguish the donor from the recipient. The two tests currently most widely used are *in situ hybridization* with six chromosome-specific probes, and typing of *variable number tandem repeat* (VNTR) polymorphisms by DNA amplication. In situ hybridization is applicable only when the donor and recipient are of the opposite sex. To successfully analyze the results of VNTR testing, it is crucial to obtain DNA samples from the donor and recipient before HSCT. Concurrent amplification of pretransplantation samples from the donor and recipient, together with a posttransplant sample, generally allows identification and minimizes confusion caused by background DNA bands.[16]

Chimerism tests are also used in a variety of other applications. Their roles are of greatest importance in patients who have inadequate marrow function and in patients who might be candidates for donor lymphocyte infusion or for a second transplant from the same donor. Genetic markers are also used in patients who have delayed engraftment or a sudden decrease in blood counts. In this situation chimeric testing can be used to predict recurrent malignancy since the presence of donor cells can sometimes be obscured by leukemic relapse or by a myelosuppressive malignant population.[86,88]

Graft Rejection

Graft rejection, the failure of the donor marrow to sustain engraftment in the recipient, is associated with (1) ineffective immunosuppression of the host; (2) damage of the microstromal environment by conditioning treatment; and/or (3) significant discordance between the donor and recipient tissue types.[74] When immunosuppression is inadequate, functional recipient immune cells are capable of recognizing the foreign T lymphocytes and destroying the graft. Graft rejection can also be associated with T-lymphocyte depletion in which those T cells that prevent graft rejection are removed indiscriminately along with those T cells that lead to aGVHD. It is believed that a subset of T cells in the donor marrow may facilitate donor engraftment by destroying residual host cells that mediate rejection.[16]

Graft Versus Leukemia

It is theorized that there is a relationship between aGVHD and disease recurrence, most specifically with the leukemias. The phenomenon is called graft versus leukemia effect. Allogeneic HSCT patients who experience some degree of acute or chronic GVHD have a lower incidence of leukemic relapse than those patients who do not.[83] This probably is related to the immunocompetent donor T lymphocytes[1] providing additional tumoricidal activity against residual leukemia cells.

Acute Graft-Versus-Host Disease

GVHD is an immune-mediated response that occurs between the donor's immunocompetent cells and the patient's immunosuppressed cells. It is the major cause of morbidity and mortality in allogeneic HSCT. This immune response is related to the genetically determined histocompatibility difference, or disparity between the tissue type of the donor and recipient. Immunocompetent donor T-lymphocyte cells are capable of mounting an immune reaction against the patient, but the patient's cells are incapable of reacting against the donor cells. The immunocompetent donor T lymphocytes become sensitized to the patient's antigens and generate cytotoxic effector cells targeted at specific host tissues, most notably those of the skin, GI tract, and liver.

Acute GVHD occurs in the first 100 days after transplant and is usually preceded by documented engraftment. The risks of aGVHD increase when there is HLA disparity, the patient is older, the recipient is male, or there is female-to-male recipi-

ent pairing. The latter is a significantly higher risk if the female donor was previously alloimmunized through pregnancy or previous blood transfusion(s). The overall grade of GVHD is based on involvement of each of the three organs affected (skin, GI tract, liver)[24] (Table 8-5).

Clinical presentation

Skin. Usually the first clinical manifestation of aGVHD is a maculopapular skin rash, commonly occurring at or near the time of the white blood cell engraftment (Figure 8-8). The early stages may be pruritic, involving the nape of the neck, ears, and the shoulders, as well as the palms of the hands and the soles of the feet. The rash resembles a sunburn.[41] From these initial areas of involvement, the rash may spread to the whole integument and become confluent. In severe GVHD the maculopapular rash forms bullous lesions with epidermal necrolysis. The progression of GVHD can be clinically divided into four stages, depending on the extent of skin involvement.[24]

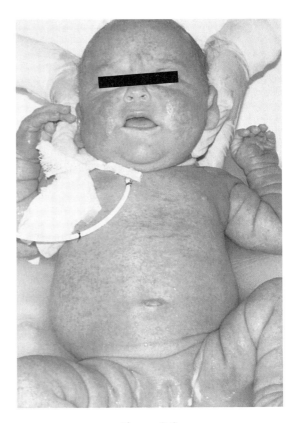

Figure 8-8

Skin rash commonly seen in aGVHD.

TABLE 8-5	GVHD Stage and Grading Systems

STAGING OF INDIVIDUAL ORGAN SYSTEM(S)

Organ	Stage	Description
Skin	+1	Maculopapular (M-P) eruption over <25% of body area
	+2	Maculopapular eruption over 25%-50% of body area
	+3	Generalized erythrodema
	+4	Generalized erythrodema with bullous formation and often with desquamation
Liver	+1	Bilirubin 2.0-3.0 mg/dl; SGOT 150-750 IU
	+2	Bilirubin 3.1-6.0 mg/dl
	+3	Bilirubin 6.1-15.0 mg/dl
	+4	Bilirubin >15.0 mg/dl
Gut	+1	Diarrhea >30 ml/kg or >500 ml/day
	+2	Diarrhea >60 ml/kg or >1000 ml/day
	+3	Diarrhea >90 ml/kg or >1500 ml/day
	+4	Diarrhea >90 ml/kg or >2000 ml/day; or severe abdominal pain and bleeding with or without ileus

OVERALL GRADING OF ACUTE GVHD

Grade	Skin Staging	Liver Staging		Gut Staging
I	+1 to +2	0		0
II	+1 to +3	+1	and/or	+1
III	+2 to +3	+2 to +4	and/or	+2 to +3
IV	+2 to +4	+2 to +4	and/or	+2 to +4

Adapted from Chao, N. J. (1999). Graft-versus-host disease (2nd ed.). Austin, TX: R. G. Landes.

Liver. The second organ most commonly affected by aGVHD is the liver. Patients will rarely have moderate to severe liver GVHD without evidence of cutaneous disease. Abnormal liver function tests indicate liver involvement, which is difficult to treat effectively. The earliest and most common abnormality is a rise in the conjugated bilirubin and alkaline phosphatase caused by damage to the bile canaliculi, which leads to cholestasis. Unfortunately a rise in the bilirubin or alkaline phosphatase is not specific enough since there are many competing factors that may also lead to abnormal liver function tests (VOD of the liver, hepatic infections, the effects of the preparatory regimen, and/or drug toxicity).

Biopsy is the definitive method to diagnose GVHD of the liver. Unfortunately, this may not be feasible because intrahepatic and extrahepatic bleeding can be a significant risk. Newer, less invasive methods, such as a transjugular approach, may reduce the bleeding hazard. The primary histologic findings are bile duct atypia and degeneration, which occasionally leads to severe cholestasis.[24,119]

Gastrointestinal tract. The third main organ affected by GVHD is the gut. Gut GVHD is often the most severe complication and frequently is the most difficult to treat. It is characterized by diarrhea and abdominal cramping. The diarrhea can be quite profuse, making it a challenge to maintain an adequate fluid balance. The crampy abdominal pain associated with severe GVHD often responds poorly to treatment. An ileus may develop from the GVHD or from the opioids used to control the physical discomfort.[23,109,119]

The diarrhea may initially be watery, reflecting primarily the salt and water reabsorption defect in the distal small bowel and colon. Frequently it then becomes bloody, requiring transfusion. It is not unusual for patients to need two units of packed red blood cells daily to keep the hematocrit in the 30% range. The stage of gut GVHD is usually graded by the volume of diarrhea. One must remember, however, that diarrhea unrelated to GVHD is a very common occurrence following HSCT. Within the first weeks diarrhea may be related to the preparatory regimen, the nonabsorbable antibiotics, or the systemic antibiotics. Later in the course of HSCT, superinfection must be considered as a cause for the diarrhea, as well as *Clostridium difficile* toxin.

In severe gut GVHD whole areas of the GI tract may be denuded, with total loss of epithelium similar to that observed in the skin. A rectal biopsy can be helpful in making the diagnosis. Colonoscopy or upper endoscopy are also usually performed. Infectious agents, most commonly CMV, may mimic the

TABLE 8-6	**TOXICITIES OF IMMUNOSUPPRESSIVE AGENTS**					
Cyclosporine	**Tacrolimus**	**Methotrexate**	**Corticosteroids**	**ATG**	**Mycophenolate Mofetil**
Nephrotoxicity	Nephrotoxicity	Mucositis	Hyperglycemia	Infection risk	
Hypertension	Hypertension	Delayed engraftment	Muscle wasting	Fever, chills	Leukopenia
Decreased magnesium	Decreased magnesium	Hepatotoxicity	Infection risk	Skin reactions	Anemia
Tremors (hand)	Tremor		GI hemorrhage		Thrombocytopenia
Neurotoxicity	Neurotoxicity		Hypertension	Hypersensitivity	Gastrointestinal effects
Hyperkalemia	Hyperkalemia			Serum sickness	Headaches
Hirsutism	HUS				
HUS					

HUS, Hemolytic uremic syndrome; *ATG,* antithymocyte globulin.

clinical, as well as the histological, features of gut GVHD.[76] Selective staining for such pathogens must be performed to rule out an infectious agent as the cause of the GI symptoms.

Acute upper GI GVHD has also been described. This form presents with anorexia, dyspepsia, food intolerance, nausea, and vomiting. This syndrome has been documented by upper endoscopic biopsies of the esophagus and stomach and seems to be more responsive to immunosuppressive treatment. If treatment for upper GI aGVHD fails, it frequently progresses to symptomatic lower GI GVHD, suggesting that this syndrome may be an earlier and perhaps more treatable form of intestinal pathology.[122,124]

Effect on the hematopoietic system. The effect of GVHD on the hematopoietic system is usually not dramatic. However, persistent thrombocytopenia is a frequent indication of GVHD. An indirect, long-term issue is decreased responsiveness to active immunization. One study suggests that immune responses to polio vaccination resulted in less protection in those patients who had GVHD.[24,55]

Staging and overall grade. The staging system for aGVHD is presented in Table 8-5. Each of the stages of involvement of each organ are combined to obtain an overall aGVHD grade. Grades II to IV aGVHD are usually defined as clinically significant. Grade I aGVHD is mild GVHD, grade II is moderate, and grades III and IV are severe. The overall grading is important in assessing response to prophylaxis or treatment, impact on survival, and graft-versus-leukemia effect. Patients with moderate to severe GVHD have a significantly higher mortality rate.[65] One difficulty with both the

organ involvement and the overall grading of GVHD is that most of the initial reports and observations occurred before the use of cyclosporine. Since cyclosporine, and other drugs added in combination, aGVHD may have a different sequence of events, even though the overall organ manifestations are the same.

The grading and diagnosis of aGVHD are difficult. In a study conducted by the International Bone Marrow Transplant Registry, six clinical vignettes were evaluated by 49 transplant physicians from 42 bone marrow transplant centers worldwide.[119] The concordance for the diagnosis of aGVHD ranged from 24% to 74%, and the concordance for grading the aGVHD was 55%. The concordance for the decision to treat for aGVHD ranged from 43% to 55%, and the concordance for assigning the primary cause of death was 71% to 100%. These results underscore the need for revision of the scoring criteria as diagnostic methods and knowledge of the disease improve.

Pharmacologic management. Effective prevention is by far the most important part of aGVHD management. Combination prophylaxis with cyclosporine as the backbone of therapy has demonstrated the reduction in the incidence of aGVHD. Tacrolimus is currently used instead of cyclosporine for unrelated donor transplants because of its proven superiority for these patients. In the matched donor setting many immunosuppressive drugs have been tested, and their toxicity profiles are included in Table 8-6. In addition to standard drugs such as methotrexate, cyclosporine, tacrolimus, and corticosteroids, new agents—mycophenolate mofetil (CellCept), tresperimus, rapamycin, and daclizumab (Zenapax)—

are now part of the immunosuppressive armamentarium. Tolerance, the establishment of a stable chimera, is a critical concept to understand and develop safer methods for allogeneic transplantation. This improved understanding of tolerance has resulted in new approaches to the prevention of GVHD.[8,27,33,56,82]

POSTTRANSPLANT PERIOD

CHRONIC GRAFT-VERSUS-HOST DISEASE

Chronic graft-versus-host disease (cGVHD) occurs either as a progression from aGVHD, de novo disease, or after a period of quiescence from acute disease. The clinical and pathologic findings of cGVHD resemble features of the autoimmune collagen-vascular diseases, such as scleroderma, systemic lupus erythematosus, and rheumatoid arthritis. Principal target organs are the skin, liver, and lung, although ocular, oral, GI, and neuromuscular involvement is also seen.[41] Chronic GVHD is the single major determinant of long-term outcome and quality of life following allogeneic HSCT. The associated morbidity and mortality remain a grave and persistent problem in the posttransplant setting.

A secondary effect of cGVHD is marked immunodeficiency. Chronic GVHD and its treatment are immunosuppressive. Chronic GVHD also causes a delay in the recovery of immune function. These patients remain immunodeficient for as long as the disease is active. T and B lymphocyte control remains dysregulated.[6] Prolonged observation of these patients will usually show recurrent infections in up to 100%. These infectious complications account for the majority of morbidity and mortality associated with cGVHD. Chronic GVHD is defined as limited or extensive, depending on the clinical presentation (Table 8-7).

Skin

The most frequent feature of cGVHD is skin involvement.[6] The lesions resemble lichen planus and scleroderma. Inflammatory changes occur first, followed by fibrotic changes. The destructive fibrosing inflammatory reactions occur around the eccrine coils and deep dermal nerves and in the subcutaneous fat. Skin biopsy specimens show dermal fibrosis and epidermal atrophy. Patchy hyperpigmented or hypopigmented changes are noted in the periorbital areas, in sites of previous trauma, in the axillas and elbows, and in undergarment areas. Affected skin becomes progressively more indurated and adheres to the underlying fascia. The dermis becomes thickened with pressure point ulcerations and the development of joint contractures[24,41,78] (Figure 8-9).

Liver

Chronic liver GVHD is also frequently observed. A biopsy specimen may show lobular hepatitis, chronic persistent hepatitis, or chronic active hepatitis. There is a reduction or absence of small bile ducts with cholestasis and primary biliary sclerosis.[24] Hepatic function tests show a predominant cholestatic obstructive picture. The degree of hyperbilirubinemia may not reflect the ultimate outcome. Patients may have persistent hyperbilirubinemia for many years before either improvement or severe hepatic failure develops.

Gastrointestinal Tract

The gut is another frequent site of cGVHD. The oral mucosa is involved in the majority of patients

TABLE 8-7	GRADING OF CHRONIC GVHD
Grade	**Organ Involvement**
Limited	Localized skin involvement and/or hepatic dysfunction
Extensive	Generalized skin involvement and any of the following: • Liver histology showing chronic progressive hepatitis, bridging necrosis, or cirrhosis • Eye involvement (Schirmer's test with <5 mm wetting) • Involvement of minor salivary glands or oral mucosa • Involvement of any other organ

Data from Klingebiel, T., & Schlegel, P. G. (1998). GVHD: Overview of pathophysiology, incidence, clinical and biological features. *Bone Marrow Transplantation, 21*(Suppl. 2), 545-549.

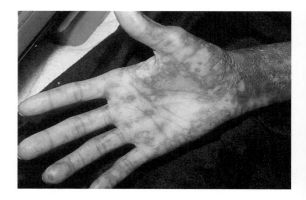

Figure 8-9

Skin cGVHD.

with extensive cGVHD. Patients develop dryness with pain secondary to ulceration. Erythema with lichenoid lesions of the buccal and labial mucosa correlates with cGVHD (Figure 8-10). Increasing oral symptoms, either increasing ulceration or pain, seem to be associated with progression of cGVHD. The esophagus is also involved, and patients may develop dysphagia, painful ulcers, and indolent weight loss.[6] If the small bowel and colon are involved, the patient will develop chronic diarrhea, malabsorption, fibrosis of the submucosa, and sclerosis of the intestine.[6,24]

Lung

Obstructive lung disease may develop in patients with cGVHD and appears to be refractory to therapy.[24] Bronchiolitis obliterans, which causes destruction of small airways, may be seen. The possible etiologies of bronchiolitis obliterans include pulmonary infections (especially viral or mycoplasma), radiation damage, toxic inhalants, connective tissue diseases, and pulmonary alveolar proteinosis.[110] It is unclear whether the lungs are a primary or secondary target in cGVHD. Clinically, patients present with dyspnea and a nonproductive cough, which usually lead to progressive respiratory failure.[24]

Other Manifestations

Manifestations of cGVHD have been observed in almost all organ systems, including ophthalmic, gynecologic, and musculoskeletal. The clinical picture is associated with fibrosis of the organ.[6,109,111]

IMMUNOLOGIC RECOVERY

Children undergoing stem cell transplantation, particularly in the allogeneic setting, have compromised immune systems for variable periods of time

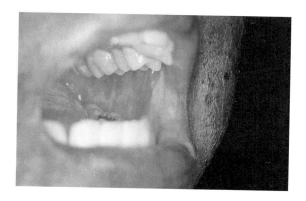

Figure 8-10

Oral mucosa cGVHD.

after hematopoietic reconstitution. This delay appears to occur irrespective of significant infections or immunosuppressive therapy.[105] The speed of immune recovery in the posttransplant period depends on the disease state before transplant, the type of transplant, and the source of stem cells. The delays in reconstitution may be increased by pretransplant myeloablative and immunosuppressive therapy, immunosuppressive therapy for active GVHD, prolonged therapy for CMV, and the presence of cGVHD.[115] Delayed immune recovery can lead to acute or chronic infections and nutritional deficiencies.

Periodic immune assessment of transplant recipients shows that each has a different rate and extent of immunologic recovery. Both cellular and humoral immunity are evaluated by laboratory tests, such as absolute lymphocyte counts, serum immunoglobulin levels, CD4+/CD8+ ratios, and mitogen studies. In general, periodic immunologic evaluations every 3 months posttransplant are recommended so that treatment can be custom tailored to each child's immunologic deficiency. Both antiviral and antifungal prophylaxis are continued until a reconstitution of both cellular and humoral responses has occurred.[60,115]

Reimmunization is performed after documented immune reconstitution, when the ability to form long-term durable memory to vaccines is present. Based on the recommendations of the Committee on Infectious Disease of the American Academy of Pediatrics, patients are usually evaluated at 12 months following HSCT for reimmunization.[87]

LONG-TERM EFFECTS

Because the use of hematopoietic HSCT has expanded and advances in supportive care have contributed to improved survival rates, a rapidly growing population of transplant survivors now exists. Knowledge of the long-term complications of HSCT is important in determining the appropriate follow-up evaluations and treatment for these patients.[34]

Many survivors return to their primary care team with occasional evaluation by the transplant team. To ensure a smooth transition, it is imperative to develop multidisciplinary teams, surveillance plans, and tested approaches that will include early detection of recurrence, recognition of late effects from transplantation, therapeutic modalities for late organ dysfunction, and appropriate counseling of transplant survivors. (Refer to Chapter 18 for additional information about late effects seen in childhood cancer survivors.) Late complications following HSCT may arise from delayed effects of pretransplant conditioning, relapse of malignancy, secondary neoplasms, or cGVHD (Box 8-6).

RELAPSE AFTER HEMATOPOIETIC STEM CELL TRANSPLANT

Relapse of the primary malignancy remains the most frequent cause of treatment failure following autologous and allogeneic HSCT. In general, risk factors predicting a poor response to chemotherapy also apply to stem cell transplantation. The presence of cytogenetic abnormalities associated with an unfavorable prognosis also predicts a higher probability of relapse after HSCT.

Relapse After Allogeneic HSCT

Allogeneic transplants are most commonly used to treat leukemia. Leukemia relapse following transplant can be systemic, and in most instances progression is rapid. Extramedullary relapses are not uncommon. There are several potential ways to treat leukemic relapses, and no single way is effective in all patients.[110]

Discontinuing immunosuppressive therapy has been successful in some patients. Cessation of immunosuppression triggers GVHD in some patients with an associated decline in leukemic cells. Without the development of GVHD the antileukemic response may be only transient. This approach has also been combined with other immunotherapy approaches (e.g., donor lymphocyte infusion) to maximize the antileukemic potential.

Second transplants have been used with variable success in an attempt to change the course of the disease. This strategy and its success depend on the time interval from HSCT to relapse, the intensity of prior therapy, the disease stage, the performance status of the patient, and the availability of a donor. Second transplants performed less than 1 year after the first transplant are associated with high mortality. The use of PBSCs instead of marrow for the second HSCT has become common practice and is presumed to confer a greater leukemic effect.[66]

To take advantage of the graft-versus-leukemia reaction, additional lymphocytes may be collected from the donor and given to relapsed patients. This is referred to as a donor lymphocyte infusion. Responses to donor lymphocyte infusions are most effective in patients with recurrent chronic myelogenous leukemia and in some patients with acute myeloid leukemia and myelodysplastic syndrome. Responses in acute lymphoblastic leukemia are rare. The major complication of donor lymphocyte infusion is GVHD, which can be modified by the depletion of CD8+ T cells from the lymphocyte concentrate or by transfusing very low numbers of cells and increasing doses in a stepwise fashion.[83]

Relapse After Autologous HSCT

Patients who relapse following autologous transplantation have a poor prognosis, with limited curative options available. Second autologous transplants have rarely been successful because of the patient's performance and/or organ status or resistance of the underlying malignancy. The use of autologous HSCT in high risk solid tumor patients has therefore centered around transplanting earlier in the disease course, improving and intensifying the preparative regimens, purging of tumor cells from the graft more efficiently, performing tandem transplants, and administering posttransplant immunotherapy in minimal residual disease.

PSYCHOSOCIAL AND ETHICAL PERSPECTIVES

Many of the ethical issues involved in HSCT are similar to those raised in other areas using advanced technologies.[31] These issues revolve around patient autonomy and informed consent, fair allocation of resources, beneficence and nonmaleficence, and fidelity or nonabandonment when the goals shift from treatment to palliation.[106] Stem cell teams have to contend with donors who are often minors, the great financial expense of the procedure, controversies around reimbursement, and the fact that transplant survivors may be cured of their primary diseases but left with other secondary chronic conditions.

Pediatric HSCT patients and their families face many psychosocial and emotional stressors throughout the transplant process. These include prolonged hospitalization, physical and emotional isolation, persistent uncertainty, role changes, financial strain, frequent invasive medical procedures, physical discomfort, changing medical status, treatment related side effects, and the possibility of infections, severe complications, relapse, or death.[128] The child's ability to cope with the psychosocial aspects of transplant depend on the child's age, cognitive level, personality, and supportive network. Refer to Chapter 15 for additional information about psychosocial support for children with cancer.

The psychologic sequelae related to transplantation reach beyond the patient and parents to the siblings. Additional stressors for the siblings include separation from the patient and at least one parent, changes in family dynamics, and increased anxiety if family HLA typing occurs. In many cases the preferred donor for the patient is a sibling. Few studies have looked at the effect on siblings, but those that have suggest much more attention is needed in this area. Siblings competing for the role of donor can feel excluded, disappointed, or relieved if not chosen. A sibling donor may experience a closer bond to the patient but also may feel guilty if the transplant is not successful. A recent study found that donor siblings had increased anxiety and lower self-esteem but showed more adaptive skills in school when compared with the nondonor siblings. Nondonor siblings exhibited more problems in school, and one third of both groups reported moderate levels of posttraumatic stress reaction.[85]

Each stage in the trajectory of the stem cell transplant process is associated with a fairly predictable set of physical and psychologic stressors. Andrykowski and McQuellon[3] organized the issues into five distinct stages: (1) the decision to undergo HSCT, (2) pre-HSCT preparation, (3) post-HSCT hospitalization, (4) hospital discharge and early post-HSCT recovery, and (5) long-term recovery.

The decision to undergo HSCT forces older children, adolescents, and parents to confront the possibility of death, manage the uncertainty of treatment outcome, and undergo an unclear informed consent process. Pre-HSCT preparation forces patients and families to maintain hope in the midst of strangers, separation from friends and siblings, participation in unfamiliar routines, and often painful procedures. Children in the acute phase may be in pain, while also coping with boredom and isolation. They must manage discouragement and impatience as they await engraftment. In the ambulatory follow-up period children and adolescents are asked to contend with frequent, long medical appointments and complex self-care guidelines and medical rituals. Continued isolation from friends and school can produce difficulties in reintegrating to social roles and can cause depression and apathy. Finally, the long-term recovery stage brings the challenges of accepting any long-term effects, assuming a nonpatient identity, and returning to school and other social roles after a prolonged absence.

Among other HSCT challenges facing patients and families are the hidden, indirect costs of transplant. Parents find they never adequately calculated for the loss of income as they take time off to stay with the child in the hospital for prolonged periods of time, and later at home, to care for the child. Transportation costs, food, lodging, and babysitting often add to the family's financial burdens. Once the child returns home, the caregivers face the physical and emotional challenges associated with the total responsibility for the child's care—caregiving demands that are difficult to objectively measure.

Comprehensive patient and family education and support remain integral to positive outcomes in transplantation. After discharge, caregivers are expected to manage all of the daily "nursing" care, determine what constitutes an emergency, develop organizational skills, deliver complex care, meet the needs of other children, and run a household. The educational plan must assess the readiness and abilities of the designated caregiver(s) and prepare the caregiver(s) for these demands.

ACUTE AMBULATORY TRANSPLANT CONCEPTS

ACUTE AMBULATORY FOLLOW-UP

The transition from acute treatment and care is no longer synonymous with moving from inpatient to outpatient. More and more patients are receiving therapies traditionally associated with inpatient hospitalization in the ambulatory or home care settings. These include multiple antibiotics, immunoglobulin, blood products, parenteral nutrition, chemotherapy, and electrolyte replacement.[18] Select conditioning regimen administration and GVHD management are now routinely done in outpatient settings. The definition of discharge criteria has undergone significant revision.

Most patients will require regular monitoring and follow-up for the first year following the transplant. Expected patient needs include symptom and toxicity management, nutritional monitoring, immunoglobulin, viral and fungal prophylaxis, routine blood test analysis, central line care, monitoring follow-up protocols, and physical assessment. The goal of outpatient care is to minimize toxicity, reduce complications, and when care has been stabilized, return patients to the care of their referring oncologist or primary physician. Typically, a recipient will remain under the care of the stem cell transplant team until there is evidence of immunoreconstitution and the patient is free of major transplant-related complications.

Advances in PBSCT have led to its increased use for autologous transplants. Because of well-established safety, efficacy, and feasibility, components of PBSCT have been increasingly performed in the outpatient setting. Certain allogeneic regimens using submyeloablative or immunoablative therapy and their posttransplant care are also shifting to the ambulatory setting. Administration of intensive conditioning chemotherapy, stem cell infusions, and PBSC harvesting can also be done in selected outpatient facilities. For the adult stem cell transplant population, posttransplant care with uncomplicated neutropenia has been widely accepted in the ambulatory setting. Until recently there was unwillingness to consider this option for pediatric patients. Misconceptions exist among pediatric oncologists and transplanters regarding the practicality of pediatric outpatient transplantation. Concerns include issues of infection, safety, limited isolation, patient compliance, facility, and staffing requirements.

Despite real or perceived concerns, the emphasis on health care cost containment has shifted much of the complex care and transplant treatment from the inpatient to the outpatient setting. In addition to the economic trends, the new therapeutic directions in stem cell transplantation—immunobiologic approaches using submyeloablative conditioning regimens with much less aplasia and therefore less risk—have also enabled more outpatient care. The combination will have significant impact on the care provided in the outpatient setting.

The success of pediatric outpatient transplantation depends on the established infrastructure that supports it. It is essential to have a seamless, integrated program that includes the ambulatory clinical facility, the apheresis center, transitional housing, and a dedicated home care provider. Other critical outpatient components are established standards of care and clinical algorithms, stringent patient selection criteria, and a system of communication and accountability. Knowledge of the actual outpatient program costs is important since resource allocation and utilization, as well as cost accounting, often become nebulous and difficult to quantify in the ambulatory care setting. Lastly, outcomes monitoring and analysis is critical not only to document clinical success and quality, but also to provide financial data to the transplant center and to payors. Creating and maintaining a program with a clear focus on both clinical and economic

---

BOX 8-7

TRANSPLANT TRANSITIONAL HOUSING: NECESSARY SERVICES AND CAPABILITIES

A transplant-oriented housing facility must be able to accommodate the following:
- Nursing assessment and patient education
- IV infusion and total parenteral nutrition (TPN) therapy
- Central venous catheters and peripherally inserted central catheter (PICC) lines
- Medication administration and counseling
- Wound care
- Respiratory therapy services
- Provision of durable medical equipment
- Individual family dwellings or rooms with separate bathroom facilities

---

outcomes will maximize the financial advantage of outpatient transplantation while guaranteeing quality care delivery.

Access to a transitional housing facility has become a necessity to most transplant programs. This type of housing can serve as an alternative to an inpatient hospitalization or repeated outpatient visits. Transitional housing can facilitate the administration of uncomplicated infusional care, monitoring of laboratory values, and ongoing physical assessment by home health care personnel. They also tend to be a source of significant patient and family satisfaction. In many centers transitional housing facilities and home care providers have formed partnerships to provide daily care outside the transplant facility (Box 8-7).

HOME CARE PARTNERSHIPS

Home health care services provide the transplant community with the opportunity to increase patient and family satisfaction while delivering quality, cost-effective patient care. McBride, Richards, Kelley, et al.[77] believe the working relationship between the transplant team and the home health care team can successfully promote continuity of care, enhance physical assessment and patient monitoring, minimize complications, and positively affect patient outcomes. When thoughtfully planned, this care can be a safe and cost-effective alternative to the hospital setting.

A successful transplant program–home care provider partnership should not include a shared financial and contractual relationship, but rather a relationship based on shared commitment, mutual benefit, and demonstrated quality and value. It is essential that both parties collaborate to develop

---

BOX 8-8

COMPONENTS OF A TRANSPLANT-ORIENTED HOME CARE PROGRAM

Specialized nursing staff
On-site transplant home health care liaison
Adequate numbers of nursing personnel to meet
    demand
IV pharmacy
Rapid turnaround time on labs/courier pick up
Frequent inventory evaluation
Clinical operating manual
Continuing education of nursing and pharmacy staff
After hours and weekend coverage capable of
    complex triage
Competency-based training and certification,
    specialty clinical training
Marketing and contracting staff
JCAHO accreditation

---

specific guidelines for patient care, patient education, therapy delivery, and communication. The partners must be able to accurately measure and monitor clinical and economic outcomes. A primary home health care provider is ideal, but usually not realistic nor competitive. With the restricted referrals of managed care, it is prudent to develop relationships with several home health care programs. Services from a transplant-oriented home health care agency should be negotiated with all payors, especially those who have limited coverage or wish to use less qualified providers. If the transplant program cannot trust the skill level of a home health care agency, it will not use home health care to the fullest extent.[63] This will result in greater inpatient and ambulatory resource use and an economic disadvantage for both payor and the clinical program. Transplant home health care partners also have a stake in the negotiations. It is in their best interest to have contracts with a wide variety of national payor networks. A well-accepted home health care program can facilitate the referral process and help all parties to negotiate rates and services more efficiently.

Transplant-associated home health care is not traditional home health care, limited to infusional care, lab draws, and nursing assessment. The level of care must be high tech with pediatric and oncologic skills, similar to the care administered in the hospital facility.[84] When selecting a home health care partner(s), the transplant program must critically analyze the clinical, administrative, operational, and data management capabilities of the selected candidates (Box 8-8).

DESIGNING A SUCCESSFUL TRANSPLANT PROGRAM: KEY OPERATIONAL ISSUES

Business Planning

Pediatric stem cell transplantation is undergoing evolution. At the same time HSCT programs are challenged by the dramatic pressures on the health care system to control costs, ensure quality of care, and curb overutilization of services. Designing a successful transplant program therefore requires a strategic business plan with the following components: (1) program and practice integration; (2) facility design or redesign and/or construction based on state-of-the-art clinical concepts; (3) operational start up/equipment procurement; (4) recruitment of qualified administrative directors; (5) analysis, outcome measures, and benchmarking; and (6) personnel role definition and development.[2,62]

Hematopoietic Stem Cell Transplant Contracting and Case Rating

The rapidly advancing field of stem cell transplant presents both challenges and opportunities for provider-side managed care. The operative concern is that the managed care contract must reflect the reality of the clinical care being administered. To accomplish this, the managed care negotiations have to continually incorporate new treatment paradigms.

Developing a mutually beneficial partnership with payors has taken on increasing importance as new stem cell protocols are being implemented. It is incumbent on the provider to assist payors to understand the newest technologies and treatment protocols. To address the educational needs, a team approach for negotiations is needed with integration of managed care and clinical expertise. Including a stem cell clinician in the negotiations will allow immediate responses and increase the ability to quickly explain the particulars of specific protocols.

Pricing and inclusion protocols are developed from clinical algorithms. The ability to define and elaborate protocol particulars to payors is critical. The provider has the responsibility to explain the new or changing models of care, the movement of care from inpatient to outpatient, and disease therapies during or after the transplant process. Experience has shown that a payor educated in the fundamentals of how and why a specific protocol is used has been more likely to support and approve the newest treatment modalities.

In addition to payor education, transplant providers must remain creative and flexible in their approach to contracts. Successfully employed techniques include contracting for case rates that are disease- or protocol-specific and case rates by age.

Negotiations in outpatient transplantation contracting have centered around single versus sequential transplants, partial versus complete approaches, and the extent of home health care involvement. Secondarily, housing and transportation support have to be secured whenever possible. Traditional pediatric stem cell transplant contracts begin with the conditioning regimen and extend through day 100. A traditional contract applied to the outpatient setting with no modifications can be in the best interest of the transplant center, assuming conscientious outpatient resource utilization. Rarely, however, is such a contract extended. More commonly, the contract is for discounted services with inpatient day limitations. Regardless of the type of contract or the payor involved, home health care can present its own distinct problem. Payors often want to include home health care in the total package, forcing transplant centers to then pay the home health care provider. Certain plans have a restricted number of home health care visits per year, which can include physical and occupational services and infusional support (e.g., parenteral nutrition, IV antibiotics). In such plans frugal use of home health care is demanded, affecting the overall outpatient transplant approach.

Effective contracting for coverage of outpatient transplant, as well as the other new therapeutic options, has resulted from adopting an integrated clinical and managed care negotiating approach. With its dual emphasis on education and flexibility, this contracting methodology has secured coverage in the current managed care environment.

Foundation for the Accreditation of Hematopoietic Cell Therapy

The Foundation for the Accreditation of Hematopoietic Cell Therapy (FAHCT) was founded in 1996 by the American Society for Blood and Marrow Transplantation (ASBMT) and the International Society for Hematotherapy and Graft Engineering (ISHAGE). The purpose of this accreditation body was to establish standards for high-quality medical and laboratory practice and to develop and implement voluntary inspection and accreditation.[37]

FAHCT accreditation has been adopted by the major cooperative research groups, comprehensive clinical programs, and payors alike. The emphasis on infrastructure, safety, quality, and standards has been especially helpful to programs under development or expansion.

STEM CELL TRANSPLANT NURSING AS A SUBSPECIALTY

Just as HSCT has undergone revolutionary changes, so have the roles and responsibilities of stem cell transplant nurses (Table 8-8). Significant influences on nursing care include the growing use of hematopoietic stem cell apheresis, outpatient transplant procedures, models that emphasize use of critical pathways and case management, and the increased use of advanced practice nurses.

Nurses working in a stem cell environment require comprehensive basic and advanced didactic and clinical training. Numerous skills are required, including an in-depth knowledge of stem cell transplant concepts, the immune and hematopoietic systems, complex treatment protocols, and a commitment to continuing education about the constantly changing technologies associated with HSCT nursing care.

Outpatient stem cell transplant patients are more acutely ill than ever before and require new treatments and therapies. Outpatient nursing roles are, therefore, adapting to meet this need. Results of a descriptive survey recently published by the Oncology Nursing Society documented that nurses working in oncology ambulatory care settings spend more than 98% of their time completing assessments and infusing chemotherapy.[127] Clearly, ambulatory stem cell transplant nursing will come to evolve as a specialty within a subspecialty practice.

A growing emphasis has been placed on defining the standards for nursing staffing ratios on stem cell transplant units, both inpatient and outpatient. Although standards for ratios or categories of personnel are not yet described in the ambulatory setting, FAHCT standards (B6.610, B6.620) outline ideal training, ratios, and staffing requirements.

A growing role in transplant care has been the use of advanced practice nurses throughout the transplant trajectory. Reductions in training of medical specialists, an increased interest in cost-effective ways of providing acute care, and rapidly growing demand in the absence of available resources have all contributed to this trend.[127]

FUTURE DIRECTIONS

With the application of HSCT in various disorders now widely accepted, the focus in this decade turns to the improvement of survival and reduction of toxicity. New uses for HSCT will also be explored. Extensive research and experimental therapeutics will be carried out worldwide on all aspects of HSCT.

Some of the theorized future directions are gene therapy, in utero HSCT, expansion of the use of cord

TABLE 8-8	**NURSING ROLES IN HEMATOPOIETIC STEM CELL TRANSPLANTATION***
Nursing Role	**Functions**
Staff nurse (inpatient, ambulatory clinic, home health care, apheresis)	Provide/coordinate physical and psychosocial care. Supervise unlicensed assistive personnel. Educate patient/family. Support patient/family. Participate in clinical research.
Coordinator	Organize patient entry into transplant program. Provide clinical consultation for community and direct care staff. Support and educate patient/family (informal and classroom). Collaborate on insurance/reimbursement issues. Collaborate on protocol and program development.
Clinical nurse specialist	Provide clinical consultation to team. Develop clinical practice standards. Conduct, review, utilize research. Orient/educate staff.
Nurse practitioner†	Perform intake history and physical assessment and develop a problem list. Write/individualize admission and daily care orders according to protocol or in collaboration with transplant team. Perform technical procedures (e.g., harvests, lumbar puncture, central line placement) according to attained competencies. Review and respond to laboratory/diagnostic tests. Assess and manage symptoms/side effects of treatment. Perform follow-up examinations. Educate/consult with other team members.
Administrator‡	Prepare/oversee program financial/budgetary issues. Manage/evaluate human resource needs. Coordinate quality assessment/improvement activities. Evaluate/reorganize programs in response to needs/demands. Acts as liaison with insurance programs. Coordinate program accreditation activities.

From Wheadon, M. B., & Fliedner, M. (1999). Nursing issues in hematopoietic cell transplantation. In E. D. Thomas, K. Blume, & S. Forman (Eds.), *Hematopoietic cell transplantation* (pp. 381-385). Malden, MA: Blackwell Science.
*Overlapping functions mandate a high degree of collaboration/communication among nursing team members.
†A developing service role on inpatient units.
‡Often a nurse or nonnurse with an advanced degree in business.

blood banking, adoptive immunotherapy, submyeloablative regimens, and the use of HSCT in nontraditional disorders (autoimmune and degenerative diseases).[22,29,35,80,104] Present therapeutic concepts will be further developed—sequential (tandem) autologous PBSC rescues in high-risk diseases, as well as related and unrelated allogeneic transplantation for the hemoglobinopathies.[46,57,98,125] Opportunities abound for the development of innovative HSCT concepts—from research, to technology, to administrative issues and business development.

ACKNOWLEDGMENT

The authors would like to thank Sandra Mattox, RN, MSN, Clinical Nurse Specialist at St. Jude Children's Research Hospital, for her careful review of the manuscript.

REFERENCES

1. Alegre, A., Diaz, M. A., Madero, L., et al. (1996). Large-volume leukapheresis for peripheral blood stem cell collection in children: A simplified single-apheresis approach. *Bone Marrow Transplantation, 17,* 923-927.
2. Alkire, K., & Shelton, B. K. (1994). Creating critical care oncology beds. *Seminars in Oncology Nursing, 10,* 208-221.
3. Andrykowski, M. A., McQuellon, R. P., Russell, G. B., et al. (1999). Quality of life and psychological distress of bone marrow transplant patients: The time trajectory to recovery over the first year. *Bone Marrow Transplant, 21,* 477-486.
4. Applegate, G. L., Mittal, B. B., Kletzel, M., et al. (1998). Outpatient total body irradiation prior to bone marrow transplantation in pediatric patients: A feasibility analysis. *Bone Marrow Transplant, 21,* 651-652.
5. Armitage, J. O. (1994). Bone marrow transplantation. *New England Journal of Medicine, 330,* 827-838.
6. Atkinson, K. (1990). Review: Chronic graft-versus-host disease. *Bone Marrow Transplantation, 5,* 69-92.

7. Attal, M., Huguet, F., Rubie, H., et al. (1992). Prevention of hepatic veno-occlusive disease after bone marrow transplantation by continuous infusion of low-dose heparin: A prospective, randomized trial. *Blood, 79,* 2834-2835.

8. Basara, N., Blau, W. I., Romer, E., et al. (1998). Mycophenolate mofetil for the treatment of acute and chronic GVHD in bone marrow transplant patients. *Bone Marrow Transplantation, 22,* 61-65.

9. Baxter-Lowe, L. A. (1994). Molecular techniques for typing unrelated marrow donors: Potential impact of molecular typing disparity on donor selection. *Bone Marrow Transplantation, 14*(Suppl. 4), S42-S50.

10. Bearman, S. I., Shen, D. D., Hinds, M. S., et al. (1993). A phase I/II study of prostaglandin E1 for the prevention of hepatic venocclusive disease after bone marrow transplantation. *British Journal of Haematology, 84,* 724-727.

11. Bensinger, W. I. (1998). Editorial: Should we purge? *Bone Marrow Transplantation, 21,* 113-115.

12. Bensinger, W. I., Weaver, C. H., Applebaum, F. R., et al. (1995). Transplantation of allogeneic peripheral blood stem cells mobilized by recombinant human granulocyte colony stimulating factor. *Blood, 85,* 1655-1658.

13. Bianco, J. A., Appelbaum, F. R., Nemunitis, J., et al. (1991). Phase I-II trial of pentoxifylline for the prevention of transplant-related toxicities following bone marrow transplantation. *Blood, 78,* 1205-1210.

14. Blume, K., & Amylon, M. (1999). The evaluation and counseling of candidates for hematopoietic cell transplantation. In E. D. Thomas, K. Blume, & S. Forman (Eds.). *Hematopoietic cell transplantation* (pp. 371-380). Malden, MA: Blackwell Science.

15. Bortin, M. M., Bach, F. H., van Bekkum, B. W., et al. (1994). 25th anniversary of the first successful allogeneic bone marrow transplants. *Bone Marrow Transplant, 14,* 211-212.

16. Bryant, E., & Martin, P. (1999). Documentation of engraftment and characterization of chimerism following hematopoietic cell transplantation. In E. D. Thomas, K. Blume, & S. Forman (Eds.), *Hematopoietic cell transplantation* (pp. 197-206). Malden, MA: Blackwell Science.

17. Buckner, C. D., Meyers, J. D., Springmeyer, S. C., et al. (1984). Pulmonary complications of marrow transplantation. Review of the Seattle experience. *Experimental Hematology, 12* (Suppl. 15), 1-5.

18. Burns, J. M., & Tierney, D. K. (1996). A daily flowsheet for an outpatient bone marrow transplant treatment center. *Oncology Nursing Forum, 23,* 1313-1314.

19. Busca, A., Vivenza, C., Vassalo, E., et al. (1992). Continuous intravenous pentoxifylline in children undergoing bone marrow transplantation. Results of a pilot study. *Blood, 80* (Suppl. 1), 237a.

20. Button, L. N., DeWolf, W. C., Newburger, P. E., et al. (1981). The effects of irradiation on blood components. *Transfusions, 21,* 419-424.

21. Cahn, J. Y., Flesh, M., Brion, A., et al. (1992). Prevention of veno-occlusive disease of the liver after bone marrow transplantation: Heparin or no heparin? *Blood, 80,* 2149-2152.

22. Champlain, R., Khourri, I., & Giralt, S. (1999). Graft-vs-malignancy with allogeneic blood stem cell transplantation: A potential primary treatment modality. *Pediatric Transplantation, 3*(Suppl. 1), 52-58.

23. Chan, C. K., Hyland, R. H., Crawford, S. W., et al. (1990). Pulmonary complications following bone marrow transplantation. *Clinics in Chest Medicine, 11,* 323-332.

24. Chao, N. J. (1999). *Graft-versus-host disease* (2nd ed., pp. 63-122). Austin, TX: R. G. Landes.

25. Chen, A. R. (1999). High-dose therapy with stem cell rescue for pediatric solid tumors: Rationale and results. *Pediatric Transplantation, 3*(Suppl. 1), 78-86.

26. Cohen, S. B. A., Dominiguez, E., Lowdell, M., et al. (1998). The immunological properties of cord blood: Overview of current research presented at the 2nd EUROCORD Workshop. *Bone Marrow Transplantation, 22*(Suppl. 1), S22-S25.

27. Deeg, H. J. (1994). Prophylaxis and treatment of acute graft-versus-host disease: Current state, implications of new immunopharmacologic compounds and future strategies to prevent and treat acute GVHD in high-risk patients. *Bone Marrow Transplantation, 14*(Suppl. 4), S56-S60.

28. Demeocq, F., Kanold, J., Chassagne, J., et al. (1994). Successful blood stem cell collection and transplant in children weighing less than 25 kg. *Bone Marrow Transplantation, 13,* 43-50.

29. Denning-Kendall, P. A., & Horsley, H. (1998). Clinical application of in vitro expansion of cord blood. *Bone Marrow Transplantation, 22*(Suppl. 1), S63-S65.

30. Dracker, R. A. (1996). Cord blood stem cells: How to get them and what to do with them. *Journal of Hematotherapy, 5,* 145-148.

31. Durbin, M. (1988). Bone marrow transplantation: Economic, ethical, and social issues. *Pediatrics, 82,* 774-783.

32. Essell, J. H., Thompson, J. M., Harmon, G. S., et al. (1992). Pilot trial of prophylactic ursodiol to decrease the incidence of veno-occlusive disease of the liver in allogeneic bone marrow transplant patients. *Bone Marrow Transplant, 10,* 367-371.

33. Fay, J. W., Wingard, J. R., Antin, J. H., et al. (1996). FK506 (tacrolimus) monotherapy for prevention of graft-versus-host disease after histocompatible sibling allogeneic bone marrow transplantation. *Blood, 87,* 3514-3519.

34. Fisher, V. L. (1999). Long-term follow-up in hematopoetic stem-cell transplant patients. *Pediatric Transplantation, 3*(Suppl. 1), 122-129.

35. Flake, A., & Zanjani, E. (1999). In utero hematopoietic stem cell transplantation: Ontogenic opportunities and biologic barriers. *Blood, 7,* 2179-2191.

36. Forte, K. (1997). Alternative donor sources in pediatric bone marrow transplantation. *Journal of Pediatric Oncology Nursing, 15,* 213-224.

37. Foundation for the Accreditation of Hematopoietic Cell Therapy (FAHCT). (1997). *Hematopoietic progenitor cell collection, processing and transplantation accreditation manual.* Omaha, NE: Foundation for the Accreditation of Hematopoietic Cell Therapy.

38. Gluckman, E., & Wagner, J. (1994). *Umbilical cord blood cells in transplantation.* Presented at the Keystone Symposium, Keystone, CO.

39. Gluckman, E., Jolivet, I., Scrobohaci, M. L., et al. (1990). Use of prostaglandin E1 for prevention of liver venoocclusive disease in leukemic patients treated by allogeneic bone marrow transplantation. *British Journal of Haematology, 74,* 277-283.

40. Gluckman, E., Rocha, V., Boyer-Chammard, A., et al. (1997). Outcome of cord-blood transplantation from related and unrelated donors. *The New England Journal of Medicine, 337,* 373-381.

41. Gonzalez Ryan, L. (1997). Topical armamentarium in the management of acute and chronic graft-versus-host disease. *Journal of Pediatric Oncology Nursing, 14,* 239-251.

42. Gonzalez Ryan, L., Van Syckle, K., Coyne, K. D., et al. (2000). Umbilical cord blood banking: Procedural and ethical concerns for this new birth option. *Pediatric Nursing, 26* (1), 105-110.

43. Gordon, B., Haire, W., Ruby, E., et al. (1997). Factors predicting morbidity following hematopoietic stem cell transplantation. *Bone Marrow Transplantation, 19,* 497-501.

44. Gordon, M. Y., & Blackett, N. M. (1995). Some factors determining the minimum number of cells required for successful clinical engraftment. *Bone Marrow Transplantation, 15,* 659-662.

45. Gorlin, J. B., Humphreys, D., Kent, P., et al. (1996). Pediatric large volume peripheral blood progenitor cell collections from patients under 25 kg: A primer. *Journal of Clinical Apheresis, 11,* 195-203.

46. Graham Pole, J., Casper, J., Elfenbein, G., et al. (1991). High dose chemoradiotherapy supported by marrow infusions for advanced neuroblastoma: A Pediatric Oncology Group study. *Journal of Clinical Oncology, 9,* 152-158.

47. Guidelines for preventing opportunistic infections among hematopoietic stem cell transplant recipients. Recommendations of the CDC, the Infectious Diseases Society of America, and the American Society of Blood and Marrow Transplantation. (2000). *Biology of Blood and Marrow Transplantation, 6,* #6A Special Issue.

48. Gururangan, S., Dunkel, I. J., Goldman, S., et al. (1998). Myeloablative chemotherapy with autologous bone marrow rescue in young children with recurrent malignant brain tumors. *Journal of Clinical Oncology, 16,* 2486-2493.

49. Hansen, J. A., Choo, S. Y., Geraghty, D. E., et al. (1990). The HLA system in clinical marrow transplantation. *Hematology/Oncology Clinics of North America, 4,* 507-515.

50. Haut, P., Cohn, S., Morgan, E., et al. (1998). Efficacy of autologous peripheral blood stem cell (PBSC) harvest and engraftment after ablative chemotherapy in pediatric patients. *Biology of Blood and Marrow Transplantation, 4,* 38-42.

51. Henslee-Downey, P. J., Parrish, R. S., MacDonald, J. S., et al. (1996). Combined in vitro T-lymphocyte depletion for the control of GVHD following haplo identical marrow transplants. *Transplantation, 61,* 738-745.

52. Horowitz, M. (1999). Uses and growth of hematopoietic cell transplantation. In E. D. Thomas, K. Blume, & S. Forman (Eds). *Hematopoietic cell transplantation* (pp. 12-18). Malden, MA: Blackwell Science.

53. Howe, C. W. S., & Radde-Stepaniak, T. (1999). Hematopoietic cell donor registries. In E. D. Thomas, K. Blume, & S. Forman (Eds). *Hematopoietic cell transplantation* (pp. 503-512). Malden, MA: Blackwell Science.

54. Hurley, C. K., & Ng, J. (1994). Interpretation of DNA-based typing of HLA and correlation with serologic types for bone marrow transplantation: A guide for transplant coordinators. (National Marrow Donor Program). Minneapolis, MN: Georgetown University Press.

55. Iwasaki, T., Fujiwara, H., Shearer, G. M., et al. (1986). Loss of proliferative capacity and T cell immune development potential of bone marrow from mice undergoing a graft-versus-host reaction. *Journal of Immunology, 137,* 3100-3108.

56. Jacobson, P., Uberti, J., & Ratanatharathorn, V. (1998). Review: Tacrolimus: A new agent for the prevention of graft-versus-host disease in hematopoietic stem cell transplantation. *Bone Marrow Transplantation, 22,* 217-225.

57. Jakacki, R. I., Jamison, C., Heifetzs, S. A., et al. (1997). Feasibility of sequential high dose chemotherapy in peripheral blood stem cell support for pediatric central nervous system malignancies. *Medical and Pediatric Oncology, 29,* 553-559.

58. Jones, R. J., Lee, K. S., Beschorner, W. E., et al. (1987). Venocclusive disease of the liver following bone marrow transplantation. *Transplantation, 44,* 778-784.

59. Kanold, J., Halle, P., Berger, M., et al. (1999). Large-volume leukapheresis procedure for peripheral blood progenitor cell collection in children weighing 15 kg or less: Efficacy and safety evaluation. *Medical and Pediatric Oncology, 32,* 7-10.

60. Kapoor, N. (1999). Immunological recovery post-hematopoietic stem cell transplantation: Role of prophylactic prevention of infection in post-transplant period. *Pediatric Transplantation, 3*(Suppl. 1), 14-18.

61. Kawano, Y., Watanabe, T., & Takaue, Y. (1999). Mobilization/harvest and transplantation with blood stem cells, manipulated or unmanipulated. *Pediatric Transplantation, 3*(Suppl. 1), 65-71.

62. Kelleher, J. (1994). Issues for designing marrow transplant programs. *Seminars in Oncology Nursing, 10,* 64-71.

63. Kelley, C. H., Leum, E. A., Randolph, S., et al. (May 1997). Transplant certification course for homecare nurses. Paper presented at the meeting of the Oncology Nursing Society, New Orleans, LA.

64. Kletzel, M., Longino, R., Rademaker, A. W., et al. (1998). Peripheral blood stem cell transplantation in young children: Experience with harvesting, mobilization and engraftment. *Pediatric Transplantation, 2,* 191-196.

65. Klingebiel, T., & Schlegel, P. G. (1998). GVHD: Overview on pathophysiology, incidence, clinical and biological features. *Bone Marrow Transplantation, 21*(Suppl. 2), S45-S49.

66. Korbling, M., & Przepiorka, D. (1995). Allogeneic blood stem cell transplantation for refractory leukemia and lymphoma: Potential advantage of blood over marrow allografts. *Blood, 85,* 1659-1665.

67. Koscielniak, E., Klingebiel, T. H., Peters, C., et al. (1997). Do patients with metastic and recurrent rhabdomyosarcoma benefit from high-dose therapy with hematopoietic rescue? Report of the German/Austrian Pediatric Bone Marrow Transplantation Group. *Bone Marrow Transplantation, 19,* 227-231.

68. Krivit, W., Lockman, L. A., Watkins, P. A., et al. (1995). The future for treatment by bone marrow transplantation for adrenoleukodystrophy, metachromatic leukodystrophy, and globoid cell leukodystrophy and Hurler syndrome. *Journal of Inherited Metabolic Disease, 18,* 398-412.

69. Kurtzberg, J., Laughlin, M. Graham, M. L., et al. (1996). Placental blood as a source of hematopoietic stem cells for transplantation into unrelated recipients. *New England Journal of Medicine, 335,* 157-166.

70. Locatelli, F., Perotti, C., Zecca, M., et al. (1998). Transplantation of peripheral blood stem cells mobilized by haematopoietic growth factors in childhood. *Bone Marrow Transplantation, 22*(Suppl. 5), S51-S55.

71. Madero, L., Munoz, A., de Toldeo, S., et al. (1998). Megatherapy in children with high-risk Ewing's sarcoma in first complete remission. *Bone Marrow Transplantation, 21,* 795-799.

72. Marolleau, J. P., Ternaux, B., Dal Cortivo, L., et al. (1998). T cell repertoire of human umbilical cord blood. *Bone Marrow Transplantation, 22*(Suppl. 1), S39-S40.

73. Marson, P., Petris, M. G., De Silvestro, G., et al. (1998). Collection of peripheral blood stem cells in pediatric patients: A concise review on technical aspects. *Bone Marrow Transplantation, 22*(Suppl. 5), S7-S11.

74. Martin, P. (1999). Overview of marrow transplant immunology. In E. D. Thomas, K. Blume, & S. Forman (Eds.), *Hematopoietic cell transplantation* (pp. 19-27). Malden, MA: Blackwell Science.

75. Matthay, K. K. (1999). Intensification of therapy using hematopoietic stem-cell support for high-risk neuroblastoma. *Pediatric Transplantation, 3*(Suppl. 1), 72-77.

76. Matthes-Martin, S., Aberle, S. W., Peters, C., et al. (1998). CMV-viraemia during allogeneic bone marrow transplantation in paediatric patients: Association with survival and graft-versus-host disease. *Bone Marrow Transplantation, 21*(Suppl. 2), S53-S56.

77. McBride, L. H., Richards R., Kelley, C., et al. (1995). Home care in transplantation: Creating a successful "partnership." *Journal of Transplant Coordination, 5,* 121-129.

78. McCann, S., & Solomon, R. (1991). Chronic graft-versus-host disease: Dermatological manifestations, nursing management, and research with extracorporeal chemophotopheresis. *Dermatology Nursing, 3,* 221-228.

79. McDonald, G. B., Hinds, M. S., Fisher, L. D., et al. (1993). Veno-occlusive disease of the liver and multiorgan failure after bone marrow transplantation: A cohort study of 355 patients. *Annals of Internal Medicine, 118,* 225-230.

80. McIvor, R. S. (1999). Gene therapy of genetic diseases and cancer. *Pediatric Transplantation, 3*(Suppl. 1), 116-121.

81. Miescher, P. A., & Jaffe, E. R. (Eds). (1990). Current approaches to the prevention and treatment of cytomegalovirus disease after bone marrow transplantation. [Special Issue]. *Seminars in Hematology, 27* (2 Suppl. 1), 1-4.

82. Mookerjee, B., Altomonte, V., & Vogelsang, G. (1999). Salvage therapy for refractory chronic graft-versus-host disease with mycophenolate mofetil and tacrolimus. *Bone Marrow Transplantation, 24,* 517-520.

83. Morecki, S., & Slavin, S. (2000). Toward amplification of a graft-versus-leukemia effect while minimizing graft-versus-host disease. *Journal of Hematotherapy and Stem Cell Research, 9,* 355-366.

84. National Association of Children's Hospitals and Related Institutions, Patient Care FOCUS Group, and the Association of Pediatric Oncology Nurses (APON). (2000). Home care requirements for children and adolescents with cancer. *Journal of Pediatric Oncology Nursing, 17,* 45-49.

85. Packman, W. L., Crittenden, M. R., Schaeffer, E., et al. (1997). Psychosocial consequences of bone marrow transplantation in donor and nondonor siblings. *Developmental and Behavioral Pediatrics, 18,* 244-253.

86. Petit, T., Raynal, B., Socie, G., et al. (1994). Highly sensitive PCR reaction methods show frequent survival of residual recipient multipotent progenitors after non T cell depleted bone marrow transplantation. *Blood, 84,* 3575-3583.

87. Peter, G. (Ed.). *2000 Red book: Report of the Committee on Infectious Diseases* (25th ed.). Elk Grove Village, IL: American Academy of Pediatrics.

88. Petz, L. D., Yam, P., Wallace, R. B., et al. (1987). Mixed hematopoietic chimerism following bone marrow transplantation for hematologic malignancies. *Blood, 70,* 1331-1337.

89. Poliquin, C. (1997). Overview of bone marrow and peripheral blood stem cell transplantation. *Clinical Journal of Oncology Nursing, 1,* 11-17.

90. Prentice, H. G., & Kho, P. (1997). Clinical strategies for the management of cytomegalovirus infection and disease in allogeneic bone marrow transplant. *Bone Marrow Transplantation, 19,* 135-142.

91. Quabeck, K. (1994). The lung as a critical organ in marrow transplantation. *Bone Marrow Transplantation, 14*(Suppl. 4), S19-S28.

92. Quan, C., & Bowden, R. A. (1993). Clinical aspects of cytomegalovirus infection in marrow transplantation. *Marrow Transplantation Reviews, 3*(2), 17-21, 32.

93. Rowe, J. M., Ciobanu, N., Thompson, H., et al. (1994). Recommended guidelines for the management of autologous and allogeneic bone marrow transplantation. *Annals of Internal Medicine, 120,* 143-158.

94. Rubinstein, P., Rosenfield, R. E., Adamson, J. W., et al. (1993). Stored placental blood for unrelated bone marrow reconstitution. *Blood, 81,* 1679-1690.

95. Sable, C. A., & Dunowitz, G. R. (1994). Infections in bone marrow transplant recipients. *Clinical Infectious Diseases, 18,* 273-284.

96. Sanders, J. E. (1999). Stem-cell transplant preparative regimens. *Pediatric Transplantation, 3*(Suppl. 1), 23-34.

97. Sanders, J., & Buckner, C. D. (1987). Experience in the marrow harvesting from donors less than two years of age. *Bone Marrow Transplant, 12,* 45-50.

98. Santana, V. M., Schell, M. J., Williams, R., et al. (1992). Escalating sequential high dose carboplatin and etoposide with autologous support in children with relapsed solid tumors. *Bone Marrow Transplantation, 10,* 47-52.

99. Schuyler, B. (1997). Progress in the use of hematopoietic stem cell. *Hemasphere, 10*(3), 1, 5-6.

100. Seber, A., Shu, X. O., DeFor, T., et al. (1999). Risk factors of severe hemorrhagic cystitis following bone marrow transplantation. *Bone Marrow Transplant, 23,* 35-40.

101. Shea, T. C., Mason, J. R., Storniolo, A. M., et al. (1992). Sequential cycles of high dose carboplatin administered with recombinant human granulocyte/macrophage colony stimulating factor and repeated infusion of autologous peripheral/blood progenitor cells: A novel and effective method of delivering multiple courses of dose intensive therapy. *Journal of Clinical Oncology, 10,* 464-473.

102. Shulman, H. M., & Hinterberger, W. (1992). Hepatic veno-occlusive disease-liver toxicity syndrome after marrow transplantation. *Bone Marrow Transplant, 10,* 197-214.

103. Slavin, S., Nagler, A., Naparstek, E., et al. (1998). Non-myeloablative stem cell transplantation and cell therapy as an alternative to conventional bone marrow transplantation with lethal cytoreduction for the treatment of malignant and non-malignant hematologic diseases. *Blood, 91,* 756-763.

104. Slavin, S., Nagler, A., Varadi, G., et al. (2000). Graft vs autoimmunity following allogeneic non-myeloablative blood stem cell transplantation in a patient with chronic myelogenous leukemia and severe psoriasis and psoriatic polyarthritis. *Experimental Hematology, 28,* 853-857.

105. Smith, F. O., & Thomson, B. (1999). T-cell recovery following marrow transplant: Experience with delayed lymphocyte infusions to accelerate immune recovery or treat infectious problems. *Pediatric Transplantation, 3*(Suppl. 1), 59-64.

106. Snyder, D. (1999). Ethical issues in hematopoietic cell transplantation. In E. D. Thomas, K. Blume, & S. Forman (Eds.), *Hematopoietic cell transplantation* (pp. 390-397). Malden, MA: Blackwell Science.

107. Speiser, D. E., Tiercy, J. M., Rufer, N., et al. (1996). High resolution HLA matching associated with decreased mortality after unrelated bone marrow transplantation. *Blood, 87,* 4455-4462.

108. Spitzer, G., Kicke, K., & Zander, A. R. (1984). High dose chemotherapy with autologous bone marrow transplantation. *Cancer, 54,* 1216-1225.

109. Sullivan, K. M. (1986). Acute and chronic graft-versus-host disease in man. *International Journal of Cell Cloning, 4*(Suppl. 1), 42-93.

110. Sullivan, K. M., & Agura, E. (1991). Chronic graft versus host disease and other late complications of bone marrow transplantation. *Seminars in Hematology, 28,* 250-259.

111. Sullivan, K. M., Witherspoon, R. P., Storb, R., et al. (1988). Alternating-day cyclosporine and prednisone for treatment of high-risk chronic graft-v-host disease. *Blood, 72,* 555-561.

112. Takaue, Y., Kawano, Y., Abe, T., et al. (1995). Collection and transplantation of peripheral blood stem cells in very small children weighing 20 kg or less. *Blood, 86,* 372-380.

113. Thomas, E. D., Storb, R., Clift, R. A., et al. (1975). Bone marrow transplantation. *New England Journal of Medicine, 292,* 832-843, 895-902.

114. Thompson, C. (1995). Umbilical cords: Turning garbage into gold. *Science, 268,* 805-806.

115. Trigg, M. E. (1999). Can we make some general recommendations regarding immune recovery after hematopoietic reconstitution preceded by ablative therapy? *Pediatric Transplantation, 3*(Suppl. 1), 45-51.

116. Trigg, M. E. (1999). Marrow transplantation in children: Current results and controversies—Meeting No. 4. *Pediatric Transplantation, 3*(Suppl. 1), 7-8.

117. Urban, C., Weber, G., Slavc, I., et al. (1990). Anesthetic management of marrow harvesting from a 7-week-old premature baby. *Bone Marrow Transplant, 6,* 443-444.

118. van Rood, J. J., & Oudshoorn, M. (1998). The quest for a bone marrow donor—optimal or maximal HLA matching? *The New England Journal of Medicine, 339,* 1238-1239.

119. Vogelsang, G. V. (1992). Acute graft-versus-host disease following marrow transplantation. *Marrow Transplantation Reviews, 2,* 49-64.

120. Wagner, J. E., Broxmeyer, H. E., Byrd, R. L., et al. (1992). Transplantation of umbilical cord blood after myeloablative therapy: Analysis of engraftment. *Blood, 79,* 1874-1881.

121. Wagner, J. E., Rosenthal, J., Sweetman, R., et al. (1996). Successful transplantation of HLA-matched and HLA-mismatched umbilical cord blood from unrelated donors: Analysis of engraftment and acute graft-versus-host disease. *Blood, 88,* 795-802.

122. Wakui, M., Okamoto, S., Ishida, A., et al. (1999). Prospective evaluation for upper gastrointestinal tract acute graft-versus-host disease after hematopoietic stem cell transplantation. *Bone Marrow Transplantation, 23,* 573-578.

123. Walters, M. C., Patience, M., Leisenring, W., et al. (1996). Bone marrow transplantation for sickle cell disease. *New England Journal of Medicine, 335,* 369-376.

124. Weisdorf, D., Snover, D., Haake, R., et al. (1990). Acute upper gastrointestinal GVHD: Clinical significance and response to immunosuppressive therapy. *Blood, 76,* 624-629.

125. Weissman, I. (2000). Translating stem and progenitor biology to the clinic: Barriers and opportunities, *Science, 287,* 1442-1446.

126. Welte, K. (1994). Matched unrelated transplants. *Seminars in Oncology Nursing, 10,* 20-27.

127. Whedon, M. B., & Fliedner, M. (1999). Nursing issues in hematopoietic cell transplantation. In E. D. Thomas, K. Blume, & S. Forman (Eds.), *Hematopoietic cell transplantation* (pp. 381-385). Malden, MA: Blackwell Science.

128. Wiley, F. M., Lindamood, M. M., & Pfefferbaum-Levine, B. (1984). Donor-patient relationships in pediatric bone marrow transplantation. *Journal of the Association of Pediatric Oncology Nurses, 1*(3), 8-14.

129. Woolfrey, A., & Anasetti, C. (1999). Allogeneic hematopoietic stem-cell engraftment and graft failure. *Pediatric Transplantation, 3*(Suppl. 1), 35-40.

9

Complementary and Alternative Treatments

Janice Post-White
Susan F. Sencer
Maura A. Fitzgerald

Children with cancer use many different types of complementary and alternative medicine (CAM). Most of these therapies are employed as adjuncts to conventional medical therapy (complementary), as opposed to those that replace standard care (alternative). Despite the prevalent use of CAM in both adults and children with cancer,[12,13] there are few published results documenting the safety and efficacy of CAM therapies in cancer care and whether they lead to improved quality of life and positive clinical outcomes.

Nurses can provide comprehensive care and healing by documenting the use of CAM by their patients and by providing an open and safe environment to discuss CAM. Parents of children with cancer often choose CAM as a way to participate in their child's care, manage side effects, cope with emotional effects, feel more hopeful,[45] and reduce the pain and suffering of their children.[49] Parents need assistance to sort out the myriad resources of varying quality and to evaluate the use of CAM in conjunction with standard cancer treatment. Many pediatric oncology nurses have also been trained in various CAM modalities, such as imagery, massage, aromatherapy, or healing touch.

DEFINITION OF COMPLEMENTARY AND ALTERNATIVE MEDICINE

Although the terms *complementary* and *alternative* are used interchangeably, there are important differences. The American Cancer Society defines complementary therapies as those methods that add to or support conventional treatments.[2] These methods do not claim to cure cancer, but rather to assist with symptom control. There are a wide variety of complementary therapies, including spiritual and psychologic approaches, energy medicine, and nutritional and pharmacologic therapies. Alternative treatments generally fall outside the main-

stream of conventional medicine. These interventions may claim to cure cancer. In general, alternative treatments have not been scientifically tested or have been tested and found to be ineffective.[2,6]

The dialogue around CAM had led to an appreciation of the need to integrate the body, mind, and spirit to promote wellness. A new entity, integrative medicine, reflects a fusion of CAM practices and conventional medicine. Integrative medicine in pediatric oncology seeks to improve the supportive care available to patients and to determine through scientific clinical trials which adjuvant CAM therapies are medically sound and compatible with conventional chemotherapy and radiation.

The National Center for Complementary and Alternative Medicine of the National Institutes of Health (NCCAM, NIH) has grouped CAM therapies into five major domains[39] (Box 9-1). This framework provides an overview of the field.

USE OF CAM IN PEDIATRIC CANCER CARE

Pediatric surveys indicate a surge in CAM use over the past 20 years.[12,13] These trends are worldwide, with 31% to 46% use in children with cancer in the Netherlands,[25] Finland,[40] British Columbia,[50] and Australia.[51] Similar rates are reported in the United States, with 59% use in the Midwest,[45] 65% in Florida,[21] and 84% in New York City.[29] The most common therapies employed are prayer and spiritual healing, nutritional supplements, vitamins, massage, and mind-body therapies.[14,21,29,45] European countries are more likely to use homeopathy, bioelectric therapies,[25] and micronutrients.[40]

Almost all families view CAM as an adjunct to conventional therapy.[14,25] Less than 2% used it without conventional care.[8] Families relied on CAM as the sole treatment most often in the face of an extremely poor prognosis.[14,25] Many families

---

BOX 9-1

NCCAM DOMAINS OF COMPLEMENTARY AND ALTERNATIVE MEDICINE

1. Alternative Medical Systems
   a. Traditional oriental/Chinese medicine—emphasizes proper balance of qi (life force energy); includes acupuncture, herbal medicine, qigong (energy based practice to cultivate one's life force to promote healing), and oriental massage
   b. Ayurveda—India's traditional medicine with the goal of restoring harmony of the body, mind, and spirit; includes diet, exercise, meditation, herbs, massage, controlled breathing, and sunlight
   c. Homeopathy—based on the principle that like cures like; use of minute doses of plant extracts to stimulate body's defenses specific to condition
   d. Naturopathy—views disease as alterations in the natural healing process—includes diet; nutrition; homeopathy; acupuncture; herbal medicine; hydrotherapy; spinal and soft-tissue manipulation; physical therapies using electric current, ultrasound, and light therapy; therapeutic counseling; and pharmacology to restore natural healing
2. Mind-Body Interventions
   a. Standard care: patient education, cognitive-behavioral therapies, and imagery/relaxation
   b. Untested interventions: meditation, certain uses of hypnosis, dance, music, art therapy, prayer, and mental healing
3. Biologic Based Therapies
   a. Natural and biologically based practices, interventions, and products
   b. Special dietary programs and herbal, orthomolecular (supplements/chemicals), and individual biologic therapies
4. Manipulative and Body-Based Methods
   a. Chiropractic manipulation of skeletal structure
   b. Osteopathic manipulation of musculoskeletal system
   c. Massage therapy manipulation of soft tissues
5. Energy Therapies
   a. Intent to direct energy fields originating within the body (biofields) or from other sources (electromagnetic fields)
   b. Qigong, reiki (practice of laying on of hands to exchange energy with the intention to heal), healing touch, therapeutic touch, and bioelectromagnetic therapies (pulsed fields, magnetic fields, alternating current, direct current fields)

Data from National Center for Complementary and Alternative Medicine, National Institutes of Health. (2000). Major domains of complementary and alternative medicine. http://nccam.nih.gov/nccam/fcp/classify/ Accessed 9/25/00.

(43% to 55%), however, did not tell their health care providers that they used CAM.[14,29,45] Some parents (18%) did not tell their child's health care provider because they were never asked.[45] In one large study 85% of children receiving CAM were simultaneously enrolled in clinical trials for primary treatment of their cancer.[29]

The push toward integrative medicine has primarily come from patients and parents, who perceive CAM as being more patient friendly and more natural. This natural approach is appealing because of the debilitating side effects of chemotherapy and radiation. However, because most pediatric cancers are curable with conventional treatment, the health care team must stress that CAM therapies may be, at best, positive adjuncts to conventional treatment. There is currently no cure for any type of cancer with complementary therapies alone, and there is little scientific evidence that CAM therapies increase survival, extend life, or improve quality of life. Nonetheless, preliminary and anecdotal evidence suggests that some therapies offer relief of symptoms associated with cancer treatment.[55,56,58]

TYPES OF COMPLEMENTARY AND ALTERNATIVE MEDICINE USED IN CANCER CARE

Specific CAM therapies have geographic variability and wax and wane in popularity. Many of the mind-body techniques considered alternative in adult practice are mainstream in pediatrics. Various studies have tested the effectiveness of hypnosis on anticipatory nausea and vomiting in children with cancer, the use of hypnosis for pain and anxiety during painful procedures (lumbar punctures and bone marrow aspirations), and imagery for symptom and pain relief in children.[28] The more novel therapies, such as herbal, nutritional, and pharmacologic agents, which may carry greater risk of side effects, have yet to undergo rigorous scientific testing. A definitive list of all therapies is beyond the scope of this chapter, but a review of some commonly used therapies is provided.

BIOLOGIC BASED THERAPIES

Biologic based therapies, primarily ingestible or injectable agents, can be herbal medicines, dietary supplements, or the more unusual pharmacologic treatments such as antineoplastons. Although these agents should be used with caution in children, it is important to remember that many current drugs, such as etoposide, vincristine, and paclitaxel, are of "herbal" origins, and that new plant-based agents will likely play an important role in future anticancer therapy. Many natural products clearly have definite biologic activity.[19,31] Some may be helpful in the treatment or prevention of cancer but may also have potentially harmful side effects or interactions. There currently are no standards for recommended dosages of nutritional supplements, and there is little formal oversight of the herbal industry, with great batch-to-batch variability and uneven quality and purity of products. Finally, herbs and supplements used to treat cancer have rarely been studied specifically in children, and therefore the use must be regarded as experimental and unproven.[32]

A debate currently rages about the appropriate role of antioxidants in the treatment of children with cancer. Although antioxidants appear to have a role in cancer prevention in adults,[37] their value is less clear in children and in patients already diagnosed. Children with newly diagnosed leukemia have low antioxidant levels and evidence of high oxidative stress.[30] However, this relationship is not necessarily causal and may reflect the effects of the cancer. Antioxidant use often is encouraged by CAM practitioners to help combat side effects of cancer therapy. However, both radiation and certain chemotherapeutic agents (e.g., anthracyclines) exert their anticancer effects by causing oxidative damage. Therefore controversy exists regarding if and when to use antioxidants during chemotherapy and radiation. There are few controlled studies, especially in children, and results are contradictory.[33] At the present time many oncologists recommend that antioxidants (above those amounts found in a children's multivitamin) not be taken during anthracycline therapies or during radiation.

"Immunostimulants" or "immune boosters" are generally natural products that have been tested using in vivo and in vitro studies and have shown to stimulate production of immune cells, in particular select lymphocytes (i.e., natural killer cells), which may have a role in cancer surveillance. Unfortunately, it is not possible to directly link increased cell numbers to actual anticancer activity. In addition,

many childhood cancers such as leukemia and lymphoma are themselves malignancies of immune cells. Immune stimulation has the theoretical possibility of stimulating the malignant clone. Nonetheless, the role of these immune modulators has intriguing possibilities and is deserving of randomized controlled clinical trials. Several agents are outlined in Table 9-1. An excellent resource for comprehensive evaluation of botanical products can be found from The Longwood Herbal Task Force website.[35]

MANIPULATIVE AND BODY-BASED METHODS: MASSAGE THERAPY

Massage is the intentional and systematic manipulation of the soft tissues of the body. Although no research on massage in pediatric oncology exists in the literature, there are related studies demonstrating that massage reduces pain in adults with cancer,[15] anxiety in children,[16-18] and caregiver stress.[37] Massage affects cancer related pain by reducing large muscle spasms and tension, improving circulation, removing pressure on adjoining tissues and nerves, and increasing blood flow, which removes fluid and toxic metabolic waste products and decreases ischemia.[38]

Anxiety heightens the perception of pain and results in increased cortisol levels in response to perceived stress. One group (The Touch Institute, Miami, Florida) has extensively studied massage therapy and found massage effective in reducing anxiety and related cortisol levels in children with chronic conditions.[16-18] In other studies massage reduced anxiety in adults with cancer[1,15] and in parents of children with cancer.[46]

Fatigue is one of the most commonly reported side effects of cancer treatment. Pain, stress, and anxiety interact to reduce a child's ability to sleep and relax, resulting in increased fatigue. After receiving massage, children generally feel more relaxed and often fall asleep. Massage also may be helpful in the treatment of nausea and vomiting, specifically anticipatory nausea that is related to anxiety. Massage helps redirect attention away from treatments and hospital routines and may be most effective when coupled with music or aromatherapy.[5,58]

Massage therapy provided by certified massage therapists is becoming a common service available to adults and children with cancer. However, health insurance coverage of massage therapy remains scattered and inconsistent. Parents can easily be taught to do gentle massage for their children, which offers a low cost intervention that can be done in the home or hospital setting. Nurses can provide simple, light massage to enhance the therapeutic effects of analgesics and anxiolytics. Al-

TABLE 9-1	**BIOLOGIC BASED THERAPIES**	
Therapy	**Components/Presumed Mechanism of Action**	**Comments/Cautions**
Essiac	Herbal tea (also Flor-Essence); combination of sorrel, burdock root, slippery elm bark, medicinal rhubarb root	No prospective RCT; not for children <2 years of age; avoid if renal stones or intestinal obstruction
Astragalus	Traditional Chinese medicine herb; increases T lymphocyte function; stimulates interferon production; enhances macrophage activity	Relatively nontoxic; no studies in children; use with caution in patients on hypoglycemic or anticoagulant medications
Antineoplastons	Organic compounds available only through Dr. Stanislaw Burzynski's clinic in Houston, Texas; may induce cell differentiation and apoptosis	Phase I/II trials in adults; no RCT; high cost; many mild side effects including the body smelling like urine
Inositol hexaphosphate (IP6)	Fiber associated component of cereals and legumes; antitumorigenic effect in cellular and animal models; may inhibit cell proliferation and enhance cell differentiation	No clinical trials; no trials in humans
Shark cartilage	Antiangiogenic properties	Phase I/II studies; current RCT funded by NCI; new, more potentially powerful antiangiogenesis agents are currently undergoing preclinical trials; caution in young children because of possible effects on organ development

Data from Kemper, K. J. (1999). Shark cartilage, cat's claw, and other complementary cancer therapies. *Contemporary Pediatrics, 16,* 101-126; Spaulding-Albright, N. (1997). A review of some herbal and related products commonly used in cancer patients. *Journal of the American Dietary Association, 97*(Suppl. 2), S208-S215; Vucenik, I., Kalebic, T., Tantivejkul, K., et al. (1998). Novel anticancer function of inositol hexaphosphate: inhibition of human rhabdomyosarcoma in vitro and in vivo. *Anticancer Research, 18,* 1377-1384.
RCT, Randomized clinical trials.

though most nurses do not have extensive massage training, simple techniques such as foot and hand massage or the "m"-technique (light touch modified massage[4]) can be done after short training periods. Some considerations when doing massage in any setting with children with cancer are summarized in Box 9-2.

ENERGY THERAPIES

Energy-based healing therapies are based on the belief that all matter is energy and that disease or illness represents an imbalance in the person's energy flow. Healing occurs when the person's energy system is without blockages and is balanced. Acupuncture and acupressure use a traditional Chinese medicine approach to stimulate unobstructed flow of energy (qi) through the meridians or channels of the body. In acupuncture thin needles penetrate the skin. Acupressure involves firm finger pressure applied to select points. Acupuncture has become so

widely accepted that it is no longer considered alternative by The National Center for Complementary and Alternative Medicine (NCCAM).

Acupuncture has successfully treated chemotherapy and anesthesia induced nausea and vomiting in adults and is among the most researched of CAM therapies, particularly for pain.[42,49,56] Acupuncture was the third most often used CAM therapy in children in a Canadian survey[54] and has been used for a variety of childhood conditions, including allergies, attention deficit disorders, enuresis, and skin rashes.[36] However, there are no reports of use of acupuncture in children with cancer, with the exception of studies reported in the Chinese literature.[26,34] Alternatives such as acupressure and needleless acupuncture (electrical stimulation of pulse points) may be preferred for children who fear needles.

Healing touch is an energy based practice that also encompasses therapeutic touch (TT). Healing touch can involve direct touch; TT generally does not (Figure 9-1.) Both therapies are useful in cancer for pain and symptom management and general relaxation and well-being.[23] The practitioner first "centers" by focusing (putting intention and attention on the patient) with the intent to promote the best possible healing, then assesses for blockages (tension or congestion of qi) using hand techniques such as unruffling. Unruffling involves hand-over-hand movement downward over the body (but not touching) to detect and release blockages.

Children have a greater ability to feel the energy field from touch therapy[20] and may respond more favorably to TT when they are unable to tolerate direct touch or physical contact. Several meta-analyses and integrative reviews of studies using TT support its role in reducing pain and anxiety in adults and promoting relaxation in children.[9,27,53,59] In contrast, Engle and Graney[11] found no evidence of relaxation and no effect on anxiety, and instead measured increased peripheral vasoconstriction in 11 adult students. However, concerns over design, methods, and reporting of in-

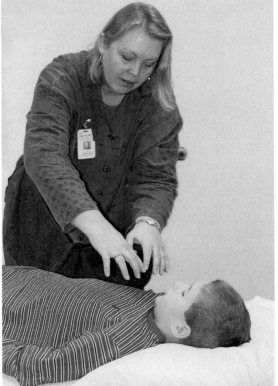

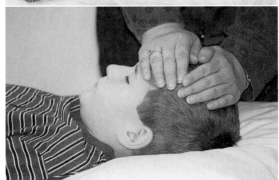

Figure 9-1

Leukemia (ALL) survivor receiving healing touch to reduce anxiety before venipuncture. **A,** Magnetic unruffling used to sweep, rake, or clear the energy field of any blockages or congestion. **B,** One of the steps of balancing and connecting the chakras, known as the chakra connection. (Courtesy Sue Hageness, RN, MA, director of Integrative Medicine Program, Children's Hospital and Clinics, Minneapolis, MN.)

dividual TT research[43] prevent generalization of findings.

Clinical aromatherapy is the therapeutic use of essential oils. Essential oils are aromatic compounds derived from plants that can be directly ap-

TABLE 9-2	QUESTIONS TO CONSIDER IN EVALUATING INFORMATIONAL RESOURCES	
Consider the Source	**Background Checks**	**Cover All Bases**
Who is promoting it, supporting it, updating it, or conducting the research, and what do they have to gain by it?	Are there research-based data with randomized, controlled clinical trials to support the information being conveyed?	Has the information been published in the scientific literature or peer-reviewed journals?
Are there pyramid schemes, indirect commercial links, questionable distributors, or unclear contact, support, or source information when tracking a product or resource?	Is it recorded, referenced, reviewed, or recommended in credible sources with respected, professional affiliations or associations?	What do peers or other experts in the field, national associations, government agencies, or competitors have to say about this source, author, or creator?
Has it earned awards, seals of approval, or merits for conduct? Are these awards from commercial vendors?	Is it related to reliable or accepted standards, practices, or protocols?	How easy is it to go straight to the source, author, or creator, and what would you like to learn from this direct contact?

plied to the skin, inhaled, or ingested. Essential oils are used singularly or in combination to reduce nausea and pain or relieve anxiety and stress.[4,48] Some essential oils are considered calming, whereas others are alerting. Many essential oils also have antiseptic properties. Indications for specific essential oils and their therapeutic effects are referenced in texts by Buckle,[4] Price and Parr,[47] Price and Price,[48] and Battaglia.[3]

Research in aromatherapy is just emerging. Three essential oils used for digestive disorders in adults and children[4,48] are currently being tested as adjuvants to serotonin inhibitors for chemotherapy-induced nausea and vomiting in children with cancer.[46] They include ginger (botanical name: *Zingiber officinale*), peppermint *(Mentha piperitae),* and spearmint *(Mentha spicata).*[3] One other study found that true lavender *(Lavandula angustifolia)* and Roman chamomile *(Chamaemelum nobile)* reduced pain perception and improved sleep patterns and relaxation in children with HIV in palliative care.[55] In adults aromatherapy, added to massage, resulted in greater improvement in psychologic and quality of life indicators.[58] These are small studies that identify areas for potential clinical benefit.

THE ROLE OF THE NURSE IN COMPLEMENTARY AND ALTERNATIVE MEDICINE

An important role of the nurse is to assess and document what patients are using. With the documented dangers of some CAM therapies, health care providers risk liability if they fail to inquire about CAM.[7,10,57] It is important to ask direct, nonjudgmental questions about what patients are us-

ing, the exact dosages, the frequency of use, and the reasons. The Oncology Nursing Society's guidelines recommend that nurses (1) assess patients for CAM use; (2) rely on credible sources and providers when giving information to patients; (3) evaluate CAM for safety, efficacy, cost, third-party payor coverage, ethics, and liability; and (4) evaluate their own personal and professional beliefs regarding CAM.[44]

Most nurse practice acts are silent on CAM; thus, they do not preclude nurses from practicing CAM modalities.[22] Many nurses seek training and certification in select CAM therapies. Additionally, many nursing programs offer electives and some programs offer graduate studies in CAM interventions. Institutional policies regarding the use of CAM should define the scope of therapies covered, address credentialing and referrals, emphasize communication between the patient and health care provider, and require informed consent and a signed assumption of risk by the patient or parent.[57] The goal is to ensure standards of care and guide the rights and obligations of health care practitioners, while also respecting patient autonomy.

Although it is not feasible to know about all CAM therapies, it is important to know how to obtain and screen CAM resources for safety and efficacy and to be alert to any adverse effects, interactions, or other changes in the patient's condition. Filtering and evaluating the quality of resources are challenging. Asking relevant questions (Table 9-2) may help to evaluate the quality of resources available. The key is to ensure that CAM therapies are not contraindicated and do not pose greater risks than do benefits. In addition, some effort should be made to ensure that any alternative practitioners in pediatric settings have experience working with children.

FUTURE ROLE OF CAM IN PEDIATRIC CANCER

"The aim of evidence-based practice is to provide the best care based on the best available research."[43] Research on CAM is needed to determine efficacy and outcomes, dosage (especially for children), provider effectiveness, cost, and mechanism of action. Pediatrics must be included in the integrative medicine research agenda. It is inaccurate to assume that studies of adult patients will be applicable to children.[52]

Many CAM therapies are effective for symptom management of terminally ill children, and CAM options for patients with advanced disease should be expanded.[24,50] Nurses make a great difference in symptom management and end-of-life care; research in these areas is especially needed.

Regardless of the level of acceptance in mainstream medicine, CAM therapies have infiltrated every aspect of health care.[50] Parents use CAM in their child's treatment for cancer and will continue to do so. These parents are educated consumers who want to assume an active role in relieving symptoms and improving the well-being of their child. As an advocate for patients and families, nurses can help parents make informed decisions and become partners in their child's care. Their satisfaction and ability to balance the demands of treatment with CAM resources can empower them on their journey. Providing integrative cancer care can nurture patients, families, and caregivers in body, mind, and spirit.

ACKNOWLEDGMENT

The authors appreciate the invaluable assistance of the Integrative Medicine team members: Pam Ahrens, MLS, Lisa Baker, OTR, CMT, NCTMB, and Sue Hageness, MA, RN, HNC, CHTP, for contributing their expertise to this chapter.

REFERENCES

1. Ahles, T. A., Tope, D. M., Pinkson, B., et al. (1999). Massage therapy for patients undergoing autologous bone marrow transplantation. *Journal of Pain and Symptom Management, 18,* 157-163.
2. American Cancer Society. (2000). *American Cancer Society's guide to complementary and alternative methods.* Atlanta, GA: American Cancer Society.
3. Battaglia, S. (1995). *The complete guide to aromatherapy.* Brisbane, Australia: Watson Ferguson.
4. Buckle, J. (1997). *Clinical aromatherapy in nursing.* London: Arnold.
5. Buckle, J. (1999). Use of aromatherapy as a complementary treatment for chronic pain. *Alternative Therapies, 5*(5), 42-51.
6. Cassileth, B. R. (1998). Overview of alternative/complementary medicine. *Cancer Practice, 6,* 243-245.
7. Cassileth, B. R. (1999). Evaluating complementary and alternative therapies for cancer patients. *CA-A Cancer Journal for Clinicians, 49,* 362-375.
8. Druss, B. G., & Rosenheck, R. A. (1999). Association between use of unconventional therapies and conventional medical services. *Journal of the American Medical Association, 282,* 651-656.
9. Easter, A. (1997). The state of research on the effects of therapeutic touch. *Journal of Holistic Nursing, 15,* 158-175.
10. Eisenberg, D. M., Davis, R. B., Ettner, S. L., et al. (1998). Trends in alternative medicine use in the United States, 1990-1997: Results of a follow-up national survey. *Journal of the American Medical Association, 280,* 1569-1575.
11. Engle, V. F., & Graney, M. J. (2000). Biobehavioral effects of therapeutic touch. *Journal of Nursing Scholarship, 32,* 287-293.
12. Ernst, E. (1999). Prevalence of complementary/alternative medicine for children: A systematic review. *European Journal of Pediatrics, 158,* 7-11.
13. Ernst, E., & Cassileth, B. R. (1997). The prevalence of complementary/alternative medicine in cancer. *Cancer, 83,* 777-782.
14. Fernandez, C. V., Stutzer, C. A., MacWilliam, L., et al. (1998). Alternative and complementary therapy use in pediatric oncology patients in British Columbia: Prevalence and reasons for use. *Journal of Clinical Oncology, 16,* 1279-1286.
15. Ferrell-Torry, A., & Glick, O. (1993). The use of therapeutic massage as a nursing intervention to modify anxiety and the perception of cancer pain. *Cancer Nursing, 16,* 93-101.
16. Field, T., Henteleff, T., Hernandez-Reif, M., et al. (1998). Children with asthma have improved pulmonary function after massage therapy. *Journal of Pediatrics, 132,* 854-858.
17. Field, T., Hernandez-Reif, M., Seligman, S., et al. (1997). Juvenile rheumatoid arthritis: Benefits from massage therapy. *Journal of Pediatric Psychology, 22,* 607-617.
18. Field, T., Schanberg, S., Kuhn, C., et al. (1998). Bulimic adolescents benefit from massage therapy. *Adolescence, 33,* 555-563.
19. Foster, S., & Tyler, E. V. (1999). *Tyler's honest herbal* (4th ed.). New York: The Haworth Herbal Press.
20. France, N. E. (1993). The child's perception of the human energy field using therapeutic touch. *Journal of Holistic Nursing, 11,* 319-333.
21. Friedman, T., Slayton, W. B., Allen, L. S., et al. (1997). Use of alternative therapies for children with cancer. *Pediatrics, 100,* 1-6.
22. Geddes, N., & Henry, J. K. (1997). Nursing and alternative medicine: Legal and practice issues. *Journal of Holistic Nursing, 15,* 271-281.
23. Giasson, M., & Bouchard, L. (1998). Effect of therapeutic touch on the well-being of persons with terminal cancer. *Journal of Holistic Nursing, 16,* 383-398.
24. Grady, P. A. (1999). Improving care at the end of life: Research issues. *Journal of Hospice and Palliative Nursing, 1,* 151-155.
25. Grootenhuis, M. A., Last, B. F., de Graaf-Nijkerk, J. H., et al. (1998). Use of alternative treatment in pediatric oncology. *Cancer Nursing, 21,* 282-288.

26. Huang, X., Chen, H., Guo, X., et al. (1993). Treatment with cone moxibustion of chemotherapeutic leukocytopenia in 114 cases. *Journal of Traditional Chinese Medicine, 13,* 266-267.

27. Ireland, M. (1998). Therapeutic touch with HIV-infected children: A pilot study. *Journal of the Association of Nurses in AIDS Care, 9,* 68-77.

28. Kelly, K. (2000). Summary of current literature. (Carol Ann's Library, Columbia University Pediatric Oncology Integrative Therapies Program, New York.) http://cpmc-net.columbia.edu/dept/pediatrics/oncology/carolann/altmed/current.html. Accessed 9/25/00.

29. Kelly, K. M., Jacobson, J. S., Kennedy, D. D., et al. Use of unconventional therapies by children with cancer at an urban medical center. *Journal of Pediatric Hematology/Oncology, 22,* 412-416.

30. Kelly, K., & Kennedy, D. (2000). Antioxidant and oxidative status of children on treatment for acute lymphoblastic leukemia. (Carol Ann's Library, Columbia University Pediatric Oncology Integrative Therapies Program, New York.) http://cpmcnet.columbia.edu/dept/pediatrics/oncology/carolann/altmed/antioxidant.html. Accessed 9/25/00.

31. Kemper, K. J. (1996). *The holistic pediatrician.* New York: Harper.

32. Kemper, K. J. (1999). Shark cartilage, cat's claw, and other complementary cancer therapies. *Contemporary Pediatrics, 16,* 101-126.

33. Lamson, D. W., & Brignall, M. S. (2000). Antioxidants and cancer therapy II. Quick reference guide. *Alternative Medicine Review, 5,* 152-163.

34. Liu, S., Chen, Z., Hou, J., et al. (1991). Magnetic disk applied on Neiguan point for prevention and treatment of cisplatin-induced nausea and vomiting. *Journal of Traditional Chinese Medicine, 11,* 181-183.

35. The Longwood Herbal Task Force. (August 14, 2000). (The Herbs and Supplements.). www.mcp.edu/herbal. Accessed 9/25/00.

36. Loo, M. (1999). Complementary/alternative therapies in select populations: Children. In J. Spencer & J. Jacobs (Eds.), *Complementary/alternative medicine: An evidence based approach* (pp. 371-390). St. Louis, MO: Mosby.

37. MacDonald, G. (1998). Massage as a respite intervention for primary caregivers. *American Journal of Hospice & Palliative Care, 15,* 43-47.

38. MacDonald, G. (1999). *Medicine hands: Massage therapy for people with cancer.* Tallahassee, FL: Findhorn Press.

39. Mayne, S. T., & Vogt, T. M. (2000). Antioxidant nutrients in cancer prevention. *Principles & Practice of Oncology Updates, 14,* 1-12.

40. Möttönen, M., & Uhari, M., (1997). Use of micronutrients and alternative drugs by children with acute lymphoblastic leukemia. *Medical and Pediatric Oncology, 28,* 205-208.

41. National Center for Complementary/Alternative Medicine, National Institutes of Health. (2000). Major domains of complementary and alternative medicine. http://nccam.nih.gov/nccam/fcp/classify/ Accessed 9/25/00.

42. NIH Consensus Conference. (1998). Acupuncture: NIH Consensus Development Panel on Acupuncture. *Journal of the American Medical Association, 280,* 1518-1524.

43. O'Mathuna, D. P. (2000). Evidence-based practice and reviews of therapeutic touch. *Journal of Nursing Scholarship, 32,* 279-285.

44. Oncology Nursing Society. (2000). Oncology Nursing Society position on the use of complementary and alternative therapies in cancer care. *Oncology Nursing Forum, 27,* 749.

45. Post-White, J., Sencer, S., & Fitzgerald, M. (2000). Complementary therapy use in pediatric cancer. *Oncology Nursing Forum, 27,* 342-343.

46. Post-White, J., Sencer, S., Fitzgerald, M., et al. (2000). *Effects of massage therapy in children with cancer and their parents.* Manuscript in preparation.

47. Price, S., & Parr, S. (1996). *Aromatherapy for babies and children.* London: Thorsons.

48. Price, S., & Price, L. (1999). *Aromatherapy for health professionals.* Edinburgh, Scotland: Churchill Livingstone.

49. Primack, A. (1999). Complementary/alternative therapies in the prevention and treatment of cancer. In J. Spencer & J. Jacobs (Eds.), *Complementary/alternative medicine: An evidence based approach* (pp. 123-169). St. Louis, MO: Mosby.

50. Richardson, M. A. (1999). Research of complementary/alternative medicine therapies in oncology: Promising but challenging. *Journal of Clinical Oncology, 17*(Suppl. 11), 38-43.

51. Sawyer, M.G., Gannoni, A. F., Toogood, I. R., et al. (1994). The use of alternative therapies by children with cancer. *Medical Journal of Australia, 160,* 320-322.

52. Sencer, S. (2000). Not little adults: Pediatrics and integrative medicine. *Minnesota Medicine, 14,* 24-25.

53. Spence, J., & Olson, M. (1997). Quantitative research on therapeutic touch. *Scandinavian Journal of Caring Science, 11,* 183-190.

54. Spigelblatt, L., Lane-Ammara, G., Pless, B., et al. (1994). The use of alternative medicine by children. *Pediatrics, 94,* 811-814.

55. Styles, J. L. (1997). The use of aromatherapy in hospitalized children with HIV disease. *Complementary Therapies in Nursing, 3,* 16-20.

56. Taylor, A. G. (1999). Complementary/alternative therapies in the treatment of pain. In J. Spencer & J. Jacobs (Eds.), *Complementary/alternative medicine: An evidence based approach,* (pp. 282-339). St. Louis, MO: Mosby.

57. Vincler, L. A., & Nicol, M. F. (1997). When ignorance isn't bliss: What healthcare practitioners and facilities should know about complementary and alternative medicine. *Journal of Health and Hospital Law, 30,* 160-178.

58. Wilkinson, S., Aldridge, J., Salmon, I., et al. (1999). An evaluation of aromatherapy massage in palliative care. *Palliative Medicine, 13,* 409-417.

59. Winstead-Fry, P., & Kijek, J. (1999). An integrative review and meta-analysis of therapeutic touch research. *Alternative Therapies, 5,* 58-67.

III

Supportive Care

10

Prevention and Treatment of Infections

Nancy E. Kline

The immune system consists of four major components: cellular immunity (involving T cells), humoral immunity (antibodies derived from B cells), phagocytic cells, and the complement system. Immune deficiency, or defects in one or more of these immune system components, can result in infection by various pathogens.[23] The immune system includes the structural elements: lymph nodes, spleen, thymus, and tonsils (see Figure 2-12 in Chapter 2). Important nonimmunologic host defense mechanisms include local mucocutaneous mechanical barriers such as the physical integrity of the skin and mucous membranes, the cough reflex, and the patency of anatomic sites of mucous drainage or other body fluid excretion (e.g., anus and urethra) (Figure 10-1). Practitioners must obtain a comprehensive health history of a cancer patient to assess for frequent infections, particularly noting recurrent, unusual, or life-threatening infections.[23] Cancer patients often lack the classic signs of infection, as the immune response that typically produces signs of infection (e.g., erythema or edema) may be blunted.[23]

Immunocompromised hosts have one or more defects in the normal defense mechanisms that protect them from infectious agents, predisposing them to increased risks of severe life-threatening infection. Combinations of host defense defects produced by cancer chemotherapy, together with the use of indwelling central venous access devices, predispose the cancer patient to a high risk of serious opportunistic infections.

Congenital (primary) immune deficiency is caused by a genetic anomaly (e.g., severe combined immune deficiency, Wiskott-Aldrich syndrome). Acquired (secondary) immune deficiency results from illness (e.g., cancer or viral infection), treatment of the illness (e.g., cytotoxic chemotherapy), or normal physiologic changes that occur during the aging process. Acquired forms of immune deficiency are more common than the congenital forms. However, some patients have underlying congenital immune deficiencies that place them at risk for developing malignancy (e.g., ataxia-telangiectasia). These patients have added infectious risks when receiving cancer therapy.[23]

One of the most important factors that increase the risk of infection among hospitalized cancer patients is the alteration of colonizing organisms. The normal flora, which are primarily aerobic gram-positive organisms, can change into aerobic gram-negative organisms within a day of hospital admission.[25,26] The use of broad-spectrum antibiotics also promotes bacterial colonization. More than 80% of documented infections that occur in patients with acute nonlymphocytic leukemia are caused by organisms that are part of the endogenous microflora.[40]

CAUSES OF IMMUNOSUPPRESSION IN THE CHILD WITH CANCER

Cancer therapy contributes to many deficiencies in local and systemic host defense (Box 10-1). Lymphocyte function can be impaired by several factors: stem cell defects preventing normal lymphocyte development and causing failure of the immune system; dysfunction of a main lymphoid organ (e.g., the spleen), preventing maturation of stem cells into T or B cells; or disruption of the final stages of B cell maturation. Alterations in the inflammatory response (e.g., chemotactic and phagocytic activities of neutrophils and macrophages) also can impair host resistance.

Chemotherapy and radiation therapy can cause decreased immunoglobulin concentrations, diminished opsonic activity (a process rendering bacteria more susceptible to phagocytosis), deficient agglutination and lysis of bacteria, and inadequate neutralization of bacterial toxins.[21] Patients with B cell defects, such as hypogammaglobulinemia, are prone to recurrent respiratory infections (both upper and lower tracts) and/or chronic gastrointestinal infections.[23] Cancer patients with immunoglobulin deficiency are susceptible to infections with encap-

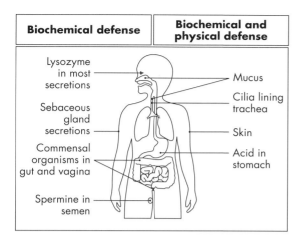

Biochemical defense	Biochemical and physical defense

Figure 10-1

Exterior defenses of the immune system.   (Adapted from Roit, I.V., Brostoff, J., & Male, D. [1989]. *Immunology.* St. Louis, MO: Mosby.)

BOX 10-1

SELECTED CAUSES OF LOCAL AND SYSTEMIC HOST DEFENSE DEFECTS

LOCAL
Central venous catheter placement
Surgery
Mucositis
Venipuncture
Ventriculoperitoneal shunt
Skin lesions

SYSTEMIC
Neutropenia
Lymphopenia
Impaired B and T cell function
Malignancy
Chemotherapy
Radiation
Splenectomy
Malnutrition

sulated organisms, *Haemophilus influenzae,* and pneumococcal bacteria.[21]

Cancer therapy causes both quantitative and qualitative defects in cellular immunity.[29] Children with T cell defects are prone to viral infections (e.g., varicella, herpes simplex, cytomegalovirus) and fungal infections (e.g., *Cryptococcus, Candida spp.*), as well as *Pneumocystis carinii.*[21,23] The risk of these infections increases with steroid use.[21] Certain malignancies such as Hodgkin's disease cause cellular immune system defects.

Many infections in cancer patients are related to the degree of neutropenia occuring during treatment. The significance of fevers during periods of neutropenia was noted in an early, landmark study of 1001 children and young adults with cancer hospitalized at the National Cancer Institute between 1975 and 1980. In a prospective analysis, 80% of fevers in these patients occurred when the neutrophil count was less than 500/mm³. Nearly 75% of these patients had infections noted by culture or on exam. In contrast, less than 20% of nongranulocytopenic febrile patients had documented infections.[36] In a later study during the 1980s only 30% to 40% of febrile neutropenic patients had a definable infection.[34] The rate of true infections was not likely decreasing, but rather, actual infections were presumably masked by the prompt use of antibiotics in the later study.[21] The duration of neutropenia is often indicative of the risk of infection. Less than 30% of patients with neutropenia with duration less than one week have evidence of infection, compared with nearly 100% of patients when the neutropenia lasts longer than 1 week.[33,35] Granulo-

cytopenia may be a result of the disease itself (e.g., acute leukemia) or metastatic disease (e.g., neuroblastoma), but it is more commonly a consequence of cytotoxic chemotherapy or radiotherapy. Steroids decrease neutrophil migration and phagocytosis.[21] Local or wide-field radiotherapy may cause myelosuppression if a large amount of bone marrow is radiated. The pelvis, spine, and long bones each contain a significant amount of the bone marrow. Radiation to any of these areas may cause neutropenia to develop.

Children who have had a splenectomy are at higher risk of certain bacterial infections. The spleen is involved in antibody formation, improves opsonization, and acts as a phagocytic filter for microorganisms.[21] Splenectomy or functional asplenia in combination with cytotoxic chemotherapy may be particularly problematic. Splenectomized patients are more likely to develop severe and fatal infections when exposed to encapsulated bacterial pathogens such as *Streptococcus pneumoniae, H. influenzae,* and *Neisseria meningitidis.*[28]

MANAGEMENT OF THE FEBRILE NEUTROPENIC CHILD

Fever is usually defined as two oral temperature elevations above 38° C during a 24-hour period or a single temperature of 38.5° C or higher.[28] Granulocytopenia increases the likelihood of an infectious cause of fever. The neutropenic individual may not be able to manifest signs of inflammation. Fever may be the only sign of an infection. Other causes of fever in children with cancer include blood transfusions, allergic reactions, and the malignancy itself (i.e., tumor fevers). Figure 10-2 outlines the care of a febrile pediatric oncology patient.

Management of the child with fever and neutropenia differs markedly from that of other patients with fever. Because of the high mortality rate associated with untreated infection, all fevers experienced by children with neutropenia are considered due to a life-threatening infection until proven otherwise. The initial clinical signs and symptoms of infection (e.g., erythema, exudate, swelling, localized adenopathy) in neutropenic patients with either unexplained fever or septicemia can be blunted or absent, as white blood cells are needed for these processes.

At the onset of fever, it is crucial to perform a careful but expeditious evaluation before initiating antibiotic therapy. The lung is the most frequent site of serious infection, followed by soft tissues, mucosa, and the blood. Urinary tract infections are less common in children than adults, and infections of the central nervous system are unusual.[17] Because the classic signs and symptoms of infection often are absent, subtle signs of inflammation must be noticed. Detailed questioning about cough, shortness of breath, tachypnea, pain with defecation, skin rashes and lesions, odynophagia (inability to swallow), sore throat, and retrosternal pain is necessary. A meticulous physical examination must be done so that any subtle signs of infection or inflammation are not missed. Blood pressure, heart rate, and respiratory rate are carefully monitored. Special attention is given to the oral cavity and posterior oropharynx for ulcers or lesions; fingers and toes for paronychia (infection of the skin around the nail); axillae and groin for rashes or lesions; perianal and vulvar areas for lesions or fissures; and sites of previous procedures such as intravenous or urinary catheters, fingersticks, and bone marrow or other biopsy sites. Relatively innocuous-appearing lesions can be the focus for bacteremia or sepsis. The nurse must remove all dressings and bandages to examine the skin beneath.

Before antimicrobial therapy is initiated, the child must have baseline laboratory studies including a complete blood count, electrolytes, blood urea nitrogen, creatinine, liver function tests, and blood cultures. If the child has an indwelling central venous catheter, cultures are obtained from each lumen. Peripheral blood cultures may also be obtained according to institutional practice, which varies between medical centers. If the child does not have central venous access, a peripheral blood culture is obtained. A chest radiograph will determine the presence of pneumonia or pleural effusion. Urine culture is necessary to diagnose urinary

tract infection, as pyuria is not often present. Skin lesions are cultured for appropriate viral, bacterial, fungal, and mycobacterial organisms. Pulse oximetry readings are obtained for any child with respiratory symptoms or evidence of poor circulation (e.g., cool extremities, weak pulse).

Once the initial evaluation is completed and blood cultures are obtained, prompt institution of antibiotic therapy is required. The nurse must take all steps to ensure that antibiotics are given quickly. Broad-spectrum antibiotic therapy is routinely administered on an empiric basis in the febrile neutropenic child. Once culture and sensitivity results are available, or when a definitive diagnosis is made, antibiotic therapy can be adjusted accordingly. Bacterial isolates and antibiotic susceptibility vary greatly among institutions, necessitating tailoring of antimicrobial regimens.

Empiric antimicrobial therapy is reassessed within 24 to 72 hours after it is instituted. During this time results of pretreatment cultures and the child's response to therapy will be discernible. If an organism is isolated, treatment can be modified based on susceptibility results. If the child has persistent bacteremia or develops new symptoms or signs of infection while receiving empiric therapy, modifications of the original antimicrobial regimen may be required (Table 10-1). It is important to note that over time bacterial sensitivities will change as antibiotic resistance develops.

Results of several studies support the concept that a child admitted for fever and neutropenia can be safely discharged once the child is clinically well, with negative cultures for at least 48 hours, afebrile, and with evidence of imminent blood count recovery (e.g., rising ANC, absolute phagocyte count, and/or platelet count), provided that the child has no risk factors for prolonged myelosuppression (e.g., positive marrow disease, concurrent marrow irradiation). In these studies the rate of hospital readmission was 0% to 6%, and all subsequent hospital courses were uncomplicated.[8,20,27,32]

TYPES OF INFECTIONS

Treatment of infections in immunocompromised children is dependent on the causative organism. Viruses, bacteria, fungi, and protozoa can all cause infection in children who are immune suppressed from cancer treatment. Specific antimicrobial agents will be discussed briefly in reference to each type of infection.

PNEUMONIA

The respiratory tract is a common site of serious infections in children with cancer.[17] Although the

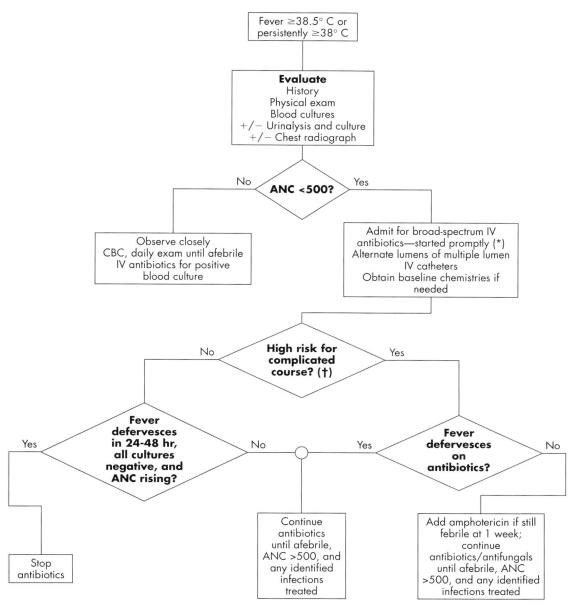

(*) If patient lives far from pediatric oncology center, may admit locally with daily follow-up with primary oncologist. If fever persists >3 days, recommend transfer to pediatric oncology center.

(†) Hypotension, uncontrolled cancer (e.g., leukemia in induction, unresponsive or metastatic cancer), impaired organ function, or mental status changes.

Figure 10-2

Algorithm for oncology patient with fever.   (Data from Freifeld, A. G., Walsh, T. J., & Pizzo, P. A. [1997]. Infectious complications in the pediatric cancer patient. In P. A. Pizzo & D. G. Poplack [Eds.], *Principles and practice of pediatric oncology* [3rd ed., pp. 1069-1114]. Philadelphia: Lippincott-Raven; Kelly, K. P. [2000]. ALL in children: A medical success story. *Advance for Nurse Practitioners, 8*[4], 57-58, 61-64, 94.)

TABLE 10-1	NEW CLINICAL SIGNS THAT MAY NECESSITATE THERAPY MODIFICATIONS IN THE FEBRILE NEUTROPENIC PATIENT	
Clinical or Laboratory Finding	**Therapy Modification**	
Catheter-associated infection	Add vancomycin and other gram-negative coverage, as needed.	
Persistent bacteremia	If gram-positive, add vancomycin; if gram-negative, change according to susceptibility data.	
Oral mucositis	Obtain viral and fungal cultures as needed; add antimicrobial agent specific for anaerobes or candida.	
Esophagitis		
Pneumonia	Start broad-spectrum antibiotics and/or trimethoprim sulfamethoxazole; consider bronchoalveolar lavage.	
Perianal tenderness	Add antimicrobial agent specific for anaerobes.	
Persistent or recurrent fever and neutropenia	Continue antibiotics; after 1 week add empiric antifungal therapy.	

majority of pulmonary complications in immunosuppressed children are due to infection, there are also noninfectious causes that may produce a similar picture (Box 10-2).

The pattern of the infiltrate on the chest radiograph and the degree of neutropenia can influence the choice of empiric therapy. If necessary, bronchoalveolar lavage may be needed for definitive diagnosis, and it is done early in the patient's course if diffuse infiltrates are present.[21] Lavage is safe and can be performed at the bedside.

The child with fever, neutropenia, and pneumonia can be infected with one of a wide array of microorganisms. Common bacterial pathogens *(H. influenzae, S. pneumoniae),* mycoplasma, and viruses (influenza, adenovirus, respiratory syncytial virus), as well as gram-negative bacteria, *S. aureus,* and fungi need to be considered (Table 10-2). Diffuse infiltrates in a neutropenic child may be caused by any of the pathogens mentioned, and results of the bronchoalveolar lavage examination may help guide therapy.

Children with bacterial pneumonia appear ill and exhibit general and localized physical findings. Signs and symptoms include fever, malaise, rapid and shallow respirations, cough, and chest pain.

A diffuse infiltrate or a normal-appearing chest radiograph in the child with tachypnea and hypoxia is an ominous finding. *Pneumocystis carinii* (a primitive fungus, with characteristics similar to a protozoa) rarely presents as a focal pneumonia, but as a more diffuse process.[6] In the early stages the chest radiograph may appear normal, but the child's clinical condition may be unstable and worsen rapidly.

Serious fungal infections are not likely to be identified at the onset of fever. However, the finding of a progressive or new infiltrate accompanied by fever, nonproductive cough or hemoptysis, and

BOX 10-2

CAUSES OF PNEUMONITIS IN THE IMMUNOCOMPROMISED CHILD

INFECTIOUS CAUSES
Respiratory syncytial virus
Influenza
Aspergillus
Parainfluenza
Adenovirus
Bacteria, various types
Mycobacterium tuberculosis
Cytomegalovirus
Pneumocystis carinii
Oral flora (aspiration)
Disseminated fungi (*Cryptococcus, Histoplasma*)
Herpes simplex

NONINFECTIOUS CAUSES
Pulmonary or interstitial fibrosis
Malignancy (primary or metastatic disease)
Radiation pneumonitis
Drug toxicity (e.g., bleomycin)
Pulmonary hemorrhage
Atelectasis

pleuritic chest pain in a persistently neutropenic patient despite the use of broad-spectrum antibiotic therapy suggests a fungal pneumonia, often caused by the *Aspergillus* species.[21] Computed tomography (CT) of the chest is essential to aid in the diagnosis of *Aspergillus.* Bronchoalveolar lavage is positive for *Aspergillus* in approximately 50% of cases; therefore the diagnosis of *Aspergillus* lung infection is often a presumptive diagnosis based on characteristic findings on CT of the chest (e.g., nodules progressing to cavitation and the CT halo sign).[21] *Aspergillus* pulmonary infection is a significant cause of morbidity and mortality in neutropenic patients.[21] Treatment includes prolonged antifungal therapy (e.g., amphotericin B). Patients must be evaluated for evidence of disseminated

TABLE 10-2	PATHOGENS THAT CAUSE PNEUMONIA AND ASSOCIATED TREATMENT
Organism	**Treatment**
H. influenzae	Cefotaxime, ceftriaxone, ampicillin
S. pneumoniae	Penicillin V, erythromycin
Mycoplasma pneumoniae	Erythromycin (<8 years of age), clarithromycin, azithromycin, tetracycline (>8 years of age)
Influenza	Supportive therapy; hydration, supplemental oxygen
Adenovirus	Supportive therapy; hydration, supplemental oxygen
Respiratory syncytial virus	Supportive therapy; hydration, supplemental oxygen, mechanical ventilation as needed
S. aureus	Nafcillin or oxacillin + vancomycin + gentamicin
P. carinii	Trimethoprim sulfamethoxazole, pentamidine
Aspergillus	Amphotericin B
Cytomegalovirus	Ganciclovir, mechanical ventilation as needed
Herpes simplex	Acyclovir

Data from Report of the Committee on Infectious Diseases. (2000). *Red Book* (25th ed.). Elk Grove, IL: American Academy of Pediatrics.

fungal infection, with attention to the liver, spleen, kidneys, and skin.

Nursing care of the child with pneumonia is primarily supportive, based on the symptomatology. A thorough respiratory assessment is necessary to determine the degree of respiratory distress and to guide interventions. Physical examination focuses on auscultation of the lungs and the presence of adventitious sounds (e.g., wheezes, rales, rhonchi); the quality of respiration (e.g., rate, depth, ease); supraclavicular, intracostal, substernal retractions; nasal flaring; pulse oximetry values, peripheral perfusion; skin color and the presence of cyanosis. Collaboration with respiratory therapists is helpful.

Antibiotics are given according to schedule, and if a cough is present, expectorants or antitussives are given only before periods of rest, sleep, or meals. To prevent dehydration, intravenous fluids are administered while the child is hospitalized. If oral fluids are allowed, they should be used judiciously, as aspiration may occur during coughing episodes. If the child is hypoxic, humidified oxygen is administered via nasal cannula or mask. If respiratory compromise occurs, mechanical ventilation may be necessary.

Frequent vital signs and pulmonary assessment are necessary to determine whether the child is responding to therapy and to detect early signs of complications. Children with an ineffective cough or with difficulty handling secretions (e.g., infants) will require suctioning to maintain a patent airway.

SKIN INFECTIONS

Cutaneous infections are common in immunocompromised patients and can be caused by viruses, fungi, or bacteria. The incidence of skin infections in children with cancer is influenced by the severity of immunosuppression, as well as the disruption of skin integrity from diagnostic or therapeutic procedures or ordinary childhood scrapes. Immunocompromised children may also develop common childhood skin infections such as impetigo.[41]

Bacterial skin infections are usually caused by staphylococci or streptococci. These often begin at the sites of skin breakdown, such as surgical or biopsy sites, or areas of prior radiation therapy. In immunocompromised patients, both gram-positive and gram-negative bacteria can be isolated from the blood or from an area of cellulitis (infection of the subcutaneous tissue). Microbiologic confirmation of the diagnosis is important, and new lesions are cultured as they appear. Treatment for presumed bacterial cellulitis includes broad-spectrum antibiotic coverage.

Fungal pathogens including *Candida* spp., *Aspergillus, Fusarium,* and *Mucor* can cause cutaneous lesions either as isolated findings or as manifestations of disseminated infection. The normal flora of the skin ordinarily acts as a defense against bacteria and fungi. However, antibiotic use alters this normal flora, causing susceptibility to fungal skin infections. Impairment of cellular immunity, as occurs with the use of steroids, increases the risk for fungal skin infections.[15] Tender, erythematous skin nodules or pustules can develop with candidal infections. Any black, rapidly progressing, necrotic eschar requires immediate evaluation for fungi (Figure 10-3). These lesions often develop at intravenous sites, particularly at areas of tape placement or other moist, occluded areas. Surgical excision is often needed.[41]

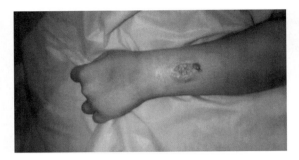

Figure 10-3

Cutaneous *Aspergillus.*

Cutaneous infections secondary to viruses are common in immunocompromised patients. Herpes simplex virus (HSV) and varicella-zoster virus (VZV) can cause painful or pruritic vesicular lesions that can become secondarily infected. Diagnosis is often made on the basis of clinical findings of typical skin lesions, but can be confirmed by obtaining a culture from a scraping from the base of a fresh vesicle.

Patients with cancer who develop primary varicella, especially those actively receiving chemotherapy, are at increased risk of serious disseminated disease, including pneumonia, encephalitis, hepatitis, and purpura fulminans.[7] Dissemination and subsequent mortality has been reduced by rapid initiation of therapy with intravenous acyclovir.[9] Immunosuppressed children who are at high risk for developing varicella infection should receive varicella zoster immune globulin (VZIG) within 96 hours of varicella exposure. Protection against varicella is optimized by giving the injection as soon as possible after exposure. Children with a history of chickenpox or herpes zoster are usually considered immune.

Immunocompromised children are at risk for the development of perirectal cellulitis. These lesions provide a focus for local cellulitis or abscess, usually with enteric bacteria, particularly gram-negative and anaerobic organisms. Manifestations of perirectal cellulitis include erythema, tenderness, warmth, and swelling. Indurated or fluctuant (fluid filled) swelling in the perirectal area may indicate the presence of a perirectal abscess. A child presenting with perianal tenderness and erythema and pain with defecation must be treated with medications effective against gram-negative and anaerobic bacteria.

Nursing care of children with perianal cellulitis includes administration of parenteral antibiotics and oral or intravenous pain medications, as well as other pain control measures such as sitz baths.

TABLE 10-3	ANTIMICROBIAL AGENTS USED IN THE TREATMENT OF CUTANEOUS INFECTIONS
Infection	**Antimicrobial Agents**
Staphylococcus	Nafcillin, oxacillin, cefazolin, vancomycin, clindamycin, ampicillin + sulbactam, cefadroxil, cephalexin, amoxicillin + clavulanate
Streptococcus	Penicillin V, erythromycin
Candida	Fluconazole, ketoconazole, nystatin, clotrimazole
Fungal	Amphotericin B
Viral	Acyclovir, valacyclovir

Data from Report of the Committee on Infectious Diseases. (2000). *Red Book* (25th ed.). Elk Grove, IL: American Academy of Pediatrics.

Daily assessment of the perirectal area must be made to determine whether the infection is worsening, persistent, or resolving. Stool softeners are administered, as the pain often makes children afraid to defecate and constipation occurs.

To assist in establishing a diagnosis of cutaneous infection, it is important for nurses to accurately describe changes in the character of the skin. The color, shape, and distribution of the lesions or wounds are important observations. Fissures or wounds are assessed for depth of tissue damage, signs of infection, and evidence of healing. The skin is palpated for temperature, moisture, texture, tenderness, and swelling. Patient history provides information regarding how the lesions initially appeared and have subsequently evolved, and the presence of pain, burning, tingling, and itching. Observing the infant or young child for restlessness and irritability may provide additional information. Treatment of skin infections is dependent on the causative organism, virus, or fungus (Table 10-3).

Supportive interventions may be required for management of pruritis or pain. Topical preparations such as hydrocortisone cream may decrease itching, as may a warm bath with colloidal oatmeal added to the bath water. Diphenhydramine or hydroxyzine are antipruritic medications that can be taken orally or intravenously. Pain associated with herpes zoster may require acetaminophen and codeine or other opioids such as morphine. If pain medications are given, a pain assessment instrument is used before administering the drug and consistently thereafter to monitor the degree of pain relief. Adjustment in dose or route, or changing pain medications, is based on the patient's assessment of pain.

Gastrointestinal Tract Infections

Gastrointestinal (GI) tract infections are common occurrences among children with cancer. The underlying diseases, cytotoxic treatments, and radiation treatments all predispose the child to alterations of the mucosal surface, leading to local infections and serving as an entry point for the microorganisms residing in the GI tract.

Mucositis and Esophagitis

Mucositis can range in severity from isolated small oral ulcers to extensive mucosal sloughing of the oral cavity and more distal GI tract. Children who have been hospitalized for prolonged periods of time or who have been treated with broad-spectrum antibiotics are predisposed to mucosal infections, as they are often colonized with gram-negative organisms or yeast. Chemotherapy-induced mucositis can also become superinfected with *Candida* or herpes simplex virus (HSV). If a scraping of a candidal lesion is suspended in potassium hydroxide (KOH) and viewed under the microscope, pseudohyphae will be evident. HSV infection can be documented by immunofluorescent staining of oral lesions or culture from a swabbing of the involved area.[21]

The infectious and noninfectious processes predisposing to mucositis in the oral cavity can also produce esophagitis. Additionally, mediastinal irradiation can produce a syndrome of esophagitis clinically similar to infectious esophagitis. Children with both types will complain of odynophagia and substernal or retrosternal chest pain. Diagnostic studies include performing a barium swallow and endoscopic visualization of the mucosa. Definitive diagnosis requires endoscopic biopsy and culture.

Nursing care of children with mucositis and esophagitis is mainly supportive. Meticulous oral hygiene is required to reduce oral pathogens and keep the mucosa clean and debrided. Oral care measures that are instituted following cytotoxic chemotherapy or during head and neck radiation may help to prevent or reduce the severity of mucositis.[10,11,19] Daily oral care, including twice daily brushing of the teeth and gums with a soft bristle brush, and consistent use of non–alcohol-based mouthwash helps to promote good oral hygiene. Children who develop severe mucositis or esophagitis will have pain associated with the lesions or ulcers. These children will require frequent pain assessment and prompt administration of pain medications.[30] Additional information regarding the management of mucositis is found in Chapter 11.

Intraabdominal Infections

The immunosuppressed child is at increased risk of intraabdominal infections because of invasion or obstruction of the bowel by tumor, distal extension of mucosal sloughing, or ulcerations due to chemotherapy, as well as alterations in the normal intestinal flora caused by antibiotic use.

Diarrhea occurs frequently in immunocompromised patients. When infection is the cause of diarrhea in these patients, the specific organism involved varies, depending on such factors as the age and sex of the child, degree of immunosuppression, geographic area, and presence of other risk factors.[31] Common infectious causes of acute diarrhea in hospitalized neutropenic patients include *Campylobacter, Salmonella,* and *Shigella* species; *Escherichia coli* O157:H7; rotavirus; and *Clostridium difficile.*[31] Cases of acute diarrhea caused by *Shigella, Salmonella, C. difficile, E. coli* O157:H7, and CMV have been associated with complications such as peritonitis, intestinal perforation, and bacteremia.[31]

Diagnostic evaluation of the immunosuppressed child with acute diarrhea includes standard stool culture, testing for occult blood, and enzyme immunoassay for rotavirus and *C. difficile.* Although parasites are a frequent cause of community-acquired diarrhea, they are an infrequent cause of nosocomial diarrhea. Thus stool cultures for ova and parasite examination are recommended only for outpatients or inpatients who have been hospitalized less than 4 days.[31] Management of the child with *C. difficile* diarrhea is described below. Additional information regarding the management of diarrhea in the child receiving cancer therapy is found in Chapter 11.

Pseudomembranous or antibiotic-associated colitis has been reported following the use of many of the antibiotics that are part of empiric therapy in febrile neutropenic patients.[31] This process is associated with the production of toxins by *C. difficile.* Chemotherapeutic agents such as methotrexate, doxorubicin, cyclophosphamide, and fluorouracil have also been associated with *C. difficile* colitis.[31] Up to one half of young infants can be colonized, although colonization decreases with age. Many patients become colonized with *C. difficile* during hospitalization but never have symptoms. Children with *C. difficile*–associated diarrhea can have symptoms ranging from mild abdominal pain to severe bloody diarrhea.[1]

Stool samples are tested for *C. difficile* toxin in children with diarrhea and neutropenia. *C. difficile* colitis usually responds to treatment with oral metronidazole or oral vancomycin, but a small percentage of patients may relapse following initial treatment. If this occurs, the child can be retreated with a second course of the same medication.[1]

Typhlitis, or neutropenic enterocolitis, is a process involving the cecum and terminal ilium. It is seen almost exclusively in children with acute leukemia or other causes of prolonged, severe neutropenia.[31] Patients with typhlitis present with acute right lower quadrant pain and fever, similar to patients with appendicitis. Surgical intervention carries many risks for the neutropenic patient and is rarely performed. Because the child is neutropenic, signs of peritonitis are not commonly observed. If not identified promptly, the bowel may perforate. If this occurs, surgical resection may be necessary. Although uncommon, spontaneous peritonitis and resulting septicemia may occur. Despite aggressive intervention, mortality rates are approximately 30% to 50%.[17]

Nursing care of children with typhlitis consists of frequent patient assessment, administration of antibiotics, and supportive care measures such as nasogastric suctioning and fluid replacement. These children need frequent monitoring of vital signs, physical assessment, and pain assessment. Bowel sounds are assessed on a regular basis, and absence of bowel sounds is reported immediately. Changes in physical condition can occur quickly, and inadequate peripheral perfusion may be the first sign of perforation and bleeding. Measurement of the child's abdominal girth at the time of admission is an important baseline parameter, and subsequent measurements are done when vital signs are obtained. Parenteral antibiotics and other medications to provide comfort, such as antipyretics and pain relief, must be administered as ordered.

One of the most problematic of the intraabdominal infections afflicting patients with cancer is hepatic candidiasis. This infection occurs primarily in the child who is recovering from a prolonged period of neutropenia. Typically the child will have had persistent fever and neutropenia that is unresponsive to broad-spectrum antibiotics. Right upper quadrant pain and tenderness may or may not be present, and alkaline phosphatase may be elevated. Until the neutrophil count recovers, diagnostic imaging studies will not identify liver abnormalities or lesions.[24] However, once the inflammatory response has recovered, ultrasonography, CT, and magnetic resonance imaging may be useful in locating areas of fungal infection within the liver. Confirmation of the diagnosis requires liver biopsy. Treatment of hepatic candidiasis is difficult, usually requiring long-term treatment with an appropriate antifungal agent.[24]

Central Nervous System Infections

Central nervous system (CNS) infections are rare in children with cancer. However, any child with cancer who has undergone a neurosurgical procedure (e.g., placement of a VP shunt or Ommaya reservoir) is at increased risk for a CNS infection. If a child with one of these devices develops fever, vomiting, headache, sleepiness, or confusion, a diagnostic work-up is needed to determine whether a CNS infection has developed.

Pediatric oncology patients are also at risk of developing meningitis, usually bacterial or fungal. These patients present with headaches, altered mental status, and fevers, often without meningeal signs (e.g., stiff neck).[17] Immunocompromised children may also develop encephalitis, presenting with fever, headache, nuchal rigidity, and altered mental status. Cranial nerve deficits or seizures may also occur. The causative agents are often bacterial, fungal, parasitic, or viral organisms.[17] Pediatric oncology patients with altered mental status often require cranial imaging (e.g., CT scan or MRI) to discriminate between infectious and malignant causes of the mental status changes. Cranial lesions noted by diagnostic imaging can be either abscesses or malignant lesions. Children with CNS infections often require physical and occupational therapy in addition to prolonged antimicrobial therapy.

SEPSIS AND BACTEREMIA

Central venous catheters, as well as other types of indwelling devices, increase the incidence of infection in children with cancer. Normal flora that reside on the skin (e.g., staphylococci), as well as nosocomial pathogens, find a portal of entry via the central venous catheter. Without parenteral antibiotic therapy these infections can spread rapidly, leading to sepsis and bacteremia.

Sepsis is defined by the clinical suspicion of infection and evidence of a systemic response (e.g., hypotension, tachycardia, tachypnea, hyperthermia or hypothermia, leukocytosis or leukopenia). Bacteremia is defined by detection of viable bacteria in blood cultures.[39]

A wide variety of etiologic agents are responsible for causing septicemia in children with cancer (Box 10-3). Optimal management of the child with sepsis has three goals: rapid eradication of bacteria with effective antimicrobial therapy, stabilization of hemodynamic status, and modulation of the harmful inflammatory response.

Prompt initiation of antimicrobial agents is essential. The choice of antimicrobial agents is based on the likely causative organism, the age of the pa-

---

BOX 10-3

COMMON PATHOGENS THAT CAUSE SEPTICEMIA IN CHILDREN WITH CANCER

GRAM-POSITIVE BACTERIA
Staphylococcus (coagulase-negative, *S. aureus*)
Streptococcus (alpha-hemolytic and beta-hemolytic)
Enterococcus spp.
Corynebacterium spp.
Listeria spp.
Clostridium difficile

GRAM-NEGATIVE BACTERIA
Enterobacteriaciae *(Escherichia coli, Klebsiella,*
   Enterobacter, Serratia)
Pseudomonas aeruginosa, Stenotrophomonas
   maltophilia (and similar oxidase-positive
   multiresistant gram-negative organisms)
Anaerobes

FUNGI
Candida spp.
Aspergillus spp.
Cryptococcus spp.

OTHER
Pneumocystis carinii
Toxoplasma gondii
Strongyloides stercoralis
Cryptosporidium spp.

VIRUSES
Herpes simplex virus
Varicella-zoster virus
Cytomegalovirus
Epstein-Barr virus
Respiratory syncytial virus
Adenovirus

From Freifeld, A. G., Walsh, T. J., & Pizzo, P. A. (1997). Infectious complications in the cancer patient. In P. A. Pizzo & D. G. Poplack (Eds.), *Principles and practice of pediatric oncology* (3rd ed., pp. 1069-1114). Philadelphia: Lippincott-Raven.

tient and the immunologic status, and how the infection was acquired (e.g., nosocomial vs. community acquired).[38,39]

Supportive care must be provided to these children during the acute phase of illness to prevent or ameliorate complications. Appropriate management of fluid and electrolyte balance is a critically important supportive measure, especially if peripheral perfusion is compromised. Early expansion of circulating blood volume may be successful in enhancing oxygen delivery and preventing shock. Crystalloid substances such as Ringer's lactate or normal saline given in bolus volumes (20 ml/kg) is needed as a first line attempt at correcting or preventing circulatory shock. If these are not successful, then a colloid solution is added. Inotropic agents such as dopamine can be given if the child remains hypotensive.

Other supportive measures, including oxygen supplementation, mechanical ventilation, and pain control, are important. Both hypothermia and hyperthermia increase the oxygen requirement. Therefore a normal body temperature must be maintained with the help of warming measures or antipyretics as needed. Chemical disturbances such as electrolyte imbalances, metabolic acidosis, hypocalcemia, hypophosphatemia, and hypoglycemia are common. Septic shock is an emergent issue and is further described in Chapter 13.

Nurses caring for children with septicemia or bacteremia need to be aware of the potential complications that may occur. Frequent patient assessment and vital signs are performed with particular attention to pulse oximetry readings, peripheral perfusion, and neurologic status. Fluid and electrolyte balance must be monitored, and any deviations from normal are reported and interventions initiated. Strict intake and output must be monitored, as oliguria and anuria are early signs of renal failure. Respiratory compromise can occur at any point; therefore pulmonary assessment is included to determine the presence of tachypnea and adventitious breath sounds. Increased respiratory effort will also cause nasal flaring, retractions, and shortness of breath. If respiratory compromise occurs or if the circulating blood volume is not corrected, cardiac complications can develop. The nurse needs to assess for tachycardia, pulse quality, and peripheral perfusion as part of the physical examination.

PREVENTING INFECTIONS

Patient education about infectious risks is an essential component in preventing infection. Patients and their families are taught to avoid crowded areas and ill contacts, particularly when the patient's neutrophil count is low. Frequent hand washing is the single most important aspect of infection prevention.[18] High-efficiency particulate air (HEPA) filters provide some degree of protection against aspergillosis.[42] Construction areas are a source of aerosolized fungi infection in immunocompromised patients and are thus avoided when feasible.[14] The patient's environments at home and in the hospital are kept as clean as possible. However, reverse isolation and food sterilization have little impact on infection rates.[37] Families are also encouraged to avoid completely sheltering the child, as the origin of many infections is the child's own endogenous flora.[40] Data are lacking on the effectiveness of many infection prevention measures, making it difficult to determine the appropriate degree of lifestyle restriction.

Some patients have hypogammaglobulinemia, noted on testing done at baseline or due to recurrent infections. For these patients, IV immune globulin (IVIG) is administered as passive immunization, often on a monthly basis.[16] Hyperimmune globulins are also available, with high levels of antibodies for a particular pathogen. Certain products are given prophylactically to patients at high risk of developing infection with the pathogen, such as CMV immune globulin and respiratory syncytial virus immune globulin. Other products are available to be administered after exposure to the pathogen, including immune globulins for varicella (VZIG), tetanus, measles, hepatitis A, hepatitis B, and rabies.[16]

Guidelines for active immunization of pediatric oncology patients vary among centers. Live-virus vaccines are routinely avoided in immunocompromised children, as they may promote infection in the recipient. Although killed vaccines can be administered safely to immunocompromised hosts, controversy surrounds the use of killed vaccines.[12] Some oncologists do not recommend administering vaccines to pediatric oncology patients during treatment, as the effectiveness of the vaccines in immunocompromised hosts is unclear. As previously mentioned, pneumococcal and meningococcal vaccines are given to asplenic children. The influenza vaccine can be safely administered to patients and household contacts.[22]

Another controversy exists in the practice of administering varicella vaccine to siblings of immunocompromised children. The vaccine type infection is spread only via direct contact, rather than by the respiratory route, with a transmission rate of approximately one fourth the rate of typical varicella infection.[22] Varicella is transmitted only when the vaccine causes a rash, occurring in less than 5% of vaccinated immunocompetent children. Although the risk is low, there are reports of children transmitting the virus to immunosuppressed patients after developing a rash following varicella immunization.[13] Thus many oncologists avoid administering the varicalla vaccine to healthy siblings or household contacts. Varicella vaccine is not currently licensed for use in immunocompromised children in the United States.[13]

Oral polio vaccine is not given to household contacts of immunocompromised children, as the poliovirus is shed in the stool after administration of the oral vaccine. The oral polio vaccine is no longer routinely administered in the United States.

ANTIBIOTIC PROPHYLAXIS

Children with cancer are often at risk for developing infection because of the immunosuppression from the therapy they receive. Standard chemotherapy diminishes the body's ability to fight infection, as does splenectomy. Children undergoing hematopoietic stem cell transplant (HSCT) are at increased risk for infection after receiving myeloablative preparative regimens or if graft-versus-host disease (GVHD) develops. Prophylactic medication regimens are useful in preventing certain infections in these patients.

Immunocompromised children with cancer are at risk for developing infection due to *Pneumocystis carinii* (PCP). PCP infection occurs primarily in the lungs but can develop systemically as well. The incidence of PCP has decreased dramatically with the use of chemoprophylaxis. Trimethoprim-sulfamethoxazole, dapsone, pentamidine, and atovaquone are agents that are used prophylactically to decrease the incidence of infection with PCP.[6]

Children who have undergone splenectomy or who have functional asplenia are at risk for developing bacteremia. The most common pathogens that cause systemic infection include *Streptococcus pneumoniae, Neisseria meningitidis,* and *Haemophilus influenzae* type b (Hib). Pneumococcal, meningococcal, and Hib vaccines are recommended for use in asplenic children. The ages at which these vaccines are given vary. Meningococcal vaccines can be given to children 2 months of age and older, whereas immunization with Hib and pneumococcus can occur on the schedule recommended for healthy young children and for all unimmunized children with asplenia who were not previously vaccinated. Antimicrobial prophylaxis with oral penicillin or amoxicillin, in addition to vaccination against pneumococcal infection, is recommended in children after splenectomy.[4]

Antifungal prophylaxis is used primarily in children who have received HSCT. Various agents are used and vary according to institutional practice and cytotoxic chemotherapy that was given. Fluconazole is often used and is most beneficial in preventing the development of systemic candidiasis. However, the use of prophylaxis with fluconazole may cause patients to develop resistance to certain species, including *Candida krusei, Candida glabrata,* and *Aspergillus.*[17]

Children who are seropositive for herpes simplex virus (HSV) may require antiviral prophylaxis with intravenous or oral acyclovir during or after high-dose chemotherapy for leukemia or if receiving HSCT. If the patient develops acyclovir-resistant HSV, foscarnet can be given.[3]

Immunocompromised children who develop infection with influenza A can become severely ill and require hospitalization. Depending on institutional policy, antiviral agents can be given for selective prophylaxis. Oral amantadine and rimantadine are used for treatment and prophylaxis of influenza A in children 1 year of age and older.[5]

HSCT recipients are particularly at risk for developing serious, invasive infection with cytomegalovirus (CMV). Cytomegalovirus IVIG is available for use in seronegative transplant recipients.[2] Alternatively, intravenous ganciclovir can be used prophylactically to decrease the incidence of CMV infection in this population. The use of ganciclovir is associated with myelosuppression, therefore limiting its usefulness in some cases.[17]

Children with immune deficiency from cancer treatment are at risk for developing many different infections. The combination of immunologic and nonimmunologic risk factors (e.g., malnutrition, mucositis, granulocytopenia, indwelling catheters, and VP shunts) increases the likelihood that serious infection will develop in these patients. The most common sites of infection are the bloodstream, lungs, skin, GI tract, oral cavity, esophagus, and central nervous system. Nurses caring for this population must be acutely aware of the predisposing factors and signs and symptoms of infection in order to make a rapid assessment of the situation and initiate appropriate interventions and supportive care measures.

REFERENCES

1. American Academy of Pediatrics. (2000). *Clostridium difficile.* In L. K. Pickering (Ed.), *2000 Red Book: Report of the Committee on Infectious Diseases* (25th ed., pp. 214-216). Elk Grove Village, IL: Author.

2. American Academy of Pediatrics. (2000). Cytomegalovirus infection. In L. K. Pickering (Ed.), *2000 Red Book: Report of the Committee on Infectious Diseases* (25th ed., pp. 227-230). Elk Grove Village, IL: Author.

3. American Academy of Pediatrics. (2000). Herpes simplex. In L. K. Pickering (Ed.), *2000 Red Book: Report of the Committee on Infectious Diseases* (25th ed., pp. 309-318). Elk Grove Village, IL: Author.

4. American Academy of Pediatrics. (2000). Immunization in special clinical circumstances. In L. K. Pickering (Ed.), *2000 Red Book: Report of the Committee on Infectious Diseases* (25th ed., pp. 54-81). Elk Grove Village, IL: Author.

5. American Academy of Pediatrics. (2000). Influenza. In L. K. Pickering (Ed.), *2000 Red Book: Report of the Committee on Infectious Diseases* (25th ed., pp. 351-359). Elk Grove Village, IL: Author.

6. American Academy of Pediatrics. (2000). *Pneumocystis carinii* infections. In L. K. Pickering (Ed.), *2000 Red Book: Report of the Committee on Infectious Diseases* (25th ed., pp. 460-465). Elk Grove Village, IL: Author.

7. American Academy of Pediatrics. (2000). Varicella-Zoster infections. In L. K. Pickering (Ed.), *2000 Red Book: Report of the Committee on Infectious Diseases* (25th ed., pp. 624-638). Elk Grove Village, IL: Author.

8. Aquino, V. M., Tkaczewski, P., & Buchanan, G. R. (1997). Early discharge of low-risk febrile neutropenic children and adolescents with cancer. *Clinical Infectious Disease, 25,* 74-78.

9. Arvin, A. M. (1997). Varicella-Zoster virus. In S. S. Long, L. K. Pickering, & C. G. Prober (Eds.), *Principles and practice of pediatric infectious diseases* (pp. 1144-1154). New York: Churchill Livingstone.

10. Beck, S. (1979). Impact of a systematic oral care protocol on stomatitis after chemotherapy. *Cancer Nursing, 2,* 185-199.

11. Borowski, B., Benhamou, E., Pico, J. J., et al. (1994). Prevention of oral mucositis in patients treated with high-dose chemotherapy and bone marrow transplantation: A randomized controlled trial comparing two protocols of dental care. *European Journal of Cancer B Oral Oncology, 30B,* 93-97.

12. Centers for Disease Control and Prevention. (1993). Use of vaccines and immune globulins in persons with altered immunocompetence: Recommendations of the Advisory Committee on Immunization Practices (ACIP). *MMWR Morbidity and Mortality Weekly Reports, 42(RR-4),* 1-18.

13. Centers for Disease Control and Prevention. (1996). Guidelines for prevention of varicella: Recommendations of the Advisory Committee on Immunization Practices (ACIP). *MMWR Morbidity and Mortality Weekly Reports, 45(RR-11),* 1-36.

14. Centers for Disease Control and Prevention. (1997). Guidelines for prevention of nosocomial pneumonia. *MMWR Morbidity and Mortality Weekly Reports, 46(RR-1),* 1-79.

15. Chapman, S. W., & Daniel, C. R. (1994). Cutaneous manifestations of fungal infection. *Infectious Disease Clinics of North America, 8,* 879-910.

16. Conway, W. C. (2001). Immunizations in the immunocompromised host. In C. C. Patrick (Ed.), *Clinical management of infections in immunocompromised infants and children* (pp. 537-561). Philadelphia: Lippincott Williams & Wilkins.

17. Freifeld, A. G., Walsh, T. J., & Pizzo, P. A. (1997). Infectious complications in the cancer patient. In P. A. Pizzo & D. G. Poplack (Eds.), *Principles and practice of pediatric oncology* (3rd ed., pp. 1069-1114). Philadelphia: Lippincott-Raven.

18. Garner, J. S., & Favero, M. S. (1986). CDC guidelines for the prevention and control of nosocomial infections: Guideline for handwashing and hospital environmental control, 1985. *American Journal of Infection Control, 14,* 110-129.

19. Graham, K. M., Pecoraro, D. A., Ventura, M., et al. (1993). Reducing the incidence of stomatitis using a quality assessment and improvement approach. *Cancer Nursing, 16,* 117-122.

20. Griffin, T. C., & Buchanan, G. R. (1992). Hematologic predictors of bone marrow recovery in neutropenic patients hospitalized for fever: Implications for discontinuation of antibiotics and early discharge from the hospital. *Journal of Pediatrics, 121,* 28-33.

21. Groll, A. H., Irwin, R. S., Lee, J. W., et al. (2001). Management of specific infectious complications in children with leukemias and lymphomas. In C. C. Patrick (Ed.), *Clinical management of infections in immunocompromised infants and children* (pp. 111-143). Philadelphia: Lippincott Williams & Wilkins.

22. Hasting, C., Goes, C., & Wolff, L. J. (1997). Immunization of the child with cancer. In A. R. Ablin (Ed.), *Supportive care of children with cancer: Current therapy and guidelines from the Children's Cancer Group* (2nd ed., pp. 13-22). Baltimore: Johns Hopkins University Press.

23. Hostoffer, R. W. (2001). Disorders of host defense. In C. C. Patrick (Ed.), *Clinical management of infections in immunocompromised infants and children* (pp. 3-32). Philadelphia: Lippincott Williams & Wilkins.

24. Jackson, M. A., & Swanson, D. S. (2000). Infectious complications in the neutropenic patient. *Seminars in Infectious Diseases, 11,* 90-96.

25. Johanson, W. G., Pierce, A. K., & Sanford, J. P. (1969). Changing pharyngeal bacterial flora of hospitalized patients: Emergence of gram-negative bacilli. *New England Journal of Medicine, 281,* 1137-1140.

26. Johanson, W. G., Woods, D. E., & Chaudhuri, T. (1979). Association of respiratory tract colonization with adherence of gram-negative bacilli to epithelial cells. *Journal of Infectious Diseases, 139,* 667-673.

27. Jones, G. R., Konsler, G. K., Dunaway, R. P., et al. (1994). Risk factors for recurrent fever after the discontinuation of empiric antibiotic therapy for fever and neutropenia in pediatric patients with a malignancy or hematologic condition. *Journal of Pediatrics, 124,* 703-708.

28. Lewis, L. L., & Pizzo, P. A. (1997). Fever and granulocytopenia. In S. S. Long, L. K. Pickering, & C. G. Prober (Eds.), *Principles and practice of pediatric infectious diseases* (pp. 640-648). New York: Churchill Livingstone.

29. Mackall, C., Fleisher, T., Brown, M., et al. (1995). Age, thymopoiesis, and CD4+ T-lymphocyte regeneration, after intensive chemotherapy. *New England Journal of Medicine, 332,* 143-149.

30. Mackie, A. M., Coda, B. C., & Hill, H. F. (1991). Adolescents use patient-controlled analgesia effectively for relief from prolonged oropharyngeal mucositis pain. *Pain, 46,* 265-169.

31. Mitchell, D. K., & Pickering, L. K. (2001). Enteric infections. In C. C. Patrick (Ed.), *Clinical management of infections in immunocompromised infants and children* (pp. 413-449). Philadelphia: Lippincott Williams & Wilkins.

32. Mullen, C. A., & Buchanan, G. R. (1990). Early hospital discharge of children with cancer treated for fever and neutropenia: Identification and management of the low risk patient. *Journal of Clinical Oncology, 8,* 1998-2004.

33. Pizzo, P. A., Commers, J. R., Cotton, D. J., et al. (1984). Approaching the controversies in the antibacterial management of cancer patients. *American Journal of Medicine, 76,* 436-449.

34. Pizzo, P. A., Hathorn, J. W., Heimenz, J. W., et al. (1986). A randomized trial comparing ceftazidime alone with combination antibiotic therapy in cancer patients with fever and neutropenia. *New England Journal of Medicine, 315,* 552-558.

35. Pizzo, P. A., Robichaud, K. J., Edward, B. K., et al. (1983). Oral antibiotic prophylaxis in cancer patients: A double-blind randomized placebo controlled trial. *Journal of Pediatrics, 102,* 125-133.

36. Pizzo, P. A., Robichaud, K. J., & Wesley, R. (1982). Fever in the pediatric and young adult patient with cancer: A prospective study of 1001 episodes. *Medicine, 61,* 153-165.

37. Pizzo, P. A., Rubin, M., Freifeld, A., et al. (1991). The child with cancer and infection. I. Empiric therapy for fever and neutropenia and preventative strategies. *Journal of Pediatrics, 119,* 679-694.

38. Powell, K. R. (2000). Sepsis and shock. In R. E. Behrman, R. M. Kliegman, & H. B. Jenson (Eds.), *Nelson textbook of pediatrics* (16th ed., pp. 747-751). Philadelphia: W. B. Saunders.

39. Sáenz-Llorens, X., & McCracken, G. H. (1997). Septicemia and septic shock. In S. S. Long, L. K. Pickering, & C. G. Prober (Eds.), *Principles and practice of pediatric infectious diseases* (pp. 102-107). New York: Churchill Livingstone.

40. Schimpff, S. S., Young, V. M., Greene, W. H., et al. (1972). Origin of infection in acute non-lymphocytic leukemia. Significance of hospital acquisition of potential pathogens. *Annals of Internal Medicine, 77,* 707-714.

41. Soloway-Simon, D., & Levy, M. (2001). Dermatologic findings with infection. In C. C. Patrick (Ed.), *Clinical management of infections in immunocompromised infants and children* (pp. 470-508). Philadelphia: Lippincott Williams & Wilkins.

42. Withington, S., Chambers, S. T., Beard, M. E., et al. (1998). Invasive aspergillosis in severely neutropenic patients over 18 years: Impact of intranasal amphotericin B and HEPA filtration. *Journal of Hospital Infection, 38,* 11-18.

Management of Disease and Treatment-Related Complications

Cheryl Panzarella
Christina Rasco Baggott
Michael Comeau
Janet M. Duncan
Valerie Groben
Debbie Woods
Janet L. Stewart

Children with cancer face many physical challenges from their illness and the complications of treatment. Nurses employ both the science and art of symptom management when caring for these children.[73] Skilled symptom management requires up-to-date knowledge of evidence-based management strategies, continual evaluation of the effectiveness of the strategies used, and both creativity and persistence in adapting strategies to the needs and experiences of individual children. Nurses must learn to overcome barriers to effective symptom management, which include "we've always done it this way" thinking, financial concerns, inadequate administrative support, lack of knowledge, professional rivalry, "old wives tales," and poor communication.[73] Nurses skilled in symptom management provide critical expertise not only to the child and family, but also to physicians and other team members who look to them for guidance.

Ideally, nursing management of the complications of disease and treatment is research-based practice, employing interventions that have been systematically tested and shown to be effective. However, few studies of symptom management have been conducted in pediatric nursing, and findings from adult studies may have limited applicability or require significant adaptation for use in children. Therefore the goal of this chapter is to review what is currently known about managing the most prevalent physical symptoms of childhood cancer and its treatment, drawing from the existing research literature and the clinical expertise of experienced clinical staff. Pediatric oncology nurses can use this information to develop and implement preventive care strategies, symptom management interventions, and child and family education, with the ultimate goal of improving the outcomes of treatment for children with cancer.

BONE MARROW SUPPRESSION

Bone marrow suppression may occur as a result of disease or treatment. Bone marrow suppression, which is the one of the most common dose-limiting toxicities of chemotherapy,[21] may result in a decrease in red blood cells (RBCs), white blood cells (WBCs), and platelets. The life span of these three types of blood varies (Table 11-1), but the nadir, or time of most profound bone marrow suppression, is approximately 10 to 14 days after myelosuppressive treatment. Previous chemotherapy and/or radiation can affect the nadir and recovery time from subsequent courses of myelosuppressive therapy.[130] A basic format that can be used in teaching about blood counts is included in Table 11-2.

LEUKOPENIA

Definition/contributing factors. Leukopenia is a decrease in the absolute number of white blood cells. Neutropenia, a decrease in the number of neutrophils that fight infection, is the most severe consequence of bone marrow suppression. The relative risk of infection is determined by the absolute neutrophil count (ANC), calculated as total WBC count $\times$ neutrophils (% polys + % bands). Children with severe neutropenia (ANC <500) are at risk for life-threatening infections, which may be bacterial, fungal, or viral.

TABLE 11-1	LIFE SPAN AND FUNCTION OF HEMATOPOIETIC CELLS	
Cell Type	Life Span	Function
Mature RBCs	120 days	Carry oxygen to cells
Neutrophils	6-8 hr	Phagocytosis
Eosinophils	5-24 hr	Allergic reactions
Lymphocytes	100-300+ days	Antibody production (B) Cellular immunity (T)
Monocytes	8 hr	Phagocytosis
Platelets	10 days	Prevent or stop bleeding

Clinical presentation. A thorough physical assessment of the febrile child is essential. Evaluation includes the following: monitoring for hemodynamic instability with assessment of peripheral pulses, skin color, perfusion, and vital signs; assessing the skin for altered integrity, erythema, swelling, or drainage, particularly at central venous access sites; auscultating the lungs for abnormal breath sounds or cough; assessing the ears, nose, throat, and mouth for signs and symptoms of infection, such as rhinorrhea, tenderness, erythema, or stomatitis; auscultating the abdomen and assessing for abdominal tenderness; monitoring the perineum for perirectal tenderness, abcesses, or fissures; and evaluating for signs of dehydration such as skin turgor and urinary output.

Treatment strategies. If fever is present with neutropenia, intravenous (IV) antibiotic treatment is imperative. Antifungal therapy is often added if fever persists with prolonged neutropenia. Respiratory compromise is minimized by encouraging incentive spirometry, increased activity, administering oxygen as ordered, and allowing the patient to assume a position of comfort. Abdominal pain or tenderness usually requires a combined approach of clinical and radiologic evaluation. Computed tomography (CT) scan is the best diagnostic method to rule out neutropenic colitis. Based on diagnostic imaging and clinical findings, the most likely approach is conservative. This may include bowel rest and parenteral nutrition, but each case is evaluated on an individual basis. Hemodynamically unstable patients are given fluid and medications to support blood pressure. Patients with altered skin integrity need close monitoring and may require surgical debridement of wounds.

Treatment with granulocyte colony stimulating factor (G-CSF) to stimulate the bone marrow and reduce the severity and length of neutropenia is often prescribed. This agent is usually given daily by subcutaneous injection beginning 24 to 36 hours after chemotherapy is completed and continuing until the white blood cell count recovers from its nadir. There is a theoretical risk that G-CSF given concurrently with chemotherapy may induce progenitor cell cycling to cause an increase in myelotoxicity.[18] Thus, the first dose of G-CSF is administered at least 24 hours after completing chemotherapy.

Most, but not all, children undergoing immunosuppressive therapy will be given prophylactic antibiotics to prevent the opportunistic infection *Pneumocystis carinii* pneumonia[56] throughout their treatment course.

Nursing role. Thorough assessment of any pediatric oncology patient with fever or other signs of infection is an essential nursing role. The nurse must communicate pertinent laboratory values and the patient's clinical condition to the treatment team and recognize subtle signs of infection and evidence of impending septic shock.

Home care instructions must clearly communicate that fever in this population can be an emergency. Parents are instructed to call if the child experiences temperatures greater than 38° C on two occasions in 24 hours or greater than 38.5° C once (or as determined by institutional policy). Families must also be instructed to report shaking chills, signs of respiratory compromise, a change in the child's level of consciousness, or any general change in the child's condition. The key to managing a febrile neutropenic patient is early assessment and intervention. Nurses must also reinforce the importance of frequent hand washing. Additional information about preventing and treating infections is found in Chapter 10. Septic shock is covered in Chapter 13.

ANEMIA

Definition/contributing factors. Anemia, or a decrease in RBCs, can occur secondary to myelosuppressive chemotherapy or radiation, blood loss, effects of chronic disease, replacement of the bone marrow by tumor cells, or by viral suppression.

Clinical presentation. Children with anemia may present with decreased energy, fatigue, pallor, tachypnea, tachycardia, and/or headache. Children often tolerate low hemoglobin concentrations well. However, if they are symptomatic, about to undergo surgery or intensive radiation treatment, or are about to enter a myelosuppressive period, then transfusion with packed red blood cells may be indicated.

TABLE 11-2	**A Basic Format That Can Be Used for Teaching About Blood Counts**	
Purpose	**Normal Values**	**Special Care for Low Values**
RED BLOOD CELLS		
Give energy to the body Provide color to the skin Carry oxygen to all parts of the body	Hemoglobin (Hgb) 13.5-17.0 g/dl Hemocrit (Hct) 34%-41% **ADEQUATE/ACCEPTABLE** Hgb >7-8 g/dl Hct >21%-24% **TRANSFUSION OFTEN NEEDED** Hgb <7 g/dl Hct <21% (or at higher values with certain circumstances—see text)	Transfusion may be necessary. Watch for increasing fatigue, headache, dizziness, pallor (particularly in conjunctiva and lips), and irritability. Provide rest between periods of activity.
PLATELETS		
Prevent bleeding Promote clotting	150,000-450,000/mm^3 **ADEQUATE/ACCEPTABLE** 50,000-100,000/mm^3 **TRANSFUSION OFTEN NEEDED** <10,000-20,000/mm^3 (or at higher values with certain circumstances—see text)	Transfusion may be necessary. Provide for safety in activity when platelets low—avoid activities that can cause injury when platelet count below 50,000-100,000/mm^3: • Clean teeth with soft toothbrush, gauze, or washcloth. • Wear helmet when bike riding. • Avoid contact sports. • Shave with electric razor only. • Avoid sexual intercourse. Know how to stop nosebleed or profuse bleeding. Watch for gum bleeding or bleeding from other sources. Prevent perirectal injury by maintaining soft stools and avoiding rectal temperatures, enemas, or suppositories. Avoid medications containing ibuprofen or aspirin, and Pepto-Bismol.
WHITE BLOOD CELLS		
Fight infection Neutrophils—type of WBC that fight bacterial infections Neutrophils also called segs and bands, polys, stabs, or granulocytes	4,500-11,500/mm^3 **ADEQUATE/ACCEPTABLE** Absolute neutrophil count (ANC) >1,000/mm^3 **WATCH CLOSELY** ANC <500/mm^3	Learn how to calculate ANC; know your child's current ANC level. Calling for fevers is the single most important activity to prevent severe complications from low ANC; children

Adapted from Waskerwitz, M. J. (1984). Special nursing care for children receiving chemotherapy. *Journal of the Association of Pediatric Oncology Nurses, 1*(1), 16-25.

Continued

TABLE 11-2	A BASIC FORMAT THAT CAN BE USED FOR TEACHING ABOUT BLOOD COUNTS—cont'd	
Purpose	**Normal Values**	**Special Care for Low Values**
WHITE BLOOD CELLS—cont'd		
		with fever are admitted for intravenous (IV) antibiotics if ANC <500/mm^3 because children can die within 12-24 hours of untreated bacterial or fungal blood infection. Do not give acetaminophen for fevers unless you have talked with the oncology team; may use for pain after checking for fever and temperature is below 100° F (one dose only). Good hand-washing is essential; avoid ill contacts. Monitor skin for signs of infection. Call if child has chills, especially after flushing IV; becomes extremely fatigued; or has other significant change in condition. Avoid rectal temperatures, enemas, and suppositories.

Adapted from Waskerwitz, M. J. (1984). Special nursing care for children receiving chemotherapy. *Journal of the Association of Pediatric Oncology Nurses, 1*(1), 16-25.

Treatment strategies. The standard transfusion volume is 10 to 20 ml/kg of leukocyte-reduced, irradiated, packed red blood cells. The hemoglobin values used as criteria for transfusion vary by institution, but usually transfusion is considered with hemoglobin values of 6 to 7 g/dl or when children develop severe fatigue, irritability, tachycardia, or lassitude. Most radiotherapists request that transfusions be given to children receiving radiation therapy to maintain a hemoglobin level of 10 g/dl or higher because well-oxygenated cells respond best to radiotherapy. Controversy exists about transfusing children with hemoglobin levels between 7 and 10 g/dl.[20] When making the decision about blood transfusion consider the clinical situation (e.g., tachycardia, concurrent respiratory infection, and concurrent radiotherapy), and whether or not the blood counts are recovering (e.g., presence of nucleated RBCs or reticulocytes). Education for family caregivers includes the signs and symptoms of anemia and strategies to support the child while anemic. Recombinant human erythropoietin may be used to boost erythropoiesis during periods of myelosuppression, particularly for those with religious objec-

tions to blood transfusions. Subcutaneous erythropoietin given three times a week will cause a 1 to 2 g/dl rise in the hemoglobin level.[163]

Nursing role. The nurse must assess the child's need for transfusion and communicate pertinent laboratory values and clinical symptoms to the health care team. When blood products are administered, monitor the patient closely for transfusion reactions. The family is taught to recognize the signs and symptoms of anemia, and the administration of erythropoietin if needed. Additional information regarding anemia is found in Chapter 14.

THROMBOCYTOPENIA

Definition/contributing factors. Thrombocytopenia is defined as fewer than 100,000/mm^3 circulating platelets, caused by malignant cells in the marrow, myelosuppressive therapy, or increased platelet consumption (e.g., disseminated intravascular coagulation [DIC]). Fever and other conditions may exacerbate thrombocytopenia. Spontaneous bleeding (i.e., without antecedent trauma) is generally associated with a platelet count of less than 5,000/mm^3.[155] The number of platelets removed randomly each day from the circulation is about 7100/mm^3, which is thought to be the number of platelets needed to repair the endothelium and prevent bleeding in many circumstances.[65]

Clinical presentation. Children may have presenting symptoms of petechiae, increased bruising, epistaxis, mucosal bleeding, or less commonly, neurologic changes secondary to intracranial bleeding. It is important to assess the child's neurologic status and the skin, mouth, nose, sclera, and output (urine, stool, emesis) for signs of microscopic or obvious bleeding.

Treatment strategies. Controversy exists regarding the transfusion of platelets and whether or not they should be given prophylactically, because of the risks of alloimmunization, transfusion reactions, and hepatitis.[20] Platelet transfusions are indicated when a child is bleeding and may be given prophylactically when a child's platelet count is 10,000 to 20,000 cells/mm^3. At least one study in adult leukemia patients has shown that the frequency of major bleeding episodes was not reduced by administering prophylactic platelet transfusions for platelet counts less than 20,000/mm^3 as compared with 10,000/mm^3.[134] Platelets may be transfused at levels higher than this for patients experiencing fevers, coagulopathies, or fresh bleeding, or before invasive procedures, although findings from a study at St. Jude Children's Research Hospital suggest that serious complications related to lumbar puncture are rare even in children with platelet counts less than 20,000/mm^3.[77] The American Society of Clinical Oncology (ASCO) performed an extensive review of the literature on platelet transfusions and recommends that the threshold for platelet transfusions in children receiving cancer therapy be set at 10,000/mm^3. This recommendation is based on prospective randomized studies in adults. However, the recommendations included considering higher thresholds for patients with signs of hemorrhage, high fever, hyperleukocytosis, rapid decrease in the platelet count, coagulation abnormalities, and those undergoing invasive procedures, as well as in neonates.[143] A standard platelet transfusion (4 random donor units of platelets per square meter) should increase a child's platelet count by 50,000/mm^3 when measured 1 hour after the transfusion.[9]

Nursing role. Nurses must assess a child's need for platelet transfusion and communicate any pertinent findings to the treatment team. When platelets are ordered, the patient is monitored for transfusion reaction. Refer to Chapter 14 for additional information about platelet transfusion. Nurses must also teach the family to recognize the signs and symptoms of low platelet count and safety measures for children and adolescents when the platelet count is low (see Table 11-2).

FATIGUE

Definition/contributing factors. Although fatigue is increasingly identified as a major complication of childhood cancer treatment, it has only recently been systematically studied. Research indicates that adult cancer patients are profoundly affected by fatigue, which affects their psychologic, physical, spiritual, and social quality of life.[51,136] However, because it has been seen as a subjective experience, the study of fatigue has been slow to emerge. Recent studies in children with cancer have brought this issue to the forefront in pediatric oncology nursing.[69,70,72]

Defining fatigue has been a major challenge, but ongoing pediatric fatigue research suggests that both children (age 7 to 12 years old) and adolescents (age 13 to 18 years old) can effectively describe fatigue in terms of physical and mental symptoms. Younger children described fatigue as feeling weak or tired, having a "dull face," or feeling mad and sad.[72] Teens were more elaborate, describing not only physical symptoms of sleepiness, nausea, dizziness, and wearing away their body, but also being mentally tired, not themselves, and feeling sorry for themselves.[72]

The causes of fatigue identified in school-age children and adolescents include treatment for cancer (surgery, chemotherapy, and/or radiation), side effects of low blood counts, fever, pain, and doing too many activities.[72] Changes in the patterns and quality of sleep are also a major cause of fatigue, particularly in the hospital when hospital staff, medical equipment, and other noises interrupt patients' sleep. Adolescents also identified worry and fears as causes of fatigue, describing being afraid to fall asleep or having concerns that prevented them from sleeping (Figure 11-1).[69] Parents and staff also noted waiting (for procedures and appointments), inadequate nutrition, and receiving cues about fatigue from others as sources of children's fatigue.[69]

Treatment strategies. Treatment strategies are varied and begin with a thorough assessment of the child, including the child's concept of the causes of fatigue. Other assessment measures include looking for correctable causes of fatigue (anemia, pain, dehydration, or poor nutrition), differentiating fatigue from depression, and evaluating the child's pattern of activity.[181]

Although in the work of Hinds et al. neither children nor adolescents saw parents or medical

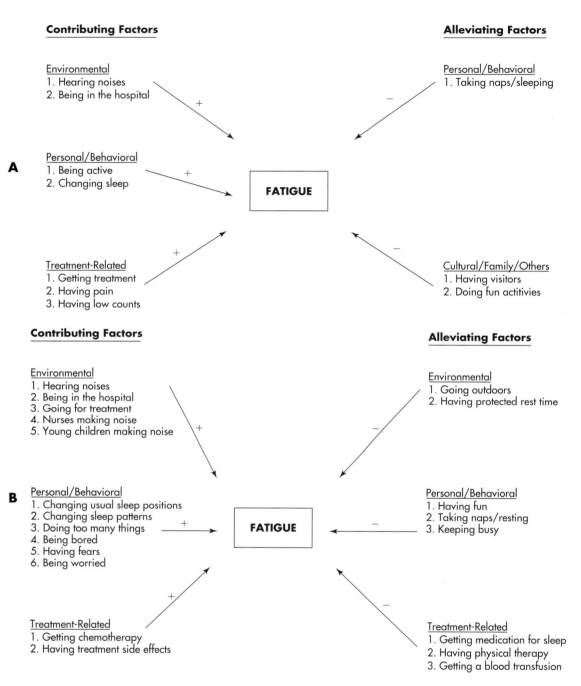

Figure 11-1

A, Factors identified by 7- to 12-year-old patients that contribute to or alleviate their fatigue. **B,** Factors identified by 13- to 18-year-old patients that contribute to or alleviate their fatigue. (From Hinds, P. S., Hockenberry-Eaton, M., Quargnenti, A., et al. [1999]. Comparing patient, parent, and staff descriptions of fatigue in pediatric oncology patients. *Cancer Nursing 22*[4], 284.)

staff as being able to help alleviate fatigue, they were able to identify many self-care strategies for managing fatigue. Children identified taking naps, having visitors, and doing fun activities. Teens listed similar activities and medication for sleep, physical therapy, and blood transfusions to relieve fatigue.[69] Family, friends, and staff may support these self-care strategies by encouraging adequate nutrition and rest, providing activities that distract from treatment or hospital life, minimizing interruptions during sleep, and encouraging participation in usual activities. Some children and adolescents may not be able to attend school for the whole day but may attend half a day, or just during lunch to interact with peers.[69,70,72]

Nursing role.   A variety of potential nursing interventions have been described by these early studies of fatigue in children with cancer. These include respecting sleep time; decreasing interruptions, noise, and waiting times; providing encouragement; and problem solving with the child about new ways to participate in activities, meet nutritional or physical needs, or receive emotional support. Education of the child and family includes information about what to expect and how to maximize energy and relaxation and providing some guidelines for modifying activities.[69] Other important nursing interventions include optimizing treatment-related strategies to prevent or alleviate fatigue by responding to the child's symptoms quickly and efficiently, initiating adequate analgesia, nutrition, and transfusions, and implementing complementary therapies with the goals of maximizing energy and well-being and decreasing fatigue.

GASTROINTESTINAL SYSTEM

The gastrointestinal system, because of its natural patterns of rapid cell division, is a prime target for toxicity from chemotherapy and radiation therapy. Nurses play a key role in prevention strategies, early detection, appropriate supportive care, and patient and family education. Typhlitis, a life-threatening gastrointestinal complication of cancer treatment, is covered in Chapter 10. The more prevalent gastrointestinal side effects include mucositis, nausea and vomiting, diarrhea and constipation, chemical hepatitis, pancreatitis, and diminished nutritional status.

Mucositis

Definition/contributing factors.   Inflammation of the oral mucosa, known as mucositis, is a common dose-limiting toxicity induced by cancer

chemotherapy, radiotherapy, and neutropenia.[115,124] Cell destruction by chemotherapy or local radiation and an inadequate production of new cells result in the loss of mucosal integrity. Estimates of the incidence of oral mucositis secondary to standard cancer chemotherapy range from 31% to 40%[119,132,160] and rise to 76% in hematopoietic stem cell transplant patients.[160] The incidence of mucositis in children is thought to be higher than that in adults, possibly related to the high mitotic rate in children's gastric mucosa.[159] Chemotherapeutic agents associated with mucositis are listed in Box 11-1. Children who lack routine dental care before cancer treatment have a greater risk for developing severe stomatitis and infectious complications than children receiving regular dental care.[119] The consequences of mucositis include painful lesions that often require opiate analgesia, and decreased oral intake and nutrition.[45,97,114,124,131] Furthermore, compromised oral mucosa provides a portal of entry for microorganisms, and when accompanied by concomitant neutropenia, can result in significant infections.[85,94] Recovery from mucositis often occurs as the white blood cell count increases after chemotherapy-induced myelosuppression.

Clinical presentation.   The onset, duration, and severity of mucositis are related to the agent, dose, and duration of chemotherapy administration.[1] Stomatitis can range from reddened areas to deep ulcerations. Other signs and symptoms include pain; difficulty swallowing; thick oral secretions; white patches; cracked, dry lips; and drooling.

Impaired tissue integrity in the oral cavity greatly increases the risk of infection. Fungal infection, commonly caused by *Candida albicans,* presents as white plaques with indurated borders. The tongue is often swollen, dry, and cracked. Herpes

---

BOX 11-1

CHEMOTHERAPEUTIC AGENTS COMMONLY ASSOCIATED WITH MUCOSITIS

Bleomycin
Cytarabine
Dactinomycin
Daunorubicin
Doxorubicin
Fluorouracil
Mercaptopurine
Methotrexate
Thioguanine

From Aitken, T. (1992). Gastrointestinal manifestations in the child with cancer. *Journal of Pediatric Oncology Nursing, 9,* 99-108.

simplex virus (HSV) presents as painful, scabbed blisters on the lips or anywhere in the oral cavity, accompanied by a yellowish-brown membrane. A viral culture must be done to ensure proper diagnosis. Patients with positive HSV titer are more likely to develop herpetic lesions.[135]

Several oral assessment tools have been validated for clinical use,[47,144,161] but these tools can be used only by health care professionals because they are complex, requiring the rating of eight or more different areas of the oral cavity. Other severity scales put both observable and functional status into one grading scale,[109,178] but they may have limited reliability because some patients with severe mucositis continue to eat and drink adequately. Because mucositis tends to occur several days after chemotherapy is administered, when many patients are at home, simpler mucositis rating systems that can be used by patients and families are needed. This will facilitate crucial data collection for research studies of the efficacy of mucositis interventions.

Treatment strategies. There are no drugs or treatments currently available that have shown consistent efficacy in preventing mucositis.[85,98,129] The treatments and/or prophylaxis for mucositis are therefore quite variable from one oncology center to another and reflect a variety of approaches.[114] Conflicting data exist on the efficacy of chlorhexidine gluconate (Peridex), a commonly used mouthwash for the prevention of mucositis.[42,52-54,177] The largest study compared prophylaxis with chlorhexidine to sterile water for adult oncology patients receiving outpatient chemotherapy and found no significant difference in the incidence, severity, or duration of mucositis between the two groups.[42] Data on reliable methods to treat existing mucositis are also limited and come primarily from adult studies. In a recent study, 200 adults with mucositis after chemotherapy were randomized to one of three treatment regimens: salt and soda, chlorhexidine, or "magic" mouthwash (lidocaine, diphenhydramine, and an antacid preparation). Resolution of mucositis was not significantly different among the three preparations.[41] Other agents used to prevent and/or treat mucositis in clinical practice also have conflicting research results, including sucralfate* and glutamine, an amino acid.[6,7,154] Research into the usefulness of these and other agents is ongoing.

Given the lack of evidence supporting the use of particular medications in the management of mucositis, the role of routine oral hygiene is criti-

cal.[85,98,129] Beck reports that when oncology patients used a systematic oral care program of toothbrushing and mouthwash after meals and at bedtime, they had less intense mucositis and decreased rates of infection when compared with controls.[10] Graham and her colleagues also noted a decrease in the incidence of severe mucositis in an oncology population after a systematic oral care regimen of brushing the teeth with a soft toothbrush and rinsing with saline after meals and at bedtime was implemented.[61] Borowski et al. also documented significantly less mucositis in hematopoietic stem cell transplant patients who had intensive dental assessment and intervention before transplant and maintained oral hygiene regimens during aplasia, as compared with those without pretransplant dental screening and with suspended toothbrushing during aplasia.[16]

Oral infections can occur concomitantly with mucositis and must be adequately treated. IV or oral acyclovir is given to treat patients with HSV infection. Many centers give prophylactic acyclovir to patients with positive HSV titers. Nystatin is used at many centers for the prevention or treatment of oral candidiasis, but its effectiveness has not been demonstrated in clinical studies.[19,38,48] Clotrimazole troches have been effective in preventing oral candidiasis in adults.[28,37]

The discomfort that accompanies mucositis may range from mild to severe. Topical agents such as lidocaine, diphenhydramine, and an antacid can be mixed and applied directly to sores. Acetaminophen is helpful, but for more severe mucositis an opioid may be necessary to control pain. A continuous opioid infusion and/or boluses can be accomplished with patient-controlled analgesia for the older child. Consider pain control before mouth care and before meals or snacks to ensure the optimal compliance of the child. Additional information on pain control is found in Chapter 12.

Nursing role. Maintaining adequate nutrition and hydration is a challenge for the child with moderate to severe mucositis. A soft diet with cool and bland foods may be most accepted. Ice chips and popsicles can be soothing and helpful in hydration and maintaining moisture in the lips and mucous membranes. The child's nutritional status must be closely monitored. Accurate recording of intake, output, and weight are necessary. If oral intake cannot be maintained, supplemental IV fluids will be necessary. For some children, parenteral nutrition may be necessary until the oral cavity heals.

Education regarding oral hygiene begins at the time of diagnosis. Routine practices are evaluated and modified as necessary. A soft toothbrush is the

---

*References 24, 26, 49, 55, 92, 96.

preferred tool to clean the teeth. Although a foam brush alone is ineffective in controlling plaque and gingivitis, a foam brush soaked in chlorhexidine may be an effective dental tool.[133] Lanolin or petroleum jelly can be applied to the child's lips routinely to maintain moisture.

Education for the child and family includes the expected time of onset for mucositis and its signs and symptoms, methods of good oral hygiene, and strategies to relieve pain, maintain nutrition, and identify potential complications such as infection, bleeding, and dehydration.

NAUSEA AND VOMITING

Definition/contributing factors. Nausea and vomiting are common side effects of cancer treatment. Nausea is a subjective symptom that is described as the recognition of the need to vomit.[75] Vomiting is the forceful expulsion of gastric contents as a consequence of the complex reflex actions initiated by the vomiting center in the medulla. Retching is the attempt at vomiting, without the expulsion of gastric contents. Nausea and vomiting are often associated with perspiration, pallor, gastric stasis, and tachycardia.[86] Because the experience of nausea may be difficult for a young child to describe, family members can be very helpful in understanding the child's special words or expressions. Nausea often occurs in conjunction with vomiting, but either can occur independently. Uncontrolled nausea and vomiting can lead to severe dehydration, electrolyte imbalances, and emotional distress.

There is a paucity of research on nausea and vomiting in children. Much of the baseline research was performed in the 1980s and has not been replicated recently with newer antiemetic and chemotherapeutic regimens. Research on adult cancer patients' experiences with nausea and vomiting is useful but must be applied cautiously because the pharmacokinetics of many drugs vary between adults and children. Additional research on antiemetics in children is greatly needed.

Vomiting occurs when central and/or peripheral neurologic pathways stimulate the vomiting center in the brainstem (also known as the emetic integrative circuitry or emetic center). The chemoreceptor trigger zone (CTZ), vagal afferents, pharyngeal afferents, midbrain afferent, and the vestibular system are some of the pathways involved (Figure 11-2).[75]

The CTZ is located in the brain at the area postrema near the fourth ventricle. Neurotransmitters such as serotonin, dopamine, histamine, prostaglandins, and γ-aminobutyric acid stimulate the CTZ, which then stimulates the vomiting center. The CTZ receives messages from locally released

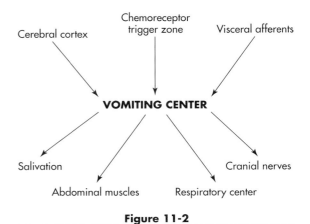

Figure 11-2

The pathway of emesis.

neurotransmitters and indirectly from peripherally released neurotransmitters in the gut via the vagal afferents. The vagal afferents can also stimulate the vomiting center directly, after detecting mechanical or chemical changes within the upper gastrointestinal tract (Figure 11-3).[75] Although the CTZ was previously considered the central mechanism of emesis, the peripheral mechanisms are gaining attention, because 80% of the body's serotonin is released from the intestinal enterochromaffin cells.[35] Stimulation of the pharyngeal afferents, such as that occurring with intense coughing, can promote vomiting. Increased intracranial pressure can also cause vomiting through stimulation of the midbrain afferent. The vestibular system causes motion-related nausea and vomiting.[75] The cerebral cortex also plays a role in nausea and vomiting. Psychologic factors such as anxiety and a patient's prior experience with nausea and vomiting can increase chemotherapy-associated nausea and emesis.[43,113]

Chemotherapy administration causes nausea and vomiting through the release of emetic neurotransmitters. In the 1980s dopamine and histamine were thought to be the primary neurotransmitters associated with chemotherapy-induced vomiting. However, further investigation lead to the discovery of serotonin as an important cause of emesis for patients receiving chemotherapy. Radiation-induced emesis is also likely related to serotonin release when treatment is directed to the abdomen. Radiation may also directly stimulate the vagus to send impulses to the CTZ. Cerebral edema is thought to be the cause of emesis for patients receiving cranial radiation.[75] Cancer patients may also experience nausea and vomiting related to increased intracranial pressure, metabolic disturbances, delayed gastric emptying, anesthetic

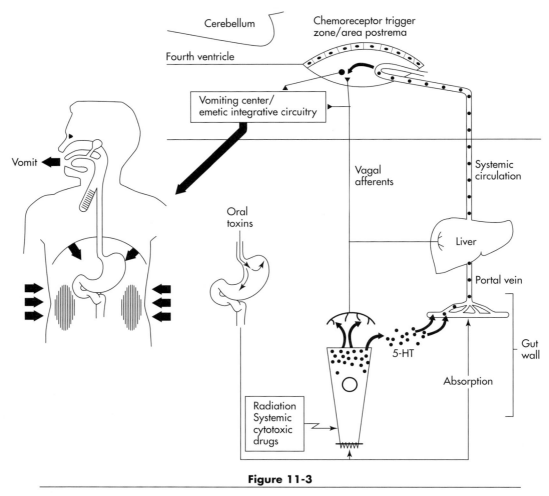

Figure 11-3

Physiologic mechanisms of nausea and vomiting. (From Hogan, C. M., & Grant, M. [1997]. Physiologic mechanisms of nausea and vomiting in patients with cancer. *Oncology Nursing Forum, 24[Suppl. 7]*, 8-12.)

agents, and opioid therapy.[75] Use careful assessment to determine the likely cause of nausea and vomiting.

Nausea and vomiting related to chemotherapy may be acute, delayed, or anticipatory. Acute emesis occurs within the first 24 hours of treatment. In a survey of emetic control among pediatric patients, girls experienced more acute nausea and vomiting than did boys, and adolescents experienced more symptoms than did children 4 to 11 years of age.[156] Delayed emesis occurs approximately 24 hours after chemotherapy administration and may last a week or longer.[75] In multiple-day chemotherapy cycles, children may experience the effects of both acute and delayed emesis simultaneously. Anticipatory nausea and vomiting (ANV) is considered to be a conditioned response and occurs

after a child has received at least one cycle of chemotherapy.

Treatment strategies. A variety of techniques are used to control or prevent nausea and vomiting. The most common is the administration of antiemetics. Principles for the use of antiemetics include the following[172]:

- Conditioned responses are more likely to occur if early chemotherapy courses are not well controlled. It is difficult to ameliorate nausea and vomiting once it becomes severe, thus prophylactic doses are given 30 to 60 minutes before chemotherapy and continued on a routine basis if prolonged nausea is expected.
- Base the antiemetic regimen on the emetogenicity of the chemotherapy given. An example of an

TABLE 11-3	EMETIC POTENTIAL		
No Emetic Potential	**Low Emetic Potential**	**Moderate Emetic Potential**	**High Emetic Potential**
Asparaginase	Cladribine	Carboplatin	Azacytidine
Bleomycin	Cyclophosphamide	Carmustine	Cisplatin
Chlorambucil	<10 mg/kg	Cytarabine <1 g/m^2	Cyclophosphamide
Corticosteroids	Etoposide	Dactinomycin	>10 mg/kg
Hydroxyurea	Fluorouracil	Daunorubicin	Cytarabine ≥ 1 g/m^2
Mercaptopurine PO	Intrathecal	Doxorubicin	Dacarbazine
Methotrexate <1 g/m^2	chemotherapy	Idarubicin	Mechlorethamine
Paclitaxel	Mercaptopurine IV	Ifosfamide	
Thioguanine	Procarbazine	Lomustine	
Vinblastine	Teniposide	Methotrexate ≥ 1 g/m^2	
Vincristine		Mitoxantrone	

Data from Fishman, M., & Mrozek-Orlowski, M. (1999). *Cancer chemotherapy guidelines and recommendations for practice.* Pittsburgh, PA: Oncology Nursing Press; van Hoff, J., Hockenberry-Eaton, M. J., Patterson, K., et al. (1991). A survey of antiemetic use in children. *American Journal of Diseases in Childhood, 145,* 773-778.

ANTIEMETIC REGIMEN

Move to the next step if patient experiences 4 hr of nausea in 24 hr or two emetic episodes in 24 hr.

Step 1: Ondansetron PO before chemotherapy Step 2: Ondansetron PO before chemotherapy and additional dose 4-6 hr later—maximum two doses per day	Step 1: Ondansetron PO before chemotherapy and × 1 after chemotherapy, given every 4-6 hr PO or IV*—maximum two doses per day Step 2: Ondansetron: increase to two doses after chemotherapy—maximum three doses per day Step 3: Add dexamethasone† Step 4: Add any of the following agents: • Promethazine‡ • Hydroxyzine • Lorazepam • Scopolamine‡ patch (use only for adolescents) • Metoclopromide with diphenhydramine‡	Step 1: Ondansetron PO or IV* before chemotherapy and × 2 after chemotherapy, given every 4-6 hr PO or IV—maximum three doses per day and dexamethasone† Step 2: Add any of agents in Step 4 of moderate emetic potential column Step 3: Add dronabinol (only for adolescents) Step 4: Stop ondansetron; start granisetron Step 5: Increase granisetron dose

*Give ondansetron IV only if patient is unable to tolerate the oral dose—comes in solution, 4-mg and 8-mg tabs (may be halved), and 4-mg and 8-mg oral disintegrating tablets (ODT).
†Dexamethasone is to be used with caution for patients with brain tumors or patients with any steroids in treatment protocol.
‡Scopolamine, diphenhydramine, and promethazine may have additive anticholinergic effects.

emetogenicity scale is included in Table 11-3. Keep the drug plan simple to avoid errors.

• Individualize the antiemetic plan. Some patients prefer to sleep all day, whereas others detest feeling drowsy. Document the plan used and the response to treatment for guidance during future chemotherapy courses.

Acute nausea/vomiting. Box 11-2 lists the antiemetic agents commonly used in children. The most frequently used drugs are the serotonin (5-HT$_3$) antagonists (e.g., ondansetron and granisetron). Serotonin is released from intestinal cells

in response to chemotherapy or radiation and binds to 5-HT$_3$ receptors, sending impulses to the CTZ and vomiting center via the vagal afferents. Serotonin antagonists block 5-HT$_3$ receptors, preventing transmission of these impulses (Figure 11-4).[35] Serotonin antagonists are nonsedating and do not cause dystonic reactions, because dopamine receptors are not affected. Multiple studies have compared various serotonin antagonists in adults, with no particular agent consistently showing superior efficacy.§ The only published trial comparing the

---

§References 59, 81, 101, 104, 117, 139.

BOX 11-2

COMMONLY USED ANTIEMETICS IN CHILDREN WITH CANCER

Serotonin antagonists
    Ondansetron
    Granisetron
    Dolasetron
Phenothiazines
    Prochlorperazine
    Chlorpromazine
    Perphenazine
    Thiethylperazine
    Promethazine
Corticosteroids
    Dexamethasone
    Methylprednisolone
Benzodiazepine
    Lorazepam
Antihistamines
    Diphenhydramine
    Hydroxyzine
Procainamide derivative
    Metoclopramide
Cannabinoid
    Delta-9-tetrahydrocannabinol (THC)

---

efficacy of serotonin antagonists in children compared ondansetron to tropisetron (a drug not currently available in the United States). Ondansetron provided superior control for children receiving mild or moderately emetogenic chemotherapy. There was no difference in the control for children receiving highly emetogenic chemotherapy.[165]

The standard dose of ondansetron (0.15 mg/kg, three times per day) was based on studies in adults. However, no randomized dose-finding studies have been performed in children. In adults, low doses of ondansetron have been as efficacious as standard or large doses in many randomized trials.[11,39,40,148,166] Hesketh et al. studied the use of a sliding-scale ondansetron dose in adults, based on emetogenicity of the chemotherapeutic agents. Emesis was completely prevented in 72% to 88% of patients.[67] A once-a-day dose of ondansetron (0.45 mg/kg) has been used in adults, but no data exists on the efficacy of this dose in children.

Cost is a significant factor in choosing 5-HT$_3$ antagonists. Oral administration of the rapidly dissolving ondansetron tablet offers a cost-effective alternative to parenteral administration[180] and may be used even with nauseated patients or for patients with oral intake restrictions before anesthesia.

Granisetron, a second serotonin antagonist, has been evaluated in children at doses varying from 10

to 40 mcg/kg daily, with conflicting evidence for the superiority of any single dosing regimen. The product insert recommends a pediatric dose of 10 mcg/kg daily.[158] In a dose-finding study, there was no significant difference in the nausea or vomiting experienced in a study of 80 children randomized to 10 mcg/kg versus 20 mcg/kg versus 40 mcg/kg.[128] Although granisetron doses of 40 mcg/kg daily were superior to 20 mcg/kg doses in children receiving chemotherapy in one study,[168] there was no significant difference between the two doses in another study.[87] Of note, there was no significant difference between a 10 mcg/kg dose of granisetron and placebo in controlling postoperative vomiting in children, yet the children receiving 40 mcg/kg doses had superior results.[30] Further research is needed to determine the ideal granisetron dose in children. Higher doses of granisetron ($\geq$20 mcg/kg) are not cost-effective at many institutions.

Dolasetron is another serotonin antagonist that offers once-daily dosing. A daily dose of 1.8 mg/kg of dolasetron was shown to be more effective than lower doses for children receiving chemotherapy, with a complete response (no emetic episodes) reported for 50% of the subjects.[33]

Until the 1990s phenothiazines were the mainstay of antiemetic treatment.[62,102] With the advent of serotonin antagonists, they are used far less frequently because of their sedative effects and potential for dystonic reactions; however, they may be useful in some situations. Phenothiazines block dopamine receptors and thus have antiemetic properties. The administration of IV phenothiazine derivatives may increase the risk of dystonic reactions, which may be limited by slow IV administration (30 minutes to 1 hour) and concurrent administration of antihistamines. Antihistamine administration must continue for 24 hours after the last phenothiazine dose. Because of the risk of sedation from phenothiazines and concomitant antihistamines, the infant or very young child must be positioned to prevent aspiration. Children must also be protected from falls, and close monitoring of respiratory rate, blood pressure, and level of consciousness may be indicated. Promethazine may be considered more of an antihistamine than a phenothiazine and does not require concurrent antihistamine dosing, because the incidence of extrapyramidal symptoms is low. Although metoclopramide is not a phenothiazine, it blocks dopamine receptors at high doses and therefore can also be used as an antiemetic with concurrent antihistamine administration.[89] Antihistamines, because they block histamine, may add some emetogenic control in addition to their use in preventing dys-

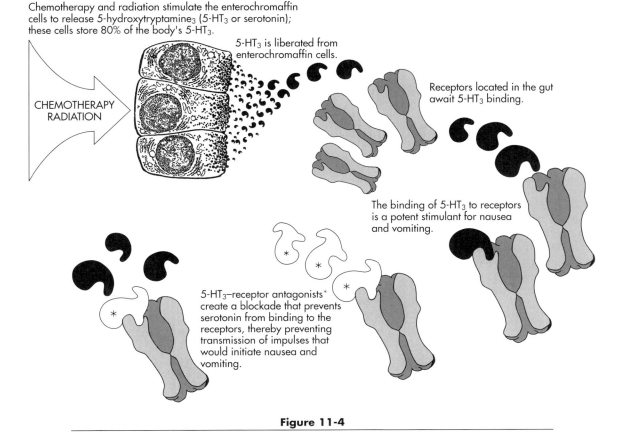

Chemotherapy and radiation stimulate the enterochromaffin cells to release 5-hydroxytryptamine$_3$ (5-HT$_3$ or serotonin); these cells store 80% of the body's 5-HT$_3$.

5-HT$_3$ is liberated from enterochromaffin cells.

CHEMOTHERAPY RADIATION

Receptors located in the gut await 5-HT$_3$ binding.

The binding of 5-HT$_3$ to receptors is a potent stimulant for nausea and vomiting.

5-HT$_3$–receptor antagonists* create a blockade that prevents serotonin from binding to the receptors, thereby preventing transmission of impulses that would initiate nausea and vomiting.

Figure 11-4

Mechanism of action of 5-HT$_3$ receptor antagonists.   (From Cunningham, R. S. [1997]. 5-HT$_3$–receptor antagonists: A review of pharmacology and clinical efficacy. *Oncology Nursing Forum 24[Suppl. 7]*, 33-40.)

tonic reactions. Rarely, these agents have the potential to cause a paradoxical hyperactivity.[172]

Corticosteroids are commonly used in conjunction with other antiemetics, although their mechanism of action is unclear. When added to commonly used single agents such as ondansetron, granisetron, and metoclopramide, emetic control may be improved.[5,68] Dexamethasone is the steroid most frequently used as an antiemetic. No research has been done to define the optimal dexamethasone dose in children. A variety of steroid dosing has been used to prevent nausea and vomiting in adults receiving chemotherapy (4 mg to 20 mg once daily, 0.3 mg/kg to 1 mg/kg, 5 to 10 mg/m^2). Although a high single dose (20 mg IV) was superior to lower doses in complete control of emesis, there were no differences in mild emesis or nausea.[82] The use of steroids is associated with many serious sequelae, including immunosuppression, decreased bone density, and avascular necrosis of joints. In addition, antiemetic steroid use is contraindicated for

many patients receiving steroids as cancer therapy, such as those on leukemia and lymphoma protocols. Steroids must also be used with caution for many brain tumor patients. Thus, further research is needed to determine the lowest effective dexamethasone dose when used as adjuvant antiemetic treatment in the pediatric population.

Benzodiazepines such as lorazepam have no antiemetic properties but have been used along with antiemetics because they can provide antegrade amnesia and euphoria.[173] These drugs typically provide benefit to patients experiencing anticipatory nausea and vomiting.[100] Caution must be used when administering other sedative antiemetics, because of the long half-life of lorazepam (up to 16 hours).

Oral cannabinoids (marijuana derivatives) have been used for nausea, particularly with adolescents and adults.[27] The method of action is thought to be central nervous system depression. The drug may cause euphoria. However, some patients dislike the somnolence or the sensation of feeling out of control that can occur with these agents.

Scopolamine, which is effective in the control of motion sickness and may have some vestibular effects against nausea and vomiting, has been used with adults in combination with other antiemetics.[108] However, scopolamine may cause tachycardia, dysphoria, and confusion and thus is used with caution. The safety of the use of scopolamine in children has not been established, and pediatric dosing is difficult because of the transdermal delivery system.

Delayed nausea/vomiting. Delayed emesis, which is theorized to have a different mechanism of action than acute vomiting, is typically less well controlled with current antiemetic agents than acute nausea and vomiting. Levels of 5-hydroxyindoleacetic acid (5-HIAA), a serotonin metabolite, were noted to increase in the first several hours after administration of emetogenic chemotherapy such as cisplatin and to decrease once serotonin antagonists were administered. However, the levels of 5-HIAA excretion 24 hours after chemotherapy administration were similar to baseline levels of the metabolite.[34] Nevertheless, adults in a large randomized trial had significantly lower emesis on days 2 through 5 after chemotherapy when receiving ondansetron as compared with placebo.[118] More effective agents are need for control of delayed chemotherapy-associated nausea and vomiting in pediatric patients, particularly for patients who lack adequate control of acute emesis.

Anticipatory nausea/vomiting. Anticipatory nausea and vomiting can occur anytime after the first treatment. As many as 59% of children may experience some degree of ANV.[169] The incidence and severity are influenced by expectations of severe postchemotherapy nausea and vomiting, degree of distress associated with nausea and vomiting, and poor control of nausea and vomiting during prior chemotherapy cycles. ANV most often begins within 2 hours before treatment and is most severe at the time of drug administration.[44]

Effective management of nausea and vomiting from the start of treatment is important to prevent ANV. The child's environment becomes particularly important. Psychogenic factors such as walking into the hospital, smelling particular odors, or the sight of a syringe can trigger nausea. A careful assessment is necessary to determine the negative associations that have developed. Lorazepam administered at bedtime the night before chemotherapy treatment and again the following morning can diminish the distress associated with triggering

factors and reduce the incidence and severity of anticipatory nausea and vomiting.[100]

Nursing role. Pediatric nurses must first make an accurate assessment of factors contributing to nausea and vomiting. Nonpharmacologic techniques can be combined with antiemetic therapy, depending on the child's age and preferences. Providing appropriate information can ameliorate anxiety. Music can be used as a distraction and a general relaxation technique. Distraction for a young child may be watching a favorite videotape or listening to a favorite story.[86] Self-hypnosis can be learned by children as young as 4 to control nausea and vomiting during chemotherapy infusion.[32,83] The nurse must work with the child and family to make the treatment environment as comfortable as possible. Child life specialists can assist in distraction and relaxation techniques.

Nurses must carefully assess fluid balance in children experiencing nausea and vomiting. Intravenous fluids may be needed for hydration in children with persistent vomiting and can often be administered in the home to avoid hospitalization.

When a successful antiemetic regimen is found, the plan is reviewed with family caregivers and carefully documented in the child's record for future treatment courses. Families should be prepared for delayed onset of vomiting and given instruction on the prolonged administration of antiemetics. Families are also given guidelines for assessing and maintaining the child's hydration status. Oral intake, one of the few areas within children's and parents' control, is possible even with mild to moderate nausea and vomiting. Small amounts of clear fluids or bland foods such as crackers can be offered when the child feels ready. Children's preferences for a specific food or drink after periods of nausea should be respected. Caregivers are encouraged to have the child gradually resume oral intake and not to overwhelm the child with too much food and drink too soon.

DIARRHEA

Definition/contributing factors. Diarrhea is defined as an abnormal increase in the quantity, frequency, or liquidity of stool.[88] Diarrhea in the child with cancer can be particularly debilitating and can quickly lead to severe dehydration, renal insufficiency, electrolyte imbalances, and impaired skin integrity. Diarrhea can delay treatment, increase the cost of care because of hospitalization, and diminish the child's overall quality of life.

To maintain bowel function, the proper balance must exist between absorption, secretion, and intestinal motility. Diarrhea occurs when a disturbance occurs in the mechanical or biochemical processes that maintain this balance between intestinal secretion and absorption of water and electrolytes.[140] The extent to which any one of these factors is affected dictates the type of diarrhea. Determining the etiology of diarrhea is of great importance in identifying the proper treatment choice.[74]

Cascinu classified diarrhea into six different types, based on the underlying cause: secretory, malabsorptive, intestinal dismotility, osmotic, exudative, or chemotherapy-induced.[25]

Secretory diarrhea is characterized by intestinal hypersecretion induced by endocrine tumors, bacterial endotoxins, or damage to the gut wall, as in the case of graft-versus-host disease (GVHD). Diarrhea may also be due to a malabsorption process resulting from factors that cause alteration in luminal or mucosal integrity of the gut, such as enzyme deficiencies and surgical resection (which may alter the amount of available absorbative surfaces, as in the case of small bowel resection). Bowel dismotility related to fecal impaction or peristaltic stimulants results in rapid transit of stool through the small and large intestine. Osmotic diarrhea is characterized by the influx of a large volume of fluid and electrolytes into the intestinal lumen, which overwhelms the intestine's absorbative capacity, such as the ingestion of enteral feeding solutions and nonabsorbable solutes. Exudative diarrhea results from the release of excessive blood and fluids into the bowel and can be caused by inflammatory and ulcerative effects of both disease and treatment, such as radiation therapy, neoplasms of the colon, and typhlitis.

Diarrhea is a well-recognized side effect of a number of chemotherapeutic agents (Box 11-3). The mechanism of chemotherapy-induced diarrhea is not fully understood but is thought to result from the interference of certain chemotherapy agents in the division of intestinal cells, producing acute damage to the intestinal mucosa, thereby resulting in a shortening of the intestinal villi and a shift in the balance between the number of absorbative and secretory cells.[176]

Diarrhea in the child with cancer can be either an acute or chronic condition and is often multifactorial. Acute diarrhea, generally lasting less than 2 weeks, is commonly associated with infections, alteration in the patient's diet, drug reactions, or fecal impaction.[74] Infectious diarrhea may be caused by viruses, bacteria, or protozoa. Due to frequent prophylactic and therapeutic antibiotic use in children with cancer, one of the most common enteropathogens inducing diarrhea in this population is the bacteria *Clostridium difficile*.[110] Radiation to the abdomen and pelvis is one of the major causes

---

BOX 11-3

ANTICANCER AGENTS COMMONLY ASSOCIATED WITH DIARRHEA

Cisplatin
Cyclophosphamide
Cytarabine
Daunorubicin
Doxorubicin
Fluorouracil
Hydroxyurea
Interferon
Interleukin-2
Irinotecan
Methotrexate
Thioguanine
Topotecan

Data from Abigerges, D., Chabot, G. G., Armand, J. P., et al. (1995). Phase I and pharmacologic studies of the camptothecin analog irinotecan administered every three weeks in cancer patients. *Journal of Clinical Oncology, 13,* 210-221; Cascinu, S. (1995). Drug therapy in diarrheal disease in oncology/hematology patients. *Critical Reviews in Oncology/Hematology, 18,* 37-50; Hogan, C. M. (1998). The nurse's role in diarrhea management. *Oncology Nursing Forum, 25,* 879-886.

---

of chronic diarrhea in the child with cancer, usually lasting for periods greater than 2 weeks. GVHD following hematopoietic stem cell transplant may also cause chronic diarrhea.[1]

Another cause of diarrhea in the child with cancer may be the presence of concurrent illnesses, such as hyperthyroidism, diabetes, or gastrointestinal disorders.[74] Medications used in the supportive care of the child with cancer may also cause diarrhea. Antibiotics are commonly associated with diarrhea because they can cause alteration in the normal flora of the gut and/or inflammation of the intestinal mucosa.[175] Other supportive drugs that may cause diarrhea include antacids, antihypertensives, antiemetics, and electrolyte supplements.[1]

Clinical presentation. The clinical presentation of diarrheal illness depends largely on the type and cause. Patients may have stool varying in consistency, water content, quantity, and frequency. They may experience dehydration, electrolyte imbalances, abdominal cramping, rectal excoriation or ulceration, hyperactive bowel sounds, fever, or blood or mucous discharge in the stool. Patients may also exhibit the clinical signs of dehydration including poor skin turgor, dry mucous membranes, weight loss, and hypotension. Quality of life may be compromised. Diarrhea can lead to increased hospitalization and isolation. Uncontrollable diarrhea may interfere with children's work and play, thus challenging their psychologic growth and development. Chronic or acute uncontrollable diarrhea can also affect the child's self-image, which may be especially problematic for adolescents with cancer.

Treatment strategies. The goal of diarrhea management is to restore normal bowel habits, maintain adequate nutrition, restore fluid and electrolyte balance, protect skin integrity, enable the patient to achieve comfort and maintain dignity, and support the patient in resuming activities of daily living.[140] The management of diarrhea is directly related to its cause, and therefore establishing the underlying cause is the first step in effective treatment. It is especially important to determine if an infectious process is present. Drugs that slow peristalsis are sometimes prescribed for diarrhea but are contraindicated in infectious diarrhea, because they would slow or prevent the elimination of pathogens from the gastrointestinal system.[175]

Intravenous fluid replacement may be necessary if the patient cannot maintain adequate oral intake or is exhibiting signs and symptoms of dehydration. Careful assessment of the patient's blood chemistry studies will guide the clinician in appropriate electrolyte supplementation if indicated. Antidiarrheal or anticholinergic medications may be used for noninfectious diarrhea. Diet must be carefully assessed and modified to meet the patient's individual needs. Age-appropriate feedings, including breast-feeding, are continued, but fatty foods and those high in simple sugars are avoided. Lactose-free diets are generally unnecessary. If no dehydration is present, age-appropriate feeding is encouraged, with oral rehydration solution (ORS) (e.g., Rehydralyte) given to replace excessive fluid loss in stool. If small amounts of ORS cannot be provided in the home, IV fluids may be necessary.[171] Because diarrhea can lead to rectal skin breakdown, the perianal area is assessed frequently. Sitz baths may be recommended both for patient comfort and for skin care. Clinicians may also consider the use of a moisture barrier ointment to prevent skin breakdown and reduce the risk of opportunistic infection.

Nursing role. In diarrhea management, the pediatric oncology nurse obtains a thorough history including the following factors: primary diagnosis; current and prior therapy; surgical history; current medications; normal diet; any recent travel or consumption of foods not common to patient's regular diet; allergies; normal bowel routine; onset of diarrhea; frequency, volume, consistency, and other characteristics of stool; complaints of pain or cramping; and an estimate of recent food and liquid intake. A thorough physical assessment focuses on evaluation of vital signs, clinical signs of dehydration, abdominal assessment (bowel sounds, abdominal girth, palpation, pain assessment), and also meticulous assessment of skin in the perianal region. If diarrhea is suspected to be an infectious process, stool cultures are obtained to isolate the infectious organism.

The nurse caring for the child with significant diarrheal illness maintains strict intake and output (I&O) measurements, obtains the patient's weight daily or more frequently as indicated, provides skin care as needed, and communicates significant changes or signs of impending complication to the health care team. The occurrence of diarrhea also presents an opportunity for patient and family education. Basic infection control principles are reinforced, with strong emphasis on hand washing and the dangers of cross contamination. The patient and family can be taught the signs and symptoms of diarrhea and the importance of an accurate intake and output record. The patient and family are also given advice about diet management, including what foods are likely to contribute to the problem and certain foods that may help correct diarrhea by adding bulk to the diet. Education also involves discussion of the psychosocial impact of diarrhea. Diarrhea may interfere with activities of daily living. Persistent loose stools may lead to regression or a feeling of loss of control. This is discussed with the family so parents can recognize the child's emotional needs and provide extra support.[1]

CONSTIPATION

Definition/contributing factors. Constipation is a decrease in the normal frequency of stool production. Constipated stool is often hard, difficult to pass, and accompanied by straining, abdominal pain or cramping, and rectal discomfort. As described by Aitken, constipation can be categorized as primary, secondary, or iatrogenic.[1] Primary constipation results from external factors such as a decrease in physical activity, improper diet, or inadequate time for defecation. In the child with cancer, periods of hospitalization and acute illness, along with general malaise and fatigue, may cause a decrease in physical activity and alterations in the child's diet, predisposing the child to primary constipation. In addition, hospitalization may compound the problem by limiting opportunities for privacy.

Secondary constipation results from pathologic changes such as intestinal obstruction, spinal cord compression, hypercalcemia, hypokalemia, or hypothyroidism. Secondary constipation in the child with cancer may result from tumor mass causing intestinal obstruction. Tumor growth can also cause spinal cord compression, interfering with innervation of the intestine.

Constipation may be iatrogenic in nature, most often due to the use of narcotic analgesics and chemotherapy agents such as the vinca alkaloids. Vinca alkaloids such as vincristine and vinblastine have a neurotoxic effect on the smooth muscle of the gastrointestinal tract, causing decreased peristaltic activity.[13] Constipation may also be promoted by decreased oral intake secondary to nausea and vomiting. When a patient has decreased oral intake, there is a decrease in peristaltic pushdown. When a patient does not eat, less stool is formed, transit time increases, and stool becomes hard, thereby interfering with normal defecation.[13] Constipation can also be caused by decreased peristalsis secondary to abdominal or pelvic surgery. Rarely do any of the above-mentioned risk factors for constipation occur independently. Rather, in the complex treatment of childhood cancer, constipation is often a multifactorial problem.

Clinical presentation.   A patient experiencing constipation may exhibit a decline in the normal production of stool, change in the characteristics of stool (hard, dry, possibly blood streaked), hypoactive bowel sounds, distended and/or firm abdomen, diffuse abdominal tenderness, decreased appetite, feeling of satiety, nausea, straining with attempted bowel movements, and pain associated with defecation.

Treatment strategies.   With early assessment and intervention, constipation in the child with cancer is a manageable and often preventable problem. It is important to obtain a baseline assessment of the patient's normal bowel habits. In anticipation of particular treatments such as vinca alkaloids or opioid medications, prophylactic measures can be taken to prevent constipation. Prophylactic stool softeners and/or laxatives, a diet high in fiber, and adequate intake of oral or intravenous fluids may prevent or alleviate constipation. In the case of bowel obstruction or compression of the intestines by a tumor mass, surgical intervention may be indicated. Nonpharmaceutical measures to prevent constipation include encouraging physical activity, promoting maintenance of normal toileting routines, and providing privacy.

Nursing role.   The pediatric oncology nurse plays an important role in the prevention, diagnosis, and treatment of constipation. A baseline assessment of the patient's bowel habits is obtained.

Accurate records are maintained including the frequency, consistency, and amount of stool output. Any variations from normal bowel routine are communicated to appropriate members of the health care team. A thorough abdominal assessment includes bowel sounds, degree of abdominal distention, and the presence of pain or cramping. Because constipation can also be associated with straining and passing hard stools, the perirectal area is thoroughly inspected for the presence of hemorrhoids, skin breakdown, rectal fissures, or bleeding.

The importance of perineal hygiene is reinforced with the patient and family. The nurse must also advocate for prophylactic measures to prevent constipation. For example, if the patient is receiving vinca alkaloid therapy, a stool softener and/or stimulant may be initiated before the onset of treatment. The nurse and nutritionist can assist the patient and family in recognizing the benefits of a high-fiber diet and identifying particular foods to aid in the prevention of constipation. To prevent any trauma to the perirectal area and the occurrence of an opportunistic infection, the use of enemas, rectal thermometers, digital examinations, or suppositories must be avoided. Parents and patients are encouraged to report any change in bowel habits or associated physical symptoms. Encouraging proper diet, activity, consistent perineal hygiene, and avoiding any rectal trauma are also important elements of the educational plan.

CHEMICAL HEPATITIS

Definition/contributing factors.   Chemical hepatitis is a nonviral inflammation of the liver that can be caused by exposure to chemical and environmental agents such as chemotherapy and radiation. The liver plays a central role in the metabolism of many chemotherapy agents and is therefore a target for drug toxicity.[80] The incidence of drug-induced liver disease appears to be increasing, reflecting the increasing number of new agents that have been introduced into the clinical setting over the past several decades.[91] Cancer treatment factors that may contribute to the occurrence of chemical or reactive hepatitis include chemotherapeutic agents, particularly asparaginase, mercaptopurine, thioguanine, methotrexate, carmustine, lomustine, vincristine, vinblastine, doxorubicin, daunorubicin, idarubicin, dactinomycin; radiation to the abdomen; surgical resection of the liver; intraarterial hepatic chemotherapy administration; and/or an underlying hepatic disease process. Several categories of supportive therapy for cancer treatment may also contribute to drug-induced hepatitis, including anticonvulsants, antimicrobials, and nonsteroidal antiinflammatory drugs (NSAIDs).[50]

Clinical presentation. The clinical presentation of chemical hepatitis varies, as does the extent of hepatic injury. Chemical hepatitis is usually identified first by abnormalities in the enzymes associated with hepatic function (e.g., alanine transaminase [ALT], aspartate transaminase [AST]). This results from the lysis of hepatocytes, which release protein into the bloodstream. The patient may also exhibit clinical signs and symptoms of hepatitis, including jaundice, pain, particularly in the right upper quadrant, fever, diaphoresis, malaise, flulike symptoms, nausea, vomiting, anorexia, and bruising or bleeding.[91] Because there is no specific test for chemical or drug-induced hepatitis, the diagnosis requires a careful medication history and documentation of the onset of symptoms, as well as the exclusion of other disorders.[50] Screening is also done to rule out infectious hepatitis. The exclusion of an infectious process may help establish the diagnosis of chemical hepatitis.

Treatment strategies. Treatment strategies for the patient experiencing chemical hepatitis are directed at isolating the cause of the hepatic injury and modifying treatment to decrease toxicity. Chemotherapeutic agents and supportive drugs that may be causing hepatotoxicity, as well as those metabolized by the liver, may be reduced in dose or discontinued.[80] Serum chemistry studies, hepatic enzyme levels, and coagulation studies are monitored as indicated. If the patient is experiencing clinical symptoms of hepatitis such as nausea and vomiting, supportive care with fluids and antiemetic medications is indicated. Patients with hyperbilirubinemia may be treated with ursodiol (Actigall). Complications of chemical hepatitis can include chronic active hepatitis, cirrhosis, and a range of extrahepatic syndromes, including associated pulmonary injury and marrow injury.[91]

Nursing role. The nurse plays an important role in the assessment and management of chemical hepatitis. The nurse may be involved with obtaining a thorough drug history, identifying any specific correlation between drug ingestion or treatment administration and the onset of clinical symptoms. A thorough physical assessment focuses on the detection of any signs and symptoms of hepatitis. The patient's comfort level is monitored, with a particular concern for abdominal pain. The patient is also monitored for any signs of bruising or bleeding. Supportive care may be indicated, including antipyretics, analgesics, and antiemetics. If the patient is experiencing pruritus related to elevation of bilirubin, antipruritics may be administered and the patient can be encouraged to take soothing baths and wear loose, soft clothing for comfort.

PANCREATITIS

Definition/contributing factors. Pancreatitis, or inflammation of the pancreas, may be categorized as acute, chronic, necrotic, hemorrhagic, or hereditary.[127] Acute pancreatitis is a self-limiting disorder that in children is commonly associated with trauma, infection, medications, anatomic variants, and metabolic disorders. Chronic pancreatitis can result in the loss of both exocrine and endocrine tissue and may be caused by congenital defects. In necrotizing, hemorrhagic pancreatitis, the inflamed gland becomes infected with bacteria and is associated with sepsis and multisystem organ failure. Hereditary pancreatitis is an autosomal dominant condition, characterized by recurrent attacks of pancreatitis, with a young age at onset.[127] In the child with cancer, one of the most common causes of pancreatitis is cancer treatment, including asparaginase therapy. The concomitant use of corticosteroids may also be a contributing factor in the development of pancreatitis.[90]

Clinical presentation. The classic clinical presentation of pancreatitis in childhood includes abdominal pain, nausea, vomiting, and anorexia. Abdominal pain may be diffuse or localized to the epigastrium and/or radiates to the back or flank.[127] Patients may experience pain and vomiting more after meals, particularly after high-fat meals. Such pain does not usually decrease after vomiting. Emesis is often characterized as bilious in nature. The patient's abdomen may be distended with guarding present on palpation and hypoactive bowel sounds. Low-grade fever is sometimes present, along with tachycardia and hypotension.[127] Pancreatitis is usually accompanied by an elevation in pancreatic enzymes, lipase and amylase. The differential diagnosis of pancreatitis requires evaluation of clinical status, review of pancreatic function, and review of various radiographic studies such as abdominal x-ray examination, CT scan, and/or ultrasonography.[127]

Treatment strategies. Treatment strategies for pancreatitis relate to supportive care.[127] Adequate hydration and nutritional intake must be maintained in the presence of nausea, vomiting, and anorexia. Intravenous fluids, antiemetics, and total parenteral nutrition are often indicated. In cases of severe pancreatitis, the patient may require bowel rest with nasogastric suction. Pain relief is essential and may be difficult to achieve in children. Opiates have been reported to worsen symptoms by increasing spasms of the sphincter of Oddi, increasing pain. Meperidine and hydromorphone have been used successfully in both acute and chronic pancreatitis.[127] The major complications that accompany pancreatitis are septic complications. These can occur when bacteria invading from the gastrointestinal tract cause pancreatic abscess, pseudocyst, or pancreatic necrosis.[127] Surgical drainage may be required if an abscess or pseudocyst develops.[2]

Nursing role.   The nursing role in caring for the child with pancreatitis involves a complete physical assessment, timely communication with the health care team, and administration of supportive treatments. On physical assessment, particular attention is given to the abdominal assessment, the level of pain, and signs and symptoms of shock. Any significant changes in a patient's condition must be quickly communicated to the health care team in an effort to intervene early in the disease process. The nurse administers antiemetics as ordered and performs good oral care. Patient and family education includes the signs and symptoms of pancreatitis. In addition, the nutritionist and the nurse can provide information on any dietary recommendations. The nurse also plays a vital role in support of both the patient and family, particularly in situations of prolonged pancreatitis, which may result in lengthy hospital stays and delays in subsequent chemotherapy administration.

NUTRITIONAL DEFICITS

Definition/contributing factors/clinical presentation.   In the treatment of cancer, nutritional support is an integral component of care that can directly affect clinical outcomes.[36] Adequate nutritional intake is critical because maintaining a positive nitrogen balance supports wound healing, enhances the immune response, provides for increased energy and a sense of well-being, and maximizes the patient's ability to tolerate cancer treatment. Malnutrition has been reported to occur in 8% to 32% of children treated for cancer.[170]

Alterations in nutrition can develop as a result of mechanical barriers, systemic or local effects of the disease process, side effects of treatment, psychosocial reactions to the disease process, or a combination of these factors.[149] Mechanical barriers may interfere with oral intake by limiting the ability to eat or chew. Radiation to the head and neck region can affect the tissues of the salivary glands, oral mucosa, muscle, and bone, resulting in xerostomia, stomatitis, dysphagia, and taste alterations.[106] Radiation to the abdomen can cause nausea and vomiting that is difficult to prevent.[142]

Chemotherapy may result in a host of side effects that interfere with nutritional status, including anorexia, nausea, vomiting, stomatitis, taste aversions, diarrhea, constipation, and pain.

Anorexia and cachexia are among the most common complications of cancer and its treatment.[167] Anorexia is defined as a decrease in appetite accompanied by a decrease in food consumption. Anorexia in cancer patients is a complex and multifactorial problem. Factors contributing to anorexia may include nausea, vomiting, taste aversions, early satiety, anxiety, depression, and environmental changes.[63] Interventions for anorexia involve counseling the patient and an individualized diet designed to promote nutritional restoration and prevent further nutritional deficits. Cancer cachexia is a syndrome that develops secondary to the progressive growth of a malignant process and limits quality of life, length of survival, and treatment options. The clinical features include muscle wasting, anorexia, weakness, anemia, and metabolic deficit.[4]

Children who perceive a lack of control over their diagnosis, treatment, and hospitalization may choose to exert power over situations that they can control, such as what they will eat. This can be frustrating to the family and challenging to the health care team. Special considerations are often necessary when planning supportive care for the pediatric oncology patient, including the child's body composition, growth and developmental needs, and treatment-related complications.[78]

Treatment strategies.   The primary goals of nutritional intervention are to restore and promote growth and development and to minimize side effects of therapy.[64] The assessment of the child's nutritional status and relative risk provides the basis for a supportive nutrition plan. Nutritional screening is an ongoing process that must take into account weights, food intake, treatment that affects nutrition, functional status, physical examination, and biochemical indicators of protein stores (e.g., albumin and prealbumin levels).[4] To prevent malnutrition and subsequent treatment complications nutritional interventions are initiated early. Nutritional management may include diet modifications, oral supplements, enteral feedings, parenteral nutrition, and medications to stimulate the appetite (e.g., megestrol [Megase]). Controversy often exists over the choice of enteral feedings versus parenteral nutrition. Unless contraindicated, the enteral approach to nutritional support is more advantageous, because continued stimulation of the gut prevents atrophy of the microvilli of the intestinal wall and minimizes the change in bacterial flora and the risk for sepsis.[14] Nasogastric feedings can be administered at about one fourth the cost of parenteral nutrition. Even in patients with intensive chemotherapy or hematopoietic stem cell transplantation, nasogastric feedings are well tolerated without complications of epistaxis or sinusitis.[126] In clinical situations where malnutrition cannot be corrected by enteral feedings, total parenteral nutrition is indicated. (e.g., severe diarrhea, radiation enteritis, chronic malabsorption, or short-bowel syndrome).[14] However, in one study of children with cancer receiving parenteral nutrition, no significant changes in weight, skinfold reserves, or serum albumin levels were seen when the therapy was administered for 9 to 14 days. Benefits were noted only after parenteral nutrition was given for at least 28 days.[137] Parenteral nutrition may suppress the hunger or thirst mechanisms. In a randomized study of adult and pediatric hematopoietic stem cell transplant recipients, patients receiving IV hydration resumed oral intake quicker than the patients given parenteral nutrition after hospital discharge.[29]

Nursing role. Nurses play a critical role in the assessment, prevention, and management of nutritional deficits in children with cancer. A baseline nutrition assessment (e.g., plotting measurements on a growth curve) is obtained at diagnosis, identifying those patients with nutritional deficits and those at high risk related to their disease and treatment. Nutritional support for the child with cancer is a complex process, best served by a multidisciplinary approach. The nurse communicates frequently with other health care team members and advocates for specific nutrition consultation as indicated. Nurses help to prevent malnutrition by providing supportive care and caregiver education. Antiemetics must be administered aggressively to control nausea and vomiting. Pain control must be provided for radiation- or chemotherapy-induced mucositis. Good oral hygiene is encouraged. The patient and family are instructed in the importance of oral hygiene and encouraged to maintain an appropriate mouth care regimen. Accurate intake and output records must be maintained and frequently reassessed, especially if the patient is experiencing vomiting and/or diarrhea. Encourage oral intake, offering small, frequent meals or snacks. Provide patients and family with information on the side effects that may cause nutritional deficits, with emphasis on the relationship between nutritional status and clinical outcomes. If necessary, patients and parents can be taught to properly administer enteral or parenteral nutrition.

CARDIOVASCULAR COMPLICATIONS

Cardiac complications related to therapy may be categorized as acute and chronic. Chronic or long-term complications are discussed further in Chapter 18. This section focuses primarily on acute cardiotoxicity related to disease and therapy.

Most cardiac complications can be categorized according to their cardiotoxic effect: decreased contractility or relaxation, ischemia, and conduction problems resulting in dysrhythmias.[23] Complications may arise as a direct result of chemotherapy (e.g., anthracyclines, cyclophosphamide, busulfan, cytarabine, carmustine), radiation to the mediastinum, or direct tumor invasion into the heart.[46,66,151]

CARDIOMYOPATHY

Anthracyclines cause both acute and long-term cardiotoxic effects. Reports in the adult literature indicate that the incidence increases rapidly in patients who receive a cumulative dose greater than 450 mg/m^2 for both doxorubicin and daunorubicin and 125 mg/m^2 for idarubicin.[80] However, there are reports of toxicity occurring at cumulative doses as low as 200 mg/m^2, and individual patients may develop toxicity at significantly lower doses than those used in standard treatment regimens.[46,80,164] Chemotherapy-induced cardiotoxicity manifests as congestive heart failure with shortness of breath, exercise/activity intolerance, chronic cough, weight gain, dependent edema, and/or frequent respiratory infections.

Daunorubicin and doxorubicin have been shown to cause immediate electrocardiographic changes, as well as acute and chronic congestive heart failure and cardiomyopathy.[57] Injury may be acute or subacute, occurring immediately after a single dose or within a week after a treatment course.[122] Manifestations of toxicity may include abnormal stress ejection fractions, impaired filling, dysrhythmias, left ventricular dysfunction, muscle atrophy, and long-term cardiomyopathy.[46,151] The cause is believed to be related to the mechanism of action of anthracycline function. Anthracyclines interrupt DNA and RNA synthesis. Doxorubicin combines with iron, forming intracellular doxorubicin-iron complexes that catalyze the production of free radicals (powerful cell-damaging oxidizing agents) and damage the myocardial cells (myocytes).[46,162,179] Cardiac biopsy specimens show fibrosis and hypertrophy of the myocytes,[46] which result in cardiac muscle atrophy with decreased contractility.[151] Mediastinal radiation increases anthracycline toxicity.[80,151] The body has a finite number of myocytes, and therefore damaged ones are not replaced. Thus the remaining myocytes must compensate for this loss of cells.

There is evidence that both short- and long-term cardiotoxicity are related to the peak plasma concentration of anthracycline.[122] Studies in adults show that decreasing the peak circulating dose by using split or lower weekly doses or continuous infusion may result in decreased cardiotoxicity.[80] Further pediatric studies must be conducted to determine if this finding extends to children receiving potentially cardiotoxic agents.

Other chemotherapeutic agents such as cyclophosphamide have been found to affect the myocytes as well. Cyclophosphamide at doses of 120 mg/kg has been associated with hemorrhagic cardiac necrosis, pericardial effusion, dysrhythmias, and heart failure in adults. Acute toxicity may occur 5 to 16 days after therapy and is thought to be more common in high-dose regimens such as those used in stem cell transplant.[151]

Treatment strategies.   Monitoring patients receiving cardiotoxic cancer therapy includes collection of interval history and physical examination, electrocardiography (ECG), echocardiography (ECHO), and/or multigaited angiography (MUGA).[164] These studies may be obtained as frequently as every or every other dose of cardiotoxic chemotherapy, particularly if the cumulative anthracycline dose is expected to exceed 300 mg/m^2.[164]

The cardioprotective agent ICRF-187 (dexrazoxane [Zinecard]), used to prevent the development of anthracycline-induced cardiotoxicity, is currently under investigation. ICRF-187 selectively binds to the iron at intracellular sites, preventing iron from binding with the anthracycline. This prevents the generation of free radical oxygen, which is believed to cause damage to the myocytes. In one pediatric study of sarcoma patients receiving cumulative doxorubicin doses of 410 mg/m^2, patients treated with ICRF-187 developed less short-term cardiotoxicity than those without the ICRF-187, with no apparent adverse effect on antitumor activity.[179] Pediatric studies are ongoing to determine the long-term benefits and side effects associated with cardioprotective agents, including any deleterious effects on disease-free survival.

PERICARDIAL EFFUSIONS

Definition/contributing   factors.   The   pericardium, the membranous sac surrounding the heart, normally contains less than 50 ml of fluid.[157] Excessive accumulation of fluid between the pericardium and the heart muscle itself may result in constriction of the heart. The lymphatic system, which normally drains the pericardium, may be blocked by tumor, or tumor may produce fluids that accumulate within the pericardium. Accumulation

may be gradual, allowing for compensation, or acute, resulting in cardiac tamponade (compression of the heart).

Clinical presentation.   Pericardial effusions can be associated with solid tumors or hematologic malignancies. Patients who have received radiation to the pericardium may be at higher risk. Signs and symptoms are related to the degree of cardiac compromise and may include chest pain, muffled heart sounds, neck vein distention, pulsus paradoxus, and hypotension.

PERICARDITIS

Definition/contributing factors.   Pericarditis is an inflammation of the pericardium. Pericarditis may be a result of radiation to the mediastinum or of the underlying malignant disease process itself. Pericarditis results in edema, thrombosis, destruction of pericardial capillaries, and fibrosis.[57]

Clinical presentation.   Symptoms of pericarditis may include fever and pleuritic chest pain.[57] The patient may be more comfortable in a forward-leaning, sitting position. A pericardial friction rub may be heard on auscultation. Diagnosis is based on physical examination, ECG, and ECHO.

Treatment strategies.   Mild symptoms can be treated with rest and salicylates, or nonsteroidal antiinflammatory drugs. Acute symptoms are treated with corticosteroids and antipyretics. Analgesics can be used to manage pain. Hemodynamically unstable patients may require pericardiocentesis to drain the pericardial sac[57] and must be monitored for the development of cardiac tamponade.

HYPOTENSION

Hypotension in the child with cancer may be related to several factors including drug therapy (e.g., amphotericin, etoposide), sepsis, dehydration, and blood loss. The management of hypotension includes fluid resuscitation and therapy directed at the underlying cause. Vasopressors are used when fluid boluses do not cause a sufficient increase in the blood pressure.

HYPERTENSION

Hypertension in the child with cancer may be the result of certain malignant diseases (e.g., Wilms tumor, adrenal masses). Medications such as cyclosporine or corticosteroids can cause accumulation of fluid leading to high blood pressure, which may require treatment with antihypertensive agents. Concurrent kidney dysfunction, obesity, and adrenal gland disorders may also affect blood pressure. Hypertension may be related to excess fluid in patients with renal compromise or those undergoing aggressive hydration therapy.

Nursing role. Nursing care of the child with or at risk for cardiac complications during or after treatment includes the assessment of risk factors, monitoring for clinical signs and symptoms of heart failure, and following the results of diagnostic tests such as ECG and ECHO. Assess for cyanosis, tachycardia, hypertension or hypotension, neck vein distention, murmurs, delayed capillary refill, cool skin, or pallor. Patient and caregiver education includes the child's relative risk for developing heart problems and the symptoms associated with cardiac complications. They must also be instructed about the potential late cardiac complications and associated prevention and early detection interventions. Refer to Chapter 18 for additional information about cardiac complications.

PULMONARY COMPLICATIONS

Pulmonary complications of pediatric cancer may be the result of the disease process, treatment, or infection. Radiation therapy and some chemotherapeutic agents such as bleomycin, dactinomycin, and methotrexate are known to cause injury to lung tissue, resulting in transient or permanent damage. The lungs may also be a site of direct invasion by tumor, bacteria, or viruses.

RADIATION PNEUMONITIS

Definition/contributing factors. Radiation pneumonitis occurs secondary to injury to the lung tissue. Damage to blood vessels results in a cascade of events leading to capillary leak and white blood cell infiltration of the alveolar spaces. Over time, the capillaries attempt to repair the damage using platelets, fibrin, and collagen. Damage to the capillary endothelium results in edema and thrombosis. Increased capillary permeability allows fluid to seep into the alveolar spaces, causing damage to the hyaline membrane, which thereby interferes with gas exchange. This process ultimately results in chronic pulmonary fibrosis. It is believed that the incidence of pneumonitis is between 5% and 15% of patients undergoing radiation therapy to the lung.[57] Factors that influence the severity of the process include the volume of lung irradiated, cumulative radiation dose, dose fractionation, prior chemotherapy, and other concurrent factors such as asthma or pulmonary disease.

Clinical presentation. Radiation pneumonitis typically develops 1 to 3 months after treatment but

may occur up to 6 months following completion of treatment. Signs and symptoms include dyspnea, dyspnea on exertion, fever, harsh nonproductive or chronic cough, changes in breath sounds, tachypnea, and cyanosis. Radiographic changes include infiltrates within the radiation field.

Treatment strategies. Treatment for pneumonitis is supportive and includes antimicrobials for secondary infections, prophylactic trimethoprim sulfamethoxazole, pentamidine, or dapsone to prevent *Pneumocystis carinii* pneumonia, and bronchodilators (albuterol) to improve breathing. Supplemental oxygen and mechanical assistance may be indicated. Treatment may also include bed rest and the use of corticosteroids.[57]

Nursing role. The goal of therapy is to improve gas exchange, promote comfort, and maintain quality of life. The nurse monitors for tachypnea, cough, quality of breath sounds, presence of rales or rhonchi, dyspnea, nasal flaring, retractions, and oxygen saturation as indicated. Nursing interventions include chest physiotherapy, administration of aerosol medications and oxygen therapy, prevention of infection, and promotion of self-care and physical activity as tolerated. Patient and caregiver education includes information about potential therapies associated with pneumonitis, the signs and symptoms of pulmonary compromise, and preparation for diagnostic tests such as measurement of blood gas levels, laboratory tests, pulmonary function tests, and oximetry.

RENAL COMPLICATIONS

Renal impairment in the child with cancer may be caused by the use of nephrotoxic medications, especially certain antibiotics and chemotherapy agents, abdominal or pelvic radiation, or the underlying disease process (Table 11-4). These complications may be transient or permanent and may be experienced acutely during treatment or as long-term sequelae to treatment. Renal complications in the child with cancer range from actual structural damage to the bladder, kidney, or ureters to varied electrolyte imbalances.

HEMORRHAGIC CYSTITIS

Definition/contributing factors. Hemorrhagic cystitis is defined as dysuria from bleeding and inflammation of the bladder with the presence of leukocytes, erythrocytes, or clots in the urine.[90] In the child with cancer, hemorrhagic cystitis is frequently seen as a complication of cyclophosphamide or ifosfamide therapy.[95] Cyclophos-

TABLE 11-4	NEPHROTOXIC CHEMOTHERAPEUTIC AGENTS	
Drug	**Possible Effect on the Kidneys/Bladder**	**Treatment Strategies**
Carmustine (BCNU) Lomustine (CCNU)	These can cause progressive damage and affect renal tubules frequently later (months or years), well after completion of therapy. Effects can be irreversible, leading to renal failure.	Monitor serum creatinine, bicarbonate, potassium, protein, pH, and glucose. Consider diuresis and furosemide.
Carboplatin	May cause renal tubular damage.	Though cleared by kidneys, carboplatin is not highly toxic to kidney itself. However, in patients with poor renal function, elimination is affected and half-life increases, producing greater myelotoxicity. Dose should be adjusted for renal dysfunction. Monitor creatinine clearance.
Cisplatin	May cause proximal and distal renal tubular damage resulting in hypomagnesemia, hyponatremia, hypocalcemia, hemolytic uremic syndrome, and decreased glomerular filtration rate (GFR). It can increase nephrotoxicity associated with ifosfamide or methotrexate. Recovery from renal tubular damage is uncertain. Deterioration may continue after therapy stops.	Provide aggressive hydration and diuresis with mannitol with cisplatin. Monitor electrolytes, magnesium, calcium, and urinalysis. Ensure adequate hydration during and immediately after administration to prevent renal damage. Monitor intake and output and maintain a urine output >2 ml/kg/hr.
Cyclophosphamide	May cause hemorrhagic cystitis (microscopic to gross bleeding). Prior radiation to bladder increases risk.	Provide aggressive hydration before and after infusion. Monitor specific gravity of urine and I&O. Maintain urine output >2 ml/kg/hr. Encourage frequent voiding.
Cyclosporine	Causes elevation in serum creatinine and hypertension. Drug-drug interactions (e.g., ketoconazole) increase plasma levels.	Monitor appropriate laboratory parameters. Decrease or discontinue if elevations severe. Change route of administration. Monitor drug levels.
Ifosfamide	May cause proximal renal tubular dysfunction (impaired reabsorption of glucose, amino acids, sodium, and phosphate). Proximal tubule effects may be more severe in younger children. Fanconi's syndrome (glucosuria, aminoaciduria, low fractional excretion of phosphate, elevated fractional excretion of sodium bicarbonate) has been noted. Though acute effects improve partially or completely between treatments, this becomes increasingly more difficult. Progression of toxicity may continue after completion of therapy.	Provide aggressive hydration before and after infusion. Monitor specific gravity of urine and I&O. Monitor electrolytes, magnesium, calcium, phosphorus, and urinalysis. Ensure adequate hydration during and immediately after administration to prevent renal damage. Maintain urine output >2 ml/kg/hr.

Data from Gootenberg, J., & Pizzo, P. (1991). Optimal management of acute toxicities of therapy: Solid tumors in children. *Pediatric Clinics of North America, 38*, 269-294; Iacuone, J., Steinherz, L., Oblender, M., et al. (1997). In A. R. Ablin (Ed.), *Supportive care of children with cancer* (2nd ed., pp. 79-111). Baltimore: Johns Hopkins University Press; Shlafer, M., (1993). *The nurse pharmacology and drug therapy: A prototype approach* (2nd ed.). Redwood City, CA: Addison-Wesley.

Continued

TABLE 11-4	NEPHROTOXIC CHEMOTHERAPEUTIC AGENTS—cont'd	
Drug	**Possible Effect on the Kidneys/Bladder**	**Treatment Strategies**
Methotrexate	Methotrexate can directly damage renal tubules or form precipitate in renal tubules or collecting ducts, causing damage to renal tubules. Methotrexate in combination with cisplatin increases risk of nephrotoxicity.	Discontinue or reduce dose if patient experiences toxicity. Ensure hydration to establish high urine flow. Alkalinize urine (difficult if in renal failure). Administer loop diuretics to increase excretion, leucovorin rescue, and high-flux hemodialysis as indicated.
Vincristine High-dose cyclophosphamide	These may result in syndrome of inappropriate antidiuretic hormone (SIADH). Vincristine affects central nervous system, and cyclophosphamide affects distal tubules and collecting ducts. Hydration for therapy results in a rapid fall in serum sodium. Urine cannot be concentrated by kidney and hyponatremia develops, which may lead to seizures, coma, and death.*	Monitor serum sodium level and for signs and symptoms of hyponatremia (e.g., excessive thirst and decreased urination)

Data from Gootenberg, J., & Pizzo, P. (1991). Optimal management of acute toxicities of therapy: Solid tumors in children. *Pediatric Clinics of North America, 38,* 269-294; Iacuone, J., Steinherz, L., Oblender, M., et al. (1997). In A. R. Ablin (Ed.), *Supportive care of children with cancer* (2nd ed., pp. 79-111). Baltimore: Johns Hopkins University Press; Shlafer, M., (1993). *The nurse pharmacology and drug therapy: A prototype approach* (2nd ed.). Redwood City, CA: Addison-Wesley.
*Gootenberg, J., & Pizzo, P. (1991). Optimal management of acute toxicities of therapy: Solid tumors in children. *Pediatric Clinics of North America, 38,* 285.

phamide and ifosfamide are metabolized to acrolein, which is excreted in the urine and can cause irritation and necrosis of the bladder lining. Necrosis subsequently exposes the submucosal blood vessels of the bladder, which can rupture, causing microscopic to gross hematuria, clot retention, and potentially life-threatening hemorrhage.[153] Hemorrhagic cystitis may occur from hours to years after therapy, and the risk of recurrence increases with additional bladder-toxic therapies. Delayed complications include bladder fibrosis, reflux, and hydronephrosis.[90] Radiation to the abdomen or pelvis can also cause hemorrhagic cystitis or increase the risk from bladder-toxic chemotherapy.[80]

Clinical presentation. Clinical symptoms of hemorrhagic cystitis include mild to severe dysuria and hematuria. The diagnosis is made by history and urinalysis. In addition, ultrasonography may reveal an edematous, hemorrhagic bladder.[90]

Treatment strategies. Bladder function is assessed by urinalysis before and during therapy. Hemorrhagic cystitis can be prevented or its severity lessened by vigorous hydration before, during, and after treatment.[80] Hypoperfusion, high drug concentration, and prolonged contact of the toxic metabolite with the bladder increase the likelihood of damage.[123] Children with cancer are particularly susceptible to factors that influence hydration status, including diarrhea, anorexia, nausea, and vomiting. Supportive measures are instituted to ensure adequate hydration. The administration of mesna during ifosfamide and high-dose cyclophosphamide therapy is effective in reducing the incidence and severity of hemorrhagic cystitis. Mesna binds with and inactivates acrolein and other urotoxic metabolites.[153]

If prophylactic measures are not successful, treatment of hemorrhagic cystitis includes aggressive hydration, bladder irrigation, and transfusions as indicated to correct anemia, thrombocytopenia, and clotting abnormalities. Medications such as oxybutynin (Ditropan) may be used to control bladder spasms.[90] If severe bleeding occurs, surgical intervention to create permanent urinary diversion may be necessary.[153]

Nursing role. Nurses have an important role in the prevention and management of hemorrhagic cystitis. Urinalysis is obtained at baseline and frequently during and after bladder-toxic therapy. Accurate assessment of the patient's intake and output is maintained during administration of bladder-toxic chemotherapy. Assess the patient for any signs and symptoms of inadequate hydration and any complaints of dysuria. Adequate hydration is maintained to promote dilute and frequent urine output, thereby decreasing the exposure time to urotoxic metabolites. When possible, encourage oral intake of fluids and encourage the patient to void frequently, approximately every 2 hours during and for 24 hours following therapy.[80] Patient and caregiver education includes the importance of hydration and frequent voiding, even during the night. The patient and family are also instructed to report dysuria or any changes in the appearance of the child's urine. Before discharge assess the child's ability to maintain adequate oral intake of fluids at home. Antiemetics may be used to control nausea and vomiting and promote adequate oral hydration. Supplemental intravenous fluids at home may be indicated to ensure adequate hydration.

RENAL TUBULAR DAMAGE

Definition/contributing factors.   A significant adverse effect of some chemotherapy agents is nephrotoxicity, which can induce renal failure or result in specific renal tubular damage. Tubular damage may lead to excessive wasting of electrolytes, particularly magnesium, potassium, bicarbonate, and phosphorus.[153] Cisplatin is associated with both proximal and distal renal tubular damage, resulting in hypomagnesemia, hyponatremia, and hypocalcemia.[80] Ifosfamide has been associated with the development of Fanconi's syndrome, a generalized dysfunction of the proximal tubule, characterized by varied degrees of phosphate, glucose, amino acid, and sodium bicarbonate wasting.[15] Generally the tubular damage resulting from chemotherapy resolves between treatment courses. However, nephrotoxicity may increase with cumulative doses, and tubular damage may persist long term, continuing to progress after the completion of treatment.[80]

Clinical presentation.   The patient experiencing tubular damage may exhibit clinical signs and symptoms related to electrolyte imbalance and wasting of amino acids and glucose in the urine. The patient may also have metabolic acidosis from excessive urinary bicarbonate losses or fluid balance disturbances.[80]

Treatment strategies.   Hydration again plays an important role in the prevention of nephrotoxicity. Adequate hydration, the maintenance of intravascular fluid balance, and the use of diuretics only after adequate intravascular hydration is achieved are necessary preventative measures.[80] If electrolyte imbalances occur, correction with oral or intravenous supplementation may be required. Monitoring for renal toxicities includes a review of current medications, assessment of nutritional status (including serum albumin), assessment of serum chemistry values and urinary creatinine clearance or glomerular filtration rate, urinalysis, and blood

pressure. Dose reduction of specific chemotherapy agents may be indicated based on clinical and diagnostic findings.[80]

Nursing role.   The nurse conducts a thorough physical assessment with particular attention to vital signs; hydration status; signs and symptoms of metabolic acidosis including tachypnea, hyperventilation, abdominal pain, vomiting, fever, and lethargy; and electrolyte imbalances. Accurate assessment of intake and output are necessary to correct fluid imbalances and prevent dehydration. Urinalysis is obtained before chemotherapy administration to evaluate urine specific gravity and pH and to check for hematuria. Adequate hydration results in urine output at a minimum of 1 to 2 ml/kg/hr or more as dictated by the chemotherapy regimen.[80] With highly emetogenic chemotherapy such as cisplatin, antiemetics may be indicated to control nausea and prevent additional fluid and electrolyte loss.

Patient and family education includes reinforcement of the importance of maintaining proper hydration, signs and symptoms of dehydration, and electrolyte supplementation as indicated. Continued emphasis is placed on monitoring the patient's hydration status and urine output at home following nephrotoxic chemotherapy, and reporting any deviations immediately to the treatment team.

ENDOCRINE COMPLICATIONS

Chemotherapy, radiation, and certain tumors may affect the endocrine system and cause hormonal imbalances. The endocrine effects of treatment are related to the agent, dose, site of radiation treatment, and the age and sex of the patient. The hypothalamus, pituitary, and thyroid glands are particularly vulnerable to the effects of radiation. Endocrine effects usually occur over time and require vigilance to understand and detect changes in growth and/or function as children grow and develop. Refer to Chapter 18 for additional information about late endocrine effects.

INSULIN INSUFFICIENCY

Insulin insufficiency may be due to the effects of medications such as corticosteroids or asparaginase. Corticosteroids cause decreased production of insulin, decreased glucose uptake, and increased gluconeogenesis (the formation of glycogen from noncarbohydrate sources, protein and fat).[31] Asparaginase causes pancreatic damage that results in hyperglycemia. The combination of asparaginase and corticosteroids increases the likelihood of the development of insulin insufficiency.[174]

The hyperglycemic effects of corticosteroids normally are balanced by increased insulin production. However, there are times when the body cannot control blood sugar, and exogenous insulin is required.[150] Certain medications such as asparaginase decrease protein synthesis,[174] and because insulin is a protein it may be produced in insufficient amounts to control blood sugar. Some patients are able to control elevated serum glucose with diet alone, but others may temporarily require exogenous insulin administration.

PRECOCIOUS PUBERTY

Cranial radiation delivered in high doses for central nervous system (CNS) tumors or in low doses for CNS involvement in leukemia or lymphoma is associated with precocious puberty. On rare occasions it is also a sign of leukemic CNS involvement. Girls are affected more than boys,[152] and the younger the age at treatment, the earlier the onset of puberty.[125] Children with precocious puberty experience rapid growth rates and development of secondary sexual characteristics. This can lead to premature sexual development, accelerated growth, and adult short stature, because the syndrome can cause accelerated skeletal maturation and premature closure of the growth plates.[107] Children with early-onset puberty and short stature may experience psychosocial problems associated with changes in body image. Referral to an endocrinologist at the earliest sign of precocious puberty is essential to prevent long-term complications associated with this disorder.

DIABETES INSIPIDUS

Diabetes insipidus (DI) is a disorder of the posterior lobe of the pituitary gland and is caused by a deficiency of antidiuretic hormone (vasopressin). Symptoms include polydipsia (excessive thirst) and polyuria (increased urine production). The etiology of DI may include trauma, malignancies, radiation, medications, and surgery. Malignancies that are associated with the development of DI include craniopharyngioma, glioma, leukemia, lymphoma, meningioma, and germinomas, as well as histiocytosis.[141] Medications associated with the development of DI include aminoglycosides, amphotericin, cisplatin, foscarnet, furosemide, gentamicin, methicillin, and vinblastine.[141]

Diabetes insipidus typically presents with dilute, waterlike urine with a low specific gravity, excessive thirst, and increased urine output, even with fluid restriction. The large amounts of urine produced can result in dehydration.[157] Diagnosis is based on fluid deprivation tests, serum vasopressin levels, and urine and plasma osmolality. The inability to increase urine specific gravity and osmolality (the concentration or number of particles in solution) is diagnostic for DI.

Treatment for DI includes providing adequate fluid replacement, administering exogenous vasopressin (Desmopressin [intranasal DDAVP]), and identifying and correcting the underlying cause when possible.[157] Nursing care of the child with DI focuses on careful monitoring of intake and output, weight, urine specific gravity, serum electrolytes, and vital signs (especially heart rate and blood pressure) and close communication with the health care team to promote early detection and prevention.

Nursing role. Nursing care of the child with endocrine problems includes assessment of sexual development by Tanner stage, assessment of structural growth with serial height and weight measurements, a careful menstrual history in girls, and monitoring and documentation of appropriate laboratory and radiographic indicators (e.g., gonadotropin-releasing hormone [Gn-RH] stimulation test, luteinizing hormone, follicle-stimulating hormone, estradiol level, and bone age). In children with growth hormone problems it is important to consider timely treatment with growth hormone. Early intervention is important because untreated children may demonstrate rapid growth, accelerated skeletal maturation, and premature closure of the growth plates, resulting in short stature. Children receiving corticosteroids and asparaginase need glucose monitoring and assessment for evidence of hyperglycemia (e.g., excessive urine output, polydipsia, and polyuria). These complex medical issues warrant early referral to an endocrinologist.

THROMBOTIC COMPLICATIONS

Thrombotic complications are uncommon in children with cancer but may be a serious consequence of disease and treatment. Thrombosis can be caused by a variety of factors (Table 11-5), including occlusion of central venous access devices, disease-related DIC, medications, or a hereditary predisposition to thrombosis. A review of the pathophysiology of the clotting process is found in Chapter 14. Catheter-related thrombosis is covered in Chapter 4.

STROKE

Definition/contributing factors. A stroke is a cerebral vascular accident (CVA) that occurs when the flow of blood to the brain is interrupted and brain cells are not oxygenated. Although the overall risk of CVA in children is 2 to 3 per 100,000 children per year, those with cancer are at an increased risk.[20,121] This risk is approximately 3% in children diagnosed with non-CNS primary malignancies, with leukemia having the greatest risk.[90] Cerebral vascular accidents may be linked to DIC, chemotherapy, primary CNS infection, advanced metastatic dis-

TABLE 11-5	CAUSES OF THROMBOSIS	
Predisposing Cause	**Location**
Disseminated intravascular coagulation*	Usually generalized
Asparaginase*	Central nervous system; large veins
Central venous access devices (external catheters and implanted ports)*	Subclavian vein, jugular vein, superior vena cava
Inherited antithrombin III, protein C, or protein S deficiency†	Large veins
Antiphospholipid (lupus-type) inhibitor†	Arteries (especially cerebral vessels) or large veins
Resistance to activated protein C (factor V mutation)†	Large veins

From Buchanan, G. R. (1997). Hematologic supportive care of the pediatric cancer patient. In P. A. Pizzo & D. G. Poplack (Eds.), *Principles and practice of pediatric oncology* (3rd ed., pp. 1051-1068). Philadelphia: Lippincott-Raven.
*Related to malignancy or its treatment.
†Unrelated to malignancy or its treatment.

ease, sepsis, or thrombocytopenia.[90,121] Procoagulants may be released as cells lyse, causing DIC and potentially a CVA, particularly in children with acute nonlymphocytic leukemia (ANLL).[20] Asparaginase, a mainstay of chemotherapy for acute lymphocytic leukemia (ALL), is known to cause an imbalance in the coagulation and anticoagulation factors that may result in cerebral hemorrhage or thrombosis.[22] Methotrexate has also been implicated in focal neurologic deficits[121] and when given intrathecally has the potential to cause a CVA.[182] Although rare, hyperleukocytosis (WBC >100,000/mm^3) may cause a life-threatening cerebral hemorrhage or thrombosis.[90] Cranial irradiation has also been implicated as causing small focal vascular occlusions at doses of 18 to 24 Gy or large vessel occlusions at doses greater than 55 Gy that may cause vascular anomalies and predispose a child to a CVA as well.[90]

Clinical presentation. Children experiencing CVA have acute symptoms such as impairment in motor or speech function accompanied by headache, seizures, and/or hemiparesis.[22,90] Strokes that occur at the beginning of treatment are most commonly due to disease-related coagulopathies. A CVA that occurs during treatment is more likely due to a chemotherapeutic agent such as asparaginase, which has been associated with venous and arterial thrombosis and sagittal or lateral sinus thrombosis.[90,121] In children with progressive disease, strokes may be due to sepsis, tumor growth, or DIC. If a CVA occurs long after treatment, it is most likely due to radiation-induced damage to the vasculature.[90]

Treatment strategies. Treatment is primarily supportive, including decreasing intracranial pressure with steroids and/or hyperosmolar agents.[90] Rapid correction of coagulation abnormalities is

essential and is achieved with the use of anticoagulants, fresh frozen plasma, platelet transfusions, or administration of antithrombin III concentrate, depending on the cause of the CVA. Once a patient is stabilized, CT scan or magnetic resonance imaging (MRI) is performed to confirm the location and extent of the clot or hemorrhage.

Nursing role. Children who suffer sequelae of CVA face additional challenges in life. Physical and mental rehabilitation may be prolonged, and referral to rehabilitation medicine with intensive physical therapy, occupational therapy, and speech therapy is often necessary to promote maximum function and prevent long-term residual effects. Most children recover to normal function. However, they may have some residual sequelae such as extremity weakness.

DEEP VEIN THROMBOSIS

Definition/contributing factors. Deep vein thrombosis (DVT) in children with cancer is rare, but the risk is greater than in children without cancer.[8] DVT may occur in the upper or lower venous system. The most common predisposing factor is the presence of a central venous catheter.[90,105] A DVT may also occur as a result of asparaginase-altered coagulation, radiation, or prolonged immobilization. Children with cancer are also susceptible to other risk factors unrelated to cancer therapy, such as immobilization secondary to surgery, use of oral contraceptives, or hereditary predisposition.

Clinical presentation. The presentation of a child with a DVT catheter-related clot is discussed in Chapter 4. DVT can also cause CVA, which was previously discussed. DVT of the lower extremity may present with unilateral leg swelling, pain, inflammation, and positive Homans' sign (pain in the calf when toes are passively dorsiflexed).

Treatment strategies. A child with a DVT is treated initially with intravenous anticoagulation therapy such as heparin, followed by oral or subcutaneous anticoagulant therapy. The duration of treatment varies but is often more than 3 months.[8] Heparin and oral anticoagulant monitoring has traditionally been challenging, and therefore low–molecular-weight (LMW) heparin is frequently employed. The primary advantage of LMW heparin is that its pharmacokinetics are more predictable and therefore it requires minimal monitoring, and LMW heparin is also less affected than warfarin by interference from other drugs or diet.[111] During treatment therapy can be easily interrupted for invasive procedures such as lumbar punctures. Currently there is minimal experience with thrombolytic agents such as tissue plasminogen activator (TPA) in children, and such agents have been used primarily to restore catheter patency.[76]

Nursing role. Assessment and prevention of DVT are key aspects of the nursing role. Adequate exercise or range-of-motion exercises of the extremities may decrease DVT caused by immobilization. Central venous access thrombosis and extremity DVT can potentially cause pulmonary embolus.[8] Safe administration of anticoagulant and antithrombolytic therapies requires close monitoring for signs of bleeding. Caregivers are instructed in these skills when the child can be managed at home. Referral to physical therapy may be warranted. Monitoring for delayed signs of postphlebitic syndrome such as pain, swelling, discoloration, ulceration, and pulmonary hypertension is important in follow-up visits.[8]

NERVOUS SYSTEM

This section on potential CNS complications focuses on the acute and intermediate side effects and management. Long-term CNS sequelae are discussed in Chapter 18. Several CNS complications are discussed in other chapters as appropriate: increased intracranial pressure and seizures in Chapter 13, posterior fossa syndrome in Chapter 21, and somnolence syndrome in Chapter 5.

CRANIAL NERVE DEFICITS

Definition/contributing factors. Cranial nerve dysfunction is caused by pressure on the nerves that arise from the brainstem.[99] Primary contributing factors are usually disease related and are associated with CNS malignancies, leukemias, lymphomas, and solid tumors that invade the cranial nerve space. Secondary factors are treatment-related complications. Surgery, radiation, chemotherapeu-

tic agents (vincristine, vinblastine, cisplatin, cytarabine, and ifosfamide), and infection can contribute to cranial nerve deficits.[93,99] Chemotherapy-induced deficits are usually dose related and occur in up to 10% of patients receiving these agents.[93]

Clinical presentation. Clinical presentation is specific to the cranial nerve involved and the extent of deficit. Table 11-6 lists the cranial nerves, their specific function, and the common causes of dysfunction. Jaw pain is considered a cranial nerve toxicity.[93] Potential complications of cranial nerve dysfunction include corneal abrasions, visual loss or deficit, facial palsy, muscle atrophy, dysphasia and aspiration, altered taste and smell, change in motor and sensory function, and deafness.[58,99]

Treatment strategies. The management of cranial nerve deficits depends on the cause (disease or treatment) and whether the condition is acute or chronic. Disease-related deficits require evaluation by history, thorough neurologic examination, and radiographic imaging. Initiation of treatment may alleviate deficits secondary to a mass. Therapy-related deficits can be minimized by early detection and intervention.[99] Toxicities are graded in severity according to the Common Toxicity Criteria (CTC), developed by the National Institutes of Health (NIH). Potential dose reductions are based on toxicity grading.[116]

Specific areas of concern are vision, nutrition, and hearing. Routine follow-up with an ophthalmologist for ongoing assessment of visual acuity is highly recommended. Functional deficits can cause corneal abrasions or changes in depth perception. Eye lubrication and protection, while awake and asleep, is necessary to maintain eye integrity.

Nutrition can be affected by changes in smell and taste, inability to properly chew or swallow, loss of sensation, and tongue weakness. Dietary counseling and speech therapy can maximize oral intake if severe deficits persist. Tube feedings (gastrostomy or nasogastric) or total parenteral nutrition (TPN) may be considered for weight maintenance and normal growth and development.

Routine audiology examinations are recommended for all patients at risk for ototoxicity. Early detection of loss is essential to prevent developmental delays. Early intervention with hearing aids can prevent loss of crucial speech development, especially in children less than 5 years old.[58]

Nursing role. A key component of nursing care for the child with cranial nerve deficits is assessment that includes presenting symptoms, acute versus chronic duration, safety issues related to the

TABLE 11-6	CRANIAL NERVE DYSFUNCTION		
Cranial Nerve	**Functions**	**Dysfunctions**	**Common Causes of Dysfunction**
I. olfactory	Sense of smell	Inability to smell, decreased sensation of smell, or distortion of smell	Head trauma; neurodegenerative disorders; frontal lobe tumors; hydrocephalus
II. optic	Sense of vision (visual acuity, peripheral vision, light reflexes)	Decreased visual acuity; decreased visual field	Lesions of frontal, temporal, parietal or occipital lobes; optic chiasm lesions; optic nerve tumors; aneurysms; migraines; third ventricular lesions; (causes are many due to nerve's widespread distribution)
III, IV, VI. oculomotor, trochlear, abducens	Extraocular movements; III—pupillary constrictions to light and accommodation; elevation of upper eyelid	Decreased extraocular motility; diplopia; nonreactive pupil; ptosis; inability to accommodate	Brainstem lesions; III—aneurysms; herniation, trauma; VI—multiple sclerosis; elevated intracranial pressure
V. trigeminal	Sensation to face, cornea, anterior scalp, nasal and oral mucosa, teeth, tongue, and portions of ear; muscles of mastication; corneal reflex	Decreased facial, mouth, and teeth sensation; impaired ability to chew; facial dysesthesia; decreased or absent corneal reflex	Tumors; trigeminal neuralgia; brainstem lesions
VII. facial	Movement of facial muscles; taste sensation anterior two thirds of tongue; salivary and lacrimal glands	Weak or paralyzed face; inability to close eye; decreased taste sensation; increased or decreased salivation and/or tearing	Bell's palsy; brainstem lesions; strokes; trauma
VIII. vestibulocochlear (acoustic)	Sense of hearing; control of balance and equilibrium	Decreased or absent hearing; dizziness; imbalance; poor spatial orientation; vertigo; tinnitus	Acoustic nerve tumors; brainstem lesions; Meniere's disease; trauma; middle and inner ear tumors
IX, X. glossopharyngeal, vagus	Taste sensation posterior third of tongue; sensation to throat, pharynx, and soft palate; elevation of pharynx; afferent limb of circulatory and respiratory reflexes (carotid sinus and carotid body); innervation of parotid gland; muscles of larynx, pharynx, and alimentary tract; secretion of gastric glands and pancreas;	Dysarthria; dysphagia; cardiac instability; respiratory difficulty	Brainstem lesions; basilar artery insufficiency

Data from Geary, S. M. (1995). Nursing management of cranial nerve dysfunction. *Journal of Neuroscience Nursing, 27,* 102-108.

Continued

TABLE 11-6	CRANIAL NERVE DYSFUNCTION—cont'd		
Cranial Nerve	**Functions**	**Dysfunctions**	**Common Causes of Dysfunction**
IX, X. glossopharyngeal, vagus—cont'd	inhibition of heart; constriction of coronary arteries; muscles of bronchial wall; respiratory, cardiac, and circulatory reflexes		
XI. spinal accessory	Elevation of shoulders; turning head side to side	Inability to shrug shoulders or to turn head to one side	Torticollis; brainstem and skull base lesions; deep neck wounds
XII. hypoglossal	Tongue movement	Dysarthria; dysphagia	Brainstem lesions; trauma

Data from Geary, S. M. (1995). Nursing management of cranial nerve dysfunction. *Journal of Neuroscience Nursing, 27,* 102-108.

deficit, learning needs, and patient and family coping mechanisms. Patient and family education focuses on symptom management to optimize activities of daily living, management of potential complications, and developmentally appropriate safety measures for the home environment. Safety measures are especially important for those with decreased visual acuity, sensation changes causing imbalance, or inability to distinguish hot and cold. Referral to speech, occupational, and/or physical therapy may be appropriate. A plan for school reentry and modifications must be in place.[58,99,112]

COGNITIVE AND BEHAVIORAL CHANGES

Definition/contributing factors. Cognitive and behavioral changes from disease or therapy may be acute or delayed. Cognitive changes refer to deficits in intellectual or developmental abilities and functioning. Behavioral changes refer to personality and social functioning.[100] Children who receive CNS therapy with radiation or chemotherapy and those with brain tumors are at an increased risk for developing behavioral-cognitive changes.[93,99,112,120,138] Chemotherapy agents associated with behavioral-cognitive changes include procarbazine, ifosfamide, high-dose cytarabine, methotrexate, cisplatin, asparaginase, fludarabine, and intrathecally administered agents. Other medications that can contribute to acute behavioral-cognitive changes are steroids, narcotics, some antiemetics, and antidepressants.[93,99,112]

Clinical presentation. Symptoms of behavioral-cognitive changes can range from mild to severe. Behavioral changes often have a more acute onset with mood swings, emotional lability, depression, fatigue, inattentiveness, poor impulse control, increased anger, or psychosis.[93] Symptoms of cognitive changes have a broader time frame for emergence. Acute manifestations are confusion or short-term memory loss. Delayed effects typically manifest as a decline in school performance in one or more subjects (often math skills), decline in abstract reasoning, failure to achieve or loss of developmental milestones, and decrease in generalized intelligence (loss of 10 to 20 IQ points). There can also be changes in visual spatial skills, speed of information processing, and verbal fluency (see Chapter 18).[71,99,112] Potential complications include leukoencephalopathy, severe permanent cognitive impairment, low self-esteem, isolation, stress, and impaired relationships.[99,112]

Treatment strategies. Management of cognitive-behavioral changes includes careful history and physical examination, radiographic studies such as CT scan, MRI, or positron emission tomography (PET) scan, and appropriate rehabilitative or therapeutic intervention. Ideally neuropsychologic testing is performed before the initiation of treatment known to contribute to cognitive deficits and repeated at regular intervals. Medications to minimize mood or depressive disorders can be considered but must be monitored closely. Proper monitoring for behavioral manifestations can provide for early detection, intervention, and prevention of severe symptoms. Cognitive changes can be monitored by thorough interval history, early identification of educational needs, and early initiation of an individualized education plan (IEP). Psychologic support offered to patients and families can minimize their risk for isolation, low self-esteem, and poor relationships.[71,99]

Nursing role. Patient and family education about potential behavioral and/or cognitive changes, typical symptoms, and strategies for management is essential. Families are educated about the short- and long-term behavioral-cognitive consequences of cancer treatment. Neuropsychologic testing results communicated to family and educators guides the plan to minimize deficits. Referral for psychologic support plays an important role in behavioral management and the prevention of psychopathology.

Long-term follow-up is directed to developmental and psychologic evaluation, symptom assessment, and anticipatory guidance for changing developmental needs. School reintegration is an ongoing role for nurses in collaboration with educators to promote the cognitive, social, and emotional well-being of children at risk of behavioral-cognitive changes.[71,99,112]

PERIPHERAL NEUROPATHY

Definition/contributing factors.   Peripheral neuropathy is a disorder of the peripheral nervous system that results in motor or sensory loss in the distribution of one or more nerves.[146] In children with cancer, disease-associated neuropathy can be caused by direct infiltration or peripheral nerve compression. Contributing factors may also include CNS tumors and solid tumors that invade the peripheral nerve compartment. The vinca alkaloids (vincristine, vinblastine) are the most common agents causing peripheral neurotoxicity, but etoposide, cisplatin, carboplatin, ifosfamide, and paclitaxel also have neurotoxic side effects.[60]

Clinical presentation.   Symptoms of peripheral neuropathy are symmetric and bilateral. One of the earliest signs may be a diminished ankle jerk reflex, with progression to tingling or numbness, pain, paresthesias, weakness, and depressed deep tendon reflexes. Areflexia (absent reflexes) can be found in up to 50% of patients with peripheral neuropathy. Children may experience stumbling, increased falls, inability to walk up stairs, or decreased ability to grasp and maintain their grip on objects. Permanent paresthesias and footdrop are potential complications.[17,93]

Treatment strategies.   Treating disease-associated neuropathy involves prompt identification of the causative agent and initiation of appropriate therapy. Patients receiving potentially neurotoxic agents need a thorough baseline neurologic evaluation, then routine neurologic examinations with subsequent follow-up. Early identification of neuropathy is essential during therapy to minimize complications.[17,93] Symptoms of peripheral neuropathy are assessed and graded by the NIH CTC, and dose reductions are considered when toxicity is severe.[116] Physical and occupational therapy are

instituted to minimize permanent sequelae and to provide adaptive strategies for maintaining independence.[17] Pain management strategies include both pharmacologic and nonpharmacologic interventions. Effective pharmacologic interventions may include nonnarcotic analgesics such as acetaminophen or nonsteroidal antiinflammatory drugs, narcotics, and the adjunctive use of antidepressants or anticonvulsants (e.g., amitriptyline, carbamazepine, gabapentin) for persistent paresthesias and pain. Dosing and administration can be guided by World Health Organization (WHO) recommendations. Nonpharmacologic interventions thought to be effective for painful neuropathies are relaxation, and imagery, distraction, and hypnosis.[84]

Nursing role.   Patient and caregiver education includes the child's relative risk for neuropathies, the symptoms of peripheral neuropathy, and strategies for managing the discomfort and compromised function. Patients and families need to be reassured that the symptoms are typically transient but can last many months. Patients and families are encouraged to pursue physical and/or occupational therapy. Safety issues include sensation changes, protection from environmental temperature extremes, helmet precautions to decrease effects of severe ataxia, and guidance for adapting to lifestyle limitations. Routine and thorough pain assessment and evaluation of the effectiveness of pain management strategies is important in nursing management of painful neuropathies.[17,84,93]

MUSCULOSKELETAL COMPLICATIONS

This section addresses acute and chronic issues involving functional limitations of the musculoskeletal system. Care following limb-sparing surgery and amputation are addressed in Chapter 27. Long-term musculoskeletal sequelae, including osteoporosis and avascular necrosis, are found in Chapter 18.

LIMITED RANGE OF MOTION

Definition/contributing factors.   Limited range of motion (ROM) is defined as any discrepancy in either the passive or active range of movement in a joint. The cause can be either musculoskeletal or neurologic and can result from either disease or treatment.[145] Contributing factors include the location of the malignancy, degree of surgical resection, site and dose of radiation, chronic use of steroids, and acute or chronic neuropathies. Patients at highest risk for limited ROM are those with bone tumors, solid tumors invading the muscles or joints, paralysis caused by central nervous system tumors, younger age at diagnosis, extended immobility, high-dose radiation to the extremities, and hematopoietic stem cell transplant patients with chronic GVHD. Conditions causing severe pain may also inhibit ROM. Limb salvage procedure or amputation can also result in functional limitations.[12,79]

Clinical presentation. Potential complications from limited ROM are muscle atrophy, fractures, asymmetry, scoliosis and kyphosis, thrombosis, altered body image and self-esteem, and decreased occupational opportunities.[12,79,103]

Treatment strategies. Treatment for limited ROM requires a multidisciplinary approach. Diseases that cause functional limitations are often treated by therapies that may or may not correct the underlying cause. Pain assessment and symptom management are important components in maximizing ROM. Physical and occupational therapy referral in both early and chronic phases are key components to achieving maximum limb use and a timely return to activities of daily living. Physical therapy may vary from basic range-of-motion exercises to vigorous strengthening activities. Prostheses, orthotics (e.g., braces, splints), and crutches can assist in joint stability. Hydrotherapy can be considered for contractures and muscle atrophy. Encouraging children to engage in activities they enjoy, such as swimming, will aid in compliance.[12] Psychologic support must be provided for children with significant and/or persistent limitations. A recent study of children surviving treatment for osteosarcoma indicated that up to 33% required professional emotional assistance when treatment included limb salvage or amputation.[79]

Nursing role. Assessment of the child with limited ROM includes musculoskeletal and neurologic examination and evaluation of functional abilities and muscle strength. Patient and caregiver education at discharge and during subsequent follow-up visits includes evaluating and reinforcing the plan for physical and/or occupational therapy. Assisting families in correctly performing ROM exercises, applying orthotics, assessing for potential safety hazards in the home environment, and adapting activities of daily living are included in self-care instructions. The use of community resources for school reintegration must be reevaluated at regular intervals. Signs and symptoms of inadequate coping, especially when severe or prolonged, are also an important assessment parameter. Families are encouraged to recognize and report symptoms of inadequate coping so that early intervention can be provided.[79,84,103]

INTEGUMENTARY SYSTEM

The integumentary system, comprising the skin and hair follicles, is the first line of defense against infection. Insults to this system in the pediatric oncology patient can be multifactorial in cause, because the integument is susceptible to a wide range of treatment-related side effects.

Definition/contributing factors. An intact integumentary system is a natural barrier to infection. Disruption of skin integrity alters an important protective barrier and increases the risk for opportunistic infection. Alterations may also result in pain and changes in body image and self-esteem.[93,147] Severe skin alterations leading to infection may also result in a delay of cancer treatment, which not only affects treatment outcomes but may also heighten a patient's and family's anxiety and stress levels. Factors contributing to the development of impaired integument include subcutaneous tumor manifestation, large radiation fields, exposure to specific chemotherapeutic agents (Table 11-7), hypersensitivity reactions to medications, malnutrition, poor hygiene, noncompliance with preventative measures such as sunscreen application, surgical procedures, poor-fitting prosthetics, diagnostic or invasive procedures such as lumbar puncture and bone marrow aspiration, prolonged immobility, trauma, or contact dermatitis. Table 11-7 identifies potential skin reactions, causative agents, and subsequent management. Table 11-7 also specifically addresses pertinent treatment and patient education for those undergoing radiation therapy.

Clinical presentation. Clinical presentation of alterations in the integumentary system may occur with a tremendous amount of variation depending on the underlying cause. Radiation effects on the skin can manifest as mild erythema and tenderness, dry desquamation, or weeping desquamation. The syndrome of radiation recall can also affect skin integrity, resulting in changes that vary from warmth and erythema at the site to severe desquamation and ulceration. Radiation can also cause temporary alopecia or permanent hair loss depending on the dose. Chemotherapy can cause alopecia as well, usually occurring several weeks after the initiation of therapy. Certain chemotherapy agents can cause skin reactions, which can alter skin integrity and cause pruritus. Chemotherapy agents (e.g., methotrexate) and supportive care drugs (e.g., trimethoprim sulfamethoxazole) can cause photosensitivity. Subcutaneous manifestations of tumor may leave the affected skin friable and prone to break down. Special care should be taken to protect these areas, which may appear as palpable nodules that

TABLE 11-7	POTENTIAL SKIN REACTIONS		
Potential Change	**Causative Agent**	**Treatment**	**Patient/Caregiver Education**
Urticaria	Asparaginase Cisplatin Etoposide Melphalan Mesna Paclitaxel Procarbazine Teniposide	Cessation of causative agent Antihistamines, steroids, epinephrine if associated with severe allergic reaction Preventive treatment with antihistamines and corticosteroids	Teach signs and symptoms of delayed allergic reaction. Reassure that rash will resolve.
Erythematous rash	Allopurinol Azacytidine Dacarbazine Hydroxyurea Leucovorin Mechlorethamine Methotrexate Procarbazine	Oral antihistamine Hydrocortisone cream	Teach signs and symptoms. Instruct in proper application of cream. Advise to avoid sun exposure, use sunscreen.
Desquamation	Radiation	Moisturizing lotion	Advise to: • Avoid sun. • Protect skin from weather extremes. • Keep skin clean. • Avoid deodorant.
Stevens-Johnson syndrome	Trimethoprim sulfamethoxazole	Cessation of drug Steroids May require hospitalization	Educate patient to report rashes and skin lesions.
Photosensitivity	Anthracyclines Cyclosporin Methotrexate Radiation Retinoic acid Trimethoprim sulfamethoxazole	Sunscreen	Advise to: • Use sunscreen. • Identify more sensitive areas. • Use protective clothing.
Alopecia (degree may vary)	Many chemotherapy agents Radiation	None Preventive measures controversial	Reassure that hair will most likely return, but may return different color. Use hats and/or wigs and/or head painting. Refer to American Cancer Society for support services.
Face flushing	Corticosteroids Dacarbazine	Cessation of causative agent	Teach potential for occurrence.
Skin peeling	Graft-versus-host disease Retinoic acid Etoposide	Creams Possible dose modification of retinoic acid	Teach potential for occurrence and importance of reporting symptoms.
Hypopigmentation	Thiotepa Radiation	None	Reassure that it could be temporary. Provide emotional support. Provide cosmetic consult with American Cancer Society.

Data from Fishman, M., & Mrozed-Orlowshi, M. (1997). *Cancer chemotherapy guidelines and recommendations for practice* (2nd ed.). Pittsburgh, PA: Oncology Nursing Society; Howard, V. (1998). Skin changes. In M. J. Hockenberry-Eaton (Ed.), *Essentials of pediatric oncology nursing: A core curriculum* (pp. 140-141). Glenview, IL: Association of Pediatric Oncology Nurses; Lindley, C., Finley, R., & LaCevita, C. L. (1995). Adverse effects of chemotherapy. In L. Young (Ed.), *Applied therapeutics: The clinical use of drugs* (6th ed., pp. 91.2-91.17). Vancouver, WA: Applied Therapeutics; Millot, F., Auriol, F., Breecheteau, P., et al. (1999). Acral erythema in children receiving high-dose methotrexate. *Pediatric Dermatology, 16,* 398-400.

Continued

TABLE 11-7	POTENTIAL SKIN REACTIONS—cont'd		
Potential Change	**Causative Agent**	**Treatment**	**Patient/Caregiver Education**
Hyperpigmentation	Bleomycin Busulfan Dactinomycin Etoposide Hydroxyurea Radiation	None Cessation of drug	Reassure that it is likely to resolve. Educate regarding this potential change.
Acne	Corticosteroids Dactinomycin	General topical acne treatments Benzyl peroxide	Teach appropriate hygiene. Prepare for potential exacerbation of acne. Reassure that it will likely diminish after drug is stopped.
Atopic dermatitis	Thioguanine Mercaptopurine	Hydrocortisone cream	Teach potential for occurrence
Radiation recall	Administration of certain chemotherapy agents following radiation therapy (anthracyclines, bleomycin, dactinomycin, mitoxantrone)	Moisturizing cream Topical steroids Oral steroids for severe symptoms	Apply cool, wet compress to acute reaction. Teach presenting symptoms of recall and signs of infection. Teach good hygiene. Instruct in proper application of any topical products. Reassure that process is temporary. Advise to use sunscreen. Avoid extreme heat and cold and sun.
Nail bed changes (Beau's lines, bluish or brown horizontal or vertical bends)	Cyclophosphamide Daunorubicin Doxorubicin Fluorouracil	None	Assess for nail bed breakdown. Teach signs/symptoms of infection. Teach good hygiene. Reassure resolution in 6-12 months.
Acral erythema (palmar-plantar erythematous skin)	Cyclophosphamide Cytarabine Doxorubicin Fluorouracil Hydroxyurea Mercaptopurine Methotrexate	Comfort measures if lesions painful Cold compresses Acetaminophen Steroid creams Pyridoxine	Reassure that condition is temporary. Observe for signs of infection. Teach importance of frequent hand washing. Elevate affected area to decrease edema.

Data from Fishman, M., & Mrozed-Orlowshi, M. (1997). *Cancer chemotherapy guidelines and recommendations for practice* (2nd ed.). Pittsburgh, PA: Oncology Nursing Society; Howard, V. (1998). Skin changes. In M. J. Hockenberry-Eaton (Ed.), *Essentials of pediatric oncology nursing: A core curriculum* (pp. 140-141). Glenview, IL: Association of Pediatric Oncology Nurses; Lindley, C., Finley, R., & LaCevita, C. L. (1995). Adverse effects of chemotherapy. In L. Young (Ed.), *Applied therapeutics: The clinical use of drugs* (6th ed., pp. 91.2-91.17). Vancouver, WA: Applied Therapeutics; Millot, F., Auriol, F., Breecheteau, P., et al. (1999). Acral erythema in children receiving high-dose methotrexate. *Pediatric Dermatology, 16*, 398-400.

are sometimes hemorrhagic (blueberry muffin syndrome). These nodules can diminish as cancer treatment is initiated but may leave areas of hyperpigmentation. Any invasive procedure creates an opportunity for infection. For example, infected bone marrow aspirate sites may appear erythematous and edematous and have drainage. Pediatric oncology patients who have decreased mobility during a long hospitalization are at additional risk for skin alteration. Skin changes in immobile patients and those wearing prostheses may begin as subtle erythema that can progress to severe ulceration. Poor nutritional status, which is not an uncommon occurrence in the pediatric oncology patient, is also associated with increased risk for infection and poor wound healing.

Treatment strategies. Protection of the integumentary system is essential, particularly in the care of the immunocompromised patient. Thorough assessment and early intervention are imperative to maintain this barrier to infection. Treatment strategies include good daily hygiene, encouraging mobility, application of antibiotic or moisture barrier ointments as indicated, and a wound and/or skin care plan specific for the patient's clinical status. Antipruritic drugs are often administered for patient comfort. Pain medications may also be necessary. Nutritional support is initiated if indicated, because good nutrition status is essential to promote wound healing.

Nursing role.   Nurses play a crucial role in the prevention and treatment of altered skin integrity. A meticulous skin assessment is an essential element of care. Particular attention is given to any break in the skin, to radiation fields, and to any potential problem areas. Both patients and families are educated in the importance of good daily hygiene and reporting skin changes in a timely manner to their health care provider. Nurses must encourage frequent mobilization and ensure that immobile patients are repositioned at least every 2 hours. Education must also be provided regarding photosensitivity and the need to avoid excessive exposure to sunlight and to use sunscreen. Because nutrition is essential to wound healing, it is also necessary for the nurse to encourage good oral intake whenever possible. In the event that the patient is unable to maintain adequate oral nutrition, the nurse should discuss other options such as supplements, nasogastric feeds, and/or parenteral nutrition with the health care team.

Pediatric oncology patients are at risk of numerous and varied complications related to their disease process or the consequences of therapy. Nurses play an integral role in ameliorating these effects and can truly make a difference in the lives of children and adolescents with cancer. Advances in supportive care have been linked to the improved survival rates and improved quality of life for pediatric oncology patients over recent decades.[3] The field of symptom management is growing, and further research is needed in many aspects of care to provide patients with optimal care.

REFERENCES

1. Aitken, T. (1992). Gastrointestinal manifestations in the child with cancer. *Journal of Pediatric Oncology Nursing, 9,* 99-108.
2. Albano, E. A., & Ablin, A. R. (1997). Oncologic emergencies. In A. R. Ablin (Ed.), *Supportive care of children with cancer* (2nd ed., pp. 175-192). Baltimore: Johns Hopkins University Press.
3. Albano, E. A., & Odom, L. F. (1993). Supportive care in pediatric oncology. *Current Opinion in Pediatrics, 5,* 131-137.
4. Alexander, H. R., Rickard, K. A., & Godshall, B. (1997). Nutritional supportive care. In P. A. Pizzo & D. G. Poplack (Eds.), *Principles and practice of pediatric oncology* (3rd ed., pp. 1167-1181). Philadelphia: Lippincott-Raven.
5. Alvarez, O., Freeman, A., Bedros, A., et al. (1995). Randomized double-blind cross-over ondansetron-dexamethasone versus ondansetron-placebo for the treatment of chemotherapy-induced nausea and vomiting in pediatric patients with malignancies. *Journal of Pediatric Hematology/Oncology, 17,* 145-150.
6. Anderson, P. M., Schroeder, G., & Skubitz, K. M. (1998). Oral glutamine reduces the duration and severity of stomatitis after cytotoxic cancer chemotherapy. *Cancer, 83,* 1433-1439.
7. Anderson, P. M., Ramsay, N. K. C., Shu, X. O., et al. (1998). Effect of low-dose oral glutamine on painful stomatitis during bone marrow transplantation. *Bone Marrow Transplantation, 22,* 339-344.
8. Andrew, M., David, M., Adams, M., et al. (1994). Venous thromboembolic complications (VTE) in children: First analyses of the Canadian registry of VTE. *Blood, 83,* 1251-1257.
9. Barnard, D. R., Feusner, J. H., & Wolff. L. J. (1997). Blood component therapy. In A. R. Ablin (Ed.), *Supportive care of children with cancer* (2nd ed., pp. 37-46). Baltimore: Johns Hopkins University Press.
10. Beck S. (1979). Impact of a systematic oral care protocol on stomatitis after chemotherapy. *Cancer Nursing, 2,* 185-199.
11. Beck, T., York, M., Chang, A., et al. (1995). Oral ondansetron 8 mg bid as effective as 8 mg tid in the prevention of nausea and vomiting associated with cyclophosphamide-based chemotherapy. *Proceedings of the American Society of Clinical Oncology, 14,* 538.
12. Binder, H., Perrin, J. C. S., & Gerber, L. H. (1997). Rehabilitation of the child with cancer. In P. A. Pizzo & D. G. Poplack (Eds.), *Principles and practice of pediatric oncology* (3rd ed., pp. 1229-1239). Philadelphia: Lippincott-Raven.
13. Bisanz, A. (1997). Managing bowel elimination problems in patients with cancer. *Oncology Nursing Forum, 24,* 679-686.
14. Bloch, A. (2000). Nutrition support in cancer. *Seminars in Oncology Nursing, 16,* 122-127.
15. Bonnardeux, A., & Bichet, D. G. (2000). Inherited disorders of the renal tubule. In B. M. Brenner & F. C. Rector (Eds.), *The kidney* (6th ed., pp. 1656-1665). Philadelphia: W. B. Saunders.
16. Borowski, B., Benhamou, E., Pico, J. J., et al. (1994). Prevention of oral mucositis in patients treated with high-dose chemotherapy and bone marrow transplantation: A randomized controlled trial comparing two protocols of dental care. *European Journal of Cancer, B Oral Oncology, 30B,* 93-97.
17. Bottomley, S. (1998). Late effects of childhood cancer. In M. Hockenberry-Eaton (Ed.), *Essentials of pediatric oncology nursing. A core curriculum.* (pp. 242-249.) Glenview, IL: Association of Pediatric Oncology Nurses.
18. Broxmeyer, H. E., Benninger, L., Patel, S. R., et al. (1994). Kinetic response of human marrow myeloid progenitor cells to in vivo treatment of patients with granulocyte colony-stimulating factor is different from the response to treatment with granulocyte-macrophage colony-stimulating factor. *Experimental Hematology, 22,* 100-102.

19. Buchanan, A. G., Riben, P. D., Rayner, E. N., et al. (1985). Nystatin prophylaxis of antifungal colonization and infection in granulocytopenic patients: Correlation of colonization and clinical outcome. *Clinical Investigative Medicine, 8,* 139-147.

20. Buchanan, G. R. (1997). Hematologic supportive care of the pediatric cancer patient. In P. A. Pizzo, & D. G. Poplack (Eds.), *Principles and practice of pediatric oncology* (3rd ed., pp. 1051-1068). Philadelphia: Lippincott-Raven.

21. Buick, N. T. (1994). Cellular basis of chemotherapy. In R. T. Dorr & D. D. Von Hoff (Eds.), *Cancer chemotherapy handbook* (2nd ed., pp. 3-14). Norwalk, CT: Appleton & Lange.

22. Bushara, K. O., & Rust, R. S. (1997). Reversible MRI lesions due to pegaspargase treatment of non-Hodgkin's lymphoma. *Pediatric Neurology, 17,* 185-187.

23. Camp-Sorrell, D. (1999). Surviving the cancer, surviving the treatment: Acute cardiac and pulmonary toxicity. *Oncology Nursing Forum, 26,* 983-990.

24. Carter, D. L., Hebert, M. E., Smink, K., et al. (1999). Double blind randomized trial of sucralfate vs placebo during radical radiotherapy for head and neck cancers. *Head & Neck, 21,* 760-766.

25. Cascinu, S. (1995). Drug therapy in diarrheal disease in oncology/hematology patients. *Critical Reviews in Oncology/Hematology, 18,* 37-50.

26. Cengiz, M., Ozyar, E., Ozturk, D., et al. (1999). Sucralfate in the prevention of radiation-induced oral mucositis. *Journal of Clinical Gastroenterology 28,* 40-43.

27. Chan, H. S. L., Correia, J. A., & MacLeod, S. M. (1987). Nabilone versus prochlorperazine for control of cancer chemotherapy-induced emesis in children: A double-blind crossover trial. *Pediatrics, 79,* 946-952.

28. Charak, B. S., Parikh, P. M., Banavali, S. D., et al. (1988). Comparison of clotrimazole with nystatin in preventing oral candidiasis in neutropenic patients. *Indian Journal of Medical Research, 88,* 416-420.

29. Charuhas, P. M., Fosberg, K. L., Bruemmer, B., et al. (1997). A double-blind randomized trial comparing outpatient parenteral nutrition with intravenous hydration: Effect on resumption of oral intake after marrow transplantation. *JPEN, Journal of Parenteral and Enteral Nutrition, 21,* 157-161.

30. Cieslak, G. D., Watcha, M. F., Phillips, M. B., et al. (1996). The dose-response relation and cost-effectiveness of granisetron for the prophylaxis of pediatric postoperative emesis. *Anesthesiology, 85,* 1076-1085.

31. Clayton, B., & Stock, Y. (1997). *Basic pharmacology for nurses,* (11th ed.). St. Louis, MO: Mosby.

32. Contanch, P., Hockenberry, M., & Herman, S. (1985). Self-hypnosis as antiemetic therapy in children receiving chemotherapy. *Oncology Nursing Forum, 12*(4), 41-45.

33. Coppes, M. J., Yanofsky, R., Pritchard, S., et al. (1999). Safety, tolerability, antiemetic efficacy, and pharmacokinetics of oral dolasetron in pediatric cancer patients receiving moderately to highly emetogenic chemotherapy. *Journal of Pediatric Hematology/Oncology, 21,* 274-283.

34. Cubeddu, L. X., & Hoffmann, I. S. (1993). Participation of serotonin on early and delayed emesis induced by initial and subsequent cycles of cisplatinum-based chemotherapy: Effects of antiemetics. *Journal of Clinical Pharmacology, 33,* 691-697.

35. Cunningham, R. S. (1997). 5-HT$_3$-receptor antagonists: A review of pharmacology and clinical efficacy. *Oncology Nursing Forum, 24* (Suppl. 7), 33-40.

36. Cunningham, R. S., & Bell, R. (2000). Nutrition in cancer: An overview. *Seminars in Oncology Nursing, 16,* 90-98.

37. Cuttner, J., Troy, K. M., Funaro, L., et al. (1986). Clotrimazole treatment for prevention of oral candidiasis in patients with acute leukemia undergoing chemotherapy: Results of a double-blind study. *The American Journal of Medicine, 81,* 771-774.

38. DeGregorio, M. W., Lee, W. M., & Ries, C. A. (1982). Candida infections in patients with acute leukemia: Ineffectiveness of nystatin prophylaxis and relationship between oropharyngeal and systemic candidiasis. *Cancer, 50,* 2780-2784.

39. Dicato, M. A. (1991). Oral treatment with ondansetron in an outpatient setting. *European Journal of Cancer, 27* (Suppl. 1), S18-S19.

40. DiPiro, C. V., Sanal, S. M., Harkness, R. M., et al. (1996). The antiemetic efficacy of intravenous ondansetron (OND) at conventional versus low dose in women with early stage breast cancer. *Proceedings of the American Society of Clinical Oncology, 15,* 540.

41. Dodd, M. J., Dibble, S. L., Miakowski, C., et al. (2000). Randomized clinical trial of the effectiveness of 3 commonly used mouthwashes to treat chemotherapy-induced mucositis. *Oral Surgery Oral Medicine Oral Pathology Oral Radiology Endodontics, 90,* 39-47.

42. Dodd, M. J., Larson, P. J., Dibble, S. L., et al. (1996). Randomized clinical trial of chlorhexidine versus placebo for prevention of oral mucositis in patients receiving chemotherapy. *Oncology Nursing Forum, 23,* 921-927.

43. Dolgin, M. J., & Katz, E. R. (1988). Conditioned aversions in pediatric cancer patients receiving chemotherapy. *Journal of Developmental and Behavioral Pediatrics, 9,* 82-85.

44. Dolgin, M. J., Katz, E. R., McGinty, K., et al. (1985). Anticipatory nausea and vomiting in pediatric cancer patients. *Pediatrics, 75,* 547-552.

45. Dreizen, S. (1990). Description and incidence of oral complications. *NCI Monograph, 9,* 11-15.

46. Dunn, J. (1994). Doxorubicin-induced cardiomyopathy. *Journal of Pediatric Oncology Nursing, 11,* 152-160.

47. Eilers, J., Berger, A. M., & Petersen, M. C. (1988). Development, testing, and application of the Oral Assessment Guide. *Oncology Nursing Forum, 15,* 325-330.

48. Epstein, J. B., Vickars, L., Spinnelli, J., et al. (1992). Efficacy of chlorhexidine and nystatin rinse in prevention of oral complications in leukemia and bone marrow transplantation. *Oral Surgery Oral Medicine Oral Pathology, 73,* 682-689.

49. Epstein, J. B., & Wong, F. L. (1994). The efficacy of sucralfate suspension in prevention of oral mucositis due to radiation therapy. *International Journal of Radiation Oncology, Biology, Physics, 28,* 693-698.

50. Farrel, G. C. (1998). Liver disease caused by drugs, anesthetics and toxins. In M. Feldman, B. Scharschmidt, M. Sleisenger., et al. (Eds.), *Gastrointestinal and liver disease: Pathophysiology, diagnosis and management.* (6th ed., pp. 1126-1228). Philadelphia: W. B. Saunders.

51. Ferrel, B. R., Grant, M., Dean, G. E., et al. (1996). "Bone tired": The experience of fatigue and its impact on quality of life. *Oncology Nursing Forum, 23,* 1539-1547.

52. Ferretti, G. A., Ash, R. C., Brown, A. T., et al. (1987). Chlorhexidine for prophylaxis against oral infections and associated complications in patients receiving bone marrow transplants. *Journal of the American Dental Association, 114,* 461-467.

53. Ferretti, G. A., Ash, R. C., Brown, A. T., et al. (1988). Control of oral mucositis and candidiasis in marrow transplantation: A prospective, double-blind trial of chlorhexidine digluconate oral rinse. *Bone Marrow Transplantation, 3,* 483-493.

54. Ferretti, G. A., Raybould. T. P., Brown, A. T., et al. (1990). Chlorhexidine prophylaxis for chemotherapy-induced stomatitis: A randomized double-blind trial. *Oral Surgery, Oral Medicine, Oral Pathology, 69,* 331-338.

55. Franzen, L., Henriksson, R., Littbrand, B., et al. (1995). Effects of sucralfate on mucositis during and following radiotherapy of malignancies in the head and neck region: A double-blind placebo-controlled study. *Acta Oncologica, 34,* 219-223.

56. Freifeld, A. G., Walsh, T. J., & Pizzo, P. A. (1997). Infectious complications in the pediatric cancer patient. In P. A. Pizzo & D. G. Poplack (Eds.), *Principles and practice of pediatric oncology* (3rd ed., pp. 1069-1114). Philadelphia: Lippincott-Raven.

57. Fristoe, B. (1998). Long-term cardiac and pulmonary complications in cancer care. *Nurse Practitioner Forum, 9,* 177-184.

58. Geary, S. M. (1995). Nursing management of cranial nerve dysfunction. *Journal of Neuroscience Nursing, 27,* 102-108.

59. Gebbia, V., Cannata, G., Testa, A., et al. (1994). Ondansetron versus granisetron in the prevention of chemotherapy-induced nausea and vomiting. *Cancer, 74,* 1945-1952.

60. Girolami, U., Frosch, M. P., & Anthony, D. C. (1994). The central nervous system. In F. J. Schoen (Ed.), *Robbins pathologic basis of disease* (5th ed., pp. 1283-1285). Philadelphia: W. B. Saunders.

61. Graham, K. M., Pecoraro, D. A., Ventura, M., et al. (1993). Reducing the incidence of stomatitis using a quality assessment and improvement approach. *Cancer Nursing, 16,* 117-122.

62. Graham-Pole, J., Weare, J., Engel, S., et al. (1986). Antiemetics in children receiving cancer chemotherapy: A double-blind prospective randomized study comparing metoclopramide with chlorpromazine. *Journal of Clinical Oncology, 4,* 1110-1113.

63. Grant, M., & Kravits, K. (2000). Symptoms and their impact on nutrition. *Seminars in Oncology Nursing, 16,* 113-121.

64. Hanigan, M. J., & Walter, G. (1992). Nutritional support of the child with cancer. *Journal of Pediatric Oncology Nursing, 9,* 110-118.

65. Hanson, S. R., & Slichter, S. J. (1985). Platelet kinetics in patients with bone marrow hypoplasia: Evidence for a fixed platelet requirement. *Blood, 66,* 1105-1109.

66. Hertenstein, B., Stefanic, M., Schmeiser, T., et al. (1994). Toxicity of bone marrow transplantation: Predictive value of cardiologic evaluation before transplant. *Journal of Clinical Oncology, 12,* 998-1004.

67. Hesketh, P. J., Beck, T., Uhlenhopp, M., et al. (1995). Adjusting the dose of intravenous ondansetron plus dexamethasone to the emetogenic potential of the chemotherapy regimen. *Journal of Clinical Oncology, 13,* 2117-2122.

68. Hesketh, P. J., Harvey, W. H., Harker, W. G., et al. (1994). A randomized, double-blind comparison of intravenous ondansetron alone and in combination with intravenous dexamethasone in the prevention of high-dose cisplatin-induced emesis. *Journal of Clinical Oncology, 12,* 596-600.

69. Hinds, P. S., Hockenberry-Eaton, M., Gilger, E., et al. (1999). Comparing patient, parent, and staff descriptions of fatigue in pediatric oncology patients. *Cancer Nursing, 22,* 277-289.

70. Hinds, P. S., Hockenberry-Eaton, M., Quargnenti, A., et al. (1999). Fatigue in 7-12 year old patients with cancer from the staff perspective: An exploratory study. *Oncology Nursing Forum, 26,* 37-45.

71. Hobbie, W., Ruccione, K., Moore, I., et al. (1993). Late effects in long term survivors. In G. V. Foley, D. Fochtman, & K. Hardin Mooney, (Eds), *Nursing care of the child with cancer* (2nd ed., pp. 466-496). Philadelphia: W. B. Saunders.

72. Hockenberry-Eaton, M., Hinds, P. S., Alcoser, P., et al. (1998). Fatigue in children and adolescents with cancer. *Journal of Pediatric Oncology Nursing, 15,* 172-182.

73. Hogan, C. M. (1997). Cancer nursing: The art of symptom management. *Oncology Nursing Forum, 24,* 1335-1341.

74. Hogan, C. M. (1998). The nurse's role in diarrhea management. *Oncology Nursing Forum, 25,* 879-886.

75. Hogan, C. M., & Grant, M. (1997). Physiologic mechanisms of nausea and vomiting in patients with cancer. *Oncology Nursing Forum, 24* (Suppl. 7), 8-12.

76. Hooke, C. (2000). Recombinant tissue plasminogen activator for central venous access device occlusion. *Journal of Pediatric Oncology Nursing, 17,* 174-178.

77. Howard, S. C., Gajjar, A., Ribeiro, R., et al. (2000). Safety of lumbar puncture for children with acute lymphoblastic leukemia and thrombocytopenia. *Journal of the American Medical Association, 284,* 2222-2224.

78. Howard, V. (1998). Nutritional complications. In M. Hockenberry-Eaton (Ed.), *Essentials of pediatric oncology nursing: A core curriculum* (pp. 142-143). Glenview, IL: Association of Pediatric Oncology Nurses.

79. Hudson, M. M., Tyc, V. L., Cremer, L. K., et al. (1998). Patient satisfaction after limb-sparing surgery and amputation for pediatric malignant bone tumors. *Journal of Pediatric Oncology Nursing, 15,* 60-69.

80. Iacuone, J., Steinherz, L., Oblender, M., et al. (1997). Modifications for toxicity. In A. R. Ablin (Ed.), *Supportive care of children with cancer* (2nd ed., pp. 79-111). Baltimore: Johns Hopkins University Press.

81. Italian Group for Antiemetic Research (1995). Ondansetron versus granisetron, both combined with dexamethasone, in the prevention of cisplatin-induced emesis. *Annals of Oncology, 6,* 805-810.

82. Italian Group for Antiemetic Research. (1998). Double-blind, dose-finding study of four intravenous doses of dexamethasone in the prevention of cisplatin-induced acute emesis. *Journal of Clinical Oncology, 16,* 2937-2942.

83. Jacknow, D. S., Tschann, J. M., Link, M. P., et al. (1994). Hypnosis in the prevention of chemotherapy-related nausea and vomiting in children: A prospective study. *Developmental and Behavioral Pediatrics, 15,* 258-264.

84. Jacox, A., Carr, D. B., Payne, R., et al. (1994). *Management of cancer pain, Clinical practice guidelines No. 9* (AHCPR Publication No. 94-0592). Rockville, MD: Agency for Health Care Policy and Research, U.S. Department of Health and Human Services, Public Health Service.

85. Karthaus, M., Rosenthal, C., & Ganser, A. (1999). Prophylaxis and treatment of chemo- and radiotherapy-induced oral mucositis: Are there new strategies? *Bone Marrow Transplantation, 24,* 1095-1108.

86. Keller, V. E. (1995). Management of nausea and vomiting in children. *Journal of Pediatric Nursing, 10,* 280-286.

87. Komada, Y., Matsuyama, T., Takao, A., et al. (1999). A randomised dose-comparison trial of granisetron in preventing emesis in children with leukemia receiving emetogenic chemotherapy. *European Journal of Cancer, 35,* 1095-1101.

88. Krejs, C., & Fordtran, J. (1983). Diarrhea. In J. Sleisenger & J. Fordtran (Eds.), *Pathophysiology, diagnosis, and management* (pp. 257-277). Philadelphia: W. B. Saunders.

89. Kris, M. G., Gralla, R. J., Tyson, L. B., et al. (1985). Improved control of cisplatin-induced emesis with high-dose metoclopramide and with combinations of metoclopramide, dexamethasone, and diphenhydramine-Results of consecutive trials in 255 patients. *Cancer, 55,* 527-534.

90. Lange, B., O'Neill, J., Jr., Goldwein, A., et al. (1997). Oncologic emergencies. In P. A. Pizzo & D. G. Poplack (Eds.), *Principles and practice of pediatric oncology* (3rd ed., pp. 1025-1049). Philadelphia: Lippincott-Raven.

91. Lewis, J. H. (2000) Drug induced liver disease. *Medical Clinics of North America, 84,* 1275-1311.

92. Lievens, Y., Haustermans, K., Van den Weyngaert, D., et al. (1998). Does sucralfate reduce the acute side-effects in head and neck cancer treated with radiotherapy? A double-blind randomized trial. *Radiotherapy & Oncology, 47,* 149-153.

93. Lindley, C., Finley, R., & LaCevita, C. L. (1995). Adverse effects of chemotherapy. In L. Young, (Ed.). *Applied therapeutics: The clinical use of drugs* (6th ed., pp. 91.2-91.17). Vancouver, WA: Applied Therapeutics.

94. Lockhart, P. B., & Sonis, S. T. (1979). Relationship of oral complications to peripheral blood leukocyte and platelet counts in patients receiving cancer chemotherapy. *Oral Surgery Oral Medicine Oral Pathology Oral Radiology Endodontics, 48,* 21-28.

95. Lopez-Beltran, A. (1999). Bladder treatment. *Urologic Clinics of North America, 26,* 535-554.

96. Loprinzi, C. L., Ghosh, C., Camoriano, J., et al. (1997). Phase III controlled evaluation of sucralfate to alleviate stomatitis in patients receiving fluorouracil-based chemotherapy. *Journal of Clinical Oncology, 15,* 1235-1238.

97. Mackie, A. M., Coda, B. C., & Hill, H. F. (1991). Adolescents use patient-controlled analgesia effectively for relief from prolonged oropharnygeal mucositis pain. *Pain, 46,* 265-269.

98. Madeya, M. L. (1996). Oral complications from cancer therapy. II. Nursing implications for assessment and treatment. *Oncology Nursing Forum, 23,* 808-821.

99. Madsen, L., (1998). Central nervous system complications. In M. J. Hockenberry-Eaton (Ed.), *Essentials of pediatric oncology nursing: A core curriculum* (pp. 124-127). Glenview, IL: Association of Pediatric Oncology Nurses.

100. Malik, I. A., Khan, W. A., Qazilbash, M., et al. (1995). Clinical efficacy of lorazepam in prophylaxis of anticipatory, acute, and delayed nausea and vomiting induced by high doses of cisplatin: A prospective randomized trial. *American Journal of Clinical Oncology, 18,* 170-175.

101. Mantovani, G., Maccio, A., Bianchi, A., et al. (1996). Comparing granisetron, ondansetron, and tropisetron in the prophylaxis of acute nausea and vomiting induced by cisplatin for the treatment of head and neck cancer: A randomized controlled trial. *Cancer, 77,* 941-948.

102. Marshall, G., Kerr, S., Vowels, M., et al. (1989). Antiemetic therapy for chemotherapy-induced vomiting: Metoclopramide, benztropine, dexamethasone, and lorazepam regimen compared to chlorpromazine alone. *Journal of Pediatrics, 115,* 156-160.

103. Marson, K. (1998). Musculoskeletal complications. In M. J. Hockenberry-Eaton (Ed.), *Essentials of pediatric oncology nursing: A core curriculum* (pp. 141-142). Glenview, IL: Association of Pediatric Oncology Nurses.

104. Martoni, A., Angelelli, B., Buaraldi, M., et al. (1996). An open randomized cross-over study of granisetron versus ondansetron in the prevention of acute emesis by moderate dose cisplatin-containing regimens. *European Journal of Cancer, 32A,* 82-85.

105. Massicotte, M. P., Dix, D., Monagle, P., et al. (1998). Central venous catheter related thrombosis in children: Analysis of the Canadian registry of venous thromboembolic complications. *Journal of Pediatrics, 133,* 770-776.

106. McGuire, M. (2000). Nutritional care of surgical oncology patients. *Seminars in Oncology Nursing, 16,* 128-134.

107. Meacham, L., Ghim, T., Crocker, I., et al. (1997). Systematic approach for detection of endocrine disorders in children treated for brain tumors. *Medical and Pediatric Oncology, 29,* 86-91.

108. Meyer, B. R., O'Mara, V., & Reidenber, M. M. (1987). A controlled clinical trial of the addition of transdermal scopolamine to a standard metoclopramide and dexamethasone antiemetic regimen. *Journal of Clinical Oncology, 5,* 1994-1997.

109. Miller, A. B., Hoogstraten, B., Staquet, M., et al. (1981). Reporting results of cancer treatment. *Cancer, 47,* 207-214.

110. Mitchell, D., & Pickering, L. (2001). Enteric infections. In C. C. Patrick (Ed.), *Clinical management of infections in imunocompromised infants and children* (pp. 418-441). Philadelphia: W. B. Saunders.

111. Monagle, P., Michelson, A. D., Bovill, E., et al. (2001). Antithrombotic therapy in children. *Chest, 119* (Suppl 1), 344S-370S.

112. Moore, I. M. (1995). Central nervous system toxicity of cancer therapy in children. *Journal of Pediatric Oncology Nursing 12,* 203-210.

113. Morrow, G. R. (1992). Behavioral factors influencing the development and expression of chemotherapy-induced side effects. *Bristish Journal of Cancer, 19,* S54-S61.

114. Mueller, B. A., Millheim, E. T., Farrington, E. A., et al. (1995). Mucositis management practices for hospitalized patients: National survey results. *Journal of Pain and Symptom Management, 10,* 510-520.

115. National Cancer Institute. (1990). US Monographs. Consensus development conference on oral complications of cancer therapies: Diagnosis, prevention and treatment. Bethesda, MD: National Institutes of Health.

116. National Cancer Institute. (1999). Common Toxicity Criteria (Version 2.0). Betheseda, MD: National Institutes of Health.

117. Navari, R., Gandara, D., Hesketh, P., et al. (1995). Comparative clinical trial of granisetron and ondansetron in the prophylaxis of cisplatin-induced emesis. *Journal of Clinical Oncology, 13,* 1242-1248.

118. Navari, R. M., Madajwicz, S., Anderson, N., et al. (1995). Oral ondansetron for the control of cisplatin-induced delayed emesis: A large, multicenter, double-blind, randomized comparative trial of ondansetron versus placebo. *Journal of Clinical Oncology, 13,* 2408-2416.

119. Niehaus, C. S., Peterson, D. E., & Overholser, C. D. (1987). Oral complications in children during cancer therapy. *Cancer Nursing, 10,* 15-20.

120. Ochs, J., Mulhern, R., Fairclough, D., et al. (1991). Comparison of neuropsychologic functioning and clinical indicators of neurotoxicity in long term survivors of childhood leukemia given cranial radiation or parenteral methotrexate: A prospective study. *Journal of Clinical Oncology, 9,* 145-151.

121. Packer, R. J., Rorke, L. B., Lange, B. J., et al. (1985). Cerebrovascular accidents in children with cancer. *Pediatrics, 76,* 194-201.

122. Pai, V., & Nahata, M., (2000). Cardiotoxicity of chemotherapeutic agents: Incidence, treatment, and prevention. *Drug Safety, 22,* 263-302.

123. Perazella, M. A. (1999). Crystal-induced acute renal failure. *American Journal of Medicine, 106,* 459-465.

124. Peterson, D. E. (1999). Research advances in oral mucositis. *Current Opinion in Oncology, 11,* 261-266.

125. Pieters, R. (1997). Side effects of radiation therapy in children and their preventive management. In A. R. Ablin (Ed.), *Supportive care of the child with cancer* (2nd ed., pp. 118-143). Baltimore: Johns Hopkins University Press.

126. Pietsch, J. B., Ford, C., & Whitlock, J. A. (1999). Nasogastric tube feedings in children with high-risk cancer: A pilot study. *Journal of Pediatric Hematology/Oncology, 21,* 111-114.

127. Pietzak, M. & Thomas, D. (2000). Pancreatitis in childhood. *Pediatrics in Review, 21,* 406-412.

128. Pinkerton, C. R. (1992). Experience with granisetron in children. *Proceedings of the 17th European Society of Medical Oncology (EMSO),* 20-23.

129. Plevova, P. (1999). Prevention and treatment of chemotherapy- and radiotherapy-induced oral mucositis: A review. *Oral Oncology, 35,* 453-470.

130. Plowman, P. N. (1983). The effects of conventionally fractionated, extended portal radiotherapy on the human peripheral blood count. *International Journal of Radiation Oncology Biology Physics, 9,* 829-839.

131. Raber-Durlacher, J. E. (1999). Current practices for management of oral mucositis in cancer patients. *Supportive Care in Cancer, 7,* 71-74.

132. Raber-Durlacher, J. E., Weijl, N. I., Abu Saris, M., et al. (2000). Oral mucositis in patients treated with chemotherapy for solid tumors: A retrospective analysis of 150 cases. *Supportive Care in Cancer, 8,* 366-371.

133. Ransier, A., Epstein, J. B., Lunn, R., et al. (1995). A combined analysis of a toothbrush, foam brush, and a chlorhexidine-soaked foam brush in maintaining oral hygiene. *Cancer Nursing, 18,* 393-396.

134. Rebulla, P., Finazzi, G., Marangoni, F., et al. (1997). The threshold for prophylactic platelet transfusions in adults with acute myeloid leukemia. *New England Journal of Medicine, 337,* 1870-1875.

135. Redding, S. W. (1990). Role of herpes simplex virus reactivation in chemotherapy induced oral mucositis. *NCI Monograph, 9,* 103-105.

136. Richardson, A., Ream, E., & Wilson-Barnett, J. (1998). Fatigue in patients receiving chemotherapy: Patterns of change. *Cancer Nursing, 21,* 17-29.

137. Rickard, K. A., Grosfeld, J. L., Kirksy, A., et al. (1979). Reversal of protein-energy malnutrition in children during treatment of advanced neoplastic disease. *Annals of Surgery, 190,* 771-781.

138. Robison, L. L., Nesbit, M. E., Sather, H. N., et al. (1984). Factors associated with IQ scores in long term survivors of childhood acute lymphoblastic leukemia. *American Journal of Pediatric Hematology/Oncology, 6,* 115-121.

139. Ruff, P., Paska, W., Pouillart, P., et al. (1994). Ondansetron compared with granisetron in the prophylaxis of cisplatin-induced emesis: A multicentre double-blind, randomized, parallel-group study. *Oncology, 51,* 113-118.

140. Rutledge, D., & Engelking, C. (1998) Cancer related diarrhea: Selected findings of a national survey of oncology nurse experience. *Oncology Nursing Forum, 25,* 861-872.

141. Saborio, P., Tipton, G., & Chan, J., (2000). Diabetes insipidus. *Pediatrics in Review, 21,* 122-129.

142. Sacks, N., & Meek, R. S. (1997). Nutritional support. In A. R. Ablin (Ed.), *Supportive care of children with cancer* (2nd ed., pp. 193-209). Baltimore: Johns Hopkins University Press.

143. Schiffer, C. A., Anderson, K. C., Bennett, C. L., et al. (2001). Platelet transfusion for patients with cancer: Clinical practice guidelines of the American Society of Clinical Oncology. *Journal of Clinical Oncology, 19,* 1519-1538.

144. Schubert, M. M., Williams, B. E., Lloid, M. E., et al. (1992). Clinical assessment scale for the rating of oral mucosal changes associated with bone marrow transplantation. *Cancer, 69,* 2469-2477.

145. Seidel, H., Ball, J., Dains, J. E., et al. (1999). The musculoskeletal system. In J. Thompson (Ed.), *Mosby's guide to physical examination* (4th ed., pp. 706-710). St. Louis, MO: Mosby.

146. Seidel, H., Ball, J., Dains, J. E., et al. (1999) The neurologic system. In J. Thompson (Ed.), *Mosby's guide to physical examination* (4th ed., pp. 755-761). St. Louis, MO: Mosby.

147. Seidel, H., Ball, J., Dains, J. E., et al. (1999). Skin, hair, and nails. In J. Thompson (Ed.), *Mosby's guide to physical examination* (4th ed., pp. 161-163). St. Louis, MO: Mosby.

148. Seyaeve, C., Schuller, J., Buser, K., et al. (1992). Comparison of the anti-emetic efficacy of different doses of ondansetron, given as either a continuous infusion or a single intravenous dose, in acute cisplatin-induced emesis: A multicentre, double-blind, randomized, parallel study group. *British Journal of Cancer, 66,* 192-197.

149. Shils, M. (1994). Nutrition and diet in cancer management. In M. Shils, J. A. Olson, & M. Shike (Eds.), *Modern nutrition in health and disease* (8th ed., pp. 1317-1348). Philadelphia: Lea & Febiger.

150. Shlafer, M. (1993). *The nurse pharmacology and drug therapy: A prototype approach* (2nd ed.). Redwood City, CA: Addison-Wesley.

151. Shuey, K. (1994). Heart, lung and endocrine complications of solid tumors. *Seminars in Oncology Nursing, 10,* 177-188.

152. Sklar, C. (1997). Growth and neuroendocrine dysfunction following therapy for childhood cancer. *Pediatric Clinics of North America, 44,* 489-499.

153. Sklar, C. A., & LaQuaglia, M. P. (2000). The long-term complications of chemotherapy in childhood genitourinary tumors. *Urologic Clinics of North America, 27,* 563-568.

154. Skubitz, K. M., & Anderson, P. M. (1996). Oral glutamine to prevent chemotherapy induced stomatitis: A pilot study. *Journal of Laboratory Clinical Medicine, 127,* 223-228.

155. Slichter, S. J. (1995). Principles of platelet transfusion therapy. In R. Hoffman, E. J. Benz, Jr., S. J. Shattil, et al. (Eds.), *Hematology: Basic principles and practice* (2nd ed., pp. 1987-2006). New York: Churchill Livingstone.

156. Small, B. E., Holdsworth, M. T., Raisch, D. W., et al. (2000). Survey ranking of emetogenic control in children receiving chemotherapy. *Journal of Pediatric Hematology/Oncology, 22,* 125-132.

157. Smeltzer, S., & Bare, B. (Eds.). (1996). *Brunner and Suddarth's textbook of medical-surgical nursing* (8th ed.). Philadelphia: Lippincott-Raven.

158. SmithKline Beecham. Product insert for granisetron.

159. Sonis, A. L., & Sonis, S. T. (1979). Oral complications of cancer chemotherapy in pediatric patients. *Journal of Pedodontistry, 3,* 122-128.

160. Sonis, S. T. (1992). Oral complications of cancer therapy. In V. T. Devita, S. Hellman, & S. A. Rosenberg (Eds.), *Cancer: Principles and practice of oncology* (3rd ed., pp. 2144-2152). Philadelphia: JB Lippincott.

161. Sonis, S. T., Eilers, J. P., Epstein, J. B. (1999). Validation of a new scoring system for the assessment of a clinical trial research of oral mucositis induced by radiation or chemotherapy. *Cancer, 85,* 2103-2113.

162. Speyer, J., Green, M., Zeleniuch-Jacquotte, A., et al. (1992). ICRF-187 permits longer treatment with doxorubicin in women with breast cancer. *Journal of Clinical Oncology, 10,* 117-127.

163. Spivak, J. L. (1994). Recombinant human erythropoietin and the anemia of cancer. *Blood, 84,* 997-1004.

164. Steinherz, L., Graham, T., Hurwitz, R. et al. (1992). Guidelines for cardiac monitoring of children during and after anthracycline therapy: Report of the Cardiology Committee of the Children's Cancer Study Group. *Pediatrics, 89,* 942-949.

165. Stiakaki, E., Savvas, S., Lydaki, E., et al. (1999). Ondansetron and tropisetron in the control of nausea and vomiting in children receiving combined chemotherapy. *Pediatric Hematology & Oncology, 16,* 101-108.

166. Sylvester, R. K., Etzell, P., Levitt, R., et al. (1996). Comparison of 16 mg vs 32 mg ondansetron and dexamethasone in patients receiving cisplatin. *Proceedings of the American Society of Clinical Oncology, 15,* 547.

167. Tisdale, M. J. (1992). Cancer cachexia. *British Journal of Cancer, 63,* 337-342.

168. Tsuchida, Y., Hayashi, Y., Asami, K, et al. (1999). Effects of granisetron in children undergoing high-dose chemotherapy: A multi-institutional, cross-over study. *International Journal of Oncology, 14,* 673-679.

169. Tyc, V. L., Mulhern, R. K., Barclay, D. R., et al. (1997). Variables associated with anticipatory nausea and vomiting in pediatric cancer patients receiving ondansetron antiemetic therapy. *Journal of Pediatric Psychology, 22,* 45-58.

170. Tyc, V. L., Vallelunga, L., Mahoney, S., et al. (1995). Nutritional and treatment related characteristics of pediatric oncology patients referred or not referred for nutritional support. *Medical and Pediatric Oncology, 25,* 379-388.

171. Ulshen, M. H. (2001). Diarrhea and steatorrhea. In R. A. Hoekelman, H. M. Adam, N. M. Nelson, et al. (Eds.), *Primary pediatric care* (4th ed., pp. 1020-1033). St. Louis, MO: Mosby.

172. Van Hoff, J. (1996). Antiemetics. In A. K. Ritchey (Ed.), *The Pediatric Oncology Group supportive care manual* (pp. III-1–III-10). Chicago: The Pediatric Oncology Group.

173. Van Hoff, J., & Olszewski, D. (1988). Lorazepam for the control of chemotherapy-related nausea and vomiting in children. *Journal of Pediatrics, 113,* 146-149.

174. Vietti, T. J. (1991). Cellular kinetics and cancer chemotherapy. In D. J. Fernbach & T. J. Vietti (Eds.), *Clinical pediatric oncology* (4th ed., pp. 173-212). St. Louis, MO: Mosby.

175. Wadle, K. (1990). Diarrhea. *Symptom Management, 25,* 901-908.

176. Wadler, S., Benson III, A. B., Engelking, C., et al. (1998). Recommended guidelines for the treatment of chemotherapy induced diarrhea. *Journal of Clinical Oncology, 16,* 3169-3178.

177. Weisdorf, D. J., Bosttrom, B., Raether, D., et al. (1989). Oropharyngeal mucositis complicating bone marrow transplantation: Prognostic factors and the effect of chlorhexidine mouth rinse. *Bone Marrow Transplantation, 4,* 89-95.

178. Western Consortium for Cancer Nursing Research. (1991). Development of a staging system for chemotherapy-induced stomatitis. *Cancer Nursing, 14,* 6-12.

179. Wexler, L., Andrich, M., Venzon, D., et al. (1996). Randomized trial of the cardioprotective agent ICRF-187 in pediatric sarcoma patients treated with doxorubicin. *Journal of Clinical Oncology, 14,* 362-372.

180. White, L., McKenna, C. J., Zhestkova, N., et al. (1998). A comparison of oral ondansetron syrup and intravenous ondansetron (OND) regimens given in combination with oral dexamethasone (DEX) for the prevention of emesis and nausea in paediatric patients receiving moderately/highly emetogenic chemotherapy. *Proceedings of the American Society of Clinical Oncology, 17,* 193.

181. Winningham, M. L., Nail, L. M., Burke, M. B., et al. (1994). Fatigue and the cancer experience: The state of the knowledge. *Oncology Nursing Forum, 21,* 23-36.

182. Yim, Y. S., Mahoney, Jr., D. H., & Oshman, D. G. (1990). Hemiparesis and ischemic changes of the white matter after intrathecal therapy for children with acute lymphocytic leukemia. *Cancer, 67,* 2058-2061.

12

Treatment of Pain

Sandy Sentivany-Collins

OVERVIEW OF PEDIATRIC PAIN MANAGEMENT

All children with cancer experience pain, and 70% experience severe pain.[33] Although the knowledge and resources exist for the safe, effective relief of pain, children's pain is often inadequately managed.[7,29]

Pain is a primary concern of families and children who are diagnosed with cancer.[11] Pain is often named by children as the most frightening part of hospitalization. Pediatric oncology patients become fearful of experiences or procedures that cause pain and can lose trust of hospitals and medical personnel. Children can become irritable, anxious, and restless in response to pain. They sometimes experience nightmares, as well as eating or sleeping problems. Children whose pain is poorly treated or untreated may feel victimized, depressed, isolated, lonely, or guilty, compromising their ability to tolerate cancer treatment.[31] Some children believe that pain is punishment for some real or imagined transgression.[20] Pediatric oncology patients report that they fear pain more than their diagnoses or anything else about their hospitalizations.[9,10,18]

Parents and family members of a child experiencing unrelieved pain can become angry and distrustful of the medical system. They may feel depressed, guilty, vulnerable, or powerless because they are not able to prevent their child's suffering.[33]

DEFINITION OF PAIN

Pain is a subjective experience. The American Pain Society defines pain as "an unpleasant sensory and emotional experience associated with actual or potential tissue damage, or described in terms of such damage."[23] This definition delineates two important points. First, a child's report of pain reflects sensory experience and affective and cognitive responses. It is essential for the nurse to consider how cognition and psychosocial factors precipitate or sustain pain and concurrently to assess the potential impact of pain on physical and psychosocial

functioning. Second, the relationship between the experience of pain and tissue damage is neither uniform nor constant.[25] Margo McCaffery's definition is "Pain is whatever the experiencing person says it is, existing whenever he says it does."[19] Objective observations such as vital sign changes, grimacing, and crying are only sometimes helpful in assessing pain. These signs are often absent in patients with pain, especially those with chronic pain.[3] Although physiologic changes associated with the stress response often accompany painful experiences, they may be equivocal in demonstrating the presence or absence of pain. A child may experience severe pain without elevated blood pressure, tachycardia, tachypnea, or palmar sweating. Conversely, those physiologic responses may indicate something other than pain, such as fear. The most reliable way of assessing a patient's pain is listening to and acknowledging the child's self-report, the single most reliable indicator of pain.[2]

Acute and chronic pain. Acute pain is defined as a pain of relatively brief duration, usually caused by a well-defined stimulus, which subsides as healing occurs. This type of pain is a primitive protective response, which may result from any acute injury such as surgery, trauma, or fractures. Acute pain is often, but not always, associated with signs of autonomic arousal, including tachycardia, hypertension, dilated pupils, and palmar sweating.[4] This physiologic stress response is generally short-lived, frequently inconsistent, and not necessarily specific to pain.

Chronic pain is not protective. It persists long beyond the initial protective function and is described as lasting 3 to 6 months or longer.[16] Chronic pain often involves long-term changes in the nervous system, including spinal "memory" for pain and molecular changes that establish a memory tracing of an injury.[22] The autonomic response seen with acute pain is often not present in children with chronic pain, even in those with known structural lesions. The child's body adapts to the stress of pain and regains a state of homeostasis. As a result, physiologic indicators, especially in children with chronic pain, are seldom helpful in assessing the existence and intensity of pain.

Cancer pain may be acute, chronic, or intermittent. It generally has an identifiable cause related to a tumor or treatment. Unlike acute cancer pain, chronic cancer pain is rarely accompanied by signs of sympathetic nervous system arousal. This lack of objective clinical signs does not necessarily indicate an absence of pain.

Nociceptive and neuropathic pain. Children experience either nociceptive or neuropathic pain. Nociceptive and neuropathic pain differ in their etiology, symptoms, and response to analgesics. They often coexist, confusing diagnosis and treatment recommendations.

Nociceptive pain results from activation of nociceptive afferent nerves in somatic or visceral structures that have been damaged. Nociceptive somatic pain is usually a consequence of direct tumor involvement caused by damage to muscle, joint, bone, or cutaneous tissues. It is often described as dull, throbbing, aching, or pressurelike pain in well-defined locations. Nociceptive visceral pain, which is often poorly localized, is a result of stretching, distention, or obstruction of thoracic or abdominal structures, causing intermittent cramping. In general, somatic and visceral pain can be well managed with cancer treatment and/or conventional analgesics such as nonsteroidal antiinflammatory drugs (NSAIDs) and opioids.

Neuropathic pain is associated with abnormal processing of sensory input by the central or peripheral nervous system. It is generally described as being like "pins and needles" or as sharp, burning, stabbing, electrical, or shooting. Response to conventional analgesics is usually poor, but anticonvulsants, antidepressants, oral and cutaneous local anesthetics, corticosteroids, clonidine, benzodiazepines, neuroleptics, and nondrug therapies are often quite helpful.[31]

TYPES OF PAIN IN CHILDREN WITH CANCER

Children with cancer experience pain caused by the disease itself, treatments, invasive diagnostic and therapeutic procedures and interventions and incidental pain from unrelated causes, as listed in Box 12-1.[33]

BOX 12-1

SOURCES OF CANCER PAIN IN CHILDREN

DISEASE RELATED
Bone (primary or metastatic); bone marrow
Central nervous system
Neuropathic
Somatic or visceral

TREATMENT RELATED
Chemotherapy
   Mucositis (multiple agents)
   Peripheral neuropathies (vinca alkaloids, cisplatin)
   Aseptic bone necrosis (corticosteroids)
   Myalgias or arthralgias (corticosteroids)
   Extravasation injuries (vinca alkaloids, anthraclines)
   Bone pain (vinca alkaloids, filgrastim)
   Typhlitis
   Pancreatitis
   Constipation or bowel obstruction
Radiation therapy
   Mucositis
   Radiation dermatitis
   Myelopathy
   Radiation fibrosis
   Osteoradionecrosis
   Radiation-induced peripheral nerve tumors
   Radiation burns
Surgery
   Acute postoperative

Postthoracotomy syndrome (numbness or neuropathic pain that can occur after thoracic surgeries)
   After amputation; stump and/or phantom pain
Infection
Graft-versus-host disease

PROCEDURE RELATED
Mildly invasive
   Finger stick
   Venipuncture
   Intravenous (IV) cannulation
   Implanted central venous device
   Venous access device removal
   Tape or dressing removal
   Suture removal
Moderately or severely invasive
   Bone marrow aspiration
   Bone marrow biopsy
   Lumbar puncture (LP)
   LP-related headache or backache

UNRELATED
Preexisting
   Migraine
Trauma
   Fractures
   Lacerations

Disease-related pain can be acute or chronic and is generally caused by direct invasion of anatomic structures, by pressure on or entrapment of nerves, or by obstruction. Malignancies, such as leukemia, lymphoma, and neuroblastoma, can cause diffuse bone and joint pain.[33]

Treatment- and procedure-related pain can be a direct result of interventions, such as lumbar punctures, bone marrow aspirations, venipunctures, or surgical procedures, or a side effect of treatments, such as radiation therapy, chemotherapy, and other medications.[33] Many children consider treatment-related pain the most difficult part of their disease experience, generally intensifying with repeated interventions.[15]

The primary goal of procedure-related pain control is to complete the procedure with adequate pain management for the child. Other goals include eliminating the fear and anxiety related to the procedure, facilitating the child's cooperation during the procedure, and promoting a prompt, safe recovery.[20] To facilitate these goals, the child must understand the procedure and the pain management plan, presented in a developmentally appropriate manner. Numerous pharmacologic and nonpharmacologic or cognitive-behavioral pain management techniques are available (Table 12-1), which are discussed in more detail later.

UNDERTREATMENT OF PAIN IN CHILDREN

An inadequate understanding of the current scientific information on pain and treatment, in addition to unfounded fears and misunderstandings, has led to ineffective pain management for children. These problems include the following:
- Insufficient knowledge about pain and treatment
- Prevalence of numerous myths about pain:
    The nervous systems of babies and young children are immature, so they do not "feel" pain the same as older children and adults do.
    If children are distractible (e.g., watching TV, reading, or talking on the telephone), they must not be in pain.
    Starting opioid pain medications too early means nothing will work if pain gets worse.
    Drug addiction is a common problem.
- Widespread lack of recognition that established methods already exist for satisfactory management of most cancer pain in children
- Inadequate understanding of the physiologic and psychologic consequences of untreated or poorly treated pain
- Misunderstanding of the pharmacokinetics and pharmacodynamics of opioid analgesics in children
- Inappropriate concern or inadequate knowledge about analgesic side effects

- Exaggerated concern over respiratory depression
- Lack of information about simple behavioral, cognitive, and supportive techniques that can be employed by children and families to decrease pain experiences
- Poor pain assessment
- Lack of understanding of the nature of children's perceptions of pain and illness
- Low priority given by physicians and nurses to pain treatment
- Inadequate reimbursement
- Restrictive regulation of controlled substances

Traditionally the use of opioid medication was discouraged because of fear of opioid addiction. Psychologic addiction is uncommon in children, occurring in less than 1% of all patients who are prescribed opioids in a controlled setting.[26,34] Tolerance and physiologic dependence, the normal, predictable consequences of long-term opioid use, are often confused with addiction (psychologic dependence).

Addiction is an acquired, chronic disease that is characterized by a persistent pattern of dysfunctional drug use for nonmedical reasons, aberrant behavior involving loss of control over drug use, and continued drug use despite adverse physiologic, psychologic, and/or social consequences.

Tolerance refers to the need for an increasing amount of a medication to achieve the same analgesic effect as the original dose. This is a normal neuroadaptive response to long-term opioid administration and must be anticipated when patients are taking opioids regularly for a prolonged period of time. The initial indication of tolerance is generally a decrease in the duration of effect. Increasing the dose, occasionally to very high levels, or switching to an alternate opioid, usually at less than an equianalgesic dose, may be needed to maintain analgesia. Tolerance does not cause addiction, nor does its presence imply addiction.[20]

Physiologic dependence refers to an altered neuroadaptive state manifested by the development of opioid withdrawal symptoms when opioids are abruptly discontinued. Like tolerance, this is a normal physiologic response. Physiologic dependence must be anticipated in patients who have been on opioids for approximately a week. To avoid withdrawal, the opioid dose is reduced slowly.

Opioid "pseudoaddiction" refers to a common iatrogenic syndrome in which patients develop certain behavioral characteristics of psychologic dependence as a consequence of inadequate pain treatment. This may occur as a result of PRN dosing during periods of continuous pain, the use of dosing intervals that are greater than the duration of action of a given analgesic, or the use of insuffi-

TABLE 12-1   PROCEDURAL PAIN MANAGEMENT INTERVENTIONS

Method	Route	Indications	Comments
PHARMACOLOGIC INTERVENTIONS			
Local anesthetics	Topical, local infiltration, intradermal, subcutaneous (SQ)	Venipuncture, suturing, bone marrow aspiration, thoracentesis	Simple, inexpensive, relatively safe
TAC (tetracaine, epinepherine [adrenaline], cocaine), LET (lidocaine, epinepherine, tetracaine)	Topical	Wound cleaning	Superficial anesthesia only
EMLA, ELA-Max	Topical	Venous, arterial, lumbar, finger, heel punctures, implanted port access, peripheral insertion of central catheters, removal of sutures, staples, cardiac catheterization lines, epicardial wires, superficial biopsies, skin grafts, intramuscular (IM) and SQ injections	Application at least 60 min before procedure required for EMLA, 20 min for ELA-Max
Iontophoresis "Numby Stuff"	Transdermal	Intravenous (IV) catheter insertions, IM and SQ injections, implantable port needle insertion	Occasionally young children frightened by sensation of the current; occasionally "burns" under Numby Stuff; onset in 10-15 min, but duration only 20-30 min
Opioids	IV (preferred), by mouth (PO), oral transmucosal, SQ, IM, per rectum (PR), epidural, intrathecal	Any	Monitoring of respiratory and sedation status necessary; may need to decrease opioid dose if benzodiazepines used
Benzodiazepines	IV, IM, PO, PR	Any requiring diminishment of skeletal muscle spasm or anxiety, or amnesia	No analgesic properties
Ketamine	IV, IM, PO	Any	Safely provides profound pain relief at subanesthetic doses; patient may experience dissociative state; agitation upon awakening possible in younger children
Propofol	IV	Any, as adjuvant to opioids	No analgesic properties; quick recovery, minimal respiratory depression when properly titrated
NONPHARMACOLOGIC OR COGNITIVE-BEHAVIORAL INTERVENTIONS			
Distraction		Any awake procedure	Variety of distraction techniques
Imagery		Any awake procedure	
Relaxation		Any awake procedure	May involve breathing, progressive muscle relaxation
Music		Any	May be used as relaxation and/or distraction; best if patient chooses music
Application of cold		Procedures that involve localized pain and/or inflammation	Application of cold pack before and after procedure

Adapted from McCaffery, M., & Pasero, C. (1999). *Pain: Clinical manual* (2nd ed.). St. Louis, MO: Mosby.

ciently potent analgesics. Patients with this syndrome must continually demonstrate their need for analgesics and are often described as difficult patients, chronic complainers, or "addicts."[31]

CONSEQUENCES OF UNTREATED OR POORLY TREATED PAIN

Pain triggers a physiologic stress response that activates the sympathetic nervous system, alerting the body to imminent or existing harm. This response causes adverse endocrine, immunologic, and metabolic changes in the body. Pain can precipitate compromise of the cardiovascular, endocrine, gastrointestinal, genitourinary, metabolic, musculoskeletal, respiratory, and immune systems.[5] The longer pain goes untreated or poorly treated, the more difficult it is to manage and the longer lasting the effects. Weinstein and Tripp reported that brief or sustained noxious stimuli can produce adverse changes within the cells of the spinal cord, which allows pain responses to be prolonged or persistent. Suppression of established pain is thus more difficult to treat, requiring increased doses of opioids for prolonged periods of time.[30] Untreated or poorly treated pain can cause significant changes in quality of life, including changes in eating and sleeping habits, alterations in self-concept, fear, anxiety, depression, and hopelessness.[20]

ASSESSMENT

Cancer pain is a complex mix of physical, emotional, and psychologic experiences that are distressing for children. Many factors, including tissue damage, developmental age, gender, culture, previous experiences with pain, familial experiences with and responses to pain, emotional and cognitive state, personality traits, and the child's fears and concerns about illness and death contribute to the child's experience of pain and suffering. Anxiety, fear, depression, and a sense of hopelessness influence a child's perception of pain. Therefore assessment includes exploration of physical, psychologic, spiritual, interpersonal, social, and financial considerations that contribute to a patient's "total pain" experience. No objective measure of pain exists. The pain experience is always subjective, and pain can never be proved or disproved. A child's report of pain must always be believed, and all reports of pain are to be taken seriously.[20] Appropriate pain management consists of a thorough assessment of the sensory characteristics of the pain (location, quality, intensity, duration), aggravating or relieving factors, cognitive response to pain, and the patient's goal for pain management.

If a child is too young, developmentally delayed, or critically ill to use a self-report method of communicating pain, validated observational tools can be used to assess pain.[12] These tools assess children's manifestations of pain such as facial expressions, body posture or guarding, vocalizations, and motor responses. One such tool, the FLACC, is valid for use in children 2 months to 7 years of age.[21] These observational tools should not act as a substitute for any child capable of using self-report measures.

Numerous tools exist for the assessment of pain in children. It is important that the scale be appropriate for the child's developmental age, that it be used consistently, and that it be introduced before the child experiences severe pain. Some of the tools recommended for use in children are listed in Table 12-2. Although the opinion of the nurse or the parent is helpful in assessing pain, many studies have demonstrated that they are often not consistent with the child's report of pain.[8,20,27]

The U.S. Department of Health and Human Services Agency for Health Care Policy and Research recommends the following clinical approach for the assessment and management of pain:

A   *Ask* about pain regularly, and *Assess* patient systematically.

B   *Believe* patient and family in their reports of pain and what relieves it.

C   *Choose* pain control options appropriate for patient, family, and setting.

D   *Deliver* interventions in a timely, logical, and coordinated fashion.

E   *Empower* patients and their families, and *Enable* patients to control their course to the greatest extent possible.[7]

Assessment of pain in infants is particularly challenging because of the subjectivity and complexity of the pain experience, the cognitive and language limitations that preclude comprehension and self-report, the variability and inconsistency of pain expression, and the dependence on others to infer the presence and intensity of pain from behavioral and physiologic indicators.[20] Some pain assessment tools for neonates are indicated in Table 12-3.

MANAGEMENT

Effective pain management is best achieved by a team approach involving patients, families, and various health care providers. The pain treatment plan must address the individual child and family, his or her diagnosis, the stage of disease, previous responses to pain and interventions, and personal preferences.[7]

TABLE 12-2	PEDIATRIC PAIN ASSESSMENT TOOLS USING SELF-REPORT	
Measure	**Description**	**Indication for Use**
Wong-Baker faces scale	Cartoon faces indicate intensity of pain.	3-8 yr
Oucher*	Photos of children's faces indicate intensity of pain. Children are asked to point to the face that represents the amount of pain they are experiencing. It is available featuring children with several racial backgrounds. A 100-point corresponding vertical scale may be used with older children.	3-12 yr
Poker chip tool†	Child chooses 1-4 chips to represent "pieces of hurt." One chip represents "a little hurt," four chips represent "as much hurt as you could ever have."	4-13 yr
Color tool‡	Children rank eight crayons to represent different pain intensity then use those colors to draw on a body outline the location and amount of their pain.	4-10 yr
Numeric rating scale	Child chooses number between 1 and 10 (or 1 and 100) to represent intensity of pain.	7 yr and older

Adapted from McCaffery, M., & Pasero, C. (1999). *Pain clinical manual* (2nd ed.). St. Louis, MO: Mosby.
*Beyer, J. E., & Wells, N. (1989). The assessment of pain in children. *Pediatric Clinics of North America, 36,* 837-854.
†Hester, N. K. (1979). The preoperational child's reaction to immunization. *Nursing Research, 28,* 250-255.
‡Eland, J. (1981). Minimizing pain associated with prekindergarten intramuscular injections. *Issues in Comprehensive Nursing, 5,* 361-372.

TABLE 12-3	NEONATAL PAIN ASSESSMENT TOOLS	
Measure	**Description**	**Indications for Use**
CRIES	Five physiologic and behavioral indicators to measure intensity of pain in infants; acronym for *C*rying, *R*equires O_2 for saturation >95%, *I*ncreased vital signs (heart rate and blood pressure), *E*xpression, *S*leeplessness	Postoperative neonates
PIPPS	A seven-indicator measure that includes physiologic, behavioral, and contextual indicators	Preterm and term neonates

Data from Krechel, S. W., & Bildner, J. (1995). CRIES: A new neonatal postoperative pain measurement score—Initial testing of validity and reliability. *Pediatric Anesthesiology, 5,* 53-61; Stevens, B., Johnston, C. C., & Petryshen, P. (1996). Premature infant pain profile: Development and initial valildation. *Clinical Journal of Pain, 12,* 13-22.

Generally a multimodal approach, using a combination of nonpharmacologic, cognitive-behavioral, pharmacologic, and other pain therapies best addresses the complex pain often experienced by pediatric oncology patients (Table 12-4). Early intervention can limit the negative effects of pain, preventing or reducing the hyperexcitability responses or memory of pain, and can reduce the total amount of medication necessary to treat pain.[12]

Primary interventions directed to the cause of the pain can significantly affect analgesia. Radiotherapy, surgical removal of tumors, and some chemotherapeutic drugs may provide pain relief (Table 12-5).

PHARMACOLOGIC INTERVENTIONS

Analgesic medications are the mainstay for the management of acute and chronic cancer pain. The three general categories of analgesic medications are NSAIDs and acetaminophen, opioids, and analgesic adjuvants.

NSAIDs and acetaminophen. Acetaminophen and NSAIDs are nonopioids. They are useful analgesics for acute or chronic, mild to moderate pain of various causes.[4] These analgesics may be used alone or in combination with one another. However, the simultaneous use of more than one NSAID is not recommended because of the increased risk of toxicity without the benefit of additional analgesia. Acetaminophen and NSAIDs have an analgesic ceiling. Doses higher than the "ceiling" do not provide additional analgesia but increase the risk of dose-related side effects and toxicity. Nonopioids are used for nociceptive and neuropathic pain. They are particularly effective

TABLE 12-4	GENERAL PRINCIPLES OF PAIN MANAGEMENT	
Principle	**Nursing Considerations**
Determine analgesic dose on individual basis.	Effective dose of analgesic medication varies considerably from individual to individual. "Correct" dose of analgesic is the one that gives an acceptable level of pain relief to patient for reasonable amount of time, with minimal or no adverse effects. Opioids have no "analgesic ceiling," so dose can be increased to whatever is required to achieve adequate pain control without unacceptable side effects. Initial choice and dose of medication is based on patient's report of pain.
For pain that is present most of the day, administer analgesics around-the-clock (ATC) rather than on PRN basis.	Around-the-clock pain requires around-the-clock analgesia. If only PRN medications are available, it may take several hours and higher doses of opioids to achieve pain relief. This practice often leads to a cycle of undermedication and pain alternating with overmedication and drug toxicity.
Anticipate and aggressively treat analgesic side effects.	Constipation, nausea, vomiting, and pruritis are common side effects of opioids that must be anticipated, monitored, and treated appropriately. Clinically significant opioid-induced respiratory depression is uncommon, especially in children who chronically receive opioids.
Do not use placebos to determine if pain is "real."	Use of placebos does not yield any helpful information for health care professionals. Use of placebos most often instills mistrust between patients and caregivers. Deceptive use of placebos and misinterpretation of placebos response discredit patient's pain report, are unethical, and should be avoided. Do not administer placebos in these circumstances even if there is a medical order.

Data from McCaffery, M., & Pasero, C. (1999). *Pain: Clinical manual* (2nd ed.). St. Louis, MO: Mosby; Rushton, C. H. (1995). Placebo pain medication: Ethical and legal issues. *Pediatric Nursing, 21,* 166-168.

TABLE 12-5	PAIN MANAGEMENT INTERVENTIONS FOR CHILDREN WITH CANCER			
Anticancer Treatments	**Analgesic Medications**	**Noninvasive Techniques**	**Neurosurgical Interventions**	**Regional Nerve Blocks**
Radiotherapy	NSAIDs	Transcutaneous	Dorsal rhizotomy	Peripheral
Chemotherapy	Acetaminophen	electrical nerve	Cordotomy	Epidural
Biologic therapy	Opioids	stimulation (TENS)	Myelotomy	Intrathecal
Surgery	Adjuvants	Physical therapy		
Hematopoietic		Hypnosis or imagery		
stem cell		Relaxation		
transplant		Biofeedback		
		Acupuncture		
		Therapeutic touch		
		Counseling		

with somatic pain such as muscle and joint pain. Acetaminophen and/or NSAIDs are often used in combination with opioids.

Acetaminophen is not an NSAID. It has analgesic and antipyretic potency, relatively few antiinflammatory effects, and no antiplatelet effects. Hepatic toxicity may occur in patients with a history of alcohol abuse or following ingestion of large doses.[31]

NSAIDs have analgesic, antipyretic, and antiinflammatory properties. Potential side effects of conventional NSAIDs include prolongation of bleeding time, gastrointestinal irritation, and renal insufficiency. The antipyretic and antiplatelet effects limit their use in patients with neutropenia or thrombocytopenia. Side effects from NSAIDs or acetaminophen can occur at any time, so patients taking these medications regularly should be monitored carefully. Of the NSAIDs, choline magnesium trisalicylate (Trilisate) has the least effect on platelet aggregation.[35] NSAIDs, especially in combination with opioids, may be particularly useful in treating moderate to severe pain.[31] NSAIDs have an opioid dose-sparing effect that helps reduce opioid side effects when given in conjunction with opioids. NSAIDs differ from one another in their analgesic effects. If a patient does not experience pain relief with one NSAID at a therapeutic dose, an alternative NSAID may be considered. Currently only ketorolac (Toradol) is available in the United States for parenteral use.

NSAIDs relieve pain by blocking production of cyclooxygenase (COX) which is an enzyme that contributes to the production of prostaglandins. Some prostaglandins help protect the body, whereas others contribute to pain and inflammation. COX-1 is released by gastric mucosa and has an important role in protection of the digestive system from its own erosive acids. COX-2 is more closely associated with prostaglandins that contribute to pain and inflammation. COX-2 inhibitors, such as celecoxib (Celebrex) and rofecoxib (Vioxx), have analgesic effects similar to traditional NSAIDs; however, they inhibit COX-2 without interfering with COX-1, thereby decreasing the potential for gastrointestinal complications such as bleeding ulcers.[13,17]

Opioids.   Opioids are the mainstay of pain management for moderate to severe pain and are safe and effective.[1] Opioids do not have an analgesic ceiling. There is no predetermined maximum or ideal opioid dose for any given patient. The appropriate dose is the one that provides optimal analgesia with minimal or no side effects. Although nurses may be reluctant to administer high doses of opioids to patients with advanced disease because of fear of side effects, the clinician's ethical duty—to benefit the patient by relieving pain—supports appropriately increasing opioid doses to achieve analgesia, even at the risk of significant side effects.[7] All opioids share similar side effects (Table 12-6).

For continuous pain, analgesics should be administered on a regular, around-the-clock (ATC) schedule to prevent loss of therapeutic serum levels between doses. PRN dosing often leads to inadequate analgesia with periods of pain and subtherapeutic drug levels alternating with periods of high drug levels and side effects. It is more appropriate to prevent pain or keep it in check, than to play "catch-up" with escalating pain.

Dose titration may be necessary because of the natural progression of the disease and/or the development of tolerance. If a child experiences dose-limiting side effects with one opioid, other opioids may be tried. As patients develop tolerance to the analgesic effects of an opioid, they also develop tolerance to the side effects, and they require more frequent dosing. Opioid dosing can be titrated up or down by 25% to 50% of the previous dose.

In general, opioid side effects can be treated in several ways. The dosing regimen or route can be changed to achieve relatively constant blood levels rather than high peak serum levels, which often cause side effects. Switching to a different opioid may be helpful. In general, all strong opioids have similar potential side effects at equianalgesic doses (Table 12-7). However, clinical experience demonstrates that individuals may have a different side-effect response to different opioids. A final option would be to add another drug to counteract the adverse effect.

Routes.   The drug, dose, and route of administration are individualized to each patient. Although the oral route is the easiest and least invasive route, it is not always possible or practical. Children may be unable or unwilling to take oral medications. Rectal administration is typically contraindicated in the neutropenic or thrombocytopenic cancer patient. The onset of action of orally or rectally administered medications may be too slow. Most opioids are available in many forms for various routes.

- Oral: This route is recommended for chronic treatment because of convenience, flexibility, and cost-effectiveness. Peak drug effect occurs 1½ to 2 hours after administration (except sustained-release tablets). Generally patients may take a second dose safely 2 hours after the first dose if the analgesic effect is not sufficient and if side effects are mild or nonexistent. However, the time to peak effect is a problem when treating rapidly fluctuating pain.
- Rectal: Although this route is generally disliked by children, it is a helpful alternative when parenteral and oral routes are unavailable. It is safe, effective, and inexpensive. Dosing is generally 1:1 with oral medication. Rectal suppositories are not recommended in neutropenic or thrombocytopenic patients or those with diarrhea, anal or rectal lesions, or mucositis.
- Transdermal: With transdermal patches, medication is readily absorbed through the skin, allowing for continuous analgesia. A short-acting opioid must be available for breakthrough pain. If frequent rescue doses are required, the transdermal dose is increased based on the daily total of rescue opioid used. Currently fentanyl is the only opioid available by this route.
- Intramuscular (IM): IM administration of analgesics is not recommended.

TABLE 12-6	OPIOID SIDE EFFECTS
Side Effect	**Nursing Considerations**
Constipation	A nearly universal complaint that does not improve with chronic opioid administration, constipation is best treated prophylactically by increasing regular exercise, oral fluids, and dietary fiber and by taking scheduled doses of a combined stool softener and mild peristaltic stimulant (e.g., Senokot).
Nausea and vomiting	Nausea and vomiting can be quite noxious and should be treated promptly and aggressively. Antiemetics can be used on a PRN or ATC basis. Changing to an alternate opioid may be appropriate. Tolerance usually develops over time.
Sedation	This is a common complaint after large doses or from accumulation of long-acting opioids. Administering lower doses or shorter-acting drugs more frequently may be helpful. Central nervous system (CNS) stimulants (e.g., caffeine, dextroamphetamine) may decrease opioid-induced sedation.
Pruritus	Itching is a relatively common side effect that may appear all over the body but is generally localized to the face, neck, and upper thorax. Antihistamines and low-dose nalbuphine (an opioid agonist-antagonist) may relieve symptoms of pruritus.
Urinary retention	This may occur with opioid delivered by any route but is most common with spinal opioids. Management may include decreasing the opioid dose or using in-and-out catheterization once or twice. Tolerance to this side effect generally occurs, although an indwelling Foley catheter may be necessary if urinary retention persists.
Respiratory depression	Respiratory depression is potentially the most serious side effect but one to which tolerance rapidly develops. Frequent monitoring of vital signs is advised if large doses are administered to opioid-naive patients. Significant respiratory depression is best treated with naloxone (Narcan) titrated in small increments to improve respiratory function without reversing analgesia.
	For respiratory depression after a moderate overdose of an opioid with a short half-life, physical stimulation may be sufficient to prevent significant hypoventilation. No patient has succumbed to respiratory depression while awake.
	Subacute overdose—more common than acute respiratory depression—is characterized by slowly progressive (hours to days) somnolence and respiratory depression. Withhold one or two doses until the symptoms have resolved, then reduce regular dose by 25%.

Data from American Pain Society (APS). (1992). *Principles of analgesic use in the treatment of acute pain and cancer pain* (3rd ed.). Glenview, IL; McCaffery, M., & Pasero, C. (1999). *Pain clinical manual* (2nd ed.). St. Louis, MO: Mosby.

- Intravenous (IV) bolus: IV bolus administration is the route providing the most rapid onset of action. Generally, if severe pain persists and side effects are minimal or nonexistent at the time of expected peak effect, another bolus may safely be given. For patients with severe acute pain or exacerbation of cancer pain, repeated IV boluses may be needed to load to therapeutic concentrations, followed by a continuous infusion.
- Intravenous infusion and bolus doses: Continuous infusions provide steady blood levels, which tend to provide the most effective analgesia with the fewest side effects. Short-acting opioids are generally more appropriate for continuous infusions. Bolus doses are often needed to supplement continuous infusions of opioids. The bolus dose is often set to the hourly dose infused. If frequent boluses are required, the infusion rate

may be increased. However, the full effects of the increased continuous infusion will not be felt until steady state is reached. Preceding a dose increase with a bolus dose will allow the patient to reach a steady-state level sooner.
- Patient-controlled analgesia (PCA): PCA helps the child maintain independence and some sense of control by matching medication delivery to analgesic need. It may be IV, subcutaneous (SQ), or epidural. Doses are used to treat breakthrough pain and to provide basis for more accurate and rapid titration upward of the continuous infusion rate. PCA medication allows children to treat breakthrough pain, to make transient changes in analgesic requirements, and to tailor medication according to their own requirements.
- Subcutaneous infusion: SQ infusions are an alternative to intravenous infusions and will produce equivalent blood levels at a steady state.

TABLE 12-7	EQUIANALGESIC DRUG DOSES IN CHILDREN			
Opioid	Equianalgesic Dose	Peak Effect (hr)	Duration (hr)	Comments
Morphine				
Intravenous (IV)	10 mg	0.5-1	3-4	Multiple routes available
Oral (PO)	30-60 mg*	1-2	3-6	
Controlled-release morphine, PO	20-60 mg*	3-4	8-12	
Sustained-release morphine, PO	20-60 mg*	4-6	24	Once to twice a day dosing
Hydromorphone (Dilaudid)				
IV	1.5 mg	0.5-1	3-4	Multiple routes available
PO	7.5 mg	1-2	3-6	
Oxycodone, PO	20-30 mg	1-2	3-6	Alone or combined with acetaminophen (Percocet)
Controlled-release oxycodone, PO	20-30 mg	3-4	8-12	Twice a day
Meperidine (Demerol)				
IV	75 mg	0.5-1	3-6	Not recommended for repeated use due to potential toxicity with metabolite, normeperidine, which can cause central nervous system (CNS) excitation and seizures
PO	300 mg	1-2		
Methadone				
Intramuscular (IM)	10	0.5-1.5	4->8	Risk of delayed toxicity from accumulation; multiple routes available
PO	20	1-2	4->8	
Fentanyl, IV	100 mcg/hr roughly equivalent to morphine 4 mg/hr			Fast acting, short half-life, but at steady state, slow elimination from tissues can lead to prolonged half-life (up to 12 hr)
Fentanyl, transdermal	100 mcg/hr roughly equivalent to morphine 4 mg/hr		48-72	Allow 10-12 hr to start working
COMBINATION OPIOID ANALGESICS (PO ONLY)†				
Hydrocodone with acetaminophen (Vicodin, Lortab)	30 mg	1-2	3-6	
Codeine with acetaminophen	200 mg	1-2	3-6	
Oxycodone with acetaminophen (Percocet)	20-30 mg	1-2	3-6	

Adapted from Cancer Pain Management Guideline Panel. (1994). *Management of cancer pain: Clinical practice guidelines.* (AHCPR Pub. No. 94-0592). Rockville, MD; McCaffery, M., & Pasero, C. (1999). *Pain: Clinical manual* (2nd ed.). St. Louis, MO: Mosby.

*Relative potency of parenteral to oral morphine of 1:6 changes to 1:2-3 with chronic dosing.

†Combination opioid analgesics will have a ceiling effect because of the acetaminophen component. Watch for acetaminophen overdosing.

However, SQ boluses have a slower onset and a lower peak effect than IV boluses.

- Spinal: Opioids and/or local anesthetics can be administered via indwelling catheters into the epidural or intrathecal space as intermittent boluses, continuous infusions, or both. Epidural or intrathecal medication can provide profound analgesia with fewer side effects than other routes. Epidural medication can be delivered continuously through a percutaneous, tunneled, or implanted catheter. A percutaneous catheter may be used for a short course such as postoperative pain management; an implanted or tunneled catheter may be used for long-term management. Pain resistant to conventional medical management can occur near the end of the child's life. At this point epidural or intrathecal pain management allows less systemic medication, with fewer side effects and better quality of life.[12] Occasionally a child with refractory pain may benefit from an epidural or intrathecal catheter, which allows for a more normal, functional lifestyle.[11]

Adjuvants.   Adjuvant medications enhance analgesia, treat concurrent symptoms, and provide independent analgesia for specific types of pain. Adjuvants are commonly used in addition to more conventional analgesics.

- Antidepressants are useful to treat neuropathic pain, some chronic pain, and pain-related sleep disturbances. These medications have some analgesic properties. They may potentiate the analgesic effects of opioids and help patients to sleep.
- Anticonvulsants are useful for neuropathic pain but should be used with caution in patients undergoing marrow-suppressive therapies, such as chemotherapy and radiation therapy.
- Corticosteroids are used in many different types of chronic pain, as well as pain associated with cancer, including bone pain, neuropathic pain, headaches, and arthralgias. Corticosteroids are helpful in cases of tumor infiltration into nerves or bone and in cases of cachexia and anorexia. They also have antiinflammatory activity, antiemetic activity, and bring about appetite stimulation. Side effects are common.
- α_2-Adrenergic agonists, such as clonidine, are sometimes helpful in some cancer pain states, chronic headaches, and nonmalignant neuropathic pain.
- Antiemetics are used primarily to control opioid-related nausea, on an as-needed or around-the-clock basis.
- Topical anesthetics are often applied to venipuncture or injection sites. Nurses must be aware

that the use of these agents may prevent the typical signs of an IV infiltration. Extravasations of vesicant drugs have been masked by the use of topical anesthetics.
- Local anesthetics, given orally (PO), IV, or epidurally are sometimes used to treat somatic and neuropathic pain.
- Psychostimulants such as Ritalin may be used to help control refractory opioid-related sedation, generally given early in the day so as not to interfere with sleep.[31]

NONPHARMACOLOGIC INTERVENTIONS AND COGNITIVE-BEHAVIORAL INTERVENTIONS

Patients should be encouraged to remain as active and functional as possible. Nonpharmacologic and cognitive-behavioral pain management interventions can be used concurrently with medications and other pain management methods during all phases of treatment. One cannot assume that if a cognitive-behavioral intervention decreases a child's experience of pain, the pain is "all in the child's head." Cognitive-behavioral interventions (e.g., blowing bubbles) merely place the painful experience at the periphery of the child's awareness and help the child focus elsewhere for a period of time (Figure 12-1). They help a child achieve a sense of mastery over stressful situations. For some types of mild pain, nonpharmacologic or cognitive-behavioral interventions alone may provide sufficient comfort. Most types of pain experienced by children with cancer require a combination of analgesics and nonpharmacologic and/or cognitive-behavioral interventions (Box 12-2). Although the experience of pain is very subjective, placebos should not be used for analgesia.[4,24,28]

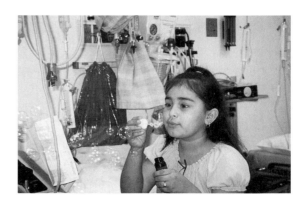

Figure 12-1

A child blowing bubbles as distraction before a medical intervention.

BOX 12-2

Nonpharmacologic and Cognitive-Behavioral Interventions for Pain Management

HEAT

Age

6 months and older

Indications

Achy or persistent muscle pain, decubiti, anorectal pain, hematoma resolution after the acute phase of bleeding has stopped

Helps relieve pain, reduce joint stiffness, relax muscles, and ease spasms; increases blood supply to the treated area; important to wrap heat source to prevent burns or keep heat source (e.g., heat lamp) far enough away to be safe

Contraindications

Contraindicated on irradiated tissue or over tumor sites

COLD

Age

6 months and older

Indications

Injury with no open wound, bruising, muscle spasms, headaches

Although generally more effective and longer lasting, often not as readily accepted as heat by patients; important to wrap cold source to prevent tissue damage and not to leave in one place for longer than 10 min

Contraindications

Contraindicated on tissue that has been damaged by radiation therapy and in patients with peripheral vascular disease

MASSAGE

Age

All ages

Indication

Achy muscles, muscle spasms, tense muscles

Usually soothing and relaxing for the body and mind; helps relax tense muscles and ease muscular spasms and aches

TENS (TRANSCUTANEOUS ELECTRICAL NERVE STIMULATION)

Age

3 years and older

Indications

Various pains, including headaches, muscle aches and spasms, incisional pain, bone metastasis, neuropathy, phantom limb pain

Delivers low-volt electrical impulses along nerves, competing with pain messages, acting as pain inhibitors

Contraindications

Caution in those with epilepsy, cardiac problems, or pacemakers; contraindicated in children with demand pacemakers

ACUPUNCTURE OR ACUPRESSURE

Age

All ages

Indications

Various pains, including some acute pains, headaches, musculoskeletal, persistent, recurrent, or chronic pain

Can be safe, effective means of relieving pain; although acupuncture must be performed only by a trained acupuncturist, acupressure can be learned and performed by others

RELAXATION

Age

7 years and older

Indications

Various acute pains, persistent achy pain, chronic pain, abdominal or limb pain

State of relative freedom from anxiety and muscle tension; may reduce distress associated with pain and stress; often involves breathing exercises and may be accompanied by other nonpharmacologic or cognitive-behavioral interventions

Progressive relaxation—focusing attention systematically on each body part, starting with the toes, relaxing and releasing tension from each area, gradually working up to the head

MUSIC

Age

All ages

Indications

Various types of acute, chronic, and procedural pain

Can provide relaxation and distraction, especially if child is able to choose his or her own music

Adapted from McCaffery, M., & Pasero, C. (1999). *Pain: Clinical Manual* (2nd ed.). St. Louis, MO: Mosby; Kuttner, L. (1996). *A child in pain: How to help, what to do.* Hartley & Marks. See Chapter 9 for additional information.

THE TERMINALLY ILL CHILD

All too often, children with terminal cancer experience considerable pain and suffering before they die.[23] A recent study demonstrated that fewer than 30% of terminally ill children had successful pain control at the time of their deaths.[32]

There are currently many barriers to effective pain control for terminally ill children. There is often a fear of "doing harm," "giving up," causing respiratory depression, or addicting a child to opioids.[12] Many nurses and physicians are concerned that giving opioid analgesia to a dying child will

BOX 12-2

Nonpharmacologic and Cognitive-Behavioral Interventions for Pain Management—cont'd

BREATHING
Age
3 years and older
Indications
Various nonacute pains, persistent achy pain,
  chronic pain, abdominal or limb pain, pain
  associated with muscle tension and/or anxiety
Slow deep, rhythmic breathing helps focus attention
  away from pain, helps muscles relax, and
  decreases anxiety

BLOWING AWAY PAIN
Age
1 year and older
Indications
Various pains, especially acute, brief pain, such as
  procedural pain
Blowing out candles, blowing bubbles, party
  blowers, blowing pinwheels, and blowing away
  the pain are all ways to help facilitate deep
  breathing and distraction.

BIOFEEDBACK
Age
3 years and older
Indications
Migraine and muscle tension headaches, persistent
  muscle pains, some pain caused by stress or
  disease
Encourages autonomy and self-sufficiency by
  teaching children that they can control aspects of
  their own behavior that they previously thought
  were beyond their conscious control; requires
  trained personnel and specialized equipment

IMAGERY
Age
3 years and older
Indications
Various types of acute, chronic, and procedural pain
  involves using one's imagination, involving as
  many senses as possible in the creation of

pleasant, therapeutic images; child may imagine
  being in a special, safe, enjoyable place and
  seeing, hearing, and feeling what is around him or
  her in this special place; focuses on altering the
  image or sensations of pain, giving child more
  control over and relief from pain
Contraindications
Patients with severe emotional problems, or
  psychiatric illness, or history of hallucinations

HYPNOSIS
Age
3 years and older
Indications
Various types of acute, chronic, and procedural pain
Refers to altered state of consciousness that is
  characterized by temporary cessation of critical
  judgement, rapid assimilation of information,
  capacity to alter sensation and perception, and
  capacity to create feelings, sensations, or ideas
  that are incongruent, congruent; hence, change in
  the child's perception of pain can be facilitated;
  more intense and purposefully directed than
  imagery
Should be guided only by qualified, trained
  individuals
Contraindications
Patients with severe emotional problems, psychiatric
  illness, or history of hallucinations

DISTRACTION
Age
10 months and older
Indications
Treatment-related pain, various types of acute and
  chronic pain
Involves any interesting, pleasant activity that
  diverts focus away from a painful procedure or
  event; most helpful with mild pain that is familiar
  to child
Methods of distraction include bubble blowing, pop-
  up books, music, video games

cause the child to stop breathing and die. Ethically and legally we, as health care providers, are obligated to offer appropriate pain management to our terminally ill patients. The ethical principle of "double effect" distinguishes between the intended effect of an action (pain relief) and the unintended

but foreseeable side effects (respiratory depression or apnea). According to this principle, giving opioids to a dying patient is appropriate, acceptable behavior as long as the intent is to relieve pain. The intent is not, as it is with euthanasia or assisted suicide, to shorten the life of the patient. The Position

Statement on Promotion of Comfort and Relief of Pain in Dying Patients of the American Nursing Association states[3]:

> Nurses should not hesitate to use full and effective doses of pain medication for the proper management of pain in the dying patient. The increasing titration of medication to achieve adequate symptom control, even at the expense of life, thus hastening death secondarily, is ethically justified.

Additional information about the care of terminally ill children is found in Chapter 17.

Many terminally ill children experience dyspnea, which can be particularly frightening and distressing for the child and family. Although all opioids may be helpful, morphine is the drug of choice for dyspnea and can be delivered orally, IV, or sublingually. There is some evidence that nebulized morphine can be safe and effective in the treatment of dyspnea. Nebulized morphine has a bioavailability of 9% to 35%, and maximum serum concentrations are reached within 10 to 45 minutes. Nebulization is not recommended for analgesia because only small amounts are actually absorbed.[20]

No child should have to suffer unnecessary pain. We have the necessary technologic, pharmacologic, and nonpharmacologic tools to alleviate most pain that children with cancer experience. It is our responsibility to be knowledgeable about pain, its adverse effects, and treatment options.

Pediatric oncology nurses are in key positions to promote good pain management for their patients. Nurses have more contact with hospitalized patients than other health care providers. They are in the position to take an active role in educating patients, families, other nurses, and physicians about pain, its effects, and proper management.

The American Pain Society has promoted the concept of pain as the fifth vital sign to increase awareness of pain and proper treatment among health care practitioners. In his presidential address to the American Pain Society in 1995, Joseph Campbell, M.D., stated: "Vital signs are taken seriously. If pain were assessed with the same zeal as other vital signs are, it would have a much better chance of being treated properly. We need to train doctors and nurses to treat pain as a vital sign. Quality care means that pain is measured and treated."[6] Many states are requiring more vigorous pain assessment. For example, California legislates that health care facilities (hospitals and nursing homes) include pain as a fifth vital sign, to be assessed at the same time other vital signs are taken.

The Joint Commission on Accreditation of Healthcare Organizations (JCAHO) has created new pain management standards with which all health care facilities are expected to comply. These standards require diligent assessment, appropriate pain management interventions, and reassessment, as well as the education of patients and families about pain and its management. As of 2000, JCAHO states that all accredited hospitals and other health care facilities will be called upon to (1) recognize the right of patients to appropriate assessment and management of pain; (2) assess the existence and, if present, the nature and intensity of pain in all patients; (3) record the results of the assessment in a way that facilitates regular reassessment and follow-up; (4) determine and ensure staff competency in pain assessment and management; address pain assessment and management in the orientation of all new staff; (5) establish policies and procedures that support the appropriate prescription and ordering of effective pain medications; (6) educate patients and their families about effective pain management; and (7) address patient needs for symptom management in the discharge planning process.[14]

Pediatric cancer patients experience pain from many sources. Children and families are not always aware of what might cause pain, the adverse impact of untreated pain, or what pharmacologic and nonpharmacologic resources are available for the management of pain. It is the professional, ethical, and legal responsibility of pediatric oncology nurses to provide optimal pain management and education to patients and families in their care. It is the right of our patients and families to expect quality pain management assessment and treatment from all professionals who provide care.

REFERENCES

1. Acute Pain Management Guideline Panel. (1992). *Acute pain management in adults: Operative procedures—Quick reference guide for clinicians* (AHCPR Pub. No. 92-0019). Rockville, MD: Agency for Health Care Policy and Research, Public Health Service, U.S. Department of Health and Human Services.
2. Acute Pain Management Guideline Panel. (1993). *Acute pain management in infants, children, and adolescents: operative procedures. Quick reference guide for clinicians.* (AHCPR Pub. No. 94-0020) Rockville, MD: Agency for Health Care Policy and Research, Public Health Service, U.S. Department of Health and Human Services.
3. American Nursing Association. (1991). *Position statement on promotion and comfort and relief of pain in dying patients.*
4. American Pain Society (APS). (1992). *Principles of analgesic use in the treatment of acute pain and cancer pain* (3rd ed.). Glenview, IL.
5. Anand, K., & Carr, D. (1989) The neuroanatomy, neurophysiology, and neurochemistry of pain, stress and analgesia in newborns and children. *Pediatric Clinics of North America, 36,* 795-817.

6. Campbell, J. (November 1995). Presidential address. Paper presented at the American Pain Society annual meeting, Los Angeles, CA.

7. Cancer Pain Management Guideline Panel. (1994). *Management of cancer pain: Clinical practice guidelines.* (AHCPR Pub. No. 94-0592). Rockville, MD.

8. Cleeland, C. S., Gonin, R., Hatfield, A. K., et al. (1994). Pain and its treatment in outpatients with metastatic cancer. *New England Journal of Medicine, 330,* 592-596.

9. Conte, P. M., Walco, G. A., Sterling, C. M., et al. (1999). Procedural pain management in pediatric oncology: a review of the literature. *Cancer Investigation, 17,* 448-459.

10. Enskar, K., Carlsson, M., Golsater, M., et al. (1997). Life situation and problems as reported by children with cancer and their parents. *Journal of Pediatric Oncology Nursing, 14,* 18-26.

11. Galloway, K., Staats, P. S., & Bowers, D. C. (1999). Intrathecal analgesia for children with cancer via implanted infusion pumps. *Medical and Pediatric Oncology, 34,* 265-267.

12. Galloway, K. S., & Yaster, M. (2000). Pain and symptom control in terminally ill children. *Pediatric Clinics of North America, 47,* 711-746.

13. Goldstein, J. L., Silverstein, F. E., Agrawal, N. M., et al. (2000). Reduced risk of upper gastrointestinal ulcer complications with celecoxib, a novel COX-2 inhibitor. *American Journal of Gastroenterology, 95,* 1681-1690.

14. Joint Commission on Accreditation of Healthcare Organizations. Pain assessment and management standards. (online) Available from URL: http://www.jcaho.org

15. Kleiber, C., & Harper, D. C. Effects of distraction on children's pain and distress during medical procedures: A meta-analysis. *Nursing Research, 48,* 44-49.

16. Kuttner, L. (1996). *A child in pain: How to help, what to do.* Hartley & Marks.

17. Leese, P. T., Hubbard, R. C., Karim, A., et al. (2000). Effects of celecoxib, a novel cyclooxygenase-2 in hibitor, on platelet function in healthy adults: A randomized, controlled trial. *Journal of Clinical Pharmacology, 40,* 124-132.

18. Ljungman, G., Gordh, T., Sorensen, S., et al. (2000). Pain variations during cancer treatment in children: A descriptive survey. *Pediatric Hematology and Oncology, 17,* 211-221.

19. McCaffery, M. (1968). *Nursing practice theories related to cognition, bodily pain, and man-environment interactions* Los Angeles: University of California at Los Angeles Students' Store.

20. McCaffery, M., & Pasero, C. (1999). *Pain clinical manual* (2nd ed.). St. Louis, MO: Mosby.

21. Merkel, S. I., Voepel-Lewis, T., Shayevitz, J. R. (1997). The FLACC: A behavioral scale for scoring postoperative pain in young children. *Pediatric Nursing, 23,* 293-297.

22. Merskey, H. (Ed.). (1986). Classification of chronic pain: Description of chronic pain syndromes and definitions of pain terms. *Pain, Suppl 3*:S217.

23. Morgan, E. R., & Murphy, S. B. (2000). Care of children who are dying of cancer. *New England Journal of Medicine, 342,* 347-348.

24. Oncology Nursing Society (ONS). *Position statements on the use of placebo for pain management.*

25. Portenoy, R. K. (1997). *Contemporary diagnosis and management of pain in oncologic and AIDS patients.* Pennsylvania: Handbooks in Health Care.

26. Porter, J., & Hick, H. (1980). Addiction rare in patients treated with narcotics. *New England Journal of Medicine, 302,* 123.

27. Romsing, J., Moller-Sonnergaard, J., Hertel, S., et al. (1996). Postoperative pain in children: Comparison between ratings of children and nurses. *Journal of Pain and Symptom Management, 11,* 42-46.

28. Rushton, C. H. (1995). Placebo pain medication: Ethical and legal issues. *Pediatric Nursing, 21,* 166-168.

29. Teoh, N., & Stjernsward, J. (1992). WHO cancer pain relief program: ten years on. *International Association for the Study of Pain Newsletter.*

30. Weinstein, J. W., & Tripp, S. D. (1993). Acute pain management. *Orthopedic Knowledge Update, #4.*

31. Weissman, D. E., Burchman, S. L., Dinndorf, P. A., et al. (1988). *Handbook of cancer pain management,* (3rd ed.). Medical College of Wisconsin and The University of Wisconsin Medical School in conjunction with The Wisconsin Cancer Pain Initiative.

32. Wolfe, J., Grier, H. E., Klar, N., et al. (2000). Symptoms and suffering at the end of life in children with cancer. *New England Journal of Medicine, 342,* 326-333.

33. World Health Organization in collaboration with the International Association for the Study of Pain. (1998). *Cancer pain relief and palliative care in children.* Geneva, Switzerland: World Health Organization.

34. Yaster, M., Kost,-Byerly, S., Berde, C., et al. (1996). The management of opioid and benzodiazepine dependence in infants, children, and adolescents. *Pediatrics, 98,* 135-140.

35. Zuckerman, L. A., & Ferrante, F. M. (1996). Nonopioid and opioid analgesics. In R. K. Portenoy & R. M. Kanner (Eds.), *Pain management theory and practice.* (pp. 111-140). Philadelphia: F. A. Davis.

13

Oncologic Emergencies

Karla D. Wilson

Pediatric oncology nurses require a broad spectrum of knowledge, because they must have proficiency in general pediatrics, oncology, critical care, and end-of-life issues. Children with cancer, regardless of their diagnosis or stage of treatment, are at risk for critical, potentially life-threatening complications. The assessment skills and clinical judgment of the nurse play an essential role in recognizing early signs of impending oncologic emergencies. All oncology nurses must develop expertise in determining the severity of the patient's condition, making both qualitative and quantitative assessments. Often the nurse's impression of how the patient looks is one of the most important aspects of physical assessment.[18]

Oncologic emergencies are life-threatening events that can occur at diagnosis or at any point during the treatment process.[51] They are related to hematologic disorders, bone marrow function, metabolic or hormonal problems or result from obstruction or pressure.[30] The treatment of these emergencies requires the knowledge of intensive care nursing along with the expertise of oncology nursing. Pediatric oncology nurses must be able to distinguish potential emergencies to provide prompt intervention, thereby reducing the morbidity and mortality experienced by pediatric oncology patients.

HEMATOLOGIC DISORDERS AND BONE MARROW FUNCTION

Hematologic emergencies are acute, life-threatening events that are directly or indirectly related to total white blood cell (WBC) count, red blood cell (RBC) volume, platelet count, and/or coagulation factors. They arise secondary to chemotherapy side effects, bone marrow replacement with cancer, or marrow aplasia.

HYPERLEUKOCYTOSIS

Hyperleukocytosis occurs when the peripheral WBC count is greater than 100,000/mm³, resulting in increased blood viscosity. The excessive number of WBCs may result in obstruction of the microcirculation, damage to vessel walls, and severe metabolic disturbances related to rapid destruction of WBCs when cytotoxic therapy is initiated. This may result in intracranial or pulmonary hemorrhage, renal failure, disseminated intravascular coagulation (DIC), and acute tumor lysis syndrome (ATLS).[22,37]

Risk factors. Hyperleukocytosis is associated with newly diagnosed or recurrent leukemias. The incidence is 9% to 13% with acute lymphocytic leukemia (ALL), 5% to 22% in acute nonlymphocytic leukemia (ANLL), and 50% to 100% during the acute phase of chronic myelogenous leukemia (CML).[25] Other risk factors associated with hyperleukocytosis include extramedullary organ involvement and either monocytic or promyelocytic subtypes of ANLL.[14]

Clinical presentation. By definition, children with hyperleukocytosis have a white blood cell count that is greater than 100,000/mm³. Initial symptoms may include fever, headache, vomiting, visual blurring, tinnitus, and oliguria or anuria. Physical examination may show papilledema, retinal vein distention, diminished lung sounds, diffuse pulmonary rales, tachycardia, hepatosplenomegaly, and priapism. The hallmark signs and symptoms arise from an accumulation of leukocytes in the microvasculature of the lungs and central nervous system (CNS). Progressive hyperleukocytosis is demonstrated by worsening tachypnea, respiratory distress, hypoxia, restlessness, ataxia, progressive mental status changes, and dizziness. If not reversed, seizures, coma, and ultimately death occur.[14,22]

Medical management. Medical management is directed to reducing the number of WBCs and preventing secondary complications. Reducing excessive leukemic cells may be done by leukapheresis, exchange transfusions, and initiating cytotoxic chemotherapy. Intravenous (IV) hyperhydration (3000 ml/m^2/day), alkalinization, and allopurinol decrease the risk of acute tumor lysis syndrome. Maintenance of a urine output of 1 to 2 ml/kg/hr, aggressive correction of metabolic abnormalities, and blood product support also are essential.[49,50] Potential secondary complications include hemorrhage, pulmonary leukostasis, metabolic alterations, renal failure, and sudden death from massive intracerebral hemorrhage. Prognosis has improved with the use of supportive care measures described above. Children with ANLL and leukemia patients with a WBC count over 250,000/mm^3 have the greatest risk for a serious intracranial bleed and death.[4] There is an increased relapse rate in children who present with hyperleukocytosis at initial diagnosis.[14]

Nursing interventions. Nursing interventions include assessment of cardiopulmonary and neurologic status and fluid and electrolyte balance. These observations are essential to identify real and potential changes so that early interventions can be implemented.[11,22]

Disseminated Intravascular Coagulation

DIC is a hypercoagulable state with an excessive stimulation of normal coagulation, causing the formation of microthrombi. This leads to consumption and use of clotting factors and platelets, resulting in simultaneous thrombosis and hemorrhage. These alterations in clotting mechanisms are manifested by (1) decreased platelets, (2) increased prothrombin, (3) decreased fibrinogen, and (4) an accumulation of fibrin degradation products, resulting in diffuse intravascular coagulation and tissue ischemia.*

Risk factors. DIC is not a primary disease, but a secondary process of clotting abnormalities that occurs during the course of many different disorders.[49] Risk factors for development of DIC are malignancies, infection, and trauma. Acute promyelocytic leukemia, any leukemia with WBC count greater than 100,000/mm^3, neuroblastoma, and disseminated malignancies are the most common pediatric oncologic conditions associated with DIC. In children with cancer, the primary cause of DIC is gram-negative sepsis.[8]

Clinical presentation. Clinical presentation includes petechiae, ecchymosis, purpuric rash, and/or diffuse bleeding. Thrombotic complications may occur in small vessels, leading to microangiopathic

hemolytic anemia, liver, kidney, and cerebral dysfunction, and gastrointestinal bleeding.[33] Laboratory values demonstrate a platelet count less than 20,000/mm^3, prothrombin time (PT) and partial thromboplastin time (PTT) 1½ to 2 times normal, fibrinogen less than 75,000 mg/dl, and elevation of fibrin degradation products determined by a D-dimer assay greater than 500 µg/L.[8,38,49]

Medical management. Medical management is focused on treatment of the acute symptoms and the underlying cause. Blood product support may include fresh frozen plasma (FFP), platelet and packed RBC transfusions, and possibly cryoprecipitate. Heparin therapy, once a mainstay of DIC treatment, is now used infrequently except for treatment of DIC associated with promyelocytic leukemia.[8,38] Transfusions of blood products and clotting factors will be of only transient benefit if the underlying cause is not ameliorated. Potential complications are irreversible end-organ damage and death. Prognosis has improved over the last 20 years because of new antileukemic agents and advancements in supportive care, including improved antibiotics, antifibrinolytic therapy, and platelet transfusions.[26,28]

Nursing interventions. Nursing interventions include monitoring the patient for bleeding and assessing for tissue perfusion and ensuring adequate circulation and oxygenation. Assessment includes observing the skin for color and petechiae, monitoring potential sites of bleeding (e.g., mucosa, sclerae, esophagus, joints, or intestines), checking urine and stools for occult blood, and evaluating mental status to monitor for intracranial bleeding. It is essential to understand and communicate laboratory values and to provide appropriate safety measures for patients at risk for bleeding. Informing and supporting the patient and family is a vital component of comprehensive nursing care during this life-threatening crisis.[11,38,50]

Septic Shock

Septic shock is a systemic response to pathogenic microorganisms in the blood, when the body fails to initiate an adequate immune response.[6] Children who have a compromised immune system from diseases such as human immunodeficiency virus (HIV), organ transplant, asplenism, or cancer chemotherapy have the greatest risk of developing septic shock. Fever is usually the first symptom of possible sepsis.[7] Frequently the febrile neutropenic child will not demonstrate clinical symptoms of sepsis until after the initiation of antibiotics. As bacteria die, they release endotoxins into the blood-

---

*References 5, 26, 28, 31, 37, 52.

stream, interfering with the uptake and transport of oxygen, leading to decreased tissue perfusion, cellular hypoxia, and death.[1] Although 60% of all septic episodes in neutropenic cancer patients are from gram-positive organisms, the organisms involved in septic shock are usually gram-negative and often arise from endogenous flora.[30,43] Septic shock is defined as sepsis with a systolic blood pressure (BP) of less than 90 mm Hg or a reduction of greater than 40 mm Hg from baseline, in spite of fluid resuscitation.[34,49] Generally the patient will also have both profound leukopenia and thrombocytopenia.

Risk factors. Risk factors include an absolute neutrophil count (ANC) less than 100/mm³, prolonged neutropenia (longer than 7 days), breaks in the integrity of the skin and mucous membranes, invasive devices such as central venous lines, malnutrition, and asplenism. Infants may be at an even greater risk due to a decreased production of T-lymphocytes and limited inflammatory response.[2,15,27]

Clinical presentation. In the presence of infection, the body mounts an inflammatory response characterized by two or more of the following conditions: hypothermia (temperature <36° C) or hyperthermia (temperature >38° C), tachycardia, tachypnea, leukocytosis, or neutropenia.[1,2,18,19,44] Table 13-1 delineates the important differences between sepsis and septic shock, because not all children with sepsis will develop shock. If untreated or unresponsive to treatment, the continuum of shock progresses through the early, intermediate, and late stages before death (Table 13-2).

TABLE 13-1	SEPSIS VERSUS SEPTIC SHOCK	
Symptoms	**Sepsis**	**Septic Shock**
Temperature	<36° C or >38° C	<36° C or >38° C
Pulse	Tachycardia	Tachycardia
Respirations	Tachypnea	Tachypnea
Blood pressure	Normal or close to normal baseline	Persistent hypotension, unresponsive to fluid resuscitation
Physical changes	Warm, flushed skin, weakness, malaise, and adequate urine output	Bilateral rales; hypoxia; cyanosis; cool, clammy skin; anasarca, and oliguria progressing to anuria
Mental status changes	Possible minor confusion and restlessness; irritability in younger children	Restlessness, confusion, agitation, lethargy, delirium, and decrease in level of consciousness

Data from Peterson, P. (1998). Sepsis and septic shock. In C. Chernecky & B. Berger (Eds.), *Advanced and critical care oncology nursing: Managing primary complications* (pp. 549-565). Philadelphia: W. B. Saunders.

TABLE 13-2	CLINICAL STAGES OF SHOCK	
Hyperdynamic Compensated Shock Early Stage	**Hyperdynamic Compensated Shock Intermediate Stage**	**Cardiogenic Uncompensated Shock Late Stage (May Be Irreversible)**
10% ↓ in blood volume	15%-20% ↓ in blood volume	>25% ↓ in blood volume
Skin warm, pink, and dry	Skin cool and mottled	Trunk cool and very mottled
Beginning ↓ in tissue perfusion	Clammy extremities	Cold extremities
Chills and fever	↑ thirst and ↓ urine output	No urine output
Normal BP, heart rate, and respiratory rate	Normal BP and heart rate and ↑ respiratory rate	↓ BP and cardiac output
Very early signs of mental confusion	↑ hypoxia and mental confusion	Delirium progressing to coma
Slightly ↓ Po₂	Pulmonary congestion	Metabolic and lactic acidosis
		Hemorrhagic lesions and DIC

Data from Hazinski, M. F. (1993). Children are different. In M. F. Hazinski (Ed.), *Nursing care of the critically ill child* (pp. 1-17). St. Louis, MO: Mosby–Year Book; Hazinski, M. F., & Barkin, R. M. (1998). Shock. In R. M. Barkin (Ed.), *Pediatric emergency medicine: Concepts and clinical practice* (2nd ed., pp. 118-155). St. Louis, MO: Mosby.

Medical management. Medical management initially focuses on maintaining cardiovascular volume and blood pressure by administering hyperhydration, vasopressors, and blood and coagulation products. If necessary, dialysis and/or respiratory ventilation may be instituted due to multisystem organ failure.[41] Identification and treatment of the underlying infection must also be initiated if the child is to survive septic shock. This includes obtaining blood cultures and initiating broad-spectrum antibiotics and possibly antifungal agents. Potential complications are related to the progression of shock, leading to extreme circulatory compromise, left ventricular dysfunction, decreased cardiac output, hypotension, and severe acidosis.[18,19] If interventions do not reverse shock and halt the progression of the underlying cause, multiorgan failure and death will occur. Prognosis is dependent on the nature of the infectious organism, timely initiation of treatment, and the individual's response to treatment. If multiple organisms are involved, mortality is reported as high as 90%.[46] In the past two decades, overall mortality for infections with gram-negative organisms in the profoundly neutropenic child has dropped from 80% to 10% to 40% with the prompt initiation of empiric antibiotics in the event of fever.[30]

Nursing interventions. Nursing interventions involve close monitoring of vital signs and physical assessment (e.g., perfusion, level of consciousness, respiratory effort), noting that changes in children's vital signs often lag behind deterioration of their physical status. Early subtle signs of impending shock are listed in Table 13-2. Obtaining blood cultures, administering IV antibiotics immediately, and managing fluids are essential, as well as prompt communication with the physician regarding the patient's status and laboratory values.[18,19,29,34,49]

TYPHLITIS

Typhlitis is a bowel inflammation, most commonly of the cecum, leading to necrotizing colitis. It is caused by bacterial invasion of the mucosa and ranges from inflammation to full-thickness infarction and/or perforation. *Clostridium septicum* and *Pseudomonas aeruginosa* are the most prevalent organisms associated with typhlitis. The cecum is most often affected because its decreased vascularity and lymphatic drainage and increased distensibility promote the possibility of infection, necrosis, and swelling, which are common in typhlitis.[30,47]

Risk factors. Patients with myelodysplastic syndrome, ALL, or ANLL who are profoundly neutropenic, with or without concurrent sepsis and/or mucositis, have the greatest risk for developing typhlitis, although any neutropenic child is at risk.[17]

Clinical presentation. Clinical presentation is usually within 7 to 14 days from initiation of chemotherapy. There is profound neutropenia and fevers with severe right lower quadrant abdominal pain and a distended abdomen. Over the course of several hours, the pain will become generalized to the entire abdomen. Fevers are persistent. Nausea, vomiting, and diarrhea, which may be bloody, are frequently present. Bowel sounds range from being high pitched or "tinkling" to being diminished or absent.[31]

Medical management. Crucial treatment of typhlitis is broad-spectrum antibiotics, supportive management, and bowel rest. Radiologic evaluation may show nonspecific gas patterns, a fluid-filled, distended cecum, with dilated small bowel loops, and decreased to absent large bowel gas.[23] Medical management is the treatment of choice. Surgical interventions may be required for (1) persistent gastrointestinal bleeding, despite resolution or correction of clotting abnormalities; (2) evidence of free intraperitoneal perforation; (3) clinical deterioration requiring support with vasopressors and hyperhydration, suggesting uncontrolled sepsis from infarction; and (4) symptoms of an intraabdominal process that would require surgical intervention in the nonneutropenic patient.[30] Potential complications are increased if surgical intervention is required, because there is an increased risk of peritonitis, sepsis, and impaired wound healing. Mortality rates are high, but prognosis has improved with earlier diagnosis and advances in supportive care, such as granulocyte colony stimulating factor, new generations of antibiotics, and imaging studies. The single most critical factor related to prognosis is the recovery of neutrophils.[30]

Nursing interventions. Nursing assessment focuses on close evaluation of the patient's abdominal size, function, and pain by monitoring vital signs, bowel sounds, tympany, abdominal tension, and girth. It is essential to provide pain management and thorough skin, oral, and perianal care. Accurate nursing assessment and timely interventions contribute to the successful outcome for children with typhlitis. The patient and family need reassurance and education regarding the diagnosis, potential for recurrence with future neutropenic episodes, and recognition of early symptoms.[47,50]

METABOLIC DISORDERS

ACUTE TUMOR LYSIS SYNDROME

ATLS, a potentially fatal metabolic condition, occurs when the rapid breakdown of a large number of malignant cells releases intracellular metabolites into the extracellular circulation. The hallmarks of ATLS are hyperuricemia, hyperkalemia, hyperphosphatemia, and hypocalcemia. These electrolyte alterations may occur individually or in combination, regardless of prophylactic measures such as hyperhydration and urinary alkalinization. They can lead to metabolic acidosis, impaired renal function, and cardiac arrhythmias.[14,30,40,42,50]

Risk factors.   Patients at risk for ATLS have cancers that have a large tumor burden. The most commonly associated malignancies are B-cell leukemia or Burkitt's lymphoma, T-cell leukemia or lymphoma, or any leukemia presenting with an initial WBC count greater than 100,000/mm^3. Rarely neuroblastoma or other bulky abdominal tumors that are associated with elevated uric acid and lactate dehydrogenase (LDH) levels will develop ATLS.[30]

Clinical presentation.   ATLS has a rapid onset, typically occurring within 24 to 48 hours after initiating cytotoxic therapy, and may last 5 to 7 days. Symptoms include generalized weakness and fatigue, abdominal pain with cramping, vomiting, fullness, and ascites. Back or flank pain may be related to kidney or ureter obstruction and be associated with oliguria and/or anuria. Cardiac arrhythmias, tachycardia, numbness, tingling, and tetany can result from mineral and electrolyte abnormalities.

Medical management.   Medical management focuses on facilitating the kidney's excretion of the metabolites by hyperhydration, urinary alkalinization, and allopurinol.[51] Intravenous hydration at 2 to 4 times maintenance fluids with sodium bicarbonate to maintain the urine pH between 7.0 and 7.5 promotes uric acid and phosphate excretion. Allopurinol inhibits xanthine oxidase, the enzyme that forms uric acid. At a pH above 7.5, hypoxanthine stones may occur; at a pH of 8 or above, calcium phosphate may crystallize within the kidney, making rigorous assessment of urine pH essential.[30] Close monitoring of fluid balance, physical status, vital signs, and electrocardiogram (ECG) values and frequent laboratory evaluations are key to the treatment of metabolic abnormalities. Laboratory evaluations include determinations of complete blood count (CBC) electrolytes, blood urea nitrogen (BUN), creatinine, uric acid, phosphate, and urine pH and urinalysis. Potassium is restricted, and medications such as furosemide, kayexalate, and insulin may be needed to facilitate potassium excretion.[42] Dialysis becomes necessary if renal failure and hyperkalemia cannot be controlled.[30]

Nursing interventions.   Nursing interventions concentrate on the accurate measurement of intake and output, patient weight, urine specific gravity, urine pH, and hematologic status. Clinical assessment includes evaluating Trousseau's (carpal pedal spasms after occlusion of arterial blood flow in the arm) and Chvostek's (facial muscle twitch) signs for symptoms of tetany resulting from decreased calcium. The ECG must be monitored for evidence of cardiac arrhythmias, which may occur secondary to hyperkalemia. Communication of the patient's laboratory values and physical status to the physician is imperative. Due to the critical status of the patient and the nursing acuity level, the patient is frequently treated in the intensive care unit (ICU).[42] The nurse must be able to provide crisis intervention, serve as a child advocate, ensure proper preparation for invasive procedures, and provide educational and emotional support to the patient and family.[21]

SYNDROME OF INAPPROPRIATE ANTIDIURETIC HORMONE

Syndrome of inappropriate antidiuretic hormone (SIADH) is characterized by a continuous release of antidiuretic hormone (ADH) regardless of plasma osmolality. It is associated with a decrease in urine output and an increase in weight without edema, leading to hyponatremia and water intoxication.[9,35,50]

Risk factors.   Patients at risk for the development of SIADH are those with CNS tumors or infections, pediatric malignancies such as Hodgkin's disease and non-Hodgkin's lymphoma, pulmonary fungal or bacterial infections, recent cessation of exogenous steroids, and treatment with drugs such as narcotics, anesthetics, thiazide diuretics, vincristine, cisplatin, and cyclophosphamide.[35] SIADH may be iatrogenic due to overhydration with a hypotonic solution such as D_5W or D_5 ¼ NS. In pediatric oncology the most common cause of SIADH is the use of vincristine and/or cyclophosphamide.[30,50]

Clinical presentation.   Clinical presentation is initially often vague or nonspecific but can progress to the development of seizures secondary to hyponatremia (sodium level <120 mEq/L).

TABLE 13-3	Symptoms Related to Serum Sodium Levels in SIADH		
	Sodium <130 mEq/L Early	Sodium <125 mEq/L Midpoint	Sodium <120 mEq/L Late
	Thirst and/or anorexia	Nausea and vomiting	Seizures
	Headache	Hyporeflexia	Coma
	Muscles cramps and/or lethargy	Confusion	Death

Data from Maxson, J. (1998). Syndrome of inappropriate antidiuretic hormone secretion. In C. Chernecky & B. Berger (Eds.), *Advanced and critical care oncology nursing: Managing primary complications* (pp. 622-636). Philadelphia: W. B. Saunders.

Symptoms (listed in Table 13-3) are related to the serum sodium level, decreased urine output, weight gain, increased urine specific gravity, and length of time over which the syndrome develops.

Medical management.   Medical management involves restricting fluids, measuring urine osmolality, correcting electrolyte abnormalities, and treating the underlying cause. Potential complications are secondary to the neurologic impairments associated with water intoxication. These are usually reversible and do not require long-term rehabilitation. When late SIADH has developed, the incidence of irreversible morbidity or mortality is increased, usually related to cerebral edema.[30] Overall prognosis is related to the underlying cause of SIADH and the rate of development of severe hyponatremia.[11]

Nursing interventions.   Nursing interventions include identifying high-risk patients and instituting appropriate screening measures, such as daily weights, accurate intake and output, and measuring urine specific gravity and serum sodium. The nurse must understand the complicated and contradictory laboratory values associated with SIADH (see Table 13-3) and observe the patient for mental status changes and seizures associated with hyponatremia and water intoxication.[35]

ANAPHYLAXIS

Anaphylaxis is an immediate systemic hypersensitivity reaction to a foreign protein, which can occur within seconds to minutes of administration or at any point during an infusion of the agent. The reaction to this antigen is potentially life threatening because the release of mast cell mediators may result in respiratory and/or cardiovascular system dysfunction.[7]

Risk factors.   Allergic reactions are most common with IV administration of medications but may occur with any delivery method. Common

TABLE 13-4	Clinical Presentation of Anaphylaxis
System	Presentation
Mental status	Anxiety, confusion, dizziness, agitation, feeling of impending doom
Cardiac	Tachycardia, hypotension
Pulmonary	Chest tightness, inspiratory stridor, wheezing
Skin	Flushed appearance, urticaria, pruritus

Data from Sullivan, T. J. (1988). Systemic anaphylaxis. In L. M. Lichtenstein & A. S. Fauci (Eds.), *Current therapy in allergy, immunology, and rheumatology* (pp. 91-98). Toronto: B. C. Decker; von Hohenleiten, C., & Webster, J. (1998). Anaphylaxis from chemotherapy. In C. Chernecky & B. Berger (Eds.), *Advanced and critical care oncology nursing: Managing primary complications* (pp. 67-83). Philadelphia: W. B. Saunders.

agents may include antibiotics, such as trimethoprim sulfamethoxazole, penicillin, and amphotericin; IV immune globulin; chemotherapy such as asparaginase, etoposide, teniposide, and phase I drugs; repeated blood product infusions, or radiologic contrast media.[30,48]

Clinical presentation.   Clinical presentation may be mild to severe and include hives, rash, swollen lips, difficulty breathing, pruritus, nausea, and vomiting. Infants and toddlers may demonstrate increased irritability. There may be a sensation of anxiety or impending doom, often preceded by a warmth or tingling sensation (Table 13-4).

Medical management.   Medical management includes preventative measures such as the administration of test doses of high-risk medications or pretreatment with diphenhydramine, cimetidine, and/or hydrocortisone. Prompt administration of diphenhydramine and hydrocortisone, epinephrine, and/or oxygen once symptoms appear may prevent progression.[45] Mild to moderate discomfort can

TABLE 13-5	PRESENTING SYMPTOMS OF MALIGNANCY-INDUCED HYPERCALCEMIA		
Gastrointestinal	**Cardiovascular**	**Neuromuscular**	**Renal**
Anorexia, nausea, and vomiting; dehydration; constipation, ileus	Sinus bradycardia, dysrhythmias, short QT interval, wide PR interval	Hypotonia, decreased deep tendon reflexes, lethargy, fatigue, apathy, depression, stupor, coma	Polyuria, nocturia, oliguria

Data from Meriney, D., & Reeder, S. (1998). Hypercalcemia. In C. Chernecky & B. Berger (Eds.), *Advanced and critical care oncology nursing: Managing primary complications* (pp. 254-269). Philadelphia: W. B. Saunders.

progress to respiratory distress and potentially death if symptoms are not controlled or reversed. The prognosis is directly related to early recognition of symptoms, discontinuation of the causative agent, and prompt emergency interventions.[7,48]

Nursing interventions. Nursing interventions begin with knowing the potential risk factors and documenting an accurate history of the patient's allergies and past reactions to medications and blood products. In the event of anaphylaxis, stop the infusion, hang normal saline wide open, notify the physician immediately, and administer emergency drugs.[48] The patient will need to be monitored closely until all symptoms abate and the vital signs are stable. Have appropriate doses of emergency drugs and easy access to the emergency cart and oxygen delivery systems available when administering agents known to cause anaphylaxis.[44,48,50] Patients receiving PEG-asparaginase should be informed that the drug has the potential for delayed or prolonged allergic reactions because of its half-life of 5 to 7 days.[3] The patient and family must be educated about allergic reactions, the need to report allergies in the future, and measures to take to treat the anaphylactic reaction.

ACUTE HYPERCALCEMIA

Normal calcium homeostasis is maintained by a balance of bone formation, bone resorption, and calcium reabsorption from the gut with the urinary excretion of calcium. Malignant hypercalcemia is thought to be related to tumors that produce parathyroid hormone–related protein, osteolytic prostaglandins, and osteoclast activating factors, which initiate a self-sustaining spiral of dehydration and rising calcium levels.[30,36] Acute hypercalcemia occurs when a patient develops a serum calcium level of greater than 10.5 mg/dl. Levels greater than 12 mg/dl can adversely affect almost all organ systems, and a level greater than 20 mg/dl is almost always fatal.

Risk factors. Although rare in pediatrics, hypercalcemia has been reported in children with ALL, non-Hodgkin's lymphoma, neuroblastoma, adolescents with rhabdomyosarcoma metastatic to bone marrow and bone, infants with rhabdoid renal tumors, and females with small cell carcinoma of the ovaries.[30] Risk factors are primarily associated with adult malignancies such as metastatic breast cancer and multiple myeloma.[36]

Clinical presentation. Clinical presentation is associated with renal, gastrointestinal, neuromuscular, and cardiovascular symptoms (Table 13-5).

Medical management. Medical management is guided by the serum calcium level. The goal is to restore the intravascular volume by facilitating renal excretion of excess calcium with saline diuresis and diuretics. Higher calcium levels may require IV fluids at 3 times maintenance and 2 to 3 mg/kg of furosemide every 2 hours. This therapy may cause significant fluid shifts, hypokalemia, and hypomagnesemia. Glucocorticoids and calcitonin may provide additional control, but these agents may take 2 to 3 days to have an effect. Treatment of the underlying cause and management of any organ dysfunction are essential. Oral phosphorus can be helpful in treating chronic, but not acute, hypercalcemia. Potential complications of hypercalcemia range from neurologic impairment, seizures, and cardiac arrhythmias to death. The prognosis for hypercalcemia is dependent on the underlying cause and the response to treatment.[30]

Nursing interventions. Nursing interventions focus on symptom management for nausea, vomiting, constipation, polyuria, and pain. The nurse must monitor the patient's ECG values, hydration status, and vital signs. Assess neurologic status, and initiate seizure precautions. Muscle weakness and mental status changes occur with elevated calcium, and appropriate safety measures must be provided. Patients are at risk for pathologic fractures and require range-of-motion and safe weight-bearing opportunities. An understanding of calcium and its role in the body are essential for effective treatment, care, and teaching.[36]

NEUROLOGIC DISORDERS

SEIZURES

Seizure activity is not a primary disease but a symptom of an underlying pathologic problem. CNS irritation causes transient involuntary alterations in the neurologic system with changes in consciousness, behavior, motor function, sensation, or autonomic function.

Risk factors.   Risk factors in pediatric oncology are either disease or treatment related. Seizure foci may be triggered by tumors within the CNS, especially supratentorial lesions; metabolic disorders; medications such as intrathecal (IT) chemotherapy, vincristine, cisplatin, and cytarabine; infection; leukoencephalopathy; and radiation necrosis.[20,30]

Clinical presentation.   Clinical presentation ranges from minimal symptoms, which may go undetected, to obvious alterations in sensory and/or motor function. Simple partial seizures are manifested by pure motor, sensory, or autonomic symptoms, which are very subtle and do not impair consciousness. Complex partial seizures are associated with a combination of minor alterations in consciousness, altered behavior, and motor or sensory symptoms that commonly last only 1 to 2 minutes. Generalized seizures are almost always tonic-clonic in nature, result in sudden loss of consciousness, and are followed by a postictal state. The ictal or clonic-tonic phase of the seizures may last from 3 to 5 minutes.

Medical management.   Medical management almost always involves the use of anticonvulsants to control the seizure activity. If the underlying cause can be eliminated, drug therapy may be short term. However, treatment of the underlying cause does not always eliminate the seizure activity, especially with temporal or parietal lesions, leukoencephalopathy, or radiation necrosis. Potential complications are related to the underlying cause and the associated long-term sequelae. Status epilepticus may result from poor compliance with anticonvulsant medication, trauma, metabolic disturbances, infections, and space-occupying lesions.

Prognosis is related to the cause of the seizure activity. If the precipitating factor was transient and controllable (e.g., electrolyte imbalance), the seizure is likely to be an isolated event. Seizures resulting from structural damage, such as radiation necrosis, or permanent residual damage from CNS infection are more likely to recur and require long-term or permanent anticonvulsant therapy.[24,30]

Nursing interventions.   Nursing interventions are focused on protection of the child during seizure activity. Documentation of the seizure pattern, including physical and sensory activity, is essential. Patient and family education should include instructions on medications and potential side effects, importance of compliance, and providing a safe environment if a seizure occurs. Whatever the cause or type of seizure, the patient and family will need psychologic support and education to overcome the fear of recurrent seizures.[24]

CEREBRAL VASCULAR ACCIDENTS

Cerebral vascular accidents (CVAs) occur when there is impaired blood supply to the brain with subsequent ischemia. The extent of damage is related to the degree of ischemia. Symptoms vary by the location of the injury and may be minimal to severe with temporary or permanent deficits. CVAs are rare occurrences in pediatric oncology and are associated with disease or metastases, treatment, infection, or underlying coagulation abnormalities.[20,30]

Risk factors.   CVAs are associated with brain tumors, leukemia (especially acute promyelocytic or monoblastic leukemias), metastases to the dura from tumors such as neuroblastoma, or leptomeningeal spread of primary CNS tumors. Other risk factors are thrombosis development associated with asparaginase or intrathecal methotrexate therapy, sepsis, DIC, bacterial or fungal meningitis, and platelet-resistant thrombocytopenia. If a CVA occurs months to years after completion of treatment, it is usually associated with large vessel occlusion or mineralizing microangiopathy from radiation therapy.[30]

Clinical presentation.   Clinical presentation of a CVA is directly related to the affected area of the brain. There is often an acute impairment in motor function or speech, with or without seizure activity. If a major CVA involves the brainstem or is the result of a sagittal sinus thrombosis, it is difficult to determine if the child is obtunded or in a postictal phase following a seizure.

Medical management.   Medical management initially involves stabilization of the child. Magnetic resonance imaging (MRI) or computed tomography (CT) scan (with and without contrast) is used to determine the area of brain involvement and severity of the damage. Supportive care may include steroids and hyperosmolar agents to decrease intracranial pressure. Anticoagulants, such as heparin, are contraindicated because they may cause extension of the venous infarct. If the CVA is thought to be related to asparaginase or profound coagulation abnormalities, infusions of antithrombin III concentrate or FFP may be indicated. Rarely is surgical intervention a feasible option based on the underlying cause of the CVA or the child's pancytopenic state. Potential complications include paralysis and sensory and motor deficits. Prognosis is dependent on the location of the injury and the underlying cause.

Nursing interventions. Nursing interventions include supportive care and education for the patient and family. Physical care requirements are determined by the clinical manifestations of the CVA. Frequently evaluation by rehabilitation services is helpful because patients may require physical, occupational, and/or speech therapy. These therapies may be short term or long term, depending on the degree and permanence of the deficit.

SPINAL CORD COMPRESSION

Spinal cord compression is a neurologic emergency that occurs in approximately 5% of patients with malignancies, either at diagnosis or at recurrence.[39] It is usually not life threatening, but prompt assessment and intervention is needed to preserve neurologic function. The spinal cord is compressed or injured as a direct or indirect result of a malignancy invading the intramedullary, intradural, extradural, or extravertebral space.[16]

Risk factors. Risk factors for spinal cord compression include primary tumors of the spinal cord, drop metastases from brain tumors, paraspinal neuroblastomas, non-Hodgkin's lymphoma, and metastatic sarcomas.[30]

Clinical presentation. Clinical presentation is typically back pain, which may be local, referred, or diffuse, and is considered the early "hallmark" sign of disease. Motor deficits include weakness, ataxia, paralysis, or muscle atrophy. Reflexes may be absent, hypotonic, or hyperreflexic. Sensory deficits can include bowel and/or bladder dysfunction, paraesthesia, and loss of pain or temperature sensation. Paralysis and sensory deficits are late symptoms and may not be reversible.

Medical management. The initial goal is stabilization or reversal of the neurologic process.

Spinal cord edema is treated with high-dose steroids. Diagnostic evaluation includes a detailed neurologic examination and an MRI or CT of the spine. Radiation therapy to the lesion may relieve or reverse the neurologic deficits. Surgical decompression may be done to preserve neurologic function and prevent further deterioration. Ultimately, the underlying disease must be treated. Prognosis is dependent on the degree of injury and the location of the lesion causing compression. If irreversible damage occurs, the child will have permanent loss of function below the level of cord compression. Patients with middle or lower thoracic lesions may have less recovery due to poor collateral blood supply in this area. Compression lesions that do not infiltrate into cord tissue have more favorable outcomes. Vertebral collapse, along with extradural tumor, is generally associated with a poorer prognosis.[13] Although many adults with paralysis from spinal cord compression are unable to regain ambulation, children frequently are able to walk again after treatment, even with severe spinal cord compression.

Nursing interventions. Back pain in a child with cancer must be carefully documented and reported. This type of pain is unusual in children and is often secondary to a space-occupying lesion. Assess the patient for sensation, pain, decreased mobility, paralysis, and diminished urinary or bowel function. Provide appropriate positioning and range of motion, safety precautions related to altered mobility, skin care, and supportive care.[16]

CARDIOPULMONARY DISORDERS
MASSIVE HEMOPTYSIS

Massive hemoptysis is defined as the expectoration of 600 ml of blood within 24 hours in the adult patient. In children, the volume is significantly less and is based on the size of the child.[30]

Risk factors. This condition is rare in children, and its occurrence is usually associated with pulmonary aspergillosis or erosion of the pulmonary vessels by tumor.[30]

Clinical presentation. Major hemoptysis is often preceded by minor episodes of bloody expectoration. Chest radiographs (CXRs) often show a nodular or cavitary lesion.

Medical management. If hemoptysis is large and unexpected, the initial management will focus on maintaining a patent airway and preventing asphyxiation. Oral intubation provides access for passage of a bronchoscope. Bronchoscopy is used to identify the location of the lesion and provides access for transcatheter embolization or occlusion of a hemorrhagic vessel with a balloon catheter. Anemia, thrombocytopenia, and other coagulopathies will need to be corrected. Occasionally surgical intervention to remove a portion of lung may be indicated. After the patient is stabilized, treatment focuses on correcting the underlying cause. Potential complications are asphyxiation and death if the bleeding or the underlying cause cannot be controlled. The incidence of hemoptysis in pulmonary aspergillosis is reported to be from 2% to 26%. Prognosis is related to the ability to halt the bleeding and successfully treat the underlying cause. In massive hemoptysis, death occurs because of blockage of the airways by blood clots and the inability to maintain adequate ventilation.[30]

Nursing interventions.   If the site of bleeding is known, the patient is positioned on the side of the hemorrhage because this will decrease blood accumulating in the normal lung. The family may require emotional support because the bleeding is often very distressing. Monitor the patient's vital signs carefully, and observe for signs and symptoms of shock. Administer blood products as indicated.

SUPERIOR VENA CAVA SYNDROME

Superior vena cava syndrome (SVCS) refers to the clinical symptoms that occur when the superior vena cava is either compressed or obstructed.[39] Venous congestion, reduced cardiac output, edema of surrounding structures, and hypoxia are the hallmark signs.[33]

Risk factors.   Primary malignancies such as non-Hodgkin's lymphoma, Hodgkin's disease, neuroblastoma, and germ cell tumors are associated with the development of SVCS. Of these malignancies, non-Hodgkin's lymphoma has the highest correlation with SVCS. The incidence of SVCS in pediatric oncology is low, only occurring in approximately 12% of all thoracic tumors. A more common cause is thrombosis secondary to a central venous catheter.[30]

Clinical presentation.   If a malignancy is the cause, symptoms will develop rapidly over hours to days. Initial symptoms may be cough, hoarseness, dyspnea, orthopnea, and chest pain. Less frequently, but more ominous, are anxiety, confusion, lethargy, distorted vision, a sense of fullness in the ears, and syncope. All symptoms may be increased when the child is supine. The face, neck, and upper extremities are usually edematous and flushed and at times are cyanotic. Venous distention is evident, and the child may be diaphoretic with stridor and/or wheezing. A CXR may show a large anterior mediastinal mass, tracheal compression, and pleural or pericardial effusions. Clinical presentation of SVCS in a clotted venous catheter is more insidious.

Medical management.   Medical management initially focuses on preventing life-threatening symptom progression. Maintenance of the airway, cardiac output, and hemodynamic status are the priority. If the obstruction or thrombosis is from a central venous catheter, thromboembolic therapy to dissolve the clot and immediate removal of the line are necessary. If a thoracic mass is present, histologic examination of a biopsy specimen before initiation of treatment is optimal. Treatment with low-dose radiation or steroids can cause rapid dissolution of the tumor. If the histologic diagnosis cannot be obtained before shrinking the mass, it may impede appropriate treatment of the underlying cause.[33] Children with SVCS usually have an excellent prognosis. Infrequently some children have significant tracheal compression, which may necessitate short-term intubation or tracheotomy to maintain airway patency. The associated malignancies respond well to therapy, and the cure rate is high. Removal of the central venous catheter and/or administration of thrombolytic therapy provide immediate resolution of the symptoms in most cases of catheter-related SVCS. A few patients will need chronic thrombolytic therapy.[30]

Nursing interventions.   Nursing interventions involve assessment of respiratory and cardiac status. Place the child in a semiupright or upright position. Offer calm and simple explanations of treatment and supportive care. Avoid sedation, which may lead to respiratory compromise. Initiate cancer therapy as quickly as possible for patients with tumor-related SVCS.

PLEURAL AND PERICARDIAL EFFUSIONS

Pleural and pericardial effusions occur when there is a fluid accumulation in the pleural space or pericardial sac. They may be caused by solid tumor or hematologic malignancies, infection, and radiation. Pleural effusions are classified as exudates or transudates. Exudates may be caused by local invasion, metastatic spread of tumor, or infection. Transudates occur as a sympathetic response to tumor in the chest or abdomen, fluid overload, heart failure, or hypoproteinemia. Pericardial effusions are frequently asymptomatic because fluid accumulates slowly within the pericardial sac. Cardiac tamponade occurs when there is a rapid accumulation of fluid in the pericardial sac, causing left ventricular failure.[10,12]

Risk factors. The incidence of malignant pleural and pericardial effusions is greater in adults, because these effusions are most frequently associated with primary and metastatic lesions to the lungs, lymphoma, and breast cancer.[30] In children, pericardial and pleural effusions, although rare, are usually related to thoracic lymphomas but have also been associated with leukemia, Wilms tumor, and rhabdomyosarcoma. Pericardial effusions are less common than pleural effusions. Although also infrequent, infection and radiation-induced pleural and pericardial effusions occur more commonly than malignant effusions.

Clinical presentation. Frequently patients with pleural and pericardial effusions are asymptomatic due to a slow accumulation of fluid, and the effusions are found on routine radiologic scans. Initial symptoms are of respiratory difficulties and cardiovascular compromise. Other signs may include cough, chest pain, dyspnea, hiccups, and nonspecific abdominal pain. Clinical findings may include decreased breath sounds, friction rubs, diastolic murmurs, and atrial arrhythmias.[12]

Medical management. The four primary options for patients with effusions are (1) eliminate the cause, (2) remove the fluid, (3) obliterate the pleural or pericardial space to prevent reaccumulation, and (4) observe asymptomatic patients. The patient's clinical status dictates which option is chosen. Management may include chemotherapy, instillation of sclerosing agents, thoracentesis and/or cardiocentesis, and major thoracic surgery. The definitive treatment is dependent on the cause, the status of the underlying malignancy, and the patient's quality of life. The prognosis is related to the cause, stage of the malignancy and responsiveness to therapy.[10,12,30]

Nursing interventions. Nursing interventions vary depending on the severity of the symptoms. Nursing assessment includes evaluating respiratory status, tissue perfusion, abdominal tenderness and ascites, and mental status changes. Additional assessments for patients with pericardial effusions include ECG monitoring and pulsus paradoxus. Promote comfort by positioning in semi-Fowler's position, providing analgesics, and administering oxygen. Providing a quiet environment, information, preparation for possible treatment, and emo-

tional support are also crucial components of nursing care.[10,12,30]

Having a child diagnosed with cancer is a devastating experience for a family. The addition of a life-threatening event after diagnosis brings added stress to a family already in crisis. As the primary provider of patient care, nurses have numerous opportunities for assessment and intervention. Excellent nursing assessment, followed by the appropriate early interventions can help to minimize the severity of oncologic emergencies. Communicating findings to other health care providers, the patient, and family members is at the core of nursing care, especially during an emergency situation. If the patient requires transfer to an ICU, the pediatric oncology nurse provides for the transition of care. In addition to the physiologic and technologic aspects of critical oncologic care, the nurse must also focus on the psychologic components. The nurse's familiarity with the patient and family influences the approaches of other members of the health care team, affording nursing a key position to furnish education, encouragement, and support through the crisis period.[32]

REFERENCES

1. Ackerman, M. H. (1994). The systemic inflammatory response, sepsis, and multiple organ dysfunction: New definitions for an old problem. *Critical Care Nursing Clinics of North America, 6,* 243-250.
2. Ackerman, M. H., Evans, N. J., & Ecklund, M. M. (1994). Systemic inflammatory response syndrome, sepsis, and nutritional support. *Critical Care Nursing Clinics of North America, 6,* 321-340.
3. Balis, F. M., Holcenberg, J. S., & Poplack, D. G. (1997). General principles of chemotherapy. In P. A. Pizzo & D. G. Poplack (Eds.), *Principles and practice of pediatric oncology* (3rd ed., pp. 215-272). Philadelphia: Lippincott-Raven.
4. Basade, M., Dhar, A., Kulkarni, S. M., et al. (1995). Rapid cytoreduction in childhood leukemic hyperleukocytosis by conservative therapy. *Medical and Pediatric Oncology, 25,* 204-207.
5. Bick, R. (1988). Disseminated intravascular coagulation and related syndromes: A clinical review, *Seminars in Thrombic Hemostasis, 14,* 229-238.
6. Brown, K. K. (1994). Septic shock. *American Journal of Nursing 94,* 94(10), 21-22.
7. Bruce, J. L., & Grove, S. K. (1992). Fever: Pathology and treatment. *Critical Care Nurse 12*(1), 40-49.
8. Buchanan, G. R. (1997). Hematological supportive care of the pediatric cancer patient. In P. A. Pizzo & D. G. Poplack (Eds.), *Principles and practice of pediatric oncology* (3rd ed., pp. 1051-1068). Philadelphia: Lippincott-Raven.
9. Carpenter, R. (1998). Fever. In C. Chernecky & B. Berger (Eds.), *Advanced and critical care oncology nursing: Managing primary complications* (pp. 156-171). Philadelphia: W. B. Saunders.
10. Collins, P. (1998). Malignant pleural effusions. In C. Chernecky & B. Berger (Eds.), *Advanced and critical care oncology nursing: Managing primary complications* (pp. 444-460). Philadelphia: W. B. Saunders.

11. Dietz, K. A., & Flaherty, A. M. (1993). Oncologic emergencies. In S. L. Groenwald, M. H. Frogge, & M. Goodman (Eds.), *Cancer nursing: Principles and practice* (pp. 800-837). Boston: Jones & Bartlett.

12. Dragonette, P. (1998). Malignant pericardial effusion and cardiac tamponade. In C. Chernecky & B. Berger (Eds.), *Advanced and critical care oncology nursing: Managing primary complications* (pp. 425-443). Philadelphia: W. B. Saunders.

13. Dyck, S. (1991). Surgical instrumentation as a palliative treatment for spinal cord compression. *Oncology Nursing Forum, 18,* 515-521.

14. Eguiguren, J., Schell, M., Crist, W., et al. (1992). Complications and outcomes in childhood lymphoblastic leukemia with hyperleukocytosis. *Blood, 79,* 871-875.

15. Ellerhorst-Ryan, J. M. (1993). Infection. In S. L. Groenwald, M. H. Frogge, & M. Goodman (Eds.), *Cancer nursing: Principles and practice* (pp. 557-554). Boston: Jones and Bartlett.

16. Forster, D. (1998). Spinal cord compression. In C. Chernecky & B. Berger (Eds.), *Advanced and critical care oncology nursing: Managing primary complications* (pp. 566-579). Philadelphia: W. B. Saunders.

17. Friefield, A. G., Walsh, T. J., & Pizzo, P. A. (1997). Infectious complications in the pediatric cancer patient. In P. A. Pizzo & D. G. Poplack (Eds.), *Principles and practice of pediatric oncology* (3rd ed., pp. 1069-1114). Philadelphia: Lippincott-Raven.

18. Hazinski, M. F. (1993). Children are different. In M. F. Hazinski (Ed.), *Nursing care of the critically ill child* (pp. 1-17). St. Louis, MO: Mosby Year Book.

19. Hazinski, M. F., & Barkin, R. M. (1998). Shock. In R. M. Barkin (Ed.), *Pediatric emergency medicine: Concepts and clinical practice* (2nd ed., pp. 118-155). St. Louis, MO: Mosby.

20. Hickman, J. (1998). Increased intracranial pressure. In C. Chernecky & B. Berger (Eds.), *Advanced and critical care oncology nursing: Managing primary complications* (pp. 371-383). Philadelphia: W. B. Saunders.

21. Hockenberry-Eaton, M., & Kline, N. (1997). Nursing support of the child with cancer. In P. A. Pizzo & D. G. Poplack (Eds.), *Principles and practice of pediatric oncology* (3rd ed., pp. 1209-1228). Philadelphia: Lippincott-Raven.

22. Holmes, W. (1998). Hyperleukocytosis in childhood leukemia. In C. Chernecky & B. Berger (Eds.), *Advanced and critical care oncology nursing: Managing primary complications* (pp. 283-297). Philadelphia: W. B. Saunders.

23. Katz, J. A., Wagner, M. l., Gresik, M. V., et al. (1990). Typhlitis: An 18 year experience and postmortem review. *Cancer, 65,* 1041-1047.

24. Kernich, C. (1998). Seizures. In C. Chernecky & B. Berger (Eds.), *Advanced and critical care oncology nursing: Managing primary complications* (pp. 536-548). Philadelphia: W. B. Saunders.

25. Kinrade, L. (1988). Typhlitis: A complication of neutropenia. *Pediatric Nursing, 14,* 291-295.

26. Kitchens, C. S. (1995). Disseminated intravascular coagulation. In M. C. Brain, P. P. Carbone, J. G. Kelton, et al. (Eds.), *Current therapy in hematology-oncology* (pp. 182-187). St. Louis, MO: Mosby.

27. Koll, B. S., & Brown, A. E. (1993). Changing patterns of infections in the immunocompromised patient with cancer. *Hematology/Oncology Clinics of North America, 7,* 753-767.

28. Kurts, A. (1993). Disseminated intravascular coagulation with leukemia patients. *Cancer Nursing, 16,* 456-463.

29. Lamb, L. (1982). Think you know septic shock? *Nursing 82, 12*(1), 34-43.

30. Lange, B., O'Neill, J., Goldwein, J., et al. (1997). Oncologic emergencies. In P. A. Pizzo, & D. G. Poplack (Eds.), *Principles and practice of pediatric oncology* (3rd ed., pp. 1025-1049). Philadelphia: Lippincott-Raven.

31. Lankiewicz, M. W., & Bell, W. B. (1993). Disseminated intravascular coagulation. In W. R. Bell (Ed.), *Hematologic and oncologic emergencies* (pp. 105-124). New York: Churchill Livingstone.

32. Lewandowski, L. A. (1993). Psychosocial aspects of pediatric critical care. In M. F. Hazinski (Ed.), *Nursing care of the critically ill child* (pp. 19-77). St. Louis, MO: Mosby–Year Book.

33. Loney, M. (1998). Superior vena cava syndrome. In C. Chernecky & B. Berger (Eds.), *Advanced and critical care oncology nursing: Managing primary complications* (pp. 603-621). Philadelphia: W. B. Saunders.

34. Mason. C. (1986). Septic shock. *Journal of the Association of Pediatric Oncology Nurses, 4*(3&4), 25-30.

35. Maxson, J. (1998). Syndrome of inappropriate antidiuretic hormone secretion. In C. Chernecky & B. Berger (Eds.), *Advanced and critical care oncology nursing: Managing primary complications* (pp. 622-636). Philadelphia: W. B. Saunders.

36. Meriney, D., & Reeder, S. (1998). Hypercalcemia. In C. Chernecky & B. Berger (Eds.), *Advanced and critical care oncology nursing: Managing primary complications* (pp. 254-269). Philadelphia: W. B. Saunders.

37. Miller, J., & Parnes, H. (1994). Hematologic problems and emergencies. In R. B. Cameron (Ed.), *Practical oncology* (pp. 77-83). Norwalk, CT: Appleton & Lange.

38. Murphy-Ende, K. (1998). Disseminated intravascular coagulation. In C. Chernecky & B. Berger (Eds.), *Advanced and critical care oncology nursing: Managing primary complications* (pp. 119-139). Philadelphia: W. B. Saunders.

39. Parisi, M. T., Fahmy, J. L., Kaminsky, C. K., et al. (1999). Complications of cancer therapy in children: A radiologist's guide. *Radiographics, 19,* 283-297.

40. Patterson, K., & Klopovich, P. (1986). Metabolic emergencies in pediatric oncology: The acute tumor lysis syndrome. *Journal of the Association of Pediatric Oncology Nurses, 4*(3&4), 19-24.

41. Peterson, P. (1998). Sepsis and septic shock. In C. Chernecky & B. Berger (Eds.), *Advanced and critical care oncology nursing: Managing primary complications* (pp. 549-565). Philadelphia: W. B. Saunders.

42. Robison, J. (1998). Tumor lysis syndrome. In C. Chernecky & B. Berger (Eds.), *Advanced and critical care oncology nursing: Managing primary complications* (pp. 637-659). Philadelphia: W. B. Saunders.

43. Rubin, R. H., & Ferraro, M. J. (1993). Understanding and diagnosing infectious complications in the immunocompromised host: Current issues and trends. *Hematology/Oncology Clinics of North America, 7,* 795-811.

44. Secor, V. H. (1994). The inflammatory/immune response in critical illnesses: Role of the systemic inflammatory response syndrome. *Critical Care Clinics of North America, 6,* 251-264.

45. Sullivan, T. J. (1988). Systemic anaphylaxis. In L. M. Lichtenstein & A. S. Fauci (Eds.), *Current therapy in allergy, immunology, and rheumatology* (pp. 91-98), Toronto: B. C. Decker.

46. Truett, L. (1991). The septic syndrome: An oncologic treatment challenge. *Cancer Nursing, 14,* 175-180.

47. Vaughn, G., & Moles, L. (1998). Typhlitis in pediatrics. In C. Chernecky & B. Berger (Eds.), *Advanced and critical care oncology nursing: Managing primary complications* (pp. 660-674). Philadelphia: W. B. Saunders.

48. von Hohenleiten, C., & Webster, J. (1998). Anaphylaxis from chemotherapy. In C. Chernecky & B. Berger (Eds.), *Advanced and critical care oncology nursing: Managing primary complications* (pp. 67-83). Philadelphia: W. B. Saunders.

49. Wiessner, W. H., Casey, L. C., & Zbilut, J. P. (1995). Treatment of sepsis and septic shock: A review. *Heart Lung, 24,* 380-393.

50. Whitlock, D., Whitlock, J., & Coates, T. (1993). Hematologic and oncologic emergencies requiring critical care. In M. F. Hazinski (Ed.), *Nursing care of the critically ill child* (pp. 803-827). St. Louis, MO: Mosby–Year Book.

51. Wilson, K. (1998). Oncologic emergencies. In M. J. Hockenberry-Eaton (Ed.), *Essentials of pediatric oncology nursing: A core curriculum* (pp. 147-152). Glenview, IL: APON.

52. Wintrobe, M. (1981). *Clinical hematology.* Philadelphia: Lea & Febiger.

14

Blood Component Deficiencies

Robbie Norville
Rosalind Bryant

As cancer treatment has become more aggressive, the use of supportive blood transfusion therapy continues to be a major strategy in pediatric oncology. The causes for blood component deficiencies in children with cancer include marrow involvement by tumor, marrow suppression resulting from intensive multidrug chemotherapy or radiation therapy, and increased peripheral destruction of blood cells. To prevent and/or minimize the morbidity and mortality associated with the management of blood component deficiencies, the pediatric oncology nurse must have knowledge of normal blood component values, blood product administration procedures, potential transfusion reactions, and methods of nursing assessment.

HEMATOPOIESIS

ANATOMY AND PHYSIOLOGY

In 1868 Neumann demonstrated that red blood cells arose from precursors in the marrow.[30] The concept of a single pluripotent stem cell with the capacity to repopulate the entire hematopoietic system in sustained hematopoiesis (blood cell production) was first demonstrated by Till and McCulloch.[30] Subsequent research has confirmed the clonal nature of the pluripotent stem cell, proving that it can differentiate to form progenitor cells for red blood cells, white blood cells, and platelets.[30] Fetal hematopoiesis first starts in the yolk sac. Blood cells are later produced in the liver. Finally, at approximately 20 weeks' gestation, hematopoiesis occurs in the bone marrow of the flat bones (sternum, ribs, vertebrae, hip, pelvic and shoulder girdles).

Whole blood is composed of cellular and plasma components. Approximately 55% is the cellular component, which includes erythrocytes (red blood cells), leukocytes (white blood cells), and platelets. The remaining 45% is plasma, the liquid portion of blood. Red blood cells (RBCs) survive approximately 120 days in the peripheral circulation. They transport oxygen and nutrients to the cells of the body and remove carbon dioxide from the tissues to the lungs.

White blood cells (WBCs) are produced in both the bone marrow and in the lymph tissue and are categorized as granulocytes and agranulocytes. The granulocytes (neutrophils, basophils, and eosinophils) are primarily phagocytic but also detoxify foreign substances and release heparin. Granulocytes survive 12 to 14 hours in the blood and approximately 5 days in the tissues. Agranulocytes (monocytes and lymphocytes) include the monocytes that function as phagocytic cells and can survive years in the tissues as macrophages. Lymphocytes regulate the immune response and also survive for years in tissue.

Platelets (thrombocytes) are cellular fragments of megakaryocytes and have an average life span of 7 to 10 days. Platelets promote the formation of thrombin and the platelet plug during the coagulation process.

Plasma is composed of greater than 90% water, 7% to 9% proteins, plus a small amount of nutrients, electrolytes, hormones, enzymes, and metabolites. Plasma proteins originate in the liver and consist of 60% albumin, which maintains blood osmotic pressure, 36% globulin, and 4% fibrinogen. Fibrinogen transports fat-soluble vitamins and aids in immunity and clot formation.[7]

COAGULATION PROCESS

The primary hemostatic mechanism of the coagulation process includes a vascular response and the formation of a platelet plug. The secondary hemostatic mechanism includes the formation of a stable fibrin clot.[10] The coagulation cascade is designed to generate thrombin, is responsible for the proteolytic cleavage of fibrinogen to form an insoluble fibrin gel, and includes the extrinsic and intrinsic pathways (Figure 14-1).[11] The coagulation pathways are primarily associated with the endothelial cells of the vessel wall, which is the site at which

Intrinsic Pathway (APTT Test)

Extrinsic Pathway (PT Test)

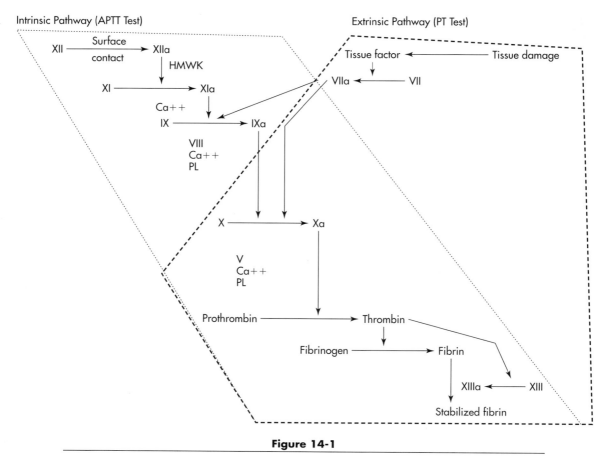

Figure 14-1

Simplified pathways of blood coagulation. The area inside the dotted line is the intrinsic pathway, measured by the activated partial thromboplastin time (APTT). The area inside the dashed line is the extrinsic pathway, measured by the prothrombin time (PT). The area encompassed by both lines is the common pathway.   (Adapted from Andreoli, T. E., Carpenter, C. C. J., Plum, F., et al. [1993]. *Cecil essentials of medicine* [3rd ed., p. 409]. Philadelphia: W. B. Saunders; Scott, J. P. [1998]. Hematology. In R. E. Behrman & R. M. Kliegman [Eds.], *Nelson's essentials of pediatrics* [3rd ed., pp. 545-582]. Philadelphia: W. B. Saunders.)

the coagulation inhibitors (antithrombin III, protein C, and protein S) function. There are 13 coagulation factors, and all but factor VIII are synthesized in the liver. The coagulation cascade can be simply described in three phases. In phase I thromboplastin is formed by the interaction of certain coagulation factors, phospholipids, and tissue factor. In phase II prothrombin (factor II) is converted to thrombin (factor IIa), and in phase III soluble fibrinogen is converted by thrombin to fibrin.[10] In contrast to clotting mechanisms, tissue plasminogen activator acts on plasminogen to initiate the clot breakdown, or fibrinolysis. This process produces plasmin, the enzyme that breaks fibrin down into split products.[29]

HISTORY OF BLOOD GROUPS

As a pioneer of blood transfusions, Landsteiner discovered the ABO blood types in 1902 and also determined that serum antibodies present on red cells cause agglutination.[7] As noted in Table 14-1, a person with a particular ABO red cell antigen (agglutinogen) possesses a corresponding serum antibody (isoagglutinin). ABO incompatibilities result from mismatched red cell antigens and serum antibodies. Blood type AB is considered the universal recipient because it possesses no serum antibodies or isoagglutinins. O is considered the universal donor because these red cells possess neither A nor B red cell antigens or agglutinogens. For example, if a supply of A red cells is not available, a type A

TABLE 14-1	ABO System Antigens and Antibodies				
Type	**Subgroups**	**Erythrocyte Antigens (Agglutinogens)**	**Serum Antibodies (Isoagglutinins)**	**Compatible RBC Type**	**Incidence in General Population**
O	None	None	Anti-A Anti-A_1 Anti-B	O	44%
A	A_1 A_2	A_1A_1 A	Anti-B	A, O	45%
B	None	B	Anti-A Anti-A_1	B, O	8%
AB	A_1B	A, A_1, B	None	O, A, B, AB	3%

From Bryant, R., & Koepke, J. (1986). Blood products. In M. J. Hockenberry-Eaton & D. K. Coody (Eds.), *Pediatric oncology and hematology* (pp. 364-379). St. Louis, MO: Mosby.

patient can be safely transfused with type O red cells because the recipient does not have serum antibodies or isoagglutinins directed against the transfused O cells.[3,18]

Wiener discovered the Rh factor and noted that 85% of individuals possess the Rh (D) antigen or agglutinogen on the surface of their red cells.[18] The remaining 15% of people do not possess the Rh (D) antigen. If Rh-negative persons receive Rh-positive cells, they almost always form antibodies to the foreign Rh (D) antigen and become immunized. For this reason blood is also tested for the Rh antigen in addition to A and B antigens.[3,18] Hundreds of blood type antigens have been described, yet the ABO and Rh systems are the only groups routinely tested before blood transfusion because they have antibodies present in the plasma without a previous exposure to an antigen.

The ability to separate the various blood components from whole blood has directed transfusion therapy toward replacement of specific component deficiencies. Several other advances have also contributed to the increased use of blood transfusions, including improved blood component preservation techniques, the establishment of blood banks, and the implementation of strict guidelines for donor centers. The introduction of plastic blood collection bags to collect each component and the discovery that each blood component possesses a different shelf life have improved blood collection and storage.

RED BLOOD CELL DEFICIENCY

Anemia is defined as a reduction in red cell mass that may be due to decreased production, increased loss, or increased destruction of RBCs. Children receiving chemotherapy and radiation therapy have diminished ability to resolve anemia because of depressed erythropoiesis (red blood cell production). Other causes of anemia include blood loss (e.g., gastrointestinal bleeding, severe epistaxis, or menorrhagia), splenic sequestration (intrasplenic pooling of blood), hemodilution (increased volume of blood plasma), hemolysis (destruction of RBCs), inflammation, infection, folate deficiency, and liver and renal disease. The clinical presentation of anemia includes signs and symptoms such as fatigue, pallor, headache, lethargy, irritability, tachycardia, hypotension, dyspnea, syncope, and possibly angina.[31-33]

TREATMENT

Anticoagulant is added to RBC units to allow storage for up to 42 days. Products containing the anticoagulant citrate phosphate dextrose adenine (CPDA-1) have a hematocrit of approximately 75% to 80%, whereas products containing an additive solution such as Adsol have a hematocrit of 55% to 60%. Because RBC units contain large numbers of leukocytes, several methods of leukocyte reduction can be used to remove or destroy the leukocytes in the product, such as saline washing, filtration, irradiation, or deglycerolization. The most commonly used method is a microaggregate filter that depletes 99.9% of the leukocytes.[4]

Children with cancer receive transfusions at varying degrees of anemia, based on institutional practice and patient conditions. Transfusions are often given to children with hemoglobin values less than 7 g/dl or those with severe fatigue, irritability, or tachycardia, but controversy surrounds the decision to give transfusions to asymptomatic children with hemoglobin values between 7 and 10 g/dl.[4] Patients receiving radiotherapy require adequate hemoglobin levels (>10 g/dl) to provide better oxygenation of the tissues being irradiated, thus theoretically increasing the effectiveness of radiation treatment.[4,13] Anemic patients undergoing surgery may also benefit from transfusion in order to tolerate anesthesia. An artificial blood substitute, perfluorochemical, is also available. This synthetic material consists of emulsified microdroplets that do not carry enough oxygen under practical conditions. It does not contain red cells and has not proved to be safe as predicted but may be indicated when there are reasons to avoid transfusion, as with Jehovah's Witness patients.[19]

NURSING IMPLICATIONS

The usual transfusion volume for children is 10 ml/kg of packed red blood cells (pRBCs) administered at a standard rate of 2 to 5 ml/kg/hr. Each unit of blood is infused over 4 hours or less. Children with severe anemia or congestive heart failure should receive repeated small aliquots of pRBCs to correct their anemia and are monitored for pulmonary congestion, tachycardia, or other signs of congestive heart failure. A helpful guide to estimate the rise in hemoglobin level after transfusion is that 10 ml/kg of pRBCs will increase the hemoglobin level by 2.5 to 3 g/dl.[4,13,14,32]

Before the transfusion, the patient's blood must be crossmatched for ABO and Rh type, and an antibody screening test must be performed. Antibody screening (Coombs' test or direct antiglobulin test) identifies antibodies in serum (indirect Coombs') and antibodies attached to the surface of the red cell (direct Coombs'). Crossmatching tests the recipient's serum against the donor's red cells to determine the presence or absence of agglutination. This testing is usually completed within 1 hour.

Whole blood transfusion is rare because separation techniques can provide the specific blood components needed. Of all the blood components the most commonly used product is pRBCs, which restores the oxygen-carrying capacity of blood with minimal volume increase. The biggest risk to the patient with chronic anemia or an extremely low hemoglobin level (<5 g/dl) is the development of congestive heart failure resulting from a rapid infusion of fluid volume. At times a partial exchange transfusion (Box 14-1) may be necessary to prevent cardiac failure and to remove damaged cells or circulating bilirubin (hyperbilirubinemia). Exchange transfusion is an attempt to replace most of the recipient's red cells and/or plasma with compatible red cells and/or plasma from donors without administration of excess fluid volume. The use of exchange transfusion for hyperleukocytosis remains controversial.

BOX 14-1

PARTIAL EXCHANGE OF PACKED RED BLOOD CELLS

INDICATIONS
Partial exchange transfusion indicated for hyperleukocytosis (controversial), sickle cell patients with acute chest syndrome, stroke, intractable pain crisis, and refractory priapism

GOAL
To reduce hemoglobin S percentage to less than 50% and to maintain hematocrit (Hct) below 35% to avoid hyperviscosity

CALCULATION
To calculate volume of pRBCs needed for double pRBC volume exchange:

$$\frac{EBV \times patient's\ Hct \times 2}{Hct\ of\ pRBCs\ (55\%\text{-}70\%)}$$

Data from Ebel, B. E., & Raffini, L. (2000). Hematology. In G. K. Siberry, & R. Iannone (Eds.), *The Harriet Lane handbook: A manual for pediatric house officers* (15th ed., p. 321). St. Louis, MO: Mosby.
EBV, estimated blood volume in milliliters (depends on age).

The nurse's role in the administration of red blood cells includes regulating the transfusion rate, critically assessing the patient, monitoring vital signs, and observing for adverse transfusion reactions. Transfusion administration policies and procedures are often institution specific. However, several key concepts are standard. The identities of the patient and blood unit are verified. The patient is observed for signs of transfusion reaction with vital signs before the administration of the pRBCs, at 10 to 15 minutes after the initiation of the transfusion, and then hourly until the completion of the transfusion. The transfusion rate is closely regulated to avoid volume overload. The use of infusion pumps for the administration of RBCs has become standard practice in many institutions. However, each infusion device must be carefully evaluated for accuracy before use. Blood warmers are in-line devices to warm the blood used on rare occasions to prevent red cell hemolysis in patients with cold agglutinins. Previously frozen blood is administered slowly, usually without warming, unless large quantities of blood are needed over a short time, in which case warming the product would prevent hypothermia and cardiac arrhythmias. Table 14-2 provides a summary of blood component therapy and nursing interventions.

Text continued on p. 354.

TABLE 14-2	BLOOD COMPONENT THERAPY AND NURSING IMPLICATIONS			
Blood Product	**Common Indications**	**Dose**	**Crossmatched**	**Nursing Implications**
Erythrocytes (packed red blood cells [pRBCs])	Renal/liver disease Myelodysplastic syndrome Hemolysis Decrease erythro- poiesis Thalassemia Splenic/liver sequestration	10-20 ml/kg of pRBCs intra- venously (IV) over 2-4 hr	ABO and Rh required	1. Assess for signs and symptoms of transfusion reactions and fluid overload (e.g., cough, tachypnea, tachycardia, weight gain, edema, dyspnea, chest pain). 2. Regulate infusion rate using micro- aggregate filter via infusion pump at 5 ml/kg/hr over 2-4 hr (usual rate). Do not use the tubing to infuse more than 1 unit of blood. 3. Monitor vital signs before trans- fusion, 15 min after initiation, then hourly until the end of transfusion. 4. Do not refrigerate blood in the nursing unit. Only the blood bank refrigerator may be used. 5. Ensure that each unit is infused in 4 hr or less. If a longer infusion time is needed, the unit must be divided. 6. Do not infuse solutions other than normal saline in the line with RBCs.
Whole blood (rarely used)	Acute massive blood loss	8 ml/kg to increase hemoglobin (Hb) 1 g/dl IV	ABO and Rh required	Measures same as for pRBCs.
Platelets (plt)	Active hemorrhage Disseminated intra- vascular coagu- lopathy (DIC) Cytotoxic therapy Irradiation Bone marrow trans- plant Thrombocytopenia (<20,000 with bleeding or as indicated by clinical status)	1 unit/10 kg IV push (IVP) or as fast as patient can tolerate	ABO and Rh preferred	1. Assess for signs and symptoms of reactions (see Table 14-3), fluid overload (see pRBCs), bleed- ing, or infection. 2. Regulate infusion rate using 170-μm micro-aggregate filter at 10 ml/kg/hr or IVP, or as fast as patient can tolerate. 3. Monitor vital signs before trans- fusion, 15 min after initiation of infusion, and at end of infusion. 4. Obtain post-platelet count 60 min to 24 hr after infusion.
Granulocyte (rarely used)	Used as adjunct to other measures for severe infections in septic neonate or high-risk patients (i.e., proven bacterial	10-15 ml/kg IV usually daily × 4 days	ABO and Rh required	1. Assess for granulocyte reactions (chills, fever, rash, and fluid overload). 2. Monitor vital signs before trans- fusion, 15 min after initiation, and at end of transfusion.

Data from Bryant, R., & Koepke, J. (1986). Blood products. In M. J. Hockenberry-Eaton & D. K. Coody (Eds.), *Pediatric oncol- ogy and hematology: Perspectives on care* (pp. 364-379). St. Louis, MO: Mosby; Buchanan, G. R. (1997). Hematologic support- ive care of the pediatric cancer patient. In P. A. Pizzo & D. G. Poplack (Eds.), *Principles and practice of pediatric oncology* (3rd ed., pp. 1051-1068). Philadelphia: Lippincott-Raven; Fitzpatrick, L., & Fitzpatrick, T. (1997). Blood transfusion: Keeping your patient safe. *Nursing, 27*(8), 34-42; Oakes, L., & Rosenthal-Dichter, C. (1998). Hematology and immunology. In M. C. Slota (Ed.), *Core curriculum for pediatric critical care nursing* (pp. 498-509). Philadelphia: W. B. Saunders.

Continued

TABLE 14-2	BLOOD COMPONENT THERAPY AND NURSING IMPLICATIONS—cont'd			
Blood Product	**Common Indications**	**Dose**	**Crossmatched**	**Nursing Implications**
Granulocyte (rarely used) —cont'd	infection in severe neutropenic patient nonresponsive to antibiotic therapy)			3. Premedicate 1 hr before transfusion —usually antihistamines, acetaminophen, steroids, or meperidine. 4. Infuse at slow rate (2-4 hr) using 170-μm blood filter 5. Recommend minimum 4-6 hr between amphotericin B and granulocyte infusions* 6. Monitor absolute neutrophil count (ANC) daily.
Fresh frozen plasma (FFP)	Deficiencies of plasma clotting factors in bleeding patients DIC, liver failure, thrombocytopenic purpura, dilutional coagulopathy, vitamin K deficiency with bleeding, and replace antithrombin III [ATIII], protein C and protein S)	10-15 ml/kg (use within 6-24 hr of thawing)	ABO required, Rh not required	1. Assess for signs and symptoms of allergic reaction, fluid overload, or infection (see Table 14-3). 2. Administer IV using microaggregate filter over 1-2 hr every 12-24 hr until hemorrhage stops,† at a rate of about 10 ml/min. 3. Monitor prothrombin time (PT) and partial thromboplastin time (PTT) levels before and after FFP. 4. May monitor other coagulation factors (e.g., fibrinogen, fibrin split products, D-Dimer, ATIII, protein C, and protein S).
Cryoprecipitate (CRYO) (rarely used)	Control bleeding in patients with DIC	4 bags/10 kg	ABO preferred, Rh not required	1. Assess for signs and symptoms of bleeding. 2. Monitor closely PT and PTT, fibrinogen, fibrinogen split products, D-Dimer. 3. Use a filter needle to draw up and administer within 15-30 min.
Intravenous immunoglobulin (IVIG)	Antibody deficiency disorders (congenital and acquired) Newborns with severe bacterial infections, posttransplant patient prophylactically, human immunodeficiency virus (HIV) infection	200-400 mg/kg IV every 3-4 wk and .5-1 g/kg in 1-2 doses for ITP patients	ABO and Rh not required	1. Assess for untoward reactions (e.g., tachycardia, flushing, fever, chills, headache). 2. Infusion rates vary, but a common guideline is to infuse slowly for first 15 to 30 min then gradually increase to maximum rate as patient tolerates.

Data from Bryant, R., & Koepke, J. (1986). Blood products. In M. J. Hockenberry-Eaton & D. K. Coody (Eds.), *Pediatric oncology and hematology: Perspectives on care* (pp. 364-379). St. Louis, MO: Mosby; Buchanan, G. R. (1997). Hematologic supportive care of the pediatric cancer patient. In P. A. Pizzo & D. G. Poplack (Eds.), *Principles and practice of pediatric oncology* (3rd ed., pp. 1051-1068). Philadelphia: Lippincott-Raven; Fitzpatrick, L., & Fitzpatrick, T. (1997). Blood transfusion: Keeping your patient safe. *Nursing97, 27*(8), 34-41; Oakes, L., & Rosenthal-Dichter, C. (1998). Hematology and immunology. In M. C. Slota (Ed.), *Core curriculum for pediatric critical care nursing* (pp. 498-509). Philadelphia: W. B. Saunders.
*Raife, T. J. (1997). Adverse effects of transfusions caused by leukocytes. *Journal of Intravenous Nursing, 20,* 238-244.
†Buchanan, G. R. (1997). Hematologic supportive care of the pediatric cancer patient. In P. A. & D. G. Poplack (Eds.), *Principles and practice of pediatric oncology* (3rd ed., pp. 1051-1068). Philadelphia: Lippincott-Raven.

TABLE 14-2	BLOOD COMPONENT THERAPY AND NURSING IMPLICATIONS—cont'd			
Blood Product	**Common Indications**	**Dose**	**Crossmatched**	**Nursing Implications**
Intravenous immuno-globulin (IVIG) —cont'd	Immunoregulatory disorders (e.g., Kawasaki disease and idiopathic thrombocytopenic purpura [ITP])			
Albumin	Used to treat patient who is both hypo-volemic and hypo-proteinemic (e.g., acute blood volume replacement, exten-sive burns, small bowel infection, acute pancreatitis)	1 g/kg = 20 ml/kg of 5% solution IV or 1 g/kg = 4 ml/kg of 25% solution IV	ABO and Rh not required	1. Assess for signs and symptoms of fluid overload and infection, chills, and rash. 2. Transfuse 5% solution 1-2 ml/min or more rapidly if patient in shock, or transfuse the 25% solution at 0.2-0.4 ml/min.
Plasma protein fraction (Plasmanate)	Volume expansion and hypoproteinemia	10-15 ml/kg per dose IV	ABO and Rh not required	1. Assess for signs and symptoms of fluid overload, infection, or sudden hypotension. 2. Infuse at 5-10 ml/min through filter provided in standard blood admin-istration set. 3. May need to slow rate if hypoten-sion develops.
Varicella zoster immune globulin (VZIG)	Immunosuppressed patients directly exposed to varicella	125 units/10 kg intramuscu-larly (IM) (maximum dose 625 units)	ABO and Rh not required	1. Assess for signs and symptoms of varicella (e.g., fever, rhinitis, maculopapular vesicular lesions). 2. Instruct parents of immunosup-pressed child at risk for varicella to notify health care provider imme-diately when child has direct vari-cella exposure (e.g., continuous household contact, direct contact with playmate or direct hospital exposure). 3. Administer IM within 96 hr after exposure to varicella. 4. Maintain strict isolation from day 10 to day 28 after exposure.

Continued

TABLE 14-2	BLOOD COMPONENT THERAPY AND NURSING IMPLICATIONS—cont'd			
Blood Product	**Common Indications**	**Dose**	**Crossmatched**	**Nursing Implications**
Rhesus D immuno-globulin 1. RhoGAM 2. Rh (D) immune globulin (Win Rho)	Rh negative mothers receive to suppress anti-antibody development Given to patients with ITP in the non-splenectomized Rh(D) positive patient	250-10,000 IV/day IM HgB >10 g/dl: 250 IU/kg/dose IV Hb <10 g/dl: 125-200 IU/kg/dose IV May repeat 125-300 IU/kg/dose IV depending on patient response	ABO and Rh not re-quired ABO not required Rh required	1. Assess for signs and symptoms of allergic reaction, which may vary from painful erythemic site to fever, chills, headache, and reduction of Hb. 2. Inspect site minimally for 1 hr after injection. 3. Administer IV doses over 3-5 min. 4. Monitor plt count day 7 and day 28 after Win Rho. 5. Do not give varicella or measles-mumps-rubella (MMR) within 3-6 mo of Rh(D) immuno-globulin (may interfere with immune response).

Follow institutional administration policies and procedures for all blood components.

Data from Bryant, R., & Koepke, J. (1986). Blood products. In M. J. Hockenberry-Eaton & D. K. Coody (Eds.), *Pediatric oncology and hematology: Perspectives on care* (pp. 364-379). St. Louis, MO: Mosby; Buchanan, G. R. (1997). Hematologic supportive care of the pediatric cancer patient. In P. A. Pizzo & D. G. Poplack (Eds.), *Principles and practice of pediatric oncology* (3rd ed., pp. 1051-1068). Philadelphia: Lippincott-Raven; Fitzpatrick, L., & Fitzpatrick, T. (1997). Blood transfusion: Keeping your patient safe. *Nursing97, 27*(8), 34-41; Oakes, L., & Rosenthal-Dichter, C. (1998). Hematology and immunology. In M. C. Slota (Ed.), *Core curriculum for pediatric critical care nursing* (pp. 498-509). Philadelphia: W. B. Saunders.

HEMATOPOIETIC GROWTH FACTORS

Rapid developments in the area of hematopoietic growth factors have led to the use of epoetin alfa (EPO), which contains an amino acid sequence identical to the endogenous serum erythropoietin. Clinical studies have demonstrated that administration of EPO significantly increases hematocrit levels and decreases transfusion requirements in patients with anemia from cancer therapy.[26]

PLATELET DEFICIENCY

Thrombocytopenia, a decrease in the number of circulating platelets, is the principal cause of bleeding in children with cancer. Thrombocytopenia may be the result of decreased platelet production, increased destruction of platelets, or sequestration of platelets in the liver or spleen.

It is uncommon for spontaneous bleeding to occur with platelet counts greater than 50,000/mm³. The risk of bleeding is increased in patients with infection, tumor lysis, hyperleukocytosis, uremia, protracted vomiting, mucositis, disseminated intravascular coagulation (DIC), or other coagulation abnormalities.[13,28] Minor bleeding episodes, evidenced by petechiae, ecchymosis, or microscopic hematuria, occur more frequently when the platelet count is less than 20,000/mm³, whereas life-threatening intracranial hemorrhage tends to occur only when the platelet count is less than 10,000/mm³.[4,14,28]

TREATMENT

Platelet transfusion in thrombocytopenic patients is indicated if there is active bleeding or if the platelet deficiency is causing or contributing to bleeding. Platelet transfusions may also be indicated for patients undergoing surgery with a platelet count of less than 50,000/mm³ or those receiving medications that interfere with platelet function, such as aspirin or ibuprofen. A threshold for transfusing platelets is sometimes set at 30,000/mm³ or 50,000/mm³ for patients with enlarging brain tumors. Controversy surrounds the issue of determining a threshold at which to transfuse platelets. The American Society of Clinical Oncology (ASCO) performed an extensive review of the literature on platelet transfusions. The review, published in 2001, recommends that the threshold for platelet transfusions in children receiving cancer therapy be set at 10,000/mm³, based on prospective randomized studies in adults. However, the recommendations included considering higher thresholds for patients with signs of hemorrhage, high fever, hyperleukocytosis, rapid decrease in the platelet count, or coagulation abnormalities, those undergoing invasive procedures, and neonates.[28] In addition to the risks for bleeding mentioned above, platelet transfusion guidelines established at each institution may also be based on the child's activity level, the presence of comorbidity such as tumor lysis syndrome, and the family's proximity to the treatment facility. Additional research in children is needed to determine the optimal use of platelet transfusions in children with thrombocytopenia in order to minimize the risk of transfusion-associated infection.

Opinion also varies about the platelet level needed before performing a lumbar puncture (LP). Administering prophylactic platelet transfusions before LPs has not been shown to reduce the risk of neurologic injury associated with LPs.[15] Lumbar punctures have been safely performed in patients with severe thrombocytopenia. In a review of 5223 LP procedures performed at St. Jude Children's Research Hospital between 1984 and 1998, there was no evidence of serious complications in 170 children undergoing LPs with a platelet count between 11,000/mm^3 and 20,000/mm^3.[15]

Platelets are obtained by centrifugation of whole blood or apheresis from a single donor and stored at 20 to 24° C for 5 days with continuous gentle agitation that prevents agglutination. They are available as pooled multiple random-donor units obtained from whole blood units or as single-donor units collected by apheresis.

Blood group–matched and Rh-compatible platelets are usually preferred. Although A and B antigens are expressed only slightly, if at all, on platelets, transfusion of incompatible platelets could result in low-grade hemolysis because of the antibodies in the plasma or the erythrocytes contaminating the platelet concentrate.[4,5] In recent years apheresis platelets have become the popular platelet source. The limited exposure to antigens in the single-donor units decreases the risk of platelet antibody production and the subsequent decrease in the effectiveness of transfused platelets.

Leukocyte depletion of platelet concentrates by filtration will further reduce the incidence of platelet refractoriness. Filtration by the newer third-generation filters removes approximately 95% of the leukocytes and can be done in the blood bank or at the bedside. Filtration also reduces the incidence of transfusion-transmitted viruses, graft-versus-host disease (GVHD), and febrile reactions. Human lymphocyte antigen (HLA)–matched platelets are recommended for patients who are thrombocytopenic and refractory to single-donor platelets.[4,5,14]

A platelet unit is defined as the number of platelets normally available in 1 unit of blood. One unit will increase the platelet count approximately 10,000 to 12,000/mm^3 in a child with a body surface area of 1 m^2.[4,14] The usual platelet dose for pediatric patients is 1 unit of random-donor platelets per 10 kg body weight.[23] The life span of the transfused platelets may be shortened by the presence of infection, fever, gross bleeding, significant splenomegaly, or platelet antibodies. Unless the child is bleeding or is at high risk for hemorrhage, platelet transfusions are avoided to decrease the likelihood of alloimmunization.

NURSING IMPLICATIONS

Nursing care includes proper administration of platelets and monitoring the patient for signs and symptoms of adverse reactions. The frequency of monitoring vital signs varies between institutions, but at a minimum they are assessed before the administration of the platelets, after 15 minutes, and at the end of the transfusion. A 1-hour or 24-hour posttransfusion platelet count is often obtained to document the effectiveness of the transfusion. Administration techniques, such as the use of infusion pumps, and infusion rates vary by institution. Several infusion devices have been studied, and no significant adverse effect on posttransfusion platelet count or corrected count increment (CCI) was noted.[20]

Recommendations for platelet infusion rates vary from IV push to over 1-hour infusions. A rapid infusion of 10 ml/kg/hr has been studied, and no adverse effects on platelet recovery or patient outcomes were noted.[21] As with any rapid infusion, the age and clinical status of the patient must be considered.

Monitoring the child's clinical condition and response to platelet transfusions includes observation for signs of bleeding or infection. The nurse must frequently assess the child's skin, stools, urine, gums, vomitus, sputum, and nasal secretions for blood. Issues for patient teaching are listed in Box 14-2.[13]

Invasive procedures such as intramuscular injections, venipuncture, lumbar puncture, and bone marrow aspirations are kept to a minimum, and puncture sites are monitored closely for bleeding, with pressure dressings applied to marrow sites. Adolescent females who experience increased bleeding during menses may need hormonal therapy to inhibit menses and minimize profound blood loss. Epistaxis occurs frequently in children, usually in the anterior nasal septum, which may be stopped with applied pressure. Nosebleeds from the posterior nasal septum are not stopped by pressure and may require nasal packing.

THROMBOPOIETIC GROWTH FACTORS

Cytokines have been shown to stimulate thrombopoiesis. In patients with temporary bone marrow failure secondary to cancer chemotherapy, the use of recombinant thrombopoietin (megakaryocyte growth factor and development factor) has been successful in initial clinical trials. Oprelvekin (Neumega) stimulates production of megakaryocyte progenitor cells and induces megakaryocyte maturation. In the near future these factors may significantly reduce the use of platelet transfusions in the cancer patient.[5]

GRANULOCYTE DEFICIENCY

Neutropenia is defined as a deficiency of circulating neutrophils with an absolute neutrophil count (ANC) less than 500/ml. Neutropenia is caused by either alteration in bone marrow production or exaggerated losses of neutrophils from the circulation. The risk of infection is inversely proportional to the ANC.[2] Nursing measures to decrease the risk of infection are included in Chapter 10. Even with the availability of several new generations of antibiotics, intravenous immunoglobulin (IVIG), and recombinant growth factors (granulocyte colony stimulating factor [G-CSF] and granulocyte macrophage colony stimulating factor [GM-CSF]), granulocyte infusions may be initiated in patients

with severe, persistent neutropenia with infection who are unresponsive to available standard therapies. Previous problems associated with granulocyte transfusions, such as the higher risk for cytomegalovirus (CMV) infection, GVHD, and acute respiratory distress syndrome (ARDS), can now be avoided with modern apheresis techniques. Although granulocyte transfusions are used very rarely, case reports suggest a beneficial role in treating fungal infections and localized infections.[34]

Indications for a course of granulocyte therapy include severe acquired neutropenia, gram-negative septicemia, and bacterial or fungal infection unresponsive after 48 to 72 hours of appropriate antibiotic or antifungal therapy. The usual granulocyte transfusion is 1 unit/day until the infection is cured, the fever resolved, and the patient's ANC is greater than 500.[14,34]

TREATMENT

Granulocyte transfusions are obtained by leukapheresis. This process separates and collects the WBCs and returns the other blood constituents to the donor. Because granulocyte concentrates contain RBC contaminants, they must be ABO and Rh compatible. To limit reactions, patients are premedicated with antihistamines, acetaminophen, steroids, and/or meperidine, and the granulocytes are infused slowly over 4 hours.[27]

Because granulocytes have a short life span, they must be infused within 24 hours of collection and are stored at 20° to 24° C until used. The usual course of granulocyte therapy consists of daily infusions (1 unit/day) for 4 to 5 days, administered as a slow infusion (2 to 4 hours) through a 170-μm filter. The administration of amphotericin B and granulocytes has been associated with respiratory distress from the sequestration of WBCs in the pulmonary vasculature. This complication can be minimized by administering them at least 4 to 6 hours apart.[23]

NURSING IMPLICATIONS

Vital signs are monitored carefully and the patient observed for chills, high fever, urticaria, and variations in pulse and respiration. If symptoms develop during the transfusion, additional diphenhydramine and/or steroids may be given intravenously. If the symptoms persist or are especially severe, the transfusion is stopped. Severe pulmonary reactions are thought to be due to the accumulation of granulocytes in the pulmonary capillaries and the activation of complement.[23] This reaction is a medical emergency that requires immediate treatment with epinephrine, antihistamines, corticosteroids, and oxygen.

GRANULOCYTE GROWTH FACTORS

With the development of colony stimulating factors such as G-CSF and GM-CSF, the need for granulocyte infusions has decreased. However, in conjunction with growth factors and other standard therapies, granulocyte infusions may lead to a more localized pyogenic reaction, which aids in the eradication of the infection.[23]

HYPOGAMMAGLOBULINEMIA

Immune deficiencies occur when one or more of the cell lines of the immune system are absent or do not function effectively. Immune deficiencies may be congenital, inherited, or acquired. These deficiencies are classified as primary when the initial condition results in an absent or inadequate functioning immune system. Secondary deficiencies are caused by another condition such as cancer or its therapy.[1] Patients with immune deficiencies present with fevers, recurrent sinus and lung infections, and other chronic infections.

IVIG is prepared from pooled plasma from at least 1000 donors and contains 95% IgG with small quantities of IgA, IgM, IgD, and IgE. IVIG enhances humoral immunity and serves as replacement therapy in both congenital and acquired immunodeficiency disorders. It has a half-life of 21 to 28 days and therefore requires repeated administration in children with chronic immunodeficiencies.[23]

TREATMENT

The gammaglobulins are commercial preparations obtained from large donor pools and therefore contain antibodies that most people have been immunized against such as measles, mumps, chickenpox, polio, diphtheria, and smallpox. They provide passive immunity because the antibodies survive 3 to 4 weeks. Therefore the gammaglobulin infusions are repeated every 2 to 4 weeks so the patient can maintain adequate immunoglobulin levels in the blood. Intravenous immunoglobulin has been approved for primary immunodeficiencies, B-cell chronic lymphocytic leukemia, idiopathic thrombocytopenic purpura, bone marrow transplant, and pediatric human immunodeficiency virus (HIV) infection.[1]

Immunoglobulin preparations are also used for prophylaxis against measles, hepatitis A, and hepatitis B. Tetanus immunoglobulin is given for prophylaxis in a nonimmunized wounded patient and rabies immunoglobulin for postexposure prophylaxis. Varicella zoster immunoglobulin (VZIG) is given for prophylaxis in an immune-suppressed patient exposed to chickenpox. IVIG is given to bone marrow transplant patients to increase immune defenses. Rh (D) immunoglobulin (RhoGAM) is given to Rh-negative mothers to suppress development of antiantibodies. Poliomyelitis immunoglobulin is given for prophylaxis in unvaccinated persons exposed to the virus.[1,13]

NURSING IMPLICATIONS

Generally the dose of immunoglobulin is 200 to 400 mg/kg every 3 to 4 weeks.[1] The infusion is started slowly and increased every 15 to 30 minutes until the maximum infusion rate is reached (most infusions run 2 to 4 hours). Infusion rate guidelines vary among brands because of the differences in the concentrations of IVIG. Because IVIG is considered a blood product, administration and monitoring is performed according to institutional policies for blood transfusions.[23]

Some common side effects of IVIG administration are flushing, headache, chills, back pain, tachycardia, nausea, and abdominal pain. Reactions are usually related to the administration rate and can often be managed by slowing the rate or briefly stopping the infusion. Premedication with antihistamines and/or steroids is common. Close assessment of the patient is required because anaphylaxis can occur.

PLASMA PROTEIN DEFICIENCY

The plasma volume expanders of choice are albumin and plasma protein fraction (PPF). Both products are heat treated, eliminating the risk of infection transmission. Albumin is used to restore or maintain blood volume in a hypovolemic patient and to correct hypoproteinemia. It is also indicated in disorders with excessive loss of albumin and/or depressed synthesis of albumin such as extensive burns.[14,23]

NURSING IMPLICATIONS

Albumin is supplied in 5% and 25% solutions; PPF in 5% solution. Dosing and administration schedules vary according to preparation. The 5% albumin solution is given at 1 g/kg, which equals 20 ml/kg, given at 1 to 2 ml/min; the 25% solution at 1 g/kg, which equals 4 ml/kg, is given at 0.2 to 0.4 ml/min. The PPF dose is 10 to 15 ml/kg given at a rate of 5 to 10 ml/min. Blood type and crossmatch are not required.[14,23]

One of the significant side effects of plasma protein administration may be sudden hypotension. To manage this side effect, slow the infusion rate until the blood pressure returns to normal. Other possible side effects of albumin administration are circulatory overload, microbial contamination, nausea and vomiting, chills, fever, and urticaria. Most can be managed with appropriate medications.

BLOOD COMPONENT TRANSFUSION REACTIONS

Any blood component can potentially cause an adverse reaction, which can range in severity from benign to fatal events. Twenty percent of all transfusions can result in an adverse reaction. This is defined as "any untoward event that happens within a few hours, weeks, or months of and as a direct result of administration of a blood product."[17] A history of multiple transfusions or prior pregnancies increases a patient's risk of developing a transfusion reaction. Table 14-3 provides a summary of the most common adverse reactions associated with transfusion therapy.

Transfusion reactions are most commonly classified as hemolytic or nonhemolytic. Hemolytic transfusion reactions usually result from infusion of blood products that are ABO or Rh incompatible. These reactions result in hemolysis of red blood cells and can be acute, delayed, intravascular, or extravascular. Nonhemolytic transfusion reactions occur more commonly and are thought to be the result of alloantibodies in the recipient's plasma reacting against HLA or other antigens on platelets and leukocytes in the transfused products. These reactions do not cause hemolysis and are usually acute in nature.[4]

HEMOLYTIC TRANSFUSION REACTIONS

The incidence of hemolytic transfusion reaction ranges from 1 per 8,300 to 1 per 33,500 with fatal hemolysis occurring in 1 per 600,000 transfusions. These reactions are especially frightening because any blood component containing red blood cells can be implicated, and the reaction can be fatal. It is estimated that 90% of all hemolytic transfusion reactions are the result of human error during collection, processing, or administration of blood components.[8,25]

Acute hemolytic transfusion reactions (AHTRs) occur when donor RBCs and recipient plasma are incompatible, and they are most commonly associated with ABO mismatch. Onset of the reaction can occur after as little as 10 to 15 ml of blood has been infused. Antibodies formed by the recipient's plasma attach to antigens on the transfused RBCs. Intravascular lysis occurs, complement is immediately activated, and lysis of the antigen is complete. When the antigen is attached, the red cell membrane to which it is bound disintegrates, producing excessive amounts of free hemoglobin resulting in hemoglobinemia. Removal of hemoglobin is accomplished primarily by the liver and kidneys. When more hemoglobin is present in the kidneys than the renal tubules can manage, hemoglobinuria (urine with a characteristic pink to port wine color)

occurs. The inflammation process is triggered, resulting in complement activation, and other processes of AHTR, including mast cell degranulation, activation of the neuroendocrine system and the clotting cascade, and organ ischemia.[8,23]

Pain at the infusion site and a "sense of impending doom" are two of the earliest symptoms of AHTR. Other clinical manifestations include fever, chills, headache, back or abdominal pain, dark urine, pallor, and jaundice. Substernal tightness, dyspnea, tachypnea, hypotension, and shock occur as the reaction becomes increasingly more severe. Early symptoms may be followed by DIC, bleeding, hemoglobinuria, and oliguria leading to acute renal failure. Abnormal laboratory results include hemoglobinuria, hyperbilirubinemia, anemia, and a positive Coombs' test or direct antiglobulin test (DAT).[4,8,23]

Prevention of this potentially life-threatening transfusion reaction is one of the most important nursing interventions associated with the administration of blood component therapy. To prevent errors resulting in this adverse reaction, two persons check the identity of the recipient and the blood product before initiating the transfusion. Information to verify includes product type, blood group, and Rh type; patient name, blood group, and Rh type; patient medical record and blood bank numbers. The patient must wear an armband including name and medical record number. The transfusion service record and labels on the bag must match for compatibility, crossmatching (if required), ABO group, unit number, expiration date of product, irradiation, CMV status, and any other information on or attached to the product. A baseline assessment of the patient, which includes vital signs, is performed before beginning the transfusion. The patient is monitored according to institutional policy. A minimum monitoring of the patient includes obtaining baseline vital signs, observing the patient for the first 15 minutes of the infusion, reassessing the patient and obtaining vital signs at the end of the first 15 minutes and then hourly until the end of the transfusion.[14]

The severity of the reaction is directly proportional to the amount of incompatible blood infused, so it is essential to stop the blood infusion immediately if a reaction is suspected. After stopping the transfusion, withdraw 3 to 5 ml of blood from the IV line for discard, flush the line with normal saline, and assess the patient's condition and vital signs. Obtain blood and urine samples for suspected blood transfusion reaction testing. Notify the physician and the blood bank of the suspected transfusion reaction. Recheck the blood bag for compatibility and the patient identification label for

Reaction	Etiology	Symptoms	Prevention	Treatment
Acute hemolytic transfusion reaction (AHTR)	Administration of incompatible blood Antibody reaction to transfused cells' antigens	Pain at infusion site, sense of impending doom, fever, chills, headache, back or abdominal pain, dark urine, pallor, jaundice, dyspnea, tachycardia, hypotension, shock, anemia	Strict adherence to institutional policy regarding administration Initiate transfusion slowly for first 15 min	Antihistamines Fluids Diuretics
Delayed hemolytic transfusion reaction	Reexposure to antigens on transfused cells	Anemia Jaundice	Strict adherence to institutional policy regarding administration	Symptomatic
Febrile nonhemolytic transfusion reaction	Recipient antibodies to granulocyte antigens	Fever Chills	Premedicate with antipyretics Leukocyte-reduced products	Antipyretics Antihistamines
Allergic reaction	Allergens in donated plasma	Urticaria Pruritus Anaphylaxis	Premedicate with antihistamines and sometimes steroids	Antihistamines Steroids Epinephrine
Bacterial contamination	Contamination during donation, processing, storage, or administration	Fever Chills Septic shock	Aseptic techniques during entire transfusion process	Antibiotics Antipyretics
Transfusion of infections	Hepatitis B and C CMV HIV	Fatigue, anorexia, right upper quadrant pain, nausea, myalgia, dark urine, jaundice Fever, splenomegaly, neutropenia Pancytopenia, opportunistic infections	Mandatory donor screening All volunteer donors Serologic testing of donated blood Leukocyte reduction by filtration	Antibiotics Antivirals Antifungals Immunoglobulins Ganciclovir
Alloimmunization	Immune response against HLA antigens	Little or no response to platelet transfusions	Leukocyte reduction by filtration Single-donor transfusions HLA-matched products	No effective treatment available
Transfusion-associated graft-versus-host disease	Proliferation of donor T lymphocytes and immune response against host cells	Fever Rash Diarrhea Hepatitis Bone marrow suppression Infection	Gamma irradiation	Symptomatic support
Circulatory overload	Excess volume	Dry cough, hypertension, dyspnea, tachycardia, sudden severe headache, edema	Volume depletion	Stop transfusion Oxygen Diuretics
Iron overload	Chronic transfusion therapy	Elevated iron levels	Judicious use of blood products	Deferoxamine mesylate

errors. Return any untransfused portion of blood to the blood bank, including the infusion tubing set. Antihistamines may be administered for signs of allergic reactions. Fluids, diuretics, and mannitol may be given to promote urine output and treat symptoms of hypotension and shock. Document the event in the patient's medical record. Documentation includes the date and time of the transfusion, unit number of the blood component, type of product and filter used, times of any filter or tubing changes, volume transfused, vital signs, observation of patient's tolerance, patient and family education provided, and any medications given to the patient.[12,14,33]

Delayed hemolytic transfusion reactions occur when RBC antibodies are present in low, undetectable levels at the time of pretransfusion testing and are stimulated to higher levels by reexposure to antigens on transfused RBCs. The higher levels of antibody can cause hemolysis of the transfused RBCs. This delayed hemolytic reaction is usually the result of previous exposure to foreign antigens through a previous transfusion or as a result of pregnancy. The inflammatory process that occurs is less severe, and complement activation is incomplete. Consequently, cell lysis does not occur intravascularly. Instead, antibody coats the cells, which are then removed to the extravascular space for destruction. These cells are sequestered in the liver, where they are lysed, causing a rise in serum bilirubin.[8] Serologic evidence of delayed transfusion reaction has been reported to occur in 0.66% of multiply transfused patients; however, clinical evidence of hemolysis occurred in only 0.12% of those patients.[25]

These delayed reactions can occur days to weeks after a transfusion and are usually self-limiting, requiring no interventions. Laboratory testing may detect a decreased hematocrit and increased bilirubin and lactic dehydrogenase (LDH) levels, and the patient may have jaundice. Side effects are rarely life threatening, and treatment is symptomatic. Meticulous verification of the patient's identification at the time of crossmatching and administration of blood products can prevent some hemolytic transfusion reactions.[8,23]

FEBRILE NONHEMOLYTIC TRANSFUSION REACTIONS

Febrile nonhemolytic transfusion reactions (FNHTRs) are the most common type of reactions associated with blood component therapy. FNHTRs are defined clinically as an elevation in body temperature of $1°C$ ($1.8°F$) or more occurring during or shortly after initiation of a blood product transfusion. These reactions make up 30% of all transfu-

sion reactions, occurring in 1% of RBC transfusions and 20% of platelet transfusions.[8,17]

The primary cause of FNHTR is the development of recipient antibodies to antigens on granulocytes and platelets in the donated product. An inflammatory process is activated, and cytokines are released. Symptoms are associated with the degranulation of white blood cells and mast cells. The release of cytokines accounts for the temperature elevation. Release of histamine and other cytokines can result in pulmonary, gastrointestinal, and cardiac symptoms. Other possible causes of FNHTR include bacterial contamination of blood products and the release of inflammatory cytokines from leukocytes contained in the plasma that accumulate in the blood product during storage.[8,16,17,24]

Although uncomfortable for the patient, FNHTRs are generally not life threatening. Clinical manifestations include fever and chills shortly after initiating a transfusion and tachycardia, hypotension, and tachypnea as the reaction progresses. Most often symptoms occur shortly after the initiation of a transfusion (within 30 minutes) but may occur up to 12 hours later.

Because fever is a sign of AHTR, any reaction that produces fever must be considered serious. Nursing interventions when fever is present include immediately stopping the transfusion, maintaining a patent IV line with normal saline, drawing blood cultures from the patient, and sending the unit and tubing to the blood bank for bacterial cultures and testing to rule out a hemolytic transfusion reaction. Antibiotics may be ordered in the neutropenic patient. Further management is symptomatic. Acetaminophen is given to decrease the fever, meperidine may be used to reduce the chills, and corticosteroids may be used to reduce the inflammatory process. Because the formation of antibodies causing the FNHTR requires previous exposure to blood products, patients with a history of febrile reactions to blood therapy and chronically transfused patients may benefit from premedication with acetaminophen with or without diphenhydramine or steroids and leukocyte-reduced products. Leukocyte-reduction by filtration has been effective in reducing the incidence of FNHTR and is recommended for patients who are candidates for chronic transfusion therapy.[8,16,17,23] Filtration of platelet products with the standard 170-μm platelet filter is not sufficient to reduce the leukocyte concentration.[8]

ALLERGIC REACTIONS

Allergic transfusion reactions are due to allergens found in the plasma of donated blood products. When transfused into a sensitive recipient, antibodies against the allergen will develop. An allergic response will then occur with the second encounter with the same allergen. The incidence of allergic reactions associated with transfusions is 1% to 3% of blood product infusions.[8] Anaphylaxis is estimated to occur in 1 per 150,000 transfusions and usually has a fatal outcome.[8,17,22]

The clinical manifestations of allergic transfusion reaction range from mild, localized skin erythema and pruritis, to severe, progressing to anaphylaxis. Symptoms include urticaria, pruritus, swollen lips, vomiting, hypotension, wheezing, laryngeal edema, anxiety, and irritability. Fever and hemolysis are not associated with allergic reactions.

Management of allergic transfusion reactions is aimed at halting the allergic process. When a patient begins to complain of itching or rash, the infusion must be stopped and an antihistamine, such as diphenhydramine, administered. If the symptoms of localized allergic reaction resolve and there is no evidence of fever, the transfusion may continue. This is the only type of transfusion reaction in which the transfusion can be continued or restarted, because symptoms of a localized allergic reaction are not dose related. If recurrent allergic reactions occur, routine premedication with an antihistamine and possibly a steroid is indicated. In addition, these patients may benefit from washed or frozen cells to remove the plasma proteins. Leukocyte reduction will not prevent this type of reaction, because filtration does not remove the plasma proteins. If bronchospasm or other life-threatening symptoms occur, the unit must be discontinued and an IV line maintained with new tubing. The immediate administration of antihistamines, steroids, and epinephrine is recommended. Respiration may be assisted with oxygen by nasal cannula or face mask. Intubation and treatment of shock may be required if the reaction progresses.[16,17,22,23]

BACTERIAL CONTAMINATION

Bacterial contamination, although a rare complication, may occur anytime during the donation, processing, storage, or administration of blood products. It is estimated that the risk of transfusion-associated bacterial sepsis is 1 per 500,000 red blood cell units transfused and 1 per 4200 platelet units transfused.[6] The infrequent incidence of bacterial contamination can be attributed to the closed blood collecting systems used during the donation process. In addition, screening donors for fever, recent dental work, and other signs of infection decreases the likelihood of bacterial contamination of blood products. Bacterial contamination is more likely to occur in products that are stored at room temperature, such as platelets, or products requiring thawing in a water bath before infusing, such as FFP.

Clinical manifestations generally occur within 30 minutes of initiation of the transfusion. Signs and symptoms include shaking chills, fever, vomiting, diffuse erythema, and hypotension leading to shock. Hemoglobinuria, acute renal failure, and DIC follow. The diagnosis is confirmed by Gram's stain and bacterial cultures of residual blood in the blood bag and/or tubing. Nursing interventions include immediately stopping the transfusion and obtaining blood samples from the patient and the product for bacterial cultures. Supportive therapy is provided to the patient in the form of broad-spectrum antibiotics, IV fluids, and vasopressors.[17,23]

TRANSFUSION OF INFECTIONS

Mandatory screening of donor blood for hepatitis B and C, HIV, and CMV has significantly decreased the risk of transmission of infectious diseases by donated blood in the United States. Standard infectious disease screening of blood in the United States includes the following tests: HIV-1 and HIV-2 antibody enzyme immunoassay (EIA), HIV-1 p24 antigen EIA, human T cell lymphotropic virus-I/II antibody EIA, hepatitis B surface antigen EIA, hepatitis C antibody EIA, anti–hepatitis B core antibody EIA, alanine transaminase (ALT), and syphilis. CMV serologic testing can be added when CMV-negative blood products are needed for immunocompromised populations.[27] Transmission of infections is greatest with paid donors, multiple transfusions, and pooled plasma products. Posttransfusion hepatitis, HIV, and CMV infection are the most serious transfusion-related diseases.

Children with cancer continue to be at risk of developing hepatitis from transfused blood. Because of their life expectancy, they may be at greater risk for serious liver disease as they age. In the past, hepatitis B was the most common type of transfusion-related hepatitis. With exclusive use of volunteer donors and more sensitive laboratory testing, the estimated risk of posttransfusion hepatitis B infection is currently 1 per 300,000 units transfused.[4,16] Hepatitis C has now replaced hepatitis B in the United States as the primary cause of transfusion-related hepatitis. Laboratory testing of donated blood has reduced the risk of acquiring hepatitis C from a single unit of donated blood to approximately 1 per 3300.[4] This testing was not readily available before July 1992. Thus long-term survivors of childhood cancer who received blood products need testing for the hepatitis C virus.

The risk of transfusion-related HIV infection is 2000-fold lower now than in the mid-1980s. This reduction in transmission rates via blood products is a direct result of nationwide serologic testing for HIV antibodies in donated blood, automatic discarding of all antibody-positive blood, diligent donor history screening, and confidential donor self-exclusion. Currently the estimated risk of HIV infection transmission is 1 for every 325,000 units of blood transfused. It is anticipated that application of newer testing methods will decrease the estimated risk to 1 in 625,000.[16]

Transfusion-acquired CMV infection is a major cause of morbidity and mortality in severely immunocompromised CMV-seronegative patients. The incidence of CMV infections in CMV-seronegative bone marrow transplant recipients has been as high as 28% in the past.[27] CMV is transmitted by blood via the lymphocytes. In the immunocompetent host, transfusion-associated CMV infection causes a mild mononucleosis type of infection about 1 month after transfusion. However, in the immunocompromised host without serologic evidence of prior CMV infection, CMV can cause a fatal systemic infection with pneumonia, hepatitis, hemolytic anemia, and thrombocytopenia.[4,16] To prevent CMV infection in seronegative bone marrow transplant recipients, CMV-negative donors are used. Unfortunately, only 30% to 50% of donors are seronegative, which makes it especially difficult for some blood banks to provide the volume of CMV-negative products needed. Removal of leukocytes by filtration has demonstrated a reduction in CMV exposure and is currently recommended to prevent CMV infection in any immunocompromised patient.[4,16,27] Other preventative measures used in bone marrow transplant patients include intravenous immunoglobulin, ganciclovir, and hyperimmune CMV globulin preparations.[4]

ALLOIMMUNIZATION

Class I and class II HLAs are cell membrane proteins that function by binding and presenting antigens for recognition by T lymphocytes. All nucleated cells and platelets express cell surface class I HLA antigens; among blood cells, only B lymphocytes express class II HLA antigens. When transfused from one individual to another, class I and class II HLA antigens on lymphocyte membranes can stimulate immune responses against HLA antigens. Graft rejection and failed responses to platelet transfusions are the major clinical complications resulting from HLA alloimmunization. Because prior sensitization to HLA antigens present on transplanted organs can lead to graft rejection, avoiding exposure to leukocyte-containing blood products is a common precaution. Failure to respond to platelet transfusions may be due to the binding of alloantibodies in transfusion recipients to class I HLA antigens present on transfused platelets. This antibody

binding leads to sequestration and destruction of transfused platelets.[24]

HLA alloimmunization is a well-recognized complication of platelet transfusions and can result in the patient becoming refractory to platelet transfusions. Studies have demonstrated that the rate of HLA alloimmunization ranges from 20% to 70% (median 35% to 40%) with the use of unfiltered blood components.[24] Refractoriness to platelet transfusions is a serious and difficult complication for patients receiving myelosuppressive therapy. If a patient does not respond to random-donor platelets, apheresis platelets from a single donor will reduce donor exposures and may decrease the risk of alloimmunization. Many studies have shown leukocyte reduction to be an effective method of decreasing the incidence of HLA alloimmunization. When platelet refractoriness is suspected, additional laboratory screening to detect antiplatelet antibodies that bind to the HLA-A and HLA-B antigens can be used to determine whether the refractoriness is due to alloimmunization. At this point, HLA-matched platelet transfusions from single donors may be required to treat the patient's thrombocytopenia. Most recently a prospective, multiinstitutional, randomized, blinded study—the Trial to Reduce Alloimmunization to Platelets (TRAP)—was conducted, comparing the rate of alloimmunization in patients with acute myelogenous leukemia (AML) receiving different types of platelet products. The TRAP study demonstrated that patients receiving either ultraviolet B (UVB) irradiated or leukoreduced products had a significantly lower rate of alloimmunization and platelet refractoriness compared with those receiving untreated platelets.[24,27,31]

Leukocyte reduction by filtration remains the most common method used to decrease the incidence of alloimmunization. The filters currently available commercially consistently reduce residual leukocyte content to less than 5×10^6 leukocytes per unit.[24]

TRANSFUSION-ASSOCIATED GRAFT-VERSUS-HOST DISEASE

Transfusion-associated graft-versus-host disease (TA-GVHD), although rare, can be life threatening in immunocompromised and immunodeficient patients. Those at risk of developing this complication include bone marrow transplant patients, patients with hematologic malignancies, premature infants, patients with congenital immunodeficiencies, and patients with advanced solid tumors receiving high-dose cytotoxic and/or immunosuppressive therapies. TA-GVHD can occur after a blood component transfusion containing viable T lymphocytes. Transfused leukocytes are recognized and cleared from the circulation by phagocytic cells in most recipients of blood transfusions. However, in the patients who develop TA-GVHD, this normal immune surveillance fails and the lymphocytes survive, proliferate, and mount an immune response against the host cells. The clinical manifestations often present 3 days to 1 month after transfusion and are usually severe. Classical symptoms include fever, maculopapular skin rash, watery diarrhea, and liver dysfunction. Pancytopenia develops as the proliferating donor lymphocytes attack the recipient's bone marrow. The mortality associated with TA-GVHD approaches 90%, with most patients dying of severe infections.[24]

Irradiation of blood products is the safest and most cost-efficient method to prevent TA-GVHD, and this has been adopted as the standard of practice. Irradiation renders the lymphocyte incapable of replication, without altering the function of the transfused cells. The currently recommended gamma irradiation dose is 25 to 30 Gy. Products are irradiated in the blood bank just before administration. Only cellular blood products and fresh plasma are irradiated, because TA-GVHD is not reported with fresh frozen plasma (frozen and thawed) or cyroprecipitate.[22,24,27]

CIRCULATORY OVERLOAD

Although any blood or fluid product may lead to circulatory overload, red cell products, plasma products, and albumin 25% are the blood components most commonly associated with this complication. Patients at greatest risk for developing circulatory overload include infants and young children, older adults, and persons with cardiac or pulmonary compromise. Transfusion volumes must be monitored closely, particularly in children weighing less than 20 kg, and must not exceed 15 ml/kg per transfusion. Circulatory overload can develop rapidly and present as an increase in systolic blood pressure (>50 mm Hg rise), the presence of rales, severe headache, dyspnea, tachycardia or a gallop, and apprehension or restlessness. Because symptoms can develop suddenly, early recognition of symptoms and close monitoring of patients at risk are important. If symptoms are observed, the transfusion must be stopped immediately. Place the patient in an upright position, and administer oxygen to support respiration. Diuretics may be ordered to aid in fluid elimination, and digitalization may improve heart contractility.[9]

IRON OVERLOAD

Iron overload is a complication of chronic transfusion therapy. Patients at risk for this complication include children with hemoglobinopathies, such as sickle cell anemia and thalassemia. The quantity of iron administered with blood transfusions is greater than that which can be excreted. This results in iron deposits in tissues throughout the body, which can ultimately lead to organ damage. The organs most often affected are the heart and liver. An iron-chelating agent, deferoxamine mesylate, prevents or may correct this complication.[23]

Despite the associated risks and expense of blood component therapy, blood product support has allowed for the delivery of intensive, curative treatments for children with cancer. Future challenges include improving hematopoietic growth factors, ensuring adequate supplies of blood components, and decreasing infection transmission risks. Blood transfusion therapy will remain a key treatment modality in the care of children with cancer. Consequently, pediatric oncology nurses must remain knowledgeable regarding current trends in practice and continue to provide meticulous nursing assessment, prompt interventions, and thorough patient education associated with blood component therapy.

REFERENCES

1. Banks, M. A. (1994). Home infusion of intravenous immunoglobulin. *Journal of Intravenous Nursing, 17,* 299-310.
2. Baebner, R. L. (1996). Neutropenia. In R. E. Behrman (Ed.), *Nelson textbook of pediatrics* (15th ed., pp. 587-591). Philadelphia: W. B. Saunders.
3. Bryant, R., & Koepke, J. (1986). Blood products. In M. J. Hockenberry-Eaton & D. K. Coody (Eds.), *Pediatric oncology and hematology: Perspectives on care* (pp. 364-379). St. Louis, MO: Mosby.
4. Buchanan, G. R. (1997). Hematologic supportive care of the pediatric cancer patient. In P. A. Pizzo & D. G. Poplack (Eds.), *Principles and practice of pediatric oncology* (3rd ed., pp. 1051-1068). Philadelphia: Lippincott-Raven.
5. Cahill, M. R., & Lilleyman, J. S. (1998). The rational use of platelet transfusions in children. *Seminars in Thrombosis and Hemostasis, 24,* 567-575.
6. Chamberland, M., & Khabbaz, R. F. (1998). Emerging issues in blood safety. *Infectious Disease Clinics of North America, 12,* 217-229.
7. Coffland, F. I., & Shelton, D. M. (1993). Blood component replacement therapy. *Critical Care Nursing Clinics of North America, 5,* 543-556.
8. Cook, L. S. (1997). Blood transfusion reactions involving an immune response. *Journal of Intravenous Nursing, 20,* 5-14.
9. Cook, L. S. (1997). Nonimmune transfusion reactions: When type-and-cross match aren't enough. *Journal of Intravenous Nursing, 20,* 15-22.

10. Corrigan, J. J. (1996). Hemorrhagic and thrombotic diseases. In R. E. Behrman (Ed.), *Nelson textbook of pediatrics* (15th ed., pp. 1422-1427). Philadelphia: W. B. Saunders.

11. Esmon, C. T. (1998). Blood coagulation. In D. G. Nathan & S. O. Oski (Eds.), *Nathan and Oski's hematology of infancy and childhood* (5th ed., pp. 1531-1556). Philadelphia: W. B. Saunders.

12. Fitzpatrick, L., & Fitzpatrick, T. (1997). Blood transfusion: Keeping your patient safe. *Nursing, 27*(8), 34-42.

13. Foley, M. K. (1993). Nursing management of the child or adolescent with blood component deficiencies. In G. V. Foley, D. Fochtman, & K. H. Mooney (Eds.), *Nursing care of the child with cancer* (2nd ed., pp. 385-396). Philadelphia: W. B. Saunders.

14. Holecek, R. (1998). Blood product support. In M. J. Hockenberry-Eaton (Ed.), *Essentials of pediatric oncology nursing: A core curriculum* (pp. 176-180). Glenview, IL: Association of Pediatric Oncology Nurses.

15. Howard, S., Gajjar, A., Ribeiro, R., et al. (2000). Safety of lumbar puncture for children with acute lymphocytic leukemia and thrombocytopenia. *Journal of the American Medical Association, 284,* 2222-2224.

16. Kevy, S. V., & Gorlin, J. B. (1998). Red cell transfusion. In D. G. Nathan, & S. O. Oski (Eds.), *Nathan and Oski's hematology of infancy and childhood* (5th ed., pp. 1784-1801). Philadelphia: W. B. Saunders.

17. Labovich, T. M. (1997). Transfusion therapy: Nursing implications. *Clinical Journal of Oncology Nursing, 1,* 61-72.

18. Luban, N. L. C. (1995). Blood groups and blood component transfusion. In D. R. Miller, & R. L. Baethner (Eds.), *Blood diseases of infancy and childhood* (7th ed., pp. 54-108). St. Louis, MO: Mosby.

19. Marelli, T. R. (1994). Use of a hemoglobin substitute in the anemic Jehovah's Witness patient. *Critical Care Nurse, 14,* 31-38.

20. Norville, R., Hinds, P., Willimas, J., et al. (1994). The effects of infusion methods on platelet count, morphology, and corrected count increment in children with cancer: In vitro and in vivo studies. *Oncology Nursing Forum, 21,* 1669-1673.

21. Norville, R., Hinds, P., Willimas, J., et al. (1997). The effects of infusion rate on platelet outcomes and patient responses in children with cancer: An in vitro and in vivo study. *Oncology Nursing Forum, 24,* 1789-1793.

22. Nugent, D. J. (1998). Platelet transfusion. In D. G. Nathan & S. O. Oski (Eds.), *Nathan and Oski's hematology of infancy and childhood* (5th ed., pp. 1802-1817). Philadelphia: W. B. Saunders.

23. Oakes, L., & Rosenthal-Dichter, C. (1998). Hematology and immunology. In M. C. Slota (Ed.,), *Core curriculum for pediatric critical care nursing* (pp. 498-509). Philadelphia: W. B. Saunders.

24. Raife, T. J. (1997). Adverse effects of transfusions caused by leukocytes. *Journal of Intravenous Nursing, 20,* 238-244.

25. Reid, M. E., & Toy, P. T. Y. (1998). Erythrocyte blood groups in transfusion. In D. G. Nathan & S. O. Oski, (Eds.), *Nathan and Oski's hematology of infancy and childhood* (5th ed., pp. 1160-1783). Philadelphia: W. B. Saunders.

26. Rieger, P. T., & Haeuber, D. (1995). A new approach to managing chemotherapy-related anemia: Nursing implications of epoetin alfa. *Oncology Nursing Forum, 22,* 71-81.

27. Rossetto, C. L., & McMahon, J. E. (2000). Current and future trends in transfusion therapy. *Journal of Pediatric Oncology Nursing, 17,* 160-173.

28. Schiffer, C. A., Anderson, K. C., Bennett, C. L., et al. (2001). Platelet transfusion for patients with cancer: Clinical practice guidelines of the American Society of Clinical Oncology. *Journal of Clinical Oncology, 19,* 1519-1538.

29. Scott, J. P. (1998). Hematology. In R. E. Behrman & R. M. Kliegman (Eds.), *Nelson's essentials of pediatrics* (3rd ed., pp. 545-582). Philadelphia: W. B. Saunders.

30. Sieff, C. A., Nathan, D. G., & Clark, S. C. (1998). The anatomy and physiology of hematopoiesis. In D. G. Nathan & S. O. Oski (Eds.), *Nathan and Oski's hematology of infancy and childhood* (5th ed., pp. 161-210). Philadelphia: W. B. Saunders.

31. The Trial to Reduce Alloimmunization to Platelets (TRAP) Study Group. (1997). Leukocyte reduction and ultraviolet B irradiation of platelets to prevent alloimmunization and refractoriness to platelet transfusions. *New England Journal of Medicine, 337,* 1861-1869.

32. Wilson, K. (1998). Bone marrow suppression. In M. J. Hockenberry-Eaton (Ed.), *Essentials of pediatric oncology nursing: A core curriculum* (pp. 120-121). Glenview, IL: Association of Pediatric Nurses.

33. Worrall, L. M., Tompkins, C. A., & Rust, D. M. (1999). Recognizing and managing anemia. *Clinical Journal of Oncology Nursing, 3,* 153-160.

34. Wuest, D. L. (1996). Transfusion and stem cell support in cancer treatment. *Hematology/Oncology Clinics of North America, 10,* 397-421.

15

Family-Centered Psychosocial Care

Carolyn L. Walker
Linda Mathis Wells
Sue P. Heiney
Debra P. Hymovich

As the number of survivors of childhood cancers has increased over the past 3 decades, there has been a corresponding increase in the awareness of the psychosocial impact of the disease and treatment on the child and family. The diagnosis typically causes fear and anxiety in the entire family. Treatments are complex and intense, often with long-term effects that must be monitored long past treatment. A multidisciplinary approach is required to attain a positive outcome. Each member of the team plays either a primary or a supportive role in facilitating positive psychological outcomes for the child and family. This involvement occurs by being aware of the child as a developing person and that all aspects of care impact the child's adjustment. Health care team members need to be knowledgeable about primary role functions of other health care professionals, especially areas of role overlap. In general, oncologists manage the physical disease; nurses implement and coordinate treatment and education; psychologists or mental health clinical nurse specialists may be needed to assist the child/family in coping; social workers may assist with financial difficulties, emotional support, and any necessary referrals; and in addition to child life workers, all of the team provide emotional support (individual or group) to the child and family.[37] In addition to this core group of multidisciplinary team members, physical and occupational therapists, teachers, school nurses, and many others may be needed during or after treatment.

Psychosocial interventions must be individualized with respect to the child's developmental stage, treatment demands, specific needs of each family member, and the family's cultural background. In general, nurses must be sensitive to cultural diversity within the American-born population and to cultural variations within families from other lands. Health care professionals need to be aware of culturally defined health beliefs and practices that may help explain nonadherence to conventional therapies, the degree and quality of parents' involvement in the child's care, and the family's relationship to the health care staff.[14] Nurses' knowledge of and respect for cultural differences guide assessment, nursing interventions, and the expression of the therapeutic relationship. Books such as *Culture and Nursing Care: A Pocket Guide*[46] provide extensive information about most cultures and are an excellent resource. Boxes 15-1 and 15-2 present questions that can guide the assessment of religious beliefs and the effects of culture on health care.

DEVELOPMENTAL THEORETICAL FRAMEWORK

Knowledge of normal growth and development throughout the life span provides the basis for communication between the nurse and the child and family. Piaget's cognitive development theory is fundamental to understand how children conceptualize events and how best to explain the disease and treatment (Table 15-1).[54] For example, when the nurse tells the child that only a "little bit" of blood is needed and then draws 10 ml of blood in several test tubes, how does a 5-year-old child conceptualize this volume? Young children perceive that amount as "a lot" of blood and fear that it is "too much." Children need an explanation that is grounded in their own experiences. Using Piagetian theory, the nurse could explain that children have approximately a half-gallon milk carton's amount of blood in their bodies and that the blood specimen is only 2 teaspoons. Since young children do not understand volume well, the nurse needs to demonstrate removing 2 teaspoons of water from an appropriate-sized container. Children would then be reassured that their body has enough blood.

Using preoperational thought, children make sense of the world through imaginative play, questions, talking, listening, and experimentation.

BOX 15-1

QUESTIONS TO ASSESS RELIGIOUS BELIEFS

GENERAL
Does the child and family practice any particular religion or faith?
How does the child and family use spirituality to cope? Is it helping?
Can you contact their faith leader?

RITUALS
Does the child/family participate in particular rituals (e.g., baptism, cleansing rituals, time/special location for prayers)?
Does the child wear special garments or jewelry (e.g., head cover, amulets)?

DIET
Are there any dietary restrictions?
Are there any periods of fasting that are required?

MEDICAL CARE
Are there any limitations or restrictions of medical or surgical procedures (e.g., blood transfusions, avoiding porcine heparin)?

Are faith healers used, or is the laying on of hands practiced?
Is there anointing of the ill?
Is illness viewed as the result of sin or error?

GENDER
Does religion affect the child's/family's views of gender roles?

DEATH
Are there special rites or practices that are required?
Is the presence of clergy/priest/religious advisor needed or desired?
Does the family believe in any afterlife?
Does religion affect the family's decisions regarding organ donation or autopsy?
Is there any particular mourning ritual?

Data from Wong, D. L. (1997). *Whaley and Wong's essentials of pediatric nursing* (5th ed., pp. 31-59). St. Louis, MO: Mosby.

BOX 15-2

QUESTIONS TO ASSESS EFFECTS OF CULTURE ON HEALTH CARE

HEALTH BELIEFS
How is the body viewed? Is illness seen as an "imbalance" in the body or in life? (Many cultures believe in a balance of "cold" and "hot.")
What impact do evil or supernatural spirits have on health?

HEALTH PRACTICES
Do you use folk healers, herbs, acupuncture, purification practices, spiritual healers, amulets, religious medals, prayer, or special diets to enhance health?

FAMILY RELATIONSHIPS
What is the role of the extended family?
What are the roles and values of each family member (especially children and elderly persons)?

COMMUNICATION PATTERNS
Who speaks for the family?
How are health care decisions made?
Is there a willingness to ask questions of those in authority?
Is it acceptable to openly express emotions?
What is the use and importance of nonverbal communication?
Is direct eye contact acceptable? desirable? prohibited?

Data from Wong, D. L. (1997). *Whaley and Wong's essentials of pediatric nursing* (5th ed., pp. 31-59). St. Louis, MO: Mosby.

Preschool-age children need opportunities to explore and gain experience with pretend objects and situations before experiencing them. This can be achieved by allowing them time for imaginative play (e.g., with dolls and syringes without needles) and by providing simple answers to their questions. The preschool-age child typically attributes life qualities to the doll (animistic thought) and through the doll acts out procedures such as dressing changes and intrusive procedures (Figure 15-1).

TABLE 15-1	JEAN PIAGET'S THEORY OF COGNITIVE DEVELOPMENT	
Stage	**Age (Years)**	**Characteristics**
Sensorimotor	0-2	Immediate perceptual and motor events dominate
		Interacts actively with environment
		Develops reflex activity into purposeful actions
		Develops hand-mouth, eye-hand coordination
		Learns that objects exist when out of sight (object permanence)
		Learns limits of own body
		Separates self as person apart from others
Preoperational	2-7	Uses language to express thinking
• Preconceptual		Begins to use symbols mentally
• Intuitive		Thinks egocentrically (e.g., "The sun follows me wherever I go")
		Uses self as a standard for others
		Subjective judgments still dominate perceptions
Concrete operational	7-11 or 12	Begins various forms of conservation (holds one-dimension invariant when changes in other dimensions of an object occur)
		Grasps reversibility of objects (water→steam→water)
		Can solve concrete problems
		Organizes objects and events into classes (classification) or along a continuum of increasing values (seriation)
Formal operational	12-15	Can deal with hypothetical-deductive situations
		Can plan and implement scientific approach to problem solving
		Systematically handles combinations

Data from Hall, M., Hardin, K., & Conaster, C. (1982). The challenges of psychosocial care. In D. Fochtman & G. Foley (Eds.) *Nursing care of the child with cancer.* Boston: Little, Brown, & Co; Schuster, C. S., Ashburn, S. S. (1992). *The process of human development: A holistic life-span approach* (3rd ed.). Philadelphia: J. B. Lippincott.

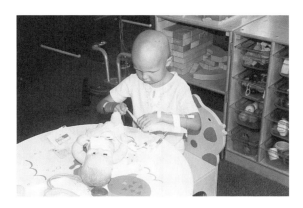

Figure 15-1

Medical play allows the child to gain experience with medical equipment and procedures.

School-age children are capable of conceptual thinking in combination with concrete images. Through memory, they integrate information about self, the problem, and the goal. Before the age of formal operations, children are not capable of abstract thought. Because most of the concepts relevant to cancer and its treatment are abstract and foreign to children, explanations must be related to their world of experience and in simple concrete terms. Blood running through a vein can be likened to water going through a garden hose. Cancer cells could be understood as an enemy army being tracked down by a good army of medicines.

Adolescents are capable of hypothetical-deductive reasoning. They usually focus on "if-then" scenarios related to desired goals: "If I complete my medical treatment, then I can graduate from school."

Erikson's psychosocial developmental theory helps nurses identify age-related developmental tasks[17] and enables them to foster the child's successful progression through each stage (Table 15-2). Erikson believed that basic resolution of each developmental task or "conflict" is built upon mastery or successful completion of the previous stage. A child must have a basic foundation of trust to be secure enough to develop autonomy. Thwarting the child's development of autonomy, for example, would lead to feelings of shame and doubt. Without a basic foundation of autonomy, children would be limited in their ability to master a sense of initiative. Because stages are seldom completely mastered, each new situation could ignite old conflicts. Nurses need to be cognizant of ways to enhance

TABLE 15-2	ERIKSON'S THEORY OF PSYCHOSOCIAL DEVELOPMENT	
Stage	**Age**	**Conflict**
Trust versus mistrust	Infancy	Learns basic trust (feeling of security with self, others, and world in general) or mistrust from person who meets needs for food, comfort, shelter
Autonomy versus shame and doubt	Toddler	Learns independent actions are acceptable (autonomy) or unacceptable (shame and doubt)
Initiative versus guilt	Preschool	Explores skills, even to the point of being intrusive (initiative) Believes tasks, questions, actions are inappropriate (guilt)
Industry versus inferiority	School-age	Seeks to master and refine physical, social, and intellectual skills learned in preschool years (industry) or if unable to excel or meet expectations, may want to quit (inferiority)
Identity versus role confusion	Adolescent	Perception of self is internally consistent (identity) or internally inconsistent (role confusion)
		Perception of self is in harmony with perception of others (identity) or is in disagreement with perception of others (role confusion)
		Tries out roles in all areas of life (e.g., moral, intellectual, sexual)
		Uses peer group for reality testing
		Condemns or ridicules those unlike self
Intimacy versus isolation	Young adult	Shares self with others in friendships and love relationships (intimacy) or keeps self uninvolved with others (isolation)

Data from Hall, M., Hardin, K., & Conaster, C. (1982). The challenges of psychosocial care. In D. Fochtman & G. Foley (Eds.) *Nursing care of the child with cancer.* Boston: Little, Brown, & Co; Schuster, C. S., & Ashburn, S. S. (1992). *The process of human development: A holistic life-span approach* (3rd ed.). Philadelphia: J. B. Lippincott.

and foster all developmental stages. For example, encouraging parental presence or performing procedures in a treatment room rather than the infant's bed can enhance an infant's development of trust. A toddler's or preschooler's autonomy can be encouraged by giving the child choices. Mastering the skills needed to perform a flush on a central venous access device can enhance a school-age child's sense of industry. Facilitating ongoing relationships and sense of connection with peers can encourage the adolescent's sense of identity.

PSYCHOSOCIAL IMPACT OF CANCER ON THE CHILD

Despite advances in the treatment of pediatric cancers and psychosocial care, children with malignancies remain at risk for psychological dysfunction. Although very few patients develop a major depression or thought disorder, adjustment disorders have been reported.[3] The focus of psychosocial nursing care is to identify periods of distress and to develop ways to mediate these issues. The long-term goal is to promote the child's mental health and development. The psychological impact on the child with cancer begins with the shock, disbelief, and inconvenience of treatment. These are overlaid with the constant stress of living with a life-threatening illness. Peak times of distress occur at diagnosis, induction, completion of therapy, and relapse. Although some problems occur or recur throughout treatment, the various stages of treatment often present different areas of concern for the patient.[4,43]

PHASES OF TREATMENT

Diagnosis and Beginning of Treatment

The child may begin to feel the impact of cancer on his or her life before diagnosis. The child may have pain and undergo multiple physical examinations, blood tests, and antibiotic therapy before a diagnosis of cancer is suspected. The child may arrive at the pediatric hematology-oncology clinic with preconceived fears and mistrust of hospital staff and treatments. During the diagnostic period, the necessary work-up, which includes multiple invasive and painful procedures, does not alleviate these fears. Instead, the child may develop procedural-related distress that makes further testing and treatment more difficult.

Before the 1970s most children were not told the diagnosis and prognosis in an effort to protect the child from additional anxiety. That strategy was not particularly successful and sometimes led to problems with trust.[42] As children lived longer, their cooperation became essential and their need to know the diagnosis increased. Children should be told about the diagnosis in consultation with the parents.[28] The child's reaction may be disbelief, anger, fear, or frustration, which is exhibited through tears, outbursts of temper, inappropriate laughter or remarks, or silence. Denial may be so great that the child physically and emotionally turns away from the discussion. Additionally, the child may have greater emotional stress if he believes that feelings of fear and apprehension must be masked to protect the parents and other family members. The child's response may change or become more intense as the physician and nurse discuss treatment issues. These emotions are even more heightened as induction, the first phase of treatment, begins. During induction the child experiences psychological distress related to treatment and side effects.[43]

Surgery

Some children will have a surgical procedure, which may be done to complete the diagnostic work-up, establish staging of the tumor, facilitate full resection of a tumor, or place a central venous access device. Regardless of the severity of surgery, the patient will experience fears and some degree of pain. Certain types of surgery, such as amputation or creation of an ostomy, can result in long-term stressors, including loss of function and changes in body image. Occasionally an adolescent's fears appear out of context to an adult. Displaying a greater reaction to the cosmetic effect of the incision (how she will look in a bathing suit) may indicate that the adolescent is more concerned with the developmental issue of body image than with the meaning of surgery or cancer.[75]

Radiation therapy

Although noninvasive and painless, radiation treatment and its side effects may cause the child considerable distress. During simulation and treatment, the child must remain very still on the treatment table. This is a difficult process, because concentration is required to prevent movement. The stress is compounded if the child worries about remaining motionless. Another emotional concern is the stigma of the radiation marks and the misconceptions about radiation (e.g., becoming "radioactive").

Chemotherapy-induced side effects

Chemotherapy-induced side effects may result in high levels of stress and anxiety throughout treatment. For example, chemotherapy-related nausea and vomiting are aversive experiences, and painful mucositis is a significant stressor. Conditioned anxiety in anticipation of the actual treatment occurs concomitantly with recurrent diagnostic and treatment procedures. It can manifest as nausea, vomiting, anorexia, withdrawal, or insomnia.[3] For example, some children become upset as soon as the nurse enters the treatment room to set up for the procedure. The best intervention for conditioned anxiety is prevention. Thus appropriate premedications to counteract treatment side effects are given before the side effect occurs.[24,63]

Hair loss is a common side effect of chemotherapy that creates anxiety for the patient, especially in the adolescent. Regardless of age, the child may develop a negative self-image and avoid contact with friends, which further increases a sense of isolation and loneliness. Even if the patient is old enough to understand intellectually that the hair will grow back, baldness is a visible reminder that the child is different from her peer group and is a major stressor.

Depending on treatment center protocol, chemotherapy-induced neutropenia and associated illnesses may require the child to stay away from friends and classmates. The child may need to avoid crowds, which means no trips to the movies, a shopping center, or even a favorite fast-food restaurant. These restrictions add to the child's loneliness and sense of isolation.[76]

Perceived vulnerability

Perceived vulnerability is associated with both the acute and chronic aspects of cancer. During periods of exacerbation, the child feels vulnerable because of hospitalization, which evokes dormant fears of death and ultimate separation from parents, friends, and familiar environment. Feelings of helplessness and the experience of repeated painful medical treatments contribute to vulnerability.[8]

Maintenance

As treatment proceeds, the child faces a different set of challenges related to emergency hospital admissions and restrictions in normal routines. An emergent medical situation, such as fever and neutropenia, requires hospitalization and may reawaken fears faced at diagnosis. For the toddler or preschooler, hospitalization may increase the normal developmental fear of separation or abandonment, whereas in the older child, the main concern related to the hospitalization may be the disruption of usual routines, especially isolation from peers. School-age children miss normal activities such as birthday parties, sporting events, and special school programs and may not be allowed to have overnight visits, go on weekend trips, or participate in social events with peers. Most children are able to return to school or day-care centers on a regular basis once maintenance therapy starts. Although young school-age children may have some concerns about reactions of peers, both the school-age children and adolescents worry about their friends' and schoolmates' reactions to the diagnosis and treatment side effects, particularly to the loss of hair or other body disfigurement. Children may also be concerned about their grades and ability to compete academically with peers.[5,74]

Developmental issues

The unpredictability of acute episodes induces considerable uncertainty about attainment of developmental tasks, such as achievement of autonomy.[45] Children with cancer must often rely on the skills and support of parents, medical and nursing staff, and the health care system, which may exacerbate the struggle for independence.[59] Lability of illness and fluctuation between acute and chronic periods create imbalance in the child's life, requiring constant redefinition of self-identity (whether to view self as an ill or healthy person). This variability also necessitates constant change in expected performance ability on the part of both the child and the parents. For example, adolescents may perceive their parents as overprotective, as trying to help too much, and as being unwilling to include them in treatment decisions, and this parental overprotectiveness may continue during periods of chronicity, when adolescents can be more autonomous.

Incongruence between the parents' perceptions of the child's ability and the child's actual performance represents a source of tension and potential conflict within families that may be attenuated through counseling. Parents are counseled to provide opportunities for children to participate in the decision making about tasks within the family and to allow graded independence and flexibility. Almost every aspect of cancer treatment has potentially negative implications related to separation-loss and control-compliance. Separation from significant people (i.e., peers, family members) and school activities may result in loss of self-identity, self-esteem, academic achievement, and attainment of developmentally appropriate interpersonal relationships. During times of acute illness, an increased dependence on parents and decreased personal control may alter family relations. However, during remission there is a resurgence of striving for autonomy and independence, often in relation to control of activities of daily living, privacy, and relationships with peers, and to management of the illness and its treatment.

Studies indicate that uncertainty about the reaction of peers to changes in physical appearance, the loss of friends, difficulty keeping up with school-work, and extreme separation anxiety all contribute to disruption in the return to school and participation in school-related activities. Side effects of treatment serve as constant reminders that the child is different. Body changes may precipitate withdrawal from peers and anxiety about performance.[76]

End of Therapy and Long-Term Follow-Up

Once the therapy has been completed, the child may be frightened each time he feels ill. Routine tests such as computed tomography (CT) scans, bone marrow aspirations, and lumbar punctures may induce apprehension about results. Long-term follow-up may also produce anxiety, because children become aware of possible late effects.[42]

Positive aspects of cancer and cancer treatment

A child's experience with cancer and treatment can result in positive outcomes for the child. These include (1) the benefits of mastery, such as becoming more confident and outgoing after completion of cancer treatment; (2) developing a sense of "I made it, I was tough, I succeeded"; (3) a sense of having emerged as a better person who can handle almost anything and who has increased sensitivity to the needs of others; and (4) becoming more religious.[21,58]

Relapse

A recurrence or relapse of disease causes an intense period of anxiety. The child's focus is on the required treatments, which may be very aggressive and require hospitalization.[33] The child may also react to parental distress and have behavioral changes, nightmares, or increased separation anxiety. The same stresses experienced at diagnosis may recur and be even more intense because of negative memories of treatment. If remission is not attained, the child faces additional stressors related to death (see Chapter 17).

PSYCHOSOCIAL PROBLEMS

Most children cope with the emotional upheaval related to having cancer, adapt, and experience positive psychosocial growth and development. However, a minority of children develop psychologic problems such as depression, anxiety, sleep disturbances, behavioral problems (including acting out), difficulties in interpersonal relationships, and nonadherence with treatment. These issues require intensive interventions by a mental health specialist. The nurse's priority is the initiation of strategies to promote adjustment.

Before initiating any particular strategy, the nurse completes an assessment to choose appropriate interventions. The overall assessment determines the child's level of emotional maturity and

TABLE 15-3	RISK FACTORS IN ASSESSMENT
Risk Factor	**Results**
Previous experience with illness, hospitalization	If good experience, then positive coping
Family dysfunction	Greater risk for poor coping
Personal ego strength	If poor self-concept, then greater risk for difficulty with coping
Cultural barriers	If unable to speak or understand language, greater difficulty with coping
Special needs, such as learning disability or low IQ	Greater risk for poor coping
Preexisting body image problems, such as severe acne	Greater risk for poor coping
Sensory/perceptual alternation due to disease	Greater risk for poor coping

his or her ability to cope with illness and treatment. These factors depend on the family situation, the child's age and stage of development, previous experience with illness, hospitalization, treatment, and personal ego strength. Table 15-3 presents major risk factors to be assessed.

Assessment Factors

The child's cultural background, family situation, and the general anxiety and distress experienced by the parents influence the child's coping abilities. Extremely stressed parents are less able to meet the child's needs and to encourage coping strategies that result in an adaptive outcome. They may have such a need for support themselves that they have difficulty giving support to the child. The child may feel insecure and act out as an expression of distress. External events may affect the family, or the child's diagnosis may reawaken a previously unresolved crisis. One or both parents may decompensate because of these circumstances. For example, a death in the family may have occurred, or the parents may be getting a divorce. Whatever the cause of the parent's anxiety and distress, the child's adjustment partially depends on the support from parents.

Assessment of psychosocial and cognitive development will suggest to the nurse particular conflicts that a child may have at a given age and the limits of the child's cognitive understanding of situations. For example, the toddler focuses on learning control, possesses very basic reasoning skills, and is beginning to play make-believe. The nurse observes the child, listens to verbal expression, and talks with the parents to obtain an accurate assessment. Integrating the assessment into normal care routines is an efficient method. For example, while checking vital signs, the nurse asks the child to explain what is being done and why. Another approach is to ask the child to tell a story. These approaches give valuable clues to the child's state of development and level of cognitive maturity.

A third factor to assess is the child's previous experiences with illness, hospitalization, and treatment. Asking the child and parent about these previous experiences helps the nurse understand the child's expectations and determine if misconceptions exist. Particularly, the nurse should ask if the child knows someone who has had cancer. The child may have known an elderly person or relative who died from cancer or who experienced severe side effects and may expect the same to happen to her. Also, if the child has had positive experiences with doctors and nurses during well-child visits or trips to the dentist, the level of fear may be decreased. The nurse might also ask if the child has seen any television programs about being sick or being in the hospital. The child's perceptions of events are important to understand as the nurse begins to select supportive strategies.

Finally, the nurse must attain an understanding of the child's personality and general ego strength. The parents are asked how the child coped in the past to new or different situations such as changing schools or moving. The nurse observes the child in unfamiliar situations. Does the child cringe and avoid the situation, or does the child ask questions, look around, and try to understand? In general, the child who has weathered stressful situations previously is better able to cope with diagnosis and treatment. The child who demonstrates problematic behavior at diagnosis, such as difficulty in school, poor peer relations, or poor impulse control, may have minimal ego strength from which to draw while coping with this crisis. Such a child may need extra support during treatment.

DIFFERENTIATING STRESS REACTIONS FROM PSYCHOPATHOLOGY

While most children experience mild adjustment reactions to the diagnosis and treatment of cancer, some children exhibit true psychopathology. The nurse has a particular advantage in the early detection of difficulty because of the intimate nature of the contact with the patient and family. Therefore the nurse must be aware of signs of psychopathology and must differentiate them from simple adjust-

TABLE 15-4	ABC ASSESSMENT FOR MENTAL HEALTH REFERRAL	
Category	Problem	Determine by
Affect	Depression or anxiety	Inquiring if the child feels "blue" or "down"
		Asking the child to draw a picture of how he or she feels
Behavior	Behavior secondary to depression, anxiety or psychosis, or conduct disorders	Observing for withdrawal; excessive outbursts or temper tantrums; poor sleeping or eating; failure to engage in usual play; signs of hallucinative behaviors such as talking to self, saying strange or unusual things, reaching into the air, or putting hands over his or her ears.
		Identifying if behaviors seem regressive or abnormal for the particular age
		Judging whether reactions are disproportionate to a situation
Cognition	Delusions and/or hallucinations	Assessing for orientation and the presence of psychotic thinking
		Asking the child if he or she is having scary thoughts or seeing things that other people do not see

ment reactions or stress responses. Stress responses are usually seen as simple regressive behaviors, such as thumb sucking, that improve over time, especially as supportive measures are instituted for the child and parents.

Psychopathologic difficulties include depression, severe anxiety, intractable nausea and vomiting, or psychosis. Problems that warrant follow-up care include severe regressive behaviors such as bed-wetting, declining grades or poor attitude in school, increased fighting with siblings or friends, and school phobia.

If the child's behavior exceeds that expected for a normal stressful experience, further assessment of the child's affect, behavior, and cognition (ABC) is warranted. This simple ABC formula easily and quickly identifies the child who needs referral to a mental health specialist.[45] Table 15-4 demonstrates the ABC assessment process. The following questions may help determine if referral is needed. Has the problem persisted longer than several weeks? Is the symptom or problem intense? Does the problem increase in the presence of anxiety-producing situations? Has the child's behavior changed significantly from the prediagnosis personality? Is the behavior at great variance from normal development? Does the ABC assessment reveal excessive sadness or the presence of abnormal thoughts? Four or five positive responses to the previous questions warrant further investigation.

A picture of dysfunction is not always easy to identify. To validate the accuracy of the assessment, consult with other team members such as the pediatric social worker or child life specialist. Their observations may add insight that will aid in assessment. After consultation the child may be referred to the mental health clinical nurse specialist, child psychologist, child psychiatrist, or behavioral pediatrician.

MEDIATING THE STRESS OF DIAGNOSIS AND TREATMENT

Patients may be overwhelmed by a myriad of stressors during the initial period of diagnosis and treatment. The goals of psychosocial support are to encourage ventilation of fears and concerns, increase cognitive understanding of the situation, provide a sense of mastery over the stressors, promote the child's self-esteem, and develop a supportive network.[4] To attain these goals, the nurse uses a variety of supportive techniques directed to the individual patient and to groups of patients. Since any single approach may not be appropriate for a specific child, the nurse must be prepared to try several until one is selected that seems to "fit" that particular child. Parents must be involved in any strategy selected for the child, using a collaborative, cooperative approach. Parents also help the child by reinforcing strategies and supporting the child in using a strategy. Serendipitously, parents themselves may benefit from using the strategies, especially relaxation training.

Individual Approaches

Selecting the appropriate strategy for a particular child depends on the assessment, the stage of treatment, and the identified problem. Effective approaches for decreasing stress and increasing adaptation include education, anticipatory guidance, and debriefing; behavioral techniques; expressive therapies such as bibliotherapy, play therapy, and art therapy; and imaginative strategies. These strategies may be used alone or in various combinations, depending on the nature of the stressor and the individual child.

Education, anticipatory guidance, and debriefing

An important element in coping is cognitive understanding of events. Therefore one must create opportunities to help the child understand what is happening. Explain medical terms, tests, and treatments in simple terms. The use of books and videotapes improves the child's understanding, especially when undergoing unfamiliar procedures. Puppets or dolls can be used to explain complicated medical procedures such as central venous access device insertion. Rehearsing procedures or at least verbally "walking the child through" a procedure enhances coping. Telling the child what to expect, clearly indicating the things the child will see, hear, smell, and feel, also provides cues for coping. For example, the nurse might say, "You will lie on a hard table and hear strange sounds." The nurse might add, "When you hear the sounds, think about something you enjoy doing." After the procedure is over, ask the child to describe what happened. This debriefing allows the child to ventilate negative and positive feelings and to identify the effective coping strategies. Also, the nurse is able to clarify areas of concern and reduce possible misconceptions resulting from the child's anxiety.[24,73]

Behavioral techniques

Behavioral strategies to reduce anxiety and increase coping are derived from behavioral psychotherapy, which posits that problematic behaviors occur as a response to stimuli and that the resulting distress is learned. Simply stated, learned behaviors may be unlearned. The use of positive reinforcement to improve coping is one example of this theory's implementation. A child who has "learned" to be anxious, to cry, and to resist is given a reward for cooperating or helping with a procedure. The reward—a coupon, sticker, toy, or trophy—is given to increase the likelihood of future cooperation. Nurses and parents can also reinforce the tangible reward with praise and positive comments.[48]

Expressive therapies

Children engage in a variety of expressive therapies to help them cope more effectively. These therapies, regardless of the specific modality, provide an outlet for the expression of feelings and release of tension. They enable the child to act out psychic problems associated with diagnosis and treatment, attain a sense of mastery and competence from facing the stressor even symbolically, and develop insight into the stressor. The child may problem-solve as he or she plays; thus problems are reworked and fears are allayed. Additionally, expressive therapies are used as a way of assessing the child's understanding and perceptions and gaining access to the child's inner world. These techniques include play therapy, art therapy, storytelling, and bibliotherapy.

Play therapy is a major modality for helping children cope with diagnosis, hospitalization, treatment, and chronic illness. Play therapy may be directive or nondirective. Typically, the child with cancer engages in play therapy to understand treatments and procedures and to work through fears and anxieties associated with the illness. A variety of material can be used in the play experience, including a play hospital with equipment and supplies, hand puppets, teaching dolls, and medically related flannel boards.[69,73]

Art therapy involves using the child's drawings as a means of communicating with the child and helping the child to express inner feelings nonverbally. Through art the child brings emotional conflicts to resolution, gains self-understanding, and experiences personality change and growth. Encourage the child to draw a picture about being in the hospital, getting treatments, and other situations that can foster self-awareness and personal growth; or simply provide art materials, paper, markers, and crayons and permit the child to draw whatever he or she wishes (Figure 15-2). This allows the child to project into the drawing fears and concerns without having to face them directly. After the drawing is complete, ask the child to "tell me about your picture" rather than asking "what is that?" Thus the child attains some emotional distance from stressful situations and in telling about the picture, may experience mastery. For children

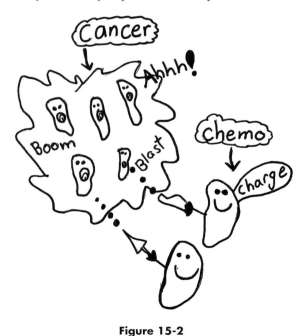

Figure 15-2

This 10-year-old's drawing depicts a tumor filled with cancer cells being attacked and destroyed by good chemotherapy.

who are more inhibited, using partially completed pictures that act as incomplete sentences may facilitate expression.[69] Music therapy is another expressive therapy that is very useful for children with cancer. Nurses may consider using musical tapes and/or singing with patients during procedures as means of distracting and relaxing children.

Expressive therapies that capitalize on both normal development and the child's imagination are bibliotherapy and storytelling. The child projects his or her own fears and concerns into fictional stories or characters in a book. The child attains mastery through symbolically acting out his or her own fears or identifying with the character in the book or story, and can learn new coping methods for dealing with a particular experience.[12,25]

Bibliotherapy involves reading the child a story that reflects some of the issues and problems confronting the child.[25] Through the telling of the story a process of identification, catharsis, and insight occurs. The theme of the story should be one similar to the difficulties the child is having and should contain positive resolution of fears or problems. The child may project his or her own concerns into the story without losing any self-esteem by admitting to the fears. Parents may be given books to read and discuss with the child at home. Often books for younger children can be used with older children by explaining that the child is too old for the book but you need his or her opinion about its usefulness for a younger child. Box 15-3 lists some books that help children cope. These well-written

---

BOX 15-3

BOOKS TO HELP CHILDREN COPE

TITLE / **AUTHOR**

SIBLING RIVALRY

Title	Author
I'll Fix Anthony	Judith Viorst
Peter's Chair	Ezra Jack Kents
That One in the Middle Is the Green Kangaroo	Judy Blume
Tales of a Fourth Grade Nothing	Judy Blume

SELF-CONFIDENCE

Title	Author
If I Were in Charge of the World	Judith Viorst
Where the Wild Things Are	Maurice Sendak
My Mama Says There Aren't Any Zombies, Ghosts, Vampires, Creatures, Demons, Monsters, Fiends, Goblins or Things	Judith Viorst
I'm Terrific	Marjorie Sharmat
There's a Nightmare in My Closet	Mercer Mayer
Is There Life on a Plastic Planet	Mildred Ames
Fifth Grade Magic	Beatrice Gormley

FEARS

Title	Author
Curious George Goes to the Hospital	Margaret & H. A. Rey
If You Are Afraid of the Dark, Remember the Night Rainbow	Cooper Edens
In the Dark	Stan & Jan Berenstain
If I Found a Wistful Unicorn	Ann Ashford
The Carrot Seed	Ruth Krauss
The Runaway Bunny	Margaret Wise Brown
Otherwise Known As Sheila the Great	Judy Blume

STRESS

Title	Author
The Bridge to Terebithia	Katherine Paterson
Alexander and the Terrible, Horrible, No Good, Very Bad Day	Judith Viorst
Will I Have a Friend	Miriam Cohen

WEBSITES LISTING CHILDREN'S BOOKS FOR ONCOLOGY PATIENTS
http://oncolink.upenn.edu/reviews/children/
http://mel.lib.mi.us/health/cancerbooks/
http://www.candlelighters.ca/res.html

books dealing with children's emotions have withstood the test of time. Numerous health-related books exist to provide children information about an illness as well as scenarios to help them emotionally. Lists of books for children with cancer can be obtained through health libraries that exist at many children's hospitals or through the websites listed in Box 15-3. Nurses must be familiar with these books to make appropriate recommendations. Books with health-related content must include current information presented in an unthreatening manner and must be written or reviewed by health care professionals. Additional resources exist to enable nurses to evaluate books for hospitalized children.[2,47]

Storytelling involves encouraging the child to make up his or her own story or telling the child stories made up by the nurse that are similar to the child's situation. Variations to telling a story include writing a television script, acting in a play, putting on a puppet show, or making a videotape.[25]

Imaginative strategies

Children have an active fantasy life and are easily engaged in techniques using their imagination. Children are less inhibited than adults and readily play "let's pretend." For this reason children as young as 3 years of age are excellent candidates for using imaginative strategies to control anxiety and pain. Relaxation, imagery, and hypnosis capitalize on the natural abilities of children to focus their concentration so strongly that they do not attend to anxiety-producing situations or even pain. Although hypnosis requires specialized training, no extensive training is needed to teach children relaxation and imagery. Children naturally move from the imaginative to the real with great ease. The idea is introduced by explaining that the nurse needs the child to do a special part of the procedure or test. Explain that the child will be in control and can take care of herself by using the special "magic" or energy that is inside each person. This magic can help the child control scary or bad feelings. The important focus is to help the child be less fearful. Once the child knows what to do to control fear, he will be more amenable to helping. The goal is to help the child relax and feel good about her ability to help.[15,24]

Relaxation is accomplished by encouraging the child to begin to breathe very slowly (i.e., breathe in to a count of 3 and breathe out to a count of 6). Children are encouraged to breathe by using blow bubbles, pinwheels, or party blowers. Most children do not like to close their eyes, viewing this as a loss of control or associating it with going to sleep. Instead, encourage the child to watch the stars float down a magic wand or look at a picture in the room. The child is directed to relax specific parts of the body in succession, using elements from progressive relaxation. Even toddlers can begin to use this strategy. As the child focuses on the breathing, the attention is directed away from the anxiety-producing event.[24]

Once the attention is engaged, the child is encouraged to relax further by playing "let's pretend" or thinking of a pleasant time such as going to the beach. The child's imagination is used even more by telling a story, taking a special trip on a magic carpet, or watching a favorite cartoon or television hero on a magic movie screen. The child is asked about favorite times or fun activities, and these can be integrated into the story. Elements of the story should incorporate strength, control, and good feelings. Similarly, the child is engaged in distracting activities to such an extent that the anxiety-producing event (e.g., venipuncture) is ignored. The nurse or parent might read a pop-up book to the child, do finger plays, sing songs, or recite nursery rhymes.[24,25,63]

Group Approaches

Participation in a support group has many benefits for the young child with cancer. The therapeutic factors of being in a group include catharsis, commonality, reality testing, interpersonal learning, and instilling hope. The group provides the child with a forum for ventilation of feelings, learning coping methods from others, decreasing loneliness and fear, and learning realistic aspects of treatment. Through group participation the child develops insight into concerns, learns new coping strategies, and acquires a sense of responsibility for behavior.[12]

Children may be involved in groups as inpatients or as outpatients. Typical goals for the group are to increase a sense of support through peer interaction, decrease the feeling of isolation, promote self-esteem, and increase ventilation of feelings. Children who especially benefit from group participation are those who are newly diagnosed, have relapsed, have a major change in treatment protocol, have undergone extensive hospitalization or surgery, have recently had a hematopoietic stem cell transplant or have problems with peer relations. The traumatic nature of these events is shared and discussed so that they become less anxiety producing. The child may learn that other children in the group have had similar feelings and experiences. Through discussion and expressive play, the child gains some mastery over the stressful nature of the events and feels more confident in her ability to cope.

PROMOTING MENTAL HEALTH AND NORMAL DEVELOPMENT

A second overall purpose of psychosocial support is to promote the child's return to normalcy through mental health promotion strategies and fostering of normal development. The nurse assists the child with attaining these goals through individual or group approaches.

Individual Approaches

The majority of pediatric cancer therapy is given in ambulatory care settings and at home; therefore the child has more opportunities to participate in age-appropriate activities. However, parents may be so focused on coping with the disease that they fail to initiate these activities or they ignore the child's need to master developmental tasks. Encourage parents to engage the child in play that stimulates development (Figure 15-3). Assess if the child is becoming independent and is learning to function separate from parents. Age-appropriate activities may be included in playroom programs. Exercise programs, music, and arts and crafts are ways to promote growth and development, even while the child is receiving treatment.[38]

Program Approaches

Recognizing the need to promote the child's reconnection with the usual events of childhood, programs have been developed that specifically promote the child's independence, mental health, and return to age-appropriate functioning. The two most prevalent programs are school reentry and summer camps.

School reentry

Because school is a major part of a child's life, the child with cancer needs to become a productive learner in school. School reentry for the child with cancer presents unique challenges for both the child and the family. These challenges include dealing with teachers who may have minimal experience with cancer and with classmates who do not understand the child's problems, and the cancer patient's own problems of dealing with a life-threatening illness and the side effects of treatment. Table 15-5 summarizes the potential impact of school reentry programs. Research studies have focused on ways to help children reenter the school system and return to their prediagnosis level of attendance and achievement. Review of these studies identifies the importance of a three-pronged approach to school reentry: communicating directly with school personnel, educating the child's classmates, and determining the child's attitude toward school.[5,51,74] This approach helps the child or teen cope with returning to school and have better peer relations. Box 15-4 lists goals and interventions for successful school reentry programs.

First, direct communication between the pediatric oncology treatment team and school personnel is critical as the child returns to school. If a school nurse or health educator is available, her partnership with the pediatric oncology nurse is critical to ensure a positive school reentry. This communication includes medical information about cancer and its effects on the child and the psychosocial impact of cancer on the child and family. Workshops incorporating this information have been successful in enhancing teachers' knowledge about cancer and decreasing their anxieties about working with students with cancer.

The second important aspect of school reentry is

TABLE 15-5	IMPACT OF SCHOOL REENTRY PROGRAMS
Teachers	Improve knowledge and comfort
Peers	Increase knowledge leading to: • Decreased fear of cancer • Decreased worry about classmate • Increased interaction with child with cancer
Child with cancer	Increased understanding and acceptance leading to: • Decreased behavior problems • Decreased anxiety/depression • Increased social competence • No impact on absences or performance

Data from Katz, E. R., Rubinstein, C. L., Hubert, N. C. et al. (1988). School and social reintegration of children with cancer. *Journal of Psychosocial Oncology, 6,* 123-140.

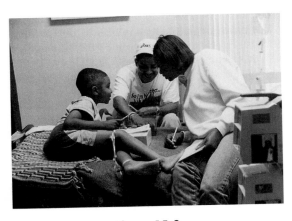

Figure 15-3

Parents promote normal development through a game of Yahtzee.

educating the child's classmates. If the classmates understand the disease and side effects of treatment, social acceptance is more likely to occur. Classmate education can be accomplished by having a member of the pediatric oncology team talk to the class, by having the cancer patient speak directly to the class about the disease, or by using puppet shows or videotapes to explain the process.[51]

Third, the child's attitude toward school attendance can contribute to the problem of reentry. Table 15-6 outlines factors that may impact the child's school attendance and performance. Changes in appearance, stamina, coordination, and sense of well-being require physical and emotional adjustment and threaten the child's developing self-image and ability to compete successfully with classmates. The child may develop a fear of rejection and/or fear of an inability to compete and may refuse to attend school. Attendance problems can be present even if the child and family are enthusiastic about the return to school. Incorporate discussions about school attendance into routine clinic visits. Detailed questions about atten-

dance, grades, peer relationships, and participation in school events can help uncover school problems that the child may be experiencing. Early recognition of problems may lead to early interventions, making school reentry an easier process for the child with cancer.

Summer camps

Returning to school is one method of normalizing the life of the child with cancer; however, the child needs other opportunities for independence and interaction with people outside the family unit. Summer camps for children with cancer provide the children with a normal childhood experience and a time to enhance their independence.[6] Goals of these camps include providing a normal camping experience for the child with cancer, a week of respite for the parents, a chance to develop a different relationship between patient and medical and nursing staff, and an informal support network for the patient. Attainment of these goals often leads to increased self-esteem, increased self-worth, and improved self-image during and after camp.[16]

The structure used to accomplish the goals varies from camp to camp, but all of the camps are designed to provide a week of fun and excitement. Regardless of the camp's structure, the majority of the campers return from camp with feelings of accomplishment and a host of new friends. Nurses involved in children's oncology camps would find the Children's Oncology Camping Association, International, a valuable resource. Contact them at 1-800-737-2667 or online at www.COCA-intl.org.

SPECIAL NEEDS OF ADOLESCENTS

Adolescence is a tumultuous time characterized by conflicts with parents and concerns over peer

---

BOX 15-4

SCHOOL REENTRY GOALS AND INTERVENTIONS

GOALS
- Establishing the importance of school to child, family, community
- Bridging the initial absence from the classroom
- Exploring the impact of the diagnosis on school peers and personnel

INTERVENTIONS
- Communication to parents and child by treatment team that school is not an option but a viable and important endeavor
- School instruction during hospitalizations whenever physically possible
- Encourage home school to send cards and notes during child's hospitalization
- School conference before return to regular classroom to provide specific information to school personnel about child's disease and treatment
- Recommend development of Individualized Education Plan (IEP) or 504 Plan
- Ongoing assessment of school attendance and performance
- Homebound instruction only when absolutely necessary, and then on an intermittent basis (exception being transplant patients)

Data from Davis, K. G. (1989). Educational needs of the terminally ill student. *Issues in Comprehensive Pediatric Nursing, 12,* 235-245; Patterson, K., & Stewart, J. (1992). *School integration for the child with cancer: Beyond re-entry.* Paper presented at the Association of Pediatric Oncology Nurses National Conference, Minneapolis, MN, October 1992.

TABLE 15-6	FACTORS IMPACTING SCHOOL ATTENDANCE AND PERFORMANCE
Physiologic	Demands of treatment schedule
	Comfort status
	Hematologic status
	Limitations on activity/mobility
Psychologic	Body image
	Behavioral response to illness
	Family response to illness
	Community response to illness
Psychophysiologic	Fatigue
	Inattention
	Cognitive and social sequelae

Data from Patterson, K., & Stewart, J. (1992). *School integration for the child with cancer: Beyond re-entry.* Paper presented at the Association of Pediatric Oncology Nurses National Conference, Minneapolis, MN, October 1992.

relations, career, and sexuality. The overall tasks of adolescence include the consolidation of identity, psychosexual differentiation, the development of life skills, and emotional separation from parents. During adolescence, peer relations and peer acceptance are of major importance, along with forming close relationships with members of the opposite sex. Even under normal circumstances, the mastery of these tasks is fraught with difficulty. When the diagnosis of cancer is superimposed on these developmental issues, difficulties in coping may arise at any point on the treatment continuum (i.e., from diagnosis through long-term follow-up).

The adolescent with cancer experiences many of the same stressors as the child diagnosed at an earlier age; yet they may be more difficult to manage because of the adolescent's need to appear normal and to be coping well. Although adolescents may experience situational anxiety, depression, and/or psychogenic reactions, particularly anticipatory nausea and vomiting, overall their adjustment and reactions are within a normal range. As with younger children, the adolescent's challenge is to cope with the many stressors while continuing to deal with normal developmental demands. Major stressors include hair loss and other body changes that may lead to negative feelings about self-image. Intrusive procedures, restrictions in activities, isolation from peers, hospitalizations, and fear of death are ongoing stressors that may cause the adolescent to feel a loss of control. These circumstances cause the adolescent, more than the younger child, to act out by being noncompliant with treatment (e.g., not taking prescribed medications); taking unnecessary risks (e.g., ignoring precautions when white blood count is low); or having conflicting interpersonal relationships with family, peers, and staff.[65] Some adolescents seem to have decreased social adjustment and lowered academic competence and may be unable to look to the future and make plans. Because of the potential for these problems in the adolescent patient, the nurse must identify problems early and initiate interventions that seek to promote the attainment of developmental tasks and adaptation to the illness. These approaches are implemented with the individual patient or in a group setting.[4,29]

Individual Approaches

Nurses may implement a variety of interventions directed to an individual patient. They include working with the family, developing a relationship with the adolescent, and promoting adaptation.

Collaboration with the family

Although adolescents are in the process of emancipation, they are viewed as part of a family system. The adolescent's need for independence must be balanced with an understanding of the influence of the family system and culture on the adolescent's behavior. Collaboration with the parents, while respecting the adolescent's emerging independence, may work best. The parents' concerns must be addressed and fears allayed while allowing the adolescent to have input into care issues. Through a collaborative approach, the nurse is modeling for the parents ways to support the adolescent and get their own parental needs met. The nurse needs to establish clear boundaries between the nurse and parent and the nurse and adolescent. For example, the nurse may indicate that the physical examination will be private. If these boundaries are identified, the adolescent will be comfortable asking questions and will not need to feel adversarial toward the parents or the nursing staff. Clear messages about the adolescent's role in decision making are given. The goal is to achieve a balance between the adolescent's and the parents' needs. This approach is particularly critical in matters involving the adolescent's sexuality.[26,29]

Anticipatory guidance and education

Although seeming self-assured, the adolescent needs information and guidance about procedures, treatment, and side effects. Additionally, the adolescent requires assistance in mentally rehearsing potentially stressful social situations and how best to handle them. For example, the adolescent may need coaching on going back to school and answering classmates' queries. The paradoxical problem is that the adolescent's competent appearance may prevent asking about the issues. Therefore the nurse may intervene by saying, "By the way, some other teens wonder about. . . ." Adolescents may benefit from watching videotapes or reading pamphlets about their illness because these activities can be done in private. Increasing the adolescent's cognitive understanding of the illness and treatment increases adaptation.

Facilitating coping with diagnosis and treatment

Assist the adolescent in overall adaptation by encouraging the ventilation of feelings and the use of adaptive coping skills. The adolescent may be hesitant to try relaxation and imagery because of concern over loss of control, misconceptions about the techniques, or fear of appearing weak. Therefore offer the skills as a way to add to the many coping skills the patient already has. Another adolescent patient might be able to introduce the idea positively and increase acceptance.

An important area to address in helping the adolescent cope is the issue of compliance with treatment protocols. As a preventive measure, when teaching is initiated at the diagnosis, help the family clarify who is responsible for administering the medication—the parent or the adolescent. Once agreement is reached, teaching will include ways to help the patient take the medicine on time (e.g., use of calendar, pillbox). Also, seek feedback about the adolescent's and parents' satisfaction with the information given. All of these strategies appear to improve compliance with adolescents.[57,64]

Promotion of community reentry and mainstreaming

The importance of school and community reentry are discussed at diagnosis so that the goal of normalcy is introduced early. The actual timing of this preparation is based on treatment protocols. Involving the adolescent in discussions and plans for return to school increases the success of this effort and decreases the stress felt by the patient and family.[18,31]

Group Approaches

The adolescent's ability to cope with the diagnosis and treatment and the reentry into school may be enhanced through group participation.[26,29] However, not all adolescents are comfortable in a group setting. Although groups when available may be an alternative or supplement to individual counseling, individual approaches such as relaxation training may still be beneficial. The adolescent support group may accomplish the following goals: (1) provide emotional support and understanding of feelings about common stressors, (2) promote the sharing of feelings and experiences among the members, (3) build self-esteem by promoting a sense of responsibility and pride in accomplishments, (4) enhance relationships with peers and family, (5) build socialization skills, (6) provide normalizing experiences, and (7) support career and adult functioning.[26,29]

Activities within a support group may range from having a pizza party to making a videotape.[29] By involving the adolescent in structured activities, anxiety is lessened. Additionally, interpersonal learning and support may emerge from activities and projects. Adolescents may write a newsletter, perform community service projects, visit newly diagnosed patients in the hospital, communicate in chat rooms or use other Internet resources, or attend weekend retreats. Usually, engaging adolescents in a variety of projects assists in maintaining their interest in the group while helping them learn concrete ways to share and reach out to one another (Figure 15-4).

PSYCHOSOCIAL IMPACT OF CANCER ON THE PARENTS

All family members are affected by the diagnosis of cancer. As discussed in Chapter 1, the child with cancer may be a part of a variety of family arrangements. It is critical for the nurse to understand who constitutes family for any particular child and who occupies the role of parent.

The child's biological mother and father may or may not be in ongoing parental roles. These adults, however, are faced with special coping burdens when their child is diagnosed with cancer. Key issues include concern that they have contributed genetic material leading to the child's cancer, questions about their lifestyle choices that may have influenced the onset of cancer, and/or concern that they have taken appropriate care of the child before the illness. The emotional intensity of these issues is great even if the biological parents continue in the parent roles. It is likely that that intensity will be magnified if there has been a break in the relationship.

In this chapter, the term *parents* denotes either a mother or father and is not meant to imply only a married couple. Parents are faced with the burden

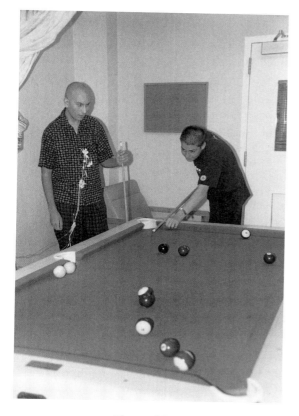

Figure 15-4

Adolescents provide mutual support while engaged in activities.

of coping with their own needs and feelings as well as those of their children. When there are two parents, the coping methods may not be congruent, thus adding to the family's stress. Nurses must assess the commonalities and differences in coping styles and abilities and provide support as necessary. Nurses are involved in helping parents meet their needs for trust, information, guidance, support, skills, and resources throughout the course of the illness. Nurses can be instrumental in helping families transition from what was before the diagnosis to a "new normal" state that involves altered daily routines, uncertainty, and a new worldview.

TREATMENT PHASES

Diagnosis

The time surrounding diagnosis is very stressful for parents. Some parents describe the time surrounding diagnosis as "waiting and not knowing."[10] Even though they may have suspected something was wrong, they are unprepared for the diagnosis of cancer. Parents usually respond with shock, grief, disbelief, anger, guilt, and numbness. It would be ideal for the physician and nurse together to tell the parents the diagnosis in private and give them the opportunity to compose themselves before they return to tell the child. Seeing the parent distraught only adds to the child's fears. The parents may need to leave the hospital to share their concerns and express their emotions before they are able to see their child. For single parents, finding someone with whom to share their initial feelings may be difficult. The nurse can help them mobilize an outside support person.

Despite receiving the information about long-term survival and even cure, many parents still equate cancer with death. Regardless of actual risks quoted, they leave the initial conference with the fear that their child's life is threatened. Although they may accept the diagnosis intellectually, they are less likely to accept it emotionally. Denial and a sense of "this can't be real" may lead them to second opinions. Having the nurse present during the diagnosis discussion facilitates the reinforcement of information after the initial conference.

While dealing with their own powerful emotions, parents must establish relationships with unknown physicians and nurses, adjust to hospitalization and hospital bureaucracy, learn medical language while making treatment decisions, and manage their family's life outside the hospital.[9] Rapid consent decisions are made regarding chemotherapy, surgery, and/or radiation. All of this is done while fearing for their child's life and fearing that they may make a wrong decision. If not treated, the child will die; if they agree to treatment, there are no guarantees, and the child will likely suffer known and unknown side effects and long-term effects of treatment.

A major parental task is to learn about their child's illness and treatment. Nurses must help them process a tremendous amount of verbal and written information about the diagnosis, treatment, and prognosis. Although parents need some information immediately, it is unlikely that they will retain much of it, and frequent repetitions will be needed. They need to be told that they are not expected to retain all of the information given and to seek clarification as often as needed from the physicians, nurses, and social workers. An offer to help explain the diagnosis and treatment to other family members is usually appreciated. Researchers are beginning to study informational needs and decision making because of the significant amount of information parents must assimilate to make treatment-related decisions.[55]

The informed consent for cancer treatment is lengthy, extensive, and involves words and concepts that are foreign to parents. Parents may not understand the technical information about treatment regimens, especially while still in a state of shock over the diagnosis. Although parents generally express satisfaction with the consent process, they find discussion with staff more helpful than the actual document.[41] Because parents are often asked to consent to procedures and treatments throughout the course of their child's illness, consent is an ongoing process rather than a single event. Nurses need to be knowledgeable about who is authorized to give consent for the child's treatment. Health care institutions often ask for copies of legal documents to ensure their compliance with court orders. Such requests may of themselves be stressful to the family.

Regardless of the degree of knowledge or acceptance, most parents are still able to fulfill their parental roles, mobilize themselves fairly rapidly, and act on their child's behalf. They are usually able and willing to continue to provide their child with comfort, food, and social experiences. Supporting the parents' strengths and pointing out how they are helping their child can foster parental self-esteem and confidence. Nurses must continue to keep the parents informed and consult with them about the child's care while facilitating their participation as members of the health care team.

Parents are faced with multiple challenges: providing special attention and care for the sick child, making frequent visits to (or remaining in) the hospital or clinic, and caring for the rest of the family. The family system becomes disorganized as plans and routines are disrupted. Frequent hospitalizations, costs of medical care, changes in the child's physical condition, and extended separation from one's spouse require alterations in the couple's role definitions. For single parents, carrying the burden alone can be very stressful. Intense emotional focus on the ill child drains energy and attention from other family members.

Although open communication from the beginning is encouraged, all parents find disclosure to the child about the diagnosis, treatment, and prognosis difficult. Nurses can assess parent-child communication through observation and by asking questions in nonthreatening ways. Parents want to share information but find it difficult, especially with young children.[11] They may benefit from learning about cognitive development in children, how they respond to emotional changes in their parents, and what research and experience has shown are the more common fears and concerns of children with cancer.

A trusting relationship between parents and the oncology team begins in the diagnostic phase and is essential throughout treatment. Parents need to trust that their child is receiving the best care possible. Patience, consideration, and acceptance of parents and their feelings are important. Open, courteous, and honest communication fosters trust and parental adaptation. Unless parents believe they can trust the staff, they will not feel free to communicate openly about their fears and feelings. Being accessible, listening, providing individualized information, and providing telephone numbers and ways parents can contact the treatment team members engenders trust. Cultural differences among families and health care providers that may create communication barriers must be recognized and bridged. All oncology team members must instill hope without giving false reassurances. Even when there is a poor prognosis, parents need reassurance that all that can be done will be done and that they and their child will not be abandoned.

Rapport that is established during this initial diagnostic period lays the foundation for support to meet future challenges. Helping parents understand the feelings they are likely to experience is useful regardless of their ability to express those feelings. Expressing your confidence that, in time, they will understand the illness and be able to work with the health care system fosters a sense of security and confidence in the parents.

Assessment of the family's available social support and social network must be done as soon as possible. Encourage continued contact with those who have been helpful in the past, but alert the family that some people will not be able to respond to their requests for help.

Virtually all cancer treatment centers provide some form of psychosocial services.[37] Nurses need to inform the family of the existence of support programs within the treatment center and community and facilitate contact if requested. Cancer support groups provide an outlet for discussing concerns and decrease a sense of isolation. However, the nurse must respect the individual decision of each family member whether to participate or not.

Ongoing assessment of parents' problem-solving skills is an important nursing role. Parents with effective problem-solving skills need to have them reinforced, whereas those with ineffective skills need additional help to enhance their abilities. Characteristics of effective problem solvers include an understanding of the nature of their child's illness; the ability to communicate their knowledge to all family members, including the ill child; expressions of appropriate concern and sadness; and tolerance for expression of feelings by others. In addition, they are able to prepare themselves for the "long haul" and to support one another throughout the illness.

Beginning the necessary teaching early allows parents time to absorb what is being taught and to perform return demonstrations of skills learned. This enhances parents' sense of control and usefulness while decreasing their sense of helplessness. While performing procedures, reinforce what was previously told and begin teaching the parents skills they will need to take care of their child. Written information (with room for notes) and a variety of audio-visual aids facilitates comprehension. Some centers use a treatment center–specific parent handbook,[27] as well as disease-specific booklets that are available through the Association of Pediatric Oncology Nurses (Box 15-5), while others use information from organizations such as the National Cancer Institute or the American Cancer Society. To decrease potential problems for two-parent and blended families, include all parents in teaching sessions. This may require considerable juggling of schedules for all involved; however, it is usually

---

BOX 15-5

APON PATIENT EDUCATION MATERIALS

(Available for purchase online at www.apon.org)
When Your Child Has Cancer (a slide orientation program)
Pediatric Tumor Series: Handbooks for Families
- Ewing's Sarcoma Family of Tumors
- Neuroblastoma
- Osteosarcoma
- Rhabdomyosarcoma
- Wilms Tumor
Cancer Treatment Fact Sheets (2nd edition, updated)
Cancer Treatment Fact Sheets (Spanish edition)

worth it in the long run. Because of early discharge policies, teaching plans should be shared between inpatient and outpatient areas. A multidisciplinary teaching documentation tool facilitates communication.[40] Oncology nurses may want to make a community or home health nurse referral to assess family adjustment and the parents' ability to care for the child in the home. They can reinforce teaching, clarify questions, and explore concerns in the less threatening home environment.

Treatment and Remission

Initial treatment is typically begun in the hospital, often within 24 hours of diagnosis. Beginning chemotherapy, having radiation, and/or having surgery are all stressful. Amid this stress, parents "search for meaning" as they try to deal with why this happened to them and their child. They search for an explanation of cause and may blame themselves. They may come to question their values and what is important in life. They may come to live one day at a time and become less materialistic and more child-centered.

Although initially concerned about their ability to care for their child at home, the family gradually increases their competence with managing the child's care. Depending on the type of cancer, the child may return home with medications, instructions about side effects of medications or radiation, a venous access device, dressings from surgery, or any number of physical limitations resulting from the cancer and its treatment. In one study, parents felt that home treatment was less stressful than hospital treatment; they coped better, felt more in control, and learned more.[34]

Parents benefit from discussions of child rearing practices throughout the treatment phase. Their natural tendency is to ease expectations and requirements of the child. Because the prognosis is good for most children, a discussion of the need for continuing discipline and limit setting with their child is important. In addition, providing guidance about the child's age-appropriate developmental tasks keeps normal developmental needs in focus and heightens a belief in the child's future.

As a result of initial treatments, the majority of children regain the external appearance of health. The parents are hopeful, because there is evidence that the treatment modalities, regardless of how intense, are working. Yet parents fear a relapse each time their child suffers from any minor symptom, particularly those first noted at diagnosis. Medical checkups and treatments, even when not physically uncomfortable, are stressful. Anxiety increases as the family awaits tests results, because they could invalidate hope that the cancer is still under control.

As time in remission lengthens, the child's cancer is seen as a chronic illness with multiple demands. Frequent trips to the treatment center continue to alter the family's daily routine. Some families must commute great distances to the treatment center, thus significantly increasing the disruption to their lives. During these visits, parents need to receive further information about the treatment plan. They are more able to assimilate information once the immediate threat to the child's life has been reduced. The health care team can solidify a strong, trusting relationship by actively listening to parents, asking how they are managing on a daily basis, expressing understanding of their difficulties, and providing support and guidance as needed.

Perceived social support is correlated with parental and child psychosocial adjustment during treatment. Well-meaning relatives and friends, however, may question the diagnosis or treatment choices, thus creating a burden of doubt for the parents. Some parents respond by isolating themselves from the people who raised their doubts. Asking parents about contacts with family and friends will facilitate discussion of these issues. Since these people are potentially a source of support for the family, it may be helpful for the nurse to offer to talk to them.

As parents become more knowledgeable about the illness and treatment, they come to realize that they are an important part of the treatment team. Most parents become skillful in interpreting their child's behavioral responses and are their child's best advocate. As they become more familiar with cancer treatment, many parents choose to use alternative and complementary therapies. One study found that 42% of families used some type of alternative or complementary therapy in conjunction with conventional medicine.[19] Refer to Chapter 9 for additional information about complementary and alternative medicine.

Parents experience major emotional challenges throughout treatment. The emotional pain involved, the threat of losing a child, and substantial practical stresses of day-to-day living affect the entire family. Parents express feelings of sadness, anger, and sometimes guilt during the first few months after diagnosis. Parents cope by seeking information; managing the child's care at home; modifying roles, routines, and plans; educating others (extended family, friends, school personnel); and for some, helping and supporting other parents of children with cancer (Figure 15-5). A certain level of temporary denial enables families to make necessary adaptations and maintain a sense of equilibrium.

Anger is another common emotion during this pe-

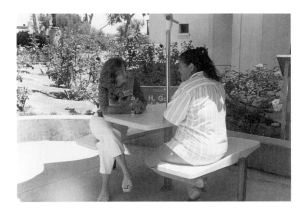

Figure 15-5

Parent-to-parent support often occurs informally at treatment centers.

riod. Anger may be directed inward or toward a biological parent or spouse, children, and/or health care providers. Nurses can listen without taking sides. When anger appears justified, encourage parents to confront the person directly with the aim of resolution.

Parents grieve for the loss of their healthy child and the way life used to be. Anticipatory grieving for the potential loss of their child is a common reaction, often beginning with diagnosis and continuing throughout treatment, especially when the prognosis is uncertain. Nurses can facilitate discussion of the parents' concerns and support and encourage their continued involvement in the child's care.

Most parents want to provide support to their children who are undergoing intrusive, painful, or frightening procedures. Nurses can assist parents with their supportive role by explaining procedures, correcting misinformation, and teaching them relaxation and distraction techniques to use with the child. Nurses must accept that for some parents, being present during the procedure is too distressing for them. Refer to Chapter 12 for additional information about procedural pain control strategies.

End of Therapy and Cure

The child's coming off therapy can be a particularly stressful time for the parents. They are faced with extreme ambivalence: glad that the long treatment phase is over, but fearful that the medication is being discontinued too soon. Now they must wait to see if the child will remain free of cancer or will develop late effects of treatment or even another cancer. Parents need anticipatory guidance before termination of therapy, and continued support. Prepare them for the feelings they are likely to experience. They may have a renewed need to protect and isolate their child, along with concern for each new minor symp-

tom. Provide frequent reassurance that their child is doing well. Although it is important to understand and support them, encourage them to move on with their lives and treat the child as normally as possible. Introducing them to other parents who have been through this phase is also useful.

Long-term survival

Parents of cancer survivors may be at increased risk for psychosocial problems. Some continue to fear that their child will die, as they do not believe the child is cured. They continue to worry about their child's ability to marry, have children, and be healthy.[35] An increase in anxiety is common when the child becomes ill or when annual checkups are scheduled. Sensitivity and respect for what the parents are feeling is essential to assist them with coming to terms with long term-survival. "Surviving Childhood Cancer: All's Well That Ends Well!?" is a helpful booklet written specifically for parents dealing with survival issues.[66] Although written for children who are survivors, *Childhood Cancer Survivors: A Practical Guide to Your Future* is also very helpful for parents.[39]

Relapse

Relapse is an extremely difficult time for parents, because it resurrects initial fears and threatens hopes for a cure. Relapse shatters illusions, especially of the curative powers of medicine. Parents fear that the oncologists will run out of treatments and that successive treatments will be even more toxic or experimental. Parents vacillate between hope for another remission and anticipatory grief. "Coming to terms" is a process parents use to limit their immediate emotional response to news of a relapse in order to take appropriate action.[32] It is not the use of denial, but one of reserved hopefulness. The nature of hope often evolves and changes focus throughout the illness.[42] As hope diminishes, depression is likely to occur. Continuing open communication with and support of parents is essential. Informing parents about available therapy and helping them deal with the implications of the relapse for the child's prognosis must be done with support, compassion, and empathy. Parents need to trust that the oncology team is doing all they can for the child. Although parents are faced with making treatment-related decisions throughout treatment, some of the most difficult decisions are faced late in the course of therapy.[33]

Terminal Phase and Death

When chemotherapy, surgery, or radiation is no longer beneficial, parents need comfort and support from all members of the team. Care of the child continues, even though it is no longer cure oriented. The delivery of high quality end-of-life care requires a multidisciplinary approach.[1]

Parents are faced with acknowledging their child's impending death while maintaining hope, meeting their daily responsibilities while dealing with disturbing emotions, and physically and emotionally caring for the child while possibly becoming emotionally detached. Parents attempt to meet their own needs and those of other children while focusing on the needs of the dying child. Most families continue to trust the medical team while accepting their limitations.

Providing care and comfort to the child is particularly supportive to the parents. Demonstrating compassion, respect, and sensitivity toward the family is generally long remembered. Parents should be informed of alternatives regarding home or hospital death. Resources regarding hospice or bereavement support groups should be identified. Greater discussion of the care of families during the terminal phase is covered in Chapter 17.

FAMILY ISSUES

Economic Stressors

Although some families have economic resources to meet the financial obligations imposed by the child's cancer, a substantial number have limited resources. For some families, medical debts continue after the child's treatment ends. Nonmedical costs are high, sometimes higher than the medical costs, as they are not covered by insurance. Nonmedical costs include transportation, parking, meals and lodging away from home, telephone calls, gifts for the sick child and siblings, and babysitting costs. Family savings may dwindle, and parents may have intangible losses such as missed work, having less time and energy to devote to career or salary advancement, or being tied to their current position for fear of losing insurance coverage. They may have to take out loans or second mortgages on their home to pay their debts.

Assess the family's third-party coverage, availability of community resources, cultural factors, and job-related issues. Even with adequate insurance, co-payment expenses may be substantial. Social work referral for financial assistance and referrals to community resources must be offered. A treatment center's financial services office may be of assistance to families in determining what is and is not covered on their health plan. Parents should be advised to keep track of out-of-pocket expenses, because some may be deductible on their income taxes.

Maintaining a Normal Family

After the initial shock of the diagnosis, the family begins to adjust to the routine of treatment and reestablish a sense of equilibrium. The parents need to normalize family life as much as possible within the limitations of the illness. Such normalization can assure well-being for the child who survives and give parents a sense that the child lived as fully as possible if death occurs. While a philosophy of normalization is intellectually acceptable, it may be difficult to put into practice. Parents tend to be more lenient and indulgent and treat the ill child differently from the other children in the family. They are often faced with the dilemma of determining the difference between drug-induced behavioral changes and normal developmental acting-out behaviors. Overindulgence and overgenerosity may lead to fear and behavior problems in the sick child and aggravate sibling jealousy.[23,42,68] Discussing age-appropriate development, discipline, and limit setting helps parents to deal with these issues and opens up communication about issues of guilt that many parents feel.

Husband and Wife Relationship

Each parent copes with the diagnosis and treatment of cancer in a unique way that is meaningful and helpful to them. It is quite usual for parents to become "out of sync" with each other.[42] Whereas one parent may cope by seeking information and openly expressing emotions, the other may be more reserved. When one parent appears controlled, focuses on activities unrelated to the illness, or has an apparent lack of emotional response, he or she appears unsympathetic to the other. This difference in coping style, or "dis-synchrony," may be viewed as a lack of empathy by the other parent. As one man said, "At a time when my wife most needed support, I was just unavailable to her. It was all I could do to hold myself together." Communicating with parents individually and together can facilitate exploration and understanding of each spouse's coping strategies and feelings.

Preexisting and/or concurrent relationship or marital difficulties and lack of mutual support places the family at greater risk for psychosocial distress. There have been conflicting reports of whether or not there is a higher divorce rate among parents of children with cancer,[36,44] with no recent research done on this topic. In light of the current high divorce rate in the general population, nurses must make every opportunity to support parents and focus on ways to foster the growth of their relationship. Even in healthy relationships, the sick child requires time and energy, thus threatening the quality and quantity of time and energy parents have for each other. Some families come out of the cancer experience with the feeling that they have lived through the worst that life can give them and are stronger as a result of it.

Parent support groups are useful in helping parents to talk out some of their feelings and establish more open communication.[30] Many parents benefit from talking to other parents of children with cancer on a less formal basis, thus gaining significant support from one another. Some communities offer a "Family Camp" weekend that is particularly helpful for parents.[72] Religion is also a source of support for some families.

Single Parent Concerns

Single parents experience many similar, and some quite different, stressors as married couples. Their shock and grief at diagnosis may be borne alone. They may have friends and other family members to talk to and gain support from; however, those people do not share the same parental bonds that a spouse would and may not be available at the times they are most needed. Nurses need to assist single parents in establishing a supportive social network.

Single parents experience even more disruption in their family life. Whereas married couples can share the workload of child care, transporting family members to clinic or other activities, and household chores, single parents must juggle their time doing everything while continuing to be the breadwinner. Additionally, most single parents have less flexibility to absorb the out-of-pocket expenses involved.

Single parents also feel the burden of making treatment decisions alone if they have sole custody, or jointly with a former spouse or the child's biological parent if a part of the former couple's legal settlement. Reestablishing communication with a former spouse or the child's biological parent may also be required. These options create additional stress. Throughout treatment the single parent may have to share precious time with their child with the former spouse and possibly a stepparent or the former spouse's family. If the former spouse or biological parent is supportive during treatment, the support is usually appreciated; however, if he or she withdraws from the situation, this withdrawal may be experienced as further abandonment. This may compound or reignite original difficulties encountered in the marriage.

Although single parents are common in our society, some may be reluctant to participate in parent support groups if the group is composed primarily of married couples. Linking them up with other single parents of children with cancer may be most appreciated.

Extended Family, Friends, and Community

Maintaining relationships with extended family members may be problematic. Although some families become closer and offer considerable comfort and support, others may be unable to face the situation and pull away, and still others want additional support for themselves and create additional stress for the parents. Grandparents tend to be either a wonderful source of support and provide additional resources to the family, or they require support for themselves.

Some grandparents question the diagnosis or treatment, thus adding more stress to the family's life. They often lack information, have limited participation in decision making, feel helpless, and have less responsibility in the child's care. All of this may ignite communication problems with the parents. Grandparents suffer two types of grief: grief for the ill grandchild and grief for their children who are suffering.

For some parents, friendships may be difficult to maintain, because they have little time and energy for social engagements. Other parents find that just when they need a social outlet, they are excluded from invitations. Friends and neighbors may withdraw for a variety of personal reasons, leading to more isolation for the parents. Others pry or make tactless comments or ask inappropriate questions. Parents may seek companionship with parents of other children with cancer, as their mutual problems and concerns provide a type of support they cannot get from friends, neighbors, or relatives.

Nurses can help parents understand the fears and concerns of others and provide suggestions for talking to friends and relatives. For example, a meeting with the grandparents may be helpful to explain the diagnosis and treatment and to explore the impact of the cancer on all family members. Providing practical ways to be of assistance (that are acceptable to the parents) may be beneficial for all involved. Sometimes neighbors ask what they can do to help. Parents need to give specific suggestions (e.g., go grocery shopping, drive a child somewhere, do laundry).

Religious affiliation can be a source of great solace and support. Families rely on religion through prayer, attending religious services, and seeking a religious explanation for what has happened. In addition, religious community members provide tangible resources such as meals, babysitting, and other needed services.

PSYCHOSOCIAL IMPACT OF CANCER ON THE SIBLINGS

Review of the research literature on siblings of children with cancer reveals somewhat conflicting results.[50,60,70] While some studies found siblings to be at risk for anxiety and emotional suffering,[60,61,68] others found minimal psychologic problems,[67,77] and still other studies identified some positive effect of the cancer experience on the siblings.[22,23] The majority of siblings exhibit behavioral changes that reflect their efforts to cope with the stress brought on by the ill child's diagnosis and treatment.[25] Precisely why some siblings do well and grow from the experience and others suffer emotionally has yet to be determined.[60] The following factors may influence the sibling's ability to cope and adapt: the degree of disruption caused by the illness, the quantity and quality of communication both within the family and between the siblings and health care providers, the type of supportive interventions provided to siblings, and the final outcome of the patient (i.e., healthy survivor, survivor with significant long-term effects, or death).

Despite the lack of conclusive research, most researchers and clinicians agree that the siblings' needs are often not met adequately, and ways to facilitate their coping need to be implemented.[49,71] In response to this need, the International Society of Pediatric Oncology (SIOP) has developed guidelines for assisting the siblings of children with cancer.[62] These guidelines are based on all the available research and clinical experience with siblings.

ISSUES WITH PARENTS

Like the patient and parents, the healthy siblings must adjust to multiple changes brought on by the diagnosis and treatment of cancer. The first adjustment is often a temporary separation from the parents and patient while the ill child is in the hospital. When the patient is first diagnosed, usually both parents are at the hospital and siblings are sent to relatives' or friends' houses to be cared for. Even when only one parent stays in the hospital, the other parent tries to manage home responsibilities, work, and hospital visits. Understandably, siblings feel varying degrees of abandonment and displacement. Siblings of all ages often experience an overwhelming sense of loss and being deprived of parental attention.[68] Developmentally, young children lack the cognitive and emotional maturity to understand that the parents' focus on the ill child is the result of medical necessity rather than a lack of love for them. Even after the patient and parents return home from the hospital, the siblings' need for parental attention often receives low priority.

Coupled with a loss of attention, siblings feel a loss of their own importance within the family. The ill child receives not only significantly more attention but may also receive many gifts from parents, grandparents, relatives, and friends. This may leave the siblings feeling left out and less valued.[60] Even when the siblings receive gifts from well-meaning relatives and friends, the gift is seen as a token and perhaps not as extravagant as the ill child's gift.

Major changes in parental roles often alter the roles of the healthy siblings. If the parent is not available to prepare meals or clean the house, one or more of the healthy siblings are asked to assume these functions. At a time when parents are often overprotective and indulgent of bad behavior in the ill child, siblings relate that the parents have increased expectations of them and a decreased tolerance for misbehaviors. Many siblings state that the patient "gets away with anything" while they must be good. The patient is seen as avoiding punishment while they are experiencing an increase in punishment.

Although siblings may not be thoroughly informed about financial changes that result from the direct and indirect costs of cancer treatment, they are aware of the impact of finances on their lifestyle. As parents' financial and emotional resources become more limited, family outings and vacations may be eliminated or severely curtailed. The vacations that do occur are planned around the treatment needs of the ill child. In many families, extra money that was spent on children's activities is now spent on the ill child. Furthermore, even when the siblings' activities continue, the parents may not be available to attend the sporting event, musical performance, or whatever the sibling is involved in.

Nurses can greatly assist the adjustment of siblings by discussing with the parents the impact of the diagnosis and treatment from the healthy siblings' perspectives. Even simple things, such as verbalizing to the siblings that the parents miss being with them as much as before and that they still love them, are valuable. To facilitate their coping, children need information and assistance in processing or understanding that information. Being apprised of the type of cancer and how it will be treated helps to foster their adaptation to all the changes within their family. Many treatment centers have videotapes, books, and pamphlets that may be helpful to initiate conversation. See Box 15-3 for books that are also helpful for siblings.

ISSUES WITH THE ILL CHILD

In all families, siblings share and compete for their parents' time, interest, and love. Sibling relationships are rarely static and display "varying degrees of loyalty, companionship, rivalry, love, hate, jealousy, and love."[70] Conflicting feelings are difficult to reconcile for young children. Siblings feel empathy and anger toward the patient and parents. They may genuinely want to help, yet feel burdened by responsibilities. They want to go out and enjoy their own activities, but sympathize with the limitations imposed on their ill brother or sister.

Siblings are often troubled by a sense of guilt that they have done or thought something that has caused the cancer. When the patient is immunosuppressed and a sibling becomes ill, the sibling experiences extreme anxiety and guilt if the patient then becomes ill. Some siblings fear that they may cause the patient's death.

Sibling arguments and fights are common in all families. In the heat of anger, one sibling may wish another dead. When that sibling is later diagnosed with cancer, memories of wishing him or her dead cause profound guilt. Feelings of guilt are rarely revealed by siblings, because they fear that the patient or parents would no longer love them if they knew what they have caused. Nurses can open communication by stating that they have known many children who have had a brother or sister with cancer and that sometimes these children think that they have done something to cause the cancer. Siblings need to know that this is never the case.

Anger toward the patient or parents is a troublesome emotion for siblings. Children are frightened by their own anger and have limited ways to express it. They are angry with the patient for taking so much of their parents' time and causing such parental anguish. Siblings may not openly share their anger for fear of making things worse. Expression of anger is hampered by an appreciation for what the patient and parents are going through. By understanding the patient's and parents' situation, siblings are unable to assign blame for the family disruption; thus they are left anxious and confused.

Personal Issues

Siblings experience loneliness from multiple sources. The patient or parents may be absent from the home, or when they return home, they are tired or preoccupied, thus leaving the siblings alone to cope with their own thoughts and feelings. When the sibling is very close to the patient (e.g., are similar in age or sex, share common friends, or share a bedroom), their loneliness is heightened. One 9-year-old boy said, "I just lie awake at night listening to him breathe. He's always so tired, we just don't do things together anymore. I miss him." Another boy said, "I know Mom needs to be with him, but I still miss her."

Many of the thoughts and feelings the siblings experience create a sense of vulnerability. Most siblings quickly realize the ill child's frailty and vulnerability to death. Fear of the patient's death may begin at diagnosis and reoccur at any point, even well after therapy has ended. Siblings also realize that their own lives are just as vulnerable. If this could happen to their brother or sister, it could happen to them. Until diagnosis, they thought their parents could protect them. The reality that their parents cannot protect them from all harm is unsettling.

Coupled with vulnerability is a sense of danger. Adolescent siblings may worry about the danger for long-term sequelae from the toxic effects of chemotherapy or radiation. During treatment, they may witness complications such as sepsis or hemorrhage. With the increased use of hematopoietic stem cell transplants and as more aggressive and toxic treatment protocols are used, the siblings' fears of dangerous effects and complications will likely increase.

Siblings who serve as bone marrow donors are caught in a particularly unsettling predicament. They are hopeful that they may be able to save their sibling's life while fearing that their marrow may not work. One study found that donors had significantly more anxiety and lower self-esteem than nondonor siblings.[53] Another interesting finding was that nondonor siblings exhibited more school problems, while the donor siblings had more adaptive skills in school. If the transplant does not work, they may feel that their "marrow wasn't good enough"[56] and that they are responsible for the patient's death and their parents' anguish.[20] Being a donor for hematopoietic stem cell transplant (HSCT) also places a sibling at risk for psychosocial problems. It has been suggested that sibling interventions of emotional support, attention, and psychosocial preparation occur throughout the HSCT process and post-HSCT, rather than as a single one-time preparation intervention.[52]

Siblings facing or experiencing the death of a brother or sister will benefit from emotional support from more than just their parents. The parents are struggling to deal with their own grief and may have little emotional energy left to assist or be supportive of the siblings. As one mother said, "In the days surrounding Andy's death, I was oblivious to everything but Andy. I knew I should be making meals and taking care of the rest of the family, but I just couldn't. It was all I could do to be with Andy. After he died, I was drowning in my own grief. I couldn't see anyone else's sorrow."

Some siblings use denial or avoidance as a subconscious attempt to cope with the painful reality of the illness. Denial can serve to provide distance from the overwhelming impact of the situation. For this reason it is prudent not to strip children of this defense mechanism before they are willing to abandon it.

Nurses can directly intervene with siblings regarding their own personal concerns during hospital and clinic visits, establishing sibling support groups or sibling camp experiences, incorporating siblings into the patients' camps, or having a "sibling day" at the treatment center. Sibling camps[7] and support groups[13] have significantly increased siblings' understanding of the illness. Nurses can provide anticipatory guidance to parents concerning sibling issues, informally during hospital or clinic visits by asking about the siblings, or formally by becoming a speaker at a parent meeting or support group. When interacting with the parents, it is important to be tactful and sensitive so as not to make them feel worse about ignoring or only partially meeting the needs of their other healthy children. Parents need to know that siblings may be hesitant to share their fears and concerns for fear of making things worse. Parents and teachers should be alerted to changes in the siblings' schoolwork. It may be a short-term effect, such as poor performance on days when the patient is going in for treatment, or long-term changes in performance.

ISSUES WITH PEERS AND THE COMMUNITY

Siblings may be caught in a double-bind situation with their peers. Some siblings do not like it when their friends do not ask how the patient is doing but also resent it when everyone is overly solicitous of the patient and ignores them.

Siblings typically feel alone and isolated with their thoughts and feelings about the cancer experience. They seldom know another child who has a brother or sister with cancer, so they often state that their friends do not appreciate what they are going through. Siblings may be highly selective about how, when, and with whom they share information about their sick sibling. They are afraid that friends or teachers will either pity them or engage in gossip. Faced with these equally undesirable alternatives, they may choose to isolate themselves by not sharing information. When siblings choose to share the experience, they receive varied reactions, from responsive empathy to disinterest. Supportive friends are appreciated, and they are angry with those who are unresponsive.

Psychosocial care of children with cancer and their family members is complex and specific to each person's needs. Nurses must assess developmental level, cultural background, need for and availability of social support, understanding of diagnosis and treatment modalities, level of emotional distress, and coping styles and strategies. Appropriate interventions are then designed to address the assessed problems. Since most families have no prior experience or knowledge with childhood cancers, extensive patient and family teaching about the disease, treatment, management of side effects of therapy, possible long-term effects, and emotional impact are included in the nursing plan.

Fifty years ago when the vast majority of children diagnosed with cancer died, psychosocial care

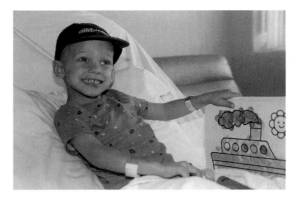

Figure 15-6

Psychosocial growth is the goal throughout the cancer experience.

was aimed at the parents to help them adapt to the inevitable loss. Parents and siblings were often studied from a perspective of psychopathology. Just as physical care of the child with cancer has advanced, so has psychosocial care. The outcome of psychosocial care is not just the resolution of problems but the psychological growth and development of each individual family member and the family unit as a whole (Figure 15-6). The role of the nurse now involves helping to prevent emotional damage to the family through an emphasis on coping, adaptation, education, and support.

REFERENCES

1. American Society of Clinical Oncology (ASCO). (1998). Cancer care during the last phase of life. *Journal of Clinical Oncology, 16,* 1986-1996.
2. Anderson, M. F. (1992). *Hospitalized children and books: A guide for librarians, families, and caregivers* (2nd ed.). Metuchen, NJ: The Scarecrow Press.
3. Baker, L. H., Jones, J., Stovall, A., et al. (1993). Workgroup # 3: Psychosocial and emotional issues and specialized support groups and compliance issues. *Cancer, 71* (Suppl.), 2419-2422.
4. Baum, B. J., & Baum, E. S. (1989). Psychological challenges of childhood cancer. *Journal of Psychosocial Oncology, 7,* 119-129.
5. Baysinger, M., Heiney, S., & Ettinger, R. (1993). An educational trajectory approach for the child and adolescent with cancer. *Journal of Pediatric Oncology Nursing, 10,* 133-138.
6. Beder, J. (2000). Training oncology camp volunteers: A developmental and strengths approach. *Cancer Practice, 8,* 129-134.
7. Carpenter, P. J., Sahler, O. J. Z., & Davis, M. S. (1990). Use of a camp setting to provide medical information to siblings of pediatric cancer patients. *Journal of Cancer Education, 5,* 21-26.
8. Chesler, M., Heiney, S., Perrin, R., et al. (1993). Principles of psychosocial programming for children and cancer. *Cancer, 71* (Suppl.), 3206-3209.

9. Clarke-Steffen, L. (1993). A model of the family transition to living with childhood cancer. *Cancer Practice, 1,* 285-292.

10. Clarke-Steffen, L. (1993). Waiting and not knowing: The diagnosis of cancer in a child. *Journal of Pediatric Oncology Nursing, 10,* 146-153.

11. Clarke-Steffen, L. (1997). Reconstructing reality: Family strategies for managing childhood cancer. *Journal of Pediatric Oncology Nursing, 12,* 278-287.

12. Coleman, B., & Heiney, S. (1992). Storytelling as a therapeutic technique in group for school age oncology patients. *Children's Health Care, 21,* 14-20.

13. Dennis, S. S. (1995). The effects of group therapy on anxiety and isolation reduction in the siblings of pediatric oncology patients. *Dissertation Abstracts International, 56-05, Section B,* 2860.

14. De Trill, M., & Kovalcik, R. (1997). The child with cancer: Influence of culture on truth-telling and patient care. *Annals of the New York Academy of Sciences, 809,* 197-210.

15. Ellis, J. A., & Spanos, N. P. (1994). Cognitive and behavioral interventions for children's distress during bone marrow aspirations and lumbar punctures: A critical review. *Journal of Pain and Symptom Management, 9,* 96-108.

16. Eng, B., & Davies, B. (1991). Effects of a summer camp experience on self-concept for children with cancer. *Journal of Pediatric Oncology Nursing, 8,* 89-90.

17. Erikson, E. H. (1963). *Childhood and society* (2nd ed.). New York: Norton.

18. Ettinger, R. S., & Heiney, S. (1993). Cancer in adolescents and young adults: Psychosocial concerns, coping strategies, and interventions. *Cancer, 71* (Suppl.), 3276-3280.

19. Fernandez, C. V., Stutzer, C. A., MacWilliams, L., et al. (1998). Alternative and complementary therapy use in pediatric oncology patients in British Columbia: Prevalence and reasons for use and nonuse. *Journal of Clinical Oncology, 16,* 1279-1286.

20. Gardner, G. G., August, C. S., & Githens, J. (1977). Psychological issues in bone marrow transplantation. *Pediatrics, 60,* 625-631.

21. Harvey, J., Hobbie, W. L., Shaw, S., et al. (1999). Providing quality care in childhood cancer survivorship: Learning from the past, looking to the future. *Journal of Pediatric Oncology Nursing, 16,* 117-125.

22. Havermans, S., & Eiser, C. (1994). Siblings of a child with cancer. *Child: Care, Health & Development, 5,* 309-322.

23. Heffernan, S. M., & Zanelli, A. S. (1997). Behavior changes exhibited by siblings of pediatric oncology patients: A comparison between maternal and sibling descriptions. *Journal of Pediatric Oncology Nursing, 14,* 3-14.

24. Heiney, S. P. (1991). Helping children cope with painful procedures. *American Journal of Nursing, 91*(11), 20-24.

25. Heiney, S. P. (1995). The healing power of story. *Oncology Nursing Forum, 22,* 899-904.

26. Heiney, S. P., Ruffin, J., Ettinger, R. S., et al. (1988). The effects of group therapy on adolescents with cancer. *Journal of the Association of Pediatric Oncology Nurses, 5*(3), 20-24.

27. Heiney, S. P., & Wells, L. M. (1995). Developing, implementing, and evaluating a handbook for parents of pediatric hematology/oncology patients. *Journal of Pediatric Oncology Nursing, 12,* 129-134.

28. Heiney, S. P., & Wells, L. M. (1996). Care of the pediatric oncology patient in cancer chemotherapy: A nursing process approach. In M. Barton Burke, G. Wilkes, & K. Ingwersen (Eds.), *Cancer chemotherapy: A nursing process approach* (2nd ed., pp. 491-518). Sudbury, MA: Jones & Bartlett.

29. Heiney, S. P., Wells, L. M., Coleman, B., et al. (1991). Lasting Impressions: Adolescents with cancer share how to cope: A videotape program. *Journal of Pediatric Oncology Nursing, 8,* 18-23.

30. Heiney, S. P., Wells, L. M., Ettinger, R. S., et al. (1989). Effects of group therapy on parents of children with cancer. *Journal of Pediatric Oncology Nursing, 6,* 63-69.

31. Heiney, S. P., Wells, L., Swygert, E., et al. (1990). Lasting Impressions: A support program for adolescents with cancer and their parents. *Cancer Nursing, 13,* 13-20.

32. Hinds, P. S., Birenbaum, L. K., Clarke-Steffen, L., et al. (1996). Coming to terms: Parents' response to a first cancer recurrence in their child. *Nursing Research, 45,* 148-153.

33. Hinds, P. S., Oakes, L., Furman, W., et al. (1997). Decision making by parents and healthcare professionals when considering continued care for pediatric patients with cancer. *Oncology Nursing Forum, 24,* 1523-1528.

34. Hooker, L., & Kohler, J. (1999). Safety, efficacy, and acceptability of home intravenous therapy administered by parents of pediatric oncology patients. *Medical and Pediatric Oncology, 32,* 421-426.

35. Hymovich, D. P., & Hagopian, G. (1992). *Chronic illness in children and adults: A psychosocial approach.* Philadelphia: W. B. Saunders.

36. Kaplan, D. M., Grobstein, R., & Smith, A. (1976). Predicting the impact of severe illness on families. *Health & Social Work, 1,* 71-82.

37. Kaufman, K. L., Harbeck, C., Olson, R., et al. (1992). The availability of psychosocial interventions to children with cancer and their families. *Children's Health Care, 21,* 21-25.

38. Keats, M., Courneya, K., Danielsen, A., et al. (1999). Leisure-time physical activities and psychosocial well-being in adolescents after cancer diagnosis. *Journal of Pediatric Oncology Nursing, 16,* 180-188.

39. Keene, N., Ruccione, K., & Hobbie, W. L. (2000). *Childhood cancer survivors: A practical guide to your future.* Sebastopol, CA: O'Reilly & Associates.

40. Kline, N. E. (1996). Implementing a computerized teaching documentation tool for pediatric oncology patients and families. *Journal of Pediatric Oncology Nursing, 13,* 232-234.

41. Kodish, E. D., Pentz, R. D., Ruccione, K., et al. (1998). Informed consent in the Childrens Cancer Group. *Cancer, 82,* 2467-2481.

42. Koocher, G. P., & O'Malley, J. E. (1981). *The Damocles syndrome: Psychosocial consequences of surviving childhood cancer.* New York: McGraw-Hill.

43. Kupst, M. J. (1994). Coping with pediatric cancer: Theoretical and research issues, In D. J. Bearison & R. K. Mulhern (Eds.), *Pediatric psycho-oncology: Psychological perspectives on children with cancer.* New York: Oxford University Press.

44. Lansky, S. B., Cairns, N. V., Hassanein, R., et al. (1978). Childhood cancer: Parental discord and divorce. *Pediatrics, 62,* 184-188.

45. Levine, M., Carey, W., Crocker, A., et al. (1999). *Developmental-Behavioral Pediatrics* (3rd ed.). Philadelphia: W. B. Saunders Company.

46. Lipson, J. G., Dibble, S. L., & Minarik, P. A. (1996). *Culture and nursing care: A pocket guide.* San Francisco: UCSF Nursing Press.

47. Manworren, R. C., & Woodring, B. (1998). Evaluating children's literature as a source for patient education. *Pediatric Nursing, 24,* 548-553.

48. McCarthy, A. M., Cool, V. A., Petersen, M., et al. (1996). Cognitive behavioral pain and anxiety interventions in pediatric oncology center and bone marrow transplant units. *Journal of Pediatric Oncology Nursing, 13,* 3-12.

49. Murray, J. S. (1995). Social support for siblings of children with cancer. *Journal of Pediatric Oncology Nursing, 12,* 62-70.

50. Murray, J. S. (1999). Siblings of children with cancer: A review of the literature. *Journal of Pediatric Oncology Nursing, 16,* 25-34.

51. Noll, R. B., Bukowski, W. M., Rogosch, F. A., et al. (1990). Social interactions between children with cancer and their peers: Teacher ratings. *Journal of Pediatric Psychology, 15,* 43-56.

52. Packman, W. L. (1999). Psychological impact of pediatric BMT on siblings. *Bone Marrow Transplantation, 24,* 701-706.

53. Packman, W. L., Crittenden, M. R., Fischer, J. B. R., et al. (1997). Siblings' perceptions of the bone marrow transplantation process. *Journal of Psychosocial Oncology, 15,* 81-105.

54. Piaget, J. (1952). *The origins of intelligence in children.* New York: International Universities Press.

55. Pyke-Grimm, K. A., Degner, L., Small, A., et al (1999). Preferences for participation in treatment decision making and informational needs of parents of children with cancer: A pilot study. *Journal of Pediatric Oncology Nursing, 16,* 13-24.

56. Rappaport, B. S. (1988). Evolution of consultation-liaison services in BMT. *General Hospital Psychiatry, 10,* 346-351.

57. Richardson, J. L., Shelton, D. R., Krailo, M., et al. (1990). The effects of compliance with treatment on survival among patients with hematologic malignancies. *Journal of Clinical Oncology, 8,* 356-364.

58. Richardson, R., Nelson, M., & Meeske, K. (1999). Young adult survivors of childhood cancer: Attending to emerging medical and psychosocial needs. *Journal of Pediatric Oncology Nursing, 16,* 126-136.

59. Schuster, C. S., & Ashburn, S. S. (1992). *The process of human development: A holistic life-span approach* (3rd ed.). Philadelphia: J. B. Lippincott.

60. Sloper, P., & While, D. (1996). Risk factors in the adjustment of siblings of children with cancer. *Journal of Child Psychology, Psychiatry and Allied Disciplines, 37,* 597-607.

61. Spinetta, J. J. (1981). The siblings of the child with cancer. In J. J. Spinetta & P. Deasy-Spinetta (Eds.), *Living with childhood cancer* (pp. 133-142). St. Louis: Mosby.

62. Spinetta, J. J., Jankovic, M., Eden, T., et al. (1999). Guidelines for assistance to siblings of children with cancer: Report of the SIOP working committee on psychosocial issues in pediatric oncology. *Medical and Pediatric Oncology, 33,* 395-398.

63. Suderman, J. (1990). Pain relief during routine procedures for children with leukemia. *Maternal Child Nursing, 15,* 163-166.

64. Tebbi, C. K. (1993). Treatment compliance in childhood and adolescence. *Cancer, 71* (Suppl.), 3441-3449.

65. Tebbi, C., Bromber, C., & Mallon, J. (1998). Self-reported depression in adolescent cancer patients. *American Journal of Pediatric Hematology Oncology, 10,* 185-190.

66. Van Dongen-Melman, J. E. W. M. (1997). Information booklet for parents of children surviving cancer. *Leukemia, 11,* 1799-1806.

67. Van Dongen-Melman, J. E. W. M., De Groot, A., Hahlen, K., et al. (1995). Siblings of childhood cancer survivors: How does this "forgotten" group of children adjust after cessation of successful cancer treatment? *European Journal of Cancer, 31A,* 2277-2283.

68. Walker, C. L. (1988). Stress and coping in siblings of childhood cancer patients. *Nursing Research, 37,* 208-212.

69. Walker, C. L. (1989). Use of art and play therapy in pediatric oncology. *Journal of Pediatric Oncology Nursing, 6,* 120-126.

70. Walker, C. L. (1990). Siblings of children with cancer. *Oncology Nursing Forum, 17,* 355-360.

71. Walker, C., Adams, J., Curry, D., et al. (1992). A delphi study of pediatric oncology nurses' facilitative behaviors. *Journal of Pediatric Oncology Nursing, 10,* 126-132.

72. Walker, C., & O'Neil, J. A. (1993). Camp Reach for the Sky: Family camp for children with cancer. *Cancer Practice, 1,* 228-232.

73. Webb, N. B. (Ed.). (1991). *Play therapy with children in crisis: A casebook for practitioners.* New York: The Guilford Press.

74. Wieder, C., Hauff, M., & Luchtman-Jones, L. (2000). The benefit of a re-entry program for school-aged children with cancer: A randomized study. *Journal of Pediatric Oncology Nursing, 17,* 98-99.

75. Woodgate, R. L. (1999). A review of the literature on resilience in the adolescent with cancer: Part II. *Journal of Pediatric Oncology Nursing, 16,* 78-89.

76. Woodgate, R. L. (1999). Social support in children with cancer: A review of the literature. *Journal of Pediatric Oncology Nursing, 16,* 201-213.

77. Zeltzer, K., Dolgin, M., Sahler, O., et al. (1996). Sibling adaptation to childhood cancer collaborative study: Health outcomes of siblings of children with cancer. *Medical and Pediatric Oncology, 27,* 98-107.

16

Home Care

Sharon Frierdich

Pediatric home health care is defined as the delivery of skilled care and support services to children in their place of residence. It encompasses a wide variety of professional and technical services. The ultimate goal of pediatric home health care is to teach family caregivers to provide independent, safe, and competent care to the child.[13] Home health care offers a unique opportunity for partnership with the family without whose cooperation home health care would not be possible.

Pediatric home health care is the fastest growing segment in the health care industry, due in part to the increased utilization of home health care services in pediatric oncology.[10] Expansion of home health care in the management of children with cancer can be attributed to multiple factors. One major factor is the improved survival rate of children.[17] More recently, increased knowledge of tumor biology, immunology, and other related sciences has lead to the development of cancer treatments such as low-dose continuous infusions, sequential days of chemotherapy, and growth factor administration after chemotherapy. These types of treatments are appropriate for delivery in the home.[22] Also, more effective interventions are available to prevent or minimize the side effects of cancer therapy that in the past often kept children in the hospital. Developments in medical technology, such as central venous lines and portable infusion pumps, have also facilitated complex care delivery in the home.[27]

Managed care and cost saving initiatives provided economic incentives for delivering care in the home. Several studies have documented the ability to safely administer intravenous therapies such as chemotherapy and antibiotics in the home setting at a cost savings compared with hospital-based care.[7,12,16,19] The initiation of prospective payment systems has shifted comprehensive home health care service to the community, especially after such treatments as hematopoietic stem cell transplants (HSCT).[18] The uncertainty of hospital bed availability, the present nursing shortage, and the concerns of infection transmission in the hospital setting are also factors that have made home care an important option in pediatric oncology.

The needs of the child and family members have contributed to the growth of home health care for children with cancer. Home health care is delivered in a familiar and nurturing environment, allowing the child to continue to engage in normal activities, thereby enhancing the child's quality of life and development. The care facilitates family cohesiveness and community interactions. It also helps to defray out-of-pocket costs typically associated with hospital and clinic visits, such as travel and parking costs, sitter fees, and work time lost.[31]

Pediatric home health care is a specialized division of home health care services, requiring a family-centered focus of care. Essential components of home health care consist of the acknowledgement of the uniqueness of each family unit as identified by its structure, culture, and support systems, and evaluation of the additional burden home care may place on all family members.[4] The transition of the child from hospital to home-based care requires interdisciplinary planning and the development of realistic measurable goals that the caregivers can successfully achieve.[1]

THE HOME HEALTH CARE PLANNING PROCESS

The home health care planning process consists of four phases: assessment, planning, implementation, and evaluation.[13,31] Planning for home care is initiated early in the child's hospital experience. The child's caregivers meet with interdisciplinary care team members, including physicians, nurses, nutritionists, therapists, social workers, teachers, and other disciplines as needed for the particular child, to identify home care needs and to establish discharge goals. The essential role of case management includes patient care coordination, facilitating the achievement of quality and cost-effective clinical outcomes, procuring resources and services needed for the child and family, and intervening at key points in the continuum of the child's care.[33] Many pediatric oncology teams have a designated case manager to plan home care and work with insurance companies. For other teams this accountability is integrated into the role of an advanced practice nurse or the primary care staff nurse. Families need to have an identified person responsible for coordinating their care and with whom they can communicate on an ongoing basis.

A comprehensive discharge plan incorporates all aspects of home health care and supportive services. This plan is crucial to achieve the optimal physical, emotional, and developmental function of the child with cancer, while minimizing adverse reactions and the financial burden on the family.

ASSESSMENT

DETERMINE THE APPROPRIATENESS OF THERAPY

Home health care agencies administer complex chemotherapy regimens, blood products, nutritional support, intravenous hydration, intravenous antimicrobial and antifungal treatment, pain management, and many other therapies. They also provide multiple services such as occupational and physical therapy. Many oncology patients have complex needs and may need all of these services, particularly patients undergoing HSCT. Additional information about the home care needs of HSCT patients is found in Chapter 8. In planning a child's discharge, the first question is not "Can this therapy be done in the home?" but rather "Should this therapy be done in the home?" Specific criteria determine the appropriateness of the home-based interventions. The first consideration is whether the child's medical condition is stable and easily managed in the home by family caregivers. A child who requires direct physician assessment and involvement or frequent close monitoring by nurses will require hospital-based care.

The therapy or service must be well defined for safe delivery in the home. A course of therapy is first administered in the hospital or clinic setting to rule out any untoward reactions before proceeding to home administration.[15] Any therapy with known or potentially deleterious or emergent complications may not be appropriate for administration in the home. Another concern is whether equipment to safely administer the therapy is available. For example, a child without a central line catheter would not be a candidate for a continuous infusion of a vesicant chemotherapeutic agent or parenteral nutrition.

The side effects of the therapy need to be managed effectively. Again, a hospital-based trial of the therapy can assist in determining the best supportive care regimen to prevent or minimize side effects of the therapy in the home setting. Any therapy that requires frequent laboratory tests and close monitoring of results during the therapy may be best performed in the hospital or clinic setting.

Is there a reasonable number of therapies the child will be receiving in the home? A caregiver can easily be instructed to give an antibiotic twice a day, but if the child is on multiple therapies with frequent administration times, home care may not be feasible.

A final consideration in determining the appropriateness of home therapy is the ability to adhere to clinical trial protocols. Protocol requirements must be observed, and if certain tests or assessments could not be performed in the home care setting, the home therapy may not be an option.

INFORMATIONAL NEEDS OF THE FAMILY CAREGIVERS

It is essential to assess the family caregivers' ability to learn and their motivation to perform needed activities in the home setting. Problem-solving and clear decision-making skills regarding the care of the child must be demonstrated. It is desirable that two members of the family be educated and capable to provide the care. This allows for internal reinforcement and respite in the home.[8] A home care contract is developed for the family caregivers listing the goals, learning objectives, and methods to demonstrate competency. Discharge from the hospital can occur upon successful completion of the care contract.[4]

The family caregivers are taught with the same equipment they will be using in their home. It is desirable for home care agencies to bring their equipment into the hospital to teach caregivers before discharge. If this is not feasible, the home care agency provides nursing support in the home for the procedure until the caregiver is independent in the task. Caregivers who have children with complex home care needs or who demonstrate insecurity or reluctance to deliver home care may benefit from a trial run before discharge. Often caregivers will develop the confidence to give complex care if they practice in the hospital for 24 to 48 hours, knowing they have the support of the hospital staff if needed.[31] A variation of this system is to discharge the child and family to a close residential facility, such as a Ronald McDonald House, and have a daily check-in with the family until their comfort and competency level is achieved. A mother of a teenage girl with acute lymphocytic leukemia stated:

> One of the most frightening aspects of Chelsea's treatment was when I was faced with the responsibility of administering her meds at home intravenously. I remember

being told I would hook her up to a portable IV pump—ensuring the medication was hung properly and the pump was infusing correctly. My first reaction was pretty negative. I was still overwhelmed with her diagnosis. I simply said I could not do it! I was assured I could, and with training at the hospital and the in-home nurse who came to check up on me, I did gain the confidence to administer her medicine.

FAMILY UNIT AND COPING ABILITIES

The center of the home care plan is the family. Therefore it is important to assess the family structure and processes before the transition to home care. This assessment will assist the health care team to create a home-based program that will empower the family system and strengthen its ability to successfully implement the home care plan. A structured family interview is conducted by the case manager or other team designate and covers the following elements.

The culture, religion, and values of the family are discussed. Often, strong family values, cultural support, and religious affiliation will be sources of strength and support.

Identify the family members who live in the household, such as parents, siblings, extended family members, and others. Many children now live in two homes because of dual custody agreements. Ideally, parents with joint custody arrangements will come to an agreement that one household is the provider of complex home care so that resources do not have to be duplicated.

Single parents often will experience unique stressors associated with home care, especially if they are employed.[24] Many parents need to apply for unpaid family leave from their jobs to stay home and care for their child or will rely on extended family members for respite.

The roles and responsibilities of each family member are assessed. It is important to identify those members employed outside the home and how household tasks are delegated. What is a typical day for the children in the household? Who has primary responsibility for the care of the child with cancer? What are the perceived changes in roles and responsibilities if home care is provided?

The case manager can help the parents examine the potential impact that home care will have on their family. The parents can then begin to determine effective reorganization strategies and identify support options.[5] Effective family adaptation is related to the family members' abilities to modify their respective roles, perform tasks essential for the continuity of family life, and redefine their personal expectations and goals.[6,21] It is recommended that the parents have a family meeting to discuss the child's return home and the special care required. The family can discuss how this plan will

impact all the family members and seek suggestions on how the family can work together and support one another in this effort.

Family Cohesiveness and Coping

Family cohesion is the emotional bond the family members have with one another.[24] Communication and interactions will enhance or restrict the cohesiveness of family members.[22] The case manager must be informed if there are problems with relationships within the family that may affect the child and the care the child receives or if there are family issues such as alcohol or drug abuse, marriage difficulties, or dysfunctional behaviors by family members.[25]

Another element of assessment is how effectively the family is coping with the crisis of cancer. Adding the responsibility of home care to the stress already imposed by the diagnosis of cancer may be overwhelming. Parents who assume responsibility for home care will have additional informational, emotional, and financial needs.[3]

The resiliency model by McCubbin and Patterson can assist the health care team to understand the family members' perceptions of crisis and their ability to cope. Families who reframe the child's illness as a challenge or an opportunity for growth appear to cope well. Families who do not adapt well to their child's chronic illness often view themselves as victims and powerless to fight the system.[20] It is important to evaluate the parents' past ability to solve problems effectively and make appropriate decisions regarding their child's health care issues. This may give the home care team information on how they may handle future unforeseen problems associated with home care.

The siblings' ability to cope with the illness is also assessed. If a sibling is already having difficulty coping, the additional attention directed to the child during home care may intensify the feelings of anger and guilt. Parents must encourage siblings to share their feelings, and they must find quality time at home to spend with the siblings.[4]

THE HOME ENVIRONMENT

An assessment of the home environment is performed early in the discharge process to determine if the child's care will require modifications in the home. Ideally, the home care nurse visits the home before the child's discharge and assists the family with preparing the home for the child's return.

An assessment of the home environment is essential to ensure care will be delivered safely and effectively. Elements to assess include general cleanliness, availability of electricity, adequate plumbing, refrigeration, and heating and cooling systems. A telephone must be easily accessible, ideally with an answering machine. The home may need modifications for adaptive equipment such as a wheelchair. Electrical outlets and wiring may need adjustment to support the medical equipment. The family's mode of transportation or access to public transportation must also be determined.[31]

The home care nurse can give suggestions for the placement of equipment and the safe storage of medicine and supplies out of reach of children and pets. The correct method for disposal of used supplies, especially used needles or other sharp objects and chemotherapy infusion equipment, is reviewed.

If the environment is unsuitable for home care for a child with cancer, the parents may need to find alternate housing. A temporary location, such as a relative's home, may be designated. If suitable housing cannot be identified, home care may not be an appropriate option.

COMMUNITY SUPPORT NETWORK

The primary care provider is notified that the child with cancer will be receiving home care, and may serve as an additional resource for the family and the hospital based oncology team. The community emergency service rescue squad and the area water, electrical, and telephone services are made aware of a child requiring complex medical care in the home. These services can then respond promptly if there is a breakdown in services to the home.[31]

If the child with cancer is attending school or a daycare facility, the principal, teacher, and school nurse are made aware of any special needs the child will have while attending school. Children who are unable to attend school will have a tutorial home-based program coordinated with the medical home care schedule.

The family and the health care team collaborate to identify community support systems.[13] Local friends, parent support groups, church groups, and other organizations may offer many types of services that can be beneficial, such as respite care, making meals, taking siblings to their routine activities, and cleaning the house. In one case, a local hardware store donated supplies, personnel, and their time to build a wheelchair ramp for a child's home.

Families can find support through a number of web sites that provide information and links to other families who are experiencing cancer.[23] In computer chat rooms, the families can share coping strategies for dealing with home care demands.

EVALUATE HOME CARE AGENCIES AND RESOURCE VENDORS

Discharge therapies and home care equipment and supplies must be identified as early as possible in the child's hospitalization. The selection of the providers for these services are often dictated by hospital joint ventures with a home care agency and preferred provider arrangements by the child's medical insurance company. These providers may not be able to meet the specialized home care needs of the child with cancer. Alternative referrals are then made. Home care nurses who have specialized knowledge in the care of children with cancer improve patient and family outcomes.[29]

The National Association of Children's Hospitals and Related Institutions (NACHRI), with endorsement by the Association of Pediatric Oncology Nurses (APON), has developed Home Care Requirements for Children With Cancer. In these guidelines the following recommendations are cited[27]:

- Pediatric health care providers, the payor, and the family must collaborate to select the most appropriate health care delivery setting based on assessment of the child and family.
- Families must be given the option to interview and select a home health care agency based on the child's specific needs and the agency's expertise (e.g., skilled care requirements, durable medical equipment).
- Home care agencies offering oncology services to children must ensure access to home care nurses and pharmacists with documented competency in pediatrics and oncology.
- Mechanisms must be established to ensure adequate and timely communication between the home care agency, payor, primary care provider, and pediatric oncology specialist about the child's long-term treatment.

NACHRI also provides an interview guide for selecting a home care agency for a child with cancer (Box 16-1).

The insurance contacts for the child and the selected providers and agencies must be easily accessible in the child's medical record to facilitate future home care planning. The family will also receive a card listing the service providers.

EVALUATE HOME CARE REIMBURSEMENT AND FINANCIAL RESOURCES

The case manager and social worker will assist the family in identifying the available financial resources for home care. They must examine the types of benefits provided by the third-party payor, whether it is a private or commercial insurance, a health maintenance organization, or a publicly supported plan such as Medicaid. Home care benefits are verified directly by contacting the insurance company and obtaining an accurate interpretation of the benefits.[32] The financial limits of the insurance policy are specified as a designated annual

BOX 16-1

INTERVIEW GUIDE FOR SELECTING A PEDIATRIC HOME CARE AGENCY

ORGANIZATION

1. Is the agency licensed by the state?
2. Is the agency Medicare/Medicaid certified?
3. By whom is the agency certified/accredited?
4. Is there a supervisory person on call 24 hours a day year-round to deal with concerns of families and staff?
5. Is there a registered nurse with pediatric and oncology experience available 24 hours a day year-round?
6. Does the agency have bilingual staff?
7. What percentage of the agency's patients are:
   - Children under 12 years of age?
   - Adolescents 12-18 years of age?
   - Older than 18 years of age?
8. How does the agency assess the patients'/families' satisfaction with services provided (e.g., follow-up phone call, written survey)?
9. Does the agency have written materials about service expectations?
10. Does the agency have a defined mechanism for families to file a grievance or appeal agency decisions?

SERVICES

1. What pediatric oncology services are provided by this agency?
   - Chemotherapy administration
   - Antibiotic administration
   - Blood product administration
   - Total parenteral nutrition
   - Hydration/fluid administration
   - Central line care and management of complications
   - Phlebotomy
   - Management of side effects
   - Skilled nursing visits
   - Hospice/end-of-life support
2. Are infusion therapy and durable medical equipment supplies provided by this agency, or are these supplies and equipment contracted through another company? Is the equipment consistent with the hospital's equipment?
3. Does the agency's staff come into the hospital/clinic to participate in teaching/caring for the patient before discharge?
4. Does a representative from the agency come to the hospital/clinic to meet regularly with the oncology team or attend patient care meetings or rounds?
5. Does the agency coordinate with the oncology team and family to develop the plan of care, changes to the plan, and outcomes from the plan? How is this done?
6. How does the agency communicate on an ongoing basis with the oncology team? Is there shared documentation following each visit with the patient?
7. How are patients' needs assessed and changes in services adjusted?
8. Are services available 24 hours a day, including weekends and holidays?
9. Does the agency have policies and procedures similar to those of the hospital/clinic? Are they available for review? Is the agency willing to use the hospital's policies and procedures?
10. Does the agency have emergency procedures outlined? Are they available for review?

PERSONNEL

1. Does the agency employ its own staff, share staff with the hospital, or subcontract for staff? If it subcontracts for staff, how is competency validated?
2. What percent of the agency's staff have experience in care for pediatric oncology patients?
3. What education, training, and experience do personnel have relevant to pediatrics and oncology?
   - RN
   - LPN
   - Home Health Aide
4. Are any of the agency's staff certified pediatric oncology nurses (CPON)?
5. What skills/competencies are validated and reassessed on an ongoing basis (e.g., chemotherapy, central line care, blood products)?
6. Does the agency have requirements for inservice training?
7. Will the same staff member be assigned for the entire length of a case? How are assignments made?

FINANCIAL

1. Does the agency accept assignment of benefits?
2. Does the agency bill the third-party payor directly, or does it require families to self-pay and then submit receipts for reimbursement?
3. Will the agency accept referrals with no source of reimbursement?
4. Will the agency negotiate rates?
5. Will the agency furnish required documentation to support a bill?

From National Association of Children's Hospitals and Related Institutions (NACHRI). (2000). Patient Care Oncology FOCUS Group: Home care requirements for children and adolescents with cancer. *Journal of Pediatric Oncology Nursing, 17,* 45-49.

ceiling amount or a maximum lifetime benefit. Parents should ask about policy deductibles for discharge medications, durable equipment, supplies, and other home care costs. Many insurance agencies will verify home health care coverage but will not guarantee payment for service. Often, only a retrospective investigation of the child's home care will determine payment. If coverage is in doubt, the physician provides a letter of medical necessity or talks directly to the insurance's medical director about the case. It is often helpful to provide a cost comparison between the hospital services and home care.[30] It is critical to determine that home health care services are authorized to be reimbursed before discharging the child from the hospital. Often these services are coordinated with insurance providers' case managers, hospital social workers, and the home care agency.

If home care is rejected by the third-party payor, the social worker may need to gather comprehensive financial information about the family's combined income, savings, and property holdings to determine if the child is eligible for local, state, or federal assistance. Application for government-based assistance programs is often tedious, and the process may take many months. Families may also seek assistance from their state's department of insurance, who will advocate for policyholders in particular cases.[9] The Department of Insurance may negotiate with insurance companies for policy exceptions as indicated, such as extending the length of stay for a child hospitalized with complex needs.

The social worker can also advise families on how to protect fund-raising donations and contributions from being taxed as family income. Placing discretionary funds in a trust under the child's name allows parents to use these funds for gaps in insurance coverage and other expenditures related to the child's health care.

PLANNING

Once a thorough assessment has been completed, planning for home care can be initiated. The planning phase involves the coordination of services and the communication of the home care plan to service providers and caregivers. A targeted discharge date is established, preferably a weekday when the health care team is available to refine any problems that may arise and to communicate directly with the home care providers.[31] All home care service providers must be appraised of the discharge timetable, especially when the child requires high-tech home care. This assures that equipment and supplies are available in the home before discharge.[8] The pharmacist must receive prescriptions for medications and IV preparations the day before discharge in order to process the order, clarify questions, or make recommendations as needed.

An initial referral is sent to the home care nursing agency before the discharge. This gives the home care nurse time to clarify orders and address any concerns before actually providing care in the home. The components of the referral are listed in Box 16-2. Any other information that may assist the home care nurse is also sent. Some institutions have a pediatric oncology care map for home care nurses that lists specific interventions and outcomes to be achieved in the home setting and can be individualized to meet a particular child's needs.[14] Any institutional policies and procedures or standardized discharge guidelines that may be helpful for home care are also shared. Often, on the day of discharge, last-minute modifications in the plan of care may be necessary, and these are communicated to the appropriate providers.

The final item in the planning phase of home care is discharge instructions to the family caregivers. This is often the time to review all home medications, procedures, and specific care needs.

Although not all families will require a home care nurse to provide direct specialized home care, many families will benefit from at least one visit by a home care nurse shortly after the child's initial diagnosis. Families receive much information (symptoms to report, medications to give, and care of the central line) while under the stress of being told the diagnosis. It is often reassuring to the family to know that a nurse will be coming to the home to reinforce the teaching and assist in problem solving. Although many families may appear comfortable with providing care at home after the diagnosis, they may gain additional benefit from the reassurance, reinforcement, and emotional support an initial nursing visit may provide.[32]

IMPLEMENTATION

The implementation phase of the home care plan begins with the initial visit by the home care nurse and service providers. The visit is set up at the convenience of the family as soon as possible after discharge.

One of the most important tools for the home care nurse is a laptop computer. Many use computerized intake assessment and documentation programs, and the data is entered at the time of the home visit. The consent for therapy, rights of the family, and an individualized plan of care or pathway can be generated on the computer. These items and daily progress reports can be shared with the

BOX 16-2

COMPONENTS OF A PEDIATRIC ONCOLOGY HOME CARE REFERRAL

1. Patient demographics
   - Name, date of birth
   - Home address and phone number(s)
   - Names of caregivers and their relationship to patient
2. Insurance details
   - Insurance carrier(s) and policy group number(s)
   - Insurance contact person
   - Home care benefits
3. Primary and secondary diagnosis (date of diagnosis)
4. Past significant medical history
   - Allergies
   - Significant medical events
5. Summary of hospitalization
   - Admission/discharge dates
   - Procedures performed
   - Significant events
6. Review of systems
   - Discharge vital signs, height, weight
   - Functional status
   - Cognitive, developmental status
   - Systems review: HEENT, integumentary, respiratory, neurologic, cardiovascular, gastrointestinal, genitourinary, musculoskeletal
   - Nutritional, pain status
7. Recent laboratory data
8. Discharge medications (dose, route, schedule)
9. Home care needs (these services require specific physician orders)
   - Teaching needs of caregivers
   - Home personnel requirements (e.g., RN, LPN, Aide) and frequency of home visits
   - Medications, parenteral fluids, nutritional supplementation to be administered in the home
   - Specific procedures to be performed in home (e.g., central line care, dressing change)
   - Daily patient assessment
   - Laboratory tests to be obtained and monitored
   - Special supplies and equipment
   - Rehabilitative therapies in the home (e.g., OT, PT)
   - Patient/family counseling services
10. Summary of family and home assessment
    - Structure of family
    - Significant aspects related to family (culture, roles and responsibilities) and family cohesion and coping ability
    - Informational needs of caregivers
    - Home environment
    - Community support and resources
    - Financial concerns
11. Other helpful information (examples)
    - Care plan map
    - Research protocol roadmap for chemotherapy administration
    - Institutional policy and procedure for central line care or other procedures
    - Discharge guidelines for hematopoietic stem cell transplants
    - Patient evaluation and therapy recommendations from hospital therapist (e.g., OT, PT)
12. Contact professionals (include emergency numbers)
    - Institutional physician
    - Team case manager (team care coordinator)
    - Community primary physician
13. Follow-up appointments
    - Dates
    - Location of appointment
    - Transportation needs

family.[26] Monitoring data such as vital signs and laboratory data can be added to the daily progress notes and faxed to the health care team for review. All phone contacts with the family and the health care team can be documented. The major purposes for complete documentation of the visit are for agency and nursing liability and for relaying information to the referring institution.

Ideally, the home care nurse contacts the institutional health care team after the initial home visit to discuss how the visit progressed. Thereafter, updates are made when the care needs of the family change, new orders are required to provide care, or an untoward or emergent event occurs in the home.

The home care nurse must have orders that provide some latitude in decision making in certain care situations, such as pain control. Giving the nurse an order for a dosage range that can be titrated in the home based on the pain assessment will allow the nurse to respond to the child's needs more quickly and effectively, as will orders for PRN supportive care drugs to administer if side effects occur.

The decision to discontinue home care services is made when the level of care required by the patient decreases, the family demonstrates safe and competent management of their child's care, or the identified outcomes of the care plan have been met by the child and family.[11] Home care services may also be suspended or terminated if the child has a change in health status requiring readmission to the hospital.[22] Many families adjust best to the discontinuation of home care when a weaning approach is implemented.[4] This method leaves the child's case open and allows the family to call the home care nurse if they require assistance.

EVALUATION

The final stage of the home care planning process is the evaluation of the plan for appropriateness and effectiveness by all members of the home care team including, the referring institution, the home care agency, service providers, and the child and family. Quality assurance programs within agencies are designed to evaluate the quality of the services that were provided. The quality of the service is routinely measured against specific outcome criteria defined by federal and organizational standards.[2]

Evaluation of the child's and family's satisfaction with the home care experience is critical. A program cannot improve without knowing how those using it evaluate its effectiveness. Without information from the consumers, efforts to deliver high-quality care will remain unsuccessful.[2]

After the child's discharge from home care the family is asked to respond to a written or telephone survey with such queries as:

- Was the plan developed to meet your child's home care needs appropriate?
- Was the coordination of all the services to provide care to your child in the home efficient and timely?
- Were you involved in the development and implementation of your child's home care plan?
- What were the benefits of home care for your child and family?
- What were the additional stressors placed on your family due to home care?
- Is there any other information you would like to share with us about your home care experience?

Any information obtained from the survey is discussed by the home care team to reinforce those service areas they do well and to initiate a discussion for changes in areas that require improvement.

Home health care is a viable system for providing care to pediatric oncology patients. It is an evolving field that continues to grow as new technologies and therapies are developed. Pediatric oncology professionals, institutions, and organizations need to recognize the community-based care and service providers as partners in the care of children with cancer. Home care planning and delivery must be incorporated in pediatric oncology education. In addition, home care providers should be invited to attend and participate in pediatric oncology educational programs, seminars, and conferences. Health care professionals must also keep abreast of

health care reform legislation and the impact policies may have on home care delivery. All children with cancer require access to high quality, comprehensive, and affordable home care that meets their special needs.[28]

REFERENCES

1. American Academy of Pediatrics. (1995). Guidelines for home care of infants, children, and adolescents with chronic disease. *Pediatrics, 96*, 161-164.
2. Applebaum, R. (2000). Assuring and improving the quality of in-home services. *Caring, 19*(6), 12-15.
3. Betz, C. L. (2000). The continual challenge of empowering children and families. *Journal of Pediatric Nursing, 15*, 61-62.
4. Chapman, D. (1998). Family-focused pediatric home care. *Caring, 17*(5), 12-15.
5. Clarke-Steffen, L. (1997). Reconstructing reality: Family strategies for managing childhood cancer. *Journal of Pediatric Nursing, 12*, 278-287.
6. Clawson, J. A. (1996). A child with chronic illness and the process of family adaptation. *Journal of Pediatric Nursing, 11*, 52-61.
7. Close, P., Burkey, E., Kazak, A., et al. (1995). A prospective, controlled evaluation of home chemotherapy for children with cancer. *Pediatrics, 95*, 896-900.
8. DiTrapons, V., & Williams, J. (1997). High-technology home care services. In M. D. Harris (Ed.), *Handbook of home health care administration* (pp. 250-270). Gaithersburg, MD: Aspen.
9. Dittbrenner, H. (1998). Recourse for pediatric denials. *Caring, 17*(5), 38-39.
10. Dittbrenner, H. (1999). Pediatric home care as a viable new service. *Caring, 18*(2), 12-13, 15.
11. Erb, J. (1997). Discharge planning. In M. D. Harris, *Handbook of home health care administration* (pp. 427-446). Gaithersburg, MD: Aspen.
12. Escalante, C. P., Rubenstein, E. B., & Rolston, K. V. (1997). Outpatient antibiotic therapy for febrile episodes in low-risk febrile neutropenic patients with cancer. *Cancer Investigation, 15*, 237-242.
13. Franco, S. M. (1997). Pediatric home care. In J. S. Spratt, R. L. Hawley, & R. E. Hoye (Eds.), *Home health care: Principles and practices* (pp. 233-252). Delray Beach, FL: GR/St. Lucie Press.
14. Frierdich, S., & Armstrong-Griffin, A. (1997). Impairment of the hematopoietic system. In W. L. Votroubek & J. Townsend, *Pediatric home care* (pp. 280-341). Gaithersburg, MD: Aspen.
15. Gorski, L. A., & Grothman, L. (1996). Home infusion therapy. *Seminars in Oncology Nursing, 12*, 193-201.
16. Holdsworth, M. T., Raisch, D. W., Chavez, C. M., et al. (1997). Economic impact with home delivery of chemotherapy to pediatric oncology patients. *Annals of Pharmacotherapy, 31*, 140-148.
17. Keene, N., Ruccione, K., & Hobbie, W. L. (2000). *Childhood cancer survivors: A practical guide to your future.* Sebastopol, CA: O'Reilly & Associates.
18. Kelley, C. H., & Randolph, S. (1998). The role of the home care nurse throughout the continuum of blood cell transplantation. *Journal of Intravenous Nursing, 21*, 361-365.
19. Lange, B. J., Burrows, B., Meadows, A. T., et al. (1988). Home care involving methotrexate infusions for children with acute lymphoblastic leukemia. *Journal of Pediatrics, 112*, 492-495.

20. McCubbin, H. I., & Patterson, J. (1983). The family stress process: The double ABCX model of adjustment and adaptation. In H. I. McCubbin (Ed.), *Social stress and the family: Advances and developments in the family stress theory and research* (pp. 7-37). New York: Haworth Press.

21. McEnroe, L. E. (1996). Role of the oncology nurse in home care: Family-centered practice. *Seminars in Oncology Nursing, 12,* 188-192.

22. McNally, J. (1997). Home Care. In S. L. Groenwald, M. H. Frogge, M. Goodmann, et al. (Eds.), *Cancer nursing: Principles and practices* (4th ed., pp. 1501-1530). Sudbury, MA: Jones & Bartlett.

23. Mercer, M., & Ritchie, J. A. (1997). Home community cancer care: Parents' perspectives. *Journal of Pediatric Nursing, 12,* 133-141.

24. Mercer, M., & Ritchie, J. A. (1997). Tag team parenting of children with cancer. *Journal of Pediatric Nursing, 12,* 331-341.

25. Messinger, R., & Dolan, K. (1997). The parent's perspective on pediatric home care. In W. L. Votroubek & J. Townsend (Eds.), *Pediatric home care* (pp. 537-560). Gaithersburg, MD: Aspen.

26. Namie, M. (1997). The value of clinical pathways in home care. *Caring, 16*(6), 42-44, 46.

27. National Association of Children's Hospitals and Related Institutions (NACHRI) Patient Care Oncology FOCUS Group. (2000). Home care requirements for children with cancer. *Journal of Pediatric Oncology Nursing, 17,* 45-49.

28. National Association of Home Care. (2000). NAHC's legislative agenda tackles mission critical issues. *Caring, 19*(5), 18-28.

29. Nemcek, M. A., & Egan, P. B. (1997). Specialty nursing improves home care. *Caring, 16*(6), 12-14, 188.

30. Seeber, S., & Baird, S. B. (1996). The impact of health care changes on home health. *Seminars in Oncology Nursing, 12,* 179-187.

31. Townsend, J. (1997). Discharge planning: Transition to home. In W. L. Votroubek & J. Townsend (Eds.), *Pediatric home care* (pp. 1-10). Gaithersburg, MD: Aspen.

32. Votroubek, W. L. (1997). Financing pediatric home care. In W. L. Votroubek & J. Townsend. (Eds.), *Pediatric home care* (pp. 25-34). Gaithersburg, MD: Aspen.

33. Zander, K. (1987). Nursing care management: A classic definition. *Center for Nursing Case Management, 2,* 1-3.

17

Palliative Care

Dianne Fochtman

Although the cure rate for childhood cancer has increased dramatically over the last three decades, the pediatric oncology nurse must approach each child newly diagnosed with cancer with optimistic honesty. No one knows at the time of diagnosis which child will live and which child eventually will succumb to the illness or to the side effects of therapy. Pediatric oncology nurses must be prepared to deal not only with issues of survivorship, but also with the care of the terminally ill child when death is inevitable. This includes learning to deal with personal feelings to help the child and family traverse the terminal phase with as much comfort, dignity, and strength as possible.

CHILDREN'S CONCEPTS OF DEATH

Helping children and their families in the terminal stages of the illness requires an understanding of how children's ideas and concepts about death develop. Social, scientific, and technologic advances over the years have produced changes that have influenced a child's experience with death. In the past, when the infant mortality rate was high and the average life expectancy was short, a child often experienced the death of siblings and/or parents. The modern child is less likely to lose a parent or sibling through death.[113] In fact, recent generations are the first known in history in which many middle-age adults have not yet experienced the death of an immediate family member.[102]

On the other hand, technologic advances and the media have exposed children to variably accurate concepts of death. Even if parents refuse to allow their child to watch "violent" television shows, they cannot completely remove the idea of death from the child's world. The mass media—television, radio, newspapers, computers, electronic games, and even books designed especially for children—expose a child to death: the bad guy gets killed; the cartoon character dies, often violently, only to be resurrected immediately or in the next sequence; war and the death it brings are presented nightly in news broadcasts; notices of death, violent and otherwise, appear daily on television broadcasts and in newspapers; and even a common bedtime prayer contains a reference to death—"If I should die before I wake . . ."

All these factors have varying consequences for the intellectual and emotional development of the child. Sooner or later children will be exposed to death—the dead animal along the highway, the death of a pet, or the death of a grandparent. Faced with these situations, children will have questions that make it necessary for parents or other adults to talk with them about death. Ideally the subject should be introduced in a nonthreatening situation, for example, when a dead animal is observed along the road, before the child has to deal with a more emotionally important death. How the subject is handled depends on many variables, one of which is the meaning of death to the child.

Early landmark studies in the development of the concept of death in children were done by Anthony[4] in prewar London (1937 to 1939) and Nagy[78] in Budapest in the 1940s. Anthony found that younger children (3 to 6 years old) in her study tended to interpret death as sleep or temporary departure. Magical thinking often pervaded. Anthony believed "that the idea of death develops in the child as intellect advances, rather than as more years increase or as personal experiences teach."[111] Almost all of the children had spontaneous death-related thoughts.

Nagy identified three stages in the development of the death concept in children: (1) death is seen as reversible separation, departure, or disappearance (3 to 5 years); (2) death is personified (either imagined as a separate person or identified with the dead), though understood as final and irreversible (5 to 9 years); and (3) death is perceived as a universal, inevitable, and final process and a cessation of body activities (9 years and older). Since the 1960s further research has added to the knowledge of how children view death at different stages of development.* Children's concepts of death

---

*References 14, 27, 49, 50, 52, 62, 87, 97, 103, 108, 114.

at various developmental stages are presented in Table 17-1.

Early studies of the development of a death concept in children proposed a series of stages, with fixed corresponding ages, during which specific kinds of behaviors and conceptual development occurred. Later studies have shown that the sequence of understanding is more reliable than ages in describing how children learn about death.[22] Life experiences, intelligence levels, family attitudes and values, self-concepts, and many other as yet unknown factors play a part in each child's individual concept of the meaning of death.

The modern consensus is that "children attain a mature concept of death through a process more dependent on developmental level than chronological age."[29] Some children, for various reasons, come to an adult understanding of death at a very early age, whereas others may not fully understand death until late childhood. Children with chronic illnesses may come face to face with death through relationships with other children in the hospital who die. Earlier researchers generally concluded that the cognitive resources necessary to conceive of death as final and inevitable were acquired near the age of 9 years.[78] However, the evidence now suggests that children between the ages of 5 and 7 years may attain a beginning understanding of these concepts.[22]

EXPLAINING DEATH TO CHILDREN

The primary social unit for children is the family, which teaches basic facts and values about self, the world, life, and death. Eventually children will ask questions about death. Answers to these questions depend on the child's age, the intensity and extent of interest, the reasons for the interest, the kind of questions asked, and the situation promoting the question. Questions should be answered clearly, directly, and as truthfully as possible without burdensome detail. Philosophic interpretations should be avoided, and adults must remember that children easily mistake the meaning of words and phrases or take literally what is only an idiom.

The parent or other adult should not attempt to hide the meaning of death with fiction that someday must be repudiated. Some unhelpful explanations of death to avoid, particularly in regard to the death of a loved one, include (1) the dead person has gone on a long journey—the child may react with anxiety and resentment at apparent desertion; (2) God took the dead person away because He wants and loves the good in heaven—the child may develop fear, resentment, and hatred against a god who capriciously took a loved one because that person was loved by God; (3) the person died because she was sick—this linking of sickness and death without any additional information (e.g., saying "The doctors could not fix it") only prolongs and intensifies the fear of death and may add new fears about illness; and (4) to die is to sleep—this explanation, besides being inaccurate, may cause a pathologic fear of sleep.

The specific answers of the adult depend very largely on (1) an understanding of the child; (2) the role of the adult in the child's life (e.g., whether the adult is the parent); (3) personal resources, attitudes, and values; and (4) the social, cultural, and religious traditions of the child and family. The adult must respond to the child's questions with genuine sincerity and conviction because what is said is important; but *how* it is said has even greater bearing on whether the child will develop anxiety and fears or will accept (within the child's capacity) the fact of death.[98] When communicating with a child, the adult must remember that words, although important, are never as important as the feelings imparted to the child.[29]

Art and play may help gain insight into the young child's feelings and may be used as a medium to share concerns and fears. Many children's books are very useful in helping children at various stages of development to understand death.[11,18] Table 17-2 reviews some books for children that deal with death. As a child matures, parents may find other books useful in helping a child understand the concept of death (e.g., *Explaining Death to Children, Talking About Death: A Dialogue Between Parent and Child,* and *Straight Talk About Death for Teenagers,* all by Rabbi Earl Grollman;[34-36] *Talking With Children and Young People About Death and Dying,*[105] *Talking With Children About Loss,*[104] *Keys to Helping Children Deal With Death and Grief,*[47] and others[37,63,90,95,96]).

The death of a loved one (e.g., a grandparent) is difficult for a child to understand and accept. Whether the death presents a barrier to appropriate psychologic development or an opportunity for development and maturation depends largely on how the adults in the child's environment handle the loved one's death. If a death is expected, the child can be gradually be prepared for the inevitable outcome. Although the death may be due to illness, the differences between a terminal illness and the routine illnesses of life must be emphasized. Feelings commonly related to someone's dying, particularly anger and sadness, should be acknowledged, with emphasis on the fact that feelings do not cause death.

TABLE 17-1	COMMON CONCEPTS OF DEATH IN CHILDHOOD	
Common Concepts of Death	**Representative Behaviors and Responses**	**Implications for Communication**
INFANCY		
No concept of death; death is experienced as separation.	Infant reacts strongly to separation from parents or caregivers and experiments with object permanence and separation with "throwaway" and "peekaboo" behaviors.	Understand strategies for dealing with separation anxiety. Help other family members cope with death so they can be available to the infant who is dying or who has experienced the death of a parent or caregiver.
EARLY CHILDHOOD		
Concepts about death are greatly influenced by attitudes of parents. The young child learns the words *dead* and *death* but understands little or nothing of their meaning. As the concept begins to form, death is viewed as temporary, gradual, reversible, and a continuation of life on a reduced level. Popular media and magical thinking may reinforce these beliefs. Egocentrism may lead the child to believe that wishes, misbehavior, or unrelated actions can cause death. Young children who have experiences related to death may have a relatively mature concept of death long before they are able to verbalize it.	Child displays increased curiosity about things related to death and spontaneity about discussing the topic. Child retains a sense of the dead person's being and may be concerned that the corpse can sense cold or discomfort or may worry about how it goes to the bathroom. Child may look forward to the dead person's return or carry on imaginary conversations with the dead person.	Expect children to be open and honest in asking questions about death if given the freedom of expression. Children may discuss death by parroting what they have heard from adults without really understanding. They often have an incomplete or erroneous understanding about death. Assess the need to correct misconceptions, especially if they are causing fear and anxiety. Help children to understand death as a part of life and to comprehend the nature of death while allowing their own positive fantasies to linger. Bereaved siblings may fear that their thoughts or feelings caused the serious illness or death of a brother or sister. Dying children need the opportunity to share concerns and ask questions of their parents. However, some parents are not able to handle the anxiety this causes, and the child may share primarily with a special nurse. Children of this age often communicate best through play. Because separation remains an important issue, dying and grieving children need special considerations to remain close to their parents.

Adapted from Miles, M. S., & Burman, S. I. (1990). Nursing care of the dying child. In S. R. Mott, S. R. James, A. M. Sperhac (Eds.), *Nursing care of children and families* (2nd ed.). Redwood City, CA: Addison-Wesley. Additional data from Betz., C. L. (1987). Death, dying and bereavement: A review of the literature, 1970-1985. In T. Krulik, B. Holaday, & I. M. Martinson (Eds.), *The child and family facing life-threatening illness.* Philadelphia: Lippincott; Fetsch, S. H. (1984). The 7- to 10-year-old child's conceptualization of death. *Oncology Nursing Forum, 11,* 52-56; Speece, M. W., & Brent, S. W. (1984). Children's understanding of death: A review of three components of a death concept. *Child Development, 55,* 1671-1686; Spinetta, J. J., & Deasy-Spinetta, P. (1981). Talking with children who have a life-threatening illness. In J. J. Spinetta & P. Deasy-Spinetta (Eds.), *Living with childhood cancer,* pp 234-253. St. Louis, MO: Mosby; Waechter, E. (1971). Children's awareness of fatal illness. *American Journal of Nursing, 71,* 1168-1172; Waechter, E. H. (1987). Death, dying and bereavement: A review of the literature. In T. Krulik, B. Holaday, & I. M. Martinson (Eds.), *The child and family facing life threatening illness* (pp. 1-31). Philadelphia: Lippincott; Wass, H. (1995). Death education for children. In I. B. Corless, B. B. Germino, & M. A. Pittman (Eds.), *A challenge for living: Dying, death and bereavement.* Boston: Jones & Bartlett.

TABLE 17-1 COMMON CONCEPTS OF DEATH IN CHILDHOOD—cont'd		
Common Concepts of Death	Representative Behaviors and Responses	Implications for Communication
MIDDLE CHILDHOOD		
The majority of children between The ages of 4½ and 8 years achieve at least some level of understanding of the universality (all living things die), irreversibility (the dead cannot be made alive again), and nonfunctionality (all life-defining functions cease) of death. Mutilation fears may be linked to death anxiety. Children may be superstitious and may view death as an unnatural event caused by random, violent, external forces. Children begin facing the fact that family members, including parents, may die.	Child asks more specific questions about death, being dead, and death-related rituals such as burial. Burial and closure rituals for coping with the death of a pet are highly important. Child may want to touch the corpse to see how it feels. Child may use play to develop further understanding of death and to cope with feelings.	Expect children in this period of development to give concrete explanations about the physical causes of death. Play may be used to facilitate a child's understanding of death and related rituals. Children may need to discuss fears about the potential loss of a parent. Siblings need opportunities to ask questions about the illness and death of a brother or sister and may need more specific information about the cause of death. Be alert to feelings of guilt in bereaved siblings and dying children. Dying children continue to need to discuss their concerns with parents and may choose a special nurse as a confidant. They are still concerned about separation and often have concerns about pain, mutilation, and other suffering that may be involved. Dying children during this developmental stage begin to worry about the impact of their death on parents and may try to protect them by closing down communication.
LATE CHILDHOOD		
Universality, irreversibility, and nonfunctionality of death are understood. Children begin to face anxiously the reality of their own mortality; personal fear of death may surface. They begin to incorporate family and cultural beliefs and attitudes about death and show an interest in exploring views about afterlife.	Child may use rituals to decrease anxiety. Reckless behavior, tough demeanor, or humor may be used to cope with sense of vulnerability and fear.	Opportunities are needed for children to verbalize fears and to understand that such fears are normal. They need more detailed explantations about why a person has died, along with opportunities to share feelings and ask questions. Children may need to discuss realistic consequences of reckless activity. Dying children need to discuss concerns with family and staff but may have difficulty in doing so. Normal emotional responses of this age may become more complex as children deal with feelings about dying. It is important to help the dying child feel that life has been important and meaningful.

Continued

TABLE 17-1	COMMON CONCEPTS OF DEATH IN CHILDHOOD—cont'd	
Common Concepts of Death	Representative Behaviors and Responses	Implications for Communication
ADOLESCENCE		
Adolescents reach an "adult" perception of death, but strong focus on "here and now" and intense search for personal identity make death emotionally unacceptable. The thrill of reckless behaviors may outweigh safety factors. Adolescents derive comfort from the concept of having a long life yet to live. They may still hold concepts from previous developmental levels depending on actual experiences and family communication. They are working through religious and philosophic views about life, death, and afterlife.	Anxiety about death may be particularly acute because body image and the emerging self-concept are threatened. Denial and avoidance of death may be used to reduce personal death anxiety.	Use opportunities in daily life to open conversation about death. Avoid assumptions of an adult understanding by assessing the adolescent's specific perceptions. Be alert to feelings of guilt, hostility, confusion, and anxiety when communicating with the adolescent. Treat the feelings and concerns with utmost respect and confidence. Be open in sharing views and concerns about death. Correct misperceptions without being judgmental. The dying adolescent and bereaved sibling may have difficulty in sharing concerns with family. The dying adolescent often feels isolated from the usual channel of communication, the peer group, and may choose a nurse as a confidant regarding concerns and fears. The adolescent needs support in maintaining self-esteem, help in gaining positive closure about the meaning of a relatively short life, and assistance in completing things undone or wishes unfilled.

Adapted from Miles, M. S., & Burman, S. I. (1990). Nursing care of the dying child. In S. R. Mott, S. R. James, A. M. Sperhac (Eds.), *Nursing care of children and families* (2nd ed.). Redwood City, CA: Addison-Wesley. Additional data from Betz., C. L. (1987). Death, dying and bereavement: A review of the literature, 1970-1985. In T. Krulik, B. Holaday, & I. M. Martinson (Eds.), *The child and family facing life-threatening illness.* Philadelphia: Lippincott; Fetsch, S. H. (1984). The 7- to 10-year-old child's conceptualization of death. *Oncology Nursing Forum, 11,* 52-56; Speece, M. W., & Brent, S. W. (1984). Children's understanding of death: A review of three components of a death concept. *Child Development, 55,* 1671-1686; Spinetta, J. J., & Deasy-Spinetta, P. (1981). Talking with children who have a life-threatening illness. In J. J. Spinetta & P. Deasy-Spinetta (Eds.), *Living with childhood cancer,* pp 234-253. St. Louis, MO: Mosby; Waechter, E. (1971). Children's awareness of fatal illness. *American Journal of Nursing, 71,* 1168-1172; Waechter, E. H. (1987). Death, dying and bereavement: A review of the literature. In T. Krulik, B. Holaday, & I. M. Martinson (Eds.), *The child and family facing life threatening illness* (pp. 1-31). Philadelphia: Lippincott; Wass, H. (1995). Death education for children. In I. B. Corless, B. B. Germino, & M. A. Pittman (Eds.), *A challenge for living: Dying, death and bereavement.* Boston: Jones & Bartlett.

DEATH SITUATIONS IN PEDIATRIC ONCOLOGY

In pediatric oncology a child's dying trajectory, or individual course of dying, may be long or short. Death may occur while the child is in remission in a sudden and unexpected way (e.g., from septic shock or intracranial hemorrhage), and death may occur unexpectedly, even when anticipated (e.g., the child with a poor prognosis at diagnosis may die from complications of therapy). Finally, there is the child in whom death is the expected outcome and it occurs at a predictable point. The child who has relapsed or for whom therapy has proven to be ineffective falls into this category.

Although no situation is without hope, there is a time when hope for cure is no longer possible and discontinuing disease-oriented therapy is appropriate.[79,83,85] When cure of the disease cannot be attained, "hope is then centered on palliative care, moving toward hope that the child will die with dignity, without pain either to the child or the significant others surviving with subsequent grief."[38] The decision-making process should be shared by the medical team, the parents, and the child, when appropriate. This shared decision making begins with open communication with the physician as the expert providing honest, clear information regarding the prognosis and the shift in goals of treatment from

Text continued on p. 410.

TABLE 17-2	BOOKS ABOUT DEATH FOR CHILDREN			
Ages	Title	Author(s)	Publisher	Comments
Younger children (4 to 8 years)	The Tenth Good Thing About Barney 1975	Judith Viorst Illustrated by Erik Blegvad	Simon & Schuster	The author succinctly and honestly handles both the emotions stemming from the loss of a beloved pet and the questions about the finality of death. An unusually good book that handles a difficult subject straightforwardly.
	Sadako and the Thousand Paper Cranes 1979	Eleanor B. Coerr Illustrated by Ronald Himler	Bantam Doubleday Dell Books	Hospitalized with the dreaded atom bomb disease, leukemia, a child in Hiroshima races against time to fold one thousand paper cranes to verify the legend that by doing so a sick person will become healthy.
	Everett Anderson's Goodbye 1983 Reprinted 1990	Lucille Clifton Illustrated by Ann Grifalconi	Henry Holt (An Owlet Book)	A picture book that goes through the stages of grief in very few words and big pictures. Everett has a difficult time coming to terms with his grief after his father dies.
	The Fall of Freddie the Leaf 1982	Leo Buscaglia	Henry Holt	Freddie and the other leaves on his tree pass through the seasons and, with the coming of winter, fall to the ground. This warm and sympathetic parable explains the delicate balance between life and death.
	The Two of Them 1987	Aliki	Morrow, William, & Co	Describes the relationship of a grandfather and his granddaughter from her birth to his death.
	When a Pet Dies 1988	Fred Rogers Jim Judkis (photographer)	Putnam	Explores the feelings of frustration, sadness, and loneliness that a youngster may feel when a pet dies.
	I'll Always Love You 1989	Hans Wilhelm	Crown Books	A boy's dog dies and the boy realizes that you never stop loving your dog, or anyone, even when they die.
	Saying Goodbye to Daddy 1991	Judith Vigna Abby Levine (Editor)	Albert Whitman	Frightened, lonely, and angry after her father is killed in a car accident, Clare is helped through the grieving process by her mother and grandfather.
	Badger's Parting Gift 1992	Susan Varley	Morrow, William, & Co	Badger's friends are sad when he dies, but they treasure the legacies he left them.
	The Saddest Time 1992	Norma Simon Illustrated by Jacqueline Rogers	Albert Whitman	Explains death as the inevitable end of life and provides 3 situations in which children experience powerful emotions when someone close dies.

Continued

Data from http://www.barnesandnoble.com.

TABLE 17-2	BOOKS ABOUT DEATH FOR CHILDREN—cont'd			
Ages	Title	Author(s)	Publisher	Comments
Younger children (4 to 8 years) —cont'd	Gentle Willow: A Story for Children About Dying 1993	Joyce C. Mills Illustrated by Michael Chesworth	American Psychological Association	Amanda is upset that she is going to lose her friend Gentle Willow, but the Tree Wizards help her understand that her memories are gifts from her friend and that there are special ways of saying goodbye.
	After the Funeral 1995	Jane Loretta Wisch Illustrated by Pamela Keating	Paulist Press	Discusses the various feelings accompanying the death of a loved one, including sadness, grief, and the fear of death itself.
	I Had a Friend Named Peter: Talking to Children About the Death of a Friend 1995	Janice Cohn Illustrated by Gail Owens	Morrow, William, & Co	When Betsy learns about the death of a friend, her parents and kindergarten teacher answer questions about dying, funerals, and the burial process.
	When a Grandparent Dies: A Kid's Own Remembering Workbook for Dealing With Shiva and the Year Beyond 1995	Nechama Liss-Levinson Karen Savary	Jewish Lights Publishing	This workbook helps children to participate in the process of mourning, and overcome the awkwardness that often accompanies their participation in grieving rituals.
	The Dead Bird 1995	Margaret Wise Brown Illustrated by Remy Charlip	Harper Collins Children's Books	When they find a dead bird, a group of children bury it in the woods, sing a song to it, and put flowers on the grave.
	Water Bugs and Dragonflies: Explaining Death to Young Children 1987	Doris Stickney Hernandez	Pilgrim Press/The United Church Press	After a water bug suddenly leaves her pond and is transformed into a dragonfly, her friends' questions about such departures are like those children ask when someone dies.
	Liplap's Wish 1997	Jonathan London Illustrated by Sylvia Long	Chronicle Books	As he builds a snowbunny, Liplap feels something is missing and wishes his grandmother who recently died was with him.
	Sophie 1997	Mem Fox Illustrated by Aminah Brenda Robinson	Harcourt	This picture book charts the cycle of life within a family as Sophie is born and grows bigger while her beloved grandfather becomes older and slower. The cycle begins again after the elderly man's death with the birth of Sophie's own child.
	When Dinosaurs Die: A Guide to Understanding Death	Laura Krasny Brown & Marc Brown	Little, Brown & Company	Explains in simple language the feelings people may have regarding the death of a loved one and the ways to honor the memory of someone who has died.

Children's Books

Title / Year	Author	Publisher	Description
Surprise 1998		Farrar, Straus & Giroux	to give him a surprise birthday party and a very special present.
Bye, Mis' Lela 1998	Dorothy Carter Illustrated by Harvey Stevenson		When Sugar Plum's friend Mis' Lela dies, she still feels the warm and lasting effect of the time they spent together. The authors capture the pace and essence of life in a small Southern town, and show how losing someone you love doesn't mean forgetting.
A Name on a Quilt: A Story of Remembrance 1999	Jeannine Atkins Illustrated by Tad Hills	Simon & Schuster	A family reminisces while gathered together to make a panel for the AIDS Memorial Quilt in memory of a beloved uncle.
Where Is Grandpa? 1999	T.A. Barron Illustrated by Chris K. Soentpiet	Putnam	As his family reminisces after his beloved grandfather's death, a boy realizes that his grandfather is still with him in all the special places they shared.
The Angel With the Golden Glow 1999	Elissa Al-Chokhachy Illustrated by Ulrike Graf	Penny Bear Company, Inc	A story about an angel's brief journey to earth. He is born with a special gift of healing. Whenever he shines his golden glow, sadness disappears and magically turns into love! He brings this gift to his family and his home overflows with love!
What's Heaven? 1999	Maria Shriver Illustrated by Sandra Speidel	Golden Books	After her great-grandmother's death a young girl learns about heaven by asking her mother all kinds of questions.
The Day I Saw My Father Cry (Little Bill Series) 1999	Bill Cosby Illustrated by Varnette P. Honeywood	Scholastic, Inc	Colorful drawings and simple language in a good attempt at teaching one of life's lessons. This is a good pick for a first book on grief/loss. The feelings are universal, and the colors are vivid.
Nana Upstairs and Nana Downstairs 2000 Reissue	Tomie dePaola	Penguin Putnam Books	Tommy loved his family's Sunday visits to his grandmother, Nana Downstairs, and his great-grandmother, Nana Upstairs. When Nana Upstairs dies, his family's closeness helps him accept her death. This is a wonderful, generational story that celebrates its 25th anniversary.

Continued

Data from http://www.barnesandnoble.com.

TABLE 17-2	BOOKS ABOUT DEATH FOR CHILDREN—cont'd			
Ages	Title	Author(s)	Publisher	Comments
Older children (5 to 11 years)	The Kids' Book About Death and Dying: By and For Kids 1986	Eric E. Rofes	Little, Brown	Fourteen children offer facts and advice to give young readers a better understanding of death.
	Claudia and the Sad Goodbye 1989	Ann Matthews Martin	Scholastic	Claudia has always been close to her grandmother, Mimi, so she needs the help of her friends in the Baby-sitters Club to deal with Mimi's death.
	The Remembering Box 1992	Eth Clifford	Houghton Mifflin	Nine-year-old Joshua's weekly visits to his beloved grandmother on the Jewish Sabbath give him an understanding of love, family, and tradition which helps him accept her death.
	When Someone Dies 1992	Sharon Greenlee Illustrated by Bill Brath	Peachtree Publishers	Explains the hurt, fear, and confusion felt by children and adults after a death has occurred. Offers suggestions for easing the pain, surviving the changes, and remembering the good times.
	I Wish I Could Hold Your Hand: A Child's Guide to Grief and Loss 1994	Pat Palmer Illustrated by Dianne O'Quinn Burke	Impact Publishers	A best friend has moved away, Dad no longer lives with the family, or a favorite pet has died. This warm, comforting book gently helps grieving children identify their feelings and learn to accept and deal with them.
	Grandpa's Berries: A Story to Help Children Understand Grief and Loss 1995	Julie Dickerson	Cherubic Press	Deals with the impact of a grandfather's death on his granddaughter.
	Don't Despair on Thursdays!: The Children's Grief-Management Book	Adolph J. Moser Nancy R. Thatch (Editor) Illustrated by	Landmark Editions, Inc	Examines, in simple text, how to deal with feelings of grief when people or pets die, or when friends move away.

Age	Title / Year	Author / Illustrator	Publisher	Description
	Anymore 1998	White Illustrated by Christine Kempf	Association	traditions and social rituals associated with death, emphasizing the child's thoughts, feelings, and memories.
	Sun and Spoon 1998 (Reprint)	Kevin Henkes	Penguin Putnam	After the death of his grandmother, 10-year-old Spoon observes the changes in his grandfather and tries to find the perfect artifact to preserve his memories of her.
	What on Earth Do You Do When Someone Dies? 1999	Trevor Romain Elizabeth Verdick	Free Spirit	Simple, insightful, and straight from the heart, this book is for any child who has lost a loved one. The author talks directly to kids about what death means and how to cope. He answers questions kids have about death—Why? How? What next? Is it my fault? What's a funeral?—in basic straightforward terms.
	Gran-Gran's Best Trick 2000	L. Dwight Holden Illustrated by Michael Chesworth	American Psychological Association	This story was written to help children deal with the loss of someone they love, and to help parents help children with the grieving process.
Teens (12 & older)	Lost and Found: A Kid's Book for Living Through Loss 1999	Marc Gellman Thomas Hartman Illustrated by Debbie Tilley	Morrow, William, & Co	Describes different kinds of losses—losing possessions, competitions, health, trust, and the permanent loss because of death—and discusses how to handle these situations.
	Beat the Turtle Drum 1994	Constance C. Greene Illustrated by Donna Diamond	Penguin Putnam	The story of how a young girl comes to terms with her sister's death.
	When a Friend Dies: A Book for Teens About Grieving and Healing 1994	Marilyn E. Gootman Pamela Espeland (Ed.)	Free Spirit Publishing, Inc	A brief guide that provides practical advice, some from teens whose friends have died. A good book for identifying and addressing feelings.

Data from http://www.barnesandnoble.com.

cure or control of disease to palliation and comfort.[117] The parents and the child share information regarding their values and beliefs, their desires for the child in terms of comfort and quality of life.[41] Together with other members of the medical team, decisions are made regarding the goals of care.[28]

Some families, and sometimes the child, are not ready to give up hope for life and feel that it is their obligation to fight death at all costs. Ethical dilemmas can develop when the desires of the parents are contrary to those of the older school-age child or adolescent or the oncology team. Because the potential exists for miscommunication and misinterpretation, it can be difficult to differentiate between denial and lack of proper information.[115] Total disclosure and open and frequent communication among all participants is necessary to attempt to support parents, child, and staff and to determine the most appropriate plan of care. Patience and understanding, offered in a nonjudgmental way, are necessary because the conflicts are often not resolved quickly.

THE CONCEPT OF PALLIATIVE CARE

Palliative care is a broad philosophy of total, compassionate care of patients whose disease no longer responds to curative treatment.[119,120] The goal is achievement of the best quality of life for these patients and their families by preventing and relieving suffering. "Pediatric palliative care is family-centered, with the child and family enwrapped in the circle of professionals addressing spiritual, social, psychological and physical needs."[43]

Palliative care affirms life and recognizes death as a normal process. It does not hasten death, nor does it postpone it.[48] It offers children with life-threatening illness the hope of living as actively as possible until death, and it offers families the support to cope during the patient's illness and in their bereavement.[46] In collaboration with the family, the objectives are to palliate physical symptoms (pain and other distressing symptoms), maintain activity and independence for as long as comfortably possible, alleviate psychologic distress (including fear, anxiety, isolation, or anger), provide for a death with as much dignity as possible, and support those who are bereaved.[3,6,8,81]

The palliative care movement was born out of the modern hospice care movement founded by Dame Cicely Saunders in 1967.[89] Hospices have since then proliferated in several countries[5] and now provide home care services, in-patient facilities, and bereavement follow-up by a specific, and separate, multidisciplinary team. Although providing a much-needed service, hospice care has frequently not met the needs of pediatric patients.

First, most hospice providers focus on adult patients with life-threatening illnesses. Few, if any, staff are prepared to deal with the medical, physiologic, emotional, and developmental issues in the dying child. Parents and the child may wish to participate in phase I or II studies at the end of life to help future families. Such "active" treatment patients often do not qualify for hospice services. Although Children's Hospice International, founded by Ann Armstrong Dailey, and advocates such as Ida Martinson[65] have increased awareness of the needs of pediatric patients, there has not been a substantive increase in pediatric hospice services. A substantial percentage of children dying of cancer in this country are still suffering, and their symptoms are not being adequately prevented or relieved.[116]

Secondly, the timing of the transition from active therapy with curative intent to hospice end-of-life care is more gradual in the pediatric patient. Because of the higher cure rates in pediatric cancers, the objective of care, even for many high-risk patients, is initially optimistic. It may be hard for both health care providers and parents to make a formal transition to non–cure-directed care.[31] Families and providers may be faced with waxing and waning palliative care needs and require recurrent discussions over time about their changing clinical status.[69] These needs "do not fit neatly into the medical, psychological, spiritual, and economic framework established for adult end-of-life care."[43] Too often, hospice care is not sought out until the very end of the child's life.

Advocates and practitioners of palliative care, on the other hand, are beginning to set the goal of incorporating this philosophy earlier in care and making it an accepted part of mainstream medicine. Pilot programs are being developed and tested, and results of studies and personal experiences and philosophies are being shared in books and journals.[88] Education for Physicians on End-of-Life Care (EPEC) is a program from the American Medical Association that has been developed to educate every physician in America about palliative care.[24] The American Academy of Hospice and Palliative Care Medicine has developed UNIPAC, a self-study program for physicians.[2] A module for pediatrics is being developed. The American Association of Colleges of Nursing (AACN) and the City of Hope Cancer Center have established the End-of-Life Nursing Education Consortium (ELNEC), an innovative initiative to bring quality end-of-life education to nursing faculty.[93] The Nursing Leadership Academy in End-of-Life Care, with representation from 22 national nursing organizations (including the Association of Pediatric Oncology Nurses and the Society of Pediatric Nurses) has been founded "to educate, train, and organize a network of nursing leaders prepared to galvanize the profession and transform end-of-life (nursing) care."[84] A list of Internet resources is included in Box 17-1. In the meantime, health care professionals must recognize some of the barriers to effective palliative care: (1) lack of training in palliative care for professionals; (2) lack of education for patients and families about palliative care; (3) delays in initiating palliative care; (4) fragmentation of palliative care; (5) inadequate relief of symptoms; (6) lack of reimbursement for palliative care; and (7) lack of sufficient research to promote evidence-based care.[43]

SYMPTOM MANAGEMENT IN THE DYING CHILD

The terminally ill child requires treatment aimed at palliation of symptoms. Interventions are defined as "palliative" by their therapeutic intent (i.e., comfort) rather than their content (e.g., surgery, radiation, or chemotherapy). For example, radiation therapy may be given to reduce the size of a tumor mass and thereby make the child more comfort-

able. Surgery and chemotherapy may be used for similar reasons. The parents and the staff must be clear that the purpose of these modalities is to make the child more comfortable, *not* to cure the child. Everyone must understand the purpose so that unrealistic expectations are discouraged.

A comprehensive review of the management of symptoms is beyond the scope of this chapter. Several texts are available that discuss these in detail.[23,41,74,75] Interventions for some of the most frequently encountered symptoms in the terminally ill child are presented in Table 17-3.

Although many children traverse the terminal phase of illness without significant discomfort, pain control is often the biggest challenge in the nursing care of the terminally ill patient. Pain control can be achieved using a variety of methods (refer to Chapter 12), including positioning and providing emotional support, massage, and cuddling. Imagery,[60] storytelling, diversion, socialization, talking through fears, and play therapy often provide comfort. Medication is used as needed in adequate doses on an appropriate schedule to relieve the pain. Multiple agents are available, varying from acetaminophen to opiates, which can be given through several routes (refer to the World Health Organization Pain Guidelines[120]).

TABLE 17-3	SYMPTOM MANAGEMENT IN PEDIATRIC PALLIATIVE CARE
Symptom	**Suggested Management**
Pain	*Pain is chronic and progressive in nature. It can be severe and permeate the patient's every thought and action, interfering with mobility, appetite, sleep, and quality of life. Pain will often require large amounts of opioid medications toward the end of life.* Give pain medicines on an around-the-clock schedule rather than PRN. Schedule doses so that patient and parents do not have to get up during the night, if possible. Choose the least traumatic and simplest route of medication administration. Include coanalgesic medications (acetaminophen, antidepressants, anticonvulsants, nonsteroidal antiinflammatory agents [NSAIDs]) as needed. Establish an alternative plan for when the pain increases or oral medication is no longer effective or possible. Initiate interventions to prevent constipation with the start of opioid pain medications. Use nonpharmacologic techniques, such as massage, distraction, music, and relaxation, when appropriate. Refer to Chapter 12 for additional information.
Fatigue	*Fatigue is expected, and the etiology is multifactorial. Possible factors include chronic anemia, pain, malnutrition, metabolic changes secondary to progressive cancer, respiratory insufficiency, disrupted sleep, inactivity, and depression.* Perform patient care activities at one time if possible to decrease frequent interruptions. Try to prevent sleep disruptions at night. Provide for additional periods of rest and sleep. Encourage enjoyable, relaxed activities as tolerated during the time of day the child reports the highest energy level. Prioritize activities. If anemia is a factor, consider blood transfusions. A decision to transfuse depends on the child's current condition and potential for improved quality of life. Refer to Chapter 11 for additional information.

Respiratory symptoms (cough, dyspnea, congestion, air hunger, breathlessness)	*Severity of respiratory symptoms varies with nature of disease process and organ involvement (e.g., decreased ventilation secondary to the presence of pulmonary or abdominal tumor or pleural effusion; decreased gas exchange due to anemia or leukemic infiltrates; altered gag reflex secondary to brain or head and neck tumors). Symptoms will be progressive in nature and are often very distressing to the patient and family.*
	Identify what exacerbates or relieves symptoms.
	Early in the terminal process the treatment objective is to improve respiratory effort; later the focus is on alleviating anxiety related to respiratory changes and shortness of breath.
	Dress the child in loose-fitting clothing.
	Raise the head of the bed 30 to 45 degrees, and use pillows to position for optimal breathing.
	Keep air in room well humidified and use a fan to circulate air.
	If tolerated, place cool compresses over cheek and temporal area (trigeminal nerve area).
	Eliminate smoke and allergens.
	Use guided imagery, relaxation, and deep-breathing exercises to reduce anxiety.
	Use oral-pharyngeal suctioning as needed.
	Administer the following:
	    Opioids for dyspnea, shortness of breath, or cough
	    Cough suppressants (dextromethorphan) with dry, nonproductive cough and expectorants (guaifenesin) with wet, productive cough secondary to infection
	    Anticholinergic medications for increased pulmonary congestion or increased oral secretions or dyspnea related to pulmonary congestion or edema
	    Bronchodilators for dyspnea, wheezing, or pulmonary congestion, to increase air exchange

Data from Hellsten, M. B., Hockenberry-Eaton, M., Lamb, D., et al. (2000). *End-of-life care for children.* Austin, TX: The Texas Cancer Council; Moldow, D. G., & Martinson, I. M. (1991). *Home care for seriously ill children: A manual for parents.* Alexandria, VA: Children's Hospice International; Yasko, J. M. (Ed.). (1983). *Guidelines for cancer care: Symptom management.* Reston, VA: Reston Publishing.

TABLE 17-3	**SYMPTOM MANAGEMENT IN PEDIATRIC PALLIATIVE CARE—cont'd**
Symptom	**Suggested Management**
Respiratory symptoms —cont'd	Diuretics for pulmonary edema Anxiolytic medications for dyspnea with anxiety Aerosolized morphine for dyspnea Administer humidified oxygen as needed. Increased fluid intake can increase pulmonary secretions; avoid excessive intravenous fluids as death nears. Severe respiratory distress due to pleural effusion or pneumothorax may require invasive interventions to increase the child's comfort (benefits should be weighed against discomfort of procedure). Refer to Chapter 11 for additional information.
Anorexia	*Anorexia can be due to medication side effects (including symptom management and palliative chemotherapy), altered taste, early satiety and decreased appetite stimulation, metabolic changes from advanced cancer, or depression. Anorexia will progress as death nears.* Identify and treat potentially reversible contributing factors such as nausea, vomiting, pain, constipation, or mouth sores. Medications may be useful in increasing appetite (megestrol acetate, dronabinol, steroids). Potential benefit for quality of life must be considered for invasive procedures associated with aggressive nutritional supplementation (e.g., total parenteral nutrition [TPN], enteral feedings). Prepare food the child chooses and likes, in small portions. Have a variety of foods available that the child likes. Feed the child slowly to decrease the risk of choking. Offer thicker liquids that are easier to swallow. Maintain good oral hygiene before and after eating. Remember that refusal to eat or drink in the last days is normal. Refer to Chapter 11 for additional information.
Nausea and vomiting	*Etiology is multifactorial and may include intestinal obstruction, increased intracranial pressure (ICP), anorexia, gastroesophageal reflux, medication side effects, especially opioids, metabolic derangements, and stress and anxiety. Treatment is directed to the cause of nausea or vomiting.* If intestinal obstruction is the cause—administer steroids, antiemetics with medication to reduce secretions (e.g., glycopyrrolate, octreotide), promethazine, nasogastric (NG) tube for decompression. If ICP is the cause—administer steroids. Administer antiemetics. Consider changing to a different opioid medication. Avoid noxious sights and odors. Increase intake of clear liquids as tolerated. Maintain good oral hygiene. Offer ice chips. Offer small portions of food, and avoid greasy or spicy foods. Use distraction techniques. Refer to Chapter 11 for additional information.
Constipation	*Patients who have no oral or enteral intake continue to produce stool. The most common cause of constipation is opioid medications used to treat pain, although other palliative care medications can cause constipation, such as anticholinergics, anticonvulsants, muscle relaxants, and antidepressants. Other causes include tumor obstruction, hypercalcemia, dehydration, and inactivity. The treatment objective is prevention.* Start a laxative regimen at the same time opioid therapy is initiated. Treat constipation promptly when it occurs.

Continued

TABLE 17-3	SYMPTOM MANAGEMENT IN PEDIATRIC PALLIATIVE CARE—cont'd
Symptom	**Suggested Management**
Constipation —cont'd	If there is no evidence of distal impaction, infection, or bowel obstruction, stimulant laxatives may be used (senna, bisacodyl, lactulose, docusate sodium).
	Mineral oil may lubricate stool to make it easier to pass.
	Glycerin suppositories or enemas can be used but should be avoided in neutropenic or thrombocytopenic patients.
	Add fruits, vegetables, and other fibers to the diet if tolerated.
	Encourage fluid intake, and increase activity level if possible.
	Encourage use of the commode 30 to 60 min after eating, and use a bedside commode instead of a bedpan if possible.
	Provide privacy for bowel movements.
	Refer to Chapter 11 for additional information.
Diarrhea	*Multifactorial causes may include tumor obstruction or treatment effects, graft-versus-host disease (GVHD), fecal impaction, high osmolarity enteral feedings or liquid medications, chronic gastrointestinal (GI) bleeding, anxiety, or stress.*
	Stop all laxatives.
	Use a high-carbohydrate diet to rest the bowel.
	Avoid milk products, fats, and protein until diarrhea stops.
	Give electrolyte solutions if tolerated.
	Manually remove fecal impaction if present.
	Use antidiarrheal medications, such as loperamide, diphenoxylate, and atropine, or tincture of opium, if appropriate.
	Refer to Chapter 11 for additional information.
Fever	*Fever is often due to progressive tumor. It can be due to infection.*
	Administer the following:
	Antibiotics for infection
	Acetaminophen
	Ibuprofen, other NSAIDs, or indomethacin (use with caution if patient is thrombocytopenic); may be more effective than acetaminophen if fever is tumor related

Data from Hellsten, M. B., Hockenberry-Eaton, M., Lamb, D., et al. (2000). *End-of-life care for children.* Austin, TX: The Texas Cancer Council; Moldow, D. G., & Martinson, I. M. (1991). *Home care for seriously ill children: A manual for parents.* Alexandria, VA: Children's Hospice International; Yasko, J. M. (Ed.). (1983). *Guidelines for cancer care: Symptom management.* Reston, VA: Reston Publishing.

The fear of pain is perhaps the greatest concern of both the parents and the child. A major nursing challenge is to give sufficient medication to relieve the child's pain while maintaining as much alertness as the child and family wish. Concerns must be allayed about addiction and the amount of pain medicine sometimes required to eliminate the pain.[26,71,72] The amount of pain medication required is whatever it takes to eliminate the pain.[94] There is no "ceiling" on the amount that eventually may be given. The family needs to know that, although the physical suffering related to a child's dying may not be totally eliminated, there is no reason the child should be in pain. The child may become drowsy once pain is controlled. Often the drowsiness is because the pain had prevented the child from sleeping and once pain is controlled

the child is able to get appropriate rest. The child may later become much more alert. If somnolence persists, there are medications to counteract this.

A terminally ill child has many of the same physical needs as any seriously ill child. Sleep deprivation can occur, particularly if the child has been in the hospital for a long period of time. It is important to set a time schedule and provide an environment conducive to sleep at the appropriate times of day or night. Administering a mild sedative may be helpful at night, although this is usually not required.

The dying child may be restless and have nightmares or frequent waking. It may be helpful to provide a night-light, keep the door open, or reinforce that loved ones are near. At home a portable intercom may give reassurance to both the parents and

TABLE 17-3	SYMPTOM MANAGEMENT IN PEDIATRIC PALLIATIVE CARE—cont'd
Symptom	**Suggested Management**
Fever—cont'd	Encourage loose-fitting clothes and a light cover.
	Prevent shivering.
	Use a fan to keep air circulating.
	Apply cool cloths to forehead and axillae.
	Refer to Chapter 10 for additional information.
Insomnia	*Insomnia is often caused by altered sleep patterns while hospitalized. Nights and days become mixed up. It can be due to anxiety, depression, or fear.*
	Insomnia due to depression is associated with early waking and inability to return to sleep.
	Attempt to maintain normal sleeping and waking routines.
	Discourage multiple daytime naps if child is awake at night.
	Give a warm bath in a relaxed atmosphere before bed.
	At home try to keep the bed a place for sleeping; if awake move to another place.
	Administer hypnotics as needed; watch for interaction with pain medications.
	Avoid giving steroids at bedtime.
	Avoid caffeinated drinks and chocolate.
	Use a night-light, keep the door open, and play relaxing music if appropriate.
	Use relaxation or guided imagery, healing touch, or massage.
	Encourage child and family to talk about child's fears, dreams, or nightmares.
Pruritus	*Pruritus is often associated with advanced cancer. The causes include release of proteolytic enzymes in the presence of tumors such as lymphoma, leukemia, and other solid tumors; release of chemical irritants from renal or liver dysfunction or hypercalcemia; and dehydration. Other causes include dry skin and opioid medications.*
	Avoid harsh, drying soaps and use mild, moisturizing soaps.
	Use oils in bath water.
	Use oatmeal or Aveeno baths.
	Regularly use moisturizing lotions.
	Dress in cotton clothing.
	Keep child cool.
	Keep fingernails trimmed and discourage scratching.

the child. As the terminal phase progresses, the child may sleep for longer and longer periods, and waking moments may be minimal. Such moments are treasured, and at this point "family time may need to be geared around the child's waking and alert moments."[39] Even when the child is "sleeping" there may still be a level of awareness that makes contact valuable during these times as well.

Nutritional status is an important consideration in the terminally ill child.[70] Oral nutrition should be maintained as long as it is physically possible and enjoyed by the child. Antiemetics may be helpful if nausea and vomiting are a problem. As the terminal stage progresses, the child's needs may be less. Oral intake should never be allowed to become a point of contention between parent and child. If the child cannot or does not want to take

adequate oral intake, the family can choose to provide no further intake or nutrition can be supplemented with tube feedings or hyperalimentation. The risks and benefits of artificial nutrition and hydration must be carefully considered. Lack of nutrition does not cause the child discomfort. Once started, artificial nutrition and hydration is very difficult to stop, and if used in the past it may be very difficult for parents to give up. In some cases the child may feel better and have increased energy from added nutrition; in other instances supplements can cause increased secretions, contribute to pulmonary edema (due to decreased absorption of fluids as death nears), or cause swelling and dyspnea (when renal failure occurs).

Problems with elimination present another important consideration in the care of the terminally ill child. Methods to deal with these problems must take into account the child's desires and comfort. For example, if the child has diarrhea, the health care professional may recommend dietary restrictions to control the diarrhea. The child, on the other hand, may have few pleasures left in life except for dietary intake. Thus the parent and child may decide how to live with the diarrhea, maintaining cleanliness and comfort, so the child can continue eating the desired foods.

For a variety of reasons, including the use of narcotics, spinal cord compression, and decreased mobility, constipation may be a problem. Dietary manipulations (aimed first at preventing this complication), the early use of laxatives, and the use of enemas may be necessary. Intermittent or continuous urinary catheterization may be necessary if urinary retention occurs.

Some children require oxygen therapy to relieve dyspnea and provide comfort. Anxiety and restlessness in the terminally ill child may be a sign of hypoxia. Oxygen therapy can be provided by a mask or cannula, in the hospital or at home. It may be required only intermittently at first, but the need for supplemental oxygen may increase as the child approaches death. Use by the child is always optional.

The decision to stop routine blood counts and transfusion of blood products when blood counts are low is difficult. In general, regular blood testing is not performed in palliative care, and the use of transfusions is based on clinical symptoms. Thrombocytopenia can result in bleeding in the terminally ill child. A low platelet count can occur because of marrow infiltration of disease or because of the intensive therapy previously received. Treatment of bleeding relates directly to the child's comfort and the degree of unpleasantness witnessed by the family. Increased bruising or petechiae may not produce discomfort in the child and may not interfere with activities of daily living; in that case a platelet transfusion is not given because it is not necessary for the child's comfort. However, in some cases a low platelet count results in severely bleeding gums or uncontrolled epistaxis. Both of these situations, and the vomiting of blood that they can produce, can increase the child's discomfort and fears. Platelet transfusions may be given in these cases to increase the comfort and decrease the fears of the child and family. Red blood cell transfusions may be given if the child is excessively fatigued and wants to remain active. However, parents must be reminded that anemia is not painful, and transfusions may not improve a child's activity level. There may come a time when red blood cell transfusions prolong the dying process.

PSYCHOSOCIAL NEEDS OF THE DYING CHILD

The terminally ill child has the same needs as any other human being approaching the last stages of life—the right to be treated with respect and to die without undue pain and suffering. Independence should be fostered and stressed as long as possible, and children should be given some degree of control (consistent with prior family dynamics and patterns) over how, where, and with whom they spend the last days of their lives.

Some children choose to attend school, even if only for a few hours a day, up until shortly before their death. "The terminally ill child needs to learn, to have the opportunity to socialize and spend time with other children, to develop increased independence and control over the environment, and to experience success."[21] Attending school can help counter boredom and depression, increase peer contacts, enhance dignity, and normalize lifestyle.

The terminally ill child may be emotionally labile for a variety of reasons (e.g., anxiety, central nervous system disease, discomfort, anger, or medication side effects).[39] Children may be irritable and act out in negative ways (e.g., being spiteful or obstinate, swearing, or throwing temper tantrums). Some children choose to touch as many lives as possible in their few remaining days or weeks, whereas others narrow their focus of relationships and interactions as death approaches. Staff and extended family may need help in understanding the child's narrowed focus of relationships as the child's energy decreases.

The child's spiritual needs must be respected.[42,121] They may intensify as death approaches, or they may diminish as the child finds peace. Discussions of God, Heaven, or an afterlife will depend on the family's beliefs, the child's beliefs, and the family's and child's openness to discussing them. Such discussions should take place only when the child indicates a willingness to participate. "Toward the end of the terminal phase, the work of the dying child (depending on his age, maturation and experience) is to center on himself, his beliefs, his concepts. He, in essence, puts his life together."[39] This is not the time for well-intentioned caregivers, family, or friends to try to impose their beliefs on the child or immediate family.

The issue of fulfilling a dying child's last or "final" wish often arises. The parents and many lay people are often willing to go to great lengths to fulfill these wishes. The desire for wish fulfillment must be tempered with a realistic expectation of children's energy level and what they can actually enjoy. For example, although children may express a desire to visit a theme park in another state, fulfillment of such a wish may really be beyond the scope of their energy and ability at that time in their life. Fulfillment of other wishes may do more to enhance the remaining weeks of their life.

The wish fulfillment issue brings to mind the advantage of introducing the concept of palliative care early. Children or adolescents can be asked early on, "What do you want to do or accomplish?" Do they want to get a driver's license, write a book, have a party, or visit a theme park? Casually bringing up the question early on, right at relapse, even as treatment commences, encourages the child to move forward with plans and dreams before the energy drain that occurs at the end of life.

In 1970 Waechter,[110] a pediatric nurse, conducted a study that demonstrated fatally ill children's awareness of death. Further studies by Spinetta, Rigler, and Karon,[101] Spinetta and Maloney,[100] and Bluebond-Langner[9] supported Waechter's findings and indicated that despite efforts to keep children with a fatal illness from becoming aware of their prognosis, children still somehow sense that their illness is not ordinary and is in fact very threatening.

Often the adults in the child's world, both the staff and sometimes the parents, are very uncomfortable if they are anticipating conversations with the child about dying, but

The dying child, depending on his age, maturation, and condition should be an active participant in his dying process. Often families (and sometimes staff) overprotect, cover-up, hedge, evade, stifle, or even lie to a terminally ill child, to make his life, short as it is, "easier." This closed approach not only makes his death more difficult, and increases the tension between family members and staff, but it disallows appropriate communication, grieving, honesty and completion of unfinished business.[39]

The most important thing to remember is that it is not so much *what* you say, as *how* you say it. However, an open approach does not mean that children are blatantly and uncaringly told they are dying. Be alert to cues, both verbal and nonverbal, from the child. As Kübler-Ross has noted, much of the child's conversation may be in symbolic language.[54] Check what the child needs, and be aware of the family's culture, religion, and previous way of dealing with these issues.[7] "Although all patients have the right to know, not all patients have the need to know."[55] In general, it is best if this information comes from the parents. Preempting this right can destroy the parents' trust in staff. Parents and caregivers need to work together to determine what is being explained to the child. There are no clear-cut guidelines on what to say and what not to say. Professionals, such as the psychologist or child

life specialist, may be helpful. Every child and every situation are different. "Children need the opportunity to complete their own unfinished business. . . . The requests are as varied as each unique child who makes them. They are usually painful for staff and family to hear, for by acknowledgement of the request we acknowledge reality."[55]

Perhaps the child's question most feared by adults is "Am I going to die?" The response to this question depends on many factors—the adult's relationship with the child and/or the family; what the adult believes the child is really asking; the child's degree of pain, discomfort, or suffering; and knowledge of the child's fears and concerns. It may be helpful if the team, together with the parents, anticipates this question ("Your child may ask . . .") and plans the response ("What we suggest is . . .") and who should deliver it. Though the response may be most appropriate from the parent, children do pick who they want to ask. Reflecting the question back to the child, "What do you think?" or "Tell me what you're asking today" will check the accuracy of the adult's understanding and perception of the child's meaning. A response such as "not right now" may suffice for the child who is not imminently dying but is afraid of going to sleep for fear of dying that night. In some cases a "no" answer is appropriate if in fact the child feels very sick but is not dying. In some situations a simple "yes" is appropriate, but be sure the parents understand that this will be your response if you are asked directly.

Older children and adolescents may question directly or indirectly if they are dying.[13,25] If they have the stamina to pose this question, they usually want and can handle the answer.[80] Some may discuss death openly with family and staff; others may want to protect their parents and choose instead to share their feelings with staff. "For the nurse who can tolerate listening to the adolescent's feelings about dying, the moments are privileged ones. They are a time to listen openly and let the patient know he will not be abandoned. They are a time to share silently, and in the silence, compassion, empathy, and humanness will be communicated."[80]

Often children need someone to listen to them and someone who is comfortable with silences with them rather than someone to talk to them. Some children work out in their own mind what their feelings are about dying, and they do not necessarily need to discuss dying with anyone. Others need help to express their feelings. Reflecting their comments or describing the feelings of other children may help them to express their concerns.

Some children have last wishes or want to "will" their possessions to a loved one. "It is during the terminal phase that the dying child completes his unfinished business. That can include delegating who gets his belongings, writing/recording letters, poems, his story, or making amends to others; essentially leaving his mark in life as he is losing his."[39] Other children have specific ideas about their funeral or burial. Some children may not realize they can express their desires, or they may be concerned about the effect such statements would have on parents or other loved ones. They need reassurance that such desires are appropriate and can be expressed, or they need to "test out" the expression of such desires on staff.

L. was a 14-year-old girl dying of leukemia. During one hospitalization she indicated a need to talk with one of the staff members at 4 o'clock in the morning. During this conversation she expressed her desire to plan her funeral. At her funeral she wanted everyone to receive a daisy because daisies to her were a sign of hope and life. Once she found that the expression of such desires was accepted by the staff person, she felt ready to explain her wishes to her mother.

Staff members who work with terminally ill children must remember to make each moment count. Even silences are moments shared. Do not make unreasonable promises, but keep promises that are made. If you promise to play a game or stop by for a short visit, do so. There may not be a tomorrow to make up for times missed.

Staff members need to come to a closure in some way. Closure may be indirectly confronted (e.g., withholding the usual "see you next week" after a clinic visit) or may involve the direct situation of saying good-bye.

L. came to clinic on what was to be her last visit. Although not in pain, she was very weak and lay quietly on the cart. While her parents discussed her terminal care with her physician, she expressed a desire to talk with the staff on the inpatient unit where she had spent so much time. With great difficulty I wheeled her around the unit and listened to her as she said her good-byes with simplicity and honesty to some very special friends. It was only as I approached the front door of the hospital with her that I realized that I, who had been so supportive to both her and the other nurses, had not said my own good-byes. With a mixture of tears and laughter and hugs, we expressed our love and caring for each other in our last conversation.

The above situations can occur only when the child's death is an expected event. When the child dies unexpectedly or in an unresponsive state such as when a child is on a ventilator, both the parents

and the staff may need to work out their feelings about not being able to share certain things with the dying child. Such feelings include guilt, anger, and disappointment. The staff must be willing to listen to the hurt and the anger in a nonjudgmental, caring way. Parents and staff should be encouraged to communicate with the child, both through touch and words, even though the child appears unresponsive. Parents must be reminded of their past everyday expressions and actions that made the child feel loved. Staff members need to remember the "good" days or moments they had with the child. Both parents and staff should be encouraged to say their good-byes.

WHEN DEATH OCCURS

In pediatric oncology nursing a child's death most often is an anticipated event. The parents, and the child, may choose to have the child die at home or in the hospital. When home is a feasible choice, caregivers have a responsibility to ensure adequate support and appropriate physical and psychosocial resources can be provided before home care is recommended for terminally ill children.[16] Home care can allow the parent and child more control over their environment, tends to keep the entire family together more easily, allows for greater sibling participation, makes it easier to attend to the needs of siblings, and allows the family to become the primary caregivers, fostering a sense of control over their environment.[59,64,109]

If the child is dying at home, ambulatory care may continue during this period to provide reassurance to the family and supportive care, or the family may chose hospice care. "Routine" clinic visits are discontinued unless the family truly needs and wants them.

Some patients, however, may require hospitalization during the final days (e.g., the child on a ventilator, the child of a single parent with complex care needs, or the child with complicated pain management). If the child is dying in the hospital, special considerations can be made for the child and family to increase comfort and decrease suffering. Laboratory tests can be eliminated or kept to a minimum; physical examinations can be scaled down and done less frequently, with awareness of what makes the child uncomfortable; monitors can be turned down or off; rules regarding visitors can be relaxed; music the child loves can be played; and the room can be made as "homelike" as possible, perhaps with a special quilt or rug or pictures on the wall and a small table lamp instead of the harsh overhead lights.

Preparing the family to take the child home to die requires extensive patient and family education.[68,75] The family must be taught how to manage pain and other side effects. Most parents wish to be prepared for any eventuality, including seizures, bleeding, or respiratory problems. Parents who are prepared for these possibilities are less likely to panic if they should occur at home.

Parents must be aware of potential changes in respiration (e.g., irregular breathing, Cheyne-Stokes respirations, or sounds of pulmonary congestion) as death approaches. If the family is not prepared for the unusual sounds of the respirations, they may become frightened. For example, the child may appear to moan loudly with each breath. However, close observation will demonstrate that the moaning sound occurs with exhalation and has nothing to do with pain or fear.

As death approaches, the child's physical appearance may change dramatically. Physical disfigurement from tumor growth may progress rapidly. The child's color may change as the child becomes more pale, bluish, mottled, and/or blotchy.

If the parents are alone with the dying child, they may have some concerns that they will not be able to know when the child has died. They must be prepared for this event, including information on things such as the final agonal breathing, described as "puffing" or "fish-out-of-water" breathing,[39] or the late reflexive "gasps" that commonly occur after a child dies.

No matter where the site of death, it is often helpful if the parents can make funeral arrangements ahead of time.[55] This is often very difficult for the parents but can make things much easier at the actual time of the child's death. Although state laws differ, if the child dies at home in many instances the funeral home personnel can come to the home and pick up the child's body if the pediatric oncologist agrees ahead of time to sign the death certificate. Some states will allow the hospice nurse to pronounce the death, others require a physician.

Parents need to know that when a child dies, it is not an emergency. Paramedics, if called, must attempt to resuscitate the child unless they have a do not resuscitate (DNR) order from a physician. It is helpful if parents have on hand a DNR letter or form declaring the DNR status of the child. On the other hand, parents do not need to call the funeral home immediately. They may spend as much time as they wish with their child. This time may include bathing, dressing, or holding their child or other family or cultural rituals. "After the last breath (gasp), there needs to be no rush for the stethoscope, but a calm period in which the family holds, prays and/or cuddles their precious child without medical intervention disrupting or validating the obvious."[39]

Whether the child dies at the hospital or in the home, the family may be asked to consent to an autopsy. They need to know that it is their right to refuse one or to request certain restrictions. However, the autopsy may be helpful if they have some unanswered questions about their child's course, or it may provide information useful to the care of other children with cancer. They may have some misconceptions that the autopsy may be mutilating or render the body not suitable for viewing. If the child dies at home, it may be more difficult to obtain an autopsy because of the cost and transportation issues. Nevertheless, it is possible in many situations to make the necessary arrangements, and the family should be assisted so that their wish for a home death does not preclude an autopsy.

Whether the child dies at home or in the hospital, the family should be given as much time as they need with the child to say good-bye and absorb the reality of the child's death. A supportive nurse, clergy member, or appropriate family friend should stay with them throughout this time to provide support, answer questions as needed, and facilitate the various procedures that must be followed. Even when death is anticipated, the family will be in shock, will be grieving, and will need compassionate support and direction.

SIBLINGS

Several studies have described the effects of childhood cancer on healthy siblings. In some families the siblings were described by parents as having problems with enuresis, depression, separation anxiety, somatic complaints, and feelings of guilt.[45,53,57] In a study by Lauer et al.,[58] children who participated in the home care of their dying brother or sister described a significantly different experience than those whose siblings died in the hospital. Data from Lauer et al. revealed multiple factors that appeared to favor more positive adjustment for the children who participated in home care. The children's reports indicated that a major advantage of home care was the opportunity for increased family communication and intimacy. Martinson, Davies, and McClowery[67] found that the self-concept ratings of bereaved siblings who had been involved in the Home Care Project[66] were significantly higher than would be expected for "normal" children. Children clearly demonstrated their desire for involvement in the ill child's care.[45,58]

Siblings of the dying child should not become the "forgotten people." In one way or another they have been a part of the child's entire illness and should be allowed to participate in the final processes of the child's life, if they wish, in a way that is comfortable for them. Siblings must be asked the extent of participation desired. It should not be assumed that they do or do not want inclusion. Parents may believe that they should protect the siblings from the reality of death; however, the sibling's fears and fantasies about the dying process may be more detrimental than the reality. If possible and if the siblings wish, they should be present when the death occurs, although their presence should not be forced. Because the parents may be overwhelmed with their own grief, the presence of a supportive adult other than the parent can help the siblings during this process. They should be allowed to participate in the funeral planning and the ceremony if they wish.

"The well siblings of terminally ill children live in houses of chronic sorrow. The signs of sorrow, illness and death are everywhere, whether or not they are spoken of."[10] When a brother or sister is terminally ill, many changes can produce role confusion and conflict and disruption of usual relationships. If siblings are not fully informed, they may feel deceived and rejected by parents. The care of the ill child may occupy so much of the parents' time and attention that the siblings are forced to take on increased responsibilities at home. The relationship between the ill child and sibling may change as death approaches and the terminally ill child withdraws.

The siblings' feelings must also be addressed, particularly those of anger, guilt, and ambivalence.[15,33,61,99] Young children particularly may have wished that their sibling would die during the child's illness. They may need help to understand that their death wish did not cause the actual death. All children have feelings of anger about the special attention and concern given to the child who is ill. They may be frustrated because they cannot express their feelings and fears to preoccupied parents.[51] Such feelings of anger and resentment may lead to feelings of guilt, particularly when the child dies. These children need a caring, nonjudgmental adult who can help them deal with these feelings. All siblings need help from their parents and other caring adults as they deal with their feelings of grief and loss.[112]

CLASSMATES

If the child has attended school, the classmates will need help to deal with their own feelings of grief and loss at the death of their classmate.[32] Many of these children will have had no experience with death, and the death of a classmate, no matter how remote from them, will be a profound life experience for them. The child's death should be confronted in an open and forthright manner, dispelling any myths or misconceptions. The classroom teacher, school nurse, school psychologist, and/or school social worker may all become involved in helping the children deal with their feelings. Voluntary attendance at the child's wake or funeral may help some children terminate the relationship and work through their feelings, but no child should be forced to attend.

STAFF

The needs of staff members working with dying patients vary according to their personal needs and their personal and professional experiences. Contrary to popular belief, one does not "get used to" working with dying children. Caregivers who have developed a wide repertoire of coping skills through exposure to previous personal and professional life stressors are probably best equipped[107] and to mentor less-experienced staff. They are alert to situations having potential for overidentification. Some staff members, for example, have difficulty caring for a patient similar in age or with characteristics reminiscent of members of their own family. Staff members who cope effectively recognize their own feelings, allow time and space for their own grieving, develop support within and outside the work situation, and gain personal satisfaction from helping the child and family throughout the child's illness and death.[20,106] Each individual develops an awareness of how best to help the child and family through the illness and dying process. Skill and compassion in dealing with death is an experience-based personal growth process.[17]

Other staff members do not cope as effectively with the dying child. They become overly involved or detach themselves as the child's death approaches. The overly involved staff member may make the dying child and family the entire focus of the staff member's life to the exclusion of personal needs. Although this happens occasionally to almost every pediatric oncology nurse, if it occurs frequently, it is often a danger signal. Frequent overinvolvement can only lead to burnout. On the other hand, the nurse who continuously backs away from the situation when death is inevitable may require as much assistance to deal with her feelings as the overly involved nurse.

For the staff "emotional adaptation involves dealing with the reality of the child's death."[12] The inevitability of death may engender feelings of anger, frustration, and depression. Efforts to support the family members in their grief and to relate to the dying child may produce feelings of helplessness and inadequacy that lead to guilt and anger. At the same time, the nurse must deal with personal feelings of sadness and grief over the loss of the child the nurse has come to know and love and the changed relationship with parents and family members with whom the nurse has established emotional bonds.

The individual nurse may choose to express these feelings in a destructive or constructive manner.[17] Destructive expressions can include counterproductive or inappropriate behavior such as distancing oneself, becoming defensive, and becoming easily upset or frustrated; overindulgence in food, alcohol, or drugs; and preoccupation with death and dying. Constructive expression includes sharing and working through feelings on a regular basis; personal sensitivity to emotional exhaustion and stress; and coming to terms with the nurse's own concept of death.

Recognizing the dying child as an independent human being "enables the nurse to work in a partnership rather than a protectorship."[17] Dealing openly and honestly with the dying child means having a willingness to be available as a confidante with whom the child can share her fears and feelings. "Availability is a physical, emotional, and spiritual presence; a willingness to respond honestly and compassionately to the child's needs at all times. Such a commitment often leads to extremely high self expectations."[17] After the child's death, nurses have a responsibility to replenish themselves. Some staff members take a physical and mental break from intense patient involvement to reevaluate, gather strength, and rekindle efforts.[1] Others use institutional resources such as psychiatric nurse clinicians or staff support groups. Still others find nonhospital friends and family the best sources for renewal. Strengthening the intellectual, emotional, and philosophic base enables a nurse to remain available day after day to children who might die.[17] Staff working as a team supporting and caring for each other can be extremely beneficial.[44,56]

With experience comes the professional maturity to deal effectively with the dying child, the child's family, and oneself.[30] Working with dying patients can help nurses face their own mortality. Each dying child and every family can teach something about life and about dying. In pediatric oncology when death is inevitable, the natural course of events cannot be changed. However, nurses can make things easier, can help alleviate pain and suffering, can facilitate coping, and can provide physical and emotional support that will make a difference.

BEREAVEMENT

Caregivers cannot provide grief support until they do their own grieving. How they support others de-

pends on how they manage their own grieving. Unresolved grief accumulates and interferes with the ability to help others. The staff's feelings must be permitted, acknowledged, felt, and expressed to others. Staff support groups are useful in helping nurses and others deal with their grief.

Parents and siblings will need support as they go through the grieving process, which will take months or even years.[86,118] Some guidelines for family and friends on being helpful and supportive are found in Table 17-4.

For parents and siblings the grieving process is long and painful.[19,76,82] "The loss of a child is the most painful of human experiences."[92] The grief of losing a child is indescribably painful, both emotionally and, at times, physically.[38,82,91,92] Physical manifestations include sleeping problems, lethargy, eating difficulties, weight fluctuations, crying, chest pain, headaches, menstrual irregularities, and muscle spasms. Emotional responses include numbness, denial, anger, sadness, depression, apathy, jealousy, insecurity, guilt, and fear. Although the probability of emotional swings is predictable, the nature and timing of these feelings are not.[92] The grieving persons may actually feel they are going crazy because of the intensity, duration, and unpredictability of their emotions. They need reassurance that they are not going crazy and that their feelings and behavior are normal.

Some may try to avoid grieving by keeping too busy to feel or by using drugs or alcohol to numb their feelings. The hard reality is that grief hurts, the painful energy of grief needs release, and "the only way beyond grief is through it."[38] Some parents and siblings have sufficient inner resources to deal with this grief on their own. Others need help from a caring supportive staff. One of the most important things that a staff member can provide is being a good listener as family members express their grief, because healing can occur only in a safe, trusting, accepting, compassionate, and nonjudgmental environment.[73] Feelings can be released through talking or writing about the experience, crying, or even screaming. Support groups may be helpful,[77] and many families draw strength from their spiritual resources. Referral can be made to community agencies for group or individual counseling. The grief of other family members (e.g., grandparents, aunts, and uncles) should also be considered.[40]

No words can take the pain away, and healing and recovery do not take place in any systematic sequence of stages. In fact, "one never gets over the loss of a loved one; one learns to live with the loss."[38] Over time the painful episodes become less intense, less frequent, and of shorter duration. Life takes on meaning again as parents and siblings

TABLE 17-4	**Do's and Don'ts for Helping Bereaved Parents**
Do's	**Don'ts**
Do let your genuine concern and caring show.	Don't let your own sense of helplessness keep you from reaching out to a bereaved parent.
Do be available—to listen, to run errands, to help with the other children, or to do whatever else seems needed at the time.	Don't avoid the parents because you are uncomfortable (being avoided by friends adds pain to an already intolerably painful experience).
Do say you are sorry about what happened to their child and about their pain.	Don't say you know how they feel (unless you have lost a child yourself, you probably do not know how they feel).
Do allow them to express as much grief as they are feeling at the moment and are willing to share.	Don't say "You ought to be feeling better by now" or anything else that implies a judgment about their feelings.
Do encourage them to be patient with themselves and not to impose any "shoulds" on themselves.	Don't tell them what they *should* feel or do.
Do allow them to talk about the child they have lost as much and as often as they want.	Don't change the subject when they mention their dead child.
Do talk about the special, endearing qualities of the child they have lost.	Don't avoid mentioning their child's name out of fear of reminding them of their pain (they have not forgotten it).
Do give special attention to the child's brothers and sisters at the funeral and in the months to come (they too are hurt and confused and in need of attention that their parents may not be able to give at this time).	Don't point out that at least they have their other children (children are not interchangeable; they cannot replace each other).
	Don't say that they can always have another child (even if they wanted to and could, another child would not replace the child they have lost).
	Don't suggest that they should be grateful for their other children (grief over the loss of one child child does not discount parents' love and appreciation of their living children).
Do reassure parents that they did everything they could and the medical care their child received was the best or whatever else you know to be *true* and *positive* about the care given their child.	Don't make any comments that in any way suggest that the care given their child at home, in the emergency room, in the hospital, or wherever was inadequate (parents are plagued by feelings of doubt and guilt without any help from their family and friends).

From Schmidt, L. (1987). Working with bereaved parents. In T. Krulik, B. Holaday, & I. M. Martinson: *The child and family facing life-threatening illness* (pp. 332-344). Philadelphia: Lippincott Williams & Wilkins.

learn to live in a world without the loved child. The hurt becomes "a muted sadness rather than a wrenching agony"[92] as the bereaved learn that, although life will never be the same, it can be good.

One of the most painful aspects of pediatric oncology nursing is learning to accept and cope with the death of a terminally ill child. It can also be one of the most personally satisfying and professionally rewarding. Nurses often begin their relationship with the child and family on a hopeful note, stressing the curability of many childhood cancers. When death becomes a probability, nurses must change course to maintain quality of life and facilitate death with dignity. The emergence of palliative care programs and teams will pave the way for a new level of care. Health care professionals may not be able change the inevitable outcome for the terminally ill child, but they can help make the child's remaining time comfortable and peaceful and help the child's parents and siblings cope with their grief.

ACKNOWLEDGMENT

The author would like to thank Joanne Hilden, MD, for her careful review and helpful suggestions for this chapter.

REFERENCES

1. Adams, J. P., Hershatter, M. J., & Moritz, D. A. (1991). Accumulated loss phenomenon among hospice caregivers. *American Journal of Hospice and Palliative Care, 8,* 29-37.

2. American Academy of Hospice and Palliative Care Medicine. (1998). *Hospice/palliative care training for physicians: UNIPACS.* Dubuque, IA: Kendall/Hunt Publishing.

3. American Academy of Pediatrics, Committee on Bioethics and Committee on Hospital Care. (2000). Palliative care for children. *Pediatrics, 106,* 351-357.

4. Anthony, S. (1940). *The child's discovery of death.* New York: Harcourt, Brace & World.

5. Aranda, S. (1999). Global perspectives on palliative care. *Cancer Nursing, 22,* 33-39.

6. Armstrong-Dailey, A., & Goltzer, S. Z. (Eds.). (1993). *Hospice care for children.* New York: Oxford University Press.

7. Backer, B. A., Hannon, N. R., & Russell, N. A. (1994). *Death and dying: Understanding and care* (2nd ed.). New York: Delmar.

8. Billings, J. A. (1998). What is palliative care? *Journal of palliative Medicine, 1,* 73-81.

9. Bluebond-Langner, M. (1978). *The private lives of dying children.* Princeton, NJ: Princeton University Press.

10. Bluebond-Langner, M. (1988). Worlds of dying children and their well siblings. *Death Studies, 13,* 1-16.

11. Bowden, V. R. (1993). Children's literature: The death experience. *Pediatric Nursing, 19,* 17-21.

12. Cairns, N., Klopovich, P., Moore, R., et al. (1980). The dying child in the classroom. *Essence, 4,* 25-32.

13. Carr-Gregg, M. R. C., Sawyer, S. M., Clarke, C. F., et al. (1997). Caring for the terminally ill adolescent. *Medical Journal of Australia, 166,* 255-258.

14. Childres, P., & Wimmer, M. (1971). The concept of death in early childhood. *Child Development, 42,* 705-715.

15. Christ, G. H. (2000). Impact of development on children's mourning. *Cancer Practice, 8,* 72-81.

16. Collins, J. J., Stevens, M. M., & Cousens, P. (1998). Home care for the dying child: A parent's perception. *Australian Family Physician, 27,* 610-614.

17. Coody, D. (1985). High expectations: Nurses who work with children who might die. *Nursing Clinics of North America, 20,* 131-142.

18. Corr, C. A. (1993). Children's literature on death. In A. Armstrong-Dailey & S. Z. Goltzer (Eds.), *Hospice care for children* (pp. 266-284). New York: Oxford University Press.

19. Davies, B. (1993). Sibling bereavement: Research-based guidelines for nurses. *Seminars in Oncology Nursing, 9,* 107-113.

20. Davies, B., & Eng, B. (1993). Factors influencing nursing care of children who are terminally ill: A selective review. *Pediatric Nursing, 19,* 9-14.

21. Davis, K. G. (1989). Educational needs of the terminally ill student. *Issues in Comprehensive Pediatric Nursing, 12,* 235-245.

22. DeSpelder, L. A., & Strickland, A. L. (1987). *The last dance.* Mountain View, CA; Mayfield.

23. Doyle, D., Hanks, G. W. C., & MacDonald, N. (Eds.). (1998). *Oxford textbook of palliative medicine* (2nd ed.). New York: Oxford University Press.

24. Emanuel, L., von Gunten, C., & Ferris, F. (1999). *The education for physicians on end-of-life care (EPEC) curriculum.* Princeton, NJ: Robert Wood Johnson Foundation

25. Faulkner, K. W. (1997). Talking about death with a dying child. *American Journal of Nursing, 97,* 64-69.

26. Ferrell, B., Virani, R., Grant, M., et al. (2000). Beyond the Supreme Court decision: Nursing perspectives on end-of-life care. *Oncology Nursing Forum, 27,* 445-455.

27. Fetsch, S. H. (1984). The 7- to 10-year-old child's conceptualization of death. *Oncology Nursing Forum, 11,* 52-56.

28. Fleischman, A. R., Nolan, K., Dubler, N. N., et al. (1994). Caring for gravely ill children. *Pediatrics, 94,* 433-439.

29. Foley, G. V., & Whittam, E. H. (1990). Care of the child dying of cancer, Part I. *CA—A Cancer Journal for Clinicians, 40,* 327-354.

30. Foley, G. V., & Whittam, E. H. (1991). Care of the child dying of cancer, Part II. *CA—A Cancer Journal for Clinicians, 41,* 52-60.

31. Frager, G. (1996). Pediatric palliative care: Building the model, bridging the gaps. *Journal of Palliative Care, 12,* 9-12.

32. Gortler, E. (1993). Lessons in grief: A practical look at school programs. In A. Armstrong-Dailey & S. Z. Goltzer (Eds.), *Hospice care for children* (pp. 154-171). New York: Oxford University Press.

33. Grogran, L. B. (1990). Grief of an adolescent when a sibling dies. *MCN, 15,* 21-24.

34. Grollman, E. A. (Ed.). (1967). *Explaining death to children.* Boston: Beacon Press.

35. Grollman, E. A. (1991). *Talking about death: A dialogue between parent and child* (3rd ed.). Boston: Beacon Press.

36. Grollman, E. A. (1993). *Straight talk about death for teenagers: How to cope with losing someone you love.* Boston: Beacon Press.

37. Gullo, S. V., Schowalter, J. E., & Patterson, P. R. (Eds.). (1985). *Death and children: A guide for educators, parents and caregivers.* Dobbs Ferry, NY: Tappen Press.

38. Gyulay, J. (1989). Grief responses. *Issues in Comprehensive Pediatric Nursing, 12,* 1-31.

39. Gyulay, J. (1989). Home care for the dying child. *Issues in Comprehensive Pediatric Nursing, 12,* 33-69.

40. Heiney, S. P., Wells, L. M., & Gunn, J. (1993). The effects of group therapy on bereaved extended family of children with cancer. *Journal of Pediatric Oncology Nursing, 10,* 99-104.

41. Hellsten, M. B., Hockenberry-Eaton, M., Lamb, D., et al. (2000). *End-of-life care for children.* Austin, TX: The Texas Cancer Council.

42. Hermann, C. P. (2001). Spiritual needs of dying patients: A qualitative study. *Oncology Nursing Forum, 28,* 67-72.

43. Hilden, J., Himelstein, B. P., Freyer, D. R., et al. (2001). Pediatric oncology end-of-life care. In K. M. Foley & H. Gelband (Eds.), *Improving palliative care for cancer.* Washington, D.C.: National Academy Press.

44. Hinds, P. S., Puckett, P., Donohoe, M., et al. (1994). The impact of a grief workshop for pediatric oncology nurses on their grief and perceived stress. *Journal of Pediatric Nursing, 9,* 388-397.

45. Iles, P. (1979). Children with cancer: Healthy siblings' perceptions during the illness experience. *Cancer Nursing, 2,* 371-377.

46. James, L., & Johnson, B. (1997). The needs of parents of pediatric oncology patients during the palliative care phase. *Journal of Pediatric Oncology Nursing, 14,* 83-95.

47. Johnson, J. (1999). *Keys to helping children deal with death and grief.* Happauge, NY: Barron's Educational Series.

48. Johnston, B. (1999). Overview of nursing developments in palliative care. In J. Lugton & M. Kindlen (Eds.), *Palliative care: The nursing role* (pp. 1-26). London: Churchill Livingstone.

49. Kane, B. (1979). Children's concepts of death. *Journal of Genetic Psychology, 134,* 141-153.

50. Kastenbaum, R. J. (1967). The child's understanding of death: How does it develop? In E. A. Grollman (Ed.), *Explaining death to children* (pp. 89-108). Boston: Beacon.

51. Kastenbaum, R. J. (2000). *Death, society and human experience* (7th ed.). New York: Allyn & Bacon.

52. Koocher, G. (1973). Childhood, death and cognitive development. *Developmental Psychology, 9,* 369-375.

53. Kramer, R. F. (1984). Living with childhood cancer: Impact on healthy siblings. *Oncology Nursing Forum, 11,* 44-51.

54. Kübler-Ross, E. (1983). *On children and death.* New York: Macmillan.

55. Kuykendall, J. (1989). Death of a child: The worst kept secret around. In L. Sherr (Ed.), *Death, dying and bereavement: An insight for carers.* Boston: Blackwell Scientific.

56. Larson, D. (1997). *The helper's journey: Working with people facing grief, loss, and life-threatening illness.* Champaign, IL: Research Press.

57. Lauer, M., Mulhern, R., Wallskog, J., et al. (1983). A comparison study of parental adaptation following a child's death at home or in the hospital. *Pediatrics, 71,* 107-112.

58. Lauer, M., Mulhern, R., Wallskog, J., et al. (1985). Children's perceptions of their siblings death at home or hospital: The precursors of differential adjustment. *Cancer Nursing, 8,* 21-27.

59. Lauer, M. E., & Camitta, B. M. (1980). Home care for dying children: A nursing model. *Journal of Pediatrics, 97,* 1032-1035.

60. LeBaron, S., & Zeltner, L. K. (1985). The role of imagery in the treatment of dying children and adolescents. *Journal of Developmental and Behavioral Pediatrics, 5,* 252-258.

61. Leder, S. N. (1992). Life events, social support, and children's competence after parent and sibling death. *Journal of Pediatric Nursing, 7,* 110-119.

62. Lonetto, R. (1980). *Children's conceptions of death.* New York: Springer.

63. Macgregor, C. (1998). *Why do people die?: Helping your child understand with love and illustrations.* Secaucus, NJ: Carol Publishing Group.

64. Martinson, I. (1976). *Home care for the dying child.* New York: Appleton-Century-Crofts.

65. Martinson, I. M. (1993). Hospice care for children: Past, present, and future. *Journal of Pediatric Oncology Nursing, 10,* 93-98.

66. Martinson, I., Armstrong, G., Geis, D., et al. (1978). Home care for children dying of cancer. *Pediatrics, 62,* 106-113.

67. Martinson, I., Davies, E., & McClowery, S. (1987). The long term effects of sibling death on self-concept. *Journal of Pediatric Nursing, 2,* 277-335.

68. Martinson, I. M., Martin, B. B., Lauer, M., et al. (1991). *Children's hospice/home care: An implementation manual for nurses.* Alexandria, VA: Children's Hospice International.

69. Masera, G., Spinetta, J. J., Jankovic, M., et al. (1999). Guidelines for assistance to terminally ill children with cancer: A report of the SIOP Working Committee on Psychosocial Issues in Pediatric Oncology. *Medical and Pediatric Oncology, 32,* 44-48.

70. Meares, C. J. (2000). Nutritional issues in palliative care. *Seminars in Oncology Nursing, 16,* 135-145.

71. Meehan, J. (1989). Pain control in the terminally ill child at home. *Issues in Comprehensive Pediatric Nursing, 12,* 235-245.

72. Milch, R. A., Freeman, A., & Clark, E. (1989). *Palliative pain and symptom management for children and adolescents.* Alexandria, VA: Children's Hospice International.

73. Miles, A. (1990). Caring for families when a child dies. *Pediatric Nursing, 16,* 346-347.

74. Miser, J. S., & Miser, A. W. (1993). Pain and symptom control. In A. Armstrong-Dailey & S. Z. Goltzer (Eds.), *Hospice Care for Children* (pp. 22-59). New York: Oxford University Press.

75. Moldow, D. G., & Martinson, I. M. (1991). *Home care for seriously ill children: A manual for parents.* Alexandria, VA: Children's Hospice International.

76. Moore, I. M., Gilliss, C. L., & Martinson, I. (1988). Psychosomatic symptoms in parents 2 years after the death of a child with cancer. *Nursing Research, 37,* 104-107.

77. Mulcahey, A. L., & Young, M. A. (1995). A bereavement support group for children. *Cancer Practice, 3,* 150-156.

78. Nagy, M. H. (1948). The child's theories concerning death. *Genetic Psychology, 73,* 2-27.

79. Nitschke, R., Meyer, W. H., Sexauer, C. L., et al. (2000). Care of terminally ill children with cancer. *Medical and Pediatric Oncology, 34,* 268-270.

80. Pazola, K. J., & Gerberg, A. K. (1990). Privileged communication—talking with a dying adolescent. *MCN, 15,* 16-20.

81. Quint Benoliel, J. C. (1988). 1988 Symposium on palliative care review lecture. In A. P. Pritchard (Ed.), *Proceedings of the 5th International Conference on Cancer Care: Cancer nursing—A revolution in care* (pp. 178-181). London: Macmillan.

82. Rando, T. A. (1983). An investigation of grief and adaptation in parents whose children have died from cancer. *Journal of Pediatric Psychology, 8,* 13-20.

83. Reimer, J. C., Davies, B., & Martens, N. (1991). Palliative care: The nurse's role in helping families through the transition of "fading away." *Cancer Nursing, 14,* 321-327.

84. Rollins, J. (Ed.). (2000). Nursing professionals unite to improve end-of-life care for patients and families. *APON Counts, 14,* 1.

85. Ross-Alaolmolki, K. (1985). Supportive care for families of dying children. *Nursing Clinics of North America. 20,* 457-466.

86. Ruden, B. M. (1996). Bereavement follow-up: An opportunity to extend nursing care. *Journal of Pediatric Oncology Nursing, 13,* 219-225.

87. Safier, G. (1964). A study in relationships between the life and death concepts in children. *Journal of Genetic Psychology, 105,* 283-294.

88. Sahler, O. J. Z., Frager, G., Levetown, M., et al. (2000). Medical education about end-of-life care in the pediatric setting: Principles, challenges, and opportunities. *Pediatrics, 105,* 575-584.

89. Saunders, C. (1993). Introduction—history and challenge. In C. Saunders & N. Sykes (Eds.), *The management of terminal malignant disease* (pp. 1-14). London: Edward Arnold.

90. Schaefer, D., & Lyons, C. (1993). *How do we tell the children?: A step-by-step guide for helping children two to teen cope when someone dies.* New York: Newmarket Press.

91. Schiff, H. S. (1978). *The bereaved parent.* New York: Penguin Press.

92. Schmidt, L. (1987). Working with bereaved parents. In T. Krulik, B. Holaday, & I. M. Martinson (Eds.), *The child and family facing life threatening illness* (pp. 332-344). Philadelphia: Lippincott.

93. Schmidt, L. M. (2000). Educating nurses in end-of-life care. *Last Acts: Care and Caring at the End of Life, 8,* 3.

94. Siever, B. A. (1994). Pain management and potentially life-shortening analgesia in the terminally ill child: The ethical implications for pediatric nurses. *Journal of Pediatric Nursing, 9,* 307-312.

95. Silverman, J. (1999). *Help me say goodbye: Activities for helping kids cope when a special person dies.* Minneapolis, MN: Fairview Press.

96. Silverman, P. R. (1999). *Never too young to know: Death in children's lives.* New York: Oxford University Press.

97. Speece, M. W., & Brent, S. W. (1984). Children's understanding of death: A review of three components of a death concept. *Child Development, 55,* 1671-1686.

98. Spinetta, J. J., & Deasy-Spinetta, P. (1981). Talking with children who have a life-threatening illness. In J. J. Spinetta, & P. Deasy-Spinetta (Eds.), *Living with childhood cancer* (pp. 234-253). St. Louis, MO: Mosby.

99. Spinetta, J. J., Jankovic, M., Eden, T., et al. (1999). Guidelines for assistance to siblings of children with cancer: Report of the SIOP Working Committee on Psychosocial Issues in Pediatric Oncology. *Medical and Pediatric Oncolog, 33,* 395-398.

100. Spinetta, J. J., & Maloney, L. J. (1975). Death anxiety in the outpatient leukemic child. *Pediatrics, 56,* 1034-1037.

101. Spinetta, J. J., Rigler, D., & Karon, M. (1973). Anxiety in the dying child. *Pediatrics, 52,* 841-849.

102. Stillion, J., & Wass, H. (1979). Children and death. In H. Wass (Ed.), *Dying: Facing the facts* (pp. 208-235). New York: Hemisphere.

103. Tallmer, M., Formanek, R., & Tallmer, J. (1974). Factors influencing children's concepts of death. *Journal of Clinical Child Psychology, 3,* 17-19.

104. Trozzi, M., & Massimini, K. (1999). *Talking with children about loss: Words, strategies, and wisdom to help children cope with death, divorce, and other difficult times.* Berkeley, CA: Berkeley Publishing Group.

105. Turner, M. (1998). *Talking with children and young people about death and dying.* London: Taylor & Francis.

106. Vachon, M. L. S. (1987). *Occupational stress in the care of the critically ill, the dying, and the bereaved.* New York: Hemisphere Publishing.

107. Vachon, M. L. S. & Parkes, E. (1985). Staff stress in the care of the critically ill and dying child. *Issues in Comprehensive Pediatric Nursing, 8,* 151-182.

108. Vianello, R., & Lucamante, M. (1988). Children's understanding of death according to parents and pediatricians. *Journal of Genetic Psychology, 149,* 305-316.

109. Vickers, J. L., & Carlisle, C. (2000). Choices and control: Parental experiences in pediatric terminal home care. *Journal of Pediatric Oncology Nursing, 17,* 12-21.

110. Waechter, E. (1971). Children's awareness of fatal illness. *American Journal of Nursing, 71,* 1168-1172.

111. Waechter, E. H. (1987). Death, dying and bereavement: A review of the literature. In T. Krulik, B. Holaday, & I. M. Martinson (Eds.), *The child and family facing life threatening illness* (pp. 1-31). Philadelphia: Lippincott.

112. Walker, C. L. (1993). Sibling bereavement and grief responses. *Journal of Pediatric Nursing, 8,* 325-334.

113. Wass, H. (1995). Death education for children. In I. B. Corless, B. B. Germino, & M. A. Pittman (Eds.), *A challenge for living: Dying, death and bereavement.* Boston: Jones & Bartlett.

114. Wenestam, C-G., & Wass, H. (1987). Swedish and U.S. children's thinking about death: A qualitative study and cross-cultural comparison. *Death Studies, 11,* 99-122.

115. Whittam, E. H. (1993). Terminal care of the dying child: Psychosocial implications of care. *Cancer, 71*(Suppl), 3450-3462.

116. Wolfe, J., Grier, H. E., Klar, N., et al. (2000). Symptoms and suffering at the end of life in children with cancer. *The New England Journal of Medicine, 342,* 326-333.

117. Wolfe, J., Klar, N., Grier, H. E., et al. (2000). Understanding of prognosis among parents of children who died of cancer. *Journal of the American Medical Association, 284,* 2469-2475.

118. Worden, J. W., & Monahan, J. R. (1993). Caring for bereaved parents. In A. Armstrong-Dailey & S. Z. Goltzer, *Hospice care for children* (pp. 122-139). New York: Oxford University Press.

119. World Health Organization. (1990). *Cancer pain relief and palliative care.* Technical report series 804. Geneva, Switzerland: World Health Organization.

120. World Health Organization & International Association for the Study of Pain. (1998). *Cancer pain relief and palliative care in children.* Geneva, Switzerland: World Health Organization.

121. Wright, K. B. (1998). Professional, ethical, and legal implications for spiritual care in nursing. *Image: The Journal of Nursing Scholarship, 30,* 81-83.

18

Care of Survivors

Wendy Hobbie
Kathy Ruccione
Jeanne Harvey
Ida M. (Ki) Moore

The vast majority of children diagnosed with cancer in the year 2000 will achieve a cure. This dramatic increase in survival is one of the twentieth century's greatest medical success stories. This achievement comes with the responsibility of caring for generations of survivors who face an uncertain future related to the long-term consequences of their treatment.[200] Education of these young people regarding optimal health behaviors and the risk factors associated with their treatment is essential. Young adults have immediate and pressing issues related to who is best able to care for them as they age. They must also deal with concerns about the emergence of unexpected late effects after a long latency period, well after they have left the supportive environment of the initial treatment center.[193]

All survivors need follow-up care that is organized, systematic, and comprehensive, including physiologic and psychosocial components. In such programs the health care team's goals are (1) to assess risk factors based on preexisting disease, the diagnosis, treatment, and acute effects; (2) to obtain a careful history (including exploration of psychosocial issues and well-being) and to provide thorough physical examination; (3) to teach health promotion and disease prevention strategies; and (4) to develop a specific plan for lifelong follow-up care that can be shared with other health care providers.[95]

Biologic cure in an individual is defined as having no evidence of disease and the same life expectancy as an individual who never had cancer. A major question for survivors of childhood cancer is, how late effects of their disease and treatment will affect life expectancy. Late effects result from a lack of nourishment of healthy cells, chronic cell injury, death of cells with subsequent loss of normal functioning tissue, and scar tissue formation. These effects manifest themselves as (1) clinically obvious effects that interfere with activities of daily living (e.g., pulmonary fibrosis resulting in respiratory distress); (2) clinically subtle effects noticeable to the trained observer

(e.g., learning impairment after treatment of the central nervous system); and (3) subclinical effects, detectable by laboratory screening or x-ray studies (e.g., elevated liver enzyme levels).[67]

The nurse caring for the long-term survivor must have comprehensive knowledge about the physiologic and psychosocial issues that face childhood cancer survivors. A description of the etiology of late effects and the necessary assessment and management are discussed. A summary of these issues is found in Table 18-1.

CENTRAL NERVOUS SYSTEM

Central nervous system (CNS) treatment for acute lymphoblastic leukemia (ALL), brain tumors, or as part of the conditioning regimen for hematopoietic stem cell transplant (HSCT) can result in a spectrum of neuropsychologic deficits, below average academic achievement, and neuroanatomic abnormalities.[*] The adverse effects of cranial radiation on cognitive and academic abilities were initially described in 1981[46] and have been replicated by numerous other investigators.[†] Higher radiation doses, such as those used for treatment of brain tumors, are generally associated with more severe neuropsychologic and academic sequelae.[62,110] However, children with ALL who are treated with lower radiation doses (e.g., 18 Gy) in combination with intrathecal chemotherapy can also experience long-term neurologic toxicities.[4,21,25,77,88,220] In an attempt to avoid these problems, intrathecal chemotherapy alone or in combination with intermediate to high dose systemic chemotherapy has now replaced radiation for CNS treatment in the majority of current ALL protocols. Several recent studies in-

---

[*]References 4, 6, 7, 9, 21, 23, 25, 31, 45, 60, 62, 65, 77, 88, 93, 102, 105, 110, 130, 145, 155, 163, 185, 220, 233.

[†]References 4, 21, 25, 77, 88, 220.

Text continued on p. 432.

Body System	Health Problem	Associated Treatment Modality	Method of Assessment	Management and Nursing Considerations
ENDOCRINE				
Ovaries	Ovarian dysfunction:	Procarbazine, cyclophosphamide, nitrogen mustard, busulfan	Careful health history and physical examination	Oophoropexy before treatment Refer to endocrinologist
	• Primary (Secondary see HPA)	4-8 Gy High risk: • Older patients • Poor nutrition • Longer length of treatment • Combination therapy	Tanner staging Serum determinations of LH, FSH, estradiol at age 12 yr if no secondary sex characteristics	Replacement hormones Refer for counseling Anticipatory teaching: • Lack of secondary sex characteristics • Loss of menses, irregularities • Decreased libido, vaginal dryness If at risk for early menopause encourage early childbearing Sperm banking at treatment
Testes	Testicular dysfunction:	Procarbazine, cyclophosphamide, nitrogen mustard, busulfan	Careful health history and physical examination	
	• Primary (Secondary see HPA)	4-6 Gy; azoospermia ≥24 Gy; Leydig cell damage High risk: • Poor nutrition • Combination therapy • Longer length of treatment	Tanner staging Testicular volumes Semen analysis Serum determination of LH, FSH if no secondary sex characteristics after 14 yr of age	Refer to endocrinologist Replacement testosterone Refer for counseling Anticipatory teaching: • Small testicles • Possible impotence • Decreased libido • Lack of secondary sex characteristics
Thyroid	Hypothyroidism: • Overt and compensatory Graves' disease	No known chemotherapy >20 Gy; overt or compensatory hypothyroidism; Graves' disease ≥7.5 Gy total body irradiation; hypothyroidism High risk: • Younger patients	Careful health history and physical examination Free T_4, TSH, T_3	Refer to endocrinologist Replacement hormones Anticipatory teaching: • Hypothyroidism or hyperthyroidism—signs and symptoms
Hypothalamic-pituitary axis (HPA)	Hypothalamic dysfunction Panhypothalamic dysfunction Panhypopituitary dysfunction	No known chemotherapy ≥24 Gy; hypothalamic dysfunction ≥40 Gy; pituitary dysfunction	Careful health history and physical examination Growth charts Tanner staging GH: stimulation tests, pulsatile tests Somatomedin-C LH, FSH, estradiol, testosterone, prolactin, Free T_4, TSH, T_3	Refer to endocrinologist Replacement hormones Bromocriptine (for hyperprolactinemia) Anticipatory teaching: • As above for ovaries and testes • Poor growth • Short stature

TABLE 18-1 **EVALUATION FOR LONG-TERM EFFECTS**

Data from Hobbie, W. L., & Schwartz, C. (1989). Endocrine late effects among survivors of cancer. *Seminars in Oncology Nursing, 5,* 14-21; Ruccione, K., & Weinberg, K. (1989). Late effects in multiple body systems. *Seminars in Oncology Nursing, 5,* 4-13.

Continued

TABLE 18-1	EVALUATION FOR LONG-TERM EFFECTS—cont'd			
Body System	**Health Problem**	**Associated Treatment Modality**	**Method of Assessment**	**Management and Nursing Considerations**
CARDIOVASCULAR				
	Cardiomyopathy	Anthracycline chemotherapy: Risk increased with • Lifetime cumulative dose ≥350 mg/m² • Mediastinal radition	ECG, echocardiogram, or MUGA History of symptoms (dizziness, palpitations, shortness of breath, or exercise intolerance) of congestive heart failure (CHF) Stress testing 24-hour Holter monitor	Effects may be subclinical Careful monitoring of anthracycline dosage to limit lifetime dose If CHF develops, supportive care with: • Referral to cardiologist • Digoxin, diuretics • Sodium restriction If pregnant will be considered high risk for cardiomyopathy
	Pericardial damage	Mediastinal radiation	Physical examination echocardiogram History of chest pain, dyspnea, fever, pulsus paradoxus, venous distension	May be subclinical If pericardial effusion develops, treatment may include: • Referral to cardiologist • Antiinflammatory drugs • Pericardial tap If restrictive pericarditis occurs, treatment may include pericardiectomy
	Early coronary artery atherosclerosis	Mediastinal radiation	ECG, echocardiogram History of chest pain with exertion, decreased exercise tolerance or symptoms such as chest or arm pain, chest pressure, heartburn, nausea, or fatigue	Referral to cardiologist Dietary restriction of fat and salt intake Program of moderate exercise If significant obstruction to coronary artery flow develops, treatment may include: • Thrombolytic drugs • Calcium channel blocking agents • Balloon dilation angioplasty • Coronary artery bypass surgery
	Atrioventricular (AV) valve tissue damage	Mediastinal radiation	Physical examination ECG, echocardiogram	Referral to cardiologist If significant AV valve insufficiency develops, treatment may include: • Diuretics • Afterload reducing agents • Surgical valve replacement
	Ventricular arrhythmias	Anthracycline chemotherapy	ECG, Holter monitor, exercise test	Referral to cardiologist If significant arrhythmias develop, treatment may include antiarrhythmic drugs

Data from Hobbie, W. L., & Schwartz, C. (1989). Endocrine late effects among survivors of cancer. *Seminars in Oncology Nursing, 5,* 14-21; Ruccione, K., & Weinberg, K. (1989). Late effects in multiple body systems. *Seminars in Oncology Nursing, 5,* 4-13.

TABLE 18-1	**EVALUATION FOR LONG-TERM EFFECTS—cont'd**			
Body System	**Health Problem**	**Associated Treatment Modality**	**Method of Assessment**	**Management and Nursing Considerations**
MUSCULOSKELETAL				
	Scoliosis, kyphosis	Radiation therapy for intrathoracic or intraabdominal tumor in which vertebrae absorb radiation unevenly	Regular physical examination May not become apparent until adolescent growth spurt	Referral to orthopedist for rehabilitative measures Instruction about normal weight maintenance to make problem less noticeable
	Spinal shortening (sitting height)	Spinal irradiation (e.g., for medulloblastoma); direct effect of radiation on growth centers of vertebral bodies	Serial measurements of sitting height (crown to rump)	Referral to orthopedic surgeon Anticipatory teaching about disproportion between shorter-than-usual trunk and normal leg length as full growth is attained; reassurance that disproportion probably will not be obvious to others but may be a problem in fitting clothing
	Increased susceptibility to fracture, poor healing, limb shortening	Irradiation to lesions in long bones (e.g., with Ewing's sarcoma)	Regular physical examination	Referral to orthopedic surgeon Teaching about protective measures such as avoiding rough contact sports
	Facial asymmetry	Surgery plus irradiation to head and neck area (e.g., for rhabdomyosarcoma), causing altered growth of facial bones	Regular physical examination	Early evaluation by reconstructive surgeon Anticipatory guidance about possible adjustment problems with visible deformity Referral to family counseling to manage or prevent adjustment and behavioral problems
	Dental problems: • Gingival irritation and bleeding, tooth loosening, migration (can lead to periodontal disease) • Delayed or arrested tooth development	Radiation therapy to maxilla and mandible Chemotherapy	Clinical observation with dental examination	Many dental problems can be minimized or prevented with: • Good oral hygiene with flossing and brushing, gingival massage, use of plaque-disclosing tablets or solutions • Pre–radiation therapy fluoride prophylaxis • Frequent dental evaluation • Extraction of damaged, nonfunctional teeth

Continued

TABLE 18-1	EVALUATION FOR LONG-TERM EFFECTS—cont'd			
Body System	**Health Problem**	**Associated Treatment Modality**	**Method of Assessment**	**Management and Nursing Considerations**
VISION				
	Cataracts	Cranial radiation Corticosteroids (long term)	Eye examination • Visual inspection • Slit-lamp examination	Ophthalmology consult Surgical removal Corrective lens fitting
HEARING				
	Hearing loss (high-tone range)	Cisplatin Increased risk: • Recurrent ear infections • Ototoxic antibiotic therapy • Radiation to auditory area	Monitor with hearing tests	Hearing aid Speech therapist consult— refer early, especially for preverbal children
RESPIRATORY				
	Pulmonary fibrosis	Lung irradiation Some chemotherapeutic agents Risk increased with: • Larger lung volume in radiation field • Dose, ≥40 Gy • Radiation-sensitizing chemotherapeutic agents	Clinical observation for dyspnea, rales, cough, decreased exercise tolerance, pulmonary insufficiency Monitor with: • Physical examination • Chest x-ray studies • Pulmonary function tests	Health education for smoking prevention or cessation Supportive care with provision of adequate rest periods Vigilance for development of pulmonary infection Pneumococcal vaccine Yearly influenza vaccination Careful oxygen administration (busulfan)
GASTROINTESTINAL				
	Chronic enteritis	Radiation therapy Risk increased with: • Dose, ≥50 Gy • Previous abdominal surgery • Radiation-sensitizing chemotherapeutic agents	Clinical observation for pain, dysphagia, recurrent vomiting, obstipation or constipation, blood or mucus-containing diarrhea, or malabsorption syndrome	Nutritional consultation for diet plan to diminish symptoms while providing adequate nutrition for growth and development and to fit family routine, ethnic, or cultural customs Dietary modifications may include low-fat, low-residue, gluten-free diet free of milk and milk products If enterostomy is performed, coordination with enterostomal therapist for patient and family teaching about stoma care

Data from Hobbie, W. L., & Schwartz, C. (1989). Endocrine late effects among survivors of cancer. *Seminars in Oncology Nursing, 5,* 14-21; Ruccione, K., & Weinberg, K. (1989). Late effects in multiple body systems. *Seminars in Oncology Nursing, 5,* 4-13.

TABLE 18-1	EVALUATION FOR LONG-TERM EFFECTS—cont'd			
Body System	**Health Problem**	**Associated Treatment Modality**	**Method of Assessment**	**Management and Nursing Considerations**
GASTROINTESTINAL—cont'd				
	Hepatic fibrosis, cirrhosis	Radiation therapy Some chemotherapeutic agents	Clinical observation for pain, hepatomegaly, jaundice Monitoring with liver function tests and liver scans may be inconclusive so periodic liver biopsy may be necessary	Supportive care with nutritional consultation
	Hepatitis C	Blood transfusion prior to July 1992	Hepatitis C antibody	If positive, will need referral to GI specialist
KIDNEY AND URINARY TRACT				
	Chronic nephritis (may lead to renal failure, cardiovascular damage)	Radiation to renal structures Risk increased with concomitant chemotherapy	Clinical observation and monitoring with: • Blood pressure readings • Urinalysis • Creatinine levels • Complete blood count (CBC)	If progressive renal failure develops, supportive care (possibly dialysis and/or transplantation)
	Chronic hemorrhagic cystitis	Chemotherapy (ifosfamide, cyclophosphamide) Risk increased with: • Pelvic irradiation • Inadequate hydration before, during, and after chemotherapy	Clinical observation for dysuria, urinary frequency, hematuria Monitoring with urinalysis, blood pressure	Ensure adequate hydration before, during, and after chemotherapy (3000 ml/m^2/24 hr) Bladder hemorrhage may be treated with formalin instillation and/or fulguration of bleeding sites
	Unilateral kidney	Nephrectomy for Wilms tumor	Clinical observation for dysuria, urinary frequency, hematuria Monitoring with urinalysis, blood pressure	Health education to avoid injury to remaining kidney (e.g., avoid contact sports) Wear kidney guard during sports If urinary tract infection develops: • Identification of causative organism • Antibiotic treatment • Urinalysis Medic-Alert identification bracelet

Continued

TABLE 18-1	EVALUATION FOR LONG-TERM EFFECTS—cont'd			
Body System	Health Problem	Associated Treatment Modality	Method of Assessment	Management and Nursing Considerations
HEMATOPOIETIC				
	Prolonged immunosup-pression	Chemotherapy (high dose, extended periods) Radiation to marrow-containing bones Splenectomy (e.g., for Hodgkin's disease)	Monitoring with: • CBC, platelet count • Tests of immune function • Bone marrow ex-aminations as indicated	Health education about infection Pneumococcal vaccine and prophylactic antibiotics for asplenic individuals Prompt treatment if infection occurs Reimmunize patient after hematopoietic stem cell transplants

Data from Hobbie, W. L., & Schwartz, C. (1989). Endocrine late effects among survivors of cancer. *Seminars in Oncology Nursing, 5,* 14-21; Ruccione, K., & Weinberg, K. (1989). Late effects in multiple body systems. *Seminars in Oncology Nursing, 5,* 4-13.

dicate that chemotherapy-based CNS treatment also may be associated with neuropsychologic deficits and academic problems.[23,45,65,105,163]

Neuropsychologic Effects of Treatment

Neuropsychologic, or cognitive, impairments are manifested as declines in IQ and academic achievement scores. In addition, specific deficits in visual spatial skills, visual motor integration, memory, attention, and motor skills usually are observed 3 to 5 years after CNS treatment, but occur earlier for some children. Several longitudinal studies indicate that neuropsychologic deficits and academic difficulties progress over time.[45,65,163] The declines in IQ scores are more commonly associated with cranial radiation; however, specific neuropsychologic and academic problems also have been reported in children who received only intrathecal or intravenous chemotherapy.[21,65,163,220] It is important to note that some studies report that children who receive only chemotherapy for CNS treatment do not experience any significant cognitive or academic problems.[25,116,119,220] Nonverbal skills (e.g., strategic planning, visual spatial abilities, sequencing, and arithmetic) are particularly vulnerable to the damaging effects of CNS treatment, and deficits in these areas often appear first.

Children who receive CNS treatment before 5 years of age are at greatest risk for cognitive late effects. This "age-at-time-of-treatment" effect is attributed to the vulnerability of the developing brain to the damaging effects of radiation and chemotherapy.[9,220,234] In addition to age, several studies report that girls are at greater risk than boys for general cognitive deficits but not for problems in language-based academic skills.[234,241]

Neuroanatomic Effects of Treatment

Diffuse brain atrophy, perfusion defects, and decreased white matter are the most common neuroanatomic abnormalities after CNS treatment.[7,9,93,182,185] Calcifications and leukoen-cephalopathy (progressive white matter destruction) occur less frequently. These structural changes can be detected by computed tomography (CT) scans, magnetic resonance imaging (MRI) studies, and single photon emission computerized tomography (SPECT) scans. Atrophy is typically seen as dilatation of the ventricles and widening of the subarachnoid space, while low-density areas in CT scans or hyperintense areas in MRI in white matter are typically used as indicators for leukoen-cephalopathy.[185]

Cranial radiation is the type of treatment most closely associated with neuroanatomic pathology, but several studies have reported widening of the ventricles and sulci as well as white matter changes in children treated only with intrathecal chemotherapy.[185,209] Perfusion defects were reported in 66% of children treated with intrathecal methotrexate but in only 23% of those treated with cranial radiation.[9] The investigators concluded that methotrexate could be responsible for the perfusion defects, because only 3 of the 11 affected patients received radiation therapy.

Efforts to link cognitive deficits with imaging changes have been largely unsuccessful. Only one study reports a significant inverse correlation between the number of abnormal imaging findings and performance on a measure of attention.[185] These findings suggest that a more comprehensive assessment may be needed to identify risk factors for cognitive and academic problems. For example, the Neurological Severity Score was inversely correlated with visual-spatial skills, memory, attention, performance IQ, and global IQ in a sample of 59 children with astrocytoma.[155] The Neurological Severity Score includes events before the diagnosis of astrocytoma, preexisting neurological deficits, perioperative events, and postoperative events due to surgery, but does not include MRI findings such as hydrocephalus or edema.[155]

Increased concentrations of biochemical markers of CNS injury in cerebral spinal fluid (CSF) may eventually be useful in identifying children at greatest risk for cognitive and academic problems. Methotrexate-induced folate deficiency has been linked to elevated levels of homocysteine (an amino acid) and excitatory amino acid neurotransmitters in the CSF of patients treated with methotrexate.[188]

Patients with the highest CSF concentrations of these amino acids were experiencing neurotoxicity at the time of sample collection.[188] Increased concentrations of CSF phospholipids, especially sphingomyelin, during CNS treatment for ALL also have been reported.[65] The increased concentration of sphingomyelin has been correlated with decreases in cognitive and academic abilities.[65] Thus CSF markers of brain injury may be more sensitive indicators of cognitive and academic outcomes in children receiving CNS treatment.

Assessment and Management

A comprehensive assessment of CNS late effects involves parental and teacher appraisal of school performance, neuropsychologic evaluation, and neuroimaging studies. The neuropsychologic evaluation consists of measures of general intelligence (e.g., Wechsler Intelligence Scale for Children–Revised) and academic achievement (e.g., Wide Range Achievement Test of Reading, Spelling and Arithmetic; or the Woodcock-Johnson–Revised Achievement Battery) as well as tests of more specific cognitive abilities, especially for those who are at high risk for CNS late effects. Baseline evaluations of cognitive and academic abilities are completed as soon as possible after diagnosis, but scheduled at an appropriate time to minimize the effects of physical and emotional stress. In addition to measures of general intelligence and academic achievement, assessment of other neuropsychologic abilities is individualized and based on the pattern of limitations, deficits, and strengths of each child.

Pediatric oncology nurses have a pivotal role in the management of children who are at risk for or who are experiencing CNS late effects. It is critical for the pediatric oncology nurse to inquire about school attendance and to encourage the child and family to participate in school reentry programs as needed. The nurse must also identify children with CNS late effects as well as those at high risk for sequelae (young age at time of treatment, and CNS treatment regimen involving cranial radiation or triple intrathecal chemotherapy in combination with intermediate- to high-dose systemic methotrexate) and refer them for neuropsychological evaluation on a regular (yearly) basis. The nurse is frequently involved in coordinating the neuropsychologic evaluation with the child's long-term follow-up assessment. Evaluation results should be summarized in a written format that can be understood by parents and school personnel.

An educational specialist or school liaison is in an ideal position to help parents and teachers use the evaluation results to develop an individualized educational program that will meet the child's needs. The educational needs of the child with CNS late effects are addressed in Public Law 94-142 and Section 504 of the Rehabilitation Act of 1973. Schools must comply with Public Law 94-142, which has categories of qualifying conditions, including "other health impaired" (which includes cancer). Additionally, Section 504 of the Rehabilitation Act of 1973 ensures that students are not discriminated against and requires that accommodations be individualized to meet the needs of the child.

Public Law 94-142 and Section 504 require that appropriate resources are provided to optimize educational outcomes. However there is limited information about effective intervention strategies to prevent or remediate cognitive and academic problems among children with cancer who have received CNS treatment. Thus future research efforts need to focus on the development and testing of appropriate interventions designed to prevent CNS late effects or to improve outcomes in children who have received CNS treatment.

ENDOCRINE SYSTEM

Dysfunction of the endocrine system can be a result of direct damage to the end organs (e.g., ovaries and testes) or the controlling hypothalamic pituitary axis.

THE HYPOTHALAMUS

Anatomically, the hypothalamus and pituitary gland are connected by the pituitary stalk. They work synergistically to maintain endocrine homeostasis. Releasing and inhibiting hormones are produced in the hypothalamus and carried to the anterior pituitary gland. The releasing and inhibitory hormones act on the anterior pituitary gland (hypophysis) to regulate production and storage of thyroid stimulating hormone (TSH), luteinizing hormone (LH), follicle-stimulating hormone (FSH), growth hormone (GH), adrenocorticotropic hormone (ACTH), and melanocyte stimulating hormone (MSH). Oxytocin and antidiuretic hormone are produced in the hypothalamus and released into the posterior pituitary gland (neurohypophysis) (Figure 18-1).[113]

Effect of Radiation

Radiation delivered to the head and neck region can cause hypothalamic-pituitary axis dysfunction. The hypothalamus is radiosensitive, and function is affected at doses of 24 Gy. The pituitary gland is radio-resistant, requiring doses greater than 40 Gy to alter function.[37] Nevertheless, its function is controlled by the hypothalamus. Damage to the hypothalamus leads to an essentially nonfunctioning pituitary gland. Other contributing factors that

impact gland function include age at diagnosis (younger children are affected more than older children), method of radiotherapy, number of fractions, fraction size, and duration of treatment.

Growth hormone deficiency is characterized by a decrease in rate of growth (less than 5 cm per year), delayed bone age (documented by x-ray), short stature, and documented low growth hormone and somatomedin C levels. Growth hormone deficiency is the most common pituitary problem following cranial radiation. Poor linear growth is the result of a combination of factors, including radiation to the head, spine, trunk, or total body; poor nutritional status; hypothyroidism; and age at diagnosis. During therapy, decreased linear growth is noted in many children. However there is a "catch-up" growth period after treatment is completed. Unfortunately for some there is permanent or continued poor growth rate.

Children treated for ALL or brain tumors with cranial radiation are at highest risk for growth hormone failure. Children treated for ALL with cranial or craniospinal radiation with 24 Gy often experience growth disturbances.[217] Children under 5 years of age at the time of treatment appear particu-

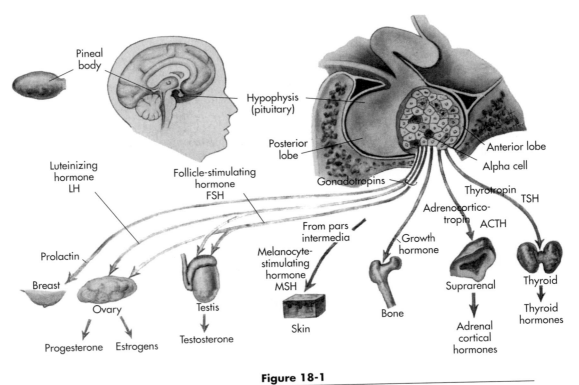

Figure 18-1

The adenohypophysis produces several hormones, some controlling the activity of other endocrine glands (thyroid, adrenal cortex, and gonads).   (From Jacob, S., Fanconi, C., & Lossow, W. (Eds.). (1982). *Structure and function in man.* Philadelphia: W. B. Saunders.

larly susceptible to these effects. Growth abnormalities have been noted in some children receiving doses as low as 18 Gy.[223] Radiation doses in excess of 35 Gy result in nearly 100% of children developing growth hormone deficiency within five years.[38]

Growth hormone failure, diminished capacity for growth secondary to epiphyseal irradiation, inhibition of vertebral growth, poor nutrition, thyroid dysfunction, and graft versus host disease (GVHD) contribute to the poor linear growth patterns in survivors of HSCT.[217] Treatment with growth hormone often results in a substandard response to therapy, most likely due to the multifactorial etiology of growth failure in these children. Recent studies have documented less growth retardation when hyperfractionated radiation doses are used or when chemotherapy preconditioning regimens are administered without radiation.[217]

There has been concern that the use of growth hormone promotes recurrences or relapse of disease, but current studies suggest that the rate of relapse or recurrence is not higher in children treated with growth hormone.[164,211] Children receiving growth hormone who also received anthracyclines in their initial treatment require close monitoring because of the risk of increased cardiac workload as the child's growth accelerates.

Growth hormone also has other important functions, including defining body composition (fat to muscle ratio), increasing muscle strength, improving cardiovascular health, and increasing immune function.[29,35] Studies have documented that adults who are growth hormone deficient are at increased risk for heart disease, decreased muscle strength, osteoporosis, and decreased lean body mass.[29,35] Therefore children who are growth hormone deficient require ongoing evaluation as they enter adulthood for continuation of replacement therapy. The problems secondary to growth hormone deficiency versus the potential or unknown risks of lifelong growth hormone replacement must be considered.

Assessment and Management

Standing height must be obtained every 6 months in children at risk for growth problems. Preferably, height is measured with a stadiometer (a device to measure linear height) and plotted on a growth chart. Sitting height also is obtained at each visit, because the spine is particularly sensitive to the effects of radiation and children with normal standing heights may have decreased sitting height (measured from top of head to rump). Diagnostic studies are ordered for any child who demonstrates deceleration in linear growth. An initial growth evaluation includes sitting and standing height, thyroid function, and bone age. Tanner staging (Tables 18-2 through 18-5)[148,149,176] is important to identify potential precocious puberty. An early growth spurt may mask a growth hormone deficiency, and premature closure of the epiphyses, which accompanies puberty, will prevent any possible effect from growth hormone replacement.[148]

There are a number of tests used to evaluate growth hormone status. Because growth hormone is secreted at intervals, stimulating tests are necessary to assess function. Drugs such as L-dopa, arginine, and insulins are a few agents used to evaluate growth hormone secretion.[139] Synthetic growth hormone replacement is given to patients with documented deficiency. Treatment generally improves final height; however there is a wide range of growth responses. Individuals treated with spinal irradiation and HCST generally have poorer responses to therapy because of the multiple factors impacting linear growth.

TABLE 18-2	STAGES OF BREAST DEVELOPMENT IN GIRLS		
		Mean Age	Range (95%)
Stage 1	Preadolescent. Only papilla is elevated.		
Stage 2	Breast bud stage. Breast and papilla are elevated as small mound. Areola diameter is enlarged.	11.2	9.0-13.3
Stage 3	There is further enlargement of breast and areola with no separation of their contours.	12.2	10.0-14.3
Stage 4	Areola and papilla project to form a secondary mound above the level of the breast.	13.1	10.8-15.3
Stage 5	Mature stage. There is projection only of papilla because of recession of the areola to the general contour of the breast.	15.3	11.9-18.8

From Marshall, W. A., & Tanner, J. M. (1969). Variation in the pattern of pubertal changes in girls. *Archives of Disease in Childhood, 44,* 291-303, as cited in Odell, W. D. (1989). Puberty. In L. J. DeGroot (Ed.). (1989). *Endocrinology* (2nd ed.). Philadelphia: W. B. Saunders.

TABLE 18-3	STAGES OF PUBIC HAIR GROWTH IN GIRLS	Mean Age	Range (95%)
Stage 1	Preadolescent vellus over pubis is no further developed than that over anterior abdominal wall (i.e., no pubic hair).		
Stage 2	There is sparse growth of long, slightly pigmented, downy hair, straight or only slightly curled, appearing chiefly along the labia.	11.7	9.3-14.1
Stage 3	Hair is considerably darker, coarser, and more curled. Hair spreads sparsely over pubic junction.	12.4	10.2-14.6
Stage 4	Hair is now adult in type, but area covered by it is still considerably smaller than in most adults. There is no spread to medial surface of the thighs.	13.0	10.8-15.1
Stage 5	Adult in quantity and type distributed as coarse triangle of classically feminine pattern. Spread to medial surface of thighs but not linea alba or elsewhere above base of triangle.	14.4	12.2-16.7

From Marshall, W. A., & Tanner, J. M. (1969). Variation in the pattern of pubertal changes in girls. *Archives of Disease in Childhood, 44,* 291-303, as cited in Odell, W. D. (1989). Puberty. In L. J. DeGroot (Ed.). (1989). *Endocrinology* (2nd ed.). Philadelphia: W. B. Saunders.

TABLE 18-4	STAGES OF GENITAL DEVELOPMENT IN BOYS	Mean Age	Range (95%)
Stage 1	Preadolescent. Testes, scrotum, and penis are about the same size and proportion as in early childhood.		
Stage 2	The scrotum and testes have enlarged; there is a change in the texture and also some reddening of the scrotal skin. Testicular length >2 cm <3.2 cm.	11.6	9.5-13.8
Stage 3	Growth of the penis has occurred, at first mainly in length but with some increase in breadth; there is further growth of the testes and scrotum. Testicular length >3.3 cm <4.0 cm.	12.9	10.8-14.9
Stage 4	The penis is further enlarged in length and breadth with development of the glands. The testes and scrotum are further enlarged. The scrotal skin has further darkened. Testicular length >4.1 cm <4.9 cm.	13.8	11.7-15.8
Stage 5	Genitalia are adult in size and shape. No further enlargement takes place after stage 5 is reached. Testicular length >5 cm.	14.9	12.7-17.1

Data from Marshall, W. A., & Tanner, J. M. (1970). Variation in pattern of pubertal changes in boys. *Archives of Disease in Childhood, 45,* 13-23, as cited in Odell, W. D. (1989). Puberty. In L. J. DeGroot (Ed.). *Endocrinology* (2nd ed.). Philadelphia: W. B. Saunders.

THYROID GLAND

Thyrotropin releasing hormone (TRH) is produced in the hypothalamus and stimulates the production and secretion of thyroid stimulating hormone (TSH) in the anterior pituitary gland. TSH stimulates the thyroid gland to produce thyroxine (T_4) and triiodothyronine (T_3). Free T_4 is unbound thyroxine and is important when evaluating thyroid gland functioning. These hormones affect oxygen consumption, carbohydrate and cholesterol metabolism, the central and peripheral nervous system, and growth and development.[139] Radiation therapy can either damage the thyroid gland directly or impact the gland's functioning by damaging the hypothalamic pituitary axis.

TABLE 18-5	STAGES OF PUBIC HAIR GROWTH IN BOYS		
		Mean Age	**Range (95%)**
Stage 1	Preadolescent. The vellus over the pubes is no further developed than that over the abdominal wall (i.e., no pubic hair).		
Stage 2	Sparse growth of long, slightly pigmented downy hair, straight or only slightly curled, appearing chiefly at the base of the penis.	13.4	11.2-15.6
Stage 3	Hair is considerably darker, coarser, and curlier and spreads sparsely over the junction of the pubes.	13.9	11.9-16.0
Stage 4	Hair is now adult in type, but the area it covers is still considerably smaller than most adults. There is no spread to the medial surface of the thighs.	14.4	12.2-16.5
Stage 5	Hair is adult in quantity and type, distributed as an inverse triangle. The spread is to the medial surface of the thighs but not up the linea alba or elsewhere above the base of the inverse triangle. Most men will have further spread of pubic hair.	15.2	13.0-17.3

Data from Marshall, W. A., & Tanner, J. M. (1970). Variation in pattern of pubertal changes in boys. *Archives of Disease in Childhood, 45,* 13-23, as cited in Odell, W. D. (1989). Puberty. In L. J. DeGroot (Ed.). *Endocrinology* (2nd ed.). Philadelphia: W. B. Saunders.

Overt and Compensated Hypothyroidism

Radiation to the head, neck, chest, and spine can result in compensated or overt hypothyroidism. Hypothyroidism is characterized by lethargy, weight gain, dry skin, anemia, hair loss, poor growth rate, and delay in intellectual development. Laboratory studies reveal an elevated TSH and a decreased T_4 and T_3. Clinically compensated hypothyroidism is demonstrated by elevated TSH levels and normal serum levels of T_3 and T_4.

It is important to identify children with compensated hypothyroidism, because there is a potential risk of secondary thyroid cancer. Overstimulation of the thyroid can cause malignant transformation in damaged cells.[42] Overt or compensated primary hypothyroidism results from radiation delivered directly to the thyroid gland. Doses greater than or equal to 26 Gy result in overt or compensated hypothyroidism in 4% to 79% of patients.[159,190] Patients receiving less than 26 Gy have an estimated rate of 17%. Dysfunction will most likely occur 3 to 5 years after treatment, although the risk is noted up to 10 years after treatment. In some cases compensated hypothyroidism has corrected without treatment 3 years after detecting an elevated TSH.[57] There is evidence that hyperfractionation of total body irradiation (TBI) may reduce the development of hypothyroidism.[218] Occasionally hyperthyroidism has been noted following radiation therapy to the thyroid gland, although the exact mechanism remains unclear.[91] Chemotherapy given alone or in combination with radiation has not been implicated in increasing the risk of thyroid dysfunction.[57]

Secondary Hypothyroidism

Secondary hypothyroidism is found in patients who receive radiation doses in excess of 55 Gy to the hypothalamic pituitary axis. These patients develop clinical and chemical signs of hypothyroidism. TSH stimulation testing confirms the diagnosis. TSH response to TRH can be used to determine whether the anterior pituitary gland is damaged (TSH level remains low) or the hypothalamus is damaged (TSH level increases).[53,139]

Assessment and Management

Annual evaluation of thyroid function (free T_4 and TSH) is performed up to 10 years after the completion of treatment. Patients with elevated TSH levels receive thyroid hormone replacement, even if free T_4 levels are normal, to suppress TSH and avoid overstimulation of the gland. Careful palpation of the gland and detailed history for symptoms of hypo- or hyperthyroidism are imperative. Any abnormalities require a referral to an endocrinologist for further evaluation and treatment.

TESTES

Testicular function is controlled by the release of FSH and LH from the pituitary gland. The gonadotrophin releasing hormone (Gn-RH) is released from the hypothalamus and controls LH and FSH secretions. The Leydig cells located in the testes produce testosterone, and the germinal epithelia produce the spermatozoa. The testosterone-producing Leydig cells affect secretion of LH and FSH via a negative feedback mechanism.[113,139] Germinal cell epithelia are very sensitive to cancer therapy and are damaged more easily than the Leydig cells. The signs and symptoms of primary testicular failure are lack of secondary sex characteristics, lack or change in libido (if Leydig cells are affected), and low sperm counts. Elevations in FSH and/or LH with possible decrease in testosterone are indicative of dysfunction.[139] Age at diagnosis, nutritional status at time of treatment, and combination therapy affect the degree of dysfunction.[151]

Radiation Effects

Radiation to the testes, directly or by scatter, can temporarily or permanently reduce sperm production. Temporary reduction in sperm count is noted with doses as low as 1 Gy.[8] The risk of permanent azoospermia increases as the dose of radiation increases. At doses between 4 and 6 Gy, azoospermia can persist after 5 years, and at doses greater than 6 Gy, the damage appears to be permanent.[8,39,201] After HSCT with 10 Gy total body irradiation, azoospermia in postpubertal males is permanent.[207] With scatter doses of 2.68 to 9.83 Gy following abdominal radiation for Wilms tumor, boys were found to have azoospermia or oligospermia in 8 out of 10 cases.[210] Leydig cells appear resistant to radiation with doses as high as 12 Gy. However with doses in excess of 20 Gy, clinical and hormonal Leydig cell failure is apparent.[219]

The testes of prepubertal males, once thought to be protected from the effects of treatment, appear to be radiosensitive as well. Prepubertal boys treated with 24 Gy of testicular radiation for ALL demonstrate low testosterone levels and delayed sexual maturation. In one study, 55% of boys treated with cranial and abdominal radiation for ALL and 17% treated with craniospinal radiation demonstrated elevated levels of FSH and a decrease in testicular volume.[219] Recovery of spermatogenesis may occur years after completion of radiation.[56] Gonadal function was evaluated in 20 males treated for Hodgkin's disease. Four out of eight treated with radiation alone who had documented azoospermia were able to father children 10 to 15 years after treatment.[180]

Chemotherapy Effects

Chemotherapy may also affect testicular function. Eighty percent to 100% of males treated for Hodgkin's disease with 5 to 6 cycles of MOPP therapy (mechlorethamine, vincristine, prednisone, and procarbazine) were found to have azoospermia 2 years after treatment.[32,213,214,239] Azoospermia was temporary in about 20% of these cases 7 years after treatment. Azoospermia with ABVD therapy (doxorubicin, bleomycin, vinblastine, and dacarbazine) appears to be about 40% while on therapy. However recovery is generally 100% following completion of treatment.[206] Cyclophosphamide as a single agent is gonadotoxic. In one study only 2 of 10 men treated with VAC (vincristine, actinomycin, and cyclophosphamide) with cumulative doses ranging between 4.7 to 31.9 g/m² had normal sperm counts. Both men with normal counts received less than 7.5 g/m² of cyclophosphamide.[123] In studies where men received 8 or more cycles of COPP (cyclophosphamide, vincristine, prednisone, and procarbazine), azoospermia was evident in 100% of subjects.[34]

Other Gonadal Effects

Surgical procedures in the pelvic region may affect gonadal function. Impotence and/or retrograde ejaculation have been noted following lymph node dissection and pelvic exenteration.[104,134] Hydroceles have been noted in survivors of Wilms tumor and Hodgkin's disease.[16]

Secondary Dysfunction

Secondary testicular dysfunction is caused by radiation to the hypothalamic pituitary axis. Doses greater than 55 Gy cause hypothalamic damage resulting in secondary testicular failure with decrease in LH, FSH, and serum testosterone levels. Secondary testicular failure is characterized by failure to progress through puberty and decreased libido. Children receiving large doses of cranial radiation are also at risk for decreased production of prolactin inhibiting factor (PIF), which causes hyperprolactinemia. This condition is characterized by decreased libido, impotence, and decreased testosterone levels. Treatment with bromocriptine can resolve these symptoms.[43] Precocious puberty has been noted following doses of cranial radiation greater than 25 Gy.[19] Survivors exhibiting early secondary sex characteristics (before age 10 for males), if untreated, will have halted growth from premature fusion of the epiphysis.[19]

Assessment and Management

Although not a life-threatening effect, gonadal dysfunction may be life-altering. Careful assessment and handling of the problem is imperative. When there is risk of azoospermia, consideration of sperm banking at diagnosis is an important aspect of pretreatment evaluation. Gonadal screening begins at about the age of 12 years or earlier if indicated. LH, FSH, and testosterone levels are assessed. Semen analysis can be helpful to definitively determine germinal damage. Referral to an endocrinologist for replacement hormones or for ongoing monitoring is recommended. If baseline studies are normal, blood work is repeated until puberty is completed and later if signs and symptoms of dysfunction are noted.

OVARIES

Ovarian function is controlled by the release of FSH and LH from the pituitary gland. The release of LH and FSH is controlled by Gn-RH from the hypothalamus. Estrogen production in the ovaries regulates the LH and FSH secretions from the hypothalamus through a negative feedback mechanism. Primary ovarian failure is characterized by lack or halt of pubertal progression, amenorrhea, decreased libido, vaginal dryness, mood swings, and hot flashes. Elevated levels of serum LH and FSH with low levels of estradiol are noted with primary ovarian failure.[113,139] Both radiation and chemotherapy can affect ovarian function. Other factors that influence the degree of dysfunction include pubertal stage at diagnosis, nutritional status, duration of therapy, and surgical procedures. Evaluating the effects of treatment on the female gonads is somewhat more difficult than on the male gonads, because the equivalent to orchidometry (measurement of testicular size) and semen analysis for germ cell function are not available for females.

Radiation Effects

The effects of radiation on the ovary are age- and dose-dependent. A prepubescent female can receive up to 15 Gy to the abdomen and retain normal function, whereas a 40-year-old woman would be rendered sterile by doses of 4 to 6 Gy.[8,144,180,224] Ovarian failure is common after pelvic irradiation (30-40 Gy) for Hodgkin's disease unless an oophoropexy is performed.[33] However oophoropexy does not protect the ovaries from systemic chemotherapy, and the manipulation of the ovary actually may cause ovarian damage due to disruption of blood flow.[74] Oral contraceptives also have been theorized to protect the ovaries by suppression of ovulation. However results of studies of the protective mechanism of oral contraceptives during therapy are mixed.[33,74] Individuals undergoing HSCT are at significant risk for ovarian failure whether a single or hyperfractionated dose of TBI is used.[38,138,207] In those patients it is difficult to determine the primary cause of dysfunction because concomitant chemotherapy is given, which

also affects ovarian function. Females who retain gonadal function posttransplant may experience premature menopause.[127,138] In one study, 50% of girls experienced ovarian failure following treatment with cranial/spinal radiation, and 93% who had additional abdominal irradiation (12 Gy) experienced delayed menses.[90]

Chemotherapy Effects

Chemotherapy also is implicated in ovarian dysfunction, but the morbidity is less than germinal dysfunction in males. Girls treated with a single alkylating agent, such as cyclophosphamide, or several cycles of MOPP are capable of achieving puberty with normal fertility.[238] Prepubertal females demonstrate the greatest chemoresistance, but these girls are not completely protected from the damaging effects. Cyclophosphamide-induced ovarian dysfunction occurs with cumulative doses of 4 g/m^2 in women over the age of 40, whereas prepubertal females can receive up to 20 g/m^2 and still progress through puberty.[129,157] However those with normal function at the completion of treatment will be at risk for early menopause because of the treatment-induced reduction of ova.[107]

Other Effects

Surgical removal of the ovaries is a rare event in pediatric oncology. Oophorectomy results in primary ovarian failure, requiring lifelong hormone replacement to achieve sexual maturation and prevent long-term consequences of estrogen depletion (e.g., osteoporosis).

Secondary Ovarian Failure

Secondary ovarian failure is caused by radiation damage to the hypothalamic pituitary axis. The fraction dose, number of fractions, and the duration of treatment are all factors affecting the degree of dysfunction. Serum studies reveal decreased LH, FSH, and estradiol levels. Higher doses of radiation ($\geq$55 Gy) to the hypothalamus decrease PIF.[16] This can cause irregular menstrual bleeding and anovulatory periods. Patients who received high doses of cranial irradiation and demonstrate these symptoms are evaluated for hyperprolactinemia. Bromocriptine is used to suppress the prolactin secretion. Precocious puberty has been noted following radiation doses greater than 25 Gy to the hypothalamus.[43] These patients begin to exhibit early secondary sex characteristics (8 years of age for females), and if untreated, halted growth may result from premature fusion of the epiphyses. Patients with early secondary sex characteristics are referred to an endocrinologist for a full evaluation and consideration for treatment.[16]

Assessment and Management

Careful monitoring of sexual development and menses is imperative for early identification of problems and for the initiation of appropriate hormonal replacement. Tanner staging and a baseline determination of LH, FSH, and estradiol levels is done at 12 years, or earlier if indicated, and annually until puberty is completed. If symptoms of ovarian failure arise, LH, FSH, estradiol, and prolactin levels are obtained. A referral to an endocrinologist is recommended for complete evaluation and consideration of hormonal replacement. Young women who currently have normal ovarian function but are at risk for early menopause are encouraged to have children before the age of 30. Furthermore, these patients should not delay obtaining an infertility referral (see Table 18-1).

REPRODUCTIVE OUTCOMES

One of the major concerns after treatment for cancer in childhood or adolescence is whether survivors will be able to have healthy children. Among the issues are actual fertility and gonadal function, pregnancy complications, congenital abnormalities, and cancer in the offspring. Although many treatments used for childhood cancer can produce reproductive toxicity, the available data are encouraging and tentatively support the conclusions that impaired fertility and adverse pregnancy outcomes are limited to select groups of survivors, and that live-born children of female and male survivors, on the whole, are not at increased risk of congenital anomalies or cancer.[15] It appears that the risk of impaired fertility is related to specific agents and dose of chemotherapy (e.g., alkylating agents are more gonadotoxic than nonalkylating agents), radiation therapy site and dose, pubertal status at the time of treatment (prepubertal children are less affected that those treated during or after puberty), and sex (girls are usually less severely affected than boys).

Reasons for concerns about pregnancy outcome data include long latency periods for some complications. Many offspring may not have had long enough follow-up to make sure they are not at increased risk.[15] Other concerns are that a majority of studies have been confined to single institution reports and retrospective cohort studies of survivors treated in an era of less intensive therapy. The large-scale design of the current Childhood Cancer Survivor Study (CCSS), a retrospective cohort study with 20,000 eligible patients and 3,000 offspring, addresses some of these concerns. As results are published in the next few years, the CCSS should provide more definitive data about past therapies. Well-designed prospective studies with long periods of follow-up and periodic evaluation are needed to better understand risks in the era of modern childhood cancer treatment.[172]

Perinatal Problems

Throughout the 1980s a number of reports of perinatal morbidity and mortality were published, and outcomes varied with cancer diagnosis and specifics of therapy. Li and colleagues reported an increased rate of intrauterine and postpartum complications in female survivors of Wilms tumor,[136] and these findings were generally confirmed and extended in three other reports, including one of survivors who received abdominal irradiation for tumors other than Wilms tumor.[27,75,98] Women at highest risk were those who received abdominal radiation (with or without chemotherapy). There was an eightfold relative risk of perinatal mortality and a fourfold relative risk of having low birth-weight infants ($<2,500$ grams) compared with the general population. It is thought that the pathogenesis may include uterine vascular insufficiency and/or radiation-induced structural changes (e.g., scoliosis or fibrosis). In addition, complications may be related to congenital genitourinary tract malformations occurring as part of the Wilms tumor complex.[15]

An early study (1978) found that Hodgkin's disease survivors (both female patients and partners of male patients) who received both chemotherapy and radiation were at increased risk of spontaneous abortion.[109] Another report also suggested that female survivors were at increased risk of pregnancy complications.[153] Other series have not confirmed these findings, but methodological problems (small size, heterogeneous population) may have limited their applicability to resolving the questions of pregnancy complications in Hodgkin's disease and Wilms tumor survivors.[15]

Congenital Abnormalities and Genetic Diseases

Exposure to ionizing radiation and chemicals designed to interfere with DNA function and replication can cause survivors significant anxiety, which may affect their decisions about childbearing. In theory many of the agents used in treatment could produce germ-cell mutations and genetic disease in the next generation. Three case series have reported an excess of congenital malformations (major and minor) in female survivors.[27,147,153] In addition, a study of 202 pregnancies in 100 survivors found 2 of 20 offspring born to 8 women treated with dactinomycin had cardiac defects.[85] More recent publications have not supported this association.[28,83] This finding requires additional study in larger numbers of survivors and their offspring.

Most studies, including the recent Five Center Study, have shown no excess of malformations.[28] The latter study is noteworthy because it was designed with a large study cohort; congenital malformations were divided into those that were likely to have resulted from germ-cell mutation and those that were not; and patients were grouped according to whether or not they had received mutagenic therapy.[71] The study found no indication that cancer chemotherapy or radiotherapy increased the risk of congenital anomalies in children subsequently conceived. The caveat, however, is that the study data are somewhat out of date; subjects were diagnosed during 1945 to 1975, and data collection concluded in 1983. Thus studies published so far cannot entirely reassure survivors. Newer, more intense treatment regimens may yet prove to be damaging to germ cells.

Cancer in Offspring

Except for single-gene inherited tumors such as retinoblastoma and cancer family syndromes, studies have not demonstrated a significantly increased overall risk of childhood cancer in offspring of survivors.[15] Studies have been hampered by the same design problems as studies of congenital anomalies, however, including heterogeneous diagnoses and treatment regimens, and small numbers of offspring. The Five Center Study analyzed cancer diagnoses in offspring by age of occurrence and found an increased risk for children less than 5 years of age.[168] In this study, male offspring of female survivors appeared to have a higher risk. A study of 5,487 offspring of 14,000 childhood cancer survivors treated in Scandinavia found fewer than 1 excess cancer diagnosis for every 1,000 offspring.[205] There was a trend toward increasing risk of cancer in children whose survivor parents were less than 10 years of age at diagnosis.

Assessment and Management

Possible reproductive effects of cancer treatment should be discussed with patients and their families as part of the process of educated consent. Some survivors of earlier eras do not recall being told that infertility was a possible consequence of treatment, and they have been overwhelmed and devastated to learn the truth after they have been through expensive and emotionally trying attempts to conceive. Information allows survivors to make informed choices. Males of appropriate age and development must be offered the option of sperm banking before receiving treatment that could affect fertility. Females at risk of early menopause are advised not to delay childbearing. Because not

all therapy causes infertility and because some patients recover fertility long after treatment is completed, couples who do not want a pregnancy are advised to use birth control methods even if fertility seems unlikely.[212]

Counseling for survivors considering pregnancy must take into account whether the survivor had a cancer that is likely to be hereditary (e.g., retinoblastoma). For those survivors (as well as survivors whose family history puts them at risk of other genetic diseases), genetic counseling, and possibly genetic testing, is offered. Referral must be made to a state-of-the-art genetic counseling program, which is the appropriate setting for professional genetic testing and counseling. Because current reports do not suggest increased risk of genetic disease in offspring, the cancer history alone is not sufficient reason to undergo invasive prenatal diagnostic procedures; however, survivors concerned about structural cardiac defects after dactinomycin therapy, as described in one report, should be offered a screening sonogram or fetal echocardiography.[85]

Female survivors may be concerned about whether their health will allow them to complete a pregnancy. Because pregnancy increases cardiorespiratory stress, survivors who had anthracycline therapy with or without radiation to the heart, as well as those who received therapy known to induce pulmonary fibrosis, should be offered cardiac evaluation and/or pulmonary function testing before pregnancy.[172] Women who received abdominal or pelvic irradiation may be at higher risk of impaired expansion of the uterus during pregnancy, leading to premature delivery. These survivors need information about their pregnancy risks before conceiving and must be under the care of a specialist in high-risk obstetrics during their pregnancies.

CARDIOVASCULAR SYSTEM

Cardiac disease is a significant source of late morbidity and mortality for childhood cancer survivors treated with anthracyclines, mediastinal radiation, and/or cyclophosphamide.[82,91] The presence or absence of acute complications does not correlate with the development of late complications. In most cases the total dose delivered, method of delivery (IV push vs. infusion), and age of the patient correlate with the development of late complications and long-term sequelae. Younger children (<2 years of age) are at risk even at lower cumulative doses. Isolated cases of cardiovascular complications with low doses of these agents and no other risk factors have been noted. Early recognition of myocardial dysfunction may improve long-term survival through early intervention.

Effects of Anthracyclines

While anthracyclines produce improved event-free survival (EFS) for childhood cancer patients, they have caused varying degrees of cardiotoxicity in many children and young adults. Up to 65% of patients who received between 228 to 550 mg/m^2 were noted to exhibit late changes in left ventricular function as measured by echocardiogram (ECHO). Further study has shown that patients who received less than 300 mg/m^2 of anthracyclines had normal left ventricular function after a median follow-up of 8 years.[175]

The left ventricular dysfunction consists of decreased contractility, elevated afterload, or both as a result of myocyte damage and loss. This leads to hypertrophy of the remaining myocytes and a decrease in the left ventricular wall thickness, creating increased afterload.[141,175] Many of these changes are noted only on echocardiogram, and the patient may have no obvious cardiac symptoms. The unanswered question is what will be the long-term implications of living with suboptimal cardiac function.[141]

Research efforts are aimed at decreasing the acute damage with cardioprotectants such as dexrazoxane (Zinecard), which could protect the heart from the toxic effects of anthracyclines.[236] While cardioprotectants have proved effective in some adult clinical trials, adequate evidence to support their widespread use in pediatrics is lacking at this time. Several large-scale randomized trials to evaluate their effectiveness are currently under way in the Children's Oncology Group (C.O.G.). Research in the use of liposomal doxorubicin to decrease cardiotoxicity in pediatric patients is currently under way.[101] Other researchers are exploring ways to improve or maintain cardiac function when damage from anthracyclines has been documented. Afterload reduction with the use of the ACE inhibitors (e.g., enalapril) is currently under study in long-term survivors.[175]

Cardiac failure can occur at times of increased cardiovascular stress, such as during anesthesia, pregnancy, after labor and delivery, with growth hormone use, prolonged illness, illicit drug use, or with heavy weight lifting or other isometric exercises. All patients who have received anthracyclines must be considered at risk for myocardial dysfunction and must be monitored carefully during activities or events that stress the cardiovascular system.

Effects of Radiation

Radiation to the chest or mediastinum generally includes radiation to the heart. Chronic effects of cardiac radiation generally do not occur until doses greater than 40 Gy are reached, although lower doses can cause toxicity in some individuals. Radiation effects on the cardiovascular system can include pericardial effusions or constrictive pericarditis, premature coronary artery disease, or valvular thickening and fibrosis.[16,91] Up to 50% of survivors may have asymptomatic cardiac changes. Symptomatic pericarditis may not appear until as late as 45 years after therapy.[14,80] In two large cohort studies involving long-term survivors of Hodgkin's disease, cardiovascular disease was the cause of death in 13% to 16% of participants who received radiation therapy.[91]

Effects of Combination Therapy

The use of radiation to the mediastinum can potentiate the toxic cardiac effects of anthracyclines. Studies have demonstrated that patients who have received both therapies have greater myocyte damage than those who received similar doses of anthracyclines without radiation.[91] Therefore careful cardiac assessment is of primary importance.

Assessment and Management

A careful review of treatment history is necessary to appreciate the survivor's risk factors for cardiac late effects. Cumulative dose of anthracycline, total radiation dose and port, and age at treatment will guide the assessment. Patient assessment includes questions regarding exercise amount and type, exercise intolerance, and any symptoms of dizziness, palpitations, or shortness of breath. It may be difficult to ascertain the patient's actual degree of dysfunction without asking specific questions about daily activities. Questions regarding household chores, yard work, stair climbing, or even taking a shower and getting dressed without difficulty may yield important information related to cardiac function.[79] Reports of cardiac symptoms such as chest or arm pain, pressure, heartburn, nausea, or fatigue should certainly raise concerns for coronary artery disease, even if the patient seems to be younger than expected for this.[91]

If the history and physical examination are normal, there are still some recommended screening tests. The guidelines are not completely clear, but most centers agree that for patients who received greater than 200 mg/m^2 of anthracylines, or a lower dose with mediastinal radiation, an electrocardiogram (ECG) and ECHO are recommended every 2 to 5 years. Multigated angiography (MUGA) scans may be performed to further evaluate cardiac function. Some centers also recommend 24-hour Holter monitors to identify arrhythmias. Regardless of the test used for evaluation, all patients at risk must be evaluated on a routine basis. Younger children, even with lower doses (<200 mg/m^2) are closely monitored. All patients are evaluated at the completion of treatment and then again after pubertal growth to assess cardiac workload.

Patients with symptoms of cardiac dysfunction, or those with evidence of subclinical decreased function, must be evaluated by a cardiologist familiar with the cardiac late effects of cancer therapy. Discussion of modifiable risk factors including smoking, alcohol and drug use, type of exercises (aerobic vs. isometric), and dietary intake are an essential part of patient education. Survivors should be aware of their history and understand when further consultation may be needed, such as before anesthesia or during pregnancy.

RESPIRATORY SYSTEM

Toxicity to the lungs and airways is caused mainly by radiation and also by some forms of chemotherapy, most notably, bleomycin. Damage occurs most often in patients who have thoracic or lung tumors, such as Hodgkin's disease, or lung metastases from a solid tumor. It can also occur in bleomycin-based treatment regimens, such as those for germ cell tumors. Two types of pulmonary injury primarily occur: radiation pneumonitis and chronic fibrosis. There may be a third pattern of injury seen in younger patients that involves restrictive lung changes related to decreased growth of the lung and chest wall.[160,242]

Acute Radiation Pneumonitis

Acute pneumonitis usually appears 3 to 6 months after therapy. Acute changes are seen in 5% to 15% of patients and generally do not develop until 30 Gy are delivered to more than 50% of the lung volume.[137,235] Clinical symptoms of pneumonitis include a dry hacking cough, sometimes with fever and/or dyspnea. These symptoms are caused by an acute phase injury consisting of local pulmonary edema with fibrin-like material deposited in the alveolar spaces.

Chronic Fibrosis

Bleomycin is the most common agent causing fibrotic changes with cough, dyspnea, and fever.[48] These changes are dose dependent. A cumulative dose of 400 units/m^2 is the accepted threshold for bleomycin. Symptoms are increased with concurrent or previous chest irradiation, cyclophosphamide, or oxygen therapy.[16] Alkylating agents such as carmustine are also thought to cause pulmonary fibrosis. Doses of greater than 800 mg/m^2 may cause toxicity, and up to 50% of patients have symptoms at doses of greater than 1500 mg/m^2.[10] Melphalan, cyclophos-

phamide, vinblastine, and methotrexate have been implicated in pulmonary fibrosis, but not with a significantly high incidence.[3,40,178]

Total body irradiation for HSCT also is associated with acute and chronic lung changes. Along with transient acute restrictive changes, obstructive changes noted on pulmonary function studies have been reported in approximately 29% of patients.[207]

Assessment and Management

Assessment of pulmonary function is made after reviewing risk factors contributing to potential injury. The treatment history must be carefully reviewed to identify thoracic radiation ports and doses, along with the cumulative doses of chemotherapeutic agents. The survivor's current health status is reviewed, focusing on any respiratory symptoms such as chronic cough, exercise intolerance, or dyspnea. Other contributory factors, such as any history of asthma and smoking history are explored. Any symptoms identified on history or physical exam must be explored further with chest radiograph (chest x-ray) and/or pulmonary function testing (PFT).

Clear guidelines on how to monitor long-term survivors for pulmonary dysfunction are not available, but some recommendations may be reasonable. Chest radiographs every 6 months to 1 year for the first 5 years after treatment, then every 2 to 5 years thereafter may be useful to identify fibrotic changes. Many programs also recommend pulmonary functional testing (PFTs) every 2 to 5 years.[94] For patients with significant symptoms or changes on chest x-ray or PFT, referral to a pulmonologist is recommended.[16,48] Patients who received bleomycin must be educated regarding the potential risks of oxygen therapy, particularly during and after surgery. Oxygen concentrations of greater than 30% should be avoided because of the risk of pulmonary edema.[78]

VISION AND HEARING

Chemotherapy, radiation, and surgery can compromise visual acuity or auditory function. Visual late effects are generally a result of radiation or surgery (enucleation) due to direct tumor involvement of the eye. Auditory changes can be a result of tumor involvement, but are usually from treatment with chemotherapy or antibiotics that are ototoxic, radiation therapy to auditory structures, or a combination of these treatments.

Effects of Treatment on the Eye

Chemotherapeutic agents such as alkylating agents, antimetabolites, steroids, plant alkaloids, and antibiotics have the potential to cause ocular toxicity, including keratitis, diplopia, blurred vision, glaucoma, and optic neuritis.[87] Most of these effects are usually acute and reversible. Survivors of childhood cancer may also have visual deficits related to the primary tumor, such as those with retinoblastoma or optic glioma.

Radiation Effects

Radiation toxicity to the eye can be varied and can affect all aspects of the eye and orbit. The lens is the most radiation-sensitive structure of the eye, and radiation damage to this area results in the development of cataracts or opacities of the lens.[1] Radiation doses of 24 Gy to the whole brain can result in cataracts in 50% of patients.[87] Doses of 10 Gy as TBI used in HSCT can cause the development of cataracts in nearly all patients treated.[1] Prolonged steroid usage, especially in combination with cranial radiation, will place patients at high risk for the development of cataracts.

Radiation to the orbital bones may cause retarded bone growth, leading to facial deformities, especially in patients who were treated at a young age.[1] Surgical removal of the eye is most commonly associated with treatment for retinoblastoma. Patients who have had an enucleation will require a prosthetic device for cosmetic purposes.

Effects of Treatment on Hearing

Hearing loss, most commonly in the high frequency ranges (6,000-8,000 Hz) may occur after the administration of ototoxic agents. These agents include platinum-based chemotherapy, aminoglycoside antibiotics, and loop diuretics.[132] All of these drugs have been shown to cause damage to the cochlear hair cells in the organ of Corti, leading to sensorineural hearing loss.[68,71,183] Cranial radiation directed at the ear, midline of the brain, or brainstem may cause atrophy of the auditory nerve as well as inner ear hair cell loss, especially when used in conjunction with other ototoxic medications.[132]

Assessment and Management

A careful review of the patient's treatment history will determine the level of risk for late effects to these senses. Assessment of vision and hearing should occur annually. A Snellen's chart eye evaluation is done annually, and all high-risk patients are examined by an ophthalmologist to evaluate for the development of cataracts or diminished vision. Vision problems may necessitate removal of cataracts or fitting with corrective lenses. After enucleation, a well-fitting ocular prosthesis enhances the cosmetic appearance of the patient and

should be resized for an appropriate fit as the child grows to decrease the risk of asymmetrical growth of the orbit.

A baseline hearing test is completed for patients treated with cisplatin or other ototoxic drugs and those who received radiation to the brain. If the results are normal, the test may be repeated every 2 to 5 years or if symptoms arise. School personnel may be able to assist with audiology testing. If abnormalities are noted, a referral to an otolaryngologist is recommended for a thorough evaluation. A hearing aid may be helpful in accommodating for the hearing loss. Depending on the age of the child when hearing loss occurs, speech therapy and special education may be necessary to accommodate for specialized learning needs caused by the hearing loss.

HEMATOPOIETIC SYSTEM

Immunosuppression and myelosuppression are possible late effects after radiation, chemotherapy, and removal of the spleen. HSCT places the patient at highest risk for hematopoietic late effects.

Immunosuppression

Total body irradiation can impair cell-mediated immunity for up to 4 years after HSCT. This effect is a result of incomplete T-cell reconstitution.[231] Total nodal irradiation in patients with Hodgkin's disease can lead to impairment of T-cell function as late as 8 years after therapy, but may also have some relationship with advanced staging and pretreatment abnormalities.[135] Splenectomized patients have impaired humoral immunity and decreases in serum levels of IgM and IgA. They are at risk of developing fulminant infections, usually from encapsulated organisms (e.g., pneumococci, *Haemophilus influenzae, Neisseria meningococcus*). Splenic atrophy after radiation (40 Gy) to the spleen results in similar infection patterns.[51]

Myelosuppression

Radiation to the bone marrow may affect lymphocytes and other bone marrow lineages. The degree of marrow damage depends on the dose and volume irradiated. After 40 Gy of total nodal radiation therapy, peripheral granulocyte counts and bone marrow reserve can be decreased up to 7 years from treatment.[111] The long-term chemotherapy effects on bone marrow function have not been well documented. However, it appears that chemotherapy given up to 3 years after radiation for Hodgkin's disease or methotrexate given up to 18 months after craniospinal radiation may result in long-term myelosuppression.[49]

Assessment and Management

Annual examinations with a detailed history to elicit symptoms of recurring infection, anemia, or bleeding disorder are important for early detection. Splenectomized survivors should receive pneumococcal vaccine, *Haemophilus* b conjugate vaccine, and meningococcal vaccine as well as annual influenza vaccine. Daily prophylaxis with penicillin or erythromycin is recommended in children, but young adult survivors may keep a prescription of penicillin at home, with instructions to take the first dose with a fever of 101° F or greater. They must then seek medical attention immediately to receive empiric treatment with antibiotics that affect encapsulated organisms.

GASTROINTESTINAL

Gastrointestinal (GI) damage usually results from fibrosis or enteritis caused by surgery or radiation. Hepatic late effects can be the result of radiation, chemotherapy, or transfusion-acquired hepatitis.

Intestinal Tract

The stomach and small intestine appear to be more radiation sensitive than other parts of the GI tract, but damage can occur anywhere within the radiation field. With radiation doses of 40 to 50 Gy, there is a 5% incidence of fibrosis that increases to 36% when doses greater than or equal to 60 Gy are given. Complications usually occur within five years of treatment, but strictures can occur up to 20 years or more after therapy and tend to be progressive or recurrent.[142,199] Fibrosis generally results in strictures of the bowel, and symptoms depend on the location. Radiation to the chest or neck can cause fibrosis and strictures of the esophagus, resulting in dysphagia.[16]

Enteropathy can result from radiation to the abdomen or pelvis, causing vascular injury, fibrosis, and mucosal ulceration, which can remain silent for many years. Symptoms include diarrhea, intestinal cramping, vomiting, weight loss, obstruction, and chronic blood loss.[94]

Hepatic

Hepatic fibrosis can result from chemotherapy such as methotrexate or from radiation to the liver, particularly in conjunction with dactinomycin. The incidence of this problem is relatively low (less than 5% with intermediate dose methotrexate) and, at least with methotrexate, appears to stabilize or improve after discontinuing the drug.[50,152]

A more concerning late effect to the liver is infection with the hepatitis C virus (HCV), usually transmitted during a blood product transfusion. Before 1993 there was no routine screening mechanism for hepatitis C in the blood supply, and a 5% to 18% rate of infection with HCV has been reported in childhood cancer survivors who received transfusions.[30,112] There are few symptoms of acute infection with HCV, and symptoms may not be detected until 2 or 3 decades after the initial infection. Chronic infection with HCV can lead to cirrhosis and liver failure or hepatocellular carcinoma; it is the leading cause of liver transplantation in the United States.[184]

Assessment and Management

A careful review of treatment history, including radiation doses and sites, chemotherapy doses, surgical interventions, and transfusion history, will determine the risk of GI late effects. History and physical exam directed at GI symptoms include information on swallowing difficulties, heartburn, bowel function, weight gain or loss, and fatigue. With a history of hepatotoxic chemotherapy or radiation to the liver, routine screening includes liver function studies every 2 to 5 years once the baseline is normal. Stool guaiac to assess for occult bleeding is performed annually if there has been any radiation to the GI tract. If there is a history of dysphagia, a barium swallow or endoscopy may be necessary to assess the degree of stricture. If there is a history of dysphagia or heartburn, a malignancy must be ruled out. Treatment is based on symptomatic relief. Any symptoms of cramping, diarrhea, or nausea are evaluated for bowel obstruction or malabsorption. A referral to a gastroenterologist would be appropriate for further evaluation and treatment.

Laboratory screening for HCV is performed if there is any history of transfusion before July 1992. Routine screening includes liver function studies with alanine aminotransferase (ALT) and a test for the presence of antibodies to HCV using either an enzyme-linked immunosorbent assay (ELISA) or recombinant immunoblot assay (RIBA). All HCV-positive patients should have further testing for the presence of HCV-RNA by polymerase chain reaction (PCR).[30,143,184] Patients who screen positive for HCV need a referral to a gastroenterologist with experience treating patients with this infection. Interventions may include therapy with interferon and/or ribavirin after pathologic confirmation.

MUSCULOSKELETAL

Cosmetic and functional changes to the bones, teeth, muscles, and soft tissue are noted following irradiation. Factors that contribute to the degree of disability include age at diagnosis, size of the port, and dose of radiation. The most common bony and soft tissue abnormalities include atrophy or hypoplasia, scoliosis, and avascular necrosis.[16]

Irradiation to vertebral bodies results in endplate irregularities, loss of vertebral height, abnormal contour, lateral wedging, atrophy of the pedicle and/or lamina, and growth arrest lines.[89] These deformities and the development of scoliosis, kyphosis, or shortened sitting height (crown to rump) are prevalent following doses of greater than 20 Gy to the spine. Studies have documented scoliosis in 67% to 80% of patients treated with 20 to 62 Gy to the spine.[41] Hypoplasia of the ilium often occurs after flank irradiation for Wilms tumor and may affect the degree of scoliosis, creating a bowstring effect across the vertebra.[229] Marked progression of scoliosis occurs during pubertal growth spurts regardless of when the child was treated. Survivors of brain tumors and ALL who receive spinal radiation experience diminished spinal growth due to direct inhibition of vertebral growth. This contributes to short stature in these populations.[16]

Radiation delivered directly to bones, epiphyses, and surrounding soft tissue dramatically affects growth. Doses of 10 to 20 Gy can cause partial growth arrest. Doses greater than 20 Gy completely arrest endochondral bone formation.[89,237] Bones, soft tissue, and blood vessels are most susceptible to damage during phases of rapid growth. Therefore the effects of radiation are most pronounced in children less than 6 years of age and during the pubertal growth spurt. In addition to decreased bone growth after irradiation, there is an associated decrease in muscle and soft tissue mass in the field of radiation. This diminished growth in soft tissue and muscle mass results in asymmetry or hypoplasia. The development of fat in irradiated areas is also compromised, which will make the asymmetry more pronounced, particularly in overweight patients.

Avascular Necrosis

Avascular necrosis (AVN) and osteoporosis are noted following the treatment of various tumors including Hodgkin's disease and non-Hodgkin's lymphoma.[16] A combination of radiation and steroids have been implicated. However, AVN following the administration of single agents, including methotrexate and cyclophosphamide, or in combination with fluorouracil has been documented.[16] AVN presents as pain in the involved joint and is often accompanied by slipped capital femoral epiphysis. AVN usually occurs during treatment or shortly thereafter; however it has been described in patients many years after treatment.[49]

In one study, 50% of children who were less than 4 years of age when treated had slipped capital femoral epiphysis, compared with 1 out of 20 patients treated between the ages of 5 and 15 years. Shielding the femoral heads during radiation therapy greatly decreases this effect.[58]

Osteoporosis

Osteoporosis, like AVN, is a result of radiation and/or steroids and occurs most prominently during treatment. Exostoses, which are outgrowths of the physis, occur in up to 18% of children treated with radiation.[2,196] The incidence is less since the development of megavoltage radiation. Other radiological findings may include growth arrest lines and epiphyseal irregularities, which are noted following radiation in children who have not achieved their final height before the completion of treatment.[196,229]

Radiation to soft tissue may produce cosmetic changes such as asymmetry. Breast tissue can be dramatically affected in the prepubertal female. Recent studies demonstrate the vulnerability of pubertal breast tissue to the risk of second tumors (see section on second malignancies). Skin pigmentation can be altered with increased nevi in the field of radiation and hyperpigmentation. Other related tissue changes include scarring secondary to extravasation, lymphedema, alopecia, chronic conjunctivitis, skin GVHD, or dry eyes and dry mouth secondary to radiation effects on the lacrimal and salivary glands.[16]

Amputation/Limb Salvage

Amputation and limb salvage procedures all have lifelong implications related to functional outcomes. Survivors who have undergone amputation, disarticulation, or limb salvage procedures may develop compensatory scoliosis, leg length discrepancies, infection, or back pain. The status of the internal prosthesis and the stump condition must be followed by orthopedic physicians.

Dental/Maxillofacial

Dental and maxillofacial changes can be significant in a growing child. Delay in tooth development has been noted with doses of 18 Gy cranial irradiation and mantle irradiation for Hodgkin's disease.[114,222] Significant changes are noted with larger doses (45-65 Gy) used in the treatment of tumors of the head and neck such as nasopharyngeal carcinoma and orbital rhabdomyosarcoma.[73,114] Facial hypoplasia and asymmetry are noted following the treatment of patients who receive greater than 35 Gy to either the orbit or the nasopharyngeal area.

Age at time of diagnosis and dose of radiation therapy will impact the degree of asymmetry.

Malocclusions, dental caries, and poor root development are common. Although radiation is the primary etiology for these problems, chemotherapy and certain antibiotics have also been implicated in discoloration, increased grooves, and other cosmetic abnormalities noted in dentition.[16] Children treated with HSCT with total body irradiation in a single fractionated dose are at risk for abnormal dentition and other skeletal changes.[127] Forty percent of children treated for leukemia with 18 to 30 Gy cranial radiation show root and crown abnormalities.[41] In addition, patients treated for leukemia with chemotherapy alone have demonstrated shortening and thinning of premolar roots.[41] Thirty-five to fifty percent of HSCT patients who receive 10 Gy of total body irradiation demonstrate impaired root development, microdentia, enamel hypoplasia, and premature apical closure.[52]

Radiation directly to the salivary glands results in decreased secretions, causing dry mouth. In one study, 40% of patients treated for head and neck sarcomas had absent secretions.[41] Forty-five percent of patients treated for Hodgkin's disease with doses of 40 Gy to the submandibular region showed decreased flow rate of secretions.[24]

Assessment and Management

Careful evaluation and physical examination should be performed on an annual basis. X-rays of the irradiated areas are recommended every 3 to 5 years to evaluate the condition of the underlying bony structure. The condition of a prosthesis must be evaluated at least annually by a prosthetist, especially during periods of rapid growth. Growing limbs require careful measurements and follow-up to evaluate for length discrepancies. Assessment by an orthopedist is recommended before a period of rapid growth. Adequate dental care and follow-up are imperative during the treatment and long-term to preserve the teeth and tissues of the oral cavity. Referral to a plastic surgeon to alter or diminish some of the asymmetry is recommended. However, the risk of suboptimal results in a field of radiation may be high because of disruption of normal blood flow and scar tissue formation in the field of radiation.[16]

URINARY TRACT

Chemotherapy, radiation, and surgery may cause functional and structural impairment of the upper and lower urinary tract. The dose of chemotherapy, field of radiation, age of the child, and surgical procedures impact the degree of dysfunction.

Radiation

The severity of radiation damage to the urinary tract is dose dependent. The risk of significant renal damage increases with doses exceeding 25 Gy to both kidneys.[16,76] These doses are reported to cause chronic nephritis, especially in patients treated for soft tissue sarcoma of the abdomen and pelvis and patients with Wilms tumor and abdominal lymphomas.[16,104,134] The signs and symptoms of chronic nephritis include fatigue, nocturia, proteinuria, anemia, hyposthenuria, edema, salt wasting, hyperuricemia with gout, and progressive renal failure. There is a 5% incidence of hemorrhagic cystitis following doses of less than 40 Gy to the bladder.[16] Larger doses of radiation to the pelvis (e.g., with pelvic rhabdomyosarcoma) can result in strictures of the urethra (which may require dilatation and bladder training), small bladder capacity requiring frequent urination, and enuresis at a late age, especially in boys.[228] Radio-enhancers such as dactinomycin can lower the threshold dose and cause earlier onset of dysfunction.[89] Combination therapy for HSCT can result in hemolytic uremic syndrome.[227] This acute assault can lead to chronic renal failure.

Chemotherapy

The chief agents affecting renal function are cisplatin and ifosfamide. Cisplatin can cause tubular and glomerular damage evidenced by elevated creatinine and decreased glomerular filtration rate (GFR).[228,232] These effects are usually dose dependent. Cisplatin-related effects typically occur within a year of completion of treatment.[191] Dysfunction following the use of ifosfamide is noted more often in younger children (less than 3 years of age) and children with prior renal dysfunction and/or nephrectomy. Fanconi's syndrome after treatment with ifosfamide can result in renal tubular damage and progress to an inability to acidify urine.[216,232] Glomerular damage may be accompanied by tubular damage and lead to a decreased GFR and an elevated serum creatinine. Poor linear growth has been noted in children with chronic renal failure. In some cases improvement in function occurs slowly after the completion of treatment.[16]

Hemorrhagic cystitis, fibrosis, and bladder shrinkage are noted following the use of cyclophosphamide and ifosfamide.[191] The by-products of these drugs (acrolein) irritates bladder mucosa. Adequate hydration and oral or IV mesna have greatly reduced the incidence of hemorrhagic cystitis.

Combination therapy can have synergistic effects. Other factors that may increase the risk of renal failure include the use of antimicrobial agents such as vancomycin, aminoglycosides, inadequate alkalization before methotrexate administration, ectopic kidneys, radiation fibrosis with subsequent hydronephrosis, and chronic urinary tract infections.[16]

Surgery

Nephrectomy results in compensatory hypertrophy of the remaining kidney. Patients with this condition must protect the remaining kidney from damage as a result of trauma or infection. Early treatment of urinary tract infection and wearing extra protection (kidney guards) during contact sports will decrease the likelihood of further damage. Hypertension following nephrectomy is not a prominent problem when the remaining kidney is unaffected by treatment.[117]

Assessment and Management

Annual evaluation of blood pressure; routine urinalysis to screen for protein, blood, and bacteria; and determination of serum urate and creatinine levels are necessary to evaluate the urinary and renal status in at-risk patients. A health history includes questions to evaluate the status of the urinary tract and any problems such as frequency, blood in urine, painful urination, or enuresis. Early detection and treatment of urinary tract infections are imperative to decrease the risk of pyelonephritis and to preserve the function of the remaining kidney. A small number of patients with severe nephrotoxicity require renal transplantation.

FATIGUE

Fatigue is a complex phenomenon, and the etiology in the posttreatment period is difficult to identify. Most of the current literature available related to fatigue is in survivors of adult cancers. Sixty percent to 75% of female survivors of breast cancer describe decreased stamina 2 to 10 years after treatment.[12] Regarding children there are reports of fatigue in children with cognitive deficits after treatment.[20,189] Anecdotally, some children experience fatigue many years after radiation delivered to the CNS or thorax or total body irradiation. Fatigue is most likely an underappreciated problem in children and adult survivors of childhood cancer. Some researchers are investigating orthostatic hypotension as the possible etiology for fatigue in childhood cancer survivors.[208] Additional information on fatigue is found in Chapter 11.

SECOND OR SUBSEQUENT NEOPLASMS

Children and adolescents cured of cancer have an increased risk of a subsequent or second malignant neoplasm (SMN), defined as a tumor whose histologic type differs from that of the first primary. The risk of SMNs is not the same for all survivors; it varies with factors such as the original type of cancer, treatment given, and genetic predisposition; and it may be affected by environmental exposures and health practices. Several of these factors may have an interactive effect, and it is, in fact, the multifactorial nature of second cancers that makes it difficult to determine the magnitude of risk and precise etiology. In contrast to studying a single factor, understanding the interaction among risk factors and the roles of modifying factors requires a large and heterogeneous population, but studies of second cancers have not always addressed this design obstacle.[197] In addition, most studies of second cancers have been confined to cancers occurring in the first decade of follow-up.[198] Clearly, risk estimates may change as studies with larger numbers of patients and follow-up into second and later decades after cure are reported. At the same time, treatment plans that have less carcinogenic potential but will not compromise cure also are being evaluated. For these reasons, ongoing observation and cohort studies are essential.

Although the fear of second cancers understandably looms large, the actual incidence is infrequent. In the current view, the risk of second cancers is higher compared to the risk of first cancers in the population at large, perhaps 10 to 20 times greater. An extremely small subset of survivors is at risk for development of a series of multiple primary cancers. Although SMNs have occurred in virtually all patient populations studied, the primary malignancies with higher risks of SMNs are retinoblastoma,[64,154] Hodgkin's disease,[11,13,17,44,244] and leukemia treated with epipodophyllotoxins[97,186,187,202] or cranial radiation.[170,195] In addition, patients with sarcomas treated with more intensive multimodality therapy have a higher rate of second leukemias and solid tumors.[103,161] The importance of recognizing these associations is to identify individuals at higher risk, focus their health surveillance, and implement prevention strategies.

Effects of Treatment

One of the main reasons that studies of childhood cancer survivors were initiated more than 30 years ago was the concern that new cancers might develop after treatment modalities and agents with presumed carcinogenic effects.[154] The risk of a second cancer is increased by the use of therapeutic radiation or intensive therapy with alkylating agents or epipodophyllotoxins, and may be potentiated when these modalities are used together.[169]

The childhood cancers most successfully treated

with radiation (lymphoma, leukemia, sarcoma, and CNS tumors) are those associated with SMNs within the radiation field. Among the most commonly reported solid SMNs are bone and soft tissue sarcomas. The risk of these tumors increases with radiation dose. They may be aggressive and poorly responsive to therapy.[70] Females treated for Hodgkin's disease have an increased risk of breast cancer, reported to be 35 to 75 times greater than that of the general population.[11,13,18,92,204,244] Age at time of treatment (when mammary cells are proliferating), dose, field, and type of energy used affect risk. Age between 10 and 16 years, doses higher than 35 Gy, higher anterior doses, axillary dose, and treatment with low-energy linear accelerator are associated with increased risk. Treatment with neck and mantle irradiation increases the risk for thyroid cancer and, less often, other head and neck cancers.[70] In a report of approximately 9,000 survivors of various childhood malignancies, Tucker and colleagues found a fifty-three-fold increased risk of thyroid cancer; 68% arose within radiation fields, and the risk increased with higher radiation dose and young age.[230] Thyroid cancer also has been reported after cranial irradiation for ALL.[230] Survivors of Ewing's sarcoma have an increased risk of second bone sarcomas, but in contrast to retinoblastoma these SMNs occur within the radiation field and usually present in adolescence or just after periods of rapid bone growth, with latency periods of at least 10 years.[154,171,225] CNS tumors have been reported as SMNs following cranial radiation as prophylaxis for CNS leukemia. At greatest risk were children exposed to radiation when less than 6 years of age.[115,146,169,195] Melanomas as SMNs are now being reported following a variety of childhood malignancies, although not always occurring within a radiation field.[47]

Chemotherapy

Leukemia following treatment with MOPP for Hodgkin's disease was among the first chemotherapy-related SMNs to be reported. Leukemia seems to be related to treatment with alkylating agents, and the degree of risk increases with increasing doses. Alkylating agents are not all equally leukemogenic. Mechlorethamine may be the most leukemogenic, and cyclophosphamide less so. The use of ABVD, either alone or in combination with MOPP or COPP, has resulted in lower rates of secondary AML or myelodysplastic syndrome (MDS) after Hodgkin's disease.[70]

The SMN risk after treatment for ALL is small, reflecting the predominant use of antimetabolites in leukemia treatment, which are not associated with the development of new leukemias. In contrast, children treated with epipodophyllotoxins for ALL do have an increased risk of secondary leukemia.[187,202] The risk is higher for children treated on a weekly or twice weekly schedule as compared with those treated every other week. Characteristic genetic abnormalities have been reported in the second leukemias related to epipodophyllotoxin exposure.[59,70] The leukemias associated with alkylating agents and epipodophyllotoxins have different features, probably related to their differing mechanisms of action. Table 18-6 summarizes these differences.

A different chemotherapy—second cancer association—has been reported recently by investigators analyzing CCSS data. They observed an increased risk of second/subsequent neoplasms in patients who had received high doses of anthracyclines.[169a] An earlier report of second malignancies following treatment for Wilms tumor showed that anthracycline (doxorubicin) increased the risk of SMN in patients who received abdominal irradiation.[19a]

Genetic Predisposition

Genetic factors may predispose individuals to both primary and secondary cancers. Preliminary data from a study of genetic risk factors for SMNs support the hypothesis that SMNs may be associated

TABLE 18-6 CONTRASTS IN SECONDARY LEUKEMIAS BY CHEMOTHERAPEUTIC AGENT	
Alkylating Agents	**Epipodophyllotoxins**
Latency period between primary and SMN long	Latency short
Dose response evident	No clear dose response, but schedule appears to be important
Complex karyotypes and deletions of chromosomes 5 and 7 common	Translocations involving 11q23 and MLL gene
No predominant subtype of leukemia	M4 and M5 phenotypes most commonly seen
Myelodysplastic phase common	
Older children and adults more affected	

Data from Friedman, D. L., & Meadows, A. T. (1999). Pediatric tumors. In A. I. Neugut, A. T. Meadows, & E. Robinson (Eds.), *Multiple primary cancers* (pp. 235-256). Philadelphia: Lippincott Williams & Wilkins.

with familial cancer syndromes.[69] Several genetic conditions are linked with an increased risk of multiple primary cancers, including hereditary retinoblastoma, neurofibromatosis, Li-Fraumeni syndrome, familial adenomatous polyposis, hereditary nonpolyposis colorectal cancer, nevoid basal cell carcinoma syndrome, and multiple endocrine neoplasia (MEN) syndrome.[70] Strong and colleagues showed that the p53 germline carriers among relatives of patients with soft tissue sarcomas are at increased risk for SMNs.[226] Table 18-7 shows selected primary cancers, their associated treatment or genetic risk factors, and the type of second cancers known to occur.

Genetic predisposition was first studied in retinoblastoma. Retinoblastoma became the paradigm for a genetically inherited cancer and provided the basis for the two-hit theory of carcinogenesis.[125] Retinoblastoma raised the red flag about the role of genetic predisposition to SMNs, when bone and soft tissue sarcomas arising in nonirradiated tissues were first reported. The prevalence of SMNs following the hereditary form of retinoblastoma is higher than that for any other pediatric malignancy. In a recent analysis, the cumulative risk of an SMN at 50 years of age was 51% for those with bilateral retinoblastoma, compared with 5% for those with unilateral disease (i.e., no different from the general population); and external beam radiation greatly increased the risk of SMNs.[243] The most common SMNs after

retinoblastoma are soft tissue and bone sarcomas; other new primaries also reported at higher-than-expected rates include leukemia, melanoma, lymphoma, and perhaps breast cancer.[61,64,243]

Genetic predisposition may be involved in the development of radiation-associated CNS tumors in children treated for leukemia. Yet to be definitively studied is the reported association between tumors of the hematopoietic system and those of the CNS. Family members of children with CNS tumors have been reported to have a greater-than-expected incidence of leukemias, lymphomas, brain tumors, and other forms of childhood cancers.[66,124,131] These may represent a familial cancer syndrome distinct from that of the Li-Fraumeni syndrome.

Lifestyle and Environmental Exposures

Survivors of childhood cancer also are at risk for the cancers generally thought of as adult cancers. Many of these are influenced by health and lifestyle choices and environmental exposures such as smoking, sun exposure, diet, and exercise.

Assessment and Management

During the routine annual evaluation, even in asymptomatic survivors, one must pay particular vigilance to survivors whose original diagnosis and treatment places them at increased risk for specific SMNs. The real key to detection of most SMNs is

TABLE 18-7	TREATMENT-RELATED AND GENETIC RISK FACTORS FOR SMNs	
Primary Cancer	**Treatment or Genetic Risk Factors**	**Second Cancer**
Hodgkin's disease	Radiation	Solid tumors, especially breast cancer, sarcoma, thyroid
	Alkylating agents	MDS and AML with deletions of chromosome 5 or 7
CNS tumors	Radiation	CNS tumors
	Gorlin's syndrome	Basal cell carcinomas
	Turcot's syndrome	Colon cancer
Leukemia	Epipodophyllotoxins	AML with 11q23 abnormality
	Cranial radiation ± alkylating agents	CNS tumors, thyroid cancer
Retinoblastoma	Germline RB1 mutation	Osteosarcoma
	Radiation therapy	Soft tissue sarcomas, melanoma
Sarcomas	Germline p53 mutation Li-Fraumeni syndrome	Various second primaries
	Radiation therapy	Osteosarcoma
	Alkylating agents	MDS and AML with deletions of chromosome 5 or 7
	Epipodophyllotoxins	AML with 11q23 abnormality

From Friedman, D. L., & Meadows, A. T. (1999). Pediatric tumors. In A. I. Neugut, A. T. Meadows, & E. Robinson (Eds.), *Multiple primary cancers* (pp. 235-256). Philadelphia: Lippincott Williams & Wilkins.
MDS, Myelodysplastic syndrome; *AML,* acute myelocytic leukemia; *CNS,* central nervous system.

education of the patient and family. Any persistent symptoms must be evaluated by a health care professional. Follow-up care of survivors provides an opportunity to teach health promotion activities for risk reduction. These include avoidance of smoking, reduced alcohol intake, a low-fat high-fiber diet, limiting excess sun exposure, and the use of simple screening methods such as testicular and breast self-examination.[63] Skin cancer screening must be performed regularly, with documentation of any freckling or pigment changes for comparison on subsequent visits. Referral to a dermatologist is indicated for abnormalities in location, size, or color.

Prospective multi-institutional studies to determine the optimal methods of surveillance for females at increased risk of breast tumors are needed. At present, monthly breast self-examination, periodic examinations by a consistent health care provider, and prudent mammographic evaluation (with screening mammography initiated at 25 years of age) have been recommended.[118] Patients with a family history of breast cancer and those with genetic mutations predisposing them to breast cancer may be considered for earlier and more intensive screening. Table 18-8 summarizes breast cancer screening guidelines for survivors who were treated with thoracic radiation.

PSYCHOSOCIAL ISSUES

Emotions and Relationships

Cancer in childhood leaves an indelible imprint on all whose lives are touched by it. Survivorship requires living with uncertainty and living with compromise.[167] Living with prolonged uncertainty is the phenomenon described by Koocher and O'Malley as the *Damocles syndrome*—a metaphor based on the ancient story of Dionysius, who wanted to teach Damocles a lesson about the perilous nature of life.[128] He invited Damocles to a grand banquet, and as Damocles was beginning to enjoy himself, he was horrified to discover a sword hanging over his head, suspended by a single hair.

Like Damocles, survivors and their families are faced with finding a reasonable balance of vigilance, enjoyment, and satisfaction in the face of an uncertain future. Most reports addressing the psychosocial adjustment and quality of life of childhood cancer survivors have indicated that the majority of the survivors are functioning as well as their peers and may actually develop increased positive affect, a greater sense of personal control, and increased intimacy.[194] Other studies suggest that a significant number of survivors have increased anxiety about their health, the possibility of disease recurrence, and—for females—concern about fertility and the health of their future children.[245] Feelings of low self-esteem, social isolation, and educational or occupational difficulties in childhood cancer survivors directly related to fears of disease recurrence have been reported.[128] Adult survivors of childhood leukemia have been reported to have increased symptoms of depression, tension, anger, and confusion compared with sibling controls.[246] Another study found that depression, alcoholism, and/or suicide attempts were higher among cancer survivors than in the general population.[133] More recently, investigators have described posttraumatic stress disorder (PTSD) in subsets of young adult survivors of childhood cancer.[106,158] PTSD was associated with poorer quality of life and increased psychological distress.

Learning how to live with compromise is a major challenge in a society that fosters the myth that after diagnosis and treatment of cancer, survivors can pick up where they left off.[36] This myth ignores the high personal price paid by cancer patients for their biologic cure and the developmental disruptions cancer causes in young people. Liv-

TABLE 18-8	BREAST SCREENING GUIDELINES FOR CHILDHOOD CANCER SURVIVORS TREATED WITH THORACIC RADIATION THERAPY	
Time of Screening	**Type of Screening**
Starting at puberty	Breast self-examination
Puberty until age 25 years	Clinical breast examination once a year
Ages 25-40 years	Clinical breast examination twice a year
	Baseline mammogram
	Repeat mammogram every 3 years until age 40 years
Age 40 years and older	Clinical breast examination twice a year
	Mammogram every year

From Kaste, S. C., Hudson, M. M., Jones, D. J., et al. (1998). Breast masses in women treated for childhood cancer. *Cancer, 82,* 784-792.

ing with compromise can have repercussions in self-concept, self-esteem, body image, and other aspects of personal life. Even those studies reporting positive emotional outcomes for survivors show areas of concern and dissatisfaction regarding relationships.[81] One might predict that survivors with marked or residual physical disability would have a more difficult adjustment. Results of studies in this area are inconclusive, however, and the literature about children with physical handicaps and other chronic illnesses does not support a straightforward association between severity and adjustment.[72,86,120,166,179,240]

Marriage and family decisions, indicators of adult adjustment, have been studied. Delayed development of adolescent sexual identity and self-esteem and delayed separation from parents have been reported in childhood cancer survivors.[126] Some studies have indicated that childhood cancer survivors may delay marriage[221] and demonstrate decreased satisfaction with relationships with partners, family, and friends.[245] Ostroff and colleagues reported that families have difficulty making the transition to not treating survivors as if they were still ill after treatment is completed.[181] Several studies have reported that survivors are less likely to marry,[84,156,174,247] although two studies reported no differences in marriage rates.[99,173] In the largest study of marriage to date, Byrne and colleagues interviewed cancer survivors and matched sibling controls.[26] They found that survivors were slightly less likely to marry than controls, with survivors of brain tumors least likely to marry. In addition, survivors who married and were not known to be infertile were only 87% as likely to report a pregnancy as controls. An interim evaluation of preliminary data from the Childhood Cancer Survivor Study[192] found a decreased likelihood of marriage among adult survivors of childhood cancer and confirms the observation of Byrne et al. that survivors of CNS tumors were least likely to marry.[26]

The psychological impact of cancer has been recognized for many years.[128] Clinical and anecdotal evidence indicates that survivors and their families grapple with fears of recurrence, anniversary reactions, grief and loss, anger, anxiety and depression, survival guilt, and post-traumatic stress. Survivors and their families also relate positive outcomes of the cancer experience: personal growth, reordering of priorities, and renewed appreciation for life. A sizable body of case reports and time-limited cross-sectional studies of psychosocial adaptation has appeared over the past 25 years; however, methodological limitations have made it very difficult to (1) predict who will function well after cancer treatment, (2) understand the impact of cancer among different age-groups, and (3) develop appropriate preventive measures for high-risk individuals.[140] As in other aspects of late effects, what is needed are well-designed prospective longitudinal studies to inform interventions.

Educational and Occupational Issues

Treatment for cancer in childhood can affect school performance. Survivors have unique needs in the educational setting due to residual neurocognitive effects of CNS therapy, numerous or lengthy hospitalizations, persistent fatigue, hearing or vision loss, fine/gross motor impairments, and impaired social skills. Several studies, mostly focused on survivors of acute leukemia and CNS tumors, have indicated an increased likelihood that survivors will require special education services.[22,55,96] Such services are the legal right of eligible childhood cancer survivors under the Individuals with Disabilities Education Act (IDEA). Children and adolescents who do not meet the eligibility requirements of IDEA may be eligible for services under Section 504 of the federal Rehabilitation Act.

Several reports have addressed survivors' likelihood of completing high school and college education. Survivors (except those diagnosed with CNS tumors) and their sibling controls had the same likelihood of graduating from high school.[122] Survivors treated with at least 23 Gy of cranial irradiation and those diagnosed before 6 years of age were less likely than their siblings to attend college.[122] Hays and colleagues also noted that survivors were less likely than their peers to be college graduates.[100]

A study of employment status of survivors found that the older subjects (who had received less-intensive treatment) had relatively similar levels of economic achievement compared with the control group; however, younger survivors had a lower range of occupational status than the controls.[100] This study excluded survivors of CNS tumors from the analysis, but another study of CNS tumor survivors found that they were at risk for a number of adverse outcomes, including unemployment.[165] Cancer survivors' right to work is better protected now by federal and state laws that address employment rights (Table 18-9). Still, some survivors do face job discrimination in finding, keeping, or changing jobs, because rights under the law are not necessarily enforced.

Insurance Issues

Several reports have indicated that survivors have significantly more difficulty obtaining both life insurance and health insurance.[101,108] According to a

TABLE 18-9	LEGAL PROTECTION AGAINST JOB DISCRIMINATION
Law	Scope
Americans with Disabilities Act (ADA) of 1990	Prohibits many types of job discrimination by employers, employment agencies, state and local governments, and labor unions
Federal Rehabilitation Act	Bans public employers and private employers that receive public funds from discriminating on the basis of disability
Family and Medical Leave Act (FMLA) of 1993	Protects job security of workers in large companies who must take a leave of absence to care for a seriously ill child, take medical leave because the employee is unable to work due to his/her own medical condition, or for birth or placement of a child for adoption or foster care

Data from Keene, N., Hobbie, W., & Ruccione, K. (2000). *Childhood cancer survivors: A practical guide to your future* (pp. 122-130). Sebastopol, CA: O'Reilly.

TABLE 18-10	LEGAL PROTECTION AGAINST INSURANCE DISCRIMINATION
Law	Scope
Comprehensive Omnibus Budget Reconciliation Act (COBRA)	Requires public and private companies employing ≥20 workers to provide continuation of group coverage for 18 months to employees if they quit, are fired, or work reduced hours. The individual pays for coverage at a rate not >2% higher than the rate set for other workers.
Employee Retirement and Income Security Act (ERISA)	Protects workers from being fired because of cancer history. Does not apply to job discrimination (denial of new job due to cancer history).
Health Insurance Portability and Accountability Act of 1996 (Kennedy-Kassebaum law)	Allows individuals to change to a new job without losing coverage if they have been insured for at least 12 months.

Data from Keene, N., Hobbie, W., & Ruccione, K. (2000). *Childhood cancer survivors: A practical guide to your future* (pp. 120-122). Sebastopol, CA: O'Reilly.

study by Holmes and colleagues, survivors are less likely than their siblings to have any health insurance coverage.[108] This is particularly troubling given the need for lifetime surveillance of potential late effects in childhood cancer survivors. Survivors encounter barriers such as insurance application rejection based on cancer history, policy reductions, policy cancellation, preexisting condition exclusions, increased premiums, or extended waiting periods. Options for health insurance include group policies, individual policies, and government health care plans (e.g., Medicaid, Medicare, Comprehensive Health Insurance Plans). No federal or state legislation mandates a person's right to health insurance, but some legal remedies to insurance discrimination do exist and are listed in Table 18-10. In addition, comprehensive long-term follow-up clinics may offer discounted fees to cash-paying patients.

Assessment and Management

Anticipatory guidance through networking, counseling, patient/family education, and advocacy can positively affect survivorship. Survivors and their families need access to a variety of resources for support to work through the complicated emotional issues raised by childhood cancer. They need to know that they are not alone in their feelings; that their feelings may ebb, resurface, and reverberate over time; and that there are resources to help. Among the possibilities are supportive loved ones and friends, peer networking or support groups (in-person or on the Internet), and/or referral to individual, private counseling. Networking and support can provide a "safe" haven for expressing feelings, learning practical lived wisdom from those who have had similar experiences, and validation that the experiences and feelings are real. To aid in assessment of psychosocial adjustment, discussion regarding difficulties with personal relationships, school, and employment should be a routine part of follow-up for cancer survivors. Comprehensive follow-up programs include a psychologist, school liaison, and social worker to help address the psychosocial, educational, and occupational concerns of survivors.

Anticipatory guidance about the disease, treatment, risk factors for late effects, and recommended monitoring must be given beginning at diagnosis. Survivors who are well informed and prepared for survivorship can advocate more effectively for the care they need to maximize health and well-being. This information will need to be reinforced and updated as young people mature and can comprehend the information at increasing levels of sophistication and as risk information changes with new information about late effects. As survivors and their families make the transition from active treatment to long-term follow-up, the evolving standard of care is to schedule a separate appointment to review the patient's history, discuss plans for the future, and provide a written health summary.[121] As survivors move or seek care from adult medicine providers, they can provide pertinent information about their health history by giving a copy of this summary to their health care providers. Comprehensive follow-up programs also provide periodic seminars or conferences for survivors, their families, and adult health care providers and third-party payors.

Advocacy can be individual—enabling survivors to get what each needs from the health care, educational, and legal systems. To advocate for themselves, survivors and their families need complete information about their health history, recommended follow-up, and available resources. Group advocacy can also be effective in enabling change at community, state, or national levels. Increasing national funding for late effects research, starting and supporting comprehensive follow-up clinics, and/or improving insurance options and antidiscrimination laws are among the possible changes. In sheer numbers, cancer survivors have the potential to be a strong and effective political voice. Participating in Cancer Survivors Day in June and other high-visibility events can help make that voice heard. Some resources for patient/family education and advocacy are listed in Table 18-11.

NURSE'S ROLE IN COMPREHENSIVE CARE

In the mid- to late-1990s three major pediatric medical organizations endorsed standards for long-term follow-up. The International Society of Pediatric Oncologists (SIOP) in 1996 published guidelines that stated: "We advocate the establishment of a specialty clinic oriented to the preventive medical and psychosocial care of long term survivors . . . The goal is to promote long-term physical, psychosocial, and socioeconomic health and productivity, not merely to maintain an absence of disease or dysfunction."[150] That same year the American Society of Pediatric Hematologists-Oncologists (ASPHO) published standards for comprehensive

TABLE 18-11	RESOURCES FOR PATIENT/FAMILY EDUCATION AND ADVOCACY
PRINT MEDIA	
Title	**Author/Publisher**
Facing Forward: A Guide for Cancer Survivors.	Bethesda, MD: National Cancer Institute (NIH Publication No. 90-2424), 1990.
Surviving Childhood Cancer: A Guide for Families.	Fromer, M. J., Washington, DC: American Psychiatric Press, 1995.
Dancing in Limbo: Making Sense of Life After Cancer.	Halvoson-Boyd, G., & Hunter, L., San Francisco: Jossey-Bass, 1995.
After Cancer: A Guide to Your New Life.	Harpham, W. S., New York: W. W. Norton, 1994.
A Cancer Survivor's Almanac: Charting Your Journey.	Hoffman, B. (ed.), Minneapolis: Chronimed, 1996.
Childhood Cancer Survivors: A Practical Guide to Your Future. (includes Personal Long-term Follow-up Guide and Treatment Record)	Keene, N., Hobbie, W., & Ruccione, K., Sebastopol, CA: O'Reilly, 2000.
The Damocles Syndrome: Psychosocial Consequences of Surviving Childhood Cancer.	Koocher, G. P., & O'Malley, J. E., New York: McGraw-Hill, 1981. (out of print, but may be available through a library)
Cancervive: The Challenge of Life After Cancer.	Nessim, S., & Ellis, J., Boston: Houghton Mifflin Co., 1991.
Life in the Shadow: Living With Cancer.	Soiffer, B., San Francisco: Chronicle Books, 1991.

TABLE 18-11	RESOURCES FOR PATIENT/FAMILY EDUCATION AND ADVOCACY—cont'd

WEBSITES

Name	Address
The American Cancer Society's Cancer Survivors' Network	http://www.cancersurvivorsnetwork.org
Cancer Survivors On Line	http://www.cancersurvivors.org
National Office of Cancer Survivorship (NIH)	http://dccps.nci.nih.gov/ocs
NCCS: The Cancer Survivor's Toolkit	http://www.cansearch.org/programs/toolbox.htm
NIH (National Institutes of Health)	http://cancernet.nci.nih.gov/facing_forward/faccont. html
Oncolink	http://www.oncolink.org
Outlook	http://www.outlook-life.org
Stanford's SURVIVING! Newsletter	http://www-radonc.stanford.edu/surviving.html
The Group Room (interactive radio talk show program focusing on cancer)	http://www.vitaloptions.org

WEB-BASED SUPPORT GROUPS

Name	Address
Association of Cancer Online Resources (maintains many support groups)	http://www.acor.org
Oncolink (has option to subscribe to cancer-related listservs)	http://www.oncolink.org/psychosocial/
Childhood ALL Network List Server (includes ALL_Off, an unmoderated discussion/support group for parents whose children have completed treatment)	http://www.all-kids.org/mailing_lists
Cancer Survivors Gathering Place	http://www.teleport.com/~jimmc

ORGANIZATIONS

Name	Address
American Brain Tumor Association	2720 River Road Des Plaines, IL 60018 (847) 827-9910
American Cancer Society	National Office 1599 Clifton Road, NE Atlanta, GA 30329 (800) ACS-2345
Cancer Legal Resource Center	919 South Albany Street Los Angeles, CA 90015-0019 (213) 736-1455
Cancervive	6500 Wilshire Blvd., Suite 500 Los Angeles, CA 90048 (310) 203-9232
Candlelighters Childhood Cancer Foundation	3910 Warner Street Kensington, MD 20895 (800) 366-CCCF or (310) 962-3520
Childhood Cancer Ombudsman Program	P.O. Box 595 Burgess, VA 22432 Fax: (804) 580-2502 or (804) 580-2304
National Cancer Institute Office of Cancer Communications	9000 Rockville Pike Building 31, Room 10A-18
Cancer Information Clearinghouse	Bethesda, MD 20205 (800) 4 CANCER [(800) 422-6237]
National Coalition for Cancer Survivorship	1010 Wayne Ave, Suite 770 Silver Spring, MD 20910-5600 (877) NCCS-YES or (877) 622-7937

long-term follow-up programs.[5] In 1997 the American Academy of Pediatrics (AAP) published guidelines that emphasized the importance of long-term follow-up with a specialist "familiar with the potential adverse effects of treatment."[203]

In keeping with these guidelines, some institutions have developed comprehensive follow-up clinics. Nurses have a vital role in the nucleus of the multidisciplinary team, which may consist of representatives from nursing, medicine, social work, psychology, and health education. A comprehensive program has close working relationships with radiologists, radiation oncologists, endocrinologists, cardiologists, survivor advocates, and adult health care providers. In these programs nurses have developed roles that encompass clinical care, patient/family education (including development of websites and other media), professional and public education, consultancy, community relations, advocacy, program development, and fundraising. Typically, nurses in comprehensive follow-up programs have considerable prior experience in acute pediatric oncology nursing, interest in working in an ambulatory setting, and competency as nurses. Nurses working with patients in the acute phase of treatment can also positively impact the lives of childhood cancer survivors when they ensure that chemotherapy or other medications are given appropriately, encourage a child to attend school, or help a child cope during therapy.

Although there is general agreement about the need for long-term follow-up of childhood cancer survivors, a recent survey of 219 institutions indicated that about 80% of survivors are not being followed on a regular basis, primarily because few programs focus on long-term follow-up needs.[177] Nurses can be instrumental in developing these programs and overcoming the barriers to care listed in Box 18-1. Networking with nurses from comprehensive follow-up programs will help with mutual problem solving and in collaboration for development of nursing research studies and educational materials. Such networking has already begun through oncology nursing organizations such as the Association of Pediatric Oncology Nurses and the Oncology Nursing Society. There will be unprecedented opportunity to further this collaboration in the recently merged Children's Oncology Group. Nurses in comprehensive follow-up programs also are precepting and mentoring students, which contributes to the development of an expanded cadre of "late effects nurses."

Nurses have led or participated in research focused on various aspects of survivorship, including insurance and employment, marriage and relationships, fatigue, and post-traumatic stress disorder. As treatment protocols evolve, the constellation of potential biologic late effects may change, as may their impact on quality of life and survivorship, and nurses are well positioned to have a leadership role in research in this area. To do this, and to provide high-quality clinical care, nurses working in long-term follow-up need to be lifelong learners. Nurses have helped build the foundation of long-term follow-up care and will continue to provide direction in this area, guided by the concept articulated by consumer advocate Grace Monaco: "Life is a hollow gift unless cancer survivors emerge from treatment as competent and worthy individuals, able to obtain insurance, equipped to earn a living, and prepared to participate in a medical surveillance program to 'keep' the life they have won."[162]

With increasing survival rates and an aging survivor population, the questions that remain are many. What will be the life-span effect on vital organ function and the actual (not relative) risk of developing other late effects or second cancers as these individuals enter the fourth and fifth decades

---

BOX 18-1
BARRIERS TO CARE

PSYCHOSOCIAL
Lack of knowledge about the importance of follow-up
Emotional difficulty in revisiting the cancer experience
Feelings that long-term effects are discounted

FINANCIAL
Lack of insurance
Third-party payors unwilling to pay for screen tests

MEDICAL
Lack of specialty clinics offering comprehensive care to survivors
Lack of adequate knowledge among primary medical doctors and specialists regarding long-term follow-up
Pediatric centers often stop seeing patients at age 21; few pediatric centers have established partnerships with adult providers

Data from Richardson, R. C., Nelson, M. B., & Meeske, K. (1999). Young adult survivors of childhood cancer: Attending to emerging medical and psychosocial needs. *Journal of Pediatric Oncology Nursing, 16,* 136-144.

of life? Who will follow these young adults to ensure that they receive adequate care?

There remains a need to gain a deeper understanding of the psychologic impact of surviving childhood cancer and the development of specific intervention programs that can assist these survivors and their families to cope with the effects of treatment and live full and productive lives. New protocols will need to incorporate questions about potential long-term issues. This strategy will ensure adequate follow-up and result in alteration of future protocols to modify treatment and diminish late effects. As Dr. D'Angio noted several decades ago, "We must have a parallel effort in oncology so that the children of today don't become the chronically ill adults of tomorrow."[54]

REFERENCES

1. Abramson, D. H., & Servodidio, C. A. (1994). Ocular complications due to cancer treatment. In C. Schwartz, W. Hobbie, L. Constine, et al. (Eds.), *Survivors of childhood cancer* (pp. 111-131). St. Louis, MO: Mosby.
2. Ackman, J. D., Rouse, L., & Johnston, C. E. (1988). Radiation induced physeal injury. *Orthopaedics, 11,* 343-349.
3. Alvardo, C. S., Boat, T. F., & Newman, A. J. (1978). Late-onset pulmonary fibrosis and chest deformity in two children treated with cyclophosphamide. *Journal of Pediatrics, 92,* 443-446.
4. Anderson, V., Smibert, E., Ekert, H., et al. (1994). Intellectual, educational, and behavioral sequelae after cranial irradiation and chemotherapy. *Archives of Disease in Childhood, 70,* 476-483.
5. Arceci, R., Reaman, G., Cohen, A. R., et al. (1996). Comprehensive pediatric hematology/oncology programs: Standard requirements for children and adolescents with cancer and blood disorders. *American Society of Pediatric Hematology Oncology News, 1,* 6-9.
6. Arvidson, J., Kihlgren, M., Hall, C., et al. (1999). Neuropsychological functioning after treatment for hematological malignancies in childhood, including autologous bone marrow transplantation. *Journal of Pediatric Hematology/Oncology, 16,* 9-21.
7. Asato, R., Akiyama, Y., Ito, M., et al. (1992). Nuclear magnet resonance abnormalities of the cerebral white matter in children with acute lymphoblastic leukemia and malignant lymphoma during and after central nervous system prophylactic treatment with intrathecal methotrexate. *Cancer, 70,* 1997-2004.
8. Ash, P. (1980). The influence of radiation on fertility in man. *British Journal of Radiology, 53,* 271-278.
9. Ater, J. L., Moore, B. D., Francis, D. J., et al. (1996). Correlation of medical and neurosurgical events with neuropsychological status in children at diagnosis of astrocytoma: Utilization of a neurological severity score. *Journal of Child Neurology, 11,* 462-469.
10. Bailey, C. C., Marsden, H. B., & Morris-Jones, P. H. (1978). Fatal pulmonary fibrosis 1, 3–bis(2-chloroethyl)–1–nitrosourea (BCNU) therapy. *Cancer, 42,* 74-76.
11. Beaty, O., III, Hudson, M. M., Greenwald, C., et al. (1995). Subsequent malignancies in children and adolescents after treatment for Hodgkin's disease. *Journal of Clinical Oncology, 13,* 603-609.
12. Berglund, G., Bolund, C., Fornander, T., et al. (1991). Late effects of adjuvant chemotherapy and postoperative radiotherapy on quality of life among breast cancer patients. *European Journal of Cancer, 27,* 1075-1081.
13. Bhatia, S., Robison, L. L., Oberlin, O., et al. (1996). Breast cancer and other second neoplasms after childhood Hodgkin's disease. *New England Journal of Medicine 335,* 352-353.
14. Billingham, M. E., Mason, J. W., Bristow, M. R. et al. (1978). Anthracycline cardiomyopathy monitored by morphologic changes. *Cancer Treatment Reports, 62,* 865-872.
15. Blatt, J. (1999). Pregnancy outcome in long-term survivors of childhood cancer. *Medical and Pediatric Oncology, 33,* 29-33.
16. Blatt, J., Copeland, D., & Bleyer, A. (1997). Late effects of childhood cancer and its treatment. In P. A. Pizzo and D. G. Poplack (Eds.), *Principles and practices in pediatric oncology* (3rd ed., pp. 1303-1330). Philadelphia: Lippincott Raven.
17. Boice, J. D. (1996). Cancer following irradiation in childhood and adolescence. *Medical and Pediatric Oncology,* (Suppl 1), 29-34.
18. Boivin, J. F., Hutchison, G. B., Zauber, A. G., et al. (1995). Incidence of second cancers in patients treated for Hodgkin's disease, *Journal of National Cancer Institute, 87,* 732-741.
19. Brauner, R., Czernichow, P., & Rappaport, R. (1984). Precocious puberty after hypothalamic and pituitary irradiation in young children (letter). *New England Journal of Medicine, 311,* 920.
19a. Breslow, N. E., Takashima, J. R., Whitton, J. A., et al. (1995). Second malignant neoplasms following treatment for Wilms' tumor: A report from the National Wilms' Tumor Study. *Journal of Clinical Oncology, 13,* 1851-1859.
20. Brouwers, P. (1987). Neuropsychological abilities of long term survivors of childhood leukemia. In N. K. Aaronsen & J. Beckmann (Eds.), *The quality of life of cancer patients* (pp. 153-165). New York: Raven Press.
21. Brown, R., Sawyer, M. B., Antoniou, G., et al. (1996). A 3-year follow-up of the intellectual and academic functioning of children receiving central nervous system prophylactic chemotherapy for leukemia. *Journal of Developmental and Behavioral Pediatrics, 17,* 392-398.
22. Brown, R. T., Madan-Swain, A., Walco, G. A., et al. (1998). Cognitive and academic late effects among children previously treated for acute lymphocytic leukemia receiving chemotherapy as CNS prophylaxis. *Journal of Pediatric Psychology, 23,* 333-340.
23. Brown, T. R., Sawyer, M. G., Antoniou, G., et al. (1999). Longitudinal follow-up of the intellectual and academic functioning of children receiving central nervous systems-prophylactic chemotherapy for leukemia: A four year final report. *Journal of Developmental and Behavioral Pediatrics, 20,* 373-377.
24. Bucher, J., Fleming, T., Fuller, L. M., et al. (1988). Preliminary observations on the effects of mantle radiotherapy on salivary flow rates in patients with Hodgkin's disease. *Journal of Dental Research, 6,* 518-521.
25. Butler, R. W., Hill, J. M., Steinberg, P. G., et al. (1994). Neuropsychologic effects of cranial irradiation, intrathecal methotrexate, and systemic methotrexate in childhood cancer. *Journal of Clinical Oncology, 12,* 2621-2629.
26. Byrne, J., Fears, T. R., Steinhorn, S. C., et al. (1989). Marriage and divorce after childhood and adolescent cancer, *Journal of American Medical Association, 262,* 2693-2699.

27. Byrne, J., Mulvihill, J. J., Connelly, R. R., et al. (1988). Reproductive problems and birth defects in survivors of Wilms' tumor and their relatives. *Medical and Pediatric Oncology, 16,* 233-240.

28. Byrne, J., Rasmussen, S. A., Steinhorn, S. C., et al. (1998). Genetic disease in offspring of long-term survivors of childhood and adolescent cancer. *American Journal of Human Genetics, 62,* 45-52.

29. Carroll, P. V., Emmanuel, C. R., Thorner, M., et al. (1998). Growth hormone deficiency in adulthood and the effects of growth hormone replacement: A review. *Journal of Clinical Endocrinology and Metabolism, 83,* 382-395.

30. Cesaro, S., Petris, M. G., Rosetti, F., et al. (1997). Chronic hepatitis C virus infection after treatment for pediatric malignancy. *Blood, 90,* 1315-1320.

31. Cetingul, N., Aydinok, Y., Kantar, M., et al. (1999). Neuropsychological sequelae in the long-term survivors of childhood acute lymphoblastic leukemia. *Pediatric Hematology and Oncology, 16,* 213-220.

32. Chapman, R. M., Rees, L. H., Sutcliffe, S. B., et al. (1979). Cyclical combination chemotherapy and gonadal function. *Lancet, 1,* 285-289.

33. Chapman, R. M., & Sutcliffe, S. B. (1981). Protection of ovarian function by oral contraceptives in women receiving chemotherapy for Hodgkin's Disease. *Blood, 58,* 848-851.

34. Charak, B. S., Gupta, R., Mandrekar, P., et. al. (1990) Testicular dysfunction after cyclophosphamide, vincristine, procarbazine and prednisone for advanced Hodgkins disease: A long term follow-up study. *Cancer, 65,* 1903-1906.

35. Chipman, J. J., Attanasio, A. F., Burket, M. A., et al. (1997). The safety of growth hormone replacement therapy in adults. *Journal of Clinical Endocrinology and Metabolism, 46,* 473-481.

36. Christ, G. H. (1987). Social consequences of the cancer experience. *American Journal of Pediatric Hematology/Oncology 9,* 84-88.

37. Cicognani, A., Cacciari, E., Veechi, V., et al. (1986). Differential effects of 18 and 24 Gy cranial irradiation on growth rate and growth hormone release in children with prolonged survival after acute lymphocytic leukemia. *American Journal of Disease Children, 141,* 550-552.

38. Clayton, P. E., & Shalit, S. M. (1991). Dose dependency of time of onset on radiation-induced growth hormone deficiency. *Journal of Pediatrics, 118,* 226-227.

39. Clifton, D. K., & Bremner, W. J. (1983). The effect of testicular x-irradiation on spermatogenesis in man. *Journal of Andrology, 4,* 387-392.

40. Codling, B. W., & Chakera, T. M. (1972). Pulmonary fibrosis following therapy with melphalan for multiple myeloma. *Journal of Clinical Pathology, 25,* 668-673.

41. Constine, L. (1991). Late effects of radiation therapy. *Pediatrician, 18,* 37-48.

42. Constine, L., Donaldson, S. S., & McDougal, I. R. (1984). Thyroid dysfunction after radiotherapy in children with Hodgkin's disease. *Cancer, 53,* 878-883.

43. Constine, L., Rubin, P., Woolf, P., et al. (1987). Hyperprolactinemia and hypothyroidism following cytotoxic therapy for CNS malignancies. *Journal of Clinical Oncology, 5,* 1841-1851.

44. Cook, K. L., Ader, D. D., Lichter, A. S., et al. (1990). Breast carcinoma in young women previously treated for Hodgkin's disease. *American Journal of Roentgenology, 155,* 39-42.

45. Reference deleted in proofs.

46. Copeland, D. R., Moore, B. D., Francis, D. J., et al. (1996). Neuropsychologic effects of chemotherapy on children with cancer: A longitudinal study. *Journal of Clinical Oncology, 14,* 2826-2835.

47. Copron, C. A., Black, C. T., Ross, M. I., et al. (1996). Melanoma as a second malignant neoplasm after childhood cancer. *American Journal of Surgery, 172,* 459-461.

48. Cossett, J., & Hoppe, R. T. (1999). Pulmonary late effects after treatment of Hodgkin's disease. In P. M. Mauch, M. O. Armitage, V. Diehl, et al. (Eds.), *Hodgkin's disease* (pp. 663-643). Philadelphia: Lippincott Williams & Wilkins.

49. Curran, R. E., & Johnson, R. B. (1970). Tolerance to chemotherapy after prior irradiation for Hodgkin's disease. *Annals of Internal Medicine, 72,* 505-509.

50. Dahl, M. G. C., Gregory, M. M., & Schever, P. J. (1971). Liver damage due to methotrexate in patients with psoriasis. *British Journal of Medicine, 1,* 625-630.

51. Dailey, M. O., Coleman, C. N., & Kaplan, H. S. (1980). Radiation induced splenic atrophy in patients with Hodgkin's disease and non-Hodgkin's lymphomas. *New England Journal of Medicine, 302,* 215-217.

52. Dahlof, G., Barr, M., Bolme, P., et al. (1988). Disturbances in dental development after total body irradiation in bone marrow transplant recipients. *Oral Surgery, Oral Medicine, and Oral Pathology, 65,* 41-44.

53. Dallas, J., & Foley, T. (1996). Hypothyroidism. In F. Lifshitz (Ed.), *Pediatric Endocrinology* (3rd ed., pp. 391-399). New York: Marcel Dekker.

54. D'Angio, G. J. (1975). Pediatric cancer in perspective: Cure is not enough. *Cancer* (Suppl.), *35,* 870-873.

55. Deasy-Spinetta, P. (1993). School issues and the child with cancer, *Cancer, 71,* 3261-3264.

56. deCuhna, M. F., Meistrich, M. L., Fuller, L. M., et al. (1984). Recovery of spermatogenesis after treatment for Hodgkin's disease with limiting dose of MOPP chemotherapy. *Journal of Clinical Oncology, 2,* 571-577.

57. Devney, R. B., Sklar, C. A., Nesbit, M. E., Jr., et al. (1984). Serial thyroid function measurements in children with Hodgkin's disease. *Journal of Pediatrics, 105,* 223-227.

58. Donaldson, S. S., & Kaplan, H. S. (1982). Complications of treatment of Hodgkin's disease in children. *Cancer Treatment Reports, 62,* 977-989.

59. Donaldson, S. S., & Lamborn, K. R. (1998). Radiation in pediatric Hodgkin's disease, *Journal of Clinical Oncology, 16,* 391-393.

60. Dowell, R. E., Jr., Copeland, D. R., Francis, D. J., et al. (1991). Absence of synergist effects of CNS treatments on neuropsychological test performance among children. *Journal of Clinical Oncology, 9,* 1029-1036.

61. Draper, G. J., Sanders, B. M., Kingston, J. E. (1986). Second primary neoplasms in patients with retinoblastoma. *British Journal of Cancer, 53,* 661-672.

62. Duffner, P. K., Cohen, M. E., & Parker, M. S. (1998). Prospective intellectual testing in children with brain tumors. *Annals of Neurology, 23,* 575-579.

63. Emmons, K. M., & Colditz, G. A. (1999). Preventing excess sun exposure: It is time for a national policy (editorial). *Journal of National Cancer Institute, 91,* 1269-1270.

64. Eng, C., Li, F. P., Abramson, D. H., et al. (1993). Mortality from second tumors among long-term survivors of retinoblastoma, *Journal of National Cancer Institute, 85,* 1121-1128.

65. Espy, K. A., Moore, I. M., Kaufmann, P. M., et al. (2001). Chemotherapeutic CNS prophylaxis and neuropsychologic change in children with acute lymphoblastic leukemia: A prospective study. *Journal of Pediatric Psychology, 26,* 1-9.

66. Farwell, J., & Flannery J. T. (1984). Cancer in relatives of children with central nervous system neoplasms. *New England Journal of Medicine, 311,* 749-753.

67. Fochtman, D., Fergusson, J., Ford, N., et al. (1982). The treatment of cancer in children. In D. Fochtman & G. Foley (Eds.), *Nursing care of the child with cancer* (pp. 177-232). Boston: Little, Brown.

68. Freilich, R. J., Kraus, D. H., Budnick, A. S., et al. (1996). Hearing loss in children with brain tumors treated with cisplatin and carboplatin-based high-dose chemotherapy with autologous bone marrow rescue. *Medical and Pediatric Oncology, 26,* 95-100.

69. Friedman, D., Thompson, S., Yassi, Y., et al. (2000). Genetic risk factors for second malignancy. Program/ Proceedings of the 6th International Conference on Long-Term Complications of Treatment of Children and Adolescents for Cancer. June 23-24, 2000. Queen's Landing, Niagra-on-the-Lake, Ontario, Canada. p. 19.

70. Friedman, D. L., & Meadows, A. T. (1999). Pediatric tumors. In A. I. Neugut, A. T. Meadows, & E. Robinson (Eds.), *Multiple primary cancers* (pp. 235-256). Philadelphia: Lippincott Williams & Wilkins.

71. Friedman, J. M. (1998). One fewer worry for survivors of childhood cancer (invited editorial). *American Journal of Human Genetics, 62,* 25-26.

72. Fritz, G. K., Williams, J. R., & Amylon, M. (1988). After treatment ends: Psychological sequelae in pediatric cancer survivors. *American Journal of Orthopsychiatry, 58,* 552-561.

73. Fromm, M., Littman, P., Raney, R. B., et al. (1986). Late effects after treatment of 20 children with soft tissue sarcoma of the head and neck experienced at a single institution with a review of the literature. *Cancer, 57,* 2070-2076.

74. Gabriel, D., Bernard, S., Lambert, J., et al. (1986). Oophoropexy and the management of Hodgkin's disease: A re-evaluation of risks and benefits. *Archives of Surgery, 121,* 1083-1085.

75. Garber, J. E., Lynch, E. A., Meadows, A. T., et al. (1990). Pregnancy outcome after therapy of childhood cancer (abstract). *Proceedings of the American Society of Clinical Oncology, 9,* 290.

76. Garnick, M. B., & Mayer, R. J. (1978). Renal failure associated with neoplastic disease and its treatment. *Seminars in Oncology Nursing, 5,* 155-165.

77. Giralt, J., Ortega, J. J., Olive, T., et al. (1992). Long-term neuropsychologic sequelae of childhood leukemia: Comparison of two CNS prophylactic regimens. *International Journal of Radiation Oncology, Biology, Physics, 24,* 49-53.

78. Goldiner, P., & Schweizer, O. (1979). The hazards of anesthesia and surgery with bleomycin treated patients. *Seminars in Oncology, 6,* 121-124.

79. Goldman, L., Cook, E. F., Mitchell, N., et al. (1982). Pitfalls in the serial assessment of cardiac functional status. How a reduction in "ordinary" activity may reduce the apparent degree of cardiac compromise and give a misleading impression of improvement. *Journal of Chronic Disease, 35,* 763-771.

80. Gottdiener, J. S., Katin, M. J., Borer, J. S., et al. (1983). Late cardiac effects of therapeutic mediastinal irradiation assessment by echocardiography and radionuclide angiography. *New England Journal of Medicine, 308,* 569-572.

81. Gray, R. E., Doan, B. D., Shermer, P., et al. (1992). Psychologic adaptation of survivors of childhood cancer. *Cancer, 70,* 2713-2721.

82. Green, D., Hyland, A., Chung, C. S., et al. (1999). Cancer and cardiac mortality among 15-year survivors of cancer diagnosed during childhood or adolescence. *Journal of Clinical Oncology, 10,* 3207-3215.

83. Green, D. M., Fiorello, A., Zevon, M. A., et al. (1997). Birth defects and childhood cancer in offspring of survivors of childhood cancer. *Archives of Pediatric and Adolescent Medicine, 151,* 379-383.

84. Green, D. M., Zevon, M. A., & Hall, B. (1991). Achievement of life goals by adult survivors of modern treatment for childhood cancer. *Cancer, 67,* 206-213.

85. Green, D. M., Zevon, M. A., Lowrie, G., et al. (1991). Congenital anomalies in children of patients who received chemotherapy for cancer in childhood and adolescence. *New England Journal of Medicine, 325,* 141-146.

86. Greenberg, H. S., Kazak, A. E., & Meadows, A. T. (1989). Psychologic functioning in 8- to 16-year old cancer survivors and their parents. *Journal of Pediatrics, 114,* 488-493.

87. Grossi, M. (1998). Management and long-term complications of pediatric cancer. *Pediatric Clinics of North America, 45,* 1637-1653.

88. Halberg, F. E., Kramer, J. H., Moore, I. M., et al. (1991). Prophylactic cranial irradiation dose effects on late cognitive function in children treated for acute lymphoblastic leukemia. *International Journal of Radiation Oncology, Biology, Physics, 22,* 13-16.

89. Halperin, E., & Constine, L. S. (1989). Second tumors and late effects of cancer treatment. In E. C. Halperin, L. E. Kuhn, L. S. Constine, et al. (Eds.), *Pediatric radiation oncology* (pp. 344-389). New York: Raven.

90. Hamre, M. R., Robison, L. L., Nesbit, M. E., et al. (1987). Effects of radiation on ovarian function in longterm survivors of childhood acute lymphoblastic leukemia: A report from the Children's Cancer Study Group. *Journal of Clinical Oncology, 5,* 1759-1765.

91. Hancock, S. (1999). Cardiovascular late effects after treatment of Hodgkin's disease. In P. M. Mauch, M. O. Armitage, V. Diehl, et al. (Eds.), *Hodgkin's disease* (pp. 647-657). Philadelphia: Lippincott Williams & Wilkins.

92. Hancock, S. L., Tucker, M. A., & Hoppe, R. T. (1993). Breast cancer after treatment of Hodgkin's disease. *Journal of National Cancer Institute, 85,* 25-31.

93. Harila-Saari, A. H., Ahonen, A. K. A., Vainionpää, L. K., et al. (1997). Brain perfusion after treatment of childhood acute lymphoblastic leukemia. *Journal of Nuclear Medicine and Allied Sciences, 38,* 82-88.

94. Harpham, W. (1998). Long-term survivorship: Late effects. In A. Berger, R. K. Portenoy, & D. E. Weissman (Eds.), *Principles and practice of supportive oncology* (pp. 889-907). Philadelphia: Lippincott-Raven.

95. Harvey, J., Hobbie, W., Shaw, S., et al. (1999). Providing quality care in childhood cancer survivorship: Learning from the past, looking to the future. *Journal of Pediatric Oncology Nursing, 3,* 117-125.

96. Haupt, R., Fears, T. R., Robison, L. L., et al. (1994). Educational attainment in long-term survivors of childhood acute lymphoblastic leukemia. *Journal of American Medical Association, 272,* 1427-1432.

97. Hawkins, M. M., Wilson, L. M., Stovall, M. A., et al. (1992). Epipodophyllotoxins, alkylating agents and radiation and risk of secondary leukemia after childhood cancer. *British Medical Journal, 304,* 951-958.

98. Hawkins, M. M., & Smith, R. A. (1989). Pregnancy outcomes in childhood cancer survivors: Probable effects of abdominal irradiation. *International Journal of Cancer, 43,* 399-402.

99. Hays, D., Landsverk, J., Sallan, S. E., et al. (1992). Educational, occupational and insurance status of childhood cancer survivors in their fourth and fifth decades of life. *Journal of Clinical Oncology, 10,* 1397-1406.

100. Hays, D. M. (1993). Adult survivors of childhood cancer: Employment and insurance issues in different age groups. *Cancer, 71,* 3306-3309.

101. Hensley, M. L., Schuchter, L. M., Lindley, C., et al. (1999). American Society of Clinical Oncology clinical practice guidelines for the use of chemotherapy and radiotherapy protectants. *Journal of Clinical Oncology, 17,* 3333-3355.

102. Hertzberg, H., Huk, W. J., Ueberall, M. A., et al. (1997). CNS late effects after ALL therapy in childhood. Part I: Neuroradiological findings in long-term survivors of childhood ALL—An evaluation of the interferences between morphology and neuropsychological performance. *Medical and Pediatric Oncology, 28,* 387-400.

103. Heyn, R., Haeberlen, V., Newton, W. A., et al. (1993). Second malignant neoplasms in children treated for rhabdomyosarcoma: Intergroup Rhabdomyosarcoma Study Committee, *Journal of Clinical Oncology, 11,* 262-270.

104. Heyn, R., Raney, R. B., Hayes, D. M., et al. (1992). Late effects of therapy in patients with paratesticular rhabdomyosarcoma. *Journal of Clinical Oncology, 10,* 614-623.

105. Hill, D. E., Ciesielski, T., Sethre-Hofstad, L., et al. (1997). Visual and verbal short-term memory deficits in childhood leukemia survivors after intrathecal chemotherapy. *Journal of Pediatric Psychology, 22,* 861-870.

106. Hobbie, W., Stuber, M., Meeske, K., et al. (2000). Symptoms of posttraumatic stress in young adult survivors of childhood cancer. *Journal of Clinical Oncology, 18,* 4060-4066.

107. Hobbie, W. L., & Schwartz, C. (1989). Endocrine late effects among survivors of cancer. *Seminars in Oncology Nursing, 5,* 14-21.

108. Holmes, B. E., Baker, A., Hassanein, R. S., et al. (1986). The availability of insurance to long-term survivors of childhood cancer. *Cancer, 57,* 190-93.

109. Holmes, G. E., & Holmes, F. F. (1978). Pregnancy outcome of patients treated for Hodgkin's disease. A controlled study, *Cancer, 41,* 1317-1322.

110. Hoppe-Hirsch, E., Renier, D., & Lellouch-Tubiana, A. (1990). Medulloblastoma in childhood: Progressive intellectual deterioration. *Childs Nervous System, 6,* 60-65.

111. Horning, S. J., Adhikari, A., & Rizk, N. (1994). Effect of treatment for Hodgkin's disease on pulmonary function: Results of a prospective study. *Journal of Clinical Oncology, 12,* 297-305.

112. Hudson, M. M., Jones, D., Boyett, J., et al. (1997). Late mortality of long-term survivors of childhood cancer. *Journal of Clinical Oncology, 15,* 2205-2213.

113. Jacob, S., Fanconi, C., & Lossow, W. (Eds.). (1982). *Structure and function in man.* Philadelphia: W. B. Saunders.

114. Jaffe, N., Toth, B. B., Hoar, R. E., et al. (1984). Dental and maxillofacial abnormalities in long-term survivors of childhood cancer: Effects of treatment with chemotherapy and radiation to the head and neck. *Pediatrics, 73,* 816-823.

115. Jankovic, M., Masera, G., Cristiani, M. L., et al. (1991). Brain tumors as second malignancies in children treated for acute lymphoblastic leukemia (ALL). *Haematologica, 76*(Suppl.), 24.

116. Kaleita, T. A., Reaman, G. H., MacLean, W. E., et al. (1999). Neurodevelopmental outcome of infants with acute lymphoblastic leukemia. *Cancer, 85,* 1859-1865.

117. Kantor, A., Li, F. P., Janov, A. J., et al. (1989). Hypertension in long-term survivors of childhood renal cancers. *Journal of Clinical Oncology, 7,* 912-915.

118. Kaste, S. C., Hudson, M. M., Jones, D. J., et al. (1998). Breast masses in women treated for childhood cancer. *Cancer, 82,* 784-792.

119. Kato, M., Azuma, E., Ido, M., et al. (1993). Ten-year survey of the intellectual deficits in children with acute lymphoblastic leukemia receiving chemoimmuno therapy. *Medical and Pediatric Oncology, 21,* 435-440.

120. Kazak, A., & Clark, M. W. (1986). Stress in families of children with myelomeningocele. *Developmental Medicine and Child Neurology, 28,* 220-228.

121. Keene, N., Hobbie, W., & Ruccione, K. (2000). *Childhood cancer survivors: A practical guide to your future.* Sebastopol, CA: O'Reilly.

122. Kelaghan, J., Myers, M. H., Mulvihill, J. J., et al. (1988). Educational achievement of long-term survivors of childhood and adolescent cancer. *Medical and Pediatric Oncology, 16,* 320-326.

123. Kennedy, L., Laufer, M., Grant, F., et al. (2000). High risk of infertility in males treated with cyclophosphamide for soft tissue sarcomas during childhood. (Abstract) Program/Proceedings of the 6th International Conference of Long Term Complications of Treatment of Children & Adolescents for Cancer. June 23-24, 2000, Niagra-on-the-Lake, Ontario, Canada.

124. Kingston, J. E., Hawkins, M. M., Draper, G. J., et al. (1987). Patterns of multiple primary tumors in patients treated for cancer during childhood. *British Journal of Cancer, 56,* 331-338.

125. Knudson, A. G., Jr. (1971). Mutation and cancer: Statistical study of retinoblastoma. *Proceedings of the National Academy of Sciences of the United States of America USA. 68,* 820-823.

126. Kokkonen, J., & Vainiopaa, L. (1996). Physical and psychological outcome for young adults with treated malignancy, *Journal of Pediatric Hematology Oncology, 14,* 223-232.

127. Kolb, H. J., & Bender-Gotze, C. (1990). Late complication after allogeneic bone marrow transplant for leukemia. *Bone Marrow Transplant, 6,* 61-72.

128. Koocher, G. P., & O'Malley, J. E. (1981). *The Damocles syndrome: Psychosocial consequences of surviving childhood cancer.* New York: McGraw-Hill.

129. Koyama, H., Wada, T., Nishizawa, Y., et al. (1977). Cyclophosphamide induced ovarian failure: Therapeutic significance in patients with breast cancer. *Cancer, 39,* 1403-1407.

130. Kramer, J. H., Crittenden, M. R., Halberg, F. E., et al. (1992). A prospective study of cognitive functioning following low-dose cranial irradiation for bone marrow transplantation. *Pediatrics, 90,* 447-450.

131. Kuijten, R., Strom, S. S., Rorke, L., et al. (1993). Family history of cancer and seizures in young children with brain tumors: A report from the Children's Cancer Group (United States and Canada). *Cancer Causes and Control, 4,* 455-464.

132. Landier, W. (1998). Hearing loss related to ototoxicity in children with cancer. *Journal of Pediatric Oncology Nursing, 15,* 195-206.

133. Lansky, S. B., List, M. A., & Ritter-Sterr, C. (1986). Psychosocial consequences of cure, *Cancer, 58,* 529-533.

134. Lawrence, W., Hays, D. M., & Moon, T. E. (1977). Lymphatic metastasis in childhood rhabdomyosarcoma. *Cancer, 39,* 556-559.

135. Levy, R., & Kaplan, H. S. (1974). Impaired lymphocyte function in untreated Hodgkin's disease. *New England Journal of Medicine, 290,* 181-186.

136. Li, F. P., Gimbrere, K., Gelber, R. D., et al. (1987). Outcome of pregnancy in survivors of Wilms' tumor. *Journal of the American Medical Association, 257,* 216-219.

137. Libshitz, H. I. & Southard, M. E. (1974). Complications of radiation therapy. *Seminars in Roentgenology, 9,* 41-49.

138. Liesner, R. J., Leiper, A. D., Hann, I. M., et al. (1994). Late effects of intensive treatment for acute myeloid leukemia and myelodysplasia in childhood. *Journal of Clinical Oncology, 12,* 916-924.

139. Lifshitz, F., & Cervantes, C. (1996). Short stature. In F. Lifshitz (Ed.), *Pediatric endocrinology* (3rd ed., pp. 1-18). New York: Marcel Dekker Inc.

140. Linuks, P. S., & Stockwell, M. L. (1985). Obstacles in the prevention of psychological sequelae in survivors of childhood cancer. *Journal of Pediatric Hematology/Oncology, 7,* 132-140.

141. Lipshultz, S. (1996). Dexrazoxane for protection against cardiotoxic effects of anthracyclines in children. *Journal of Clinical Oncology, 14,* 328-330.

142. Localio, S. A., Stone, A., & Friedman, M. (1969). Surgical aspects of radiation enteritis. *Surgical Gynecology and Obstetrics, 129,* 1163-1172.

143. Locasciulli, A., Testa, M., Pontisso, P., et al. (1997). Prevalence and natural history of hepatitis C infection in patients cured of childhood leukemia. *Blood, 90,* 4628-4633.

144. Lushbaugh, C. C., & Casarett, G. W. (1976). The effects of gonadal irradiation in clinical radiation therapy: A review. *Cancer, 37,* 1111-1125.

145. MacLean, W. E., Noll, R. B., Stehbens, J. A., et al. (1995). Neuropsychological effects of cranial irradiation in young children with acute lymphoblastic leukemia 9 months after diagnosis. *Archives of Neurology, 52,* 156-160.

146. Malone, M., Lumley, H., & Erdohazi, M. (1986). Astrocytoma as a second malignancy in patients with acute lymphoblastic leukemia. *Cancer, 57,* 1979-1985.

147. Marradi, P., Schaison, G., Alby, N., et al. (1982). Les enfants new de parents leucemiques. A propos de 23 enfants. *Nouvelle Revue Francaise d Hematologic, 24,* 75-80.

148. Marshall, W. A., & Tanner, J. M. (1969). Variations in patterns of pubertal changes in girls. *Archives of Disease in Childhood, 44,* 291-303.

149. Marshall, W. A., & Tanner, J. M. (1970). Variations in patterns of pubertal changes in boys. *Archives of Disease in Childhood, 45,* 13-23.

150. Masera, G., Chesler, M., Jankovic, M., et al. (1996). SIOP Working Committee on Psychosocial Issues in Pediatric Oncology: Guidelines for care of long-term survivors. *Medical and Pediatric Oncology, 27,* 1-2.

151. Matuse-Ridley, M., Nicosia, S., & Meadows, A. T. (1985). Gonadal effects of cancer therapy in boys. *Cancer, 55,* 2353-2363.

152. McIntosh, S., Davidson, D. L., O'Brien, R. T., et al. (1977). Methotrexate hepatotoxicity in children with leukemia. *Journal of Pediatrics, 90,* 1019-1021.

153. McKeen, E. A., Mulvihill, J. J., Rosner, F., et al. (1979). Pregnancy outcome in Hodgkin's disease. *Lancet, 2,* 590.

154. Meadows, A. T., Baum, E., Fossati-Bellani, F., et al. (1985). Second malignant neoplasms in children: An update from the Late Effects Study Group, *Journal of Clinical Oncology, 3,* 532-538.

155. Meadows, A. T., Massari, D. J., Fergusson, J., et al. (1981). Declines in I.Q. scores and cognitive dysfunction in children with acute lymphocytic leukaemia treated with cranial irradiation. *Lancet, 2,* 1015-1018.

156. Meadows, A. T., McKee, K., & Kazak, A. E. (1989). Psychosocial status of young adult survivors of childhood cancer: A survey, *Medical and Pediatric Oncology, 17,* 466-470.

157. Meadows, A. T., & Silber, J. (1985). Delayed consequences of therapy for childhood cancer. *CA:A Cancer Journal for Clinicians, 35,* 271-286.

158. Meeske, K. A., Stuber, M. L., & Ruccione, K. S. (2001). Posttraumatic stress, quality of life, and psychological distress in young adult survivors of childhood cancer. *Oncology Nursing Forum, 28,* 481-489.

159. Mefferd, J., Donaldson, S., & Link, M. (1989). Pediatric Hodgkin's disease: Pulmonary, cardiac and thyroid function following combined modality therapy. *International Journal of Radiation Oncology, Biology, Physics, 16,* 679-685.

160. Miller, R. W., Fusner, J. E., Fink, R. J., et al. (1986). Pulmonary function abnormalities in long-term survivors of childhood cancer. *Medical and Pediatric Oncology, 14,* 202-207.

161. Miser, J. (1997). Treatment-related leukemia following rhabdomyosarcoma. Presented at the annual meeting of the *American Society of Clinical Oncology,* Los Angeles, May 1997.

162. Monaco, G. (1992). The partnership of empowerment: Caregivers and survivors. *Journal of Psychosocial Oncology, 10,* 121-133.

163. Moore, I. M., Espy, K. A., Kaufmann, P., et al. (2000). A research program investigating cognitive consequences of treatment for childhood ALL: Cell membrane damage and intellectual and academic abilities in children receiving central nervous system treatment. *Seminars in Oncology Nursing, 16,* 279-290.

164. Moshang, T., Rundle, A. M., Graves, D. A., et al. (1996). Brain tumor recurrence in children treated with growth hormone. The National Cooperative Growth Study experience. *Journal of Pediatrics, 128,* 4-7.

165. Mostow, E. N., Byrne, J., Connelly, R. R., et al. (1991). Quality of life in long-term survivors of CNS tumors of childhood and adolescence. *Journal of Clinical Oncology, 9,* 592-599.

166. Mulhern, R. K., Wasserman, A. B., Friedman, A. G., et al. (1989). Social competence and behavioral adjustment of children who are long-term survivors of cancer. *Pediatrics, 83,* 18-25.

167. Mullen, F. (1984). The educational needs of the cancer survivor. *Health Education Quarterly, 10* (Suppl), 88-94.

168. Mulvihill, J. J., Myers, M. H., Connelly, R. R., et al. (1987). Cancer in offspring of long-term survivors of childhood and adolescent cancer. *Lancet, 2,* 813-817.

169. Neglia, J. P. (1994). Childhood cancer survivors: Past, present, and future (editorial). *Cancer, 73,* 2883-2885.

169a. Neglia, J. P., Friedman, D. L., Yasui, Y., et al. (2001). Second malignant neoplasms in five-year survivors of childhood cancer: Childhood Cancer Survivor Study. *Journal of the National Cancer Institute, 93,* 618-629.

170. Neglia, J. P., Meadows, A. T., & Robison, L. L. (1991). Second neoplasms after acute lymphoblastic leukemia. *New England Journal of Medicine, 325,* 1330-1336.

171. Newton, W. A. J., Meadows, A. T., Shimada, H., et al. (1991). Bone sarcomas as a second malignant neoplasm following childhood cancer. *Cancer, 67,* 193-201.

172. Nicholson, H. S., & Byrne, J. (1993). Fertility and pregnancy after treatment for cancer during childhood and adolescence. *Cancer, 71*(Suppl.), 3392-3399.

173. Nicholson, H. S., Mulvihill, J. J., & Byrne, J. (1992). Late effects of therapy in adult survivors of osteosarcoma and Ewing's sarcoma. *Medical and Pediatric Oncology, 18,* 304-310.

174. Novakovic, B., Fears, T. R., Horowitz, M. E., et al. (1997). Late effects of therapy in survivors of Ewing's sarcoma family tumors. *Journal of Pediatric Hematology/Oncology, 19,* 220-225.

175. Nysom, K., Holm, K., Lipshultz, S. R., et al. (1998). Relationship between cumulative anthracycline dose and late cardiotoxicity in childhood acute lymphoblastic leukemia. *Journal of Clinical Oncology, 16,* 545-550.

176. Odell, W. D. (1989). Puberty. In L. J. DeGroot (Ed.), *Endocrinology* (2nd ed., p. 1860), Philadelphia: W. B. Saunders.

177. Oeffinger, K. C., Eshelman, D. A., Tomlinson, G. E., et al. (1998). Programs for adult survivors of childhood cancer. *Journal of Clinical Oncology, 16,* 2864-2867.

178. Oliner, H., Fords, R., Rubio, F., et al. (1961). Interstitial pulmonary fibrosis following busulfan therapy. *American Journal of Medicine, 31,* 134.

179. O'Malley, J. E., Koocher, G., Foster, D., et al. (1979). Psychiatric sequelae of surviving childhood cancer. *American Journal of Orthopsychiatry, 49,* 608-616.

180. Orton, T. T. S., Shostak, C. A., & Donaldson, S. S. (1990). Gonadal status and reproductive function following treatment for Hodgkin's disease in childhood: The Stanford experience. *International Journal of Radiation Oncology, Biology, Physics, 19,* 873-880.

181. Ostroff, J., & Steinglass, P. (1995). Psychosocial adaptation following treatment: A family systems perspective on childhood cancer survivorship. In I. Baider, C. I. Copper, A. Kaplan DeNour (Eds.), *Cancer and the family* (pp. 129-148). New York: John Wiley & Sons.

182. Paakkoe, E., Vainionpää, L., Phytinen, J., et al. (1996). Minor changes on cranial MRI during treatment in children with acute lymphoblastic leukaemia. *Neuroradiology, 38,* 264-268.

183. Parsons, S. K., Neault, M. W., Lehmann, L. E., et al. (1998). Severe ototoxicity following carboplatin-containing conditioning regimen for autologous marrow transplantation for neuroblastoma. *Bone Marrow Transplantation, 22,* 669-674.

184. Powell, D. W., Abramson, B. Z., Balint, J. A., et al. (1997). Management of hepatitis C. *National Institute of Health Consensus Development Statement, 15,* 3.

185. Prassopoulos, P., Cavouras, D., Golfinopoulos, S., et al. (1996). Quantitative assessment of cerebral atrophy during and after treatment in children with acute lymphoblastic leukemia. *Investigative Radiology, 31,* 749-754.

186. Pui, C-H., Raimondi, S. C., & Crist, W. M. (1992). Secondary leukemias after epipodophyllotoxins. *Lancet, 340,* 672-673.

187. Pui, C-H., Ribeiro, R. C., Hancock, M. L. et al. (1991). Acute myeloid leukemia in children treated with epipodophyllotoxins for acute lymphoblastic leukemia. *New England Journal of Medicine, 325,* 1682-1687.

188. Quinn, C. T., Griener, J. C., Bottiglieri, T., et al. (1997). Evaluation of homocysteine and excitatory amino acid neurotransmitters in the CSF of children who receive methotrexate for the treatment of cancer. *Journal of Clinical Oncology, 15,* 2800-2806.

189. Radcliffe, J., Packer, R. J., Atkins, T. E., et. al. (1992). Three and four year cognitive outcomes in children with non cortical brain tumors treated with whole brain radiotherapy. *Annals of Neurology, 32,* 551-554.

190. Ramsay, N., Kim, T., Coccia, P., et al. (1978). Thyroid dysfunction in pediatric patients after mantle field radiation therapy for Hodgkin's disease. *Proceedings of the American Society of Clinical Oncology, 19,* 331.

191. Raney, B., Heyn, R., Cassady, R., & Marks, L. (1994). Late effects of cancer therapy on the genitourinary tract in children. In C. Schwartz, W. Hobbie, L. Constine, & K. Ruccione (Eds.), *Survivors of childhood cancer: Assessment and management* (pp. 245-262). Philadelphia: Mosby.

192. Rauck, A. M., Green, D. M., Yasui, Y., et al. (1999). Marriage in the survivors of childhood cancer: A preliminary description from the Childhood Cancer Survivor Study. *Medical and Pediatric Oncology, 33,* 60-63.

193. Deleted in proofs.

194. Richardson, R. C., Nelson, M. B., Meeske, K. (1999). Young adult survivors of childhood cancer: Attending to emerging medical and psychosocial needs. *Journal of Pediatric Oncology Nursing, 16,* 136-144.

195. Rimm, I. J., Li, F. C., Tarbell, N. J., et al. (1987). Brain tumors after cranial irradiation for childhood acute lymphoblastic leukemia: A 13-year experience from the Dana-Farber Cancer Institute and the Children's Hospital. *Cancer, 59,* 1506-1508.

196. Riseborough, E. J., Grabias, S. L., Burton, R. I. & Jaffe, N. (1976). Skeletal alterations following irradiation for Wilms' tumor. *Journal of Bone and Joint Surgery. American Volume, 58,* 526-536.

197. Robison, L. L. (1993). Survivors of childhood cancer and risk of a second tumor. *Journal National Cancer Institute, 85,* 1102-1103.

198. Robison, L. L. (1996). Methodologic issues in the study of second malignant neoplasms and pregnancy outcomes. *Medical and Pediatric Oncology, Supplement 1,* 41-44.

199. Roswit, B. (1974). Complications of radiation therapy: The alimentary tract. *Seminars in Roentgenology, 9,* 51-63.

200. Rourke, M., Stuber, M., Hobbie, W., et al. (1999). Posttraumatic stress disorder: Understanding the psychosocial impact of surviving childhood cancer into young adulthood. *Journal of Pediatric Oncology Nursing, 3,* 126-135.

201. Rowley, M. M., Leach, D. R., Warner, G. A., et al. (1974). Effects of graded doses of ionizing radiation on the human testes. *Radiation Research, 59,* 665-678.

202. Rubin, C. M., Arthur, D. C., Woods, W. G., et al. (1991). Therapy-related myelodysplastic syndrome and acute myeloid leukemia in children: Correlation between chromosomal abnormalities and prior therapy. *Blood, 78,* 2982-2988.

203. Sanders, J., Glader, B., Cairo, M., et al. (1997). Guidelines for the pediatric cancer center and role of such centers in diagnosis and treatment. American Academy of Pediatrics Section Statement. Section on Hematology/Oncology. *Pediatrics, 99,* 139-141.

204. Sankila, R., Garwicz, S., Olsen, J. H., et al. (1996). Risk of subsequent malignant neoplasms among 1,641 Hodgkin's disease patients diagnosed in childhood and adolescence: A population-based cohort study in the five Nordic countries. Association of the Nordic Cancer Registries and the Nordic Society of Pediatric Hematology and Oncology. *Journal of Clinical Oncology, 14,* 1442-1446.

205. Sankila, R., Olsen, J. H., Anderson, H., et al. (1998). Risk of cancer among offspring of childhood cancer survivors. *New England Journal of Medicine, 338,* 1339-1344.

206. Santoro, A., Bonadonna, G., Valagussa, P., et al. (1987). Long-term results of combined chemotherapy-radiotherapy approach in Hodgkin's disease: Superiority of ABVD plus radiotherapy versus MOPP plus radiotherapy. *Journal of Clinical Oncology, 5,* 27-37.

207. Saunders, J. (1994). Late effects after bone marrow transplant. In C. Schwartz, W. Hobbie, L. S. Constine, et al. (Eds.), *Survivors of childhood cancer: Assessment and management* (pp. 293-318). Philadelphia: Mosby.

208. Schwartz, C., Ruble, K., Rowe, P. (2000). Orthostatic intolerance in survivors of childhood cancer (abstract). Program/Proceedings of the 6th International Conference on Long Term Complications of Treatment of Children and Adolescents for Cancer. June 23-24, 2000. Queen's Landing, Niagra-on-the-Lake, Ontario, Canada.

209. Seidel, H., Nygaard, R., Haave, I., et al. (1996). Magnetic resonance imaging and neurological evaluation after treatment with high-dose methotrexate for acute lymphocytic leukaemia in young children. *Acta Paediatrica, 85,* 450-453.

210. Shalet, S. M., Beardwell, C. G., Jacobs, H. S., et al. (1978). Testicular function following irradiation of the human pre-pubertal testes. *Journal of Clinical Endocrinology & Metabolism, 9,* 483-490.

211. Shalet, S. M., & Brennan, B. D. (1998). Growth and growth hormone treatment for children with leukemia. *Hormone Research, 50,* 1-110.

212. Shalet, S. M., Vaughan Williams, C. A., Whitehead, E., et al. (1985). Pregnancy after chemotherapy induced ovarian failure. *British Medical Journal Clinical Research Ed., 290,* 898.

213. Sherins, R. J., & DeVita, V. T. (1973). Effects of drug treatment for lymphoma on male reproduction capacity. *Annals of Internal Medicine, 79,* 216-220.

214. Sherins, R. J., Olweny, C. L. M., & Ziegler, J. L. (1978). Gynecomastia and gonadal dysfunction in adolescent boys treated with combination chemotherapy for Hodgkin's disease, *New England Journal of Medicine, 299,* 12-16.

215. Siris, E. S., Leventhal, B. G., & Vaitukaitis, J. L. (1976). Effects of childhood leukemia and chemotherapy on puberty and reproductive function in girls. *New England Journal of Medicine, 294,* 1143-1146.

216. Skinner, R., Pearson, A. D., Price, L. et al. (1990). Nephrotoxicity after ifosfamide. *Archives of Disease in Childhood, 65,* 732-738.

217. Sklar, C. (1995). Growth following therapy for childhood cancer. *Cancer Investigation, 13,* 511-516.

218. Sklar, C., Kim, F., & Ramsey, N. (1982). Thyroid dysfunction among long term survivors of bone marrow transplantation. *American Journal of Medicine, 6,* 688-694.

219. Sklar, C. A., Robison, L. L., Nesbit, M. E., et al. (1990). Effects of radiation on testicular function in long-term survivors of childhood acute lymphoblastic leukemia: A report from the Children's Cancer Study Group. *Journal of Clinical Oncology, 8,* 1981-1987.

220. Smibert, E., Anderson, V., Godber, T., et al. (1996). Risk factors for intellectual and educational sequelae of cranial irradiation in childhood acute lymphoblastic leukemia. *British Journal of Cancer, 73,* 825-830.

221. Smith, K., Ostroff, J., Tan, C., et al. (1991). Alterations in self-perceptions among adolescent cancer survivors. *Cancer Investigation, 9,* 581-588.

222. Sonis, A. L., Tarbell, N., Valachovic, R. W., et al. (1990). Dentofacial development in long-term survivors of ALL. *Cancer, 66,* 2645-2652.

223. Starceski, P. J., Lee, P. A., Blatt, J., et al. (1987). Comparable effects of 1800 and 2400 rad (18- and 24-Gy) cranial irradiation on height and weight in children treated for acute lymphocytic leukemia. *American Journal of Diseases in Children, 141,* 550-552.

224. Stillman, R. J., Schinfeld, J. S., Schiff, I., et al. (1981). Ovarian failure in long-term survivors of childhood malignancy. *American Journal of Obstetrics and Gynecology, 139,* 62-66.

225. Strong, L. C., Herson, J., Osborne, B. M., et al. (1979). Risk of radiation-related subsequent malignant tumors in survivors of Ewing's sarcoma. *Journal of National Cancer Institute, 62,* 1401-1406.

226. Strong, L. C., Williams, W. R., & Tainsky, M. A. (1992). The Li-Fraumeni syndrome: From clinical epidemiology to molecular genetics. *American Journal of Epidemiology, 135,* 190-199.

227. Tarbell, N. J., Guinan, E. C., Niemeyer, C., et al. (1988). Late onset of renal dysfunction in survivors of bone marrow transplantation. *International Journal of Radiation Oncology, Biology, Physics, 15,* 99-104.

228. Tefft, M., Lattin, P. B., Jerab, B., et al. (1976). Acute and late effects on normal tissue following combined chemotherapy and radiotherapy of childhood rhabdomyosarcoma and Ewing's sarcoma. *Cancer, 37,* 1202-1213.

229. Thomas, P. R. M., Griffith, K. D., Fineberg, B. B., et al. (1983). Late effects of treatment for Wilms' tumor. *International Journal of Radiation Oncology, Biology, Physics, 9,* 651-657.

230. Tucker, M. A., D'Angio, G. J., Boice, J. D. J., et al. (1991). Therapeutic radiation at a young age is linked to secondary thyroid cancer. *Cancer Research, 51,* 2885-2888.

231. Ueda, M., Harada, M., Shiobara, S., et al. (1984). T lymphocyte reconstitution in long-term survivors after allogeneic and autologous marrow transplantation. *Transplantation, 37,* 552-556.

232. Vogelzang, N. J. (1991). Nephrotoxicity from chemotherapy: Prevention and management. *Oncology, 5,* 97-112.

233. Waber, D. P., Tarbell, N. J., Fairclough, D., et al. (1995). Cognitive sequelae of treatment in childhood acute lymphoblastic leukemia: Cranial radiation requires an accomplice. *Journal of Clinical Oncology, 13,* 2490-2496.

234. Waber, D. P., Tarbell, N. J., Kahn, C. M., et al. (1992). The relationship of sex and treatment modality to neuropsychologic outcome in childhood acute lymphoblastic leukemia. *Journal of Clinical Oncology, 10,* 810-817.

235. Wara, W. M., Phillips, T. L., Margolis, L. W., & Smith, V. (1973). Radiation pneumonitis: A new approach to the derivation of time-dose factors. *Cancer, 32,* 547-552.

236. Wexler, L. H., Andrich, M. P., Venzon, D. et al. (1996). Randomized trial of the cardioprotective agent ICRF-187 in pediatric sarcoma patients treated with doxorubicin. *Journal of Clinical Oncology, 14,* 362-372.

237. Wharam, M. D. (1983). Radiation therapy. In A. J. Altman & A. D. Schwartz (Eds.), *Malignant disease of infancy, childhood and adolescence*. Philadelphia: W. B. Saunders.

238. Whitehead, E., Shalet, S., Blockledge, G., et al. (1983). The effects of combination chemotherapy function in women treated for Hodgkin's disease. *Cancer, 52,* 988-993.

239. Whitehead, E., Shalet, S. M., Jones, P. H., et al. (1982). Gonadal function after combination chemotherapy for Hodgkin's disease in childhood. *Archives of Disease in Childhood, 57,* 287-291.

240. Whitt, J. K. (1984). Children's adaptation to chronic illness and handicapping conditions. In M. G. Eisenberg, L. C. Sutkin, & M. A. Jansen (Eds.), *Chronic illness and disability through the life span: Effects on self and family* (pp. 69-102). New York: Springer-Verlag.

241. Wilson, D. A., Nitschke, R., Bowman, M. E., et al. (1991). Transient white matter changes on MR images in children undergoing chemotherapy for acute lymphocytic leukemia: Correlation with neuropsychologic deficiencies. *Radiology, 180,* 205-209.

242. Wohl, M. E., Griscom, N. T., Traggis, O. G., et al. (1975). Effects of therapeutic irradiation delivered in early childhood upon subsequent lung function. *Pediatrics, 55,* 507-516.

243. Wong, F. L., Boice, J. D., Jr., Abramson, D. H., et al. (1997). Cancer incidence after retinoblastoma: Radiation dose and sarcoma risk, *Journal of the American Medical Association, 278,* 1262-1267.

244. Yaholom, J., Petrek, J. A., Biddinger, P. W., et al. (1992). Breast cancer in patients irradiated for Hodgkin's disease: A clinical and pathologic analysis of 45 events in 37 patients. *Journal of Clinical Oncology, 10,* 1674-1681.

245. Zeltzer, L. K. (1993). Cancer in adolescents and young adults: Psychosocial aspects for long-term survivors. *Cancer, 71,* 3463-3468.

246. Zeltzer, L. K., Chen, E., Weiss, R., et al. (1997). Comparison of psychologic outcome in adult survivors of childhood acute lymphoblastic leukemia versus controls: A cooperative Children's Cancer Group and National Institutes of Health study. *Journal of Clinical Oncology, 15,* 547-556.

247. Zevon, M. A., Neubauer, N. A., Green, D. M. (1990). Adjustment and vocational satisfaction of patients treated during childhood or adolescence for acute lymphoblastic leukemia. *American Journal of Pediatric Hematology/ Oncology, 12,* 454-461.

IV

Diseases

19

Acute Lymphoblastic Leukemia

Susan K. Westlake
Kathy L. Bertolone

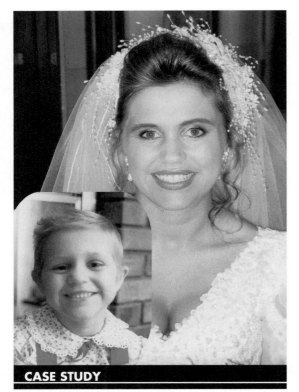

CASE STUDY

Five-year-old Melissa was seen by her pediatrician after a 2-week history of decreased appetite, pallor, and a questionable history of increased bruising in May 1979. Her parents reported no other symptoms such as fever, bone pain, or increased fatigue. The pediatrician noted her pallor and sent her to a local hospital for an anemia work-up to include a blood transfusion. An adult hematologist/oncologist reviewed the complete blood count (CBC), which revealed a white blood count (WBC) of 5,000/mm³, hemoglobin 5.5 g/dl, and a platelet count of 95,000/mm³. A bone marrow biopsy was performed and was diagnostic of acute lymphoblastic leukemia (ALL). The parents requested a second

opinion, so Melissa was transferred to a children's hospital with a pediatric hematology-oncology subspecialist. Before the transfer she received 100 ml of packed red blood cells.

On admission to children's hospital, a repeat CBC showed a WBC of 3,600/mm³, hemoglobin now 7.3 g/dl, and a platelet count of 95,000/mm³. The physical exam revealed a well-appearing, pale, white female, with a 1.5- to 2-cm left anterior, nontender cervical node, grade I-II/VI systolic murmur heard best at the left sternal border, liver tip palpable at the right costal margin, spleen down 2 cm at left costal margin, and a few scattered bruises on her extremities.

A repeat bone marrow aspiration was obtained for chromosomes and cell surface markers. Melissa had normal chromosomes and B-cell precursor lymphoblasts. A lumbar puncture was performed, which revealed only one white blood cell and no lymphoblasts. The pediatric oncologist recommended treatment on the Children's Cancer Group (CCG) low-risk ALL protocol. After informed consent was obtained from the parents, Melissa was started on induction therapy, consisting of vincristine, prednisone, and asparaginase, per CCG 161 protocol. Melissa was randomized to receive maintenance vincristine/prednisone pulses and no cranial irradiation. Her hospital course was unremarkable, and she was discharged to go home on hospital day 4, to be followed in the outpatient pediatric hematology/oncology clinic.

In 1979 ALL protocols requested bone marrow aspirates on days 14 and 28 of induction therapy, at the end of consolidation, then every 3 months until the completion of therapy. Melissa had achieved bone marrow remission (<5% lymphoblasts) by day 14 and completed 3 years of therapy in April 1982.

Melissa is currently married and has two healthy children. She enjoys a healthy life with no apparent effects from her chemotherapy. She did not receive cranial irradiation or anthracyclines, which are known for potential long-term side effects. She works full time in the convention and exposition industry and travels throughout the United States.

The term *leukemia,* from the Greek "white blood," refers to cancers of the blood-forming or hematopoietic tissues and includes a group of disorders characterized by the uncontrolled proliferation of abnormal, immature blood cells. Figure 19-1 depicts the hematopoietic pathway from its point of origin at the pluripotent stem cell to the endpoints of mature, differentiated blood cells. Leukemia can occur anywhere along this path. The leukemic disorders are categorized primarily by the specific blood cell lineage (lymphoid or myeloid) and the stage of maturity where the disruption in the hematopoietic process occurs. In this chapter, acute lymphoblastic leukemia (ALL), which affects cells along the lymphoid path of hematopoietic maturation and differentiation, will be discussed. Acute nonlymphocytic leukemia (ANLL) is discussed in Chapter 20.

Acute lymphoblastic leukemia is a heterogeneous disease that can originate in lymphoid cells of B- or T-cell lineage at any point in the process of normal lymphoid differentiation,[72] shown in Figure 19-2. As the mutant leukemic cells proliferate and fill the bone marrow, they compete and interfere with normal hematopoiesis and spread beyond the marrow to other tissues and organs. The presenting signs and symptoms of the child with ALL are due to the failure of normal hematopoiesis and to the extent of extramedullary leukemic disease.

Fifty years ago the child with ALL invariably died, generally within a matter of months. Today the majority of children with ALL will survive their disease. The overall 5-year survival rate has reached 80%.[128] This success is due primarily to the development of effective treatment strategies through large cooperative group clinical trials and the systematic investigation of the pathobiology of childhood ALL. Childhood ALL provides a paradigm for the successful treatment of malignancies of all types and for the conduct of cancer research.[72,93,97]

EPIDEMIOLOGY

ALL is the most common malignancy in children, accounting for nearly 25% of all cancer diagnosed in children less than 15 years of age[109] and occurring at an annual rate of 29.2 per million.[128] Approximately 2400 children and adolescents are diagnosed with ALL in the United States each year, and the disease accounts for three fourths of all leukemia diagnosed in childhood. Incidence rates for ALL vary across childhood. There is a sharp peak in children ages 2 to 3 years of age.[128] The shape of the age-incidence curve for ALL is

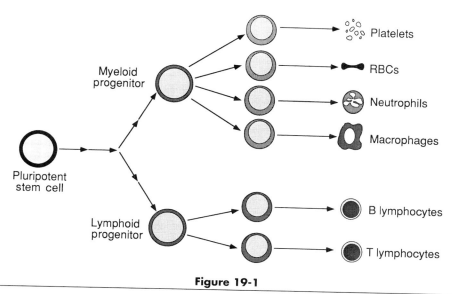

Figure 19-1

Cell lineages of the hematopoietic system showing common pluripotent stem cell and lineage-committed intermediates. Hematopoietic malignancies are identified by the nomenclature of this system. (Adapted from Sawyers, C. L., Denny, C. T., & Witte, O. N. [1991]. Leukemia and the disruption of normal hematopoiesis. *Cell, 64,* 337-350. © Cell Press.)

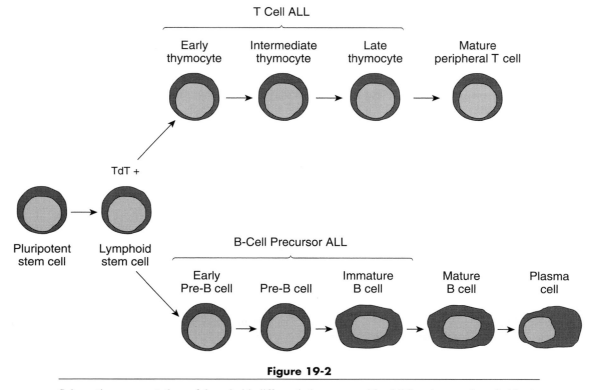

Figure 19-2

Schematic representation of lymphoid differentiation seen with childhood acute lymphoblastic leukemia.

described by a mathematical model that assumes childhood ALL results from two events required for full malignant transformation. The first of these is believed to occur in utero.[127]

The incidence of ALL is considerably higher for white children than for black children.[128] Sex-specific differences also are apparent, with ALL incidence consistently higher in males in children younger than 15 years of age (M/F = 1.2) and nearly 2 times higher in males 15 to 19 years of age.[128]

There are substantial worldwide geographic variations in the incidence of childhood ALL, thought to reflect variability in genetic susceptibility and/or environmental factors.[8,43,85] In general the incidence is higher in industrialized countries than in developing countries. This may reflect the prominence of infectious diseases, death from other causes, and underdiagnosis in developing countries, as well as exposure to leukemogens in industrialized countries.[22,70] These differences also have been attributed to different patterns of exposure to infectious agents.[41,129] A delayed pattern of exposure to common infections in more advantaged populations may leave the immune system unprepared for eventual infections and lead to an abnormal immunologic response and an increased risk of leukemia.[8]

The cumulative incidence of childhood ALL increased approximately 20% between 1977 and 1995, with a peak noted in 1989, and with rates 5% to 10% below this peak value in subsequent years.[128] The overall increase, which in part may reflect refinements in diagnostic classification, has been attributed to child or parental exposure to a variety of environmental hazards, none of which has been conclusively linked to the development of ALL.[115] The increase also may represent changes in population characteristics in specific geographic areas sampled, such as the higher incidence of ALL in Hispanic children in the Los Angeles area, where the Hispanic population has increased.[128]

Since the 1970s survival for children with ALL has improved markedly, with the overall 5-year survival for all children with ALL now at 80%,[128] as shown in Figure 19-3. The major obstacle to cure in children with ALL is bone marrow and/or extramedullary (e.g., central nervous system [CNS] or testicular) relapse. Nearly all children with ALL achieve an initial remission, but relapse can occur during treatment or following completion of therapy. The likelihood of cure following relapse is generally poor, particularly for those with marrow relapse following a short period of remission.[33] Increased survival is attributed to improvements

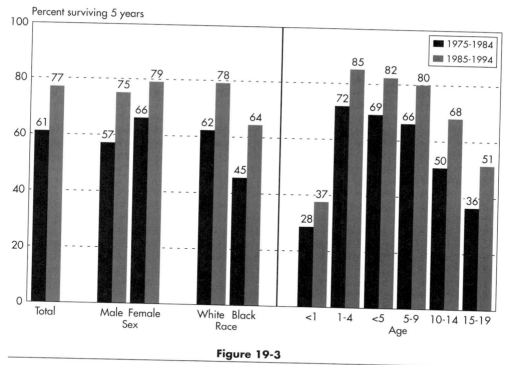

Figure 19-3

ALL 5-year relative survival rates by sex, race, age, and time period, SEER (9 areas), 1975-84 and 1985-94.   (From Smith, M. A., Ries, L. A. G., Gurney, J. G., et al. [1999]. Leukemia. In L. A. G. Ries, M. A. Smith, J. G. Gurney, et al. [Eds.], *Cancer incidence and survival among children and adolescents: United States SEER Program, 1975-1995* [p. 27]. [SEER pediatric monograph, NIH Publication 99-4649]. Bethesda, MD: National Cancer Institute.)

in CNS prophylaxis and in treatment intensification for selected groups of patients.[72]

Survival in children with ALL is strongly related to age at diagnosis. Five-year survival rates for the years 1985-1994 were highest for the 1 to 4 year age-group (85%) and the 5 to 9 year age-group (80%), followed by the 10 to 14 year age-group (68%) and the 15 to 19 year age-group (51%). Infants have the poorest survival rate (37%) (see Figure 19-3). The more favorable prognosis for children 1 to 9 years of age is attributed to the relatively high proportion of children in this age-group with favorable biologic subtypes. Infants, older children, and adolescents with less favorable biologic subtypes have more unfavorable outcomes.[128] Five-year survival rates were slightly higher for females than males (79% vs. 75%) and lower for black children than white children (64% vs. 78%). The poorer outcome in black children with ALL has been attributed to several factors, including differences in access to health care, differences in pharmacokinetics or pharmacodynamics of the drugs used for ALL, and the relative scarcity in black children of the more favorable ALL subtypes.[128]

GENETICS

Genetic abnormalities are presumed to play a significant role in the cause of ALL.[72] These include chromosomal gains (hyperdiploidy) or losses (hypodiploidy); chromosomal translocations, involving the formation of transforming genes or the dysregulation of gene expression; and deletion or inactivation of tumor-suppressor genes.[98] These abnormalities most often are acquired rather than inherited and are associated with specific biologic subtypes of ALL.[8] Acquired genetic abnormalities are found in the blast cells of 60% to 75% of patients with ALL[98] and have important prognostic and treatment implications.

Approximately 5% of acute leukemias (ALL and acute myelogenous leukemia [AML]), however, are associated with inherited genetic syndromes.[133] These include Down syndrome, where there is a ten- to twentyfold increased risk of both ALL and AML,[29,113] and Bloom syndrome, neurofibromatosis, Shwachman syndrome, and ataxia telangiectasia.* In addition, the occurrence of familial aggregation of childhood leukemia has been

---

*References 5, 36, 48, 62, 75, 144.

reported, which may represent an inherited predisposition and/or shared environmental factors. Siblings of children with ALL have a two- to fourfold higher risk of developing leukemia compared with children in the general population.[93] A high degree of concordance of leukemia also has been noted among twins, particularly monozygotic, which is highly age-dependent, occurring mostly in infants. Although this suggests a genetic predisposition, there is evidence that the leukemia develops in one fetus and spreads to the other via the shared placental circulation versus being an inherited mutation.[30]

ETIOLOGY AND RISK FACTORS

Acute lymphoblastic leukemia is believed to originate from a mutation in a single hematopoietic lymphoid progenitor cell, capable of indefinite self-renewal, which is subsequently passed on to all of its descendents.[8,72,97] The clonal expansion of the mutated cell leads to a proliferation of poorly differentiated (or malignant) hematopoietic precursor cells that crowd out normal hematopoietic cells in the bone marrow and compete for nutrition. The common clonal origin of the leukemic cells is documented by the identical patterns of immunoglobulin and T-cell receptor (TCR) gene rearrangements observed at both diagnosis and relapse.[72]

B-cell leukemia is considered to originate in the bone marrow in most cases and subsequently spread to other parts of the body. In patients who present with an anterior mediastinal mass, ALL is thought to originate in the thymus, and in the intestine in those with an ileocecal tumor.[97] The process of malignant transformation is regarded as complex and multifactorial. Spontaneous mutation in lymphoid cells of B- or T-cell lineage occur during normal lymphoid cell development. These cells are at high risk because of the intrinsic, regulated mutagenic activity occurring during the process of differentiation and the high rate of proliferation of these cells.[39,42]

Regulating genes in a lymphoid cell population undergoing significant proliferation are thought to spontaneously mutate, but the exact nature of these leukemogenic mutations has yet to be determined.[40] Alterations in master regulator proteins that control hematopoietic growth and differentiation activate proto-oncogenes that promote malignancy and inactivate genes whose proteins suppress leukemia. These genetic alterations are thought to endow the cell with a proliferative advantage or prevent its normal differentiation and programmed cell death (apoptosis).[93]

The specific causes that trigger the genetic mutations in leukemia are not known.[8] Increased risk has been associated with a number of factors. Table 19-1 summarizes current information about risk factors for ALL. Known or more generally accepted risk factors include exposure to ionizing radiation and several predisposing genetic syndromes, in addition to the age, gender, and racial risk factors observed in the incidence of childhood ALL. Exposure to low-energy electromagnetic fields, such as those from residential electrical power lines and electrical appliances, has been postulated to be leukemogenic. A recent large case-control study conducted by CCG showed little evidence to support this hypothesis,[63] and the controversial issue is being evaluated in ongoing epidemiologic studies.[128] Although a subject of intense interest, there is also no direct evidence for an infectious etiology in childhood leukemia.[8,81]

It is important to note that ALL is a heterogeneous disease with a number of biologic subtypes. Specific leukemic subgroups may have distinct etiologies, with particular subgroups associated with specific causal mechanisms. The multistage process of leukemogenesis may involve separate etiologic factors operating at the various stages.[8] The heterogeneous nature of ALL also has made it difficult to accrue study samples with sufficient statistical power to examine risk factors in these discrete subtypes. An important initiative in childhood ALL epidemiologic research is the need to investigate environmental and genetic risk factors in well-defined homogeneous biologic subgroups of the disease.[8]

CLINICAL PRESENTATION

Children with leukemia are usually symptomatic from 1 to 6 weeks before diagnosis, but some report symptom duration for months. The signs and symptoms are quite variable and reflect the degree to which bone marrow has been replaced with leukemic lymphoblasts and the extent of extramedullary disease.[97] The most common symptoms and clinical findings reflect the failure of normal hematopoiesis: fever, fatigue, bone pain, bleeding, anorexia, petechiae, purpura, pallor, lymphadenopathy, hepatosplenomegaly, and evidence of infection[97] (Table 19-2). Young children may present with complaints of bone and/or joint pain and refuse to walk. This pain is related to leukemic infiltration of the bony periosteum, causing expansion of the marrow cavity.[97] Fever, the most common finding at diagnosis, is usually due to the leukemic process, including neutropenia, and generally resolves within 72 hours from the start of induction therapy.

The work-up includes a thorough physical examination, CBC with manual differential, bone marrow aspiration (BMA) and/or biopsy, chemistry panel, uric acid, serum lactate dehydrogenase

TABLE 19-1	RISK FACTORS FOR CHILDHOOD ACUTE LYMPHOBLASTIC LEUKEMIA, BY DEGREE OF CERTAINTY
Degree of Certainty	**Acute Lymphoblastic Leukemia**
Generally accepted risk factors	Males
	Age (2-5 years)
	High socioeconomic status
	Race (whites > blacks)
	In utero x-ray exposure
	Postnatal radiation (therapeutic)
	Down syndrome
	Neurofibromatosis type I
	Bloom syndrome
	Shwachman syndrome
	Ataxia telangiectasia
Suggestive of increased risk	Increased birth weight
	Maternal history of fetal loss
Limited evidence	Parental smoking before or during pregnancy
	Parental occupational exposures
	Postnatal infections
	Diet
	Vitamin K prophylaxis in newborns
	Maternal alcohol consumption during pregnancy
	Electric and magnetic fields
	Postnatal use of chloramphenicol
Probably not associated	Ultrasound
	Indoor radon

Adapted from Bhatia, S., Ross, J., Greaves, M. F., et al. (1999). Epidemiology and etiology. In C-H. Pui (Ed.), *Childhood leukemias* (pp. 38-49). New York: Cambridge University Press.

(LDH), chest x-ray, and, after the diagnosis is established, a lumbar puncture to determine if lymphoblasts are present in the cerebral spinal fluid (CSF).[72,84] Liver, spleen, and lymph nodes are the most common sites of extramedullary involvement. Painless scrotal enlargement can be a sign of testicular leukemia, hernia, or hydrocele and may require a biopsy if clinical findings are equivocal. Approximately 25% of male patients have biopsy-proven microscopic testicular leukemia at diagnosis. However, routine testicular biopsy is no longer recommended, because these patients rarely have residual leukemia cells in their testes after remission induction therapy. Testicular biopsy is reserved to document relapse or residual disease for patients with persistently enlarged testes.[134]

In approximately 50% of childhood ALL, the initial WBC is within normal limits for age. In others, the WBC may be either decreased or elevated, but neutropenia is generally present. Lymphoblasts usually are detected when a carefully performed leukocyte differential is done. Anemia (hemoglobin <10 g/dl) is present in 80% of cases at diagnosis. Mild elevations in liver function tests may also be noted. Other common laboratory findings include hyperuricemia, elevated LDH, hyperkalemia, and hyperphosphatemia, which are related to lysis of lymphoblasts.[97] Approximately 5% to 10% of patients have an anterior mediastinal mass noted on chest x-ray. CNS involvement ($\geq$5 WBCs/mm^3 with lymphoblasts present) occurs in less than 5% of cases.[72]

DIAGNOSTIC EVALUATION

The definitive diagnosis of ALL is confirmed when the bone marrow reveals at least 25% lymphoblasts. Other bone marrow characteristics such as morphology, immunophenotype, and cytogenetics provide essential diagnostic and treatment stratification criteria. Box 19-1 summarizes all tests performed on the initial bone marrow specimen for treatment and prognostic stratification.

Presently, lymphoblasts are categorized by morphology and immunophenotype. In 1976 the French-American-British (FAB) Cooperative Group classification of lymphoblasts (as L1, L2, or L3) provided the worldwide standard for morphologic assessment of lymphoblasts. This cytological feature is defined by the amount of cytoplasm, cell

TABLE 19-2	PRESENTING CLINICAL AND LABORATORY FEATURES OF 2209 CHILDREN WITH NEWLY DIAGNOSED ALL TREATED CONSECUTIVELY AT ST. JUDE CHILDREN'S RESEARCH HOSPITAL (1962-1996)
Feature	**% of total**
Age (yr)	
• ≤1	2
• 2-9	73
• ≥10	25
Male	56
Black race	15
Symptoms[a]	
• Fever	53
• Fatigue	50
• Bone or joint pain	40
• Bleeding	38
• Anorexia	19
• Abdominal pain	10
Liver edge below costal margin	
• 1-4 cm	39
• ≥5 cm	32
Spleen edge below costal margin	
• 1-4 cm	29
• ≥5 cm	32
Mediastinal mass	10
Central nervous system leukemia	5
Leukocyte count[b]	
• <10,000/mm³	45
• 10,000-24,000/mm³	20
• 25,000-49,000/mm³	12
• 50,000-99,000/mm³	9
• ≥100,000/mm³	14
Hemoglobin (g/dl)[c]	
• <8	52
• 8-10	26
• >10	22
Platelet count[d]	
• <10,000/mm³	9
• 10,000-49,000/mm³	39
• 50,000-100,000/mm³	20
• >100,000/mm³	32

From Pui, C-H., & Crist, W. M. (1999). Acute lymphoblastic leukemia. In C-H. Pui (Ed.), *Childhood leukemias* (pp. 288-312). New York: Cambridge University Press.
[a]Based on 500 patients.
[b]Median (range), 12.1 (0.3-1512).
[c]Median (range), 7.8 (1.4-17.6).
[d]Median (range), 53 (1-1400).

size, vacuolation, and nucleoli present in the lymphoblast.[47] Although FAB morphology is used to define lymphoblasts, immunophenotyping provides more prognostic and treatment stratification value.[97]

BOX 19-1	
DIAGNOSTIC MARROW EVALUATION	

MORPHOLOGIC SLIDES
FAB Classification (% of L1, L2, L3)
• L3 denotes mature B-cell
Blast percentage
Cytochemistry (special stains)
• Nonspecific esterase stain—NASD (negative or weakly positive)
• Myeloperoxidase stain (negative in lymphoblasts, positive in myeloblasts)
• Sudan black (negative in lymphoblasts, positive in myeloblasts)
• Periodic acid schiff—PAS (positive in ALL)

IMMUNOPHENOTYPE
T- or B-lymphoid origin

CYTOGENETIC ANALYSIS
Chromosomal number or ploidy, DNA index
Structure (translocations, deletions, rearrangements)

BONE MARROW STATUS
M1: <5% blasts regardless of number of mature lymphocytes
M2: 5%-25% blasts
M3: >25% blasts (induction therapy begins)

Data from Margolin, J. F., & Poplack, D. G. (1997). Acute lymphoblastic leukemia. In P. A. Pizzo & D. G. Poplack (Eds.), *Principles and practice of pediatric oncology* (3rd ed., pp. 409-462). Philadelphia: Lippincott-Raven; Pui, C-H., & Crist, W. M. (1999). Acute lymphoblastic leukemia. In C-H. Pui (Ed.), *Childhood leukemias* (pp. 288-312). New York: Cambridge University Press.

Immunophenotyping of lymphoblasts is essential to establish the correct diagnostic subtype of ALL. Monoclonal antibodies (MoAbs) are used to identify cell surface antigens of hematopoietic cells associated with B-cell, T-cell, and myeloid lineages of malignant cells. The two lineages identified in ALL are B-cell and T-cell (see Figure 19-2), with four distinct subtypes of the B-cell lineage. These include the three B-cell precursor or progenitor subtypes (early pre-B, pre-B, and immature B-cell), and mature B-cell. Although T-lineage can be subclassified, for therapeutic purposes one need only distinguish T-cell and mature B-cell cases from those originating in B-cell precursors.[6,98]

The distinction between children with B-cell ALL and those with Burkitt's lymphoma with bone marrow involvement is based on the degree of marrow infiltration. Patients with less than 25% bone marrow replacement with lymphoblasts are considered to have Burkitt's lymphoma, whereas those with more extensive marrow involvement are diagnosed with B-cell ALL. The cytologic examination of lymphoblasts obtained from bone marrow, malignant ascites, or pleural fluid of patients with B-cell ALL or Burkitt's lymphoma typically identifies FAB L3 morphology; immunophenotype of mature B; expression of cluster designation (CD) groupings CD19, CD20, CD21; absence of terminal deoxynucleotidyl transferase (TdT), with t(8;14) (q24;q32) identified in approximately 85% of cases.[116]

MoAbs are identified by their CD groupings; antibodies within each CD group recognize the same cellular antigen. Specific patterns of lymphoblast antigen expression hold clinical and prognostic relevance. For example, the leukemic cells of B-cell precursor ALL express surface CD19, CD24, CD22, and HLA-DR. In 90% of these cases, CD10, also known as CALLA-common acute lymphocytic leukemia antigen, and TdT are expressed.[6] Children with ALL lymphoblasts that express these antigens usually present with anemia, neutropenia, and thrombocytopenia, and have a favorable prognosis. Over 90% of T lymphoblasts express CD2, CD5, and/or CD7 and TdT, and 40% to 45% of cases express CD10 and/or CD21. In patients with T-cell ALL, having cells positive for CD2 appears to confer a favorable prognosis, whereas having CD7+, CD2-, and CD5- leukemia infers a less favorable prognosis. Many children with T-cell leukemia present with normal red blood cells and platelets, along with extramedullary disease.[6,97] ALL of infancy is associated with a high leukocyte count, hepatosplenomegaly, and CNS involvement. The immunophenotype is generally immature B-lineage precursors, characterized by lack of CD10 expression with coexpression of myeloid-associated antigens (Table 19-3). This finding suggests that the classic form of infant ALL originates in a stem cell that has not fully committed to lymphoid differentiation.[9]

Intense focus has also been placed on the cytogenetic abnormalities in ALL. Aberrations in chromosome number (ploidy) and/or structure (translocations, deletions, rearrangements) occur in over 90% of childhood ALL cases, and many are of prognostic significance.[54,72] Diploid cells have 46 chromosomes. Hyperdiploid cells can be classified into those with 47 to 50 chromosomes and those with more than 50 chromosomes. Leukemia cells can also be described as pseudodiploid (46 chromosomes with structural or numeric rearrangements), hypodiploid (<46 chromosomes), and near tetraploid (82-84 chromosomes). Hyperdiploid leukemia cells accumulate increased amounts of methotrexate and active metabolites and are particularly susceptible to undergoing apoptosis.[7] Hyperdiploidy can be evaluated by measuring the DNA

content of cells (DNA index) or by karyotyping. Those patients with greater than 50 chromosomes per cell, or DNA index greater than 1.16, have a good prognosis, with approximately 85% cured with conventional therapy. Hyperdiploidy with 47 to 50 chromosomes is associated with an intermediate outcome, whereas pseudodiplody, hypodiploidy, and near tetraploidy are predictive of poor outcome.[102]

The most prevalent translocation in 17% to 25% of B precursor ALL is t(12;21), also known as the *TEL-AML1* fusion gene. It is associated with long-term disease-free survival in greater than 90% of patients.[13] Its prognostic importance exceeds that of age and WBC count at diagnosis, the gold standards of risk classification.[13,67] Poor prognostic chromosomal abnormalities include the Philadelphia chromosome (t[9;22] *BCR-ABL* fusion gene), occurring in 3% to 5% of children with ALL; and the infant ALL chromosomal abnormality (t[4;11] *ALL1/MLL/HRX* fusion gene) located on cytogenetic band (11q23) and rearranged in greater than 60% to 70% of infants with ALL.[9] Infants with t(4;11) generally present with a high WBC count, are more likely than other children with ALL to have CNS disease at diagnosis, and have a poor initial response to therapy.[9] These prognostic markers indicate a requirement for hematopoietic stem cell transplantation (HSCT) in first bone marrow remission. The cure rate of children with t(9;22) and infant t(4;11) leukemia with current chemotherapy regimens is approximately 20% without stem cell transplant.[2]

The *E2A-PBX1* chimera t(1;19) may occur as either a balanced translocation or as an unbalanced translocation. The balanced t(1;19) distinguishes an important subgroup of children with B-cell precursor leukemia who have suboptimal responses to antimetabolite chemotherapy. Studies have shown that there is improved outcome for patients with the unbalanced t(1;19) with intensive therapy.[67,138] The t(8;14) is associated with B-cell leukemia, a systemic manifestation of Burkitt's lymphoma with early treatment failure on standard ALL protocols. These children need intensified short-term protocols that are discussed in the treatment section.[104,116]

TREATMENT

HISTORY

Early reported attempts to treat leukemia date to 1865 and involved the use of arsenic chemicals[66] and irradiation.[59,120] Over the next 100 years a variety of chemotherapeutic agents were developed, many of which are used today, including mercaptopurine,[16] corticosteroids,[25] methotrexate,[26] cy-

TABLE 19-3   CLINICAL AND BIOLOGIC FEATURES OF THE MORE COMMON GENETIC SUBTYPES OF CHILDHOOD ALL

Subtype	Frequency %	Molecular Genetic Alterations	Associated Features	Estimated 5-yr Event-Free Survival (%)
Hyperdiploidy >50 chromosomes	27-29	Unknown	Predominant B-cell precursor phenotype; age between 1 and 10 yr; low leukocyte count; favorable prognosis with antimetabolite-based therapy	80-90
t(12;21)(p12-13;q22)[a]	20-25	ETV6-CBFA2 fusion (also termed TEL-AML1)	B-cell precursor phenotype; pseudodiploidy; age 1 to 10 yr; favorable prognosis with antimetabolite-based therapy	85-90
t(1;19)(q23;p13)	5-6	E2A-PBX1 fusion	Pre-B phenotype; pseudodiploidy; increased leukocyte count; black race; CNS leukemia; improved outcome with intensive therapy	70-80
t(4;11)(q21;q23) and other 11q23 translocations	4-8	MLL-AF4 fusion (MLL rearrangements)	CD10-/CD15± B-cell precursor phenotype; infant age group predominantly; hyperleukocytosis; CNS leukemia; dismal outcome	10-30
t(9;22)(q34;q11)	3-4	BCR-ABL fusion	Predominant B-cell precursor phenotype; older age; increased leukocyte count; dismal outcome in the subgroup with leukocyte counts $\geq 25 \times 10^9$/L	20-35
t(8;14)(q24;q32.3), t(2;8)(p12;q24), or t(8;22)(q24;q11)	2	Associated MYC overexpression with IGH, IGK, or IGL rearrangement	B-cell phenotype; L3 morphology; male predominance; bulky extramedullary disease; favorable prognosis with short-term intensive chemotherapy with high-dose methotrexate plus cytarabine plus cyclophosphamide	70-85
t(1;14)(p34;q11) and TAL recombination[b]	3-4	TAL (SCL) rearrangements	CD10- T-cell phenotype; male predominance; hyperleukocytosis	60-70
dic(9;12)(p11-12;?p12)	1	Unknown	B-cell precursor phenotype; male predominance; excellent outcome with antimetabolite-based therapy	80-90

From Pui, C-H., & Crist, W. M. (1999). Acute lymphoblastic leukemia. In C-H. Pui (Ed.), *Childhood leukemias* (pp. 288-312). New York: Cambridge University Press.

[a]Cryptic translocation requiring molecular detection.

[b]A local DNA deletion requiring molecular detection.

clophosphamide,[27] and vincristine.[55] However, these produced only temporary remissions, and patients invariably died of their disease. The general notion among pediatricians and hematologists was that the most one could expect from leukemia chemotherapy was temporary remission, with hopefully some extended period of survival in comfort.[90]

A shift from palliative to curative treatment occurred in the 1960s as investigators grappled with a number of identified obstacles to the cure of childhood ALL.[89] These included initial and acquired drug resistance, meningeal relapse, overlapping toxicities of agents, and the lingering pessimism that cure was not possible. Subsequently, the four treatment phases that prevail today were identified: remission induction, intensification or consolidation, preventive meningeal treatment, and prolonged continuation therapy.[35,88] Treatment was further refined in clinical trials, and additional antileukemic drugs were introduced, including cytarabine (1968), daunorubicin (1967), and asparaginase (1970). By 1970 the curability of childhood ALL had been confirmed by many institutional and collaborative groups.[95]

In the intervening years, effective multidrug regimens in well-documented clinical trials have continued to improve the cure rate of childhood ALL. Clinical trials for children with ALL are designed to compare the current standard of treatment with a potentially better treatment approach that may improve survival outcomes and/or diminish toxicity. Interestingly, the cure rate improved from 40% in the 1970s to more than 90% in the 1990s without the addition of any new front-line agents[125] but with optimization of drug combinations and doses.[11] Additionally, enhanced understanding of the biology of ALL and the recognition of disease subtypes has led to the selection and tailoring of treatment based on a child's risk of relapse. Risk-directed therapy ensures that patients with high-risk disease receive intensive treatment while those with lower-risk features receive less toxic therapy.[58] The continuing development of supportive therapy (e.g., transfusion therapy, metabolic management, and anti-infective prophylaxis and therapy) also contributed to the improved outcomes.[90]

RISK-DIRECTED THERAPY

The determination of risk status has been a major concern of investigators. In 1993 representatives from major cooperative groups and treatment centers met at a National Cancer Institute–sponsored conference to identify more uniform criteria for risk-based treatment assignment for children with ALL in order to increase the efficiency of future ALL clinical research.[126] Using outcome data from ALL clinical trials, participants determined the following risk categories. For patients with B-cell precursor ALL, the standard-risk category (4-year event-free survival [EFS] ~ 80%) was determined to include patients 1 to 9 years of age with a WBC count at diagnosis of less than 50,000, with high-risk status (4-year EFS ~ 65%) reserved for all other patients. For patients with T-cell ALL, there was no consensus on risk assignment. Some groups or institutions chose to classify these patients as high-risk, while others chose to use the aforementioned criteria of age and initial WBC as determining factors. The participants agreed that a patient's risk category might be modified by factors in addition to age and WBC count. They recommended that in future studies a common set of prognostic indicators be uniformly obtained and used to make treatment decision. These included DNA index, cytogenetics, early response to treatment, immunophenotype, and CNS status.

The Children's Oncology Group (C.O.G.) continues to refine criteria for risk-based treatment stratification in current and proposed studies. Biologic properties that are identified and defined as clinically relevant will drive future protocol development. Table 19-4 lists the current risk group criteria for the CCG, the POG, and proposed C.O.G. studies. The general structure of risk group assignment for proposed ALL studies is divided into two parts. Initial induction therapy is based on the NCI criteria of age and WBC risk group definitions for standard and high risk. Day 28 consolidation and maintenance therapy is based on specified leukemia cell genetic findings and the rapidity of response, in conjunction with the age and WBC. Risk stratification on day 28 can change a child from standard risk to low or from high risk to standard by favorable laboratory characteristics. Unfavorable laboratory characteristics or slowness of response can raise a child from standard to high risk. There are certain clinical or laboratory characteristics that imply very high risk, regardless of presenting age and WBC. These include presence of the Philadelphia chromosome, *MLL* rearrangement, hypodiploidy (<45 chromosomes), and induction failure. Proposed C.O.G. risk group designations for B-cell precursor ALL diagnosed at greater than 12 months of age are defined in Box 19-2.

Once considered to have very poor prognosis, children with mature B-cell ALL now enjoy a 75% to 85% survival after approximately 6 months of very intense treatment.[116] A recent French study of 102 children with mature B-cell ALL/non-Hodgkin's lymphoma (NHL) treated

TABLE 19-4	PROGNOSTIC FACTORS IN CHILDHOOD ALL	
Factor	Favorable	Unfavorable
Age	1-9 years	<1 year or ≥10 years (<6 months least favorable)
White blood count at diagnosis	Low (<50,000/mm^3)	High (≥50,000/mm^3)
Response to therapy	Rapid early response (RER) Day 7 and/or 14 BM (M1) "Good prednisone response"	Slow early response (SER) ≥Day 28 BM (M3) "Poor prednisone response"
Biologic properties of leukemic blasts	B-cell precursor ALL t(12;21) TEL-AML1 gene Hyperdiploidy >50 Chromosomes CALLA CD19, HLA-DR, CD22, 34 TdT Trisomy 4, 10, 17 (p12-13;q22) DNA index (DI >1.16)	t(9;22) BCR-ABL Infant t(4;11) MLL (11q23) Hypodiploidy <45 Chromosomes MRD postinduction Abnormal 9p t(1;19) balanced Induction failure DI <0.95 E2A-PBX1 CNS 3 (varies by protocol) Testicular involvement (varies by protocol)

Data from Biondi, A., Cimino, G., Pieters, R., et al. (2000). Biological and therapeutic aspects of infant leukemia. *Blood, 96*(1), 24-33; Pui, C-H., & Crist, W. M. (1999). Acute lymphoblastic leukemia. In C-H. Pui (Ed.), *Childhood leukemias*. New York: Cambridge University Press; Smith, M., Arthur, D., Camitta, B., et al. (1996). Uniform approach to risk classification and treatment assignment for the children with acute lymphoblastic leukemia. *Journal of Clinical Oncology, 14*, 18-24.
CALLA, Common acute lymphocytic leukemia antigen; *TdT*, terminal deoxynucleotidyl transferase; *MRD*, minimal residual disease.

BOX 19-2

PROPOSED C.O.G. RISK GROUP DESIGNATIONS B-PRECURSER ALL >12 MONTHS

STANDARD RISK DEFINITIONS
NCI consensus (age 1-9 yr.; WBC <50,000)
Favorable trisomies 4, 10, 17
DNA index >1.16
Rapid early responder (RER)
No adverse translocations *(MLL, BCR/ABL, E2A-PBX-1)*
No CNS-3 or testicular involvement
TEL/AML-1 (awaiting intense review)

HIGH RISK DEFINITIONS
NCI consensus (age >10 yr; WBC >50,000/mm^3)
Does not have trisomies 4, 10, 17
Standard risk—slow early responder (SER)
MLL rearrangement

VERY HIGH RISK DEFINITIONS
t(9;22) *BCR/ABL*
Hypodiploidy (<45 chromosomes)
DNA index <0.95
Induction failure

---

with a seven-drug regimen including methotrexate, cytarabine, ifosfamide, and etoposide had a cure rate of 85%.[86] Children with mature B-cell ALL and Burkitt's lymphoma will be treated on the same protocol in C.O.G. using a very intense regimen of fractionated high-dose cyclophosphamide, high-dose methotrexate, and cytarabine (+/− ifosfamide, etoposide).[72,97]

Pediatric oncologists have treated children with T-cell ALL on the same regimens as B-cell precursor ALL or as high stage T-cell NHL. Several studies have demonstrated that patients with T-cell ALL can be successfully treated on the same protocol as B-cell precursor ALL when agents and schedules previously demonstrated to be effective for T-cell ALL are administered, such as methotrexate at doses greater than 5 g/m^2, anthracyclines, cytarabine, and cyclophosphamide.[77,138] A specific T-cell MoAb is being investigated in a current pilot study. If successful, it may be included in future T-cell protocols.

A variety of treatment regimens for infant ALL have been tested, generally yielding EFS rates of 20% to 35%.[9] More recent clinical trials have used high-dose methotrexate, high-dose cytarabine, and intensive consolidation/reinduction therapy. These

TABLE 19-5	COMMONLY USED AGENTS FOR THE TREATMENT OF CHILDHOOD ALL
Treatment Phase	**Potential Agents**
Induction	Vincristine
	Prednisone or dexamethasone
	Asparaginase (*E. coli,* Erwinia, or PEG)
	Daunorubicin or doxorubicin
Intensification or consolidation	Methotrexate
	6-mercaptopurine or 6-thioguanine
	Vincristine
	Prednisone or dexamethasone
	Asparaginase (*E. coli,* Erwinia, or PEG)
	Daunorubicin or doxorubicin
	Cyclophosphamide
	Cytarabine
Maintenance	Methotrexate
	6-mercaptopurine
	Vincristine
	Prednisone or dexamethasone

From Bleyer, W. A. (2000). Therapy of cancer in children. Continuing Medical Education, M. D. Anderson Cancer Center, Houston, TX.
PEG, Polyethylene glycol.

trials appear to have improved clinical outcomes, but only a small number of patients have been enrolled.[24,103,124] Both cooperative groups (CCG, POG) shared a common induction, intensification, and reinduction, but differed in the use of high-dose methotrexate and 1 versus 2 years of treatment. There was a high early morbidity/mortality rate, especially in infants less than 3 months of age, thought to be due to the combined use of dexamethasone and anthracycline during induction.[24] New strategies are needed for treating infant ALL that balance the need for the intense therapy required to treat this high-risk disease with prevention of the morbidity and mortality associated with treating young infants with intense chemotherapy.

The successful treatment of children with ALL requires systemic combination chemotherapy, including treatment of sanctuary sites, particularly the CNS. ALL treatment regimens involve four main components: remission induction, consolidation or intensification, maintenance therapy, and CNS sanctuary therapy generally given throughout therapy. Table 19-5 lists the commonly used agents for the treatment of childhood ALL. Therapy typically lasts between 2 and 3 years. Clinical trials have shown that when therapy is continued beyond 3 years, there was no proven survival advantage.[18,73]

CNS TREATMENT

The importance of treating the CNS to prevent the development of meningeal leukemia has been recognized since the mid-1960s.[3,4] Preventive CNS therapy is based on the premise that the CNS pro-

vides a sanctuary site in which leukemic cells, undetected at diagnosis, reside protected from the action of systemic chemotherapy by the blood-brain barrier.[72] Treatment of subclinical CNS leukemia is essential to increase the chance of cure and reduce the morbidity resulting from CNS relapse and the need for consequent intensive therapy.[97] Although only 3% of patients have detectable CNS involvement at diagnosis ($\geq$5 WBC/mm^3 with lymphoblasts present, also known as CNS 3), 50% or more of children will eventually develop overt CNS leukemia unless specific therapy, such as intrathecal medication, cranial irradiation, and high-dose systemic chemotherapy with methotrexate or cytarabine, is directed toward the CNS. Accordingly, all children with ALL receive some form of CNS prophylaxis. Patients with documented CNS leukemia at diagnosis receive intrathecal therapy followed by cranial radiation with or without spinal radiation.[79] Some patients are noted to have blasts present in the spinal fluid, but have less than 5 WBC/mm^3. These patients are classified into the CNS 2 category. When this occurs at diagnosis, most protocols include weekly intrathecal doses during induction, without changes in subsequent treatment.

Clinical trial efforts have been directed toward discerning which CNS therapy is most effective, least toxic, and most appropriate for each risk group. In the 1970s cranial irradiation at a dose of 24 Gy plus intrathecally (IT) administered methotrexate, given after the induction of complete remission, was the cornerstone of ALL therapy.[97] Concerns about the adverse late effects of this approach, including altered neurocognitive and neuroendocrine function, and efforts to improve CNS disease control led to treatment modifications and new strategies of CNS-directed treatment.[91] CCG investigators found that 18 Gy cranial irradiation plus IT methotrexate was as effective as 24 Gy craniospinal irradiation or 24 Gy cranial irradiation plus IT methotrexate,[82] and that improved results were obtained with IT doses based on age-specific CSF volumes rather than body surface area.[12] POG investigators showed that triple IT treatment with methotrexate, hydrocortisone, and cytarabine, along with effective systemic chemotherapy, yielded results comparable to those produced by cranial irradiation.[131]

More recent investigations have demonstrated that intensive IT therapy given early during the remission induction and consolidation periods, and continued into the continuation phase, is effective therapy for subclinical CNS leukemia, even for patients with intermediate-risk ALL.[20,76,99,136] Cranial radiation is reserved for patients with overt CNS leukemia or those at high risk for CNS relapse, such as in T-cell leukemia with presenting leukocyte counts greater than 100,000/mm^3.[97] The current view is that cranial irradiation may not be necessary in up to 85% of patients with ALL.[21,76,99,135]

INDUCTION

The goal of induction therapy is to achieve a complete remission within 4 weeks and reestablish normal hematopoiesis as quickly as possible.[11] Remission is defined as the absence of clinical signs of disease, a reduction of lymphoblasts in the bone marrow to less than 5% with normal cellularity (M1) and near normal peripheral blood values. A three-drug regimen using vincristine, dexamethasone or prednisone, and asparaginase (native *E. coli*/polyethylene glycol [PEG]) in conjunction with IT chemotherapy results in complete remission rates greater than 95%.[98] An anthracycline is added to the three-drug regimen for high-risk patients.

Recent data suggest that the substitution of dexamethasone for prednisone in children 1 to 9 years of age significantly reduced the risk of CNS relapse because of an increased penetration into cerebrospinal fluid and longer half-life when used in induction and continuation regimens.[14,98] Dexamethasone use in adolescents has been associated with an increased incidence of steroid-induced aseptic necrosis.[83] Further study is needed in this age-group to refine optimal steroid recommendations.

There are several forms of asparaginase. Native *(E. coli)* is most commonly used. PEG-asparaginase (polyethylene glycol) has a longer half-life and appears to maintain adequate asparaginase activity for up to 21 days in patients not previously exposed to native asparaginase. PEG requires a single intramuscular dose compared with 6 to 9 doses of native asparaginase.[50] A recent report suggests that PEG-asparaginase may facilitate a more rapid response to induction therapy.[50]

Previous studies have defined early marrow response as an important prognostic indicator for children with ALL. A rapid early response (RER) to induction therapy (<5% blasts in the bone marrow at day 7 of induction) was a significant favorable prognostic factor among all risk groups.[32,130] Poor outcome was generally observed for patients of all risk groups who had a slow early response (SER), defined as M3 marrow status (>25% blasts) at either day 7 or day 14 of induction therapy.[32,78] Low- or standard-risk patients with M3 marrow status at day 14 of induction had a 3.4-fold higher risk of treatment failure compared with patients who achieve M1 (<5% blasts) by day 14.[32] Failure of induction therapy occurs in less than 5% of patients with current regimens, defined as M3 (>25% blasts on day 28). Improved supportive care (transfusions, antibiotics, and prevention of acute metabolic complications) has decreased the mortality rate to less than 3% during induction therapy.[72,97] Although greater than 95% of children will achieve complete remission within 4 weeks, they still harbor as many as 1×10^{10} leukemia cells, as illustrated in Figure 19-4. Therefore continued therapy is required.[72,97]

CONSOLIDATION

Consolidation/intensification therapy is given to strengthen remission and give direct treatment to CNS and sanctuary sites. The intensity of post-induction chemotherapy varies per patient risk group, but all involve systemic treatment for the CNS. Chemotherapy agents used during this phase may include cyclophosphamide, cytarabine, weekly IT methotrexate, asparaginase, IV methotrexate, mercaptopurine, thioguanine, and epipodophyllotoxins.

Some treatment regimens use an "interim maintenance" phase that follows consolidation. This "interim maintenance" phase uses intermediate-dose (100 mg/m^2 up to 1000 mg/m^2) methotrexate with vincristine, asparaginase, and prednisone. Several protocols use the Berlin-Frankfurt-Munster (BFM) regimen, following interim maintenance with delayed intensification (DI). This phase is given to eradicate residual or resistant leukemia and improve the outcome for children with standard-risk ALL.[10,108,135,142] The delayed intensification phase is an anthracycline-based (reinduction) regi-

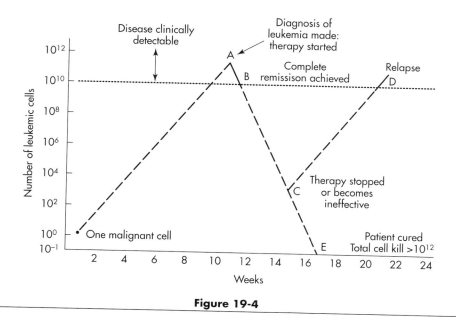

Figure 19-4

Schematic representation of the results of therapy in a patient with leukemia.   (Adapted from Valeriote, F., & Vietti, T. J. Cellular kinetics and conceptual basis of chemotherapy. In W. W. Sutow, T. J. Vietti, D. J. Fernback (Eds.), *Clinical pediatric oncology.* St. Louis, MO: CV Mosby.)

men and a cyclophosphamide-containing (reconsolidation) regimen that occurs approximately 3 to 4 months after remission induction. High-risk patients receive augmented BFM therapy that includes two courses of DI, with intensified repeated courses of IV methotrexate (without leucovorin) given with vincristine and asparaginase.[72,97] This consolidation/intensification phase lasts 20 to 28 weeks before maintenance therapy begins. The agents and schedule appear in Table 19-6. This treatment approach is under current review for future C.O.G. trials.

MAINTENANCE

Maintenance therapy is designed to provide a prolonged period of continuation therapy to eliminate all residual leukemia cells. The backbone of maintenance therapy is based on continuous antimetabolite therapy. This includes daily doses of oral mercaptopurine or thioguanine and weekly doses of methotrexate. Dosing methotrexate and mercaptopurine to the limit of tolerance (low leukocyte count) has been associated with improved clinical outcome.[18,98] Intermittent pulses of vincristine and dexamethasone or prednisone with the antimetabolite therapy are often used in maintenance and are associated with a reduced incidence of relapse.[18]

New discoveries have been made regarding antimetabolite pharmacokinetics. Oral mercapto-

purine and methotrexate given in the evening may improve EFS.[117] Children with inherited deficiency of thiopurine S-methyltransferase (TPMT), an enzyme that inactivates mercaptopurine, thioguanine, or azathioprine, require lower-than-standard doses (50-75 mg/m^2/day) than those conventionally used. Patients that are TPMT-deficient accumulate excessive thioguanine metabolites in hematopoietic tissues, which leads to severe and possibly fatal myelosuppression.[145] The diagnosis of TPMT deficiency can be made by polymerase chain reaction (PCR)-based methods on approximately 100 μl of whole blood, to prospectively identify patients who require a reduction in thiopurine doses to avoid life-threatening hematopoietic toxicity.[145]

Treatment assignment for specific patient populations is based on the risk for treatment failure. Several methods of risk-based treatment are currently undergoing intense clinical investigation. Subgroups of patients who have a poor prognosis, infants with *MLL* gene rearrangement t(4;11) and children with the Philadelphia chromosome t(9;22), need intensive chemotherapy and allogeneic HSCT in first remission.[2] High doses of methotrexate (5 g/m^2) may improve outcomes of T-cell ALL.[103] Augmented BFM therapy may be useful for patients with high-risk clinical characteristics.[78,103,112] The use of granulocyte colony stimulating factor (G-CSF) can shorten hospital

TABLE 19-6	BERLIN-FRANKFURT-MUNSTER (BFM) REGIMEN
Delayed Intensification (DI) Phase	
Vincristine	Days 0, 7, 14, 42, 49
Dexamethasone	Days 0-6, 14-20
PEG asparaginase	Days 3, 42
Doxorubicin	Days 0, 7, 14
Cyclophosphamide	Day 28
6-thioguanine	Days 28-41
Cytarabine	Days 28-31, 35-38
Methotrexate (IT)	Days 0, 28
Interim Maintenance	
Methotrexate escalating dose	Days 0, 10, 20, 30, 40
Vincristine	Days 1, 10
PEG-asparaginase	Days 1, 21
Methotrexate (IT)	Days 0, 30
Augmented BFM—High Risk Patients	

Induction
(Days 14-35)
↓
Consolidation
(9 weeks)
↓
Interim Maintenance 1
(2 months)
↓
Delayed Intensification
(2 months)
↓
Interim Maintenance 2
(2 months)
↓
Delayed Maintenance 2
(2 months)
↓
Maintenance

Data from Children's Cancer Group BFM protocols.
PEG, Polyethylene glycol; *IT,* intrathecal.

days for febrile neutropenia after remission induction or intensive therapy, but does not improve EFS.[65,94]

In theory, cancer chemotherapy would be curative if early treatment were sufficient to eradicate malignant cells before they acquire drug resistance. Age, immunophenotype, and cytogenetic rearrangements reflect or cause differences in drug-resistance factors. Future trials will continue to test these hypotheses to further refine classification and treatment to improve outcomes for childhood ALL.

RELAPSE/RECURRENT DISEASE

A better understanding of patient-specific risk factors is needed to design effective initial therapy to prevent relapse. The poor drug sensitivity of leukemia cells early in the clinical course as demonstrated at the day 7 or 14 bone marrow results and detection of minimal residual disease (MRD) after induction and consolidation are associated with an increased risk of subsequent relapse.[31,141] Technological advances, including PCR analyses and flow cytometry, have enabled detection of MRD during complete remission (less than 5% blasts in the bone marrow).[31,123] Several clinical trials monitor patients with ALL for MRD by both flow cytometry and PCR during treatment. In one study, patients previously considered low-risk by presenting features who had evidence of leukemic blasts and MRD greater than or equal to 10^{-4} by flow cytometry or PCR amplification after 6 weeks of induction therapy were assigned to receive augmented therapy similar to other high-risk patients.[17,123]

Bone marrow is the most common site of relapse in ALL. Current approach to therapy suggests that allogeneic HSCT is the treatment of choice for patients who develop hematologic relapse during front-line therapy or within 6 months of therapy. These patients, as well as patients with relapsed T-cell ALL, have approximately a 10% to 20% likelihood of long-term survival. However, if relapse occurs more than 1 year after discontinuing initial therapy, approximately 40% to 65% long-term disease-free survival is achieved with aggressive salvage chemotherapy.[33,74,111,139] The frequency of CNS or testicular relapse has decreased to less than 5% with effective CNS-directed and systemic therapy.[96] About two thirds of patients with isolated CNS relapse without prior CNS irradiation can achieve a second complete long-term remission with aggressive systemic and IT therapy combined with craniospinal irradiation. The 5-year disease-free survival rate drops from approximately 70% to 10% to 30% with prior irradiation exposure.[56,107,110]

Historically, only one third of patients with early testicular relapse, and two thirds who relapse after completion of therapy, became long-term survivors with salvage chemotherapy and bilateral testicular irradiation. It is unknown if modern intensive chemotherapy will change overall incidence and retrieval. New studies are evaluating the use of very-high-dose methotrexate (>12 g/m^2) instead of radiotherapy.[28,143]

Children who experience repeated relapses have a difficult time being reinduced into clinical remission. Length of remission decreases with each relapse, most likely because of the development of drug resistance in the leukemic cells. Careful cytochemical, immunophenotypic, and cytogenetic studies are necessary at time of relapse to determine lymphoblast characteristics and to evaluate for the possibility of therapy-induced AML. Children treated with epipodophyllotoxins have a cumulative risk of AML of 3.8% at 6 years.[34] The risk of second malignancy in children with ALL is 1/500 per year and includes secondary leukemia and CNS tumors.[34,80,122] The trend toward intensifying already aggressive therapy may reach a point where the benefits are outweighed by the damage to normal tissues.[92]

LATE EFFECTS

Each year approximately 1500 children with ALL in the United States become long-term survivors. Intensification of ALL treatment has significantly improved cure rates during the past 30 years. Long-term effects specifically associated with ALL therapies are: (1) cardiomyopathy associated with anthracycline use (especially in young girls and in patients with high cumulative doses)[64]; (2) brain tumors, thyroid cancer, neuropsychologic deficits, and endocrine dysfunction (obesity, short stature, precocious puberty, osteoporosis) after CNS irradiation[80,106]; (3) AML after intense treatment with epipodophyllotoxins (related to treatment schedule and concomitant use of other drugs)[100]; and (4) osteopenia and avascular necrosis of bone after extensive use of steroids and methotrexate.[44] Therapy changes that have had a significant impact on the development of long-term effects in the past 30 years include: (1) reduction of prophylactic cranial irradiation from 24 Gy to 18 Gy, with many children receiving IT therapy only; (2) increased use of dexamethasone, anthracyclines, cyclophosphamide, and etoposide; (3) reduction of treatment duration from 5 years to 2 to 3 years; and (4) more intensive therapy together with allogeneic HSCT in children with very high-risk, recurrent, or refractory ALL.[122]

PROGNOSIS

A number of clinical and laboratory features predict outcome of children with ALL. These prognostic factors (see Table 19-4) include initial WBC count, age, presence of cytogenetic abnormalities in the lymphoblasts, and response to therapy. Current approach to therapy is based on the child's risk of relapse.

Those children defined as having good-risk ALL are between 1 and 9 years of age, have an initial WBC count less than 50,000,[126] have t(12;21),

have hyperdiploidy (>50 chromosomes or DNA index >1.16), and achieve an M1 marrow by day 7 or 14.[32,61,130] These children have an EFS rate of greater than 80%.[128] High-risk patients include infants (<1 year), age greater than 10 years, WBC count greater than 50,000,[126] presence of *MLL* rearrangement,[9] and/or an M2/M3 marrow on day 7 or 14.[23,24] The EFS rate for high-risk ALL is approximately 65%.[128] A new category recently defined by the C.O.G., very-high–risk ALL, includes patients with one of the following: Philadelphia chromosome t(9;22), hypodiploidy (<45 chromosomes), DNA index less than 0.95, and induction failure (see Box 19-2). Subgroups of patients such as infants with t(4;11) and *MLL* rearrangement and children with t(9;22) require intensive chemotherapy to control the disease, followed by an HLA-matched, related donor HSCT if possible.[2,9] The prognostic significance of CNS disease at time of diagnosis, presence of *TEL/AML* rearrangement,[13,121] and trisomies 4,10,17[121] continue to be studied. The negative prognostic impact of CNS disease at diagnosis may diminish with the use of intensive systemic and CNS-directed therapy.[76,77]

As treatment regimens improve, various biologic and clinical indicators may decrease in their importance. For example, T-cell and B-cell ALL, once associated with a very poor prognosis, now have a long-term disease-free survival rate of 70% to 85% with use of intensive chemotherapy.[1,77,116] Many of the improvements in therapy that have led to improved survival rates for children with ALL have been made through nationwide clinical trials.[11]

NURSING IMPLICATIONS

The care of the child and family experiencing childhood ALL presents nurses with considerable challenges and rewards. It is indeed a privilege to walk beside these children and their families as they follow the path that unwinds before them. Nurses bring to the pediatric oncology care team not only their clinical knowledge and expertise but also a particular sensitivity and regard for the day-to-day needs, concerns, and lived experience of those for whom they care. Nurses play an important role in assisting children and families to acquire the knowledge and skills that will be required of them and in providing the support that is essential to them along their journey. Key components of the nursing role are discussed below.

CORE NURSING STRATEGIES

Hinds and Gattuso have identified five essential strategies pediatric oncology nurses use in caring for children with leukemia and their families.[49]

These include (1) patient and family education, (2) providing a supportive presence, (3) actively monitoring and anticipating, (4) being technically competent, and (5) serving as an advocate for patients and families. These strategies are framed within an interactive model that specifies three environmental spheres or levels of influence and operation in which patient needs, responses, and outcomes can be assessed and understood, and on which nursing care is focused. These include (1) the internal environment, representing the patient's genetic, physical, and psychologic characteristics; (2) the intermediate environment, representing the influence of family members and health care providers on the patient's response to the care provided; and (3) the institutional level, representing the influence of health care and social systems and broader society as a whole.

Hinds and Gattuso's framework specifies seven distinct phases in the care of children with ALL and their families (Table 19-7). As nurses provide care across this continuum, they can inquire thoughtfully within the environmental levels to determine appropriate strategies that are tailored to the unique circumstances of each patient and family for whom they care and to the particular treatment phase involved. For example, Table 19-7 identifies relevant patient and family education content appropriate to each possible phase of care. This content, however, reflects more than pertinent educational focus areas; indeed, it represents a comprehensive overview of the illness-related demands in ALL for which pediatric oncology nurses implement the essential nursing strategies identified. The discussion below highlights several key focus areas in the care of children with ALL and their families. A number of these are addressed in detail in Part III (Supportive Care) of this text.

MYELOSUPPRESSION

Children with ALL are at risk for potentially life-threatening effects of bone marrow suppression as a result of their disease and its treatment. Signs and symptoms of neutropenia, anemia, and thrombocytopenia frequently are present at diagnosis, reflecting the degree to which leukemic lymphoblasts have infiltrated the bone marrow. In addition, these conditions often develop as a consequence of chemotherapy and radiation treatment. As such, their management is necessary across the continuum of ALL care and requires ongoing nursing vigilance to detect early signs of sepsis, bleeding, and compromised cardiovascular status that is anemia-related. Skills in complicated central venous catheter (CVC) management involving administration of blood products and complex medication regimens are also necessary. In addition, it is criti-

cal that nurses provide patients and families with the education and support they need to monitor for signs of myelosuppression, as well as with clear information about how, when, and for what reasons they are to contact the health care team. Education about infection prevention and safety measures (such as careful hand washing, proper central venous line care, oral hygiene, and avoidance of high-risk activities) is very important in helping children and families reduce the risk of adverse events and maximize well-being.

MANAGEMENT OF TREATMENT SIDE EFFECTS

Children receiving treatment for ALL may experience a number of nonmyelosuppressive side effects. During induction, the metabolic breakdown of leukemic cells may result in tumor lysis syndrome. Careful monitoring of fluid and electrolyte status, aggressive hydration, and administration of allopurinol or other uric acid–reducing therapy are required. Procedural pain related to bone marrow aspirations, lumbar punctures, venous access, and intramuscular injections requires that nurses implement pharmacologic and nonpharmacologic measures, such as topical anesthetics, procedural sedation, and distraction and relaxation, to minimize children's distress. It is essential that atraumatic care begin with initial procedures to avoid the development of conditioned negative responses.

Antiemetic therapy is readily administered to prevent the occurrence or reduce the distress associated with chemotherapy-induced nausea and vomiting often related to cyclophosphamide, anthracycline, cytarabine, or intrathecal therapy. Nutritional guidance to avoid or reduce foods high in salt, sugar, and fat is important for a healthy diet and to help minimize weight gain, possible hypertension, and/or hyperglycemia that may develop as a result of steroid stimulation of excessive appetite. Although not permanent, changes in body appearance related to weight gain and moon facies, as well as chemotherapy-induced alopecia, may trigger considerable distress for both the child and family. The provision of supportive listening and information about wigs, hats, and scarves, as well as affirmation of positive personal characteristics, is important in reducing this distress. The neurotoxicity associated with vincristine may cause constipation, requiring dietary and pharmacologic intervention. Rectal interventions are avoided because of the potential for infection and bleeding. Ongoing assessment for peripheral neuropathies, including tingling in digits, decreased deep tendon reflexes, and difficulty walking, is important to determine whether vincristine dose reduction and physical and occupational therapy are indicated.

PSYCHOSOCIAL CARE

The psychosocial impact of the ALL experience on children and families begins from the first suspicion that the child has a serious illness. As the nature of that illness is determined and treatment is initiated, children and families must confront a number of difficult tasks and challenges as they move through the experience. A key component of their experience involves uncertainty—not knowing what lies before them, what is expected of them, how they will deal with the demands of the illness, how they will manage everything else in their life in the face of the illness. The illness triggers a life transition.[19,119] Their present reality is fractured, and they must reconstruct a new reality that integrates the ALL experience, with the desired outcome of emerging from the experience as whole and intact.

Essential coping tasks of the child and family in the various phases of the cancer experience, along with related nursing interventions, have been identified[46] and are discussed in Chapter 15 of this text. The normal developmental tasks of the child and family also must be taken into account.[51-53,68,69] A particular aspect of ALL is the long-term nature of the treatment. Children and families face several years of active treatment in which the experience intrudes upon their lives. Although the intensity of treatment diminishes across time, routine outpatient care and the occurrence or possibility of untoward events requiring hospitalization, such as episodes of fever and neutropenia, pertain across the continuum of treatment and must be integrated within daily life. When the experience involves the occurrence of relapse or the eventual determination of irreversible treatment failure, present reality is again shattered and must be reconstructed in the light of such grave developments.

Nurses have a crucial role in educating and supporting children with ALL and their families. They need to carefully assess the unique needs and abilities of each child and family in order to determine appropriate teaching strategies and tools that will support their learning.[57] Basic disease and treatment information must be provided, as well as guidance about infection risk reduction and other safety measures. Treatment protocols and roadmaps, medication side effects, and "when to call" directives need to be reviewed regularly, along with instructions about medication schedules and home CVC care. In addition, information about the responses of others to the ALL experience may be helpful in normalizing the experience. The awareness that others have successfully faced the same situation and endured, and have shared similar responses with them, can be reassuring and comforting. For this same reason, child and parent peer support contacts can be very meaningful and should be explored and encouraged if agreeable to those involved.

Successful treatment of childhood ALL cannot occur without the cooperation and involvement of the child and family.[58] The creation of a therapeutic alliance with the child and family is essential. Through their supportive presence,[49] nurses convey a nonjudgmental regard for patients and families, provide a safe "listening" for their expression of feelings and fears, and are attuned to their lived experience. This enables nurses to appreciate the demands of the situation and explore approaches to problems, as well as the meaning made of the experience. Nurses are in a unique position to assess and support the coping responses of patients and families, by virtue of their frequent interaction over the long course of ALL treatment.

FUTURE DIRECTIONS

Dramatic treatment advances have been achieved in childhood ALL over the past 50 years with 80% to 85% EFS. However, 15% to 20% of these children relapse and die. Present and future challenges to ensure improved survival rates for all children with ALL include: (1) understanding of the genetic susceptibility of childhood ALL, which may lead to intervention and preventive measures; (2) identifying specific risk-directed treatment for biologically defined subgroups of ALL; (3) understanding individual variations in pharmacokinetics or pharmacodynamics of antileukemic agents; (4) providing reliable in vitro information regarding chemosensitivity of leukemic cells; (5) improving detection of MRD; (6) developing strategies to circumvent drug resistance; (7) overcoming acute and long-term toxicity of current therapy; (8) using immunotherapy to enhance antileukemic effect during HSCT; (9) using antibodies and molecular-based purging techniques to increase the role for autologous HSCT; and (10) monitoring compliance with oral chemotherapeutic agents.[72,93,98,114]

The new "genome prospecting" using DNA microarray technology can quantitate expression of approximately 6800 human genes. This provides a new tool for diagnosis and generates an undetermined amount of new information of unknown clinical significance. When this technology is applied to normal B-cell precursors, the beginning of a complete "fingerprint" of comparative gene expression will serve as a database to help us understand the regulation of cell function in normal and abnormal B-cell development.[37,60,101]

Numerous important biologic and therapeutic

TABLE 19-7 TOPICS FOR INCLUSION IN PATIENT AND FAMILY EDUCATION EFFORTS, BY PHASE OF CARE

Content Area	Diagnosis/Induction	Consolidation/Intensification	Continuation	Hematopoietic Stem Cell Transplantation	Completion of Therapy	Recurrence	Terminal Care
Disease process	Diagnosis defined Causes Incidence	Bone marrow function Response to treatment		Ablative therapy Engraftment of donor marrow	Follow-up importance	Diagnosis defined Prognosis	Progressive disease symptoms described
Diagnostic procedures	BMA, LP Venipuncture Laboratory tests X-rays		Periodic BMA, LP		Physical exams Diagnostic imaging Laboratory tests		
Treatment protocol	Sedation/conscious sedation Meaning of protocol Roadmap/schema Informed consent			Type of transplant defined Preparative regimen Informed consent	Health promotion Well child care	Roadmap/schema Clinical trials/experimental agents Best clinical management Informed consent	Palliative care
Treatment devices/modalities	Surgery Antineoplastic agents Intrathecal therapy	Radiation therapy Antibiotics	Venous access device	Total body irradiation High-dose chemotherapy		Biological agents	Infusion devices
Symptom management	Fever Blood counts Neutropenia Infection prevention Pain control Blood products	Nutrition Anorexia Constipation Diarrhea Nausea/vomiting Mucositis Skin care	Pheresis Rehabilitation	Dry mouth Pain Graft vs. host disease	Height/weight History (e.g., school or social problems)	Pain control	Pain control Nutrition Anorexia Elimination Skin care Parental fatigue

Psychosocial issues	Hopefulness Employment (parental)	Loneliness Impact on siblings Coping strategies Reaction of peers	Establishing routines Family relationships Sexuality Late effects Body image	Isolation Hopefulness Anxiety Irregular school attendance	Fertility Growth/development Insurability School success Late effects	Monitoring Preparing Fears Grieving	Decision-making Do not resuscitate status Grieving Emotional withdrawal
Treatment setting/staff	Introduction of staff/roles Telephone contacts Maps Routines of care setting	Support groups Educational and supportive resources	Introduction of staff/roles	Introduction of staff/roles	Continued access to staff/roles		Introduction of hospice/home care staff and roles Telephone contacts Continued access to hospital staff

From Hinds, P. S., & Gattuso, J. S. (1999). Nursing care. In C.-H. Pui (Ed.), *Childhood leukemias* (pp. 542-552). New York: Cambridge University Press.

BMA, Bone marrow aspiration; *LP*, lumbar puncture.

questions remain to be answered. Scientists and researchers are currently investigating arabinosyl-guanine use in T-cell ALL patients,[97] the use of interleukin-4,[71] tyrosine kinase inhibitors,[137] immunotoxins,[140] tumor-specific cytolytic cells for targeted immunotherapy,[45] cell-permeable small molecules designed to inhibit the transcription of specific genes,[38] antisense oligonucleotides or ribozyme to disrupt oncogene expression, and the introduction of genes encoding cytokines and human leukocyte antigens that could induce immune responses against leukemic cells.[15] It is now known that ALL is angiogenic, so the use of antiangiogenic drugs may be effective in this disease.[87]

Clinical trials represent the best standard of care. There are currently approximately 40% of children with cancer who are not enrolled in clinical trials, especially in the subgroup of 15- to 19-year-old adolescents.[132] Until every child with ALL is cured, all children throughout the world, including teenagers, must be enrolled in research-based clinical trials. These children and their families will need competent, skilled, compassionate pediatric oncology nurses who can walk beside them on their journey of childhood leukemia.

REFERENCES

1. Arico, M., Basso, G., Mandelli, F., et al., for the Associazione Italiana Ematologia Oncologia Pediatrica (AIEOP). (1995). Good steroid response in vivo predicts a favorable outcome in children with T-cell acute lymphoblastic leukemia. *Cancer, 75,* 1684-1693.
2. Arico, M., Valsecchi, M. G., Camitta, B., et al. (2000). Outcome of treatment in children with Philadelphia chromosome-positive acute lymphoblastic leukemia. *New England Journal of Medicine, 342,* 998-1006.
3. Aur, R. J. A., Hustu, H. O., Verzosa, M. S., et al. (1973). Comparison of two methods of preventing central nervous system leukemia. *Blood, 42,* 349-357.
4. Aur, R. J. A., Simone, J., Hustu, H. O., et al. (1971). Central nervous system therapy and combination chemotherapy of childhood lymphocytic leukemia. *Blood, 37,* 272-281.
5. Bader, J. L., & Miller, R. W. (1978). Neurofibromatosis and childhood leukemia. *Journal of Pediatrics, 92,* 925-929.
6. Behm, F. G., & Campana, D. (1999). Immunophenotyping. In C-H. Pui (Ed.), *Childhood leukemias* (pp. 111-144). New York: Cambridge University Press.
7. Berman, E. (2000). Recent advances in the treatment of acute lymphoblastic leukemia. *Current Opinions in Hematology, 7,* 205-211.
8. Bhatia, S., Ross, J. A., Greaves, M. F., et al. (1999). Epidemiology and etiology. In C-H. Pui (Ed.), *Childhood leukemias* (pp. 38-49). New York: Cambridge University Press.
9. Biondi, A., Cimino, G., Pieters, R., et al. (2000). Biological and therapeutic aspects of infant leukemia. *Blood, 96,* 24-33.
10. Bleyer, W. A. (1990). Acute lymphoblastic leukemia in children: Advances and prospectus. *Cancer, 65,* 689-695.
11. Bleyer, W. A. (2000). Acute lymphoblastic leukemia. In C. E. Herzog & C. B. Pratt (Cochairs), *Therapy of cancer in children* (pp. 9-10). Houston: The University of Texas M. D. Anderson Cancer Center.
12. Bleyer, W. A., Coccia, P. F., Sather, H. N., et al. (1983). Reduction in central nervous system leukemia with a pharmacokinetically derived intrathecal methotrexate dosage regimen. *Journal of Clinical Oncology, 1,* 317-325.
13. Borkhardt, A., Harbott, J., & Lampert, F. (1999). Biology and clinical significance of the TEL/AML 1 rearrangement. *Current Opinions in Pediatrics, 11,* 33-43.
14. Bostram, B., Gaynon, P. S., Sather, H., et al (1998). Dexamethasone (DEX) decreases central nervous system (CNS) relapse and improves event-free survival (EFS) in lower risk acute lymphoblastic leukemia (ALL). *Proceedings of the American Society of Clinical Oncology, 17,* 527A.
15. Braun, S. E., Chen, K., Battiwalla, M., et al. (1997). Gene therapy strategies for leukemia. *Molecular Medicine Today, 3,* 39-46.
16. Burchenal, J. H., Murphy, M. L., Ellison, R. R., et al. (1953). Clinical evaluation of a new anti-metabolite, 6-mercaptopurine, in treatment of leukemia and allied diseases. *Blood, 8,* 965-999.
17. Campana, D., VanDongen, J. S., & Pui, C-H. (1999). Minimal residual disease. In C-H. Pui (Ed.), *Childhood leukemias* (pp. 413-439). New York: Cambridge University Press.
18. Childhood ALL Collaborative Group (1996). Duration and intensity of maintenance chemotherapy in acute lymphoblastic leukaemia: Overview of 42 trials involving 12,000 randomized children. *Lancet, 347,* 1783-1788.
19. Clarke-Steffen, L. (1993). A model of the family transition to living with childhood cancer. *Cancer Practice, 1,* 285-292.
20. Conter, V., Arico, M., Valsecchi, M. G. et al. (1995). Extended intrathecal methotrexate may replace cranial irradiation for prevention of CNS relapse in children with intermediate-risk acute lymphoblastic leukemia treated with Berlin-Frankfurt-Munster–based intensive chemotherapy. *Journal of Clinical Oncology, 13,* 2497-2502.
21. Conter, V., Schrappe, M., Arico, M., et al. (1997). Role of cranial radiotherapy for childhood T-cell acute lymphoblastic leukemia with high WBC count and good response to prednisone. *Journal of Clinical Oncology, 15,* 2786-2791.
22. Desch, M. D., & Bleyer, W. A. (1994). Amended long-term trends in cancer incidence rates in children [letter]. *Journal of the National Cancer Institute, 86,* 1481-1482.
23. Dordelmann, M., Harbott, J., Reiter, A., et al. (1999). Prednisolone response is the strongest predictor of treatment outcome in infant acute lymphoblastic leukemia. *Blood, 94,* 1209-1217.
24. Dreyer, Z. E., Steuber, C. P., Bowman, W. P., et al. (1998). High-risk infant ALL—improved survival with intensive chemotherapy. *Proceedings of the American Society of Clinical Oncology, 17,* A-2032, 529a.
25. Farber, S. (1950). The effect of ACTH in acute leukemia in childhood. In J. R. Mote (Ed.), *First clinical ACTH conference* (p. 325). New York: Blakiston.
26. Farber, S., Toch, R., Sears, E. M., et al. (1956). Advances in chemotherapy of cancer in man. *Advances in Cancer Research, 4,* 1-71.
27. Fernbach, D. J., Sutow, W. W., Thurman, W. G., et al. (1962). Clinical evaluation of cyclophosphamide. A new agent for the treatment of children with acute leukemia. *Journal of the American Medical Association, 182,* 30-37.

28. Finkelstein, J., Miller, D., & Feusener, J. (1994). Treatment of overt isolated testicular relapse in children on therapy for acute lymphoblastic leukemia. A report from the Children's Cancer Group. *Cancer, 73,* 219-223.

29. Fong, C. -T., & Brodeur, G. M. (1987). Down syndrome and leukemia: Epidemiology, genetics, cytogenetics, and mechanisms of leukemogenesis. *Cancer Genetics and Cytogenetics, 28,* 55-76.

30. Ford, A. M., Ridge, S. A., McCarthy, K. P., et al. (1993). In utero rearrangements in the trithorax-related oncogene in infant leukemias. *Nature, 363,* 358-360.

31. Foroni, L., Harrison, C. J., Hoffbrand, A. V., et al. (1999). Investigation of minimal residual disease in childhood and adult acute lymphoblastic leukemia by molecular analysis. *British Journal of Haematology, 105,* 7-24.

32. Gaynon, P. S., Desai, A. A., Bostrom, B. C., et al. (1997). Early response to therapy and outcome in childhood acute lymphoblastic leukemia. *Cancer, 80,* 1717-1726.

33. Gaynon, P. S., Qu, R. P., Chappell, R. J., et al. (1998). Survival after relapse in childhood acute lymphoblastic leukemia: Impact of site and time to first relapse—the Children's Cancer Group Experience. *Cancer, 82,* 1387-1395.

34. Geetha, N., Dip, N. B., Lali, V. S., et al. (1999). Late recurrence of childhood acute lymphoblastic leukemia. *American Journal of Clinical Oncology, 22,* 191-192.

35. George, P., Hernandez, K., Hustu, O., et al. (1968). A study of "total therapy" of acute leukemia in children. *Journal of Pediatrics, 72,* 399-408.

36. German, J., Bloom, D., & Passarge, E. (1979). Bloom's syndrome. VII. Progress report for 1978. *Clinical Genetics, 15,* 361-367.

37. Golub, T. R., Slonim, D. K., Tamayo, P., et al. (1999). Molecular classification of cancer: Class discovery and class prediction by gene expression monitoring. *Science, 286,* 531-537.

38. Gottesfeld, J. M., Neely, L., Tranuger, J. W., et al. (1997). Regulation of gene expression by small molecules. *Nature, 387,* 202-205.

39. Greaves, M. (1986). Differentiation-linked leukemogenesis in lymphocytes. *Science, 234,* 697-704.

40. Greaves, M. (1988). Speculations on the cause of childhood acute leukemia. *Leukemia, 2,* 120-125.

41. Greaves, M. (1997). Aetiology of acute leukemia. *Lancet, 349,* 344-349.

42. Greaves, M., & Chan, L. (1986). Is spontaneous mutation the major "cause" of childhood acute lymphoblastic leukemia? *British Journal of Haematology, 64,* 1-13.

43. Greaves, M. F., Colman, S. M., Beard, M. E. J., et al. (1993). Geographic distribution of acute lymphoblastic leukemia subtypes. Second report of the Collaborative Group Study Group. *Leukemia, 7,* 27-34.

44. Hanif, L., Mahmoud, H., & Pui, C-H. (1993). Avascular femoral head necrosis in pediatric cancer patients. *Medical and Pediatric Oncology, 21,* 655-660.

45. Hart, I., & Colaco, C. (1997). Fusion induces tumour rejection. *Nature, 388,* 626-627.

46. Harvey, J. (1998). Family systems. In M. J. Hockenberry-Eaton (Ed.), *Essentials of pediatric oncology nursing: A core curriculum* (pp. 189-193). Glenview, IL: Association of Pediatric Oncology Nurses.

47. Head, D. R., & Pui, C-H. (1999). Diagnosis and classification. In C-H. Pui (Ed.), *Childhood leukemias* (pp. 19-37). New York: Cambridge University Press.

48. Hecht, F., & Hecht, B. K. (1990). Cancer in ataxia-telangiectasia patients. *Cancer Genetics and Cytogenetics, 46,* 9-19.

49. Hinds, P. S., & Gattuso, J. S. (1999). Nursing care. In C-H. Pui (Ed.), *Childhood leukemias* (pp. 542-552). New York: Cambridge University Press.

50. Holcenberg, J., Sencer, S. F., Cohen, L. J., et al. (1999). Randomized trial of PEG-vs-native asparaginase in children with newly diagnosed acute lymphoblastic leukemia (ALL): CCG study 1962. *Blood, 94* (10 pt 1-2), A2790.

51. Hooke, C. (1998). Development of infants (Birth to 1 year). In M. J. Hockenberry-Eaton (Ed.), *Essentials of pediatric oncology nursing: A core curriculum* (p. 182). Glenview, IL: Association of Pediatric Oncology Nurses.

52. Hooke, C. (1998). Development of preschoolers (4-6 years). In M. J. Hockenberry-Eaton (Ed.), *Essentials of pediatric oncology nursing: A core curriculum* (pp. 183-184). Glenview, IL: Association of Pediatric Oncology Nurses.

53. Hooke, C. (1998). Development of toddlers (1-3 years). In M. J. Hockenberry-Eaton (Ed.), *Essentials of pediatric oncology nursing: A core curriculum* (pp. 182-183). Glenview, IL: Association of Pediatric Oncology Nurses.

54. Kanarek, R. (1998). Facing the challenge of childhood leukemia. *American Journal of Nursing, 98* (7), 42-47.

55. Karon, M. R., Freireich, E. J., Frei, E., III. (1962). A preliminary report on vincristine sulfate: A new active agent for the treatment of acute leukemia. *Pediatrics, 30,* 791-796.

56. Kumar, P., Kun, L. E., Hutso, H. O., et al. (1995). Survival outcome following isolated central nervous system relapse treated with additional chemotherapy and craniospinal irradiation in childhood acute lymphoblastic leukemia. *International Journal of Radiation Oncology, Biology, Physics, 31,* 477-483.

57. Landier, W. (1998). Teaching by developmental level. In M. J. Hockenberry-Eaton (Ed.), *Essentials of pediatric oncology nursing: A core curriculum* (pp. 212-215). Glenview, IL: Association of Pediatric Oncology Nurses.

58. Landier, W. (2001). Childhood acute lymphoblastic leukemia: Current perspectives. *Oncology Nursing Forum, 28,* 823-833.

59. Lawrence, J. H. (1940). Nuclear physics and therapy: Preliminary report on a new method for the treatment of leukemia and polycythemia. *Radiology, 35,* 51-60.

60. LeBein, T. W. (2000). Fates of human B-cell precursors. *Blood, 96,* 9-23.

61. Lilleyman, J. S. (1998). Clinical importance of speed of response to therapy in childhood lymphoblastic leukaemia. *Leukemia and Lymphoma, 31,* 501-506.

62. Linet, M. S. (1985). *The leukemias: Epidemiologic aspects.* New York: Oxford University Press.

63. Linet, M. S., Hatch, E. E., Kleinerman, R. A., et al. (1997). Residential exposure to magnetic fields and acute lymphoblastic leukemia in children. *New England Journal of Medicine, 337,* 1-7.

64. Lipshultz, S. E., Lipsitz, S. R., Mone, S. M., et al. (1995). Female sex and drug dose as risk factors for late cardiotoxic effects of doxorubicin therapy for childhood cancer. *New England Journal of Medicine, 332,* 1738-1742.

65. Lishner, M. (2000). Oral antibiotics for febrile patients with neutropenia due to cancer chemotherapy. *New England Journal of Medicine, 342,* 55-58.

66. Lissauer. H. (1865). Zwei falle von leucaemie. Berl Klin Wochenschr, 2, 403-404, as cited in D. Pinkel, (1999), Historical perspective. In C-H. Pui (Ed.), *Childhood leukemias* (pp. 3-18). New York: Cambridge University Press.

67. Look, A. T. (1997). Oncogenic transcription factors in the human acute leukemias. *Science, 278,* 5340, 1059-1064.

68. Madsen, L. (1998). Development of adolescents (13-18). In M. J. Hockenberry-Eaton (Ed.), *Essentials of pediatric oncology nursing: A core curriculum* (pp. 187-189). Glenview, IL: Association of Pediatric Oncology Nurses.

69. Madsen, L. (1998). Development of school-age children (7-12). In M. J. Hockenberry-Eaton (Ed.), *Essentials of pediatric oncology nursing: A core curriculum* (pp. 185-187). Glenview, IL: Association of Pediatric Oncology Nurses.

70. Magrath, I., O'Connor, G., & Ramot, B. (Eds.). (1984). *Pathogenesis of leukemias and lymphomas: Environmental influences.* New York: Raven.

71. Manabe, A., Coustan-Smith, E., Kumagai, M., et al. (1994). Interleukin-4 induces programmed cell death (apoptosis) in cases of high-risk acute lymphoblastic leukemia. *Blood, 83,* 1731-1737.

72. Margolin, J. F., & Poplack, D. G. (1997). Acute lymphoblastic leukemia. In P. A. Pizzo & D. G. Poplack (Eds.), *Principles and practice of pediatric oncology* (3rd ed., pp. 409-462). Philadelphia: Lippincott-Raven.

73. Miller, D. R., Leikin, S., Albo, V., et al. (1989). Three versus five years of maintenance therapy are equivalent in childhood acute lymphoblastic leukemia: A report from the Children's Cancer Study Group. *Journal of Clinical Oncology, 7,* 316-325.

74. Moussalem, M., Esperou, B. H., Devergie, A., et al. (1995). Allogeneic bone marrow transplantation for childhood acute lymphoblastic leukemia in second remission: Factors predictive of survival, relapse and graft-versus-host disease. *Bone Marrow Transplantation, 15,* 943-947.

75. Mulvihill, J. J. (1975). Congenital and genetic diseases. In J. F. Fraumeni (Ed.), *Persons at high risk of cancer* (pp. 3-31). San Diego: Academic Press.

76. Nachman, J., Sather, H. N., Cherlow, J. M., et al. (1998). Response of children with high-risk acute lymphoblastic leukemia treated with and without cranial irradiation: A report from the Children's Cancer Group. *Journal of Clinical Oncology, 16,* 920-930.

77. Nachman, J., Sather, H. N., Gaynon, P. S., et al. (1997). Augmented Berlin-Frankfurt-Munster therapy abrogates the adverse prognostic significance of slow early response to induction chemotherapy for children and adolescents with acute lymphoblastic leukemia and unfavorable presenting features: A report from the Children's Cancer Group. *Journal of Clinical Oncology, 15,* 2222-2230.

78. Nachman, J. B., Sather, H. N., Sensel, M. G., et al. (1998). Augmented post-induction therapy for children with high-risk acute lymphoblastic leukemia and a slow response to initial therapy. *New England Journal of Medicine, 338,* 1663-1667.

79. National Cancer Institute. (2000, July 7). Childhood acute lymphocytic leukemia (PDQ), treatment-health professionals. http://cancernet.nci.nih.gov.

80. Neglia, J. P., Meadows, A. T., Robison, L. L., et al. (1991). Second neoplasm's after acute lymphoblastic leukemia in childhood. *New England Journal of Medicine, 325,* 1330-1336.

81. Neglia, J., & Robison, L. (1988). Epidemiology of the childhood leukemias. *Pediatric Clinics of North America, 35,* 675-692.

82. Nesbit, M. E., Jr., Sather, H. N., Robison, L. L., et al. (1981). Presymptomatic central nervous system therapy in previously untreated childhood acute lymphoblastic leukemia: Comparison of 1800 RAD and 2400 RAD. A report for Children's Cancer Study Group. *Lancet, 1,* 461-466.

83. Ojala, A. E., Lanning, F. P., Paakko, E., et al. (1997). Osteonecrosis in children treated for acute lymphoblastic leukemia: A magnetic resonance imaging study after treatment. *Medical and Pediatric Oncology, 10,* 1787-1794.

84. O'Reilly, R., Pui, C-H., Kernan, N. (1996). NCCN pediatric acute lymphoblastic leukemia practice guidelines. *Oncology, 10,* 1787-1794.

85. Parkin, D. M., Stiller, C. A., Draper, G. J., et al. (1988). The international incidence of childhood cancer. *International Journal of Cancer, 45,* 511-520.

86. Patte, C. (1998). Non-Hodgkin's lymphoma. *European Journal of Cancer, 34,* 359-363.

87. Perez-Atayde, A. R., Sallan, S. E., Tedrow, U., et al. (1997). Spectrum of tumor angiogenesis in the bone marrow of children with acute lymphoblastic leukemia. *American Journal of Pathology, 150,* 815-821.

88. Pinkel, D. (1971). Five-year follow-up of "total therapy" of childhood lymphocytic leukemia. *Journal of the American Medical Association, 216,* 648-652.

89. Pinkel, D. (1987). Curing children of leukemia. *Cancer, 59,* 1683-1691.

90. Pinkel, D. (1999). Historical perspective. In C-H. Pui (Ed.), *Childhood leukemias* (pp. 3-18). New York: Cambridge University Press.

91. Pinkel, D., & Woo, S. (1994). Prevention and treatment of meningeal leukemia in children. *Blood, 84,* 355-366.

92. Pui, C-H. (1995). Childhood leukemias. *New England Journal of Medicine, 332,* 1618-1630.

93. Pui, C-H. (1997). Acute lymphoblastic leukemia. *Pediatric Clinics of North America, 44,* 831-846.

94. Pui, C-H., Boyett, J. M., Hughes, W. T., et al. (1997). Human granulocyte colony-stimulating factor after induction chemotherapy in children with acute lymphoblastic leukemia. *New England Journal of Medicine, 336,* 1781-1787.

95. Pui, C-H., & Crist, W. M. (1994). Biology and treatment of acute lymphoblastic leukemia. *Journal of Pediatrics, 124,* 491-503.

96. Pui, C-H., & Crist, W. M. (1995). Treatment of childhood leukemias. *Current Opinions in Oncology, 7,* 36-44.

97. Pui, C-H., & Crist, W. M. (1999). Acute lymphoblastic leukemia. In C-H. Pui (Ed.), *Childhood leukemias* (pp. 288-312). New York: Cambridge University Press.

98. Pui, C-H., & Evans, W. E. (1998). Acute lymphoblastic leukemia. *The New England Journal of Medicine, 339,* 605-615.

99. Pui, C-H., Mahmoud, H. H., Rivera, G. K., et al. (1998). Early intensification of intrathecal chemotherapy virtually eliminates central nervous system relapse in children with acute lymphoblastic leukemia. *Blood, 92,* 411-415.

100. Pui, C-H., Relling, M. V., Rivera, G. K., et al. (1995). Epipodophyllotoxins-related acute myeloid leukemia: A study of 35 cases. *Leukemia, 9,* 1990-1996.

101. Raetz, E. A., & Carroll, W. L. (2000). Gene expression profiling of childhood leukemia. *Children's Oncology News, 1* (2), 6-11.

102. Raimondi, S. C. (1999). Cytogenetics of acute leukemias. In C-H. Pui (Ed.), *Childhood leukemias* (pp. 168-196). New York: Cambridge University Press.

103. Reaman, G. H., Sposto, R., Sensel, M. G., et al. (1999). Treatment outcome and prognostic factors for infants with lymphoblastic leukemia treated on two consecutive trials of the Children's Cancer Group. *Journal of Clinical Oncology, 17,* 445-455.

104. Reis, A. (1999). Genetics and B-cell leukaemia. *Lancet, 353,* 3.

105. Reiter, A., Schrappe, M., Ludwig, W., et al. (1994). Chemotherapy in 998 unselected childhood acute lymphoblastic leukemia patients: Results and conclusions of the multicenter trial ALL-BFM 86. *Blood, 84,* 3122-3133.

106. Relling, M. V., Rubnitz, J. E., Rivera, G. K., et al. (1999). High incidence of secondary brain tumour after radiotherapy and antimetabolites. *Lancet, 354,* 34-39.

107. Ribeiro, R. C., Rivera, G. K., Hudson, M., et al. (1995). An intensive re-treatment protocol for children with an isolated CNS relapse of acute lymphoblastic leukemia. *Journal of Clinical Oncology, 13,* 333-338.

108. Richards, S., Burrett, J., Hann, I., et al. for the Medical Research Council Working Party on Childhood Leukaemia. (1998). Improved survival with early intensification: Combined results from the Medical Research Council childhood ALL randomized trials, UKALL X and UKALL XI. *Leukemia, 12,* 1031-1036.

109. Ries, L. A. G., Percy, C. L., & Bunin, G. R. (1999). Introduction. In L. A. G. Ries, M. A. Smith, J. G. Gurney, et al. (Eds.), *Cancer incidence and survival among children and adolescents: United States SEER Program 1975-1995* (NIH Publication No. 99-4649, pp. 1-15). Bethesda, MD: National Cancer Institute, SEER Program.

110. Ritchey, A. K., Pollock, B. H., Lauer, S. J., et al. (1999). Improved survival of children with isolated CNS relapse of acute lymphoblastic leukemia: A Pediatric Oncology Group study. *Journal of Clinical Oncology, 17,* 3745-3752.

111. Rivera, G. K., Hudson, M. M., Liu, Q., et al. (1996). Effectiveness of intensified rotational combination chemotherapy for the late hematologic relapse of childhood acute lymphoblastic leukemia. *Blood, 88,* 831-837.

112. Rivera, G.K., Pinkel, D., Simone, J.V., et al. (1993). Treatment of acute lymphoblastic leukemia: 30 years experience at St. Jude Children's Research Hospital. *New England Journal of Medicine, 329,* 1289-1295.

113. Robison, L. L., & Neglia, J. P. (1987). Epidemiology of Down syndrome and childhood acute leukemia. *Progress in Clinical and Biological Research, 246,* 19-32.

114. Rubnitz, J. E., Behm, F. G., Wichlan, D., et al. (1999). Low frequency of TEL/AML 1 in relapsed acute lymphoblastic leukemia supports a favorable prognosis for this genetic subgroup. *Leukemia, 13,* 19-21.

115. Sandler, D. P. (1995). Recent studies in leukemia epidemiology. *Current Opinions in Oncology, 7,* 12-18.

116. Sandlund, J. T., & Magrath, I. T. (1999). B-cell acute lymphoblastic leukemia and Burkitt lymphoma. In C-H. Pui (Ed.), *Childhood leukemias* (pp. 313-321). New York: Cambridge University Press.

117. Schmieglow, K., Glomstein, A., Kristinsson, J., et al. (1997). Impact of morning versus evening schedule for oral methotrexate and 6-mercaptopurine on relapse risk for children with acute lymphoblastic leukemia. *Journal of Pediatric Hematology/Oncology, 19,* 102-109.

118. Schrappe, M., Arico, M., Harbott, J., et al. (1998). Philadelphia chromosome positive (Ph+) childhood acute lymphoblastic leukemia: Good initial steroid response allows early prediction of a favorable treatment outcome. *Blood, 92,* 2730-2741.

119. Selder, F. E. (1989). Life transition theory: The resolution of uncertainty. *Nursing and Health Care, 10,* 436-440, 449-451.

120. Senn, N. (1903). The therapeutic value of the Roentgen ray in the treatment of pseudoleukemia. *New York Medical Journal, 77,* 665-668.

121. Shuster, J. J., Camitta, B. M., Pullen, J., et al. (1999). Identification of newly diagnosed children with acute lymphoblastic leukemia at high risk for relapse. *Cancer Research, Therapy and Control, 9,* 101-107.

122. Shusterman, S., & Meadows, A. T. (2000). Long-term survivors of childhood leukemia. *Current Opinions in Hematology. 7,* 217-222.

123. Sievers, E. L., & Radich, J. P. (2000). Detection of minimal residual disease in acute leukemia. *Current Opinions in Hematology, 7,* 212-216.

124. Silverman, L. B., McLean, T. W., Gelber, R. D., et al. (1997). Intensified therapy for infants with acute lymphoblastic leukemia: Results from the Dana-Farber Cancer Institute Consortium. *Cancer, 80,* 2285-2295.

125. Simone, J. V., & Lyons, J. (1998). The evolution of cancer care for children and adults. *Journal of Clinical Oncology, 16,* 2904-2905.

126. Smith, M., Arthur, D., Camitta, B., et al. (1996). Uniform approach to risk classification and treatment assignment for children with acute lymphoblastic leukemia. *Journal of Clinical Oncology, 14,* 18-24.

127. Smith, M., Chen, T., & Simon, R. (1997). Age-specific incidence of acute lymphoblastic leukemia in U. S. children: In utero initiation model. *Journal of the National Cancer Institute, 89,* 1542-1544.

128. Smith, M. A., Ries, L. A. G., Gurney, J. G., et al. (1999). Leukemia. In L. A. G. Ries, M. A. Smith, J. G. Gurney, et al. (Eds.), *Cancer incidence and survival among children and adolescents: United States SEER Program 1975-1995* (NIH Publication No. 99-4649, pp. 17-34). Bethesda, MD: National Cancer Institute, SEER Program.

129. Smith, M. A., Simon, R., Strickler, H. D., et al. (1998). Evidence that childhood acute lymphoblastic leukemia is associated with an infectious agent linked to hygiene conditions. *Cancer Causes and Control, 9,* 285-298

130. Steinherz, P. G., Gaynon, P. S., Breneman, J. C., et al. (1996). Cytoreduction and prognosis in acute lymphoblastic leukemia—the importance of early marrow response: Report from the Children's Cancer Group. *Journal of Clinical Oncology, 14,* 389-398.

131. Sullivan, M. P., Chen, T., Dyment, P. G., et al. (1982). Equivalence of intrathecal chemotherapy and radiotherapy as central nervous system prophylaxis in children with acute lymphatic leukemia: A Pediatric Oncology Group study. *Blood, 60,* 948-958.

132. Susman, E. (2000). New merged Children's Oncology Group takes first steps. *Oncology Times, 22* (6), 1, 54-56.

133. Taylor, G. M., & Birch, J. M. (1996). The hereditary basis of human leukemia. In E. S. Henderson, T. A. Lister, & M. F. Greaves (Eds.), *Leukemia* (6th ed., pp. 210-245). Philadelphia: W. B. Saunders.

134. Trigg, M. E., Steinherz, P. G., Chapell, R., et al. (2000). Early testicular biopsy in males with acute lymphoblastic leukemia: Lack of impact on subsequent event-free survival. *Journal of Pediatric Hematology Oncology, 22,* 27-33.

135. Tubergen, D. G., Gilchrist, G. S., O'Brien, R. T., et al. (1993). Improved outcome with delayed intensification for children with acute lymphoblastic leukemia and intermediate presenting features: A Children's Cancer Group phase III trial. *Journal of Clinical Oncology, 11,* 527-537.

136. Tubergen, D. G., Gilchrist, G. S., O'Brien, R. T., et al. (1993). Prevention of CNS disease in intermediate-risk acute lymphoblastic leukemia. Comparison of cranial radiation and intrathecal methotrexate and the importance of systemic therapy: A Children's Cancer Group report. *Journal of Clinical Oncology, 11,* 520-526.

137. Uckun, F. M., Evans, W. E., Forsyth, C. J., et al. (1995). Biotherapy of B-cell precursor leukemia by targeting geinstein to CD19-associated tyrosine kinases. *Science, 257,* 886-891.

138. Uckun, F. M., Sensel, M. G., Sun, L., et al. (1998). Biology and treatment of childhood T-lineage acute lymphoblastic leukemia. *Blood, 91,*735-746.

139. Underzo, C., Valsecchi, M.G., Bacigalupo, A., et al. (1995). Treatment of childhood acute lymphoblastic leukemia in second remission with allogeneic bone marrow transplantation and chemotherapy: Ten-year experience of the Italian Bone Marrow Transplantation Group and the Italian Pediatric Hematology Oncology Association. *Journal of Clinical Oncology, 13,* 352-358.

140. Vallera, D. A. (1994). Immunotoxins: Will their promise be fulfilled? *Blood, 83,* 309-317.

141. Van Dongen, J. J., Pongers-Willemese, M. J., Biondi, A., et al. (1999). Prognostic value of minimal residual disease in acute lymphoblastic leukaemia in childhood. [Correspondence]. *Lancet, 353,* 752-753.

142. Veerman, A. J. P., Halen, K., Kamps, W. A., et al (1996). High cure rate with a moderately intensive treatment regimen in non-high-risk childhood acute lymphoblastic leukemia: Results of protocol ALL VI from the Dutch Childhood Leukemia Study Group. *Journal of Clinical Oncology, 14,* 911-918.

143. Woodford, M. M., Smith, S. D., Shuster, J. J., et al. (1992). Treatment of occult or late overt testicular relapse in children with acute lymphoblastic leukemia: A Pediatric Oncology Group Study. *Journal of Clinical Oncology, 10,* 624-630.

144. Woods, W. G., Roloff, J. S., Lukens, J. N., et al. (1981). The occurrence of leukemia in persons with Shwachman's syndrome. *Journal of Pediatrics, 99,* 425-428.

145. Yates, C. R., Krynetske, E. Y., Loennechen, T., et al. (1999). Molecular diagnosis of thiopurine S-methyltransferase deficiency: Genetic basis for azathioprine and mercaptopurine intolerance. *Annals of Internal Medicine, 126,* 608-614.

Myeloid Diseases

Wendy Landier

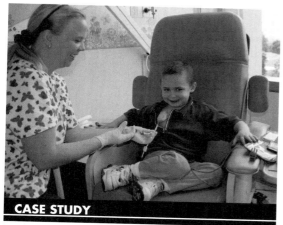

CASE STUDY

Nathan was in his usual state of excellent health until the age of 4½ years when he developed ptosis of his right eyelid. Over the next 5 weeks he developed increasing mucoid nasal discharge and congestion affecting only the right naris. He was seen by his pediatrician, who prescribed a course of antibiotics. However, the symptoms progressed, and he was referred to an ear, nose, and throat specialist. A magnetic resonance imaging (MRI) scan was performed, revealing a mass involving the right orbit and right sphenoid sinus. Results of a biopsy of the involved area were positive for granulocytic sarcoma (chloroma), suggestive of acute nonlymphocytic leukemia (ANLL). A complete blood count (CBC) revealed a white blood count of 8,300/mm³, hemoglobin of 11.2 g/dl, and platelet count of 214,000/mm³. White blood cell differential revealed 6% segs, 64% lymphocytes, 28% blasts, and 1% myelocytes. Nathan was admitted to the hospital and underwent bone marrow aspiration and biopsy; the results were positive for acute myeloblastic leukemia (AML) with maturation, FAB M2 classification. Bone marrow cytogenetics revealed a translocation involving chromosomes 8 and 21. Results of a lumbar puncture were negative for leukemic cells. Nathan was afebrile, and physical examination was negative with the exception of ptosis of the right eye-

lid and hepatomegaly extending 4 to 5 cm below the right costal margin.

He received induction chemotherapy with intensively timed idarubicin, cytarabine, etoposide, thioguanine, dexamethasone, and daunorubicin, followed by granulocyte colony stimulating factor (GCSF) support. His bone marrow was in remission by day 14 of induction therapy. Because Nathan's only sibling was not a human leukocyte antigen (HLA)–identical match, it was recommended that he proceed on with intensive chemotherapy rather than have an alternative donor stem cell transplant. His consolidation therapy consisted of idarubicin, fludarabine, and cytarabine, again with G-CSF support. He also received 20 Gy of radiation to the chloroma. This was followed with intensification therapy consisting of high-dose cytarabine, asparaginase, and intrathecal cytarabine. He then received immunomodulation with interleukin-2. Nathan's initial therapy lasted a total of 6 months, and he had no major complications.

He remained in good health for the next several months, with the exception of recurrent episodes of sinusitis. Unfortunately, 8 months following the completion of treatment Nathan was noted to have 4% blasts on his peripheral blood smear. Results from bone marrow aspiration and biopsy were confirmatory for relapse of his ANLL, again FAB-M2 morphology with t(8;21). He was reinduced with idarubicin, fludarabine, and cytarabine followed by a second course of fludarabine and cytarabine with G-CSF support. An HLA-identical unrelated donor was identified, and he went on to receive a matched unrelated hematopoietic stem cell transplant (HSCT). His preparative regimen consisted of total body irradiation in 11 fractions for a total dose of 13.2 Gy and cyclophosphamide 60 mg/kg/day for 2 days. His posttransplant course was uncomplicated, and he achieved engraftment by day +15. He received prophylaxis for graft-versus-host disease (GVHD) with tacrolimus (FK506), methylprednisolone, and methotrexate. Results from a bone marrow aspirate and biopsy performed on day +30 revealed normal hematopoiesis without evidence of leukemia. Nathan was discharged home on day +33 post-transplant and continues to be followed closely in the outpatient clinic.

Disorders of myeloid hematopoiesis are a consequence of aberrant myeloid cell line production by the bone marrow, resulting in several distinct and potentially fatal illnesses in children. The acute and chronic myeloid leukemias, myelodysplastic syndromes, and myeloproliferative disorders are all considered myeloid diseases.

CHILDHOOD ACUTE NONLYMPHOCYTIC LEUKEMIA

Childhood acute nonlymphocytic leukemia (ANLL) encompasses all acute leukemias arising from the myeloid cell lineage (Figure 20-1). These leukemias can affect the neutrophil, monocyte, erythrocyte, and megakaryocyte cell lines. ANLL results from malignant transformation of a myeloid progenitor cell that subsequently produces leukemic blasts. Expansion of these leukemic blasts in the marrow eventually causes failure of normal hematopoiesis, resulting in the anemia, thrombocytopenia, and neutropenia characteristically present at diagnosis.

EPIDEMIOLOGY

ANLL represents 17% of all childhood leukemia cases.[5] The incidence rate in the United States is 7.6 per million, with approximately 550 children and adolescents under 20 years of age diagnosed annually. Childhood ANLL rates are highest in the first 2 years of life, gradually diminishing during the school-age years, and then slowly increasing in adolescence.[33] ANLL is slightly more common in males than females, and the incidence is increased for Hispanics and whites compared with black children. Worldwide, rates of childhood ANLL are highest in Asia.[5]

Known risk factors for ANLL include treatment with alkylating agents and topoisomerase II inhibitors, exposure to ionizing radiation in utero, and constitutional disorders including Down syndrome, neurofibromatosis, ataxia-telangiectasia, Bloom syn-

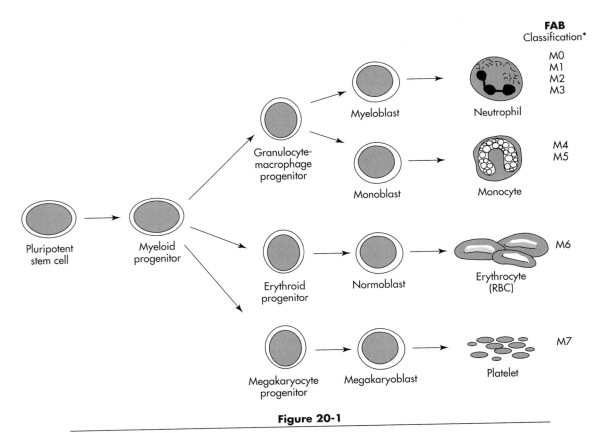

Figure 20-1

Myeloid cell lines in ANLL.
*French-American-British classification system.

drome, and Fanconi's anemia.[33] The risk is also increased for the identical twin of a child diagnosed with ANLL.[5] Suspected environmental risk factors include prenatal exposure of either parent to pesticides, prenatal exposure of the father to solvents or petroleum products, and postnatal exposure of the child to household pesticides.[6]

CLINICAL PRESENTATION

Children with ANLL typically have symptoms related to bone marrow failure, including pallor, fatigue, weakness, bleeding, fevers, and infections (Table 20-1). Infiltration of the marrow space by leukemic blasts may result in bone or joint pain. Other symptoms may be caused by leukemic infiltration of organs and tissues, such as ptosis related to an orbital chloroma or mouth discomfort due to gingival hypertrophy. Hepatosplenomegaly is present in about half of children at diagnosis, but lymphadenopathy is relatively uncommon. Testicular involvement in childhood ANLL is very rare. Symptoms related to ANLL typically begin a median of 6 weeks before diagnosis, with a range from 2 days to 12 months.[12,23,36]

Some symptoms occur more commonly with particular subtypes of ANLL defined by the French-American-British (FAB) Classification System (Table 20-2).

Chloromas are collections of leukemic cells located outside of the bone marrow. They can occur in the orbital area, bones, soft tissues, brain, and spinal cord and are most common in the FAB M2, M4, and M5 subtypes. Leukemic infiltrates can also present as bumps or rashes involving the skin (leukemia cutis) or infiltration of the gingiva, and are most often associated with the monocytic subtypes of ANLL. Central nervous system (CNS) involvement is most likely to occur in infants, those with high white blood counts, and those with FAB M4 and M5 subtypes. Signs and symptoms include headache, vomiting, cranial nerve palsies, and papilledema.[12]

The white blood count (WBC) at diagnosis is usually elevated (median $24,000/mm^3$); most patients are neutropenic (ANC $<1000/mm^3$); and peripheral blasts are detectable on the blood smear in 90% of cases. Almost all patients have some degree of anemia and thrombocytopenia, and about half exhibit a hemoglobin lower than 8 g/dl and a platelet count less than $50,000/mm^3$ at the time of diagnosis.[23,36] An exaggerated bleeding tendency is associated with the FAB M3 subtype, commonly referred to as acute promyelocytic leukemia (APL).

DIAGNOSTIC EVALUATION

Children with suspected ANLL require a thorough history and physical examination. A bone marrow aspiration and biopsy are generally the only diagnostic tests needed to confirm the diagnosis. In childhood ANLL the marrow is usually hypercellular and composed of 80% to 100% blasts, with a minimum of 30% blasts required to establish the diagnosis.[4] A diagnostic lumbar puncture is also performed to determine if there is CNS involvement.

The classification of childhood ANLL relies on assessment of the morphologic, cytochemical, and cytogenetic features of the leukemic blasts. The French-American-British (FAB) classification system (Table 20-2) is used to categorize childhood ANLL into eight distinct subtypes, M0 through M7.[4,19,23] In this classification system, "M" represents "myeloid" and is not to be confused with the M1, M2, M3 (M representing marrow) rating system that is used to quantify the percentage of blasts in the bone marrow. Classification is based on the cell line involved and the stage at which cellular maturation is arrested by neoplastic transformation (see Figure 20-1).

Certain cytochemical stains, including myeloperoxidase, Sudan black B, and esterases, are usually positive in ANLL and negative in acute lymphocytic leukemia (ALL) and may be helpful in differentiating between cell types.[23] Immunophenotyping is used to measure antibody response to antigens located on the surface of leukemic blasts. Common myeloid-associated antibodies include

TABLE 20-1	COMMON FINDINGS AT DIAGNOSIS IN CHILDHOOD ANLL
Finding	**% of Patients**
Hepatosplenomegaly	50
Fever	30-34
Bleeding	33
Pallor	25
Anorexia/weight loss	22
Weakness/fatigue	19
Sore throat	18
Bone or joint pain	18
Lymphadenopathy	13-20
Gastrointestinal symptoms	13
Swollen gingiva	9-15
Chest pain	5
Leukemia cutis	4-9
Recurrent infection	3
Chloroma	2-16

Data from Golub, T. R., Weinstein, H. J., & Grier, H. E. (1997). Acute myelogenous leukemia. In P. A. Pizzo & D. G. Poplack (Eds.), *Principles and practice of pediatric oncology* (3rd ed., pp. 463-477). Philadelphia: Lippincott-Raven; Pui, C-H., & Behm, F. G. (1999). Pathology of acute myeloid leukemia. In J. S. Lilleyman, I. M. Hann, & V. S. Blanchette (Eds.), *Pediatric hematology* (2nd ed., pp. 369-385). London: Churchill Livingstone.

TABLE 20-2	CLASSIFICATION OF ANLL SUBTYPES			
FAB Subtype	**Classification**	**Frequency (%)**	**Description**	**Clinical Features**	**Associated Cytogenetic Abnormalities**

FAB Subtype	Classification	Frequency (%)	Description	Clinical Features	Associated Cytogenetic Abnormalities
M0	Acute nonlymphocytic leukemia without maturation	2	Least differentiated myeloid leukemia; large agranular blasts; at least one myeloid antigen expressed (e.g., CD13 or CD33).	Bleeding, anemia, infection (frequently seen in all subtypes of ANLL)	Trisomy 8, del(5), del(7) (associated with all subtypes)
M1	Acute nonlymphocytic leukemia with poor maturation	10-18	Poorly differentiated myeloblasts, occasional Auer rods	Bleeding, anemia, infection	t(8;21)
M2	Acute nonlymphocytic leukemia with maturation	27-29	Differentiation of myeloblasts resembling very immature neutrophils; prominent Auer rods may be visible	Most common type of childhood ANLL; presentation may include chloromas involving orbit, brain, or spinal cord	t(8;21), inv(16)
M3	Acute promyelocytic leukemia (APL)	5-10	Hypergranular blasts usually contain bundles of Auer rods; grooved or bilobed nucleus often present	Exaggerated bleeding tendency, DIC common at diagnosis or following initiation of chemotherapy	t(15;17)
M4	Acute myelomonocytic leukemia	16-25	20%-80% monoblasts; some myeloblasts may be present; M4Eo variant positive for >5% eosinophilic precursors	More common in infants; extramedullary leukemia and gingival infiltration are common presentations	inv(16), t(9;11), t(11;19), 11q23 rearrangements
M5	Acute monocytic leukemia	13-22	>80% monoblasts, promonocytes, or monocytes	Often presents with gingival hypertrophy, extramedullary involvement, or leukemia cutis; common in very young infants and as secondary (therapy-related) ANLL	t(9;11), t(11;19), 11q23 rearrangements
M6	Erythroleukemia	1-3	>50% erythroblasts and >30% myeloblasts	Occurs more often in children with Down syndrome	
M7	Acute megakaryocytic leukemia	4-8	>30% megakaryoblasts; bone marrow fibrosis common	Associated with Down syndrome and preleukemic myelodysplasia	t(1;22)

Data from Bennett, J. M., Catovsky, D., Daniel, M. T., et al. (1985). Proposed revised criteria for the classification of acute myeloid leukemia: A report of the French-American-British Cooperative Group. *Annals of Internal Medicine, 103,* 626-629; Lilleyman, J. S. (2000). *Childhood leukaemia: The facts* (2nd ed.). New York: Oxford University Press; Pui, C-H., & Behm, F. G. (1999). Pathology of acute myeloid leukemia. In J. S. Lilleyman, I. M. Hann, & V. S. Blanchette (Eds.), *Pediatric hematology* (2nd ed. pp. 369-385). London: Churchill Livingstone; Weinstein, H. J. (1999). Acute myeloid leukemia. In C-H. Pui (Ed.), *Childhood leukemias* (pp. 322-335). New York: Cambridge University Press.

CD11b, CD13, CD14, CD15, CD33, and CD36. At least one of these antibodies is expressed in more than 90% of ANLL cases.[14] There are ranges of typical immunophenotypes but no absolute correlation with any one subtype of ANLL. For this reason immunophenotyping is used in conjunction with morphology, cytochemistry, and cytogenetics to diagnose childhood ANLL and is most useful in confirming the M0, M6, and M7 subtypes.[23]

Cytogenetic abnormalities are found in the leukemic cells of 80% to 90% of children with ANLL. Common cytogenetic abnormalities associated with the various morphologic subtypes are listed in Table 20-2. These cytogenetic abnormalities not only have prognostic significance, some have therapeutic implications as well. For instance, children with t(15;17) show a favorable response to regimens that include retinoic acid and anthracyclines, and those with t(8;21) have improved outcomes with regimens containing high-dose cytarabine.[22]

TREATMENT

Treatment for childhood ANLL has improved significantly since the first effective therapies were introduced in the 1970s. Five-year survival rates have risen from less than 5% in 1970 to 43% today as a result of treatment intensification, the incorporation of hematopoietic stem cell transplant (HSCT) into primary therapy, and enhanced supportive care strategies.[13] Unfortunately, compared with other childhood cancers, ANLL remains one of the most refractory to treatment. Current barriers to cure include heterogeneity of the disease, limited availability of effective treatment strategies, and high rates of treatment-related mortality.[16]

Chemotherapy

The most active agents for remission induction in childhood ANLL are cytarabine and the anthracyclines. Classic induction therapy for ANLL is the "7+3" strategy, combining continuous infusion cytarabine at 100 mg/m^2/day for 7 days and daunorubicin at 45 to 60 mg/m^2/day for 3 days.[16] In many current induction regimens, cytarabine and daunorubicin are combined with other agents such as thioguanine, dexamethasone, or etoposide. Daunorubicin is replaced by mitoxantrone or idarubicin in some protocols.[12,28] Timing of cytotoxic drug administration in induction may play an important role in improving outcomes. In a recent trial, intensive timing of chemotherapy in induction was shown to be superior to standard timing by decreasing the incidence of induction failure and improving overall survival rates.[39]

The most common type of postremission therapy for childhood ANLL involves very intense, short-term treatment for approximately 6 months. An allogeneic HSCT during this phase is usually recommended for children who have a matched sibling donor. Children without a sibling donor receive intensive postremission chemotherapy regimens, such as very-high-dose cytarabine combined with asparaginase (Capizzi II therapy).[38] Additional agents commonly used in postremission therapy include etoposide, thioguanine, anthracyclines, mercaptopurine, and amsacrine. High-dose chemotherapy followed by autologous HSCT has not proven superior to intensification with chemotherapy alone in childhood ANLL.[26] This may be due to lack of GVL effect or contamination of the autologous marrow cells with residual leukemia.[14]

CNS prophylaxis is delivered with intrathecal (IT) methotrexate, cytarabine, or both, often combined with hydrocortisone. For children with leukemic involvement of the CNS at diagnosis, IT chemotherapy combined with systemic therapy including high-dose cytarabine may be sufficient to prevent relapse. In some cases CNS radiation is also used.[16]

Biological Response Modifiers

Stimulating the immune system by administration of interleukin-2 (IL-2) may provide a survival advantage in children with ANLL. Trials of IL-2 are currently under way, with the goal of eradicating residual leukemia following the cessation of chemotherapy. Side effects can be significant and include fever, vascular leak, and hypotension.[32]

Hematopoietic Stem Cell Transplant

Myeloablative therapy followed by allogeneic HSCT from an HLA-identical sibling donor is superior to continuation chemotherapy for children with ANLL in first remission. Exceptions include children with APL and children with Down syndrome, who have an excellent outcome with chemotherapy alone.[16] When a matched sibling donor is available (usually in 25% to 30% of patients), the child with ANLL is referred for transplant as soon as possible after attaining remission. Preparative regimens typically include cyclophosphamide combined with either busulfan or total body irradiation. In seven large biologically randomized studies, disease-free survival at 3 to 5 years ranged from 51% to 72% for matched sibling transplants, compared with 27% to 50% for chemotherapy alone.[21]

Recurrent Disease

Salvage therapy for children with refractory or recurrent ANLL generally relies on a high-dose cytarabine-containing regimen. Remission reinduction rates range from 28% to 80%.[16] When a child with ANLL relapses after treatment with chemotherapy alone, an allogeneic HSCT is usually recommended because it represents the only true possibility of cure. Generally, these children lack a matched sibling donor. Potential alternative sources of stem cells include matched unrelated, related mismatched, or cord blood donors. Transplant-related mortality is significantly higher for children receiving transplants from an alternative donor compared with those from an HLA-identical sibling.[34] Children who relapse following an allogeneic transplant may benefit from a second transplant from the same or an alternative donor, but unfortunately, survival rates in this setting are quite low.[24]

Down Syndrome

Children with Down syndrome who develop ANLL have a high incidence of the megakaryocytic (M7) subtype and a more favorable response to treatment than other children, with survival rates reported between 69% and 100%.[17,25] Unacceptably high mortality rates occur in Down syndrome patients who undergo intensively timed induction regimens or HSCTs. Current clinical trials are evaluating the efficacy of less intensive therapy for these children.[17]

Acute Promyelocytic Leukemia

Up to 80% of children with APL have evidence of severe coagulopathy at the time of diagnosis. The bleeding problem is caused by the release of procoagulants (enzymes capable of activating blood clotting proteins) from the promyelocytic blasts as they lyse. As blood clotting proteins are activated, clots form in the microvasculature. Clotting factors and platelets are consumed during the production of these clots, resulting in increased bleeding. Cytotoxic chemotherapy causes massive lysis of promyelocytic blasts, increasing the amount of procoagulants released, often resulting in disseminated intravascular coagulation (DIC). Children with APL are at high risk of life-threatening hemorrhage (often involving the brain or lungs), with a 15% to 30% mortality rate for patients who experience this complication during initial therapy.[18]

Fortunately, all-*trans*-retinoic acid (ATRA), a naturally occurring isomer of retinoic acid, is an effective differentiating agent in APL.[18] Oral administration of ATRA allows maturation of promyelocytic blasts, usually resulting in rapid resolution of the coagulopathy. ATRA is not curative in APL, and therapy with cytotoxic chemotherapy must also be given. Close monitoring during ATRA therapy is

required. Complications include psuedotumor cerebri, hyperleukodcytosis, and the retinoic acid syndrome, potentially fatal rapid-onset pulmonary failure with associated capillary leak.[9] Regimens using ATRA in combination with chemotherapy are improving long-term survival and reducing morbidity in patients with APL.[18]

Prognosis

WBC at diagnosis is the most reliable clinical prognostic factor in childhood ANLL. Increasing WBC correlates with adverse prognosis, with particularly poor outcomes for patients presenting with WBC over 100,000/mm³. Cytogenetic features are also emerging as prognostic indicators in childhood ANLL. The t(8;21), t(15;17), and inv(16) correlate with a more favorable outcome, while monosomy 7, t(1;22), and 11q23 rearrangements correlate with a poor outcome.[14,23] Children with Down syndrome tend to have a more favorable response to treatment.[17] Survival rates in children with APL are also superior, except for the excessive hemorrhagic-related mortality during induction.[18] Secondary ANLL occurring as a result of prior cancer therapy (exposure to alkylating agents or topoisomerase II inhibitors) is very resistant to treatment. Prognosis is uniformly poor in this group of patients, and allogeneic HSCT offers the best chance of cure.[7]

Nursing Implications

Induction therapy for ANLL has a high potential for morbidity, and mortality rates range from 6% to 20%.[16] Potential early complications include tumor lysis syndrome, leukostasis, hemorrhage, DIC, and sepsis.[14] Those with high white cell counts and bulky disease are at greatest risk of complications related to tumor lysis. Preventive measures, including vigorous intravenous hydration, urinary alkalinization, and administration of allopurinol, begin before induction chemotherapy is initiated. Close monitoring of intake and output, serum electrolytes, and creatinine occurs during the initial induction period. Children with initial WBCs greater than 200,000/mm³ are at risk of complications related to leukostasis (particularly CNS and pulmonary infarcts) and may require exchange transfusion or therapeutic leukapheresis to lower the WBC to a safe range. Nonessential packed red blood cell transfusions are avoided in these children because blood viscosity is already high, placing patients at risk of respiratory failure and CNS bleeding. Platelet transfusions are given to keep the platelet count above 20,000/mm³, because spontaneous hemorrhage is a significant threat.[1] For patients in DIC plasma transfusions may be necessary. In children with APL, coagulopathies usually improve rapidly once ATRA therapy is initiated.

Infectious complications are a constant threat during the prolonged periods of pancytopenia that commonly occur with childhood ANLL therapy. These children are particularly susceptible to bacteremia caused by alpha hemolytic streptococci.[10] Infection with these organisms is associated with a high incidence of morbidity, including shock and respiratory distress, and can progress rapidly to a fatal outcome. Special care must be taken to provide early empiric coverage for alpha hemolytic streptococci (preferably with intravenous vancomycin) in any child with ANLL who presents with fever and neutropenia or suspected bacteremia.[10] Hematopoietic growth factors, including G-CSF and granulocyte macrophage colony stimulating factor (GM-CSF), are used in some protocols in an attempt to reduce infectious complications by shortening the period of neutropenia. Clinical trials in patients with ANLL have shown that use of these growth factors following cytotoxic therapy reduces the duration of neutropenia[30] without increased incidence of relapse.[11]

Families of children with ANLL require intensive nursing support to assist them in coping with the extended hospitalizations and typically difficult course throughout their child's illness. Many of these children require hospitalization for weeks to months at a time. Some proceed directly from intensive induction and consolidation therapy to transplant. Many of these children continue to require intensive supportive care at home. Nurses can be instrumental in introducing these families to hospital and community resources and in providing anticipatory guidance to help them plan for and cope with their child's ongoing care requirements.

FUTURE DIRECTIONS

Attempts to target therapy toward molecular mechanisms of leukemogenesis have been successful in APL, using retinoic acid to promote differentiation of malignant blasts into nonmalignant forms. A new targeted therapy, gemtuzumab ozogamicin, appears to have broader application to all forms of ANLL. This novel immunoconjugate combines an anti-CD33 monoclonal antibody with a potent chemotherapeutic agent (calicheamicin). Results of preliminary clinical trials with this agent appear promising.[31] In the future, it is hoped that molecularly targeted therapies will provide more effective and less toxic curative regimens than those available today.

Other future strategies will involve improvements in chemotherapy regimens, particularly related to timing, dose intensification, and modula-

tion of multidrug resistance with agents such as cyclosporine or cytokines.[22] Several new agents, including 2-chlorodeoxyadenosine and homoharringtonine, are currently being tested and may be incorporated into future front-line therapy.[37] In addition, improvements in transplant technologies, immunomodulation, and supportive care regimens also offer hope for increased survival in childhood ANLL.

MYELODYSPLASTIC SYNDROMES OF CHILDHOOD

Myelodysplastic syndromes (MDSs) are a rare group of childhood hematologic disorders characterized by ineffective hematopoiesis. These syndromes are sometimes referred to as "preleukemia" because of their tendency to progress to frank ANLL. Predisposing conditions include Down syndrome and other constitutional chromosomal aberrations, disorders associated with defective DNA repair such as Fanconi anemia, and prior exposure to mutagenic agents.[2,7] Familial clusters have been noted, often associated with monosomy 7. Approximately 32% of children with MDS will go on to develop ANLL.[20] Children treated with alkylating agents, especially those who received high-dose chemotherapy followed by autologous stem cell rescue, are at increased risk of developing therapy-related MDS. Typical onset is 4 to 5 years following treatment with the alkylating agent, and progression to ANLL occurs within a mean of 11 months.[7]

Children with MDS typically present with signs and symptoms of hematopoietic failure, including pallor, petechiae, and bleeding. Cytopenias are evident on the peripheral blood smear. The bone marrow is hypercellular and dysplastic with fewer than 30% blasts.[2,7] Because MDS is rare in children, there are few pediatric clinical trials and a lack of general agreement regarding optimal therapy.[20] However, all children require supportive care, including blood products and aggressive management of infectious complications. Cytotoxic regimens in MDS are associated with higher rates of toxicity, lower remission rates, and shorter remission duration when compared with chemotherapy-based treatment for ANLL. For most patients, HSCT currently offers the only curative therapy.[7]

JUVENILE MYELOMONOCYTIC LEUKEMIA

Children with bone marrow dysplasia and peripheral blood monocytosis associated with hemorrhage, lymphadenopathy, infection, and skin rash have previously been included in the diagnostic classification known as Juvenile Chronic Myelogenous Leukemia (JCML). This group of disorders has recently been reclassified as "Juvenile Myelomonocytic Leukemia" *(JMML)* and categorized as a myelodysplastic syndrome.[2] Children with JMML lack evidence of the Philadelphia chromosome t(9;22) in their bone marrow, have a hypercellular marrow with less than 20% blasts, and have a peripheral monocyte count greater than 1,000/mm³. In addition, most children with JMML have elevated levels of hemoglobin F (>10%) and peripheral blood leukocytosis (WBC >10,000/mm³). Some also have blasts on the peripheral blood smear. Patients with JMML are more likely to be male and are usually younger than 4 years of age, with 40% of cases occurring before age 12 months.[3] Clinical features at presentation typically include hepatosplenomegaly (>90%), lymphadenopathy (75%), pallor (69%), fever (61%), and skin rash (39%).[2] Prognosis is best in children under 2 years of age at the time of diagnosis. Unfavorable prognostic features at presentation include an increased level of hemoglobin F, older age, and thrombocytopenia. The natural course of the disease is variable, with some younger untreated patients surviving with stable disease for up to 10 years.[3] Allogeneic HCST is currently the only curative therapy known in JMML[15] and is often recommended in children with poor prognostic features. Because of the risks associated with allogeneic transplant, preferred initial treatment for children with lower-risk features may consist of supportive care alone or low-intensity therapy with mercaptopurine, thioguanine, or isotretinoin.[3]

MYELOPROLIFERATIVE DISORDERS OF CHILDHOOD

The myeloproliferative disorders of childhood all reflect an intrinsic abnormality in the hematopoietic stem cell manifested by clonal proliferation involving some portion of the myeloid cell line. Although each disorder is unique, they share many common characteristics, including the propensity to evolve into acute leukemia.

CHRONIC MYELOID LEUKEMIA

Biology and Epidemiology
Chronic myeloid leukemia (CML) arises from malignant transformation of a single multipotent hematopoietic stem cell. The cause of the neoplastic transformation is unknown, but in at least 95% of cases there is a characteristic translocation between the long arms of chromosomes 9 and 22, resulting in a structurally shortened 22 known as the Philadelphia chromosome. CML is rare in childhood. About 100 children are diagnosed annually

in the United States, more than 60% of whom are at least 6 years of age. Other than an association with ionizing radiation, no other causal relationships for CML in childhood have been established.[27]

Clinical Presentation and Diagnostic Classification
CML is classified into phases, based on symptomatology and analysis of peripheral blood and bone marrow characteristics (Table 20-3). The disease usually presents in the chronic phase, and children often experience excellent quality of life throughout this stage. Eventually, the disease undergoes a period of metamorphosis known as the accelerated phase and finally enters the terminal or blastic phase.

Treatment
Children with WBCs greater than 200,000 to 300,000/mm³ are at significant risk for complications related to hyperviscosity and leukostasis of the blood. Intravascular clumping of blasts in the circulation can result in cerebral and retinal hemorrhages, tachypnea, hypoxia, and priapism. Treatment includes vigorous hydration, leukapheresis or exchange transfusions, and initiation of chemotherapy. Because of the risks of increased blood viscosity, transfusion of packed red blood cells is generally avoided until the WBC is lowered. Oral chemotherapy with hydroxyurea is effective in controlling leukocytosis and resolving anemia in children with chronic phase CML. Resolution of symptoms is generally attained within a few days of initiating therapy, and quality of life may be significantly improved. Hydroxyurea is titrated to keep the WBC less than 10,000/mm³ and is often used as initial therapy, allowing time for decision making regarding long-term treatment options.[27] Alpha-interferon and cytarabine are also used for treatment of chronic phase CML.[29] The most recent addition to the armamentarium against CML is a new class of drugs known as "cytostatics," engineered to attack at the molecular level.[35] A novel agent, imatinib mesylate, formerly known as STI-571, selectively inhibits the oncogenic protein tyrosine kinase produced by the Philadelphia chromosome. This oral drug selectively targets CML cells and so has few toxic effects. Imatinib mesylate has had astonishing successes in clinical trials. In phase I adult clinical trials, 100% of patients achieved hematologic responses at higher dose ranges.[8] In phase II studies, imatinib mesylate demonstrated effectiveness in all phases of CML, suggesting that this agent may play a role in reducing blasts in the bone marrow for patients who are transplantation candidates.[21a]

For children who have an HLA-matched sibling

TABLE 20-3	PHASES OF CHRONIC MYELOID LEUKEMIA			
Phase	**Presentation**	**Duration**	**Peripheral Blood Characteristics**	**Bone Marrow Characteristics**
Chronic	Weight loss, fatigue, malaise, bone and joint pain, fevers, night sweats, abdominal fullness or pain; 40% of children are asymptomatic; lymphadenopathy uncommon, mild hepatomegaly may occur, splenomegaly evident in 80%-95% of cases	Several months up to >10 years (mean = 3 years)	Marked leukocytosis (WBC >100,000 in over 80% of patients); predominance of granulocytes (neutrophils, bands) and granulocytic precursors (metamyelocytes, myelocytes, promyelocytes); <5% blasts; platelet count normal or slightly elevated; mild to moderate anemia common; reduced leukocyte alkaline phosphatase activity (low LAP score); reduced serum B_{12} level; uric acid level often elevated	Marked hypercellularity of myeloid cell lines; <5% blasts; Philadelphia chromosome present in 95% of patients; virtually all cases positive for *BCR-ABL* fusion gene
Accelerated	Increasing splenomegaly, weakness, bleeding, bruising, chloromas	6-12 months	Thrombocytopenia or marked thrombocytosis (platelet count >1 million/mm³); increasing leukocytes, basophils, and eosinophils; increasing blasts; progressive anemia	Increasing numbers of blasts; biopsy may exhibit myelofibrosis; additional cytogenetic abnormalities may occur, including second Philadelphia chromosome, trisomy 8, trisomy 19, and/or isochromosome 17
Blastic	Resembles acute leukemia (myeloid type in >60%, lymphoid type in 20%-30%, mixed or undifferentiated in remainder)	2-12 months	Resembles acute leukemia with rapidly rising white blood count, >30% blasts, anemia, and thrombocytopenia	Marrow contains at least 30% blasts; many cytogenetic abnormalities may occur, resembling those in acute leukemia; abnormalities in tumor-suppressor genes (e.g., *p53* or *RB*), or proto-oncogenes (e.g., *myc* or *ras*) may be present

Data from Roberts, I. A. G., & Dokal, I. S. (1999). Adult-type chronic myeloid leukemia. In J. S. Lilleyman, I. M. Hann, & V. S. Blanchette (Eds.). *Pediatric hematology* (2nd ed., pp. 403-416). London: Churchill Livingstone; Sawyers, C. L. (1999). Chronic myeloid leukemia. *New England Journal of Medicine, 340*, 1330-1340.

donor, allogeneic HSCT in the chronic phase within 1 year of diagnosis results in long-term leukemia-free survival of 80% to 90%.[27] Relapse rates for syngeneic transplants are 2 to 3 times higher than for HLA-matched nonidentical siblings, accentuating the importance of the graft-versus-leukemia (GVL) effect resulting from allogeneic transplant in CML.[29] For children without sibling donors, an alternative donor transplant (e.g., mismatched related, matched unrelated, or cord blood) may be performed. However survival rates are lower than for matched sibling transplants, with transplant-related mortality of 25% to 40%.[27] Myeloablative therapy, usually combining cyclophosphamide with busulfan or total body irradiation, is followed by stem cell infusion. Infectious complications, toxicities related to myeloablative therapy, and graft-versus-host disease (GVHD) are the most common causes of morbidity and mortality. Relapse following allogeneic transplant in patients with CML is infrequent (15%-20%). When it does occur, infusion of donor lymphocytes with or without alpha-interferon therapy often restores durable remission.[29] Patients transplanted in the accelerated or blastic phases have a poorer rate of survival (26%-43% and 10%-20%, respectively) compared with those transplanted in the chronic phase. Therefore transplantation in the chronic phase within one year of diagnosis is strongly recommended for patients with an allogeneic donor.[27]

Prognosis

The natural course of CML is uniformly fatal, and although chemotherapy and immunotherapy may extend survival times and improve quality of life, the only known cure is allogeneic HSCT.

Future Directions

Because current treatment strategies for childhood CML rely on allogeneic HSCT as the only curative option, improvements in stem cell transplantation will ultimately improve outcomes for children with CML. Additionally, novel strategies such as molecularly targeted therapy, including the unique class of tyrosine kinase inhibitors, may eventually modify the role of transplant in CML and open up new, less toxic therapeutic options for children with this disease.

Other Myeloproliferative Disorders of Childhood

Polycythemia Vera

Polycythemia vera is a disorder resulting in increased red cell mass. The familial form is an autosomal inherited disorder and may be either dominant or recessive. Presenting symptoms reflect hyperviscosity and may include headache, weakness, dizziness, weight loss, ruddy complexion, thrombosis, splenomegaly, and pruritus. Treatment involves reducing the red cell mass by phlebotomy or erythrocytopheresis to maintain the hematocrit below 45%. In some cases, hydroxyurea may also be employed.[2,14]

Essential Thrombocythemia

Essential thrombocythemia is characterized by a platelet count greater than $600,000/mm^3$ in the absence of other systemic or myeloproliferative disorders. Symptoms may include weakness, headache, dizziness, paresthesias, hemorrhage, or thrombosis, although some children are asymptomatic. In mild cases, observation alone is indicated. Treatment may include aspirin, anagrelide, hydroxyurea, or alpha-interferon.[2]

Idiopathic Myelofibrosis

Idiopathic myelofibrosis is characterized by fibrotic proliferation within the marrow spaces. Hepatosplenomegaly may occur secondary to extramedullary hematopoiesis. Affected children develop symptoms of bone marrow failure, and the disease frequently evolves into acute leukemia. Treatment is supportive and may involve splenectomy, splenic radiation, androgens, corticosteroids, and chemotherapy. In refractory cases, HSCT offers the only realistic chance of cure.[2,14]

Transient Myeloproliferative Syndrome

Transient myeloproliferative syndrome may develop in some neonates with Down syndrome and is characterized by leukocytosis, anemia, thrombocytopenia, blasts in the peripheral blood smear, and hepatosplenomegaly. A large population of undifferentiated blasts may also be evident in the bone marrow. This condition usually resolves spontaneously without treatment within weeks to months. Close follow-up of these infants is important, however, because approximately 30% will go on to develop ANLL before their third birthday.[36]

Disorders of myeloid hematopoiesis continue to present substantial challenges to nurses caring for affected children. In the future, improved understanding of the biology of these disorders may lead to less toxic therapies and increased cure rates. In the meantime, these children and their families will continue to require expert nursing care and support throughout the course of their illness.

REFERENCES

1. Albano, E. A., & Ablin, A. R. (1997). Oncologic emergencies. In A. R. Ablin (Ed.), *Supportive care of children with cancer* (2nd ed., pp. 175-192). Baltimore: Johns Hopkins University Press.

2. Arico, M., & Biondi, A. (1999). Myelodysplastic syndromes and chronic myeloproliferative disorders. In C-H. Pui (Ed.), *Childhood leukemias* (pp. 336-353). New York: Cambridge University Press.

3. Arico, M., Biondi, A., & Pui, C-H. (1997). Juvenile myelomonocytic leukemia. *Blood, 90,* 479-488.

4. Bennett, J. M., Catovsky, D., Daniel, M. T., et al. (1985). Proposed revised criteria for the classification of acute myeloid leukemia: A report of the French-American-British Cooperative Group. *Annals of Internal Medicine, 103,* 626-629.

5. Bhatia, S., & Neglia, J. P. (1995). Epidemiology of childhood acute myelogenous leukemia. *Journal of Pediatric Hematology/Oncology, 17,* 94-100.

6. Buckley, J. D., Robison, L. L., Swotinsky, R., et al. (1989). Occupational exposures of parents of children with acute nonlymphocytic leukemia: A report from the Children's Cancer Study Group. *Cancer Research, 49,* 4030-4037.

7. Chessells, J. M. (1999). Myelodysplastic syndromes. In J. S. Lilleyman, I. M. Hann, & V. S. Blanchette (Eds.), *Pediatric hematology* (2nd ed., pp. 83-101). London: Churchill Livingstone.

8. Druker, B. J., & Lydon, N. B. (2000). Lessons learned from the development of an Abl tyrosine kinase inhibitor for chronic myelogenous leukemia. *The Journal of Clinical Investigation, 105,* 3-7.

9. Frankel, S. R., Eardley, A., Lauwers, G., et al. (1992). The "retinoic acid syndrome" in acute promyelocytic leukemia. *Annals of Internal Medicine, 117,* 292-296.

10. Gamis, A. S., Howells, W. B., DeSwarte-Wallace, J., et al. (2000). Alpha hemolytic streptococcal infection during intensive treatment for acute myeloid leukemia: A report from the Children's Cancer Group study CCG-2891. *Journal of Clinical Oncology, 18,* 1845-1855.

11. Ganser, A., & Heil, G. (1997). Use of hematopoietic growth factors in the treatment of acute myelogenous leukemia. *Current Opinion in Hematology, 4,* 191-195.

12. Golub, T. R., Weinstein, H. J., & Grier, H. E. (1997). Acute myelogenous leukemia. In P. A. Pizzo & D. G. Poplack (Eds.), *Principles and practice of pediatric oncology* (3rd ed., pp. 463-477). Philadelphia: Lippincott-Raven.

13. Greenlee, R. T., Murray, T., Bolden, S., et al. (2000). Cancer statistics, 2000. *CA—A Cancer Journal for Clinicians, 50,* 7-33.

14. Grier, H. E., & Civin, C. I. (1998). Myeloid leukemias, myelodysplasia, and myeloproliferative diseases in children. In D. G. Nathan & S. H. Orkin (Eds.), *Nathan and Oski's hematology of infancy and childhood* (5th ed., pp. 1286-1321). Philadelphia: W. B. Saunders.

15. Krance, R. A. (1999). Hematopoietic cell transplantation for juvenile myelomonocytic leukemia. In E. D. Thomas, K. G. Blume, & S. J. Forman (Eds.), *Hematopoietic cell transplantation* (2nd ed., pp. 817-822). Malden, MA: Blackwell Science.

16. Lange, B. J., & Bunin, N. J. (1999). Therapy of acute myeloid leukemia. In J. S. Lilleyman, I. M. Hann & V. S. Blanchette (Eds.), *Pediatric hematology* (2nd ed., pp. 387-402). London: Churchill Livingstone.

17. Lange, B. J., Kobrinsky, N., Barnard, D. R., et al. (1998). Distinctive demography, biology, and outcome of acute myeloid leukemia and myelodysplastic syndrome in children with Down syndrome: Children's Cancer Group studies 2861 and 2891. *Blood, 91,* 608-615.

18. Lemons, R. S., Keller, S., Gietzen, D., et al. (1995). Acute promyelocytic leukemia. *Journal of Pediatric Hematology/Oncology, 17,* 198-210.

19. Lilleyman, J. S. (2000). *Childhood leukaemia: The facts* (2nd ed.). New York: Oxford University Press.

20. Lunda-Fineman, S., Shannon, K. M., Atwater, S. K., et al. (1999). Myelodysplastic and myeloproliferative disorders of childhood: A study of 167 patients. *Blood, 93,* 459-466.

21. Margolis, D. A., & Casper, J. T. (1999). Allogeneic transplantation for acute myeloid leukemia in children. In E. D. Thomas, K. G. Blume, & S. J. Forman (Eds.), *Hematopoietic cell transplantation* (2nd ed., pp. 835-848). Malden, MA: Blackwell Science.

21a. Parmar, K., & King, R. S. (2001). Imatinib mesylate: A new pill for chronic myelogenous leukemia. *Cancer Practice.* In press.

22. Pui, C-H. (1995). Childhood leukemias. *The New England Journal of Medicine, 332,* 1618-1630.

23. Pui, C-H., & Behm, F. G. (1999). Pathology of acute myeloid leukemia. In J. S. Lilleyman, I. M. Hann, & V. S. Blanchette (Eds.), *Pediatric hematology* (2nd ed., pp. 369-385). London: Churchill Livingstone.

24. Radich, J. P., Sanders, J. E., Buckner, C. D., et al. (1993). Second allogeneic marrow transplantation for patients with recurrent leukemia after initial transplant with total body irradiation-containing regimens. *Journal of Clinical Oncology, 11,* 304-313.

25. Ravindranath, Y., Abella, E., Krischer, J. P., et al. (1992). Acute myeloid leukemia (AML) in Down's syndrome is highly responsive to chemotherapy: Experience on Pediatric Oncology Group AML study 8498. *Blood, 80,* 2210-2214.

26. Ravindranath, Y., Yeager, A. M., Chang, M. N., et al. (1996). Autologous bone marrow transplantation versus intensive consolidation chemotherapy for acute myeloid leukemia in childhood. *The New England Journal of Medicine, 334,* 1428-1434.

27. Roberts, I. A. G., & Dokal, I. S. (1999). Adult-type chronic myeloid leukemia. In J. S. Lilleyman, I. M. Hann, & V. S. Blanchette (Eds.), *Pediatric hematology* (2nd ed., pp. 403-416). London: Churchill Livingstone.

28. Sackmann-Muriel, F., Zubizarreta, P., Felice, M. S., et al. (1996). Results of treatment with an intensive induction regimen using idarubicin in combination with cytarabine and etoposide in children with acute myeloblastic leukemia. *Leukemia Research, 20,* 973-981.

29. Sawyers, C. L. (1999). Chronic myeloid leukemia. *The New England Journal of Medicine, 340,* 1330-1340.

30. Schiffer, C. A. (1996). Hematopoietic growth factors as adjuncts to the treatment of acute myeloid leukemia. *Blood, 88,* 3675-3685.

31. Sievers, E. L., Appelbaum, F. R., Spielberger, R. T., et al. (1999). Selective ablation of acute myeloid leukemia using antibody-targeted chemotherapy: A phase I study of an anti-CD33 calicheamicin immunoconjugate. *Blood, 93,* 3678-3684.

32. Sievers, E. L., Lange, B. J., Sondel, P. M., et al. (1998). Feasibility, toxicity, and biologic response of interleukin-2 after consolidation chemotherapy for acute myelogenous leukemia: A report from the Children's Cancer Group. *Journal of Clinical Oncology, 16,* 914-919.

33. Smith, M. A., Ries, L. A. G., Gurney, J. G., et al. (1999). Leukemia. In L. A. G. Ries, M. A. Smith, J. G. Gurney, et al. (Eds.), *Cancer incidence and survival among children and adolescents: United States SEER Program 1975-1995* (NIH Publication No. 99-4649, pp. 17-34). Bethesda, MD: National Cancer Institute.

34. Szydlo, R., Goldman, J. M., Klein, J. P., et al. (1997). Results of allogeneic bone marrow transplants for leukemia using donors other than HLA-identical siblings. *Journal of Clinical Oncology, 15,* 1767-1777.

35. Vastag, B. (2000). Leukemia drug heralds molecularly targeted era. *Journal of the National Cancer Institute, 92,* 6-8.

36. Weinstein, H. J. (1999). Acute myeloid leukemia. In C-H. Pui (Ed.), *Childhood leukemias* (pp. 322-335). New York: Cambridge University Press.

37. Wells, R. J., & Arndt, C. A. S. (1995). New agents for treatment of children with acute myelogenous leukemia. *Journal of Pediatric Hematology/Oncology, 17,* 225-233.

38. Wells, R. J., Woods, W. G., Lampkin, B. C., et al. (1993). Impact of high-dose cytarabine and asparaginase intensification on childhood acute myeloid leukemia: A report from the Children's Cancer Group. *Journal of Clinical Oncology, 11,* 538-545.

39. Woods, W. G., Kobrinsky, N., Buckley, J. D., et al. (1996). Timed-sequential induction therapy improves postremission outcome in acute myeloid leukemia: A report from the Children's Cancer Group. *Blood, 87,* 4979-4989.

Central Nervous System Tumors

Janis Ryan-Murray
Mary McElwain Petriccione

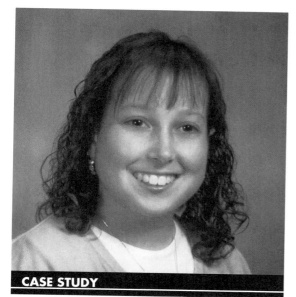

CASE STUDY

In October 1986 at 8½ years of age, Melissa was diagnosed with a medulloblastoma. At presentation, an astute ophthalmologist detected papilledema and referred her to a neurologist. The tumor was visualized on a computed tomography (CT) scan. A complete resection was performed yielding no postoperative deficits. She received 35 Gy craniospinal irradiation with a 15 Gy boost to the posterior fossa. Chemotherapy consisting of lomustine and vincristine was given from February 1987 to August 1988.

Therapy-related problems included Pneumocystis carinii pneumonia in December 1987. She continued to have mild pulmonary symptoms and was treated in 1989 for restrictive lung disease. Melissa developed endocrine late effects including growth hormone deficiency treated with growth hormone from 1989 to 1993, gonadotropin deficiency, and primary hypothyroidism. Her daily medications include levothyroxine, estrogen, and progesterone. Neuropsychologic testing revealed mild neurocognitive dysfunction, particularly with math and verbal learning. This testing was done sequentially so that Melissa was able to receive the necessary academic guidance in high school and in college. This included academic interventions such as tutoring and untimed tests. All follow-up CT and magnetic resonance imaging (MRI) scans have been negative for disease.

Melissa is now 22 years old. She has one semester left in her college career. Currently she is enjoying an internship at Disney World. She is independent, socially active, and involved with her close-knit family. Melissa's life goal is to work with children.

Melissa has been challenged on many levels as a result of her disease and its treatment. She is very cognizant of these difficulties and has always sought appropriate interventions. Her quiet determination and understated manner, however, have helped her to surmount difficult moments while recognizing and enjoying the countless happy moments. She has chosen not to let the sequelae of her illness govern her life. Rather, she continues to strive to reach her professional goal of working with children. Melissa is an inspiration to those who have known her over the years. She will be an inspiration to those who have yet to meet her.

Central nervous system (CNS) tumors are second in frequency to leukemia and are the most common cause of cancer death in children.[9] For 1998 it was estimated that 2961 children would be diagnosed with a CNS tumor.[16,17] CNS tumors are a heterogeneous mix of tumors with a wide variety of treatments and outcomes. They require aggressive, multimodal therapy that in turn leads to significant long-term difficulties and late effects. Although progress in curing children with CNS tumors has been frustratingly slow, the increasing emphasis of treating children on clinical trials may help improve length and quality of survival. Many new and innovative approaches are likely over the next decade.

EPIDEMIOLOGY

As a group, invasive tumors involving the CNS are the most common solid tumor in childhood. They are the second most frequently occurring cancer, comprising approximately 16.6% of all childhood malignancies and affecting approximately 2,200 children younger than 20 years of age each year[9,35] (Table 21-1).

The incidence of brain cancer in children has increased over the past two decades. It is not clear whether this upward trend is due to changes in environmental exposures or to diagnostic improvements in brain imaging.[35,36] A recent analysis of incidence data from 1975 to 1995 revealed significant increased incidence around 1984 to 1985, corresponding with the advent of magnetic resonance imaging (MRI) scanning.[35] These rates have not returned to that of the pre-MRI era in the ensuing decade, which sustains the MRI hypothesis.[9] The incidence of primary CNS malignancies was 29.1 per 1 million children under the age of 20 for the years 1990 to 1995. These malignancies occur more often in males (30.0 per million) than in females (24.2 per million). The increased incidence in males is more pronounced for primitive neuroectodermal tumor (PNET)/medulloblastoma and ependymoma. White children have a higher incidence than black children (28.5 per million compared with 24.2 per million). This difference is most pronounced during infancy.[35] Survival rates for children with malignant CNS tumors have not improved as dramatically as other types of pediatric cancers. Overall, 5-year survival has increased from 55% (1974-1976) to 64% (1989-1995).[33] These survival rates vary greatly depending on the age of the child (Figure 21-1) and the histologic type of tumor (Table 21-2). In 1995 nearly one quarter of childhood cancer deaths was due to invasive CNS tumors.[35]

The cause of childhood CNS tumors is largely unknown. Certain familial and hereditary syndromes are associated with the occurrence of brain tumors. Children with neurofibromatosis type I have an increased risk of developing optic gliomas. Neurofibromatosis type II is associated with acoustic neuroma, typically occurring in adults. Children with tuberous sclerosis develop subependymal giant cell astrocytomas. Bilateral retinoblastoma is associated with the development of pineoblastoma a condition known as trilateral retinoblastoma. There have been several reports of families with more than one child developing a CNS neoplasm. Brain tumors are associated with the Li-Fraumeni syndrome (see Chapter 2).[35]

Exposure to ionizing radiation can increase the risk of developing a brain tumor. This observation was made in children receiving low doses of scalp irradiation for tinea capitis and in children who develop a secondary malignancy after receiving cranial irradiation.[75] Environmental agents, such as industrial and chemical toxins, have been postulated as risk factors in the development of brain tumors.[35] Associations have been made between certain parental occupations, particularly those of the father—such as working in the aircraft or agricultural industries; electronic manufacturing; and

TABLE 21-1	DISTRIBUTION OF CENTRAL NERVOUS SYSTEM NEOPLASMS IN CHILDHOOD					
	Age					
	<5	5-9	10-14	15-19	<15	<20
PERCENTAGE OF ALL CHILDHOOD CANCERS						
Astrocytoma	6.7	14.2	11.8	6.0	10.0	8.7
Medulloblastoma/PNET	4.3	6.3	3.1	1.0	4.5	3.3
Ependymoma	2.6	1.3	1.1	0.5	1.9	1.4
Other glioma	2.2	5.0	2.9	1.5	3.1	2.6
Misc. intracranial and intraspinal neoplasms	0.2	0.3	0.3	0.3	0.3	0.3
Unspecified intracranial and intraspinal neoplasms	0.5	0.6	0.4	0.2	0.5	0.4
Total (all sites—number of cases)	9,402	5,024	5,419	9,814	19,845	29,659

Data from Ries, L. A. G., Percy, C. L., & Bunin, G. R. (1999). Introduction. In L. A. G. Ries, M. A. Smith, J. G. Gurney, et al. (Eds.), *Cancer incidence and survival among children and adolescents: United States SEER Program 1975-1995* (NIH Pub. No. 99-4649, pp. 2). Bethesda, MD: National Cancer Institute, SEER Program.
NOTE: Data represent percentage of all childhood cancers.

exposure to paint, ionizing radiation, solvents, and electromagnetic fields—and an increased incidence of CNS tumors.[35]

CLASSIFICATION OF CNS TUMORS

The diagnosis of a brain tumor includes a wide range of pathologic categories. Each tumor is

uniquely different in the histologic diagnosis, degree of anaplasia, initial location, and dissemination within and beyond the CNS. Given this diversity, attempts at developing classification systems have been only moderately successful. One of the earliest classification systems was developed by Bailey and Cushing in 1926.[6] Table 21-3 provides a comparison of the most commonly recognized classification systems.

Classification systems are helpful only if the histologic descriptions aid in predicting a specific tumor's clinical behavior. This has proven to be difficult for brain tumors. Without such a system it is impossible to compare accurately clinical strategies used to treat similar tumor types. Future attempts to provide a universally accepted system must combine current knowledge with the growth of new information stemming from advancements in the histogenetic and molecular approaches to the study of these tumors.[8]

The majority (approximately 60%) of pediatric brain tumors develop in the posterior fossa; the remaining 40% are supratentorial. The tentorium is composed of the dura mater, a flap of membrane that is a part of the meninges that separates the cerebrum from the cerebellum. The supratentorium is above the tentorium and contains such structures as the cerebral hemispheres and ventricles. The infratentorium or posterior fossa is below the tentorium and contains the cerebellum and brainstem (Figure 21-2). Another approximately 4% to 10% of CNS tumors occur as primary spinal cord tumors.[51]

More than half of all pediatric brain tumors are malignant. The most common histologic type diagnosed during childhood and adolescence is the glioma. Gliomas are tumors that arise from the

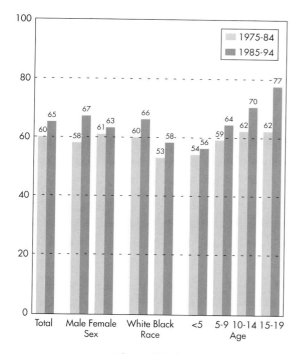

Figure 21-1

CNS tumor survival rates.

TABLE 21-2	FIVE-YEAR RELATIVE SURVIVAL RATES FOR CNS CANCER BY TYPE AND AGE GROUP, ALL RACES, BOTH SEXES, SEER, 1986-94				
	Age				
ICCC† Group	<1	1-4	5-9	10-14	15-19
All CNS cancer	45%	59%	64%	70%	77%
Astrocytoma	69%	79%	70%	75%	75%
Other glioma	*	51%	43%	64%	79%
Ependymoma	25%	46%	71%	76%	*
PNET	19%	46%	69%	57%	75%

From Gurney, J. G., Smith, M. A., & Bunin, G. R. (1999). CNS and miscellaneous intracranial and intraspinal neoplasms. In L. A. G. Ries, M. A. Smith, J. G. Gurney, et al. (Eds.), *Cancer incidence and survival among children and adolescents: United States SEER Program 1975-1995* (NIH Pub. No. 99-4649, pp. 51-63). Bethesda, MD: National Cancer Institute Program.
*Less than 20 cases.
†International Classification of Childhood Cancer (ICCC).

World Health Organization (Modified for Pediatrics)	Russell and Rubinstein	Kernohan and Associates	Bailey and Cushing
GLIAL TUMORS	**TUMORS OF GLIAL SERIES**		
1. Astrocytic astrocytoma Anaplastic astrocytoma Subependymal giant cell tumor Giagnatocellular glioma	I. Astrocytic astrocytoma Astroblastoma	1. Astrocytoma grades I-IV	1. Astrocytoma 2. Astroblastoma
2. Oligodendroglial tumors Oligodendroglioma Anaplastic oligodendroglioma	II. Oligodendroglial tumors Oligodendroglioma	2. Oligodendroglioma grades I-IV	3. Oligodendroglioma
3. Ependymal tumors Ependymoma Anaplastic ependymoma Myxopapillary ependymoma	III. Tumors of the ependyma and its homologs Ependymoma	3. Ependymoma grades I-IV	4. Ependymoma 5. Ependymoblastoma
4. Choroid plexus tumors Choroid plexus papilloma Anaplastic choroid Plexus tumor	Colloid cyst Choroid plexus papilloma		6. Choroid plexus papillomas
5. Mixed gliomas			
6. Glioblastoma multiforme	IV. Glioblastoma multiforme	(Astrocytoma IV)	7. Glioblastoma multiforme
NEURONAL TUMORS	**TUMORS OF THE NEURON SERIES**		
1. Gangliocytoma 2. Ganglioglioma 3. Anaplastic ganglioglioma	1. Ganglioneuroma 2. Ganglioglioma 3. Neuroblastoma	4. Neuroastrocytoma grades I-IV	8. Ganglioglioma 9. Neuroblastoma
PRIMITIVE NEUROECTODERMAL TUMORS (PNET)			
1. PNET not otherwise specified 2. PNET with differentiation (astrocytic, ependymal, neuronal); oligodendroglial, mixed	4. Medulloblastoma	5. Medulloblastoma	10. Medulloblastomas
3. Medulloepithelioma	5. Medulloepithelioma	(Ependymoma IV)	11. Medulloepithelioma
PINEAL CELL TUMORS	**PINEAL PARENCHYMAL TUMORS**		
1. Pineocytoma 2. PNET (pineoblastoma)	1. Pineocytoma 2. Pineoblastoma		12. Pinealoma

From Heideman, R. L., Packer, R. J., Albright, L. A., et al. (1997). Tumors of the central nervous system. In P. A. Pizzo & D. G. Poplack (Eds.), *Principles and practice of pediatric oncology* (3rd ed., pp. 633-697). Philadelphia: Lippincott-Raven.

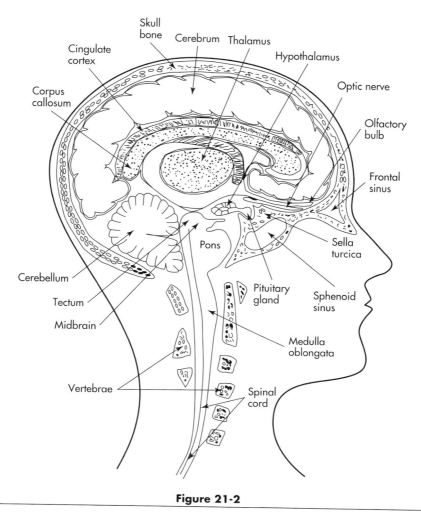

Figure 21-2

Parts of the brain.   (From American Brain Tumor Association. [1998]. *A primer of brain tumors: A patient's reference manual.* Des Plaines, IL: Author.)

glial tissue of the brain and include astrocytomas, ependymomas, oligodendrogliomas, and mixed tumors with two or more different cell types. Embryonal tumors, formed by poorly differentiated neuroepithelial cells, occur most commonly in the cerebellum and are called medulloblastomas. Tumors that are histologically similar but occur above the tentorium in the cerebrum are referred to as supratentorial primitive neuroectodermal tumors (PNET). Despite the use of common protocols, there are significant prognostic differences between the two entities.[80] Neuronal tumors arise from ganglia, which are groups of nerve cells. Included in this category is the ganglioglioma, which is composed of both nerve and supportive cells. Craniopharyngioma, a histologically benign, congenital tumor, can have a malignant course if it is

not surgically accessible and/or invades adjacent healthy structures. Midline tumors, including craniopharyngiomas, pineal region tumors, germ cell tumors, optic gliomas, and hypothalamic gliomas, range from low-grade to highly malignant lesions and are difficult to treat because of location.

Some childhood brain tumors are low-grade lesions characterized by a very slow rate of progression. Others are high-grade or anaplastic lesions that can grow rapidly, are invasive, can recur in a short time period, and sometimes metastasize. These aggressive lesions are treated with intensive protocols involving irradiation and, frequently, chemotherapy. With certain histologic types, such as astrocytomas, there is a grading system, with grade I indicating a benign lesion and grade IV indicating a highly anaplastic or malignant lesion.

Location is a critical factor in pediatric brain tumors. A low-grade tumor located in a surgically inaccessible area such as the brainstem may not have a favorable outcome. Both histology and location of the tumor determine a tumor's clinical course.[8]

CLINICAL PRESENTATION

Presenting signs and symptoms of a brain tumor are related to the location and histologic grade of the tumor and the age of the child. Brain tumors can grow as discrete masses, causing pressure on adjacent structures, and by infiltrating and destroying normal brain tissue. They may also block the flow of cerebrospinal fluid (CSF) (Table 21-4).

Posterior fossa tumors involve the fourth ventricle, the cerebellum, and the brainstem. These tumors can exert pressure on the fourth ventricle and obstruct the flow of CSF, causing hydrocephalus and symptoms of increased intracranial pressure (ICP). Children may present with the classic symptoms of increased ICP: headache, vomiting, and lethargy. Headaches may be vague or severe. Headaches that wake the child at night are usually concerning. Although typically described as morning headache and vomiting, these symptoms can occur at any time.[38]

Tumors that involve or exert pressure on the cerebellum can cause disturbances in balance. Children may complain of diplopia (double vision) and may present with nystagmus, a rhythmic movement of the eyes directed toward the side of the lesion. Brainstem tumors can manifest multiple cranial nerve findings. Again, children may complain of diplopia or have paresis of gaze (an inability to move the eyes past midline). Head tilt can occur from pressure exerted on the fourth cranial nerve. Facial droop or palsy can occur from involvement of the seventh cranial nerve. Lower cranial nerve involvement may be manifest by difficulty with speech or swallowing. Long-tract signs include hemiparesis, spastic gait, and hyperreflexia with upgoing toes (positive Babinski sign).

Supratentorial tumors present with a variety of symptoms, depending on the lobe and hemisphere involved. Increased ICP is the result of direct pressure on brain tissue or obstruction of CSF flow. Focal losses such as hemiparesis, a partial sensory loss, or visual disturbances can also occur. Tumors that involve the temporal lobe can produce focal seizures. Temporoparietal tumors may lead to aphasia if they occur in the dominant hemisphere. Lesions in the frontal lobe are often associated with changes in personality, or disinhibition. Occipital lobe tumors can lead to visual loss. Tumors that occur midline in the supratentorium, such as germ cell tumors, craniopharyngioma, and optic glioma, can cause endocrine abnormalities such as diabetes insipidus, thyroid dysfunction, and precocious puberty, as well as visual losses. Tumors arising in the pineal region can present with Parinaud's syndrome, which includes the inability to move the eyes upward, retraction nystagmus (eyes appear to bounce back [retract] when child looks medially toward the nose), and difficulty with accommodation. Children with primary spinal cord tumors can often have back pain, paralysis, or paresis. If CSF flow is blocked, symptoms of increased ICP may occur.

Age and developmental stage are also important factors in the symptoms associated with childhood brain tumors. Infants may present with delay or loss of developmental milestones, or failure to thrive. The child who was previously beginning to stand may only be able to creep. Enlarging head circumference may indicate hydrocephalus secondary to a brain tumor. Infants with optic nerve tumors may present with nystagmus or shimmery eye movements or may have a limited ability to fix and follow objects. Infants with brain tumors may also display generalized irritability. School-age children and adolescents may present with a history of personality changes or decline in school performance. Often parents may note deterioration in handwriting or a change in handedness.

DIAGNOSTIC EVALUATION

The diagnosis of a CNS neoplasm begins with a detailed health history, with special attention given to the duration of symptoms. A child presenting with rapidly progressive symptoms over a short time period is more likely to have a highly malignant tumor. A thorough physical and neurologic evaluation is done. If a tumor is suspected, neuroimaging of the head is then performed. MRI of the head is the optimal choice for several reasons. The images are clearer and are obtained in multiple phases. There is minimal risk of allergic reaction to the contrast medium, gadolinium diethylenetriamine pentaacetic acid (DTPA), and there is no radiation exposure.[64] If MRI is not available or if the child is too ill to successfully complete this evaluation, a quick but less sensitive computed tomography (CT) scan, without and with the iodinated contrast, is performed. A CT scan may be the preferred choice for a very young or fearful child who would require general anesthesia for the MRI study. An MRI of the spine may be ordered because of symptoms or as part of the metastatic work-up for tumors that are known to disseminate throughout the spinal axis. A lumbar puncture may be performed

TABLE 21-4	**GLOBAL PRESENTING SIGNS AND SYMPTOMS OF CHILDHOOD BRAIN TUMORS ACCORDING TO LOCATION**

GENERAL

Headache	These come and go, can be worse in the AM and sometimes improve during the day; worsen with cough, exercise, or bending/kneeling; can waken child at night.
Seizures	Generalized or focal depending on tumor location.
Mental status changes	May have problems with memory, speech, communication, and/or concentration. Behavior changes or changes in temperament or personality can also occur. In extreme cases, somnolence can lead to coma.
Increased intracranial pressure (ICP)	Due to tumor growth, hydrocephalus, edema. Symptoms include nausea and vomiting, drowsiness, vision problems, headache, mental changes, papilledema, decreased level of consciousness (LOC).

Tumor Location	Normal Function	Common Symptoms
POSTERIOR FOSSA (CONTAINS THE FOURTH VENTRICLE, CEREBELLUM, BRAINSTEM)		
Brainstem	Controls basic life functions (BP, HR, RR). Reticular formation controls consciousness, eating and sleep patterns, drowsiness, and attention.	Vomiting, clumsy uncoordinated walk, cranial nerve palsies, headache, head tilt, drowsiness, hearing loss, personality changes. Long track signs (hemiparesis, spastic gait, and hyperreflexia with upgoing toes—positive Babinski sign). Late development of increased ICP.
Cerebellum	Together with the thalamus and cerebrum controls intricate muscular coordination including walking and speech.	Headache secondary to tumor or headache, nausea and vomiting, and papilledema secondary to increased ICP. Clumsy uncoordinated walk, swaying, staggering. Dizziness, tremors, difficulty with coordinated speech, double vision. Nystagmus toward the involved hemisphere.
CEREBRAL HEMISPHERES		
Frontal lobe	Controls voluntary movement on the opposite side of the body. Dominant hemisphere controls language and writing (left in right-handed people, right in left-handed people). Intellectual function, thought processes, behavior, memory.	One-sided paralysis, seizures, short-term memory loss, impaired judgment, personality and mental changes (disinhibition), urinary frequency and urgency, gait disturbances, communication problems.
Occipital lobe	Understanding visual images and meaning of written words.	Visual disturbances, seizures.
Parietal lobe	Receive and interpret sensation including pain, temperature, touch, pressure, size, and shape. Body part awareness. Hearing, reasoning, memory.	Seizures, language disturbances if dominant hemisphere, loss of ability to read, spatial disorders, loss of ability to do math (can read numbers but cannot do calculations). Difficulty knowing left from right.
Temporal lobe	Understanding sounds and spoken works. Emotion and memory. Depth perception and sense of time.	Seizures, loss of ability to recognize sounds or source of sounds. Visual impairments, emotional lability.

Data from American Brain Tumor Association. (1998). *A primer of brain tumors: A patient's reference manual.* Des Plaines, IL: Author; Duffner, P. K., Cohen, M. F., & Freeman, A. (1985). Pediatric brain tumors: An overview. *Cancer, 35,* 287-301.

Continued

TABLE 21-4	GLOBAL PRESENTING SIGNS AND SYMPTOMS OF CHILDHOOD BRAIN TUMORS ACCORDING TO LOCATION—cont'd	
Tumor Location	**Normal Function**	**Common Symptoms**
MIDLINE TUMORS		
	Where the two cerebral hemispheres meet, including the optic chiasm, hypothalamic area, and pineal region.	Headache, nausea and vomiting, papilledema secondary to increased ICP. Abnormal eye movements, visual loss. Alteration of personality or consciousness. Impairment of hypothalamic/pituitary function: delayed or accelerated growth. Precocious puberty. Water balance (diabetes insipidus, SIADH). Increased or decreased appetite. Failure to thrive.
SPINAL CORD		
		Symptoms depend on location: • Thoracic—"girdle pain" in chest that worsens with cough or sneezing and when lying down. • Cervical or lumbar—neck, arm, back, leg pain, weakness, muscle wasting or spasms, sensory changes, altered bowel or bladder function. • Progression of symptoms can result in paralysis.

Data from American Brain Tumor Association. (1998). *A primer of brain tumors: A patient's reference manual.* Des Plaines, IL: Author; Duffner, P. K., Cohen, M. F., & Freeman, A. (1985). Pediatric brain tumors: An overview. *Cancer, 35,* 287-301.

to detect malignant cells in the CSF. It can also detect "tumor markers" such as α-fetoprotein (AFP) or β subunit of human chorionic gonadotropin (β-hCG), which are diagnostic for germ cell tumors. A bone scan, bone marrow aspirate, or bone marrow biopsy may be necessary when systemic dissemination is possible in tumors such as medulloblastomas. Determining the extent of disease at diagnosis is imperative because it influences both the plan of care and the overall prognosis.[5]

A variety of other neuroimaging techniques can be used to evaluate treatment response or to help determine disease recurrence. The positron emission tomography (PET) scan measures metabolic activity and is useful to evaluate recurrent tumor. Malignancy is characterized by hypermetabolism, while areas of necrosis or injury present with reduced metabolism.[64] Single-photon emission computed tomography (SPECT) may be useful for localizing tumor, predicting tumor grade, and differentiating necrosis from tumor. MRI spectroscopy is a noninvasive, potentially useful monitor of brain metabolism that is increasingly available in conjunction with current MRI imaging equipment. It will further help to differentiate be-

tween active tumor and necrotic or injured brain tissue. The magnetic resonance angiography uses the MRI to visualize blood supply to the brain. Functional MRI can help to tailor intraoperative strategies in patients with lesions located in critical areas of function. Sedation of a young child for this procedure will not interfere with results.[77]

TREATMENT

SURGERY

Surgery is the first step in the treatment of childhood brain tumors. The goal is to obtain the most extensive resection feasible while preserving neurologic function or to obtain a biopsy for tissue diagnosis if resection is impossible. Stereotactic procedures make it possible to perform a biopsy safely on almost any area of the brain.[64] One notable exception is the diffuse pontine brainstem lesion. Biopsy of these lesions can cause clinical deterioration without significantly altering the diagnosis or prognosis. However, neurosurgical techniques can be used in certain areas of the brainstem, especially when there is an exophytic (an area of tumor extending outside of the brainstem) component to the tumor.[25] Certain germ cell tumors can be diagnosed without surgery by the presence of specific tumor markers in the blood or CSF.

Often, symptomatic relief will occur once the tumor is resected. If hydrocephalus persists postoperatively, the surgical placement of a ventriculoperitoneal (VP) shunt will be necessary. If the obstruction to the CSF drainage is located in or around the fourth ventricle, a surgical option called a third ventriculostomy can be performed. Using endoscopy, the neurosurgeon creates a new drainage pathway through the floor of the third ventricle.[81]

Intricate surgical procedures using the neuroimaging techniques described previously, such as the functional MRI, make it feasible to debulk larger tumors with less morbidity.[71] Occasionally, a complete surgical resection can cure low-grade tumors such as a juvenile pilocytic astrocytoma if the tumor has a clearly demarcated plane.[51,60] When complete resection is not a viable option, the most extensive resection possible is performed. In certain types of tumors, such as an anaplastic astrocytoma or medulloblastoma, the degree of original resection affects prognosis. Although the exact mechanism is unknown, adjuvant therapy appears to be more effective when there is a lesser tumor burden.

Surgery may be necessary at various times during therapy. A second surgical resection of the tumor is considered when the disease progresses or recurs. Neurosurgical procedures such as the placement of an Ommaya reservoir can facilitate the delivery of therapy directly into the CSF. The neurosurgical operating microscope allows safer retraction of healthy brain tissue so that the surgeon has better access to the tumor. Endoscopic surgery is used to work inside the cerebral ventricles and in hypovascular tumors. Technical advances such as the development of smaller multichannel endoscopes that allow the passage of surgical instruments needed for tumor dissection, suction, and irrigation have significantly improved usefulness.

A frameless stereotactic system is a coordinated mapping system that helps the neurosurgeon to plan the approach.[60] However, this system cannot take into account the intraoperative changes that occur as a result of tumor removal, osmotic changes, or ventricular drainage. Ultrasound can further enhance navigation during the surgical procedure by defining tumor margins. A two-dimensional technique is now in use, but a three-dimensional system is currently being developed. Improvements in functional brain mapping have been crucial to identify the eloquent cortex, areas of brain that, if removed, would result in significant

clinical deficits.[77] This makes it possible for more intricate removal of tumors without causing significant postoperative morbidity.

The ultrasonic surgical aspirator uses ultrasonic energy to break up the interstitial cellular matrix of the tumor so that it can then be suctioned, thereby debulking more effectively.[60] The laser, which is used in limited situations with large tumors, has proven to be too bulky for intricate surgical procedures.[51]

Postoperative care for the child who has had a craniotomy requires careful medical and nursing observation for 2 to 3 days. Often a 24- to 48-hour stay in an intensive care setting is required. Because increased ICP can develop, frequent assessment of neurologic and mental status as well as vital signs is important.

An MRI is done within 72 hours of the surgery so that an exact estimate of residual tumor can be determined without interference from postoperative edema or artifact. Children who present preoperatively with significant hydrocephalus or edema surrounding the tumor will begin steroids 48 to 72 hours before surgery to alleviate some of the pressure on normal brain tissue. A tapering schedule starts approximately 72 hours postoperatively. These children need to be monitored for problems such as headache, vomiting, and mental status changes that may indicate increased pressure or steroid tapering done too rapidly.

Seizure activity is treated with anticonvulsants, and therapeutic serum levels need to be maintained. Meticulous monitoring of fluid balance and serum and urine sodium levels is important, particularly in children who have hypothalamic, pituitary, or other suprasellar lesions. The development of diabetes insipidus or the syndrome of inappropriate secretion of antidiuretic hormone (SIADH) is very likely in these children.[74]

Posterior fossa syndrome, a complication after surgery for posterior fossa tumors, including mutism, ataxia, nerve palsies and hemiparesis, is not completely understood. The mutism usually resolves, but the child is left with some range of neurologic deficits in most instances. Early recognition of this syndrome helps the child, family, and staff understand and cope with the associated neurologic deficits and the need to begin rehabilitation promptly.[20]

RADIATION THERAPY

Radiation therapy has long been the gold standard for treating brain tumors. As early as 1930 improved survival rates were seen in children who received radiation therapy after surgical resection of high-grade tumors. During the late 1980s and early

1990s many trials were done to minimize or even avoid radiation therapy in very young children (age less than 5 years) with brain tumors by using more intensive surgery or even myeloablative chemotherapy with bone marrow rescue. Unfortunately, many of these children developed recurrent tumors without much improvement in survival. More recent trials have focused on safer ways to give radiation to these children. There are many concerns when irradiating the developing brain; consequently, much work has been done to minimize the dose and extent of radiation for children with brain tumors.[26,29,42,54,65]

Stereotactic radiotherapy and conformal field radiation therapy are two techniques used to minimize the amount of normal tissue in the radiation field. These techniques use three-dimensional planning and complex physics to aim the radiation beam from multiple directions, so that the full dose falls on the tumor but the dose from each beam through normal tissue is minimal. This is an improvement over the more traditional radiation techniques, in which the beam is aimed from three directions. Radiosurgery, a technique that uses a single high-dose fraction of highly focal radiation, is also being used for certain patients.[65]

Hyperfractionated radiation therapy is another technique used to minimize damage to normal tissue. Rather than administer a standard dose once a day (e.g., 1.8 Gy), a smaller dose (e.g., 1 Gy) is administered twice a day with a 4- to 6-hour rest in between. The theory is that normal brain tissue repairs itself within the 4- to 6-hour rest period, while tumor cells do not. This technique allows a much higher total dose of radiation to the tumor. Hyper-fractionated radiation for children with brain tumors was initially tried in children with brainstem glioma. The technique allowed total doses in excess of 70 Gy, where more traditional therapy allowed doses in the range of 54 Gy to 60 Gy. At least for children with brainstem glioma, hyperfractionated radiation has not improved long-term survival.[24,44,56] It has also been tried in other tumor types, such as PNET, without clear advantage.[62]

CHEMOTHERAPY

Multiple studies by the major pediatric cooperative study groups have proven the efficacy of chemotherapy in certain brain tumors. Chemotherapy is usually part of a multimodal treatment plan. It can be administered before, during, and after radiation therapy and if the tumor progresses or recurs.[64] An important use in the very young child is to avoid or delay radiation therapy. The most commonly used chemotherapeutic drugs for brain tumor patients are alkylating agents, such as the nitrosoureas, and the platinum compounds, such as cisplatin or carboplatin.[63] They may be used as single agents but are most commonly used in combination with other chemotherapeutic agents. Table 21-5 lists the most commonly used chemotherapeutic agents.

The blood-brain barrier is controlled by tight junctions between endothelial cells and influences the penetration of drugs into the CNS. The blood-brain barrier is disrupted within areas of greatest tumor bulk, especially in the high-grade tumors, while remaining intact in other areas of the tumor.[64] The water-soluble chemotherapeutic agents can penetrate the disrupted areas of the blood-brain

TABLE 21-5	CHEMOTHERAPEUTIC DRUGS COMMONLY USED IN CENTRAL NERVOUS SYSTEM TUMORS
Drug	**Mechanism**
Nitrosoureas (Carmustine, Lomustine)	DNA crosslinks, carbamoylation of amino groups
Procarbazine	DNA alkylation, interference with protein synthesis
Carboplatin	Chelation via intrastrand crosslinks
Cisplatin	
Cyclophosphamide	DNA alkylation, carbonium ion formation
Ifosfamide	
Paclitaxel	Microtubule function inhibitors
Vincristine	
Etoposide	Topoisomerase II inhibitors
Teniposide	
Topotecan	Topoisomerase I inhibitors
Irinotecan (CPT-11)	
Tamoxifen	Protein kinase C inhibitor (at high doses)

From Prados, M. D., Berger, M. S., Wilson, W. B. (1998). Primary central nervous system tumors. Advances in knowledge and treatment. *CA: A Cancer Journal for Clinicians, 48*, 349.

barrier, while the more liposoluble agents may be more efficient in penetrating the intact areas.[37]

Conventional doses of chemotherapy are being evaluated in varying treatment schemas and at various times in the course of the illness: preoperative; before, during, and after irradiation; and at recurrence or progression. High-dose chemotherapy followed by autologous hematopoietic stem cell transplantation (HSCT) or peripheral blood stem cell (PBSC) reinfusion has shown some promise in treating newly diagnosed highly malignant tumors such as glioblastoma multiforme.[34] This innovative approach is labor intensive and carries with it significant, life-threatening toxicity.[22,34] As with all treatment protocols, it should be conducted only in major pediatric oncology centers that are equipped to monitor and treat all possible acute and chronic side effects.

Chemotherapy is used initially to treat infants and young children, those less than 3 years of age, with the goal of avoiding or delaying radiation therapy until the child is older.[45] Recurrent or progressive disease can also be treated with intensive chemotherapy protocols followed by PBSC rescues.[21,32] The use of single agents such as oral etoposide in the treatment of progressive or recurrent disease is under investigation.[52] Improvements in the use of antiemetic therapy has lessened the nausea and vomiting associated with such intensive protocols.[67]

There are several areas of clinical research undergoing intense investigation at this time. New drugs currently in phase I or II studies include temozolomide, which has demonstrated activity against recurrent disease and is now being tested in patients with newly diagnosed tumors such as brainstem gliomas.[63] Inhibitors of angiogenesis such as TNP-470 and thalidomide (alone or with cyclophosphamide) are in phase I and II studies.[64] Tamoxifen, used now for recurrent disease, is under evaluation as an initial agent in high doses.[11] Children's Oncology Group clinical trials are in development, which will evaluate innovative combinations of chemotherapy and radiotherapy as well as biologic investigations. Research funded by the American Brain Tumor Association (ABTA) from the present through the year 2002 includes, among others, the biologic study of cell death and mechanisms of enhanced tumor cell growth. A proposed combination of immune therapy (IL-2) and chemotherapy (BCNU) is under investigation.[15] Studies involving gene therapy include investigations of tumor-suppressor genes such as *INK4a, p53,* and *PTEN* in an effort to understand their ability to define tumor formation. Genetically engineered *p53* peptides that appear, in laboratory studies, to be able to destroy cells that have the *p53* defect

are also being investigated in research funded by the ABTA.[15] *p53* is one of the most common genetic abnormalities associated with malignant gliomas.[15,64]

Future treatment goals include the improvement of present protocols to increase survival rates and the development of new treatment strategies for resistant tumors. Clinical trials are underway to determine the efficacy of tailoring radiation fields as well as decreasing the total dose to decrease long-term sequelae. In tumors with dismal outcome, such as brainstem gliomas, research studies are looking at new agents, improving delivery of available drugs, and innovative combination protocols. The quality and quantity of laboratory research, particularly in the area of molecular biology, has been translated into new clinical trials looking at novel ways of treating malignant CNS tumors.[7]

The multidisciplinary approach to the treatment of a child with a CNS neoplasm is crucial. Typically this team is made up of nurses; oncologists; neurologists; neurosurgeons; radiation oncologists; neuropsychologists; educators; physical, occupational, and speech therapists; and social workers. Care should be given in a childhood cancer center, preferably under the direction of a neurooncologist. Participation in clinical trials will ensure that the child is monitored during treatment and in long-term follow-up care in addition to adding vital information to a central research database that will help clinicians improve both the survival rates and the quality of life for these children.

PROGNOSIS

Prognosis varies greatly among brain tumors. For example, a child with a completely resected juvenile pilocytic astrocytoma has a near 90% chance of cure, while a child with a pontine brainstem glioma has a life expectancy of approximately 1 year.[8,27] Even among tumors of the same histology, the disease may be classified as either low risk or high risk based on certain indicators, and the overall prognosis varies accordingly. Prognostic indicators and survival rates for specific tumors are discussed separately.

COMMON PEDIATRIC CNS TUMORS
Astrocytomas

The largest category of pediatric brain tumors are the astrocytomas. They can occur at any age and in various areas of the brain. They are classified according to the degree of anaplasia. Grade I tumors are the pilocytic astrocytomas; grade II tumors are the low-grade fibrillary astrocytomas; grade III consists of the anaplastic astrocytomas; and grade IV is the glioblastoma multiforme. There are, therefore, wide variations in treatment options and prognoses for this group of tumors.

Low-Grade Cerebellar Astrocytoma

Low-grade cerebellar astrocytomas account for between 10% and 20% of pediatric brain tumors and occur most commonly in the first decade of life.[37] More than 80% of all childhood cerebellar gliomas are pilocytic astrocytomas. Although rare, there have been cases of direct extension into the brainstem. Also unusual is the possibility of an aggressive clinical course with either progressive recurrent disease or leptomeningeal spread of the disease. The diffuse or fibrillary astrocytoma is the second variety of cerebellar astrocytoma and comprises approximately 15% of cerebellar astrocytomas. This tumor is more cellular and infiltrative and is more likely to have malignant transformation.[37]

Children with low-grade cerebellar astrocytomas present with headache, vomiting, ataxia, hemiparesis, and irritability. Total surgical resection is crucial and is possible in most juvenile pilocytic tumors. The diffuse cerebellar astrocytoma are a more difficult surgical challenge. No further therapy is necessary if the resection is complete. Controversy surrounds the treatment of patients with residual disease because the tumor's growth rate is slow.[12] Radiation therapy can be given for residual disease, although most oncologists will use this only if there is tumor progression. Chemotherapy has proven to be effective in controlling newly diagnosed, progressive, low-grade gliomas in young children.[55] Children who relapse after surgery alone will undergo a second surgical resection, if feasible. Localized radiation therapy is then the next treatment option, except in the very young child for whom chemotherapy would be given initially in an effort to delay radiation therapy. If there is recurrence in an unresectable area after irradiation, chemotherapy is the treatment of choice.

Prognosis differs dramatically between pilocytic and diffuse or fibrillary astrocytomas.[37] Although overall prognosis depends on tumor location, 5-year survival rates for cerebellar pilocytic astrocytomas is 85% to 95%.[8] The diffuse or fibrillary astrocytomas generally have a more dismal outcome.[37] A consistently poor prognostic indicator in cerebellar astrocytomas is the presence of brainstem involvement.[14]

Low-Grade Cerebral Astrocytoma

Supratentorial low-grade astrocytomas are a diverse group of tumors. The pilocytic and fibrillary types are usually seen in children. Anaplastic transformation is not as common in children as in adults, although fibrillary lesions have a greater tendency to anaplasia.[76] Children with these tumors can present with nonlocalizing signs related to increased ICP, seizures, and specific symptoms related to tumor location, such as focal motor deficits. Hypothalamic tumors may cause endocrine abnormalities, while tumors in the optic chiasm may cause optic atrophy. The midline diencephalic tumors can cause emesis, cachexia, and euphoria in children under 3 years of age, known as the diencephalic syndrome. The MRI reveals a hypodense lesion with poor contrast uptake; however, most low-grade lesions enhance.

Surgery is the treatment of choice, with the goal of removing as much tumor as possible with the least morbidity. Completely resected tumors do not require further treatment. With residual or recurrent disease, options include close observation, second resection, radiation, and/or chemotherapy. Localized radiation therapy is typically used after tumor progression. Low-grade tumors have shown response to some chemotherapy agents, such as carboplatin.[55] Chemotherapy may delay radiation therapy for the very young child.

Several factors that indicate a favorable prognosis include tumor histology, grade, young age (as compared with adults, but a toddler will fare worse than a school-age child), location, and in some studies, extent of resection. Five-year survival rates for children with a complete resection is as high as 90%.[76] Children with an incomplete resection will benefit from the addition of chemotherapy or radiation therapy if there is local tumor progression.[61]

High-Grade Astrocytomas

About 10% of all childhood brain tumors are high-grade astrocytomas.[76] Approximately 66% occur in the frontal, temporal, or parietal lobes of the cerebral hemispheres, 20% in the midline (diencephalon), and 15% in the posterior fossa, including the brainstem.[37] The high-grade astrocytomas, such as the anaplastic astrocytoma and glioblastoma multiforme, are classified as astrocytomas grade III and IV respectively and are the most common malignant glial neoplasms.[37] These high-grade gliomas can invade the surrounding normal brain tissue with occasional leptomeningeal dissemination that can involve the spinal cord. Systemic dissemination is rare.[41]

Children with high-grade astrocytomas present with symptoms related to tumor location. These symptoms can include headache, vomiting, seizures, speech difficulties, weakness or paralysis, visual disturbances, and personality changes. An MRI of these high-grade tumors will typically show an irregularly shaped mass with a heterogeneous, mixed density pattern, usually with mass effect, a helpful feature in distinguishing edema from tumor. Surgery is the treatment of choice, with a complete resection and low morbidity as the ultimate goal. At the very least, a biopsy is needed. The extent of tumor resection is an important prognostic factor in childhood malignant gliomas, more so with the anaplastic astrocytoma than with the glioblastoma multiforme.[79] Postoperative local or wide-field irradiation improves survival rates somewhat. Stereotactic radiotherapy is under investigation to increase doses delivered locally to the tumor.

Chemotherapy can improve 5-year survival rates slightly in high-grade gliomas, especially in children with extensive surgical resections.[46] High-dose chemotherapy, both single agents and combination modalities, followed by autologous bone marrow or stem cell reinfusions are now being studied in newly diagnosed patients.[34] The very young child is treated with high-dose chemotherapy in an effort to avoid, or at least delay, radiation therapy. Recurrent disease will be treated surgically if the tumor location and child's clinical status warrant. In patients previously irradiated, high-dose chemotherapy protocols followed by HSCT will be considered.

Overall, the prognosis for these high-grade gliomas is dismal. The anaplastic astrocytomas (grade III) have a slightly better outcome than the glioblastoma multiforme (grade IV). Five-year survival rates are 29% for patients with anaplastic astrocytoma and 18% for those with glioblastoma multiforme.[66]

MEDULLOBLASTOMA/PRIMITIVE NEUROECTODERMAL TUMOR (PNET)

Medulloblastoma/PNET accounts for approximately 20% to 25% of all childhood brain tumors.[30,31] It is a small, round, blue cell tumor, which is usually very fast growing. Medulloblastoma, by definition, occurs in the posterior fossa, usually in the midline sometimes in the cerebellar hemispheres as well. If the tumor arises in the cerebral hemispheres, it is usually called a supratentorial PNET. Although the histology looks very similar under the microscope, biologically it is not clear that medulloblastoma (posterior fossa PNET) and supratentorial PNET are the same tumor. Supratentorial PNET comprise less than 6% of all childhood brain tumors and tend to have poorer outcomes than medulloblastoma (posterior fossa PNET).[39,80]

Because of its rapid growth, medulloblastoma commonly presents with acute onset of symptoms. The posterior fossa location frequently causes ob-

struction of CSF outflow from the fourth ventricle. Thus signs of increased ICP, including vomiting, headache, and blurred vision, are common. These children can also manifest gait disturbances, truncal ataxia (unsteadiness), and dysmetria (incoordination). Infants may present with enlarging head circumference.

Approximately 30% of children with medulloblastoma will have disseminated disease, and therefore imaging of the spine as well as examination of the CSF is critical.[30,37,42] Lumbar puncture may be postponed to the postoperative period if there is concern that a spinal tap in the presence of increased ICP may cause downward herniation. Medulloblastoma/PNET is one of the few CNS tumors that can spread to the bone and bone marrow, so bone marrow aspiration and a biopsy may be performed as part of the initial work-up. However, the rate of bone marrow involvement at diagnosis is very low.[50] Surgical resection is undertaken both to confirm the diagnosis and to remove as much tumor as possible. Depending on the size of the tumor, degree of hydrocephalus, and age of the patient, a ventriculoperitoneal (VP) shunt may be placed. This is more common in young patients with moderate to severe preoperative hydrocephalus and large tumors.[43] Often, surgical resection of the tumor obviates the need for permanent shunting.

Once the diagnosis is established, staging evaluation is done to confirm the extent of disease. A postoperative enhanced MRI is obtained, ideally within 72 hours after surgery. This early timing is to help differentiate between residual tumor and postoperative changes. If not done preoperatively, a contrast (gadolinium) enhanced MRI of the spine is obtained as well.

Children with medulloblastoma may be categorized into two risk categories: (1) patients greater than 3 years of age who underwent subtotal or partial resection and who had brainstem invasion and metastatic disease (high risk); and (2) patients greater than 3 years of age who underwent gross total resection and had no metastatic disease (average risk). Children less than 3 years of age may be considered at very high risk and are typically treated on age-specific protocols.[30] The presence of metastatic disease at diagnosis is the greatest risk factor for children with medulloblastoma. Other indicators thought to be associated with a poor prognosis, such as age at diagnosis, tumor size at diagnosis, tumor location within the posterior fossa, extent of resection, and histopathology, have not consistently borne out in all studies.[31,40,50]

Treatment for children with medulloblastoma/PNET is multimodal. Surgical resection is the first step. Children over 3 years of age are usually treated with craniospinal radiation therapy with a boost to the posterior fossa. It has been proposed that the reason survival rates for children under 3 years of age have historically been very poor is the omission or reduction of craniospinal radiation because of its deleterious neurocognitive effects.[40] Radiation dose to the posterior fossa appears to be an important prognosticator, because patients receiving less than 50 Gy to the posterior fossa tend to have decreased survival.[31]

Chemotherapy plays a very important role for children with medulloblastoma.[42] Early studies found that in children with high-risk disease who were treated with chemotherapy, survival improved dramatically.[57] For children with standard-risk disease, chemotherapy can allow reduced doses of craniospinal radiation, and in infants, chemotherapy can help delay or possibly obviate the need for radiation therapy. In all children, chemotherapy is important to prevent or treat systemic dissemination.[42] Over the past several years the combination of chemotherapy with radiation therapy has become the standard approach for children with medulloblastoma, with long-term survival rates greater than 80% in some studies.[58]

BRAINSTEM TUMORS

Brainstem tumors represent approximately 10% to 15% of childhood brain tumors and occur most frequently in children under 10 years of age.[27,35] Brainstem tumors can be subcategorized into focal or diffuse infiltrative lesions. Fifteen percent to 20% of brainstem lesions are low-grade astrocytomas, while 80% are the more familiar, and more life-threatening, diffuse intrinsic pontine lesions. Histologically, these lesions can range from low-grade glioma to anaplastic astrocytoma to malignant glioblastoma multiforme.[13] These tumors often will dedifferentiate into more malignant forms when they recur or progress. Other types of tumors, such as PNET or medulloepithelioma, can also arise in the brainstem, but this is less common.[2]

Children with diffuse intrinsic brainstem tumors present with multiple cranial nerve findings, as well as diplopia, ataxia, and long tract signs including hemiparesis. Personality changes, such as irritability or depression, can also occur. Headaches and vomiting are also possible, but these are less common in brainstem tumors. Children with more focal tumors are more likely to present with unilateral cranial nerve involvement and contralateral hemiparesis. Cervicomedullary tumors are likely to present with neck pain, vomiting, lower cranial nerve dysfunction, and paresis.

The duration of clinical symptoms can offer some insight into the grade of the tumor and can have prognostic value. Children who present with a long history of vague headaches or single cranial nerve dysfunction are more likely to have a focal or exophytic, slow-growing lesion. Children who present with rapid onset of multiple cranial nerve deficits are most likely to have an aggressive, diffuse, infiltrating brainstem glioma.

Diagnosis of a brainstem tumor is made by MRI scan with and without gadolinium enhancement. A CT scan is inadequate for accurately viewing brainstem lesions.[68] PET or MRI spectroscopy may also aid in diagnosis and can be particularly helpful in follow-up to differentiate between tumor recurrence and tumor necrosis secondary to therapy. Dissemination of brainstem tumors throughout the neuraxis is not uncommon.[25]

Diffuse, intrinsic brainstem lesions are not amenable to surgery. Advances in stereotactic procedures have made fine-needle biopsy of intrinsic pontine lesions possible, the histology does not always correlate with the clinical course and does not alter outcome. Therefore biopsy is not performed on children with the typical MRI appearance and clinical presentation of an intrinsic pontine lesion.[13,24,25,27,68] The majority of children will have an initial response to treatment and subsequent resolution of symptoms with conventional radiation therapy. This response is short-lived, however, and most tumors recur within the first year of therapy. Attempts to increase the dose of radiation to the tumor using hyperfractionated radiotherapy were initially promising,[54] but subsequent studies have not shown any advantage.[25,44,56] The long-term survival for children with malignant brainstem lesions is near zero.

Over the past decade several trials have investigated the use of chemotherapy before, concurrent with, or immediately following radiation therapy. To date, results have been very disappointing.[2,27,68] Biologic response modifiers such as recombinant interferon-β have also been tried with limited success.[1] Newer therapies such as antiangiogenic agents, blood-brain barrier disrupters, and gene therapy have also been proposed. Because survival averages 6 months following progression of the tumor, chemotherapy at the time of progression may be considered,[27,53] but current agents and techniques appear inadequate.

Children with focal lesions, exophytic lesions, cystic lesions, or cervicomedullary lesions may have a more optimistic outlook. Frequently these patients present with a longer history of headache, ataxia, nystagmus, hemiparesis, or other isolated cranial nerve deficit. Depending on the type of tumor, the treatment center, and the skill of the pediatric neurosurgeon, a biopsy and tumor debulking or resection may be possible for children with long clinical histories and single, unilateral deficits.[25,73] Because of the location of these tumors, surgery carries many risks. Postoperative edema can intensify preoperative deficits and create new deficits. Although these neurologic deficits can improve as postoperative edema resolves, permanent deficits can result from intraoperative manipulation. Radiation therapy and/or chemotherapy may be used to treat low-grade tumors that either are incompletely resected or demonstrate progression.[27,68]

Children with brainstem gliomas frequently require high doses of corticosteroids to help manage symptoms. Edema from the tumor, surgical manipulation, or tissue destruction from chemotherapy or radiation therapy can cause an increase in neurologic symptoms. Steroids are weaned gradually once neurologic symptoms have diminished as the tumor initially responds to therapy. Many children, however, will require prolonged therapy with high dose steroids, especially once the tumor progresses.

EPENDYMOMAS

Approximately 10% of all pediatric brain tumors are ependymomas.[76] They come from ependymal cells lining the ventricles of the brain and the central canal of the spinal cord.[64] Approximately 65% occur infratentorially, 25% supratentorially, and 10% in the spinal cord, particularly in the lumbosacral area.[8] Ependymomas vary from well-differentiated, low-grade tumors with no anaplasia to high-grade anaplastic lesions with high mitotic activity, cellular pleomorphism, anaplasia, and necrosis.[8] Ependymomas are invasive tumors that spread into adjacent brain tissue. They rarely metastasize to liver, lung, and bone.

Children usually present with symptoms such as headache and vomiting. Supratentorial lesions often cause seizures and focal deficits, while posterior fossa tumors lead to cerebellar difficulties and cranial nerve involvement. Symptoms in the child with a spinal cord lesion will depend on the exact location of the lesion. The degree of surgical resection is the single most important prognostic factor in this neoplasm.[10,59,72] Invasion of the brainstem is a poor prognostic factor, as is young age. Tumors that arise within the ventricles have a greater tendency to spread through the subarachnoid space, resulting in disseminated disease. Therefore a spine MRI and a lumbar puncture for cytology is done.

Infratentorial ependymomas with localized disease at diagnosis receive focal radiation therapy to the posterior fossa. If there is evidence of dissemination into the CSF, craniospinal irradiation will be administered. Despite neuraxis spread, cranio-spinal irradiation may also be recommended for anaplastic ependymomas or those adjacent to the ventricular lining; however, this treatment approach is controversial.[47] Most patients are treated with focal radiotherapy if there is no evidence of dissemination at diagnosis.

Local recurrence is most common. Subsequent neuraxis dissemination is thought to be due to a lack of local control.[64] Malignant supratentorial ependymomas receive focal irradiation to the tumor area. Radical surgery alone is considered a reasonable treatment option by a few physicians in cases in which the postoperative MRI confirms a complete resection—particularly in cases in which the tumor is not located near critical areas of the brain[59] (Figure 21-3). Adjuvant chemotherapy does not appear to be advantageous in newly diagnosed disease, except in the young child. Children under 3 years of age receive chemotherapy to avoid radiotherapy.[45] Surgical options will first be explored in the case of recurrent disease. If radiotherapy has already been given, chemotherapy may produce short-term results but is unlikely to result in a cure.

Patients with spinal cord ependymomas are a distinct entity. The myxopapillary ependymoma of the caudae equina has a better prognosis. Patients who have had a complete resection of an intramedullary spinal cord ependymoma may not need local or spinal axis irradiation.[72]

Difficulties with consistent identification of the anaplastic variants of this tumor, as well as the statistical difficulties that arise because of the rarity of occurrence, have contributed to the lack of universally accepted prognostic paramaters. Those that have been examined include age (older than 5 to 7 years at diagnosis favorable), location (spinal cord primary favorable), resectability (gross total fare better than subtotal resections), and use of radiation therapy (use of radiation therapy improves prognosis). Histologic factors such as the number of mitoses, indices of proliferation markers (Ki-67 and proliferating cell nuclear antigen), and cell density are also reliable predictors of prognosis.[72] Use of radiotherapy and improved surgical techniques have increased 5-year survival rates to 40% to 60%.[72]

GERM CELL TUMORS

CNS germ cell tumors are relatively rare. The peak onset is during the second and third decades of life. The majority of these tumors occur in the pineal region (45%) or the suprasellar region (35%).[19] Up to 20% are disseminated along the neuraxis.[23]

Germ cell tumors are classified as either pure germinomas or nongerminomatous germ cell tumors (NGGCTs), depending on their histology.

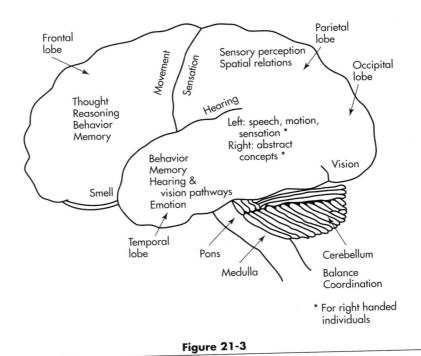

Figure 21-3

Lobes of the brain with neuro controls. (From American Brain Tumor Association. [1998]. *A primer of brain tumors: A patient's reference manual.* Des Plaines, IL: Author.)

NGGCTs are made up of cells resembling those in the earliest stages of embryogenesis. The earlier the stage, the more malignant the tumor. For example, cells resembling the trophoblast (choriocarcinoma) are the least differentiated and the most malignant, whereas cells representing the primordial cell (germinoma) are the most highly differentiated and least aggressive. Yolk sac tumors, embryonic carcinomas, endodermal sinus tumors, and teratomas are other examples of NGGCTs. Some tumors have mixed histology. The 5-year survival for intracranial germ cell tumors ranges from 80% to 100% for pure germinomas to 20% to 56% for NGGCTs.[19] Tumors of mixed histology have survival rates dependent on the predominant histology of the lesion. Those composed of pure germinoma and mature teratoma have a significantly higher survival rate than those with some elements of malignant tumors. Tumors with primarily pure malignant elements fared worse.[19,70] The presentation of children with germ cell tumors depends on the tumor location. For patients with pineal region tumors, Parinaud's syndrome (upward gaze, paresis, retraction nystagmus) is the most frequent presenting sign.[18] Symptoms of increased ICP are common. Endocrinopathies, such as diabetes insipidus,

and visual disturbances can also occur when there is involvement of the hypothalamus.

Diagnosis of intracranial germ cell tumors is made by clinical history, MRI findings, and assessment of tumor markers. Both serum and CSF are sent for AFP and β-hCG. Tumor markers are often, but not always, elevated in the NGGCTs. Some germinomas can also produce low levels of β-hCG in the CSF (secreting germinomas), which is considered an early sign of dissemination. The presence of these tumor markers in the CSF or serum combined with the presence of an intracranial mass on MRI is diagnostic of a germ cell tumor.[78]

Historically, patients with the suspicion of a pure germinoma were initially treated with radiation therapy because of the tumor's exquisite sensitivity to radiation. As neurosurgical techniques improved, however, patients with pineal lesions were initially resected, while suspected germinoma in other areas was again treated with empiric radiation. Over the past decade performing a biopsy to confirm histology became the norm before treatment with radiation and/or chemotherapy. For patients with NGGCTs surgical biopsy and resection were advocated before initiating therapy.[70] The role of surgery is somewhat controversial. Some centers recommend aggressive resection, others recommend biopsy only; some centers advocate second look surgery after initial treatment with radiation or chemotherapy for patients who have residual disease, others do not. If tumor markers have normalized during chemotherapy but a residual or progressive tumor mass remains, resection of the lesion reveals either necrosis or teratoma. If the pathology is pure teratoma, then complete surgical resection can be considered curative.[78]

Radiation therapy alone has been the standard therapy for germinoma of the central nervous system. Over the past decades, efforts to minimize the dose and volume of radiation by the addition of chemotherapy have been successful, although attempts to completely replace radiation with chemotherapy have not.[18,48] Current consensus is that unless there is evidence of tumor dissemination by CSF cytology, myelography, or spinal MRI, focal radiation is sufficient and craniospinal prophylaxis is unnecessary. The addition of chemotherapy to lower the dose of radiation, or to delay the timing of radiation in very young patients, appears to be beneficial.[23]

SPINAL CORD TUMORS

Approximately 4% to 10% of primary CNS tumors arise in the spine neurons, supporting glial cells and the meninges.[51] They can occur throughout childhood. Sixty percent of intramedullary tumors are astrocytomas. Most are low grade; approximately 30% are ependymomas; and about 4% are developmental tumors such as teratomas.[51] Primary tumors may compress the cord through expansion. Leptomeningeal metastases occur by diffuse or multifocal seeding along the meninges.

Children who present with spinal cord tumors have a variety of symptoms, depending on the tumor's location. These symptoms can include pain, weakness, gait problems, sensory disturbances, and sphincter dysfunction.[8,51] Chronic back pain in a child must be regarded with a high level of suspicion for tumor. The onset of symptoms is slower for patients with low-grade lesions. MRI is used to visualize the entire spine in multiple planes. Astroctyomas will have heterogeneous enhancement, whereas ependymomas usually demonstrate homogeneous enhancement.

Surgery is the first step, with as extensive a resection as possible while still preserving clinical function. These tumors are best approached using imaging techniques such as ultrasonography and evoked potential monitoring.[51] Postoperative morbidity and degree of neurologic recovery depend on the extent of neurologic deficits at presentation, the amount of disease, and the neurosurgeon's exper-

tise. Completely resected ependymomas will not need further therapy unless there is progression. Ependymomas have survival rates of 50% to 100% at 5 years but also experience a high rate of local disease progression when there is an incomplete resection.[37]

Controversy surrounds the management of completely resected low-grade gliomas because of their known insidious biologic behavior. Radiation therapy can be given, although many neurosurgeons choose observation alone. Patients with subtotal resections of low-grade astrocytomas may receive radiation therapy postoperatively or, in some cases, be monitored closely for disease progression. If the tumor progresses, further surgical options would be explored, followed by radiation therapy. Low-grade astrocytomas with various degrees of resection experience 66% to 70% 5-year survival rates, with local recurrence rates as high as 33% to 86%.[37]

Radiation therapy is administered to all high-grade lesions, and in most cases chemotherapy is used as salvage therapy.[51] Preoperative chemotherapy may be beneficial in shrinking tumor size.[49] However, most patients with high-grade tumors usually die within a short time period from rapid tumor progression.[49]

NURSING IMPLICATIONS

Caring for children with brain tumors is challenging. Because of the many disciplines involved, the nurse is often the pivotal point person for coordination of very complex care. Frequently the children treated for CNS tumors have aggressive disease, with a low likelihood of cure. Although the overall survival rate for all children with CNS tumors approaches 60%, many tumors, such as high-grade astrocytoma, brainstem glioma, and posterior fossa or subtotally resected ependymoma, have a far poorer prognosis.[35]

The many stressors associated with having a child with cancer can be multiplied if the child has a brain tumor. Families may suffer a double loss if the child's personality or prior abilities are also altered. The 18 month old who was toddling independently may only be able to creep. The 17-year-old track star may be hemiparetic and barely able to ambulate independently. In addition, there is always the threatened loss due to death from the tumor. Unlike several other childhood cancers, where 5-year disease-free survival means the likelihood of cure, brain tumors can recur very late.[3]

The multimodal treatment of childhood brain tumors frequently involves cranial irradiation. Neurocognitive sequelae and vocational issues can be very serious for those children who do survive. Even older children and adolescents who undergo cranial radiation therapy have to work significantly harder to achieve academically at their premorbid level.

Nursing care of the child with a brain tumor requires astute observational skills. Subtle changes in eye movements or gait can be indicative of changes in tumor status. Children with visual field deficits can benefit from being oriented in a room so that their "good side" is toward the hallway. For example, a child with a deep left-sided visual field cut will not see objects or people to the left of midline. If the hallway is to his left, he will not be able to see the activity going on around him and could become even more withdrawn while in the hospital. Children with diplopia may benefit from wearing a patch on alternate eyes to minimize the discomfort and headaches associated with double vision. Because many children with CNS tumors receive corticosteroids, particularly dexamethasone, a thorough knowledge of steroid side effects and management is important. For example, good oral hygiene will minimize the development of oral candidiasis, and monitoring for hyperglycemia and blood pressure changes is required. Lesions of the brainstem can affect swallowing ability. Some children have a decreased or absent gag reflex but can still swallow and protect their airway. Others may require nasogastric or gastrostomy feedings. Speech and occupational therapy staff can assist in the assessment of the child's ability to swallow and facilitate rehabilitation and recovery of oral feeding abilities.

Up to 30% or 40% of children with brain tumors will require placement of a permanent VP shunt. Nurses caring for these children must be familiar with the mechanics of shunt catheters and the possible complications and interventions related to shunt placement. When chemotherapy requiring aggressive hydration is administered, these children must be observed for signs of increased ICP as well as shunt malfunction. The challenge is to balance the risks of increased ICP with the risks of increased chemotherapy side effects from inadequate hydration. If fever and neutropenia occur in a child who has a VP shunt, the possibility of a shunt infection must be considered. Erythema of the shunt tract and incisions, abdominal tenderness or swelling, and meningismus may indicate the need to culture the shunt fluid. Shunt cultures are not routinely done for children with benign exams.[69]

Accurate measurement of input, output, and daily weights and frequent mental status assessment are important. Sedation from medications (e.g., antiemetic regimens using phenothiazines) must be distinguished from lethargy due to SIADH, shunt malfunction, or increased ICP. Subtle changes in neurologic status must be documented and communicated to the physician or advanced practice nurse.

Patient and family education is also critical. A recent study of families of children with brain tumors by Freeman, O'Dell, and Meola found that most parents and patients did not feel sufficiently informed about the child's tumor. During the varying stages of illness, from diagnosis to relapse, cure, or death, parents noted concerns about the lack of lay information—related to specific tumors, postdischarge care, side effects, treatment options and outcomes, and terminal care planning.[28] The American Brain Tumor Association (ABTA) offers excellent resources for families as well as professionals (www.abta.org).[4]

FUTURE DIRECTIONS

All professionals involved with the care of children and adolescents with cancer are working toward achieving a cure while preserving the highest quality of life possible. Children and adolescents with CNS neoplasms must be treated in pediatric oncology centers by multidisciplinary teams who are knowledgeable about all facets of CNS tumors and subsequent neurologic, physical, and emotional sequelae. Following completion of therapy, these children and adolescents need continued expert follow-up care to address residual long-term issues. Vocational counseling may be necessary.

It is crucial to continue to heighten public awareness so that research programs will be adequately funded. Despite the overall positive survival trend with certain types of these neoplasms, too many brain tumors are still resistant to treatment. More research is needed to understand these tumors so that innovative treatment strategies can be devised. Research is needed to determine the causality of CNS neoplasms so that effective preventive measures can be formulated and implemented.

ACKNOWLEDGMENT

The authors would like to thank Paul Fisher, MD, for his careful review of this chapter.

REFERENCES

1. Allen, J. C., Packer, R. J., & Bleyer, A. (1991). Recombinant interferon-beta: A phase I-II trial in children with recurrent brain tumors. *Journal of Clinical Oncology, 9,* 783-788.
2. Allen, J. C., & Siffert, J. (1996). Contemporary chemotherapy issues for children with brainstem gliomas. *Pediatric Neurosurgery, 24,* 98-102.

3. Amagasaki, K., Yamazaki, H., Koizumi, H., et al. (1999). Recurrence of medulloblastoma 19 years after the initial diagnosis. *Child's Nervous System, 15,* 482-485.

4. American Brain Tumor Association. (1998). *A primer of brain tumors: A patient's reference manual.* Des Plaines, IL: Author.

5. Ater, J. (1998). Treatment of brain tumors in children: An overview. *Journal of Care Management, 4,* 96-108.

6. Bailey, C., & Cushing, H. (1926). *Classification of tumors of the glioma group on a histogenic basis with a correlated study of prognosis.* Philadelphia: J. B. Lippincott.

7. Balmaceda, C. (1998). Advances in brain tumor chemosensitivity (Review). *Current Opinion in Oncology, 10,* 194-200.

8. Becker, L. E. (1999). Pathology of pediatric brain tumors. *Neuroimaging Clinics of North America, 9,* 671-690.

9. Bleyer, W. A. (1999). Epidemiologic impact of children with brain tumors. *Child's Nervous System, 15,* 758-763.

10. Bouffet, E., Perilongo, G., Canete, A., & Massimino, M. (1998). Intracranial ependymomas in children: A critical review of prognostic factors and a plea for cooperation (Review). *Medical and Pediatric Oncology, 30,* 319-329.

11. Broniscer, A., Leite, C. C., Lanchote, V. L., et al. (2000). Radiation therapy and high-dose tamoxifen in the treatment of patients with diffuse brainstem gliomas: Result of a Brazilian cooperative study. Brainstem Glioma Cooperative Group. *Journal of Clinical Oncology, 6,* 1246-1253.

12. Campbell, J. W., & Pollack, I. F. (1996). Cerebellar astrocytomas in children. *Journal of Neuro-Oncology, 28,* 223-231.

13. Cartmill, M., & Punt, J. (1999). Diffuse brain stem glioma—A review of stereotactic biopsies. *Child's Nervous System, 15,* 235-237.

14. Castello, M. A., Schiavetti, A., Varrasso, G., et al. (1998). Chemotherapy in low-grade astrocytoma management. *Child's Nervous System, 14,* 6-9.

15. Cavenee, W. (2000). Introduction to the new ABTA research awards. *Message Line of the American Brain Tumor Association, 27(2),* 1-20.

16. CBTRUS. (1998). *1997 Annual report.* Chicago, IL: Central Brain Tumor Registry of the United States.

17. CBTRUS. (2000). *Statistical report: Brain tumors in the United States, 1992-1997.* Chicago, IL: Central Brain Tumor Registry of the United States.

18. Choi, J. U., Kim, D. S., Chung, S. S., et al. (1998). Treatment of germ cell tumors in the pineal region. *Child's Nervous System, 14,* 41-48.

19. Diez, B., Balmaceda, C., Matstani, M., et al. (1999). Germ cell tumors of the CNS in children: Recent advances in therapy. *Child's Nervous System, 15,* 578-585.

20. Doxey, D., Bruce, D., Sklaar F., et al. (1999). Posterior fossa syndrome: Identifiable risk factors and irreversible complications. *Pediatric Neurosurgery, 31,* 131-136.

21. Dunkel, I. J., Boyett, J. M., Yates, A., et al. (1998). For the Children's Cancer Group: High-dose carboplatin, thiotepa, and etoposide with autologous stem cell rescue for patients with recurrent medulloblastoma. *Journal of Clinical Oncology, 16,* 222-228.

22. Dunkel, I. J., & Finlay, J. L. (1996). High-dose chemotherapy with autologous stem cell rescue for patients with medulloblastoma. *Journal of Neuro-oncology, 29,* 69-74.

23. Fouladi, M., Grant, R., Baruchel, S., et al. (1998). Comparison of survival outcomes in patients with intracranial germinomas treated with radiation alone versus reduced-dose radiation and chemotherapy. *Child's Nervous System, 14,* 596-601.

24. Freeman, C. R. (1996). Hyperfractionated radiotherapy for diffuse intrinsic brain stem tumors in children. *Pediatric Neurosurgery, 24,* 103-110.

25. Freeman, C. R., & Farmer, J. P. (1998). Pediatric brain stem gliomas: A review. *International Journal of Radiation Oncology, Biology, and Physics, 40,* 265-271.

26. Freeman, C. R., Farmer, J. P., & Montes, J. (1998). Low-grade astrocytomas in children: Evolving management strategies. *International Journal of Radiation Oncology, Biology, and Physics, 41,* 979-987.

27. Freeman, C. R., & Perilongo, G. (1999). Chemotherapy for brain stem gliomas. *Child's Nervous System, 15,* 545-553.

28. Freeman, K., O'Dell, C., & Meola, C. (2000). Issues in families of children with brain tumors. *Oncology Nursing Forum, 27,* 843-848.

29. Fuss, M., Hug, E. B., Schaefer, R. A., et al. (1999). Proton radiation therapy (PRT) for pediatric optic pathway gliomas: Comparison with 3D planned conventional photons and a standard photon therapy. *International Journal of Radiation Oncology, Biology, and Physics, 45,* 1117-1126.

30. Gajjar, A., Kuhl, J., Epelman, S., et al. (1999). Chemotherapy of medulloblastoma. *Child's Nervous System, 15,* 554-562.

31. Giordana, M. T., Schiffer, P., & Schiffer, D. (1998). Prognostic factors in medulloblastoma. *Child's Nervous System, 14,* 256-262.

32. Graham, M. L., Herndon, J. E., III, Casey, J. R., et al. (1997). High-dose chemotherapy with autologous stem cell rescue in patients with recurrent and high-risk pediatric brain tumors. *Journal of Clinical Oncology, 15,* 1814-1823.

33. Greenlee, R. T., Murray, T., Bolden, S., et al. (2000). Cancer Statistics, 2000. *CA: A Cancer Journal for Clinicians, 50(1),* 7-33.

34. Grovas, A. C., Boyett, J. M., Lindsley, K., et al. (1999). Regimen-related toxicity of myeloablative chemotherapy with BCNU, thiotepa and etoposide followed by autologous stem cell rescue for children with newly diagnosed glioblastoma multiforme. A report from the Children's Cancer Group. *Medical and Pediatric Oncology, 33,* 83-87.

35. Gurney, J. G., Smith, M. A., & Bunin, G. R. (1999). CNS and miscellaneous intracranial and intraspinal neoplasms. In L. A. G. Ries, M. A. Smith, J. G. Gurney, et al (Eds.), *Cancer incidence and survival among children and adolescents: United States SEER program 1975-1995* (NIH Pub. No. 99-4649, pp. 51-63). Bethesda, MD: National Cancer Institute, SEER Program.

36. Gurney, J. G., Davis, S., Severson, R. K., et al. (1996). Trends in cancer incidence among children in the U.S. *Cancer, 78,* 532-541.

37. Heideman, R. L., Packer, R. J., Albright, L. A., et al. (1997). Tumors of the central nervous system. In P. A. Pizzo & D. G. Poplack (Eds.), *Principles and practice of pediatric oncology* (3rd ed., pp. 633-697). Philadelphia: Lippincott-Raven.

38. Honig, P. J., & Charney, E. B. (1982). Children with brain tumor headaches: Distinguishing features. *American Journal of Diseases of Children, 136,* 121-124.

39. Jakacki, R. I. (1999). Pineal and nonpineal supratentorial primitive neuroectodermal tumors. *Child's Nervous System, 15,* 586-591.

40. Jenkin, D., Al Shabanah, M., Al Shail, E., et al. (2000). Prognostic factors for medulloblastoma. *International Journal of Radiation Oncology, Biology, and Physics, 47,* 573-584.

41. Johnson, J. H., & Phillips, P. C. (1996). Malignant gliomas in children. *Cancer Investigation, 14,* 609-621.
42. Kuhl, J. (1998). Modern treatment strategies in medulloblastoma. *Child's Nervous System, 14,* 2-5.
43. Lee, M., Wisoff, J. H., Abbott, R., et al. (1994). Management of hydrocephalus in children with medulloblastoma: Prognostic factors for shunting. *Pediatric Neurosurgery, 20,* 240-247.
44. Mandell, L. R., Kadota, R., Freeman, C., et al. (1999). There is no role for hyperfractionated radiotherapy in the management of children with newly diagnosed diffuse intrinsic brainstem tumors: Results of a Pediatric Oncology Group phase III trial comparing conventional vs. hyperfractionated radiotherapy. *International Journal of Radiation Oncology, Biology, and Physics, 43,* 959-964.
45. Mason, W. P., Grovas, A., Halpern, S., et al. (1998). Intensive chemotherapy and bone marrow rescue for young children with newly diagnosed malignant brain tumors. *Journal of Clinical Oncology, 16,* 210-221.
46. McCowage, G. B., Friedman, H. S., Moghrabi, A., et al. (1998). Activity of high-dose cyclophosphamide in the treatment of childhood malignant gliomas. *Medical and Practice Oncology, 30,* 75-80.
47. McLaughlin, M. P., Marcus, R. B., Jr., Buatti, J. M., et al. (1998). Ependymoma: Results, prognostic factors and treatment recommendations (Review). *International Journal of Radiation Oncology, Biology, Physics, 40,* 845-850.
48. Merchant, T. E., Sherwood, S. H., Mulhern, R. K. et al. (2000). CNS Germinoma: Disease control and long-term functional outcome for 12 children treated with craniospinal irradiation. *International Journal of Radiation Oncology, Biology, and Physics, 46,* 1171-1176.
49. Merchant, T. E., Nguyen, D., Thompson, S. J., et al. (1999). High-grade pediatric spinal cord tumors. *Pediatric Neurosurgery, 1,* 1-5.
50. Modha, A., Vassilyadi, M., George, A., et al. (2000). Medulloblastoma in children—The Ottowa experience. *Child's Nervous System, 16,* 341-350.
51. Nadkarni, T. D., & Rekate, H. L. (1999). Pediatric intramedullary spinal cord tumors: Critical review of the literature. *Child's Nervous System, 15,* 17-28.
52. Needle, M. N., Molloy, P. T., Geyer, J. R., et al. (1997). Phase II study of oral etoposide in children with recurrent brain tumors and other solid tumors. *Medical and Pediatric Oncology, 29,* 28-32.
53. Packer, R. J. (1996). Brain stem gliomas: Therapeutic options at time of recurrence. *Pediatric Neurosurgery, 24,* 211-216.
54. Packer, R. J., Allen, J. C., Goldwein, J. L., et al. (1990). Hyperfractionated radiotherapy for children with brainstem gliomas: A pilot study using 7,200 cGy. *Annals of Neurology, 27,* 167-173.
55. Packer, R. J., Ater J., Allen J., et al. (1997). Carboplatin and vincristine chemotherapy for children with newly diagnosed progressive low-grade gliomas. *Journal of Neurosurgery, 86,* 747-754.
56. Packer, R. J., Boyett, J. M., Zimmerman, R. A., et al. (1993). Hyperfractionated radiation therapy (72 Gy) for children with brain stem gliomas: A Children's Cancer Group phase I/II trial. *Cancer, 72,* 1414-1421.
57. Packer, R. J., Sutton, L. N., Goldwein, J. W., et al. (1991). Improved survival with the use of adjuvant chemotherapy in the treatment of medulloblastoma. *Journal of Neurosurgery, 74,* 433-440.
58. Packer, R. J., Sutton, L. N., Elterman, R., et al. (1994). Outcome for children with medulloblastoma treated with radiation and cisplatin, CCNU, and vincristine chemotherapy. *Journal of Neurosurgery, 81,* 690-698.
59. Palma, L., Celli, P., Mariottini, A., et al. (2000). The importance of surgery in supratentorial ependymomas: Long-term survival in a series of 23 cases. *Child's Nervous System, 16,* 170-175.
60. Pollack, I. F. (1999). The role of surgery in pediatric gliomas. *Journal of Neuro-Oncology, 42,* 271-288.
61. Pollack, I. F., Claassen, D., Al-Shloul, Q., et al (1995). Low grade gliomas of the cerebral hemispheres in children: An analysis of 71 cases. *Journal of Neurosurgery, 82,* 536-547.
62. Prados, M. D., Edwards, M. S. B., Chang, S. M., et al. (1999). Hyperfractionated craniospinal radiation therapy for primitive neuroectodermal tumors: Results of a phase II study. *International Journal of Radiation Oncology, Biology, and Physics, 43,* 279-285.
63. Prados, M. D., & Russo, C. (1998). Chemotherapy of brain tumors. *Seminars in Surgical Oncology, 14,* 88-98.
64. Prados, M. D., Berger, M. S., & Wilson, C. B. (1998). Primary central nervous system tumors: Advances in knowledge and treatment. *CA: A Cancer Journal for Clinicians, 48,* 331-360.
65. Raco, A., Raimondi, A. J., D'Alonzo, A., et al. (2000). Radiosurgery in the management of pediatric brain tumors. *Child's Nervous System, 16,* 287-295.
66. Rivlin, K. A., & Finlay, J. L. (1996). High-grade astrocytomas in children. *Critical Review in Neurosurgery, 6,* 110-113.
67. Roila, F., Aapro, M., & Stewart, A. (1998). Optimal selection of antiemetics in children receiving cancer chemotherapy. *Supportive Care in Cancer, 6,* 215-220.
68. Rubin, G., Michowitz, S., Horev, G. et al. (1998). Pediatric brain stem gliomas: An update. *Child's Nervous System, 14,* 167-173.
69. Ryan, J. A., & Shiminski-Maher, T. (1995). Hydrocephalus and shunts in children with brain tumors. *Journal of Pediatric Oncology Nursing, 12,* 223-229.
70. Sawamura, Y., Ikeda, J., Shirato, H., et al. (1998). Germ cell tumours of the central nervous system: Treatment consideration based on 111 cases and their long-term clinical outcomes. *European Journal of Cancer, 34,* 104-110.
71. Sawaya, R., Hammoud, M., Scmoppa, D., et al. (1998). Neurosurgical outcomes in a modern series of 400 craniotomies for the treatment of parenchymal tumors. *Neurosurgery, 42,* 1044-1055.
72. Schiffer, D., & Giordana, M. T. (1998). Prognosis of ependymoma (Review). *Child's Nervous System, 14,* 357-361.
73. Shiminski-Maher, T., Abbott, R., Wisoff, J. H., et al. (1991). Current trends in the management of brainstem tumors in childhood. *Journal of Neuroscience Nursing, 23,* 356-362.
74. Shiminski-Maher, T., & Shields, M. (1995). Pediatric brain tumors: Diagnosis and management. *Journal of Pediatric Oncology Nursing, 12,* 188-198.
75. Shore, R. E., Albert, R. E., & Pasternack, B. R. (1976). Follow-up study of patients treated by x-ray epilation for tinea capitis: Resurvey of post-treatment illness and mortality experience. *Archives of Environmental Health, 31,* 21-28.

76. Siffert, J., Greenleaf, M., Mannis, R., et al. (1999). Pediatric Brain Tumors. *Child and Adolescent Psychiatric Clinics of North America, 8,* 879-902.

77. Souweidane, M. M., Kim, K. H. S., McDowall, R., et al. (1999). Brain mapping in sedated infants and young children with passive-functional magnetic resonance imaging. *Pediatric Neurosurgery, 30,* 86-92.

78. Weiner, H. L., & Finlay, J. L. (1999). Surgery in the management of primary intracranial germ cell tumors. *Child's Nervous System, 15,* 770-773.

79. Wisoff, J. H., Boyett, J. M., Berger, M. S., et al. (1998). Current neurosurgical management and the impact of the extent of resection in the treatment of malignant gliomas of childhood: A report of the Children's Cancer Group trial no. CCG-945. *Journal of Neurosurgery, 89,* 52-59.

80. Yang, H. J., Nam, D. H., Wang, K. C., et al. (1999). Supratentorial primitive neuroectodermal tumor in children: Clinical features, treatment outcome and prognostic factors. *Child's Nervous System, 15,* 377-383.

81. Youmans, J. R. (Ed.). (1996). *Neurological surgery: A comprehensive reference guide to the diagnosis and management of neurosurgical problems* (4th ed., pp. 2493-3187). Philadelphia: W. B. Saunders.

Hodgkin's Disease

Patricia Liebhauser

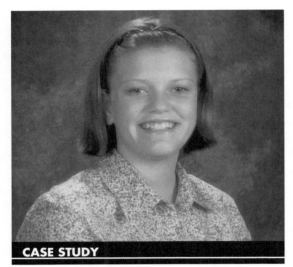

CASE STUDY

Stephanie is a 13-year-old who came to her primary care physician in July 2000 with a 1-year history of a right neck mass. The mass had increased in size over the previous 3 weeks. Her family had recently moved back to the United States after living in Italy. Her mother, an Air Force nurse, had returned to the area to complete coursework toward a master's degree in nursing.

Stephanie was referred to the local children's hospital. Initial evaluation by the pediatric oncologist revealed a negative review of systems. Specifically, she had no history of the classic B symptoms associated with Hodgkin's lymphoma of fever, weight loss, malaise, or night sweats. Physical examination was normal except for a 4 × 4 cm hard, nontender, fixed lower anterior cervical and supraclavicular mass. Diagnostic imaging, including computed tomography (CT) and gallium scan, revealed right cervical and mediastinal adenopathy and multiple, bilateral lung nodules.

A lymph node biopsy specimen showed nodular sclerosing Hodgkin's lymphoma. A lung biopsy specimen revealed granulomas consistent with past *Histoplasmosis* infection. The family has several pet birds in the home. In addition, Stephanie has lived in the Mississippi valley, known to be endemic for *Histoplasmosis* infection.

After the diagnosis was established, treatment options were discussed with Stephanie and her family. They agreed to participate in the current Pediatric Oncology Group (POG) protocol for stage IIA Hodgkin's lymphoma. This protocol is designed to evaluate a shorter and less toxic treatment regimen. Her treatment consisted of doxorubicin, bleomycin, vincristine, and etoposide. She was randomized to receive dexrazoxane before chemotherapy. This agent is being evaluated for its efficacy to reduce cardiopulmonary toxicity associated with doxorubicin and bleomycin. After two cycles, imaging studies revealed marked reduction in the adenopathy and a negative gallium scan. Because of this excellent response, she proceeded to involved-field radiation therapy consisting of 25.5 Gy given to a "minimantle" field. Completion of therapy work-up revealed no evidence of disease, and Stephanie was taken off all treatment. She then began the posttherapy follow-up phase consisting of monthly examinations and periodic imaging studies.

Stephanie tolerated her therapy well with minimal physical or psychologic sequelae. Despite having to start a new junior high school with no hair, and the multiple absences associated with intensive chemotherapy, Stephanie adjusted well to her diagnosis and treatment. Her personal strength and family support helped her to cope well with the typical stresses associated with childhood cancer and treatment. She recently participated in a school project with several classmates who filmed a documentary about childhood cancer and Stephanie's experiences.

Hodgkin's disease or lymphoma is a malignancy of the lymphoid system first described as an entity by Thomas Hodgkin in 1832.[24] It differs from the other lymphomatous diseases in its histologic characteristics, behavior, and response to treatment. Hodgkin's disease occurs at all ages and is common in adults, but the peak age incidence and histologic type vary with geography and socioeconomic status. Uniformly fatal before 1960, Hodgkin's disease was one of the first cancers found to be highly curable with multiagent chemotherapy and radiation therapy. Treatment protocols specifically for the management of children with Hodgkin's disease were implemented in the 1970s.[12,26]

EPIDEMIOLOGY

In the United States, Hodgkin's disease accounts for 5% of malignancies diagnosed in children under 15 years of age with approximately 6.2 per million in white children and 4.7 per million in black children.[20] It has been reported in infants and very young children but is considered rare before the age of 5 years.[20,35,56,65] The number of cases increases significantly in the second decade of life in the United States.[65] Hodgkin's disease occurs more frequently in boys (7.0 per million) than girls (3.9 per million), especially in children under 10 years of age.[20,43] This preponderance in boys diminishes in adolescence, when the incidence is approximately equal for boys and girls.

The highest incidence rates of Hodgkin's disease have been observed in adolescents and young adults from industrialized Western countries. The highest rates among children occur in less developed countries. Overall, the highest incidence of Hodgkin's disease is in the United States, Latin America, Africa, and Israel.[56]

The cause of Hodgkin's disease is unknown, but epidemiologic studies suggest different causes for disease diagnosed at different ages. In industrialized countries, there is a bimodal age-incidence curve, with an early peak occurring in the middle to late 20s and a second peak after age 50 years. MacMahon theorized that this bimodal curve suggests dual causes, where Hodgkin's disease in the young is the result of an infectious process and disease in older adults has a cause similar to that of other lymphomas.[43] This landmark observation launched the era of epidemiologic investigation of the causes of cancer. The bimodal curve could reflect a variation in response over age to a single causative process.[47] Whether Hodgkin's disease has one or more different etiologic processes remains unresolved.

In young children and adults, age distribution patterns vary with geographic location and socioeconomic condition. In industrialized countries or higher socioeconomic groups, the overall incidence

of Hodgkin's disease is higher, but it is rare in early childhood, increases in adolescence, and peaks in young adulthood. The most frequent histologic type in these populations is nodular sclerosis (NS).[47,48] In developing countries or lower socioeconomic groups, the overall incidence of Hodgkin's disease is lower but peaks before 15 years of age. Mixed cellularity (MC) and lymphocytic depletion (LD) are the most frequent histologic types in these populations.[47,48,65] These patterns suggest an infectious cause with social class factors affecting when exposure occurs.[21,47]

Studies have reported an increased risk of Hodgkin's disease in close relatives, especially same-sex siblings and twins.[19,41,47,55] This higher risk may be related to common exposure to an etiologic agent or genetic predisposition associated with immune competence. Studies of clusters of cases involving siblings and cousins suggest an increased association of Hodgkin's disease with specific human leukocyte antigen types.[25,26] Hodgkin's disease is more common in persons with immune deficiency, both genetic (e.g., ataxia-telangiectasia, Wiskott-Aldrich syndrome) and infectious (e.g., human immunodeficiency virus [HIV]).[26,59]

Epstein-Barr virus (EBV) has been investigated for a role in the pathogenesis of Hodgkin's disease. Associations between EBV and Hodgkin's disease include case reports of Hodgkin's disease in patients with primary EBV infection, increased incidence of Hodgkin's disease in persons with a history of infectious mononucleosis, and elevated EBV titers for several years preceding the diagnosis of Hodgkin's disease.[1,3,47] Antigens associated with EBV have been demonstrated in tumor tissue.[22] Studies implicate EBV as a potential cofactor in the etiology of Hodgkin's disease, but the relationship is not yet clearly understood.[1]

Studies suggest that tumor cells originate from a B lymphocyte, and cells may express surface markers consistent with this lineage.[22] Antigenic marker CD15 is found in a high proportion of patients with NS, MC, and LD histologic findings.

Occupational risk factors have not been established for Hodgkin's disease. Exposures to woodworking, herbicides, and other chemicals are suspected for increasing the risk of Hodgkin's disease, but additional studies are needed to confirm an etiologic role.[47,48]

CLASSIFICATION OF HODGKIN'S LYMPHOMA

The description of a characteristic giant cell by Sternberg in 1898 and Reed in 1902[54] was an important step in distinguishing Hodgkin's disease from the other lymphomatous diseases. The histologic diagnosis of Hodgkin's disease is determined by the presence of these Reed-Sternberg cells, which have distinctive nucleolar shapes (e.g., lobulated, multinucleated, large prominent nucleolus). The cells have been described as "owl's eyes." The presence of Reed-Sternberg cells alone is not diagnostic because similar cells have been identified in reactive lymphoid hyperplasias (such as infectious mononucleosis) and other neoplastic diseases.

Hodgkin's disease is classified by the predominating cells. A modification of the Lukes and Butler classification was adopted at the 1965 symposium on Hodgkin's disease held in Rye, New York, and is currently used.[40] The histologic classification of Hodgkin's disease is described in Table 22-1.

Strum and Rappaport[66] examined sequential biopsy specimens and demonstrated a histologic progression in Hodgkin's disease. Disease may remain unchanged or evolve from lymphocytic predominance (LP) to mixed cellularity (MC) to lymphocytic depletion (LD). A reversal of this progression was not found. The nodular sclerosis (NS) type does not follow this evolution, and untreated patients with NS show a progressive depletion of lymphocytes.

The LP histologic type is diagnosed in 10% to 15% of children with Hodgkin's disease. It is more common in males and younger patients and usually presents as clinically localized disease.[12,26,33] The MC type is seen in 30% of children, is more common in children 10 years of age or younger, and frequently presents as advanced disease.[9,12] LD is rare in children. These patients often have widespread disease involving bone and bone marrow. Nodular sclerosis is the most common histologic type, diagnosed in 40% of younger patients and 70% of adolescents, and often presents in lower cervical, supraclavicular, and mediastinal lymph nodes.[12,26]

CLINICAL PRESENTATION

The presenting sign of Hodgkin's disease is cervical or supraclavicular adenopathy, occurring in 60% to 90% of cases.[26,68] The lymph nodes are characteristically painless, firm, and movable in the surrounding tissue. More than half of the patients with cervical adenopathy will also have mediastinal involvement, which can cause pressure on the trachea or bronchi and symptoms of airway obstruction.

TABLE 22-1	HISTOLOGIC CLASSIFICATION OF HODGKIN'S DISEASE
Histologic Type	**Description**
Lymphocytic predominance	Numerous small benign-appearing lymphocytes and/or reactive histiocytes
	Nodular or diffuse
	Necrosis not present
	Fibrosis usually not present
	Reed-Sternberg cells rare and difficult to find
Nodular sclerosis	Collagen bands divide lymphoid tissue into nodules
	Nodules contain atypical histiocytic cells lying in clear spaces (lacunar cells)
	Eosinophils usually present
	Necrosis frequently present
	Reed-Sternberg cells difficult to find
Mixed cellularity	Intermediate between lymphocytic predominance and lymphocytic depletion
	Variety of histologic components (eosinophils, plasma cells, mature neutrophils, lymphocytes, histiocytes, and Reed-Sternberg cells)
	Necrosis may be present
	Fibrosis may be present
Lymphocytic depletion	Decreased number of lymphocytes
	Diffuse fibrosis with decreased number of all other cells against a background of disorderly connective tissue OR reticular type with atypical histiocytes and increased number of Reed-Sternberg cells
	Necrosis commonly present

Data from Hudson, M. M., & Donaldson, S. S. (1997). Hodgkin's disease. In P. A. Pizzo & D. G. Poplack (Eds.), *Principles and practice of pediatric oncology* (3rd ed., pp. 523-543). Philadelphia: Lippincott-Raven; Lukes, R. J. (1971). Criteria for involvement of lymph node, bone marrow, spleen, and liver in Hodgkin's disease. *Cancer Research, 31,* 1755-1767; Lukes, R. J., Craver, L. F., Hall, T. C., et al. (1966). Report of the Nomenclature Committee. *Cancer Research, 26,* 1311.

Axillary or inguinal adenopathy is an unusual presenting sign. The spleen is infiltrated in 30% to 40% of patients, but spleen size may not correlate with the degree of involvement.[26] Liver size is also a poor indicator of disease involvement. Infiltration of non-lymphoid organs is rare. When unexplained lymph-adenopathy persists after a trial of antibiotic therapy, further evaluation and biopsy are indicated.

Anorexia, weight loss, and fatigue are commonly seen in children. Approximately 30% of children have fever, with intermittent elevations of 1° to 2° C. Unlike adults, children rarely complain of night sweats and pruritus.

Certain systemic symptoms significantly alter prognosis. Patients with unexplained weight loss of more than 10% of body weight in the previous 6 months, unexplained persistent or recurrent fever (temperatures >38° C), or night sweats are classified B in the staging process.[8,38] The absence of these symptoms is the A classification. Approximately one third of children staged for Hodgkin's disease have B classification.[26,68] The percentage of children with the B classification increases with advanced disease. Pruritus does not have prognostic significance and is not included as a B symptom.

DIAGNOSTIC EVALUATION

Evaluation begins with a thorough history and physical examination. Particular attention is directed to the peripheral lymph nodes and abdomen. The presence of small, soft lymph nodes may be misleading in children. Only lymph nodes that have been increasing in size or are significantly enlarged are considered important in estimating involvement. Retroperitoneal disease cannot usually be palpated.

Laboratory studies in the diagnostic work-up include a complete blood count with differential, erythrocyte sedimentation rate (ESR), renal and liver function tests, including alkaline phosphatase and lactate dehydrogenase levels. Anemia may indicate advanced disease. Hemolysis and impaired mobilization of iron stores are causes of anemia in patients with Hodgkin's disease.[26] The white blood cell count is markedly decreased only in advanced disease. Abnormal liver function tests suggest liver involvement. Although nonspecific for Hodgkin's disease, results of tests such as ESR, serum copper, and ferritin may be elevated at diagnosis and relapse, reflecting activation of the reticuloendothelial system.[27,69,73]

Patients with Hodgkin's disease frequently have a cellular immune deficiency with altered functioning of T and B lymphocytes. Patients demonstrate decreased, delayed hypersensitivity reactions to skin test antigens such as tuberculin, diphtheria toxoid, streptokinase-streptodornase, and *Candida albicans*.[58,75] Total anergy (a complete lack of reactivity) may occur in advanced disease. Decreased T-lymphocyte counts may be found in patients with marked lymphocytopenia, systemic symptoms, or advanced disease.[58] A reduced number of circulating T-helper cells has been found in patients with initial or advanced disease. Patients with advanced disease and lymphocytopenia may have a decreased number of T-cytotoxic or suppressor cells.[58] Lymphocytes show impaired proliferation when stimulated by T-cell mitogens.

Antibody responses may remain intact until disease is advanced. B-lymphocyte counts are normal in most patients.[58] Antibody production may be normal or decreased. Impaired antibody production results in decreased resistance to infections. Increased serum immunoglobulin levels and elevated serum titers of antiviral antibodies (EBV and cytomegalovirus) have been reported.[58]

A chest x-ray film may show mediastinal or hilar node involvement. CT is useful for evaluating mediastinal, pulmonary, and upper abdominal disease but is only 40% sensitive in detecting abdominal adenopathy.[5] CT scan of the chest, abdomen, and pelvis is done with images at 1-cm intervals.[38] Lymph nodes greater than 1 cm in diameter on CT scan are considered abnormal. CT scan can detect enlarged nodes but cannot visualize lymph node architecture or differentiate reactive hyperplasia from tumor. Magnetic resonance imaging (MRI) and CT may show spleen or liver involvement or areas of abnormal density.[26] MRI may provide better information on abnormal lymph nodes below the diaphragm compared with CT.[23] Ultrasound imaging of the neck and abdomen can determine bulky tumor margins, spleen size, and liver masses. Gallium-67 (^{67}Ga) scan is useful in evaluating supradiaphragmatic nodes. Increased uptake is demonstrated in 60% to 70% of patients with untreated disease,[26] and persistent gallium uptake after treatment may indicate residual disease.[72] Technetium-99m bone scan can confirm the extent of involvement at a site in a child with bone pain, elevated serum alkaline phosphatase level, or extranodal disease.[26,38]

A lymphangiogram (LAG) may be done to evaluate retroperitoneal involvement. LAG can visualize lymph node size and internal architecture and can evaluate nodes too small to be visualized by CT or MRI. Specific nodes can be identified for biopsy, and it may be helpful for designing radiotherapy treatment fields. LAG has demonstrated unsuspected involvement in patients and has an overall accuracy over 70% in pediatric patients.[15] Radiopaque dye is retained in the lymph nodes for several months, and follow-up radiographs can monitor residual nodes for response to treatment. LAG is technically difficult to perform in small children, and some centers elect to omit it, especially when advanced disease has been documented or treatment will be unaffected by results.

The diagnosis is determined by biopsy of a lymph node and histologic classification by the pathologist. Needle biopsies and frozen section diagnoses, which distort or do not reveal the normal architecture of the lymph node, are contraindicated.

Staging is the determination of the extent of disease at the time of diagnosis. A standardized staging system was developed for Hodgkin's disease at the Rye symposium in 1965, modified at the Ann Arbor conference in 1971, and further defined at a meeting held in the Cotswolds, England, in 1988.[8,38,39] The clinical and pathologic staging of Hodgkin's disease is described in Table 22-2.

At the time of diagnosis approximately 60% of children with Hodgkin's disease present with pathologic stage I or II disease.[26,31,68] Pathologic stage III or IV disease is diagnosed in the remaining 40% of children.[26,68] In clinically staged children 66% have advanced-stage unfavorable disease, defined as stages I to II with large mediastinal mass and stages III to IV A or B.[12]

Laparotomy with splenectomy was initially used to validate LAG findings and search for disease in the abdomen and pelvis.[18,45] Children

TABLE 22-2	STAGING OF HODGKIN'S DISEASE	
Staging Notation	**Criteria**
CLINICAL OR PATHOLOGIC STAGE*	
I	Involvement of a single lymph node region or lymphoid structure†(I) Or a single extralymphatic site (I_E)
II	Involvement of two or more lymph node regions or lymphoid structures on the same side of the diaphragm; number of anatomic regions involved indicated by a subscript (e.g., II_3)
III	Involvement of lymph node regions or lymphoid structures on both sides of the diaphragm; may be subdivided into stage III_1 (spleen or splenic, hilar, celiac, or portal node involvement) or stage III_2 (para-aortic, iliac, or mesenteric node involvement)
IV	Diffuse or disseminated involvement of one or more extralymphatic sites with or without associated lymph node enlargement‡
SYMPTOMS	
A	Asymptomatic
B	Symptoms include the following: Unexplained weight loss of ≥10% of body weight in 6 months before initial staging Unexplained, persistent or recurrent fever with temperatures >38° C during previous month Recurrent drenching night sweats during previous month
SUBSCRIPTS	
X	Bulky disease: ≥10 cm at maximal dimension
E	Extranodal extension: involvement of extralymphatic tissue by limited direct extension from an adjacent nodal site or a single extranodal deposit consistent with extension from a regionally involved node
PS* sites	PS at a given site is indicated by a subscript: *D,* skin; *H,* liver; *L,* lung; *M,* bone marrow; *O,* bone; *P,* pleura

Data from Carbone, P. P., Kaplan, H. S., Musshoff, K., et al. (1971). Report of the committee on Hodgkin's disease staging classification. *Cancer Research, 31,* 1860-1861; Lister, T. A., Crowther, D., Sutcliffe, S. B., et al. (1989). Report of a committee convened to discuss the evaluation and staging of patients with Hodgkin's disease: Cotswolds meeting. *Journal of Clinical Oncology, 7,* 1630-1636.

*Stages are designated as *clinical stage (CS)* when extent of disease is determined by history, physical examination, radiologic and other imaging studies, laboratory tests, and initial biopsy results. *Pathologic stage (PS)* is designated when a staging laparotomy provides histologic confirmation of the presence or absence of involvement of specific sites.

†Lymphoid structures are the spleen, thymus, Waldeyer's ring (nasopharynx, tonsil, base of tongue), appendix, and Peyer's patches.

‡Liver involvement is always considered diffuse and therefore stage IV disease. Multiple extranodal disease is designated stage IV disease.

whose spleens have been removed are at increased risk for overwhelming bacterial infections, especially by encapsulated organisms such as *Streptococcus pneumoniae* and *Haemophilus influenzae.* Investigators determined that abnormal pulmonary hilar nodes visualized on CT scan were reliable predictors of abdominal involvement and developed criteria to avoid laparotomy and splenectomy while obtaining comparable clinical results.[61,63] The increased use of combined-modality therapy, in which the precise localization of disease is less crucial, and a desire to avoid the potential complications of surgery and immunosuppressive effects of splenectomy have resulted in an increased use of clinical staging, omitting laparotomy with splenectomy. Laparotomy with splenectomy is indicated only if the findings will alter the choice of therapy and has been abandoned in most pediatric centers. When comparing treatment results, clinically staged patients cannot be directly compared with patients who were staged by laparotomy.

The staging laparotomy includes a splenectomy and multiple lymph node biopsies. Splenic involvement is usually focal, beginning with small nodular infiltrates only a few millimeters in diameter, so the entire spleen is removed. The spleen is examined at 1- to 3-mm intervals to determine the presence or absence of tumor.[26] Liver biopsies include a wedge biopsy of each lobe. A bone marrow biopsy is obtained from the iliac crest in patients with clinical stage III or IV disease or B symptoms.[26] Oophoropexy may be performed in girls, repositioning the ovaries to a midline location to minimize exposure from abdominal radiotherapy. When an LAG is done, an abdominal radiograph obtained during surgery can verify that suspicious lymph nodes have been removed. Silver clips are left to mark the splenic pedicle and sites of lymph node biopsies, to assist in planning radiotherapy fields and evaluating possible recurrence.

TREATMENT

The goal of treatment is the cure of disease with minimal treatment-related toxicity and sequelae. Children who have localized disease may be treated with radiotherapy alone. Most children are treated with combined-modality therapy regimens alternating multiagent chemotherapy and low-dose involved-field radiotherapy.

Children with early-stage disease limited to the upper neck or inguinal lymph nodes have been successfully treated with involved-field radiotherapy alone.[14,31] Other patients with stage I to III disease may be treated with extended-field (EF) radiotherapy.[13,14] In EF radiotherapy, treatment is given to lymph nodes with known disease and adjacent uninvolved lymph nodes regions. Radiotherapy treatment fields used for Hodgkin's disease are shown in Figure 22-1. Total nodal irradiation (TNI), which includes the mantle field plus the inverted-Y field, may be done in more unfavorable situations. Radiotherapy to areas of bulky or residual disease is optional in stage IV disease.

Radiation doses of 35 to 40 Gy result in tumor response with a risk of recurrence of 10% or less. The tumor dose is given at a rate of 1.5 to 2 Gy per day five times a week.[16,26] Radiation doses depend on the extent of tumor involvement and whether chemotherapy will also be used. Dosages may be reduced in young children to prevent retardation of bone growth and soft tissue development.[16]

The MOPP (mechlorethamine [nitrogen mustard], Oncovin [vincristine], procarbazine, and prednisone) chemotherapy regimen produces effective disease control but has potential late risks of

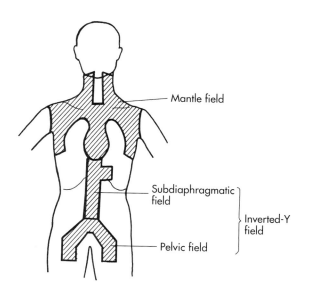

Figure 22-1

Radiotherapy treatment fields used for Hodgkin's disease. The mantle field consists of the submandibular, submental, cervical, supraclavicular, infraclavicular, axillary, mediastinal, and hilar lymph nodes. The mini-mantle field treats cervical, supraclavicular, infraclavicular, or axillary lymph nodes. Irradiation to the subdiaphragmatic field includes the para-aortic lymph nodes and the splenic pedicle or spleen. The pelvic field consists of the common iliac, external iliac, and inguinal-femoral lymph nodes. The inverted-Y field combines the subdiaphragmatic and pelvic fields. Total nodal irradiation includes the mantle field plus the inverted-Y field.

infertility and secondary leukemia. The ABVD (Adriamycin [doxorubicin], bleomycin, vinblastine, and dacarbazine) regimen was originally developed to treat MOPP-resistant disease and avoid MOPP-associated sequelae, but this has a dose-related risk of cardiopulmonary dysfunction. Alternating non–cross resistant regimens (e.g., MOPP and ABVD) produces enhanced antineoplastic activity while reducing life-threatening toxicity by limiting exposure to alkylating agents, doxorubicin and bleomycin.[12,26,28,29,71] Chemotherapy regimens used in the treatment of children with Hodgkin's disease are listed in Table 22-3. The number of chemotherapy cycles given in these regimens varies between series and protocols. Chil-

dren with advanced disease receive chemotherapy as their primary treatment.

The development of combined-modality therapy has been guided by the identification of late effects in long-term survivors.[27,60] The goals of these regimens are to limit the cumulative doses of the most toxic drugs and reduce the dose and volume of radiotherapy while obtaining comparable cure rates. Radiotherapy may be administered before chemotherapy or alternated with courses of chemotherapy. The administration of chemotherapy before radiotherapy reduces bulky disease, permitting the use of smaller radiotherapy fields and lower radiation doses.[14] Receiving radiotherapy limits the amount of chemotherapy that can be given and vice

TABLE 22-3	CHEMOTHERAPY REGIMENS USED IN THE TREATMENT OF CHILDREN WITH HODGKIN'S DISEASE
Regimen	**Chemotherapy Agents**
ABVD	Adriamycin (doxorubicin), bleomycin, vinblastine, dacarbazine
AOPE	Adriamycin (doxorubicin), Oncovin (vincristine), prednisone, etoposide
ChlVPP	Chlorambucil, vinblastine, procarbazine, prednisolone
CHOP	Cyclophosphamide, Adriamycin (doxorubicin), Oncovin (vincristine), prednisone
COMP	Cyclophosphamide, Oncovin (vincristine), methotrexate, prednisone
COPP	Cyclophosphamide, Oncovin (vincristine), procarbazine, prednisone
CVPP	Cyclophosphamide, vincristine, prednisone, procarbazine
DBVE-PC/DZR	Doxorubicin, bleomycin, vincristine, etoposide, prednisone, cyclophosphamide/dexrazoxane
EVAP	Etoposide, vinblastine, cytosine arabinoside, cis-platinum
MOPP	Mechlorethamine (Mustargen), Oncovin (vincristine), procarbazine, prednisone
OEPA	Oncovin (vincristine), etoposide, prednisone, Adriamycin (doxorubicin)
OPA	Oncovin (vincristine), prednisone, Adriamycin (doxorubicin)
OPPA	Oncovin (vincristine), prednisone, procarbazine, Adriamycin (doxorubicin)
VAMP	Vinblastine, Adriamycin (doxorubicin), methotrexate, prednisone
VBVP	Vinblastine, bleomycin, etoposide (VP-16), prednisone
VEEP	Vincristine, epirubicin, etoposide, prednisolone
VEPA	Vinblastine, etoposide, prednisone, Adriamycin (doxorubicin)

Data from Donaldson, S. S., Hudson, M. M., Link, M. P., et al. (1995). Treatment of children with early stage and favorable Hodgkin's disease: A model of success. *Proceedings of American Society of Clinical Oncology, 14,* 408 (abstract); Donaldson, S. S., Hudson, M., Oberlin, O., et al. (1999). Pediatric Hodgkin's disease. In P. M. Mauch, J. O. Armitage, V. Diehl, et al. (Eds.), *Hodgkin's disease* (pp. 531-562). Philadelphia: Lippincott Williams & Wilkins; Hudson, M. M., & Donaldson, S. S. (1997). Hodgkin's disease. In P. A. Pizzo & D. G. Poplack (Eds.), *Principles and practice of pediatric oncology* (3rd ed., pp. 523-543). Philadelphia: Lippincott-Raven; Hudson, M. M., & Donaldson, S. S. (1997). Hodgkin's disease. *Pediatric Clinics of North America, 44,* 891-906; Hutchinson, R. J., Fryer, C. J., Davis, P. C., et al. (1998). MOPP or radiation in addition to ABVD in the treatment of pathologically staged advanced Hodgkin's disease in children: Results of the Children's Cancer Group Phase III Trial. *Journal of Clinical Oncology, 16,* 897-906; Landman-Parker, J., Pacquement, H., Leblanc, T., et al. (2000). Localized childhood Hodgkin's disease: Response-adapted chemotherapy with etoposide, bleomycin, vinblastine, and prednisone before low-dose radiation therapy: Results of the French Society of Pediatric Oncology Study MDH90. *Journal of Clinical Oncology, 18,* 1500-1507; Schellong, G. (1998). Pediatric Hodgkin's disease: Treatment in the late 1990s. *Annals of Oncology, 9* (Suppl 5), 115-119; Schellong, G., Bramswig, J. H., & Hornig-Franz, I. (1992). Treatment of children with Hodgkin's disease: Results of the German Pediatric Oncology Group. *Annals of Oncology, 3* (Suppl. 4), 73-76; Schellong, G., Potter, R., Bramswig, J., et al. (1999). High cure rates and reduced long-term toxicity in pediatric Hodgkin's disease: The German-Austrian multicenter trial DAL-HD-90. The German-Austrian Pediatric Hodgkin's Disease Study Group. *Journal of Clinical Oncology, 17,* 3736-3744; Vecchi, V., Pileri, S., Burnelli, R., et al. (1993). Treatment of pediatric Hodgkin's disease tailored to stage, mediastinal mass and age: An Italian (AIEOP) multicenter study on 215 patients. *Cancer, 72,* 2049-2057.

versa.[14,44] Current pediatric protocols include six cycles of multiagent chemotherapy and radiotherapy at a dose of 25 Gy to an involved field.[12,26,32] In early-stage Hodgkin's disease, studies indicate limiting chemotherapy to three or four cycles when given with low-dose radiotherapy produces comparable cure rates with reduced treatment-related toxicity.[14,36,44,49,70] Children with B symptoms are treated with combined-modality therapy because of their poor prognosis when treated with only one modality.

In the Children's Oncology Group (C.O.G.), the goals for treatment in Hodgkin's disease are to maintain good outcomes while minimizing late effects. The major focus is using "response-based" therapy to improve efficacy. This entails identifying patients who have a good response at the beginning of therapy and minimizing their therapy and keeping those who are slow responders on more intensive therapy.

Relapses historically have occurred within the first 3 years after treatment, but the risk of relapse is present up to 10 years after diagnosis. Patients with early-stage disease previously treated with radiotherapy alone have survival rates of 50% to 80% after treatment with multiagent chemotherapy, with or without additional radiotherapy.[12,26] Although there are fewer relapses in early-stage disease treated with combined-modality therapy, their response rate to salvage therapy is lower than that of patients who received radiotherapy alone.[14,16] Both chemotherapy and radiotherapy are used for new or recurrent disease in advanced-stage disease. Localized relapse is more responsive to salvage treatment than widespread relapse.[12] Radiotherapy may be used for disease outside the previous radiotherapy fields. Salvage chemotherapy can be administered using regimens with non–cross resistant drug combinations. Complete response rates in the range of 25% to 50% have been obtained in patients with relapsed disease.[74] Patients who never achieve a complete remission, have early relapse (<12 months), or multiple relapses after one or more chemotherapy regimens have disease-free survival rates of only 10% to 20%.[26] Autologous hematopoietic stem cell transplantation can increase cure rates in these patients to 20% to 30%.[2,4,74]

PROGNOSIS

Clinical presentations with an advanced stage of disease (stage III or IV) and the presence of systemic symptoms (B symptoms) at the time of diagnosis are adverse prognostic indicators. Localized extralymphatic disease that can be treated defini-

tively with radiotherapy does not adversely affect survival rates.[8]

Tumor bulk is an adverse factor. A lymph node or nodal mass is described as "bulky" when the largest dimension is 10 cm or greater.[38] A mediastinal mass is described as bulky when the maximal width seen on a chest radiograph is one third of the mediastinal diameter at the level of T5-6.[38] Patients with stage I or II disease with a large mediastinal mass have an increased incidence of relapse when treated with radiotherapy alone.

Certain clinical presentations have a favorable prognosis in children. They include stage I nonbulky upper neck disease of any histologic type except LD, stage I nonbulky inguinal disease of any type, and stage I massive mediastinal disease of NS type.[14,16]

The prognostic significance of histologic type has declined with continued overall improvement in survival rates. Historically LP and NS types have a more favorable prognosis than the MC and LD types.[14,17] The NS type has been classified into two grades. NS grade 2 contains areas of lymphocyte depletion and has a less favorable prognosis than NS grade 1, which does not have such areas.[17]

Certain laboratory test results are associated with prognosis. Patients who have an elevated ESR at diagnosis have a higher chance of relapse.[30,69] High soluble CD8+ antigen levels have been found in children with advanced disease, B symptoms, and MC histologic findings and are significantly associated with an increased probability of treatment failure.[53] Soluble CD30+ antigen levels correlate with disease activity. High serum interleukin-2 levels correlate with poor prognosis in children.[52]

High survival rates have been obtained in children with Hodgkin's disease using different treatment strategies. Children with stage I or II disease have 5-year disease-free survival rates of 85% to 95%.* Five-year survival rates in children with advanced-stage disease treated with combined-modality therapy are 70% to 90%.† Generally, children with B symptoms do less well than those without symptoms.[62]

LATE EFFECTS

Aggressive treatment has increased long-term survival rates but also carries the inherent risk of long-term sequelae. Dose-related thyroid abnormalities,

---

*References 11, 16, 28, 37, 57, 60, 61.
†References 26, 28-30, 61, 62, 67, 68, 71.

including hypothyroidism, hyperthyroidism, and thyroid nodules, developed in 34% of young adult survivors of childhood Hodgkin's disease, especially females treated with high doses of radiation to the neck.[64] Cardiac dysfunction, including coronary artery disease, cardiomyopathy, constrictive pericarditis, and valvular disease, can be induced by radiotherapy, although contemporary regimens have modified treatment to decrease the incidence of these sequelae.[12,26] Anthracycline chemotherapy is associated with the development of cardiomyopathy and rhythm disturbances leading to congestive heart failure. Mediastinal radiation increases the risk for development of late cardiac toxicities. Pulmonary dysfunction such as fibrosis or pneumonitis can occur in patients who received pulmonary radiotherapy or chemotherapy, especially bleomycin. Impaired growth and diminished adult height are late effects of radiotherapy and chemotherapy. Pediatric patients treated for Hodgkin's disease have a small decrease in their final height, especially patients who were younger or treated with higher radiotherapy doses.[50] Both chemotherapy and radiotherapy can cause ovarian and testicular dysfunction and/or infertility.[42,51] Cryopreservation of semen should be considered for adolescent males who face possible sterility from treatment.[34]

The risk of developing a second cancer after treatment for Hodgkin's disease has been calculated at 7% for any cancer and 4.1% for a solid tumor after 15 years. After 30 years the risk is 14.4% for any cancer and 8.2% for a solid tumor.[10] Myelodysplastic syndrome and/or acute myeloid leukemia and non-Hodgkin's lymphoma have occurred within 5 years after chemotherapy treatment for Hodgkin's disease.[6,76] The risk of developing secondary leukemia is significantly greater if the patient received alkylating agents. Solid tumors usually occurred more than 10 years after treatment. The most common solid tumors were female breast, thyroid, bone, brain, colorectal, and stomach.[6,46,76] Actuarial risk of breast cancer in females is 9.2% at 20 years.[76]

NURSING IMPLICATIONS

Contemporary treatment of children with Hodgkin's disease incorporates a multidisciplinary approach from the time of diagnosis, and the nurse is an integral member of the team. Nurses educate patients and families about the diagnosis, the diagnostic evaluation, and treatment at each phase of care. Patients and families may need assistance in understanding how clinical trials work and the benefits of participating in pediatric cooperative group protocols. With reduced hospitalizations much of

this teaching and care may take place in the outpatient setting. The nurse may also coordinate care between the multiple departments involved and function as an advocate for school issues.

The development of late effects adversely affects the life expectancy of survivors of Hodgkin's disease. Survivors of childhood Hodgkin's disease require continuous follow-up throughout their lives. Long-term survivors followed by a multidisciplinary team concerned with late effects have the greatest likelihood of having all late effects recognized and optimally managed.[12] Nurses participate in the monitoring of patients for late effects. Patients and their families must be educated about the potential problems they face. Nurses can also educate patients about the importance of adopting healthy lifestyles so they do not place themselves at further risk. And if adverse effects develop, nurses will be there to provide the care required.

FUTURE DIRECTIONS

Treatment goals are to continue the disease-free survival rates in clinically staged children and to improve the outcome for advanced stage disease.[12] Future studies must determine when cure can be achieved with fewer cycles of chemotherapy and when radiotherapy can be safely omitted. Prognostic factors must be identified for children at risk for treatment failure who would benefit from more intensive therapy.[27]

Adolescents with cancer have been underrepresented in the national pediatric cancer cooperative groups and have lower-than-expected cure rates. More than 75% of adolescents 15 to 19 years of age have not been enrolled by any cooperative group sponsored by the National Cancer Institute.[7] This is especially important in Hodgkin's disease because of the increased incidence in this age group. In collaboration with the National Cancer Institute, the C.O.G. is making a concerted effort to address this "adolescent gap" to ensure that adolescents obtain the same cure rates as younger children.

New approaches with immunotherapeutic agents are being investigated in adult patients with advanced refractory disease. Clinical trials have been initiated with interleukin-2, bispecific antibodies, immunotoxins, and radioimmunoconjugates.[75] These agents may have a future role in the treatment of children with Hodgkin's disease.

Children treated for Hodgkin's disease will require continued observation for adverse late effects. The development of clinical trials with equivalent or better survival rates and reduced potential for late effects will further improve the prognosis for children with Hodgkin's disease.

ACKNOWLEDGMENT

The author acknowledges and expresses thanks to Lona Roll, RN, MSN, for her assistance in the preparation of this chapter.

REFERENCES

1. Ambinder, R. F., & Weiss, L. M. (1999). Association of Epstein-Barr virus with Hodgkin's disease. In P. M. Mauch, J. O. Armitage, V. Diehl, et al. (Eds.), *Hodgkin's disease* (pp. 79-98). Philadelphia: Lippincott Williams & Wilkins.

2. Armitage, J. O., Bierman, P. J., & Vose, J. M., et al. (1995). Autologous bone marrow transplantation for Hodgkin's disease. *Journal of Hematotherapy, 4,* 61-62.

3. Armstrong, A. A., Alexander, F. E., & Paes, R. P. (1993). Association of Epstein-Barr virus with pediatric Hodgkin's disease. *American Journal of Pathology, 142,* 1683-1688.

4. Baker, K. S., Gordon, B. G., Gross, T. G., et al. (1999). Autologous hematopoietic stem-cell transplantation for relapsed or refractory Hodgkin's disease in children and adolescents. *Journal of Clinical Oncology, 17,* 825-831.

5. Baker, L. L., Parker, B. R., Donaldson, S. S., et al. (1990). Staging of Hodgkin's disease in children: Comparison of CT and lymphography with laparotomy. *AJR. American Journal of Roentgenology, 154,* 1251-1255.

6. Bhatia, S., Robison, L. L., Oberlin, O., et al. (1996). Breast cancer and other second neoplasms after childhood Hodgkin's disease. *New England Journal of Medicine, 334,* 745-751.

7. Bleyer, W. A., Tejeda, H., Murphy, S. B., et al. (1997). National cancer clinical trials: Children have equal access, adolescents do not. *Journal of Adolescent Health, 21,* 366-373.

8. Carbone, P. P., Kaplan, H. S., Musshoff, K., et al. (1971). Report of the committee on Hodgkin's disease staging classification. *Cancer Research, 31,* 1860-1861.

9. Cleary, S. F., Link, M. P., & Donaldson, S. S. (1994). Hodgkin's disease in the very young. *International Journal of Radiation Oncology, Biology, Physics, 28,* 77-83.

10. Donaldson, S. S., & Hancock, S. L. (1996). Second cancers after Hodgkin's disease in childhood. *New England Journal of Medicine, 334,* 792-794.

11. Donaldson, S. S., Hudson, M. M., Link, M. P., et al. (1995). Treatment of children with early stage and favorable Hodgkin's disease: A model of success. *Proceedings of American Society of Clinical Oncology, 14,* 408 (abstract).

12. Donaldson, S. S., Hudson, M., Oberlin, O., et al. (1999). Pediatric Hodgkin's disease. In P. M. Mauch, J. O. Armitage, V. Diehl, et al. (Eds.), *Hodgkin's disease* (pp. 531-562). Philadelphia: Lippincott Williams & Wilkins.

13. Donaldson, S. S., & Link, M. P. (1987). Combined modality treatment with low-dose radiation and MOPP chemotherapy for children with Hodgkin's disease. *Journal of Clinical Oncology, 5,* 742-749.

14. Donaldson, S. S., Whitaker, S. J., Plowman, P. N., et al. (1990). Stage I-II pediatric Hodgkin's disease: Long-term follow-up demonstrates equivalent survival rates following different management schemes. *Journal of Clinical Oncology, 8,* 1128-1137.

15. Dudgeon, D. L., Kelly, R., Ghory, M. J., et al. (1986). The efficacy of lymphangiography in the staging of pediatric Hodgkin's disease. *Journal of Pediatric Surgery, 21,* 233-235.

16. Gehan, E. A., Sullivan, M. P., Fuller, L. M., et al. (1990). The Intergroup Hodgkin's disease in children. A study of stages I and II. *Cancer, 65,* 1429-1437.

17. Glimelius, B. (1989). Prognostic factors including clinical markers. In W. A. Kamps, G. B. Humphrey, & S. Poppema (Eds.), *Hodgkin's disease in children: Controversies and current practice* (pp. 89-96). Boston: Kluwer Academic Publishers.

18. Green, D. M., Ghorrah, J., Douglass, H. O., Jr., et al. (1983). Staging laparotomy with splenectomy in children and adolescents with Hodgkin's disease. *Cancer Treatment Reviews, 10,* 23-38.

19. Grufferman, S., Cole, P., Smith, P. G., et al. (1977). Hodgkin's disease in siblings. *New England Journal of Medicine, 296,* 248-250.

20. Gurney, J. G., Severson, R. K., Davis, S., et al. (1995). Incidence of cancer in children in the United States: Sex-, race-, and 1-year age-specific rates by histologic type. *Cancer, 75,* 2186-2195.

21. Gutensohn, N. M., & Shapiro, D. S. (1982). Social class risk factors among children with Hodgkin's disease. *International Journal of Cancer, 30,* 433-435.

22. Haluska, F. G., Brufsky, A. M., & Canellos, G. P. (1994). The cellular biology of the Reed-Sternberg cell. *Blood, 84,* 1005-1019.

23. Hanna, S. L., Fletcher, B. D., Boulden, T. F., et al. (1993). MR imaging of infradiaphragmatic lymphadenopathy in children and adolescents with Hodgkin's disease: Comparison with lymphography and CT. *Journal of Magnetic Resonance Imaging, 3,* 461-470.

24. Hodgkin, T. (1832). On some morbid appearances of the absorbent glands and spleen. *Medical-Chirurgical Society Transactions, 17,* 69-97.

25. Hors, J., & Dausset, J. (1983). HLA and susceptibility to Hodgkin's disease. *Immunological Reviews, 70,* 167-192.

26. Hudson, M. M., & Donaldson, S. S. (1997). Hodgkin's disease. In P. A. Pizzo & D. G. Poplack (Eds.), *Principles and practice of pediatric oncology* (3rd ed., pp. 523-543). Philadelphia: Lippincott-Raven.

27. Hudson, M. M., & Donaldson, S. S. (1997). Hodgkin's disease. *Pediatric Clinics of North America, 44,* 891-906.

28. Hudson, M. M., Greenwald, C. G., Thompson, E., et al. (1993). Efficacy and toxicity of multiagent chemotherapy and low-dose involved-field radiotherapy in children and adolescents with Hodgkin's disease. *Journal of Clinical Oncology, 11,* 100-108.

29. Hunger, S. P., Link, M. P., & Donaldson, S. S. (1994). ABVD/MOPP and low-dose involved-field radiotherapy in pediatric Hodgkin's disease: The Stanford experience. *Journal of Clinical Oncology, 12,* 2160-2166.

30. Hutchinson, R. J., Fryer, C. J., Davis, P. C., et al. (1998). MOPP or radiation in addition to ABVD in the treatment of pathologically staged advanced Hodgkin's disease in children: Results of the Children's Cancer Group Phase III Trial. *Journal of Clinical Oncology, 16,* 897-906.

31. Jenkin, D., Doyle, J., Berry, M., et al. (1990). Hodgkin's disease in children: Treatment with MOPP and low-dose extended field irradiation without laparotomy—Late results and toxicity. *Medical and Pediatric Oncology, 18,* 265-272.

32. Jenkin, D., & Greenberg, M. (1993). Hodgkin's disease in childhood: Early treatment results in clinically staged patients utilizing MOPP/ABV (3 cycles) and extended field radiation treatment (1500 cGy). *Medical and Pediatric Oncology, 21,* 542 (abstract).

33. Karayalcin, G., Behm, F. G., Gieser, P. W., et al. (1997). Lymphocyte predominant Hodgkin disease: Clinico-pathologic features and results of treatment—The Pediatric Oncology Group experience. *Medical and Pediatric Oncology, 29,* 519-525.

34. Kliesch, S., Behre, H. M., Jurgens, H., et al. (1996). Cryopreservation of semen from adolescent patients with malignancies. *Medical and Pediatric Oncology, 26,* 20-27.

35. Kung, F. H. (1991). Hodgkin's disease in children 4 years of age or younger. *Cancer, 67,* 1428-1430.

36. Kung, F. H., Behm, F. G., Cantor, A., et al. (1993). Abbreviated chemotherapy vs. chemoradiotherapy in early stage Hodgkin's disease of childhood. *Proceedings of American Society of Clinical Oncology, 12,* 414 (abstract).

37. Landman-Parker, J., Pacquement, H., Leblanc, T., et al. (2000). Localized childhood Hodgkin's disease: Response-adapted chemotherapy with etoposide, bleomycin, vinblastine, and prednisone before low-dose radiation therapy—Results of the French Society of Pediatric Oncology Study MDH90. *Journal of Clinical Oncology, 18,* 1500-1507.

38. Lister, T. A., Crowther, D., Sutcliffe, S. B., et al. (1989). Report of a committee convened to discuss the evaluation and staging of patients with Hodgkin's disease: Cotswolds meeting. *Journal of Clinical Oncology, 7,* 1630-1636.

39. Lukes, R. J. (1971). Criteria for involvement of lymph node, bone marrow, spleen, and liver in Hodgkin's disease. *Cancer Research, 31,* 1755-1767.

40. Lukes, R. J., Craver, L. F., Hall, T. C., et al. (1966). Report of the Nomenclature Committee. *Cancer Research, 26,* 1311.

41. Mack, T. M., Cozen, W., Shibata, D. K., et al. (1995). Concordance for Hodgkin's disease in identical twins suggesting genetic susceptibility to the young-adult form of the disease. *New England Journal of Medicine, 332,* 413-418.

42. Mackie, E. J., Radford, M., & Shalet, S. M. (1996). Gonadal function following chemotherapy for childhood Hodgkin's disease. *Medical and Pediatric Oncology, 27,* 74-78.

43. MacMahon, B. (1966). Epidemiology of Hodgkin's disease. *Cancer Research, 26,* 1189-1201.

44. Maity, A., Goldwein, J. W., Lange, B., et al. (1992). Comparison of high-dose and low-dose radiation with and without chemotherapy for children with Hodgkin's disease: An analysis of the experience at the Children's Hospital of Philadelphia and the Hospital of the University of Pennsylvania. *Journal of Clinical Oncology, 10,* 929-935.

45. Mendenhall, N. P., Cantor, A. B., Williams, J. L., et al. (1993). With modern imaging techniques, is staging laparotomy necessary in pediatric Hodgkin's disease?—A Pediatric Oncology Group study. *Journal of Clinical Oncology, 11,* 2218-2225.

46. Metayer, C., Lynch, C. F., Clarke, E. A., et al. (2000). Second cancers among long-term survivors of Hodgkin's disease diagnosed in childhood and adolescence. *Journal of Clinical Oncology, 18,* 2435-2443.

47. Mueller, N. E. (1987). The epidemiology of Hodgkin's disease. In P. Selby & T. J. McElwain (Eds.), *Hodgkin's disease* (pp. 68-93). Boston: Blackwell Scientific Publications.

48. Mueller, N. E., & Grufferman, S. (1999). The epidemiology of Hodgkin's disease. In P. M. Mauch, J. O. Armitage, V. Diehl, et al. (Eds.), *Hodgkin's disease* (pp. 61-77). Philadelphia: Lippincott Williams & Wilkins.

49. Oberlin, O., Leverger, G., Pacquement, M. A., et al. (1992). Low-dose radiation therapy and reduced chemotherapy in childhood Hodgkin's disease: The experience of the French Society of Pediatric Oncology. *Journal of Clinical Oncology, 10,* 1602-1608.

50. Papadakis, V., Tan, C., Heller, G., et al. (1996). Growth and final height after treatment for childhood Hodgkin's disease. *Journal of Pediatric Hematology/Oncology, 18,* 272-276.

51. Papadakis, V., Vlachopapadopoulou, E., Van Syckle, K., et al. (1999). Gonadal function in young patients successfully treated for Hodgkin's disease. *Medical and Pediatric Oncology, 32,* 366-372.

52. Pui, C. H., Ip, S., Thompson, E., et al. (1989). High serum interleukin-2 levels correlate with a poor prognosis in children with Hodgkin's disease. *Leukemia, 3,* 481-484.

53. Pui, C. H., Ip, S. H., Thompson, E., et al. (1989). Increased serum CD8 antigen level in childhood Hodgkin's disease relates to advanced stage and poor treatment outcome. *Blood, 73,* 209-213.

54. Reed, D. M. (1902). On the pathological changes in Hodgkin's disease, with special reference to its relation to tuberculosis. *John Hopkins Hospital Report, 10,* 133.

55. Robertson, S. J., Lowman, J. T., Grufferman, S., et al. (1987). Familial Hodgkin's disease: A clinical and laboratory investigation. *Cancer, 59,* 1314-1319.

56. Robison, L. L. (1997). General principles of the epidemiology of childhood cancer. In P. A. Pizzo & D. G. Poplack (Eds.), *Principles and practice of pediatric oncology* (3rd ed., pp. 1-10). Philadelphia: Lippincott-Raven.

57. Rock, D. B., Murray, K. J., Schultz, C. J., et al. (1996). Stage I and II Hodgkin's disease in the pediatric population: Long-term follow-up of patients staged predominantly clinically. *American Journal of Clinical Oncology, 19,* 174-178.

58. Romagnani, S., Maggi, E., & Parronchi, P. (1989). The immune derangement and strategies for immunotherapy. In W. A. Kamps, G. B. Humphrey, & S. Poppema (Eds.), *Hodgkin's disease in children: Controversies and current practice* (pp. 53-88). Boston: Kluwer Academic Publishers.

59. Safai, B., Diaz, B., & Schwartz, J. (1992). Malignant neoplasms associated with human immunodeficiency virus infection. *CA: A Cancer Journal for Clinicians, 42,* 74-95.

60. Schellong, G. (1998). Pediatric Hodgkin's disease: Treatment in the late 1990s. *Annals of Oncology, 9* (Suppl. 5), 115-119.

61. Schellong, G., Bramswig, J. H., & Hornig-Franz, I. (1992). Treatment of children with Hodgkin's disease: Results of the German Pediatric Oncology Group. *Annals of Oncology, 3* (Suppl. 4), 73-76.

62. Schellong, G., Potter, R., Bramswig, J., et al. (1999). High cure rates and reduced long-term toxicity in pediatric Hodgkin's disease: The German-Austrian multicenter trial DAL-HD-90. The German-Austrian Pediatric Hodgkin's Disease Study Group. *Journal of Clinical Oncology, 17,* 3736-3744.

63. Schellong, G. M. (1989). The German cooperative therapy studies: An approach to minimize treatment modalities and invasive staging procedures. In W. A. Kamps, G. B. Humphrey, & S. Poppema (Eds.), *Hodgkin's disease in children: Controversies and current practice* (pp. 277-292). Boston: Kluwer Academic Publishers.

64. Sklar, C., Whitton, J., Mertens, A., et al. (2000). Abnormalities of the thyroid in survivors of Hodgkin's disease: Data from the Childhood Cancer Survivor Study. *Journal of Clinical Endocrinology and Metabolism, 85,* 3227-3232.

65. Spitz, M. R., Sider, J. F., Johnson, C. C., et al. (1986). Ethnic patterns of Hodgkin's disease incidence among children and adolescents in the United States, 1973-1982. *Journal of the National Cancer Institute, 76,* 235-239.

66. Strum, S. B., & Rappaport, H. (1973). Consistency of histologic subtypes in Hodgkin's disease in simultaneous and sequential biopsy specimens. *Journal of the National Cancer Institute Monographs, 36,* 253-260.

67. Sullivan, M. P., Fuller, L. M., Berard, C., et al. (1991). Comparative effectiveness of two combined modality regimens in the treatment of surgical stage III Hodgkin's disease in children: An 8-year follow-up study by the Pediatric Oncology Group. *American Journal of Pediatric Hematology/Oncology, 13,* 450-458.

68. Tan, C. T. C. (1989). Hodgkin's disease in children and adolescents: Experiences from the Memorial Sloan-Kettering Cancer Center. In W. A. Kamps, G. B. Humphrey, & S. Poppema (Eds.), *Hodgkin's disease in children: Controversies and current practice* (pp. 291-302). Boston: Kluwer Academic Publishers.

69. Tubiana, M., Henry-Amar, M., Burgers, M. V., et al. (1984). Prognostic significance of erythrocyte sedimentation rate in clinical stages I-II of Hodgkin's disease. *Journal of Clinical Oncology, 2,* 194-200.

70. Vecchi, V., Pileri, S., Burnelli, R., et al. (1993). Treatment of pediatric Hodgkin's disease tailored to stage, mediastinal mass and age: An Italian (AIEOP) multicenter study on 215 patients. *Cancer, 72,* 2049-2057.

71. Weiner, M. A., Leventhal, B., Brecher, M. L., et al. (1997). Randomized study of intensive MOPP-ABVD with or without low-dose total-nodal radiation therapy in the treatment of stages IIB, IIA$_2$, IIIB, and IV Hodgkin's disease in pediatric patients: A Pediatric Oncology Group study. *Journal of Clinical Oncology, 15,* 2769-2779.

72. Weiner, M. A., Leventhal, B. G., Cantor, A., et al. (1991). Gallium-67 scans as an adjunct to computed tomography scans for the assessment of a residual mediastinal mass in pediatric patients with Hodgkin's disease: A Pediatric Oncology Group Study. *Cancer, 68,* 2478-2480.

73. Wilimas, J., Thompson, E., & Smith, K. L. (1978). Value of serum copper levels and erythrocyte sedimentation rates as indicators of disease activity in children with Hodgkin's disease. *Cancer, 42,* 1929-1935.

74. Wimmer, R. S. (1989). Salvage treatment for patients with multiply relapsed Hodgkin's disease. In W. A. Kamps, G. B. Humphrey, & S. Poppema (Eds.), *Hodgkin's disease in children: Controversies and current practice* (pp. 187-194). Boston: Kluwer Academic Publishers.

75. Winkler, U., Engert, A., & Diehl, V. (1999). Novel techniques in Hodgkin's disease. In P. M. Mauch, J. O. Armitage, V. Diehl, et al. (Eds.), *Hodgkin's disease* (pp. 409-431). Philadelphia: Lippincott Williams & Wilkins.

76. Wolden, S. L., Lamborn, K. R., Cleary, S. F., et al. (1998). Second cancers following pediatric Hodgkin's disease. *Journal of Clinical Oncology, 16,* 536-544.

23

Non-Hodgkin's Lymphoma

Margaret Ryan Hussong

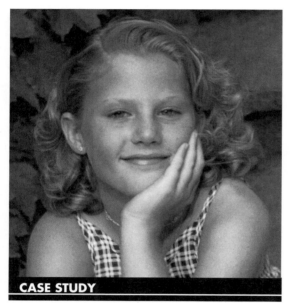

CASE STUDY

Andrea was almost 8 years old, enjoying her summer vacation in 1996, when she noticed a bump just below her left nipple. The swelling, approximately the size of a penny, was red and itchy. She showed it to her mother, who thought it was a bug bite. When there was no change after 2 weeks, the family consulted a friend who happened to be a dermatologist. The lesion was believed to be an infection, and Andrea was started on a 14-day course of cephalexin. Again there was no change in the size of the lesion, though it appeared to be darker.

A biopsy of the lesion was performed on August 22, 1996. Histopathologic examination revealed a dense dermal infiltrate consisting of lymphocytes with occasional histiocytes. The infiltrate was atypical, more because of its density than its cellular characteristics. Immunoperoxidase staining showed that the lymphocytes were predominantly T cells with scattered B cells. A few of the larger cells showed positive membrane staining for CD30 (Ki-1). Gene rearrangements indicated a clonal population of T cells. Andrea was given the diagnosis of large cell lymphoma.

Review of systems and metastatic work-up consisting of a bone marrow aspirate and biopsy, cerebrospinal fluid (CSF) analysis, chest x-ray examination, bone scan, and computed tomography (CT) of chest, abdomen, and pelvis were negative.

Andrea was treated with chemotherapy consisting of doxorubicin, cyclophosphamide, vincristine, and prednisone (A-COP). Her treatment, planned for 6 weeks, lasted 9 weeks. She tolerated therapy well with the exception of significant constipation that delayed her therapy and required aggressive intervention.

Andrea has been off therapy for 4 years. She is currently in the sixth grade and plays competitive soccer, basketball, and softball.

Non-Hodgkin's lymphomas (NHLs) are a diverse collection of malignant neoplasms of lymphoid origin.[14] Most cancers are neoplastic proliferations of a specific organ or tissue and therefore originate in a circumscribed anatomic location. They spread from their original site by local invasion or by metastasis. Like the leukemias, malignant lymphomas differ from this pattern. They are neoplasms of the constituent cells of the immune system, cells that are located throughout the body and normally circulate throughout the body to fulfill their functions. Thus this malignancy can arise anywhere and should be considered a generalized disease from the outset with patterns of spread that mimic the migration patterns of normal lymphoid cells.[24]

DESCRIPTION

Childhood NHL is distinguished from adult NHL by differing frequencies of immunohistopathologic types, by their generally more aggressive behavior, and by the relatively greater occurrence of extranodal presentations. Low-grade lymphomas and follicular lymphomas constitute a large fraction of adult lymphomas but are essentially unknown in childhood.[25] Most childhood non-Hodgkin's lymphomas are thought to arise from lymphocyte precursors in the bone marrow and thymus[3] and can be categorized into three main types: small noncleaved cell, lymphoblastic, or large cell (Table 23-1).

Small noncleaved cell lymphomas are B-cell cancers that include Burkitt and non-Burkitt subtypes. These tumor cells express surface immunoglobins and B-cell specific antigens.[10] Recurring chromosomal translocations of 8q24 are characteristic of these cells.[17] This type of lymphoma accounts for 40% to 50% of all childhood NHL. At least 90% of small noncleaved cell lymphomas arise in the abdomen.[29] B-cell lymphoma is distinguished from B-cell acute lymphocytic leukemia (ALL) by the percentage ($>$25%) of malignant cells in the bone marrow.

Lymphoblastic lymphomas are composed of immature lymphoid cells, the majority of which are T cell in origin and have the enzyme terminal deoxynucleotidyl transferase (TdT).[9,16] Chromosomal translocations at 14q11.2 or 7q34 frequently occur.[12] Lymphoblastic lymphoma is very similar to acute lymphoblastic leukemia. It is distinguished from leukemia by the percentage of blast cells present in the bone marrow; children with greater than 25% blasts are arbitrarily classified as having leukemia.[9,27] Patients with this type of NHL commonly have mediastinal disease with or without thoracic involvement and peripheral nodal disease.[27]

The large cell lymphomas are heterogeneous. One third are of B-cell origin, one third are of T-cell origin, and the final third are of indeterminate origin. The recently described Ki-1 anaplastic large cell lymphoma, the majority of which are of T-cell origin, constitute 30% to 40% of large cell lymphomas.[20] Translocation of chromosomes t(2;5)(p23;q35) has been described. Extranodal sites such as skin, lung, bone, and brain are common locations for large cell lymphoma.[27]

EPIDEMIOLOGY

The overall incidence of NHL in the general population in the United States is increasing significantly for unknown reasons; however, the rate among children has not changed greatly in the past two decades.[21] The frequency of NHL varies in different geographic regions. In Africa approximately 50% of childhood cancers are lymphomas, with Burkitt being the most common.[6,9,14,25] In the United States malignant lymphomas are the third most common malignancy in children under the age of 15, exceeded only by leukemia and brain tumors.[6,9,14] Lymphoma accounts for 12% of all pediatric cancers, of which 40% to 45% are Hodgkin's disease and 55% to 60% are non-Hodgkin's lymphoma.[9,19] NHLs are rare under the age of 2 years, but the frequency steadily increases through-

TABLE 23-1	COMMON CHARACTERISTICS OF NON-HODGKIN'S LYMPHOMA IN CHILDREN		
Histologic Classification	Immunologic Findings	Chromosomal Translocations	Common Sites of Involvement
Small noncleaved cell	B cell	8q24	Abdomen (90%) Mediastinum
Lymphoblastic	T cell	14q11.2 7q34	Mediastinum Thoracic involvement Peripheral nodes Bone marrow
Large cell	B cell T cell Indeterminant	t(2;5) (p23;q35)	Peripheral nodes Skin Lung Bone Brain

Data from Hutchinson R., Murphy S., Fairclough D., et al. (1989). Diffuse small non-cleaved cell lymphoma in children, Burkitt's versus non-Burkitt's types. *Cancer, 64,* 23-34; Kurtzberg, J., & Graham, M., (1991). Non-Hodgkin's lymphoma, biological classification and implication for therapy. *Pediatric Clinics of North America, 38,* 443-456; Magrath, I. T. (1987). Malignant non-Hodgkin's lymphoma in children. *Hematology Oncology Clinics of North America, 1,* 577-602; Magrath I. T. (1990). Small noncleaved cell lymphoma. In I. T. Magrath (Ed.), *The non-Hodgkin's lymphomas* (pp. 246-278). London: Edward Arnold; Murphy S. B. (1994). Pediatric lymphomas: Recent advances and commentary on Ki-1-positive anaplastic large cell lymphomas of childhood. *Annals of Oncology, 5*(s-1), 31-33; Non-Hodgkin's lymphoma. (1999). In E. C. Halperin, L. S. Constine, N. J. Tarbell, et al. (Eds.). *Pediatric radiation oncology,* (3rd ed., pp 233-244). Philadelphia: Lippincott Williams & Wilkins; Smith, S. D., Rubin, C. M., Horvath, A., et al. (1990). Non-Hodgkin's lymphoma in children. *Seminars in Oncology, 17,* 113-119; Van Syckle, K. (1998). Non-Hodgkin's lymphoma. In M. J. Hockenberry-Eaton (Ed.), *Essentials of pediatric oncology nursing: A core curriculum* (pp. 20-23). Glenview, IL: Association of Pediatric Oncology Nurses.

out childhood and peaks at age 7 to 11 years.[8,9] Males are affected more often than females (3:1), and white children are affected twice as often as nonwhites.[6,8,9,14,29]

There is an increased incidence of NHL among patients with compromised immune systems. Children with underlying syndromes and diseases such as Wiskott-Aldrich syndrome, Chédiak-Higashi syndrome, X-linked lymphoproliferative disorder, and ataxia-telangiectasia have a substantially higher risk of developing NHL. Children who have undergone organ transplant are at risk for developing non-Hodgkin's lymphoma because of long-term immunosuppressive therapy.[23,26]

The etiology of non-Hodgkin's lymphoma is largely unknown. Epstein-Barr virus has been associated with the African type of Burkitt's lymphoma.[25] Recent investigations indicate that NHLs result from the uncontrolled proliferation of immature lymphoid precursors that have lost the capacity to differentiate further and that accumulate progressively in the host.[14] Available evidence further suggests that these lymphomas are clonal proliferations; the neoplastic cells appear to represent the progeny of a single damaged progenitor cell. Childhood lymphomas generally grow rapidly because of high growth fractions and short doubling times (12 hours to a few days).[14]

CLINICAL PRESENTATION

The clinical presentation of a patient with non-Hodgkin's lymphoma directly correlates with the histologic classification of the cell. Symptoms leading to diagnosis are usually of short duration and relate to the location of the primary tumor. The initial clinical manifestations are often indistinguishable from those of a variety of common childhood illnesses. However, the rapid evolution of the disease soon removes all doubt of a malignancy. Constitutional symptoms of fever, weight loss, and night sweats common in Hodgkin's lymphoma are unusual in children with NHL.[14] In general, approximately 25% of children with non-Hodgkin's lymphoma have mediastinal disease (usually lymphoblastic histologic classification with T-cell markers), 30% have abdominal tumors (usually undifferentiated or small noncleaved histologic classification), and 20% to 30% have head and neck as primary sites. The remainder of patients have miscellaneous primary sites, including bone, breast, skin, epidural space, or noncervical lymph nodes.[9]

Children with mediastinal disease very often have presenting symptoms of malaise, cough, stridor, wheezing, and shortness of breath, evolving to

respiratory distress, and respiratory failure. Supraclavicular and axillary lymphadenopathy often accompany the respiratory symptoms. In addition, children may have pleural effusions and complain of chest pain. Swelling of the neck, face, and upper limbs results from superior vena cava obstruction. These fast-growing tumors are usually T-cell lymphoblastic lymphomas and have a propensity for rapid spread to the bone marrow, central nervous system (CNS), and gonads. The majority of these cases occur in adolescents with a marked male preponderance. Their presentation may pose a medical emergency.[9,25,27,29]

The majority of abdominal lymphomas are small noncleaved cell (Burkitt or non-Burkitt type). Children with a primary abdominal mass may have pain mimicking appendicitis or intussusception, accompanied by nausea, vomiting, and a change in bowel habits. They sometimes have gastrointestinal bleeding and rarely intestinal perforation. Ascites and abdominal distention, if present, indicate diffuse and massive peritoneal involvement. Metastases to the bone marrow and CNS are common. Because of rapidly dividing cell populations, these children are at significant risk of tumor lysis and often present with symptoms of tumor lysis syndrome. In these cases treatment to prevent the complications of tumor lysis syndrome should be initiated urgently before definitive diagnosis or treatment.[9,14,25]

Children with head and neck as primary sites frequently have rapidly enlarging cervical lymph nodes. If Waldeyer's ring (a circle of lymphoid tissue composed of tonsils and adenoids) is involved, children often complain of nasal stuffiness, tonsillar enlargement, and earache or hearing loss.[9,14,25] Overt CNS involvement is frequent in children with head and neck primary sites.[9]

In equatorial Africa the predominant site of Burkitt's lymphoma is the jaw, especially in patients younger than 5 years of age. Abdominal sites, which are very common in the United States and Europe, are uncommon in Africa. Bone marrow involvement is more usual in patients in the United States and Europe, and CNS involvement is more common in Africa.[25]

A small number of children have tumors in unusual extranodal sites such as skin, bone, or the epidural space. Cutaneous lymphomas frequently present in the scalp region and appear as enlarging discolored masses. Lymphoma localized to bone may present with pain, be associated with a soft tissue mass, and mimic bone tumors. These lymphomas are typically large cell and generally do not metastasize to the bone marrow or CNS. Primary lymphomas of the CNS are unusual and are observed primarily in children with inherited or acquired immunodeficiency syndromes and in patients receiving immunosuppressive therapy.[14]

DIAGNOSTIC EVALUATION

A complete history and physical examination is the initial step in determining a diagnosis. The presenting symptoms, onset, duration, and rate of progression of the clinical manifestations are elicited. Any history of an underlying illness, previous organ transplant, immunodeficiency, or immunosuppressive therapy is explored. Physical examination includes assessment of the chief complaint with additional attention to any lymphadenopathy, abdominal masses, or respiratory symptoms.

Laboratory evaluation includes a complete blood count with differential, platelet count, erythrocyte sedimentation rate, and reticulocyte count. Routine blood chemistry studies with determinations of electrolytes, uric acid, and lactate dehydrogenase (LDH) and tests of liver and renal function are also obtained.[9] Other laboratory studies such as levels of α-fetoprotein (AFP), CA 125, or urinary catecholamines may be helpful to rule out other diagnoses. Bone marrow aspirate and biopsy specimens are obtained. A lumbar puncture with examination of the cerebral spinal fluid is also necessary.[9]

Imaging studies include a chest x-ray, a bone scan, and occasionally a gallium scan. Abdominal, thoracic, and head and neck CT scans and/or MRI scans are obtained depending on the presenting site.[9]

Surgical biopsy establishes the diagnosis. The most suspicious node is selected for excisional biopsy. Needle biopsy is discouraged because it often will not obtain an adequate tissue sample to establish the diagnosis. Histologic analysis was once the primary tool to obtain definitive diagnosis and was the main determinant of therapy. Today morphologic analysis is supplemented by immunophenotype, enzymatic, and cytogenetic studies.[9,14,25] Staging laparotomy is unnecessary because it does not influence treatment or prognosis and is performed only for abdominal presentations requiring surgical intervention.[9]

Histologic classification of non-Hodgkin's lymphoma is based on the identification of the neoplastic cell of origin to predict the biologic tumor behavior and allow for selection of appropriate therapy.[14] Staging systems reflect the tumor volume, primary site, and extent of spread. They are used in determining therapy. The system used for some years at the National Cancer Institute (NCI) was originally devised as a staging system for African patients with Burkitt's lymphoma (Uganda Cancer Institute Staging System) and reflects characteristics of NHL

common in that country. This model is not applicable to patients with lymphoblastic lymphoma and is suboptimal for U.S. patients with small noncleaved cell lymphoma.[25]

The system most widely accepted today is the St. Jude Children's Research Hospital Staging System for Non-Hodgkin's Lymphoma (Box 23-1). This system is based on the Ann Arbor staging system for Hodgkin's disease and was originally devised by

---

BOX 23-1

ST. JUDE CHILDREN'S RESEARCH HOSPITAL STAGING SYSTEM FOR NON-HODGKIN'S LYMPHOMA

STAGE I

A single tumor (extranodal) or single anatomic area (nodal) with the exclusion of mediastinum or abdomen

STAGE II

A single tumor (extranodal) with regional node involvement

Two or more nodal areas on the same side of the diaphragm

Two single (extranodal) tumors with or without regional node involvement on the same side of the diaphragm

A primary gastrointestinal tract tumor, usually in the ileocecal area, with or without involvement of associated mesenteric nodes only

STAGE III

Two single tumors (extranodal) on opposite sides of the diaphragm

Two or more nodal areas above and below the diaphragm

All the primary intrathoracic tumors (mediastinal, pleural, and thymic)

All extensive primary intraabdominal disease*

All paraspinal or epidural tumors, regardless of other tumor site(s)

STAGE IV

Any of the above with initial central nervous system or bone marrow involvement†

---

*A distinction is made between apparently localized gastrointestinal tract lymphoma and more extensive intraabdominal disease. Stage II disease typically is limited to a segment of the gut plus or minus the associated mesenteric nodes only, and the primary tumor can be completely removed grossly by segmental excision. Stage III disease typically exhibits spread to para-aortic and retroperitoneal areas by implants and plaques in mesentery or peritoneum or by direct infiltration of structures adjacent to the primary tumor. Ascites may be present, and complete resection of all gross tumor is not possible.

†If marrow involvement is present initially, the number of abnormal cells must be 25% or less in an otherwise normal marrow aspirate with normal peripheral blood picture.

Dr. Sharon Murphy.[25] Unlike the Ann Arbor system, the St. Jude classification recognizes pediatric patterns of NHL spread and can be used for all classifications of pediatric non-Hodgkin's lymphomas. It takes into account the site and extent of disease and can be performed with a minimum number of standard imaging studies and invasive procedures. This staging system has proven successful in distinguishing children with a favorable prognosis (lower stage, localized; stages I and II) from those children with a less favorable prognosis (more extensive or disseminated disease; stages III and IV).[14]

TREATMENT

HISTORY

The prognosis for children with NHL has improved dramatically in the past two decades, resulting from the recognition that NHL is a rapidly disseminating systemic disease. In the 1960s, fewer than 10% of children with NHL became long-term survivors. Therapeutic interventions in the 1970s improved that number to approximately 30%, though dissemination to the bone marrow and subsequent leukemic transformation (usually within 6 months of diagnosis) occurred in approximately 30% of patients.[9,25] The identification of the similarities between childhood NHL and childhood leukemia led to the application of systemic antileukemic chemotherapy in addition to radiotherapy to control dissemination. The success of this approach established the efficacy of acute lymphoblastic leukemia type of systemic therapy and has since been the backbone of treatment for children with non-Hodgkin's lymphoma.[14] Refinement of therapy using multiagent chemotherapy has increased the overall survival of children with NHL to greater than 80%.[18,25]

RISK CATEGORIES

With the advent of the staging system and the improved ability to identify NHL subtypes, tumor-specific chemotherapy regimens have been developed. Children with B-cell tumors are usually treated with intensive, repetitive, short-duration therapy. Children with T-cell tumors are treated with chemotherapy similar to ALL for 18 to 24 months. All high-grade lymphoma regimens incorporate treatment to prevent CNS disease.[25]

Several studies throughout the past decade have identified factors that are associated with poor outcomes. Researchers have demonstrated that visceral involvement, mediastinal involvement, and an elevated LDH level at presentation were associated with a higher risk of treatment failure.[5,11] Bone marrow or CNS involvement have also been associated with a poor prognosis.[14] However, newer, more intensive therapies appear to have resulted in significantly improved outcomes for these patients.[1,4]

SPECIAL CONSIDERATIONS

Before therapy is initiated, measures must be taken to treat any acute problems that may be present. Children with a mediastinal mass often experience respiratory distress because of airway compression or vena cava obstruction. Masses in the nasopharynx or oropharynx may also result in respiratory compromise. Once a diagnosis is confirmed, appropriate chemotherapy is initiated immediately. If there is a delay in confirming the diagnosis, emergent radiation therapy may be needed following biopsy.

Patients with bulky disease and/or advanced disease often have acute tumor lysis syndrome (ATLS) because of the rapid cell turnover and resulting hyperuricemia, hyperphosphatemia, hypocalcemia, and hyperkalemia. If left untreated, ATLS can lead to renal failure and even death. It is imperative to immediately initiate measures to maintain a brisk urine output and to reduce levels of serum uric acid with the combination of urinary alkalinization and the administration of allopurinol. Vigilant treatment of this syndrome needs to continue after therapy for the lymphoma is initiated because chemotherapy will cause further cell lysis (refer to Chapter 13).[14]

CHEMOTHERAPY

All non-Hodgkin's lymphomas respond to chemotherapy, partly because of their high rate of growth.[25] Research has demonstrated that even children with localized disease have microscopic metastatic disease, and therefore regardless of their stage and histologic classification, all are treated with chemotherapy.[1,9] Treatment strategies are initially based on stage, with further stratification designated by histologic classification for patients with advanced stage disease. Patients with localized stage I or II disease have an excellent prognosis with a 9-week chemotherapy course, regardless of classification (Figure 23-1).[22]

Small noncleaved cell lymphoma. Chemotherapy is the primary treatment for small noncleaved cell lymphoma (SNCC). Successive treatment cycles are administered as soon as possible to prevent tumor regrowth. Most protocols used today to treat SNCC consist of short duration (6 weeks to 6 months), intensive, alkylating agent therapy.[25]

Children with limited disease (stages I and II) have an excellent prognosis and require less intensive treatment than patients with more extensive disease.[13,15,25] Therapy for these patients con-

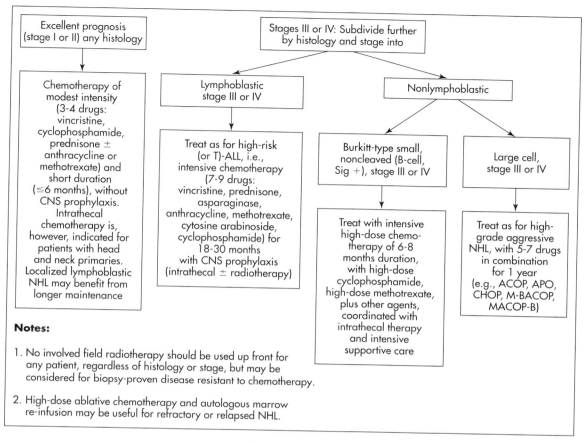

Figure 23-1

Treatment strategies in non-Hodgkin's lymphoma.   (From Murphy S. B. [2000]. Non-Hodgkin's lymphoma and Hodgkin's disease. In C. Herzog & C. Pratt [Eds.], *Therapy of cancer in children* [p. 12]. Houston, TX: University of Texas M. D. Anderson Cancer Center.)

sists of cyclophosphamide, prednisone, vincristine, and methotrexate or doxorubicin (COMP or A-COP).[9,13,25] Radiation therapy is of no benefit in this population.[15] Research efforts for patients with limited disease involve determining how little treatment can be given without reducing the excellent survival rate.[25]

In patients with extensive disease, both with and without bone marrow involvement (stages III and IV), the inclusion of high-dose methotrexate into the standard therapy of COMP or A-COP, as well as the addition of agents such as ifosfamide, etoposide, and high-dose cytarabine, has improved survival.[4,25,28] Due to the significant risk of CNS disease, intrathecal therapy is also employed.[4,28]

Patients who have central nervous system disease at diagnosis usually also have extensive disease with bone marrow involvement. Survival in this cohort of patients has improved significantly

with the addition of high-dose cytarabine and high-dose methotrexate, both of which have good CNS penetration.[25] The role of radiation therapy in these patients remains controversial.

Lymphoblastic lymphoma.   Patients with extensive lymphoblastic lymphomas often have complications at presentation and diagnosis that require immediate intervention. In some cases, such as airway compromise or organ obstructions, it may be necessary to initiate limited radiation therapy or corticosteroids before starting chemotherapy. Close attention to signs of acute tumor lysis syndrome is imperative.

The duration of therapy necessary for best outcomes for higher stage lymphomas is unknown, but research has shown that treating less than 6 months is associated with a higher rate of relapse.[15,22,25] At this time children are treated for 18 to 24 months.

Most chemotherapy regimens for lymphoblastic lymphoma are based on childhood ALL therapy.[25] LSA$_2$L$_2$ therapy originally developed by Wollner[31] and the German Berlin-Frankfurt-Munster (BFM) protocols have been the most widely used and effective regimens to treat this type of lymphoma.[1,25a] These are intensive regimens using 8 to 10 different agents during three phases of therapy: induction, consolidation, and maintenance. Prophylactic intrathecal chemotherapy, and in some cases cranial irradiation, is given.[1,25,25a] Studies by the pediatric cooperative groups have demonstrated that this therapy has been less effective in patients with mediastinal masses than those with other sites of disease.[2,25] Subsequent studies have built upon this work by intensifying the regimens and have improved therapy with the introduction of high-dose methotrexate and more recently high-dose asparaginase.[2,25a]

The duration of therapy for limited disease (localized stage 1 and 2) has been investigated in recent clinical trials. These patients have an excellent prognosis with a 9-week chemotherapy course. A small proportion of these low stage patients may benefit from additional months of maintenance therapy after achieving a complete remission.[15,21]

Large cell lymphoma. Treatment strategies for large cell lymphomas are less well defined, though most patients are cured.[25] Because this is a relatively newly defined type of NHL in the pediatric population, the best treatment has yet to be determined.[14] The Berlin-Frankfurt-Munster (BFM) trials have successfully treated large cell lymphoma with methotrexate, cytarabine, prednisone, cyclophosphamide, vincristine, doxorubicin, etoposide and ifosfamide.[24] It remains to be determined if the BFM treatment is too intensive and if less chemotherapy will result in the same good outcomes. Other studies have compared treatment with doxorubicin, prednisone, and vincristine (APO) with cyclophosphamide, vincristine, methotrexate, and prednisone (COMP) with essentially equal outcomes.[13,25]

All protocols for anaplastic large cell lymphomas include intrathecal prophylactic therapy with intrathecal methotrexate and cytarabine, combined with IV intermediate- or high-dose methotrexate and/or high-dose cytarabine.[25] The role for prophylactic radiation therapy has not been demonstrated.

RADIATION

As chemotherapy regimens have become more effective, the role of radiation therapy in treating non-Hodgkin's lymphoma has diminished significantly. Numerous studies throughout the pediatric

cooperative groups have demonstrated that chemotherapy alone is effective and that the addition of radiation therapy does not increase survival.[9,13,18,19,25] Children treated with chemotherapy and radiation have significantly more toxicities than those treated with chemotherapy alone.[12] Intrathecal chemotherapy alone has been shown to be efficacious for prophylaxis of CNS disease. These factors, in addition to the risk of secondary malignancies, have led investigators away from using radiation. However, radiation therapy in conjunction with chemotherapy is still under investigation for those situations, such as CNS disease at presentation, where additional data are needed to determine the optimal treatment.

There are situations in which emergency radiation therapy is necessary to treat a child with NHL. Radiation therapy may be necessary for superior vena cava syndrome, acute airway compromise, organ obstruction, or spinal cord compression.[9] It is sometimes used initially in conjunction with chemotherapy in patients who present with bulky disease to maximize the rate of response.[14] It is indicated in the treatment of patients who are not in complete remission after induction chemotherapy or for palliation of pain or mass effect. Radiation therapy is also used for consolidation to regions of local disease before or following hematopoietic stem cell transplant (HSCT) in patients with recurrent disease.[9]

SURGERY

Surgery is primarily used for diagnostic purposes. A laparotomy is indicated only for treatment of abdominal emergencies, such as intussusception, intestinal perforation, or serious gastrointestinal bleeding.[25]

HEMATOPOIETIC STEM CELL TRANSPLANT

Refractory or relapsed non-Hodgkin's lymphoma in children is an ominous situation that is associated with high mortality. High-dose chemotherapy followed by allogeneic or autologous HSCT for "rescue" from myelotoxicity has been employed. Patients with responsive relapse (disease that initially improves with therapy) have a much better prognosis than those with resistant relapse (disease that persists or progresses despite therapy).[11,14,23]

LYMPHOPROLIFERATIVE DISEASE

Lymphoproliferative lymphoma, also known as posttransplant lymphoproliferative disorder (PTLD), is a type of lymphoma that is associated with the immunosuppressive drugs used to prevent rejection of solid organs such as heart, kidney, and lung. This is a relatively new entity that is increasing in frequency with the increase in the number of solid organ transplants performed. Masses or enlarged nodes in these patients are often first treated with a reduction in immunosuppressive therapy. If this approach is unsuccessful, patients are given chemotherapy.[23,26] Whether this type of lymphoma will respond to therapy in the same way as other forms of NHL remains to be seen. The challenge for scientists and clinicians is to eradicate this disorder while maintaining the viability of the solid organ in the recipient.[23,26] Research in this area is in its infancy.

NURSING IMPLICATIONS

Close observation and frequent assessments are necessary because lymphomas in children generally grow rapidly. Children with mediastinal disease need to be observed for respiratory compromise such as cough, stridor, wheezing, or shortness of breath, which can lead to respiratory failure. Symptoms such as decreased breath sounds or complaints of chest pain may be indicative of a pleural effusion. Facial and/or neck swelling are signs of superior vena cava syndrome. Patients with head and neck primary sites often have nasal stuffiness or cervical adenopathy, which raise concern for tracheal deviations or obstruction.

A child with an abdominal mass will be at risk for intestinal obstruction or hydronephrosis. Complaints of pain with nausea and vomiting in the presence of a distended abdomen and/or decreased bowel sounds may require emergent surgical or radiation treatment.

Tumor lysis syndrome is a significant problem for children with non-Hodgkin's lymphoma, especially Burkitt's and T-cell lymphoblastic lymphoma. Some patients will present with this syndrome. Others are at risk for developing tumor lysis once treatment is initiated. Tumor lysis can cause severe metabolic derangements and renal failure.[9] Close observation of intake and output and results of serum chemistry studies are required. Intravenous hydration with alkalinization and the use of allopurinol is the standard of care.[29] Chapter 13 details treatment of this oncologic emergency.

Nurses play a significant role in educating the patient and the family about the disease, treatment, and side effects of therapy. Preparing the patient for procedures (lumbar punctures, bone marrow aspirates, and/or biopsies, etc.), teaching management of the logistics surrounding chemotherapy and its side effects, and arranging follow-up radiologic evaluations and laboratory studies all are important nursing responsibilities.

Last, but certainly not least, the nurse provides emotional support and guidance for both the patient and family. Parents need help to understand their child's illness and guidance to help their children cope. This assistance extends to the classmates of the child and the child's siblings as requested by the family.

FUTURE DIRECTIONS

Research into new approaches to diagnosis and therapy are under way. Better identification of prognostic and genetic factors is a major focus of investigation. Studies are being undertaken using more aggressive therapy, with the addition of growth factors to limit adverse effects, for children with poor prognostic factors. Agents such as pentostatin (an inhibitor of adenosine deaminase that is concentrated in lymphoid tissue) and Rituximab (a monoclonal antibody directed against the CD20 antigen found on B lymphocytes) have shown some efficacy in refractory or relapsed disease[7,30] and offer hope for more specific targeted therapies.

REFERENCES

1. Anderson, J. R., Jenkin, R. D. T., Wilson, J. F., et al. (1993). Long-term follow-up of patients treated with COMP or LSA$_2$L$_2$ therapy for childhood non-Hodgkin's lymphoma: A report of CCG-551 from the Children's Cancer Group. *Journal of Clinical Oncology, 11*, 1024-1032.
2. Asselin, B., Shuster, J., Amylon, M., et al. (2001 abstract). Improved event-free survival (EFS) with high dose methotrexate (HDM) in T-cell lymphoblastic leukemia (T-ALL) and advanced stage lymphoblastic lymphoma: Results of Pediatric Oncology Group (POG) study #9404. ASCO Program/Proceedings 2001 abstracts, 20, 1464.
3. Bernard, A., Boumsell, L., Reinherz, E. L., et al. (1981). Cell surface characterization of malignant T-cells from lymphoblastic lymphoma using monoclonal antibodies. Evidence for phenotypic differences between malignant lymphoma. *Blood, 57,* 1105-1110.
4. Bowman, W. P., Shuster, J. J., Cook, B., et al. (1996). Improved survival for children with B-cell acute lymphoblastic leukemia and stage IV non-cleaved cell lymphoma. A Pediatric Oncology Group study. *Journal of Clinical Oncology, 14,* 1252-1261.
5. Brugieres, L., Deley, M. C., Pacquement, H., et al. (1998). CD30$^+$ anaplastic large-cell lymphoma in children: An analysis of 82 patients enrolled in two consecutive studies of the French Society of Pediatric Oncology. *Blood, 92,* 3591-3598.
6. Diller, L., & Li, F. P. (1998). Epidemiology of cancer in childhood. In D. G. Nathan & S. H. Orkin (Eds.), *Nathan and Oski's hematology of infancy and childhood* (pp. 1071-1091). Philadelphia: W. B. Saunders.
7. Drapkin, R. (2000). Pentostatin and rituximab in the treatment of patients with B-cell malignancies. *Oncology, 14*(s-2), 25-29.
8. Gurney, J. G., Severson, R. K., Davis, S., et al. (1995). Incidence of cancer in children in the United States. *Cancer, 75,* 2186-2195.

9. Halperin, E. C., Constine, L. S., Tarbell, N. J., et al. (Eds.) (1999). Non-Hodgkin's lymphoma. In *Pediatric radiation oncology* (3rd ed., pp. 233-244). Philadelphia: Lippincott Williams & Wilkins.

10. Hutchison, R., Murphy, S., Fairclough, D., et al. (1989). Diffuse small non-cleaved cell lymphoma in children, Burkitt's versus non-Burkitt's types. *Cancer, 64,* 23-34.

11. Johnston, L. J., & Horning, S. J. (1999). Autologous hematopoietic cell transplantation in non-Hodgkin's lymphoma. *Hematology Oncology Clinics of North America, 13,* 889-1018.

12. Kurtzberg, J., & Graham, M. (1991). Non-Hodgkin's lymphoma, biological classification and implication for therapy. *Pediatric Clinics of North America, 38,* 443-456.

13. Lanzkowsky, P. (Ed.) (1995). Non-Hodgkin's lymphoma. In *Manual of pediatric hematology and oncology* (2nd ed., pp. 375-396). New York: Churchill-Livingstone.

14. Link, M. P., & Donaldson, S. S. (1998). The lymphomas and lymphadenopathy. In D. G. Nathan & S. H. Orkin (Eds.), *Nathan and Oski's hematology of infancy and childhood* (pp. 1323-1358). Philadelphia: W. B. Saunders.

15. Link, M. P., Shuster, J. J., Donaldson, S. S., et al. (1997). Treatment of children and young adults with early-stage non-Hodgkin's lymphoma. *The New England Journal of Medicine, 337,* 1259-1266.

16. Magrath, I. T. (1987). Malignant non-Hodgkin's lymphoma in children. *Hematology Oncology Clinics of North America, 1,* 577-602.

17. Magrath, I. T. (1990). Small non-cleaved cell lymphoma. In I. T. Magrath (Ed.), *The non-Hodgkin's lymphomas* (pp. 256-278). London: Edward Arnold.

18. Magrath, I. (1997). Limiting therapy for childhood non-Hodgkin's lymphoma. *The New England Journal of Medicine, 337,* 1304-1306.

19. Miller, R. W., Young, J. L., & Novakovic, B. (1994). Childhood cancer. *Cancer, 75,* 395-405.

20. Murphy, S. B. (1994). Pediatric lymphomas: Recent advances and commentary on Ki-1-positive anaplastic large cell lymphomas of childhood. *Annals of Oncology, 5*(s-1), 31-33.

21. Murphy, S. B. (1999). Modern trends in non-Hodgkin's lymphoma. *Journal of Pediatric Hematology Oncology, 21,* 87-88.

22. Murphy, S. B. (2000). Non-Hodgkin's lymphoma and Hodgkin's disease. In C. Herzog & C. Pratt (Eds.), *Therapy of cancer in children* (pp. 11-13). Houston, TX: University of Texas M. D. Anderson Cancer Center.

23. Praghakaran, K., Wise, B., Chen, S., et al., (1991). Rational management of post-transplant lymphoproliferative disorder in pediatric recipients. *Journal of Pediatric Surgery, 34,* 112-115.

24. Reiter, A., Schrappe, M., Tiemann, M., et al. (1994). Successful treatment strategy for Ki-1 anaplastic large cell lymphoma of childhood: A prospective analysis of 62 patients enrolled in 3 consecutive BFM group studies. *Journal of Clinical Oncology, 12,* 899-908.

25. Shad, A., & Magrath, I. (1997). Malignant non-Hodgkin's lymphomas in children. In P. A. Pizzo, & D. G. Poplack (Eds.), *Principles and practice of pediatric oncology* (3rd ed., pp. 545-587). Philadelphia: Lippincott-Raven.

25a. Shad, A., & Magrath, I. (1997). Non-Hodgkin's lymphoma. In M. P. Link (Ed.), *Pediatric Clinics of North America, 44,* 863-890.

26. Sheil, A. G., Disney, A. P., Mathew, T. H., et al. (1997). Lymphoma incidence, cyclosporine and the evolution and major impact of malignancy following organ transplantation. *Transplantation Proceedings, 29,* 825-827.

27. Smith, S. D., Rubin, C. M., Horvath, A., et al. (1990). Non-Hodgkin's lymphoma in children. *Seminars in Oncology, 17,* 113-119.

28. Sullivan, M. P., Brecher, M., Ramirez, I., et al. (1991). High-dose cyclophosphamide, high-dose methotrexate with coordinated intrathecal therapy for advanced non-lymphoblastic lymphoma of children: Results of a POG study. *American Journal of Pediatric Hematology Oncology, 9,* 288-295.

29. Van Syckle, K. (1998). Non-Hodgkin's lymphoma. In M. J. Hockenberry-Eaton (Ed.), *Essentials of pediatric oncology nursing: A core curriculum* (pp. 20-23). Glenview, IL: Association of Pediatric Oncology Nurses.

30. Verstovsek, S., Cabanillas, F., Dang, N. H., et al. (2000). CD26 in T-cell lymphomas: A potential clinical role? *Oncology, 14*(s-2), 17-23.

31. Wollner, N., Burchenal, J. H., Liebermann, P. H., et al. (1976). Non-Hodgkin's lymphoma in children: A comparative study of two modalities of therapy. *Cancer, 37,* 123-134.

24

Neuroblastoma

Gaye Dadd

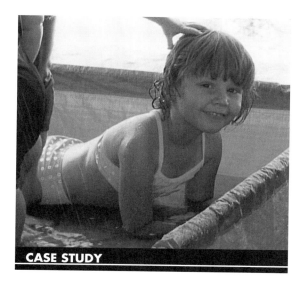

CASE STUDY

This hypothetical case illustrates a common disease course for a child diagnosed with high risk neuroblastoma. The child in the picture is Katie, who has recently relapsed after treatment for stage 4 neuroblastoma.

Brett, a 5½-year-old boy, presented in March 1996 with a 6-week history of anorexia, intermittent abdominal pain, lethargy, and weight loss. A mass was felt in the left upper abdomen, and a node was felt in the left supraclavicular region. A computerized tomography (CT) scan confirmed a large calcified mass in the position of the left adrenal gland. A bone scan showed a metastatic lesion in the thoracic spine at T7. Levels of urinary catecholamines, homovanillic acid (HVA), and vanillylmandelic acid (VMA) were elevated. A biopsy of the left neck lymph node proved to be metastatic neuroblastoma of unfavorable histologic classification. There was no evidence of disease in the bone marrow. Levels of serum ferritin (11,500 ng/l), lactate dehydrogenase (LDH) (1,688 units/l), and neuron-specific enolase (NSE) (28,000 mg/l) were all elevated. The proto-oncogene *MYCN* was not amplified. A diag-

nosis of high-risk neuroblastoma was made on all these factors.

Brett was treated on a Children's Cancer Group (CCG) high-risk neuroblastoma protocol. Chemotherapy agents were etoposide, cisplatin, doxorubicin, cyclophosphamide, and ifosfamide. Because Brett had already had 5% weight loss, a dietary consult was obtained, and a decision was made to insert a nasogastric tube and commence an overnight feeding regimen to maintain nutritional status.

Before the fifth cycle of chemotherapy second-look surgery was planned. A left nephrectomy was performed. Radiotherapy was then given to the left renal bed and to T7 spine.

Brett completed his intensive therapy in December 1996. Assessment of disease status was performed, which was negative. One month after completing chemotherapy, a 6-month course of retinoic acid was begun twice a day for 14 days, every 28 days for a total of six courses. Brett developed a dry face and lips and mild angular cheilosis after the first 14 days but had no further side effects on later cycles.

Brett returned to school and was an active, healthy 7-year-old boy until May 1998, when three nodes in the postcervical chain were noted, and he began complaining of right hip pain. A full disease evaluation was performed, revealing a mass in the para-aortic vertebral column and a metastatic lesion in the right femur. He was treated on a phase II trial using topotecan and cyclophosphamide. Within 1 week of starting treatment his pain had resolved, and he returned to school. Brett completed treatment in May 1999. In June 1999 his evaluation showed a thoracic mass. He had begun to complain of generalized pain and was lethargic. His levels of serum markers and urinary catecholamines were elevated. Bone marrow aspirates were now positive for neuroblastoma.

Brett was given palliative care in his own home, where he died quietly in the care of his parents in August 1999. The parents have had three postbereavement counseling sessions.

Neuroblastomas are the most common extracranial tumors of childhood. They are derived from primordial neural crest cells that develop into the sympathetic nervous system.[3,9,10,31,36] The neuroblastic tumors include neuroblastoma, ganglioneuroblastoma, and ganglioneuroma. These tumors demonstrate diverse biologic and clinical behavior, ranging from relatively benign tumors in infants to very aggressive, malignant tumors in older children.

Risk groups are established in part by histopathologic pattern, biologic features, and patient age.[7,21] Treatment is tailored to the risk for relapse as defined by risk-group assignment. The majority of children diagnosed with neuroblastoma have excellent survival rates with one significant exception. The majority of children with high-risk disease have poor survival rates that have proved challenging to improve.[3]

EPIDEMIOLOGY

Neuroblastomas arise from any area of the sympathetic chain including the adrenal medulla and sympathetic ganglia.[3,10,31,33] The most common site is the abdomen, specifically the adrenal gland.[10] Approximately 30% originate in the cervical, thoracic, and pelvic chains. Tumors originating in the bladder, sciatic nerve, and tissues adjacent to the testis have been reported, and there may be multiple primary sites. Approximately two thirds of children will present with metastatic disease to the bone marrow, bone, liver, and lymph nodes.[3,7,10,22]

Neuroblastoma is the most common tumor in infants less than 1 year and the second most common solid tumor in childhood, accounting for 8% to 10% of all childhood cancers.[3,10,33] The incidence is 8.7 per million per year before the age of 15 years, which is approximately 550 new cases per year in the United States.[3,10,21,33] The ratio of males to females is 1.2:1. Children often develop neuroblastoma at young ages, with 60% of cases presenting before the age of 2 years and 97% of cases presenting before the age of 10 years.[3,7,10,16,21]

In Japan, where nationwide screening of infants has been in place for over 20 years, the prevalence has doubled primarily with tumors of favorable features. Because the prevalence of tumors in children older than 1 year has not increased, researchers theorize that infant screening may detect neuroblastomas that would spontaneously regress. These findings lead to a debate whether population-based screening in infancy results in overdiagnosis and/or overtreatment.[1,7]

Neuroblastoma is rarely seen in adults and children older than 10 years. The disease in this group of patients appears to have different biologic features with an indolent course. The outcome is ultimately poor.[15]

There is no known cause for neuroblastoma. Because most patients are very young at diagnosis it is possible that causative effects may occur prenatally or very early in life.[7,10] A number of single studies have suggested that there may be a possible increased risk from maternal exposure to alcohol, neurally active drugs, diuretics, and hair coloring and paternal exposure to electromagnetic fields. These studies have not been confirmed.[3,10,21] Other studies have suggested a common genetic origin, possibly a recessive gene.[10] There is a subset of patients who appear to have a predisposition to develop neuroblastoma following an autosomal dominant pattern.[3]

The tumor cells of neuroblastoma show a number of genetic abnormalities that are unique to the disease and have prognostic significance. The pathogenesis of neuroblastoma may be caused in part by suboptimal response to the signals that regulate differentiation.[7] Chromosomal abnormalities, proto-oncogene amplification, alterations in DNA content of the tumor, and cellular markers of differentiation are genetic changes identified with neuroblastoma.[3,7,21]

The first genetic mutation identified in neuroblastoma was deletion of the short arm of chromosome 1 (1p del); 70% of neuroblastomas have this abnormality. It is associated with advanced disease and a poor prognosis.[3,21] Karyotyping of the neuroblastoma tumor cell that shows this deletion may represent a deletion of a tumor suppressor gene. Karyotyping also shows double minute chromatin bodies and homogeneously staining regions that may indicate amplification of *MYCN*, a proto-oncogene.[7] If constitutional DNA is compared to tumor DNA, loss of heterozygosity at one or more loci of chromosome 1 may be identified, which correlates with advanced poor prognosis disease.[21]

MYCN (or *n-MYC*) is a proto-oncogene found on the distal arm of chromosome 2.[3,7,21] Gene amplification (having multiple copies of the gene) of the *MYCN* is found in 30% of neuroblastomas. *MYCN* amplification is highly predictive of outcome and is strongly associated with advanced disease and poor prognosis.[7,19,21,25,38]

Tumor cells often display abnormal DNA content or chromosomal ploidy. The normal DNA index or content (DI) is diploid, equal to 1, an index often seen in advanced stage disease. Tumors that are hyperdiploid or near triploid have a DI greater than 1 and are more likely to be a low stage. This has prognostic value. Tumors that are near diploid or pseudodiploid have near normal DNA but have structural chromosome aberrations including *MYCN* amplification. Hyperdiploid or near triploid tumors are more common in infants that lack 1p del or *MYCN* amplification.[3,21]

There are three histopathologic patterns of neuroblastic tumors, with varying degrees of differentiation and maturation. Ganglioneuroma is at the benign end of the spectrum and is fully differentiated. Ganglioneuroblastoma consists of both primitive undifferentiated neuroblastoma and differentiated ganglioneuroma. Neuroblastoma is the malignant, primitive undifferentiated tumor.[3]

Neuronal differentiation is regulated by several cellular receptors known as neurotrophins. Three neurotrophins and their associated tyrosine kinase receptor genes (TRKs), which encode the primary receptors for the neurotrophins, have been studied in relation to neuroblastoma. The neuroblastoma cell's malignant transformation may be due to inadequate response to inducers of neuronal differentiation.[21] TRKs encode primary receptors for nerve growth factor (NGF), *TRK-A;* brain-derived nerve growth factor (BDNF), *TRK-B;* and neurotrophin-3 (NT-3), *TRK-C;* all of which have prognostic significance. The proto-oncogene TrkA is expressed in infants less than 1 year of age with early stage neuroblastoma but is strongly down regulated with *MYCN* amplification in advanced stage disease.[7,26]

CLINICAL PRESENTATION

Neuroblastoma can arise anywhere along the sympathetic nerve pathway. Signs and symptoms at presentation vary, depending on disease site and metastatic spread. Primary location and patterns of metastases are associated with age. Seventy percent of primary tumors arise within the abdomen. The incidence of adrenal masses is higher in children older than 1 year of age (40%) when compared with children less than 1 year of age (25%).[3,7]

Thoracic tumors are often detected incidentally through imaging of the chest for suspected infection or trauma.[7,10] Dyspnea and spinal cord compression can occur because of intraspinal extension of a primary tumor in the paraspinal area.[3,7,10]

Children with cervical tumors can present with a palpable mass, Horner's syndrome (unilateral ptosis, myosis, and anhidrosis), heterochromia of the iris (a range of colors), and occasionally superior vena cava syndrome.[3,7,10,21] Infants less than 1 year of age have a higher incidence of thoracic and cervical tumors.[3,7,10]

Primary abdominal and pelvic tumors are associated with complaints of fullness, discomfort, and pain. A hard, fixed mass can be palpated, and spinal cord compression may be evident. Bladder and bowel symptoms due to compression may occur when the primary tumor arises from the organ of Zuckerkandl (para-aortic bodies). Compression of the venous and lymphatic drainage systems can lead to scrotal and lower extremity edema.[3,7]

Metastatic dissemination occurs through lymphatic and hematogenous spread. Hematogenous spread results in bone, bone marrow, liver, and skin infiltration with related signs and symptoms. Involvement of regional lymph nodes may be noted with seemingly localized tumors. Patients with disseminated disease have tumor spreading to lymph nodes outside the cavity of origin.[3] Metastases to the brain and lung are rare (<5%) and are usually seen at relapse or at end-stage disease.[7,11] Metastatic disease can cause systemic symptoms such as low-grade fever, weight loss, fatigue, Hutchison syndrome (limping and irritability), pallor, and pain related to bone and bone marrow infiltration. Orbital metastatic disease produces proptosis and the characteristic periorbital ecchymosis of the upper eyelids (raccoon eyes) (Figure 24-1). Lymphadenopathy with palpable cervical nodes and hepatomegaly can cause respiratory distress and subsequent symptoms of obstruction.[7,10] Infants less than 1 year of age with stage 4S disease may have skin involvement seen as nontender, bluish subcutaneous nodules (blueberry muffin appearance). These nodules are seen exclusively in this age and group. Table 24-1 summarizes the signs and symptoms of neuroblastoma, and Table 24-2 presents the syndromes seen in neuroblastoma.

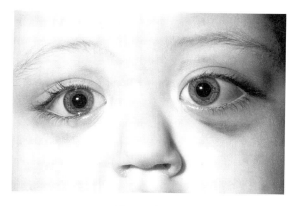

Figure 24-1

Ecchymosis (raccoon eyes) can be a presenting feature of stage 4 neuroblastoma.

TABLE 24-1	NEUROBLASTOMA SIGNS AND SYMPTOMS
Primary cervical tumor	Cervical mass
	Horner's syndrome
	Heterochromia of the iris
	Superior vena cava syndrome
Primary thoracic tumor	Dyspnea
	Spinal cord compression
Primary abdominal tumor	Abdominal mass
	Spinal cord compression
	Abdominal pain
Primary pelvic tumor	Pelvic mass
	Spinal cord compression
	Hip and/or leg pain
Metastatic tumor	Lymphadenopathy
	Hepatomegaly
	Pallor
	Exophthalmos
	Eyelid ecchymosis
	Skull mass
	Bone pain
	Skin nodules
	Purpura
Systemic symptoms	Fever
	Weight loss
	Fatigue
	Hypertension
	Intractable diarrhea
	Opsoclonus/myoclonus

From Cohn, S., Meitar, D., & Kletzel, M. (1997). Neuroblastoma: Solving a biological puzzle. *Cancer Treatment and Research, 92,* 125-162.

DIAGNOSTIC EVALUATION

A diagnosis of neuroblastoma requires an initial thorough history and physical examination. Measurement of neuroblastoma tumor markers such as urine catecholamine metabolites (VMA, HVA, and dopamine), ferritin (>142 ng/ml), NSE (>100 mg/ml), LDH ($>1,500$ units/l), and the ganglioside GD2 are useful in both making a diagnosis and monitoring the disease.

Urinary catecholamines are excessively produced in 90% of neuroblastomas. A level greater than 3.0 standard deviations above the mean creatinine level for the age is considered elevated.[10,14,21] Levels of serum ferritin (a major iron-binding protein in blood and tissue), NSE (an enzyme produced by neuronal tissue), and LDH are often elevated in patients with neuroblastoma and aid in diagnosis and follow-up of treatment, though they lack sensitivity and specificity.[10,21] Gangliosides are sugar-containing lipid molecules present on the surface of tumor cells. The ganglioside GD2 is present in large quantities on the surface of human neuroblastoma cells. It is shed by tumor cells; therefore detection of GD2 on the tumor cell surface or in the circulating blood can be a useful diagnostic tool. GD2 is also a target for novel treatments.

Neuroblastoma is part of the group of "small, round blue cell" tumors, which includes Ewing's sarcoma, non-Hodgkin's lymphoma, primitive neuroectodermal tumors (PNET), and undifferentiated soft tissue sarcomas. Initially surgical staging is recommended to obtain a tissue sample and/or to remove the bulk of the primary tumor if this can be

TABLE 24-2	PRESENTING SYNDROMES ASSOCIATED WITH NEUROBLASTOMA
Eponym	**Syndrome Features**
Pepper syndrome	Massive involvement of the liver with metastatic disease with or without respiratory distress.
Horner's syndrome	Unilateral ptosis, myosis, and anhidrosis associated with a thoracic primary tumor. Symptoms do not recover with tumor removal.
Hutchison syndrome	Limping and irritability in the young child associated with bone and bone marrow metastases.
Opsomyoclonus	Myoclonic jerking and random eye movement, with or without cerebellar ataxia. May be associated with a differentiated, favorable outlook tumor, but symptoms may or may not resolve after tumor removal.
Kerner-Morrison syndrome	Intractable secretory diarrhea associated with a biologically favorable tumor that secretes vasointestinal peptides. Symptoms always resolve with tumor removal.
"Raccoon eyes"	Noted when there is periorbital hemorrhage secondary to metastatic tumor.

From Castleberry, R. P. (1997). Biology and treatment of neuroblastoma. *Pediatric Clinics of North America, 44*(4), 919-937.

accomplished without threatening patient safety or vital organs. Surgical staging is also used to assess lymph node involvement.[3,6,7]

Immunohistochemical, cytogenetic (1p del), and molecular analysis *(MYCN)* are required to differentiate neuroblastoma from other small round cell tumors. Diagnosis is made by examination of the biopsy specimen of the tumor or by examination of the bone marrow. Histologic grading and molecular genetic studies are essential for diagnosis and treatment.[3,7,10,21] Conventional histology staining is not difficult, especially if features are suggestive of neuronal differentiation, such as the presence of neurofilaments.[3,11,21] However, neuroblasts may exhibit few features of differentiation, and electron microscopy is required to confirm the diagnosis along with the genetic features already mentioned.[14] Pathologic analysis combined with elevated levels of urine catecholamines confirms the diagnosis of neuroblastoma.

In 1994 the International Neuroblastoma Pathology Committee proposed a classification system for neuroblastoma based on the Shimada classification system.[31,32] This has been incorporated into the International Neuroblastoma Staging System (INSS). INSS criteria for diagnostic confirmation of neuroblastoma is either (1) an unequivocal pathologic diagnosis made from tumor tissue by light microscopy with or without immunohistologic analysis, electron microscopy, or increased level of urinary catecholamines or (2) a bone marrow aspirate or biopsy that contains unequivocal tumor cells and increased level of urinary catecholamines.[3,4,7]

The INSS recommends diagnostic imaging studies to evaluate the extent of primary and metastatic disease (Table 24-3), which include plain film, CT, magnetic resonance imaging, bone scintigram, and an iodine-131-metaiodobenzylguanidine (MIBG) scan (Figure 24-2).[3,7,21,31] MIBG is a guanethidine analog, which is selectively taken up by adrenergic tissue. This tissue specificity allows a diagnosis of neuroblastoma to be made and an assessment of both soft tissue and bone involvement. Because of the radioactive iodine, the thyroid cells must be protected against radiation damage. The patient must take Lugol's solution (saturated solution of potassium iodide [SSKI]) 24 to 48 hours before and 3 days after the injection of MIBG.[30]

The INSS, ratified in 1987, standardizes the definitions of diagnosis and staging and guides therapeutic management (see Table 24-3). This international staging system now establishes a stable clinical background to refine biologically based risk groups through multivariate analysis.[4,7]

TREATMENT

Treatment is based in part on the stage identified by the INSS Staging System. Because of the biologic and age-related differences in prognosis, recent trials have developed risk groups to guide therapy. Neuroblastoma is now divided into three risk categories: low, intermediate, and high (Table 24-4). Multimodal therapy includes surgery, chemotherapy, radiotherapy, peripheral blood stem cell transplant (PBSCT), and immune modulators.

Surgery plays an important role in diagnosis and local control of neuroblastoma. With the initial pro-

TABLE 24-3	INTERNATIONAL NEUROBLASTOMA STAGING SYSTEM
Stage 1	Localized tumor confined to the area of origin; complete gross excision, with or without microscopic residual disease; identifiable ipsilateral and contralateral lymph nodes negative microscopically.
Stage 2A	Unilateral tumor with incomplete gross excision; identifiable ipsilateral and contralateral lymph nodes negative microscopically.
Stage 2B	Unilateral tumor with complete or incomplete gross excision; with positive ipsilateral regional lymph nodes; identifiable contralateral lymph nodes negative microscopically.
Stage 3	Tumor infiltrating across the midline with or without regional lymph node involvement; or, unilateral tumor with contralateral regional lymph node involvement; or, midline tumor with bilateral regional lymph node involvement.
Stage 4	Dissemination of tumor to distant lymph nodes, bone, bone marrow, liver, and/or other organs (except as defined in stage 4S).
Stage 4S	Localized primary tumor as defined for stage 1 or 2 with dissemination limited to liver, skin, and/or bone marrow.

From Brodeur, G. M., Seeger, R. C., Barrett, A., et al. (1988). International criteria for diagnosis, staging, and response to treatment in patients with neuroblastoma. *Journal of Clinical Oncology, 6,* 1874-1881.

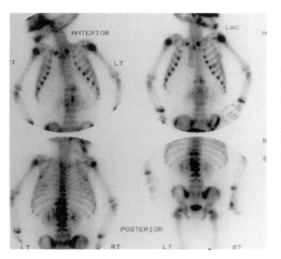
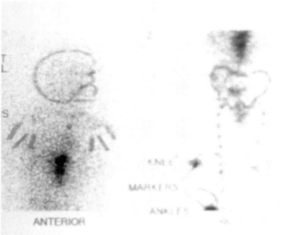

Figure 24-2

Bone scintigram and MIBG scan of stage 4 neuroblastoma.

TABLE 24-4	RISK-BASED TREATMENT FOR NEUROBLASTOMA
Risk Group	**Treatment**
LOW	
INSS stage 1, 2, 4S unless unfavorable biologic features Single copy *MYCN* Favorable Shimada DNA index >1	Stage 4S: Supportive care only; infants especially <6 wk old with either respiratory or liver complications may need cytotoxic therapy. Stages 1 and 2: surgery only.
INTERMEDIATE	
Stage 3 Stage 2, age >1 yr Favorable Shimada Single copy *MYCN* Infants, stage 4, *MYCN* nonamplified	Current therapies use the following cytotoxic agents: carboplatin, etoposide, cyclophosphamide, doxorubicin; four cycles for favorable biology and eight cycles for unfavorable biology. Surgery is used to establish a diagnosis, provide tissue for prognostic markers, stage the disease, and resect the primary tumor if feasible. Radiotherapy is used only when there is clinical deterioration.
HIGH	
Stage 4, age >1 Stage 3, age >1, *MYCN* amplified Unfavorable Shimada Stage 2, age >1, *MYCN* amplified	Surgery, radiotherapy, and chemotherapy are used. Dose intensification of cytotoxic agents such as cisplatin, carboplatin, etoposide, doxorubicin, cyclophosphamide, and ifosfamide with peripheral stem cell transplant followed by biologic modifiers such as *cis*-retinoic acid.

Data from Katzenstein, H. M., & Cohn, S. L. (1998). Advances in diagnosis and treatment of neuroblastoma. *Current Opinion in Oncology, 10,* 43-51.

cedure the surgeon typically establishes the diagnosis, gains material for biologic studies, stages the tumor, and resects the primary tumor if there is no risk to vital organs.[3,6,7,28] INSS low-risk patients with localized tumor may be successfully treated with complete resection of the primary tumor alone combined with careful follow-up and further treatment if the disease recurs. Aggressive surgery in advanced-stage disease is no longer recommended. Tumor rupture, inferior vena cava injury, and emergency nephrectomy were complications of surgery seen in 5% to 25% of patients with advanced disease. Such complications delay chemotherapy. Second-look surgery after several courses of chemotherapy removes residual disease and allows assessment of response to therapy without compromising patient safety.[3,6,7,28] In infants with INSS stage 4S, resection of tumor at diagnosis does not improve outcome compared with no surgery, probably due to the multifocal nature of the disease.[17,22]

Chemotherapy regimens use drug combinations that take advantage of synergism to prevent resistance. Drug combinations of agents that are not cell cycle specific (e.g., cyclophosphamide, ifosfamide, and platinum-based agents) are combined with cell cycle–specific agents (e.g., doxorubicin and the epipodophyllotoxins).[37] Myeloablative chemotherapy with peripheral blood stem cell rescue is used in high-risk patients.

Radiotherapy was historically used in the multimodal management of residual disease, bulky unresectable tumors, and disseminated disease.[3] With dose-intensive chemotherapy regimens radiotherapy is now indicated only for residual disease after second-look surgery or hematopoietic stem cell transplant and in stage 4S patients who have respiratory distress secondary to hepatomegaly.[3,7] Total body irradiation (TBI) was used in conditioning regimens for autologus hematopoietic stem cell transplants for stage 4 disease in the mid-1990s. This has not shown any improvement in survival; therefore the next generation of treatments will not include TBI.*

Low-risk disease (see Table 25-4) requires surgery alone, even if some tumor remains after surgery. The survival rate for this group of patients is greater than 90%.[3,19,21] Patients can be salvaged with chemotherapy in the event of tumor recurrence. Infants with stage 4S disease may show spontaneous regression. Extensive liver metastases in infants with stage 4S disease may cause massive abdominal distention with compression of the lungs leading to respiratory failure.

These patients may require intervention with chemotherapy.[3,7,19,21,36]

Intermediate-risk therapy currently consists of a 9-month course of chemotherapy, surgery, and local radiotherapy to residual disease and has a 3-year event-free survival (EFS) of 96%.[6,21-23] The future treatment plans for this group of patients with favorable biology is a shortened course of chemotherapy over 12 weeks. Those with unfavorable biology will have a longer course of therapy (24 weeks).[3,21-23] Complete biologic information must be obtained about the tumor to safely administer less intensive therapy and achieve cure. The ability to reduce therapy in this group of patients will reduce costs, improve quality of life, and reduce late effects.

Infants with INSS stage 3 disease, stage 4S, and stage 4 neuroblastoma with amplified *MYCN* (high-risk disease) require aggressive therapy to induce remission as do all children more than 1 year of age with stage 4 disease. Current therapy uses dose intensification with myeloablative therapy and peripheral blood stem cell (PBSC) support. PBSCs have recently replaced bone marrow as a source of hematopoetic stem cells because engraftment is more rapid and there is the theoretical possibility that PBSCs contains fewer cancer cells than bone marrow.[12,13,21,35] The Children's Oncology Group (C.O.G.) is currently undertaking a randomized clinical trial comparing purged and unpurged PBSCs with tandem hematopoietic stem cell transplants in this high-risk group.

The high-risk group uses an additional biologic modifier, 13-*cis*-retinoic acid, at the end of treatment for minimal residual disease, which decreases proliferation and induces differentiation in neuroblastoma cell lines and has been shown to improve EFS after autologous bone marrow transplant.[24] Despite improved remission rates and prolonged time to recurrence, the prognosis for this group of patients remains poor, with approximately 30% survival.[3,24] With the introduction of these novel therapies and longer remission duration, other complications may need to be evaluated.[27]

With the current treatment modalities for high-risk neuroblastoma, patients are gaining longer remission times, which creates opportunities for novel therapies targeted to minimal residual disease. With a recurrence rate of 50% in these patients, newer therapies need to be explored to improve the overall survival. Differentiating agents such as *cis*-retinoic acid and fenretinide, which causes growth arrest and apoptosis, are currently being used in phase III and phase I trials, respectively.[10,12,22] Variable responses in phase I trials have been noted in treatments including (1) tar-

---

*References 7, 12, 13, 21, 27, 34.

TABLE 24-5	PROGNOSTIC FACTORS IN NEUROBLASTOMA	
Prognostic Factor	**Favorable**	**Unfavorable**
Clinical factors		
Stage	1,2A,2B,4S (INSS)	3,4 (INSS)
Age	≤12 months	>12 months
Tumor markers		
Ferritin	<142 ng/ml	>142 ng/ml
LDH	<1500 IU/l	>1500 IU/L
NSE	<100 ng/ml	>100 ng/ml
Biologic factors		
DNA Index	>1.0	1.0
MYCN	Normal	Amplified
Chromosome 1p	Normal	Deleted
TrkA	High levels of expression	Low levels of expression
MRP	Low levels of expression	High levels of expression
CD44	High levels of expression	Low levels of expression
Vascularity	Low vascularity	High vascularity
Pathology		
Shimada classification	Favorable	Unfavorable
Joshi classification	Low-risk	High-risk

From Cohn, S., Meitar, D., Kletzel, M. (1997). Neuroblastoma: Solving a biological puzzle. *Cancer Treatment and Research, 92,* 125-162.

geted therapy and immunologic modulators using monoclonal antibodies to the GD2 ganglioside with or without cytokines (i.e., granulocyte macrophage colony stimulating factor [GM-CSF] with interleukin-2 [IL-2]) and (2) radiolabeled iodine-131-MIBG.[7,8,10,21,22]

Neuroblastoma cells are resistant to T lymphocytes but sensitive to natural killer (NK) cells. In vitro studies show that IL-2 and gamma interferon stimulate a broad range of immune cells, but initial clinical trials with IL-2 alone have not shown a high response rate in neuroblastoma.[9,20] Gene therapy that targets the up regulation of *TRK-A, TRK-C,* and the down regulation of *TRK-B* is in the early stages of study. In addition, gene therapy directed toward the *bcl-2* gene (a powerful protector of survival in neuronal cells) is aimed at inducing apoptosis and decreasing cell growth. Although these therapies are in their infancy, they have the ability to be more efficient and specific than current therapies.[9,15] Phase II studies using topoisomerase inhibitors such as topotecan are currently under way.[3]

PROGNOSIS

The two most important clinical risk factors for predicting outcome in neuroblastoma are age and stage of disease at diagnosis.* Age less than 1 year con-

fers the most favorable prognosis, and the pelvis and thorax are the most favorable sites.[21] Dramatic survival differences exist between low and high stages of the disease (98% survival for stages 1 and 2[29] and 22% for stage 4[30]). The importance of biologic factors such as *MYCN* is evident in the survival rates of infants—without amplification, 93%, and with amplification, 17%.[32]

The prognosis in neuroblastoma depends on the age at diagnosis and stage of disease, and there is marked survival differences between prognostic groups. Five-year survival is 88% to 90% in low-risk disease. Three-year event-free survival is 98% in the intermediate-risk group. Five-year survival in high-risk disease is only 22% to 30%.[21,31] Another predictor of poor outcome is highly expressed multidrug resistance (MDR) gene.[2] Biologic factors such as tumor histology, serum markers (ferritin, LDH, NSE), and genetic features (*MYCN* amplification, DNA index, 1p del) all contribute to prognostic grouping (Table 24-5).

NURSING IMPLICATIONS

Because of the diverse range of treatments for neuroblastoma, each child and family will require different nursing interventions. When stage 4S patients are treated with observation only, this evokes anxiety in families who will require education and emotional support to understand that having no treatment is appropriate. Education of all parents

*References 5, 7, 10, 18, 21, 36.

on side effects of treatment, home care, and long-term effects is paramount.

A family with a child with stage 4 disease needs support and counseling for the long-term outcome and the intensive treatment that is required to gain a remission in this aggressive disease. Nurses need to be cognizant of the side effects of chemotherapeutic agents and the nursing care required of an infant or child undergoing myeloablative therapy. This is similar to nursing a child receiving high-dose chemotherapy.[37] The predominant side effects are infection, bleeding, mucositis, and malnutrition. At relapse, psychosocial support mechanisms need to be in place.

With the introduction of new immune modulators and targeted gene therapy the nurse needs to understand the biology of the disease and the side effects of these new agents to administer them safely to the patient. In addition, nurses will need to develop novel educational strategies to educate the families in these innovative treatment options. The families need to understand the nature of phase I and phase II trials. Ultimately the agents being used in these trials may not actually change the final outcome of this aggressive stage of neuroblastoma.

FUTURE DIRECTIONS

Scientists are only beginning to understand the molecular pathogenesis of neuroblastoma, and future therapies will use targeted gene therapy, which may be more effective and less toxic than the current megatherapy used in front-line studies. Newer therapy strategies and further understanding of the disease may come with the identification of the suppressor genes on 1p, 14q, and/or other sites.[3]

High-risk neuroblastoma continues to challenge us to find treatments that will improve the outcome of this very poor prognosis group. The future will be in further defining biologic markers and discovering what influences proto-oncogenes and their receptors to be turned on or off. This will define the use of immune modulators to enable manipulation of the neuroblastoma cell either to mature or to die.

REFERENCES

1. Bessho, F. (1998). Colloquy on neuroblastoma mass screening: Is there a future for neuroblastoma screening? *Medical and Pediatric Oncology, 31,* 106-110.
2. Bordow, S. (1998). Prognostic significance of *mycn* oncogene expression in childhood neuroblastoma. *Journal of Clinical Oncology, 16,* 3286-3294.
3. Brodeur, G. M., & Castelberry, R. (1997). Neuroblastoma. In P. A. Pizzo & D. G. Poplack (Eds.), *Principles and practices of pediatric oncology* (3rd ed., pp. 761-797). Philadelphia: Lippincott-Raven.
4. Brodeur, G. M., Seeger, R. C., Barrett A., et al. (1988). International criteria for diagnosis, staging, and response to treatment in patients with neuroblastoma. *Journal of Clinical Oncology, 6,* 1874-1881.
5. Brodeur, G. M., Swada, T., Tsuchida, Y., et al. (Eds.). (2000). *Neuroblastoma.* New York: Elsevier.
6. Canete, A., Jovani, C., Lopez, A., et al. (1998). Surgical treatment for neuroblastoma: Complications during 15 years experience. *Journal of Pediatric Surgery, 33,* 1526-1530.
7. Castleberry, R. (1997). Biology and treatment of neuroblastoma. *Pediatric Clinics of North America, 44,* 919-937.
8. Cheung, N-K., Kushner, B., Cheung, Y., et al. (1998). Anti-GD2 antibody treatment of minimal residual stage 4 neuroblastoma diagnosed at more than 1 year of age. *Journal of Clinical Oncology, 16,* 3053-3060.
9. Cohen, P., & Thiele, C. (1997). The Matthay article reviewed. *Oncology, 11,* 1870-1872.
10. Cohen, S., Mietar, D., & Kletzel, M. (1997). Neuroblastoma: Solving a biological puzzle. *Cancer Treatment and Research, 92,* 125-162.
11. D'Angio, G., Sinniah, D., Meadows, A., et al. (Eds.). (1992). *Practical pediatric oncology.* London: Edward-Arnold.
12. Degar, B., Harrington, R., Rappeport, J., et al. (1998). 13-cis-retinoic acid induced eosinophilia following autologous bone marrow transplantation for neuroblastoma. *Medical and Pediatric Oncology, 31,* 113-115.
13. Eguchi, H., Takaue, Y., Kawano, Y., et al. (1998). Peripheral blood stem cell autografts for the treatment of children over 1 year old with stage IV neuroblastoma: A long term followup. *Bone Marrow Transplantation, 21,* 1011-1014.
14. Evans, A., Biedler, J., Brodeur, G., et al. (Eds.). (1994). *Progress in clinical and biological research: Vol 385. Advances in neuroblastoma research 4.* New York: Alan R. Liss.
15. Evans, A., D'Angio, G., Knudson, A., & Seeger, R. (Eds.). (1988). *Progress in clinical and biological research: Vol. 271. Advances in neuroblastoma research 2.* New York: Alan R. Liss.
16. Franks, L., Bollen, A., Seeger, R., et al. (1997). Neuroblastoma in adults and adolescents: An indolent course with poor survival. *Cancer, 79,* 2028-2035.
17. Guglielmi, M., DeBernardi, B., Rizzo, A., et al. (1996). Resection of primary tumor at diagnosis stage IV-S neuroblastoma: Does it affect the clinical course? *Journal of Clinical Oncology, 14,* 1537-1544.
18. Katzenstein, L., Bowman, L., Brodeur, G., et al. (1998). Prognostic significance of age, *MYCN* oncogene amplification, tumor cell ploidy and histology in 110 infants with stage D(S) neuroblastoma: The Pediatric Oncology Group experience—a Pediatric Oncology Group Study. *Journal of Clinical Oncology, 16,* 2007-2017.
19. Kushner, B., Cheung, N-K., LaQuaglia, M., et al. (1996). International staging system stage 1 neuroblastoma: A prospective study and literature review. *Journal of Clinical Oncology, 14,* 2174-2180.
20. Lode, H., Xian, R., Dreier, T., et al. (1998). Natural killer cell mediated eradication of neuroblastoma metastases to bone marrow by targeted interleukin-2 therapy. *Blood, 91,* 1706-1715.
21. Matthay, K. K. (1997). Neuroblastoma: Biology and therapy. *Oncology, 11,* 1857-1875.
22. Matthay, K. K. (1998). Stage 4S neuroblastoma: What makes it special? *Journal of Clinical Oncology, 16,* 2003-2006.

23. Matthay, K. K., Perez, C., Seeger, R., et al. (1998). Successful treatment of stage III neuroblastoma based on prospective biologic staging: A Children's Cancer Group study. *Journal of Clinical Oncology, 16,* 1256-1264.

24. Matthay, K. K., Villablanca, J., Seeger, R., et al. (1999). Treatment of high risk neuroblastoma with intensive chemotherapy, radiotherapy, autologous bone marrow transplantation and 13-cis-retinoic acid. *The New England Journal of Medicine, 341,* 1165-1173.

25. Meitar, D., Crawford, S., Rademaker, A., & Cohn, S. (1996). Tumor angiogenesis correlates with metastatic disease, N-*myc* amplification and poor outcome in human neuroblastoma. *Journal of Clinical Oncology, 14,* 405-414.

26. Nakagawara, A. (1998). The NGF story and neuroblastoma. *Medical and Pediatric Oncology, 31,* 113-115.

27. Neve, V., Foot, A., Michon, J., et al. (1999). Longitudinal clinical and functional pulmonary follow-up after megatherapy, fractionated total body irradiation and autologous bone marrow transplantation for metastatic neuroblastoma. *Medical and Pediatric Oncology, 14,* 405-414.

28. Nuchtern, J. G. (1997). The Matthay article reviewed. *Oncology, 11,* 1869-1870.

29. Perez, C., Matthay, K., Atkinson, J., et al. (2000). Biological variables in the outcome of stages I and II neuroblastoma treated with surgery as primary therapy: A Children's Cancer Group study. *Journal of Clinical Oncology, 18,* 18-26.

30. Perkins, A. C. (1995). *Nuclear medicine science and safety.* London: John Libbey.

31. Powell, J., Esteve, J., Mann, J., et al. (1997). Neuroblastoma in Europe: Differences in the pattern of disease in the U.K. *The Lancet, 3652,* 682-687.

32. Schmidt, M., Likens, J., Seeger, R., et al. (2000). Biologic factors determine prognosis in infants with stage IV neuroblastoma: A prospective Children's Cancer Group study. *Journal of Clinical Oncology, 18,* 1260-1268.

33. Shimada, H., Ambros, I., Dehner, L., et al. (1999). Terminology and morphologic criteria of neuroblastic tumors: Recommendations by the International Neuroblastoma Pathology Committee. *Cancer, 86,* 349-363.

34. Shimada, H., Ambros, I., Dehner, L., et al. (1999). The International Pathology Classification (the Shimada system). *Cancer, 86,* 364-372.

35. Shuster, J. J. (1996). The role of autologous bone marrow transplantation in advanced neuroblastoma. *Journal of Clinical Oncology, 14,* 2413-2414.

36. Van Noesel, M., Hahlen, K., Hakvoot-Cammel, F., et al. (1997). Neuroblastoma 4S: A heterogenous disease with variable risk factors and treatment strategies. *Cancer, 80,* 834-843.

37. Vaux, Z. (1996). Peripheral stem cell transplant in children. *Pediatric Nursing, 8,* 20-22.

38. Zalzen, Y., Taniguchi, S., & Suita, S. (1998). The role of cellular motility in the invasion of human neuroblastoma cells with or without N-myc amplification and expression. *Journal of Pediatric Surgery, 33,* 1765-1770.

25

Rhabdomyosarcoma

Carol Zinger Kotsubo

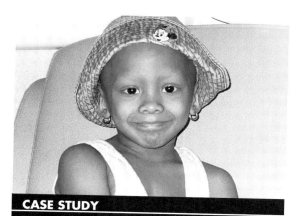

CASE STUDY

Kelsey is a 3-year-old part-Hawaiian girl who came to her pediatrician with some swelling over her left labial region. An ultrasound examination revealed a heterogenous mixed cystic solid mass. The mass was thought to be located at the posterior portion of the labium and to extend to the lower vagina. During her preoperative examination under anesthesia, the mass was measured as 3 × 7 × 8 cm. It appeared to be oblong and well circumscribed. The tumor could be felt up the entire length of the vagina and was fixed to the pubic ramus.

Although rare in this age-group, the surgeon determined that the mass was most likely an infected Bartholin cyst and a vaginal approach was used to remove it. The frozen section during the surgery revealed a malignancy, most likely a rhabdomyosarcoma. The tumor had to be removed piecemeal, and at the end of the procedure there was surgical spillage. The surgeon was convinced that he had removed the entire tumor. The pediatric oncologist was consulted during the surgical procedure, and a Hickman catheter was placed to facilitate venous access. A bone scan, bone marrow biopsy, and computed tomography (CT) scan of the chest done to rule out metastatic disease were negative. Pathologic findings revealed the tumor to be a poorly differentiated rhabdomyosarcoma, embryonal subtype. The tumor node metastasis (TNM) stage was III, based on the

site and the tumor size of greater than 5 cm. The Clinical Group was II. This was a localized tumor with gross total resection and microscopic residual. Kelsey was registered on POG 9602 (Intergroup Rhabdomyosarcoma Study [IRS] V) low risk rhabdomyosarcoma and assigned to subgroup B.

The treatment consisted of vincristine, actinomycin, and cyclophosphamide, and radiation therapy beginning at week 3. The total dose of radiation was 36 Gy. The initial chemotherapy was tolerated very well with only a 24-hour inpatient admission to guarantee hydration following the high dose cyclophosphamide. During the course of radiation therapy, Kelsey developed severe radiation burns to her perineum. The radiation therapy was delayed for 2 weeks and the dose of actinomycin at week 9 had to be omitted. The perineal area healed slowly but completely. Unfortunately this led to a period of chronic constipation caused by fear of pain on defecation. A bowel regimen consisting of generous daily doses of mineral oil and regular toileting was begun.

Weight loss also became a problem following the course of radiation therapy that was administered concomitantly with the chemotherapy. Initially a large child who weighed 25 kg at diagnosis, Kelsey lost weight until she weighed 18 kg at about week 12. A nutrition consult revealed that she was in the 95th percentile of weight for age even after the weight loss. Her mother was given instructions on increasing calories and protein. Kelsey's weight by the end of therapy had stabilized to about 20 kg, which is more appropriate for her size.

The soft tissue sarcomas constitute a heterogeneous group of malignant tumors with a common origin in primitive mesenchyme. Rhabdomyosarcoma is the most common soft tissue sarcoma in childhood.[21] Mesenchymal cells normally mature into skeletal muscle, smooth muscle, fat, fibrous tissue, bone, and cartilage. Rhabdomyosarcoma is thought to arise from immature mesenchymal cells that are committed to skeletal muscle lineage, but these tumors can arise in tissues where striated muscle is typically not found, such as in the urinary bladder. Undifferentiated sarcoma also arises from mesenchymal cells but is so primitive that it does not resemble any mature tissue type.[44]

EPIDEMIOLOGY

Approximately 250 new cases of rhabdomyosarcoma are diagnosed in the United States each year. The annual incidence of rhabdomyosarcoma is estimated as four to seven cases per million children under the age of 15 years. It is the fourth most common solid tumor in children. There are two age peaks for rhabdomyosarcoma. Sixty-five percent of the tumors occur in children under the age of 6 years. Most of the remaining cases occur in 10- to 18-year-olds. Age distribution varies significantly with site. Almost three fourths of genitourinary, bladder, and prostate primaries occur in children under the age of 5 years. Paratesticular and extremity primaries are more common in older adolescents. There is a slight male predominance with a male to female ratio of 1.5:1 in all rhabdomyosarcomas. The distribution of males and females varies by site with a high of 3.3:1 male to female ratio in genitourinary tumors. Orbital and extremity rhabdomyosarcomas are slightly more common in females, with a 0.79:1 and 0.88:1 male to female ratio, respectively.[37] In the United States, the incidence of rhabdomyosarcoma for black females was found to be only half that for white females, whereas the rate for males was similar in both groups. The incidence of rhabdomyosarcoma appears to be lower in Asian countries than in Western countries with primarily white populations.[44]

Sixty institutions in the United States, Canada, and Western Europe formed the first Intergroup Rhabdomyosarcoma Study Group (IRSG) in 1972. Since that time, four successive studies—IRS I (1972 to 1978), IRS II (1978 to 1984), IRS III (1984 to 1991), and IRS IV (1991 to 1997)—have generated data on approximately 3000 patients with rhabdomyosarcoma and undifferentiated sarcoma. Over 85% of children diagnosed with rhabdomyosarcoma in the United States are treated on IRSG protocols. The IRSG has conducted a multidisciplinary assault on rhabdomyosarcoma that has resulted in major advances in defining the biology, diagnosis, treatment, and survival of children and adolescents.

Like most childhood cancers, the primary cause of rhabdomyosarcoma is still unknown. It has been associated with familial syndromes such as neurofibromatosis and the Li-Fraumeni syndrome (LFS) or cancer family syndrome. LFS is associated with germ-line mutations in the tumor suppressor gene *p53*.[14,44] Relatives of a child with rhabdomyosarcoma may be diagnosed with breast cancer, brain tumors, osteosarcoma, or certain other cancers at a young age in this syndrome. Even though a mutant *p53* gene may not be demonstrated, the mother of a child with rhabdomyosarcoma should be alerted to her increased risk of breast cancer. This risk has been shown to be 3 to 13.5 times higher than that of control subjects.[37] At autopsy, 37 of 115 (32%) children with rhabdomyosarcoma had one or more congenital anomalies. The majority of these anomalies were minor, such as bilateral hydroceles or ovarian cysts. These data suggest that prenatal events may promote oncogenesis in the developing fetus. Epidemiologic studies of rhabdomyosarcoma have demonstrated an increased incidence of parental smoking and exposure to environmental chemicals and increased ingestion of animal organs in families with rhabdomyosarcoma.[44] Continued epidemiologic investigations are needed to clarify the importance of these findings and to identify other risk factors associated with the development of rhabdomyosarcoma and undifferentiated sarcoma.

CLINICAL PRESENTATION

Presenting symptoms vary according to the anatomic location of the primary tumor, metastases, and the age of the child (Table 25-1). Only 25% of children will have distant metastasis, and of these the majority are a single site.[44] Rhabdomyosarcoma and undifferentiated sarcoma metastasize by way of the blood and lymphatic systems. The primary site of metastasis is the lung, followed by bone marrow, bone, and adjoining lymph nodes. Rarely does rhabdomyosarcoma metastasize to the visceral organs at the time of diagnosis.

ORBIT

The most common site for rhabdomyosarcoma is the head and neck (35% to 40%). Of the head and neck tumors, 25% are located in the orbit of children less than 6 years of age. Tumors in the orbital region grow rapidly and are usually detected early because of the obvious physical changes they produce.[44] Parents may note a developing ptosis, with or without lid swelling. Exophthalmos, or proptosis, may also occur. Occasionally orbital cellulitis is present because of tissue necrosis.

OTHER HEAD AND NECK SITES

The parameningeal area is the most common other head and neck site. This includes sites adjacent to

TABLE 25-1   PRIMARY SITES OF RHABDOMYOSARCOMA AND UNDIFFERENTIATED SARCOMA

Primary Site	Relative Frequency (%)	Regional Spread and Distant Metastatic Sites
Head and Neck	40	
• Orbit	10	Nodes rarely involved; rare lung metastasis
• Parameningeal	20	Regional spread to bone, meninges, brain; lung and bone metastasis
• Other	10	Nodes rarely involved; lung metastasis
Genitourinary Tract	20	
• Bladder, prostate	12	Nodes rarely involved; metastasis to lung and bone marrow
• Vagina, uterus	2	Nodes rarely involved; metastasis to retroperitoneal nodes (mainly from uterus)
• Paratesticular	6	Retroperitoneal nodes in 30% of cases; metastasis to lung and bone
Extremities	20	Nodes involved in 20% of cases; metastasis to lung, bone marrow, CNS
Trunk	10	Nodes rarely involved; metastasis to lung and bone
Other	10	Nodes rarely involved; metastasis to lung, bone, and liver

From Lanzkowsky, P. (1995). *Manual of pediatric hematology and oncology.* New York: Churchill Livingstone.

the meninges at the base of the skull such as the nasopharynx, middle ear, paranasal sinuses, and infratemporal and pterygopalatine fossae.[21] A tumor in the paranasal sinuses may cause nasal obstruction, chronic sinusitis, epistaxis, swelling, or local pain. Signs and symptoms of tumors involving the nasopharynx include epistaxis, nasal obstruction and discharge, visible polypoid masses in the nasopharyngeal cavity, and serous discharge. Chronic otitis media is common with rhabdomyosarcoma in the middle ear. Other possible symptoms include mucopurulent and sometimes sanguinous drainage from the affected ear, facial nerve palsy, and conductive hearing loss.

An important clinical feature of parameningeal head and neck primary tumors is an approximately 25% to 35% incidence of central nervous system (CNS) involvement that may be present at diagnosis.[21] Multiple cranial nerve palsies may occur if the tumor invades the neurovascular sheath. The tumor may cross through multiple foramina and fissures and grow toward the epidural space. Intracranial spread can cause an increase in intracranial pressure (ICP), producing headache, morning vomiting, and/or diplopia. Respiratory difficulty may be caused by brainstem invasion. Intracranial extension drastically reduces the overall survival rate. These tumors can also spread distantly, primarily to the lungs and bones.[44]

GENITOURINARY

Genitourinary tumors constitute the second most common form of rhabdomyosarcoma. These usually occur in very young children and arise most frequently low on the posterior wall of the bladder or in the prostate. Presenting symptoms of bladder tumors include urinary retention, straining to void, hematuria, or passage of tissue in the urine. A prostate tumor may occur as a large pelvic mass resulting in urinary frequency, retention, or constipation if significant compression of the bladder, urethra, or intestinal tract occurs.[14]

Paratesticular tumors usually occur as asymptomatic, nontender masses in the scrotum, lying above and separate from the testes. These tumors most commonly appear with multiple lymph node involvement because of the rich lymphatic system of this region.

Until tumor growth is extensive, tumors of the retroperitoneal area are usually asymptomatic. At diagnosis, the child may complain of vague abdominal pain and/or symptoms of bowel or genitourinary obstruction. A palpable mass may or may not be present. Metastasis to local lymph nodes is commonly observed.

Vaginal rhabdomyosarcoma is associated with abnormal vaginal bleeding or mucosanguinous discharge. This tumor occurs in very young girls and often has an unusual presentation of a mass that resembles a cluster of grapes protruding from the vagina or cervical opening, thus the name *sarcoma botryoides*. Botryoides is a Greek word for grape cluster.[21] This tumor rarely spreads by direct extension to the pelvic structures. If this does occur, pain will be a presenting symptom because of interference with bowel and bladder function.

EXTREMITY

Tumors originating in the extremities are usually deep-seated, often tender palpable masses with soft to firm consistency. These tumors may be mistaken for a traumatic hematoma, especially in school-age children. Extremity rhabdomyosarcoma is most common in the adolescent age-group.[14] Because injuries to the extremities are frequent in this age-group, delays in correct diagnosis can occur.[44] Extremity tumors are relatively fixed to the underlying musculature and occasionally involve the skin. Regional lymph node enlargement may be present, most commonly with alveolar rhabdomyosarcoma.

METASTASIS

Involvement of the bone by rhabdomyosarcoma can produce symptoms similar to those of a bone tumor and/or leukemia (e.g., pain, swelling, and/or limping). Bone marrow metastasis can produce symptoms of pancytopenia, resulting in anemia, bleeding, and/or infection. Most children with bone marrow involvement present with an extremity or trunk rhabdomyosarcoma and have concomitant metastases to bone, lung, and/or lymph nodes. Primary lesions of the prostate and maxillary sinus are highly associated with bone marrow metastasis. Less than 10% of children with bone marrow involvement achieve long-term survival.[37]

DIAGNOSTIC EVALUATION

The diagnostic evaluation begins with a complete history and physical examination. Sarcomas are usually nontender and impart no unusual hue to the overlying skin or subcutaneous tissue. The physical examination is performed with particular attention to regional lymphatic structures and surrounding tissues.[44]

Careful presurgical measurement of the primary tumor size by magnetic resonance imaging (MRI) and by physical examination is critical for TNM stage assignment.[37] Regional lymph node areas that drain the tumor site are thoroughly examined and may be evaluated by CT scan or MRI. The MRI may have value in predicting the extent and probability of surgical resection for extremity, abdominopelvic, and retroperitoneal tumors because of its enhanced ability to differentiate tumor from normal surrounding tissue as compared with CT. The MRI is useful for evaluating spinal cord involvement with retroperitoneal or paraspinal tumors.[21] Positron emission tomography (PET) is used increasingly in soft tissue sarcomas to differentiate aggressive from benign lesions.[37]

Evaluation also includes a complete blood count (CBC), platelet count, urinalysis, and renal and liver function studies. Imaging studies of the chest, skeletal surveys, and bone and liver scans also aid in the determination of primary and metastatic tu-

mor spread.[38] Bone marrow aspiration and biopsy are necessary to assess the presence of bone marrow involvement by malignant cells.

Rhabdomyosarcoma of the head and neck frequently extends through the adjacent bones of the skull into the cranial cavity. A lumbar puncture is performed as part of the evaluation of all parameningeal tumors to examine the cerebrospinal fluid (CSF) for the presence of malignant cells, increased protein, and decreased glucose, indicating signs of meningeal seeding.

Other neoplasms such as neuroblastoma, Wilms tumor, or lymphoma must be ruled out in children with abdominal disease. Imaging studies, lab evaluations such as homovanillic acid (HVA) and vanillylmandelic acid (VMA), and biopsy will aid in the differential diagnosis.

Growth of a nontender mass, especially without a clear-cut history of trauma, should always alert the examiner to consider biopsy, especially if expansion is confirmed by repeated observation over 1 to 2 weeks. A mass within a body cavity can produce obstruction or discharge. Both mandate a biopsy.[44] Whenever possible, a wide excisional biopsy with sufficient margins of normal tissue is performed early. Wide excisional biopsies should be undertaken only in areas in which complete removal will not result in major cosmetic or functional impairment.[47] Biopsy of suspicious lymph nodes is also performed. Biopsy results are important determinants of treatment and prognosis. When the child is referred to a pediatric cancer center and registered on a frontline IRSG protocol, tumor tissue and other positive biopsy specimens are sent to the Pediatric Division of the Cooperative Human Tissue Network (CHTN) in Columbus, Ohio. A rapid review is done to confirm the histologic subtype of the tumor. In addition the tumor is analyzed for the incidence of t(1;13) and t(2;13), resulting in the fusion genes *PAX 7-FKHR* and *PAX 3-FKHR,* commonly seen in alveolar rhabdomyosarcoma. These fusion genes possibly act as oncoproteins, resulting in a dysregulation of cell growth and transformation.[31] At present no specific gene translocation has been identified for embryonal rhabdomyosarcoma. This research is being conducted to further promote the risk-based therapy that is designed to improve survival.

PATHOLOGY

The history of the histologic classification of rhabdomyosarcoma is confusing, and there has been no uniformly accepted classification scheme. In 1995 investigators around the world agreed to unify classification systems so that studies would be comparable.[28] Previously, the most widely used classification for rhabdomyosarcoma was that of Horn and Enterline consisting of four histologic subtypes: embryonal, botryoid subtype of embryonal, alveolar, and pleomorphic.[28] The National Cancer Institute (NCI) Cancer Therapy Evaluation Program at the National Institutes of Health (NIH) supported a landmark study to assess the available classification systems for rhabdomyosarcoma. The interrelationship between prognosis, patient survival, and histology was evaluated.

The NCI classification proposed the following categories be used by all pathologists in making the diagnosis: botryoid, spindle cell, embryonal, alveolar, and undifferentiated sarcoma. A tumor with characteristics of both embryonal and alveolar would automatically be classified as alveolar. Thus a tumor with any amount of alveolar tissue is considered to have a poor prognosis because all alveolar rhabdomyosarcomas fall into an unfavorable category. Approximately 80% of all newly diagnosed cases were classified as embryonal (60%) or alveolar (20%), and the remainder as undifferentiated or miscellaneous.[31]

Rhabdomyosarcoma belongs to the category of small round cell tumors of childhood. There are many small round cell tumors and the differential diagnosis can be difficult (Table 25-2). These tumors are primitive or embryonal in appearance. They also often occur in misleading clinical situations, such as bone marrow metastasis.[42] Referral to a pediatric cancer center with experienced pathologists is essential to ensure the correct diagnosis. Rhabdomyosarcoma is further classified both by conventional light microscopic techniques and by newer immunohistochemical, electron microscopic, and molecular genetic techniques.[45]

By light microscopy, rhabdomyosarcoma may exhibit cross-striation characteristic of skeletal muscle or rhabdomyoblasts. The two major subtypes of rhabdomyosarcoma, embryonal and alveolar, each have a characteristic histologic appearance. Alveolar rhabdomyosarcoma exhibits small, round, densely appearing cells lined up along spaces reminiscent of pulmonary alveoli, giving rise to the term *alveolar rhabdomyosarcoma*. The embryonal subtype is characterized by spindle-shaped cells with a stroma-rich appearance.[14]

Immunohistochemical staining is a useful and reliable adjunctive means of identifying skeletal muscle and muscle-specific proteins or genes.[16] These proteins include muscle-specific actin and myosin desmin, myoglobin, Z-band protein, and MyoD.[44]

Electron microscopy can provide additional information if light microscopy and immunohistochemistry results are ambiguous. The finding of actin-myosin bundles or Z-band material on electron microscopic analysis provides strong support for a diagnosis of rhabdomyosarcoma.[44]

Somatically acquired genetic changes underlie all forms of cancer; however, until recently, the genetic characteristics of rhabdomyosarcoma were largely unknown. With improved cytogenetic techniques, it is now clear that the chromosomes of this tumor contain both numerical and structural abnormalities.[13,34] More specific classification of rhab-

TABLE 25-2	CLASSIFICATION OF SMALL ROUND CELL TUMORS OF CHILDHOOD
Traditional	**Revised**
1. Ewing's sarcoma	1. pPNETs* (bone and soft tissue)
2. Neuroblastoma	a. Ewing's sarcoma
3. Rhabdomyosarcoma	b. Peripheral neuroepithelioma
4. Lymphoma	c. "Askin" tumor of chest wall
	d. PNET of bone
	e. "Extraosseous" Ewing's (neural)
	2. Round cell bone tumors
	a. Small cell osteosarcoma
	b. Mesenchymal chondrosarcoma
	c. Primitive sarcoma of bone
	3. Round cell soft tissue sarcoma
	a. Poorly differentiated rhabdomyosarcoma†
	b. "Extraosseous" Ewing's (nonneural)
	4. Metastatic neuroblastoma (rarely a diagnostic problem)
	5. Extranodal lymphoma

From Triche, T. J. (1997). Pathology and molecular diagnosis of pediatric malignancies. In P. A. Pizzo & D. G. Poplack (Eds.), *Principles and practice of pediatric oncology* (3rd ed., pp. 141-185). Philadelphia: Lippincott-Raven.
*pPNET, Peripheral primitive neuroectodermal tumor.
†Generally alveolar rhabdomyosarcoma, lacking an alveolar pattern ("solid alveolar").

TABLE 25-3	CLINICAL GROUP SYSTEM EMPLOYED IN INTERGROUP RHABDOMYOSARCOMA STUDIES I THROUGH III	
Clinical Group	**Extent of Disease and Surgical Result**	
I	A. Localized tumor, confined to site of origin, completely resected	
	B. Localized tumor, infiltrating beyond site of origin, completely resected	
II	A. Localized tumor, gross total resection, but with microscopic residual disease	
	B. Locally "extensive" tumor (spread to to regional lymph nodes), completely resected	
	C. "Extensive" tumor (spread to regional lymph nodes), gross total resection, but with microscopic residual disease	
III	A. Localized or locally extensive tumor, gross residual disease after biopsy only	
	B. Localized or locally extensive tumor, gross residual disease after "major" resection ($>50\%$ debulking)	
IV	Any size primary tumor, with or without regional lymph node involvement, with distant metastases, irrespective of surgical approach to primary tumor	

From Wexler, L. H., & Helman, L. J. (1997). Rhabdomyosarcoma and the undifferentiated sarcomas. In P. A. Pizzo & D. G. Poplack (Eds.), *Principles and practice of pediatric oncology* (3rd ed., pp. 799-829). Philadelphia: Lippincott-Raven.

domyosarcoma is being linked to chromosomal abnormalities. Embryonal and alveolar tumors are further distinguished by structural chromosomal changes.[41] Although embryonal tumors lack tumor-specific translocations, they may undergo inactivation of one or more tumor-suppressor genes, as indicated by the consistent loss of heterozygosity for multiple closely linked loci at chromosome 11p15.[31] Alveolar rhabdomyosarcoma is characterized by specific genetic structural abnormalities, the most common being t(2;13)(q35;q14), which is seen in 70% of cases. The genes fused by t(2;13) are the *PAX3* gene on chromosome 2 and the *FKHR* gene on chromosome 13.[19] Less commonly, alveolar rhabdomyosarcomas have a variant t(1;13)(p36;q13), which fuses *FKHR* to *PAX7*.[1,2]

In the current IRS V, these advances in molecular techniques are being used to detect occult bone marrow and peripheral blood metastases, evaluate the margin of resection at diagnosis in patients with no microscopic residual disease, and assess tumor margins at second look operation.[37] Ultimately this approach to tumor diagnosis will augment current methods and lead to improved understanding of these malignancies, including complex tumors, which before were poorly defined.[28]

STAGING

Histologic and clinical staging is done after completion of diagnostic tests and excisional biopsy or surgical excision of the tumor. The histology of the tumor is an indicator of how the tumor will behave and respond to treatment. Clinical staging guides the choice of therapy and is an important determinant of prognosis. The goal of a uniform staging and classification system is to enable institutions with different treatment regimens to compare results and to determine more effective forms of

treatment. Various staging systems have been used in clinical studies of sarcomas, making comparisons among studies extremely difficult. IRS I devised a clinical staging system based on the extent of surgical tumor removal (Table 25-3). This clinical staging system has been used for over 25 years in IRS I, IRS II, and IRS III.[37]

Because of criticism that surgical staging may vary with operative techniques and excludes other important prognostic factors such as tumor size and site, the IRSG committee in 1992 adopted a modification of the TNM system. The TNM system relies on pretreatment assessment of disease extension.[31] This site-based, preoperative TNM staging system has been retrospectively evaluated by numerous investigators and shown to be highly predictive of outcome.[44] The current IRS trial (IRS V) incorporates the most significant prognostic variables (size <5 cm versus >5 cm, invasiveness, lymph node involvement, and primary site) into a TNM staging system (Table 25-4). The grouping system is retained, however, to define the parameters of radiation therapy.[21]

TREATMENT

Before the combined use of radiation and chemotherapy, the overall prognosis for children with rhabdomyosarcoma and undifferentiated sarcoma was poor. Complete surgical excision of the tumor was the most successful treatment available. For most pediatric patients complete excision was not an option because up to 18% had metastasis at the time of diagnosis and the tumors were often nonresectable.[39] The addition of radiation therapy in the 1950s and chemotherapy in the 1960s greatly improved the overall prognosis for children with rhabdomyosarcoma. By using current multidisci-

TABLE 25-4	**TNM STAGING OF RHABDOMYOSARCOMA: TNM PRETREATMENT STAGING CLASSIFICATION FOR IRS IV***				
Stage	**Sites**	**T invasiveness**	**T size**	**N**	**M**
1	Orbit Head and neck† Genitourinary‡	T1 or T2	a or b	N0 N1 or Nx	M0
2	Bladder/prostate Extremity Cranial parameningeal Other§	T1 or T2	a	N0 or Nx	M0
3	Bladder/prostate Extremity Cranial parameningeal Other§	T1 or T2 T1 or T2	a b	N1 N0 N1 or Nx	M0 M0
4	All	T1 or T2	a or b	N0 or N1	M1

From Wexler, L. H., & Helman, L. J. (1997). Rhabdomyosarcoma and the undifferentiated sarcomas. In P. A. Pizzo & D. G. Poplack (Eds.), *Principles and practice of pediatric oncology* (3rd ed., pp. 799-829). Philadelphia: Lippincott-Raven.
*T (tumor): T1, confined to anatomic site of origin; T2, extension; a, <5 cm in diameter; b, >5 cm in diameter. N (regional nodes): N0, not clinically involved; N1, clinically involved; Nx, clinical status unknown. M (metastasis): M0, no distant metastases; M1, distant metastasis present.
†Excluding parameningeal.
‡Nonbladder/nonprostate.
§Includes trunk, retroperitoneum, and so on.

plinary approaches, involving a judicious blend of surgery, radiotherapy, and multiagent chemotherapy, it is anticipated that approximately 70% of all children with newly diagnosed nonmetastatic rhabdomyosarcoma will be alive 5 years later and the vast majority of them will be tumor free.[1]

CHEMOTHERAPY

The use of adjuvant chemotherapy has markedly improved the overall survival rate for children with operable and inoperable rhabdomyosarcoma. Chemotherapy is now recommended for all children with or without evidence of metastasis at the time of diagnosis. Results of the previous IRS trials suggest that the three most effective drugs against rhabdomyosarcoma are vincristine, actinomycin, and cyclophosphamide (VAC). They form the basis of the VAC regimens that have been progressively intensified by increasing the dose of cyclophosphamide and increasing the frequency of administration of vincristine.[1]

Risk-based therapy is designed to tailor the chemotherapy to the incidence of failure or success. Thus only vincristine and actinomycin are given to children with Clinical Group I disease of embryonal or botryoid histology. The majority of children with rhabdomyosarcoma have gross residual disease (Clinical Group III) and present the problem of attempting to increase cure rates while minimizing toxicity. A comparison of cyclophosphamide with agents such as ifosfamide and etopo-

side was studied in IRS III, but no significant improvement was demonstrated (Figure 25-1).[36]

In IRS IV an analysis of subgroups of patients demonstrated that patients with embryonal tumors arising at favorable sites had a significant improvement in outcome largely because of the increased dose intensity of the alkylating agents.[3] However, patients with embryonal tumors occurring at unfavorable sites with gross residual disease and those with alveolar rhabdomyosarcoma had no improvement in outcome on IRS IV. Furthermore, a significant increase in the dose intensity of the alkylating agents over the 2.2 g/m² cyclophosphamide dose initially used in IRS IV was shown to have unacceptable gastrointestinal toxicity, and thus is not an option to pursue for this group of patients.[37] Consequently, the development of new agents to be added to the already existing VAC regimen is the object of study for children with Clinical Group III disease or intermediate risk. Also, because toxic deaths were significantly increased in children under 3 years of age in the earlier IRS IV pilot, the IRSG is now using a per kilogram dosing in the children who are under 3 years of age or who have a body surface area of less than 0.6 m².[1,5]

Treatment of children with metastatic rhabdomyosarcoma at diagnosis continues to be a major challenge. Clinical Group IV patients have not done well on any of the IRS trials. Five-year survival rates range from 20% on IRS I to 27% on IRS III. Intensification of VAC therapy by the addition

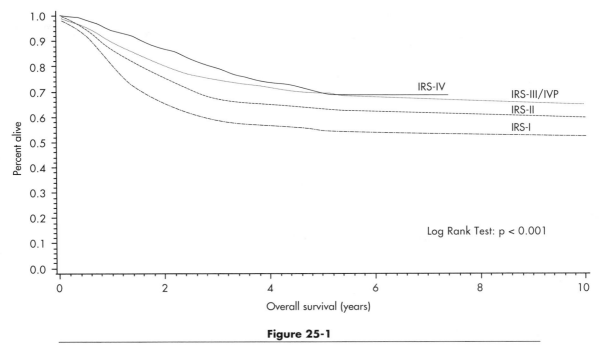

Figure 25-1

Overall survival rate by study for patients enrolled on IRS I through IV.   (From The Soft Tissue Sarcoma Committee of the Children's Oncology Group [William Crist, MD, Chairman]).

of doxorubicin, etoposide, or cisplatin has not produced results superior to those for VAC alone.[1] More recently "megatherapy" followed by autologous stem cell rescue has been investigated. Most megatherapy protocols have included high dose melphalan, which has demonstrated activity against rhabdomyosarcoma in vitro and in vivo.[11] Other strategies have included high-dose chemotherapy with or without total body irradiation.[20] Hybrid treatments with intense induction therapy followed by high-dose chemotherapy have not, however, improved the outcome of patients with metastatic disease.[37] These results suggest that novel therapies are urgently needed for the majority of patients with metastatic rhabdomyosarcoma.[4] These new strategies may include the use of biologic response modifiers, antibody targeting of immunotoxins to tumor cells, and the evaluation of a vaccine against rhabdomyosarcoma that is designed to elicit T-cell immunity with specificity for tumor-specific fusion peptides. However, until these newer therapeutic strategies are available, identification of additional active chemotherapeutic agents continues to be the best alternative available to improve outcome for these children.[7] Ongo-

ing clinical trials are investigating the use of new agents against recurrent or refractory solid tumors, including rhabdomyosarcoma. The agents in these trials include irinotecan, rebeccamycin, temozolamide and O^6-benzylguanine, vinorelbine, and docetaxel.

IRS V, which is currently ongoing, is designed to evaluate risk-based therapies as described below. The low-risk group is composed of tumors of embryonal or botryoid histology only. The sites may be favorable with complete resection, microscopic residual, or gross residual. Unfavorable sites that have been completely resected or have microscopic residual are also included. This group is further divided into subgroup A and subgroup B. Children in subgroup A, with more favorable sites will receive only vincristine and actinomycin, and no radiotherapy if there is complete resection. Because of the excellent prognosis of children with tumors of the orbit, even if there is gross residual disease these children are classified as subgroup A. Children in subgroup B, with more unfavorable sites and/or incomplete resections will receive the standard VAC therapy with or without radiation therapy. Any child who had a complete resection will not receive radiation regardless of subgroup assignment.[47] The intermediate risk group is defined as any alveolar or undifferentiated histology Clinical Group I, II, or III tumor, in addition to Clinical Group III embryonal or botryoid histology. Because of improved survival, children with metastatic disease of embryonal histology under the age of 10 years are also classified as intermediate risk. A randomization to VAC or VAC alternating with vincristine, topotecan, and cyclophosphamide (VTC) builds on the encouraging responses observed by the IRSG in two phase II "up-front" windows.[26,37,43] The high-risk group includes all patients with metastatic disease and alveolar or undifferentiated histology. Children over the age of 10 years with metastatic disease and embryonal or botryoid histology are also included. The study features an up-front window using irinotecan, a camptothecin, topoisomerase I inhibitor with promising activity against rhabdomyosarcoma. This is followed by VAC with or without vincristine and irinotecan depending on initial response.

SURGERY

The optimum surgical management is complete tumor excision while preserving vital and/or functionally useful organs. The goal is wide resection of the primary tumor with an adequate margin of normal tissue.[8] If the margins are not tumor free, primary reexcision may be beneficial, especially for trunk or extremity tumors.[1,12,40] In sites such as the vagina and urinary bladder and most head and neck sites, incisional biopsy for diagnosis may be the only feasible surgical procedure because of proximity to vital blood vessels and nerves, cosmetic considerations, or both.[9,15,22,44]

Assessment of regional node involvement is recommended in all sites where imaging studies suggest a lymph node larger than 1 cm. In extremity sites, the relatively high incidence of nodal spread demands at least a surgical sampling.[27,37] In the recent IRS IV study an attempt was made to eliminate lymph node dissection with paratesticular tumors. However, there was an increase in the relapse rate compared with the previous IRSG study.[46] Therefore in IRS V unilateral lymph node dissection will be required for paratesticular tumors.

In previous IRSG studies, a second-look surgery was used to (1) pathologically verify the response indicated by imaging, and (2) resect any viable tumor cells that survived after induction chemotherapy and local irradiation.[44] The status of three fourths of group III patients changed from partial to complete pathologic response as a result of the surgery, either because no viable tumor was found or because it was then completely excised. Those patients who obtained a complete response after second-look surgery had a better survival rate than the patients who did not obtain a complete response or who did not undergo surgery.[1] An additional benefit of second-look resection is radiotherapy dose reduction. In the ongoing IRS V study for intermediate risk patients, a second-look operation is being considered in lieu of radiotherapy at week 12 as an elective local control strategy.[37] The local control guidelines of this study are designed to use second-look resection for patients with primary sites that have an increased risk of local failure despite radiotherapy.

RADIOTHERAPY

Radiation therapy is a major tool in the treatment of children with rhabdomyosarcoma and undifferentiated sarcoma. However, rhabdomyosarcoma is only moderately radiosensitive and high doses of radiation are required for tumor cell kill.[21] Radiation therapy protocols have evolved with sequential intergroup clinical trials. Early guidelines recommended doses as high as 55 to 60 Gy to the primary tumor site.[14] With the use of aggressive adjuvant chemotherapy, the doses of radiation therapy have been decreased. Doses are also no longer modified for patient age and tumor size. Now, clinical grouping, site, and histology are the primary determinants of timing and dose.

Several important facts regarding radiation therapy have been learned from previous clinical trials such as IRS I through IV and the German Cooperative Soft Tissue Sarcoma Study Group. An important finding was that patients with alveolar and undifferentiated sarcoma who were treated with intensive chemotherapy, surgery, and radiation therapy fared better than similar patients who did not receive radiation therapy.[47] Another finding was that the more aggressive primary surgical approach could be replaced by primary radiation therapy, which allows for preservation of organ function and a better quality of life.[10,17]

In IRS IV children in Clinical Group III were given hyperfractionated radiotherapy concurrently with aggressive chemotherapy to test the effectiveness of this method to decrease late effects. It was possible to treat children in this manner, but data on the long-term effectiveness are still being analyzed.

IRS V recommends lower radiation therapy doses for certain sites because of results from previous studies. The rationale is that the lower dose will cause fewer or less severe late effects. The timing of radiation therapy in relation to chemotherapy has been variable. For patients with parameningeal tumors and evidence of meningeal involvement, data show that delaying radiation therapy until week 6 or 9 diminishes local and regional control, and survival.[45] Consequently, radiation therapy is now employed as soon as possible after diagnosis. The goal of detailed surgery and radiotherapy planning based on site, response to induction chemotherapy, preservation of organ function, and histology is to reduce the ultimate risk of local failure. Soft tissue sarcomas infiltrate so widely that without wide excision, radiation therapy, and chemotherapy, local recurrence rates approach 75%.[44] Except in patients with completely excised tumors, radiation therapy given before or at week 15 appears to have the best chance of preventing local relapse.[6,37]

RECURRENT DISEASE

Thirty percent of children with rhabdomyosarcoma will relapse. Fifty to ninety-five percent of these patients ultimately die of progressive disease. The identification of prognostic factors for patients with relapsed or progressive disease would allow the development of risk-directed therapies. Clinical features identified at the time of initial diagnosis can be combined with tumor characteristics and, in some cases, the site(s) of recurrence to reliably define prognostic subgroups.[30] The retrieval therapy is then specifically designed for the aggressiveness of the recurrent tumor.

Recurrence must be documented by biopsy or fine needle aspiration. At a minimum, imaging studies are performed to evaluate the lungs, site of primary tumor, and any sites suggested by the history and physical examination. After pathologic verification of recurrent disease, factors considered in the formulation of a treatment plan include the timing of the recurrence relative to completion of therapy, the extent of disease at recurrence, the extent of disease at diagnosis, and the nature of prior therapy.[44]

Pappo and colleagues[30] studied the records of children who had relapsed on three successive IRSG protocols, IRS III, IRS IV pilot, and IRS IV. Their findings indicated that (1) the median time to treatment failure was 1.1 years; 95% of all failures occurred within 3 years from the start of treatment; (2) the median survival time from first recurrence or progression for the entire relapse population was 0.82 years, with an estimated 5-year survival rate from first recurrence of 17%; (3) both stage and group at the time of initial diagnosis were significantly associated with outcome in children with embryonal tumors; and, (4) except for the small number of patients with group I tumors, no other sets of favorable outcomes were identified for patients with alveolar or undifferentiated histology. They concluded that these findings justify an aggressive

retreatment approach to improve unfavorable outcomes.

When rhabdomyosarcoma recurs, the clinician must choose agents that have known activity against the disease but have not been used extensively in the initial therapy, such as the anthracyclines, ifosfamide with or without etoposide, and topoisomerase I inhibitors.[30] The best chance for survival occurs when a complete surgical resection can be accomplished followed by adjuvant postoperative radiotherapy and effective chemotherapy. Experimental therapies may be appropriate for children with metastatic disease at recurrence.[24] There is a lack of knowledge about the role for marrow transplantation with recurrent rhabdomyosarcoma. Further investigation is needed to better define the role for this therapy in relapsed disease. Other strategies that have been tried include the use of growth-factor-supported autologous peripheral blood progenitor cell transfusions to permit repetitive monthly cycles of myeloablative chemotherapy.[44]

LATE EFFECTS

The cure of children with rhabdomyosarcoma comes with a high cost. As more children survive, more delayed toxicities are observed and many are related to the aggressive multimodal therapy. Cataracts, hormonal imbalance, fibrosis, growth retardation, bowel obstruction, and hematuria can be attributed to local irradiation.[18,31,34] Loss of function, including bladder dysfunction, retrograde ejaculation, lymphedema, and palsies, has occurred following surgical resection of a primary tumor. Escalating doses of chemotherapy have increased survival rates but have also increased late effects such as infertility, renal tubular dysfunction, and most devastating of all, second malignancies such as acute leukemia and osteosarcoma.[29] Chapter 18 describes in depth the problems facing survivors of childhood cancer.

PROGNOSIS

The most important prognostic factors in the survival of children with rhabdomyosarcoma are the (1) extent of disease at diagnosis (clinical group and stage[27]), (2) histology of tumor, (3) primary site, and to some extent, (4) age of the child at diagnosis. Complete resection of the primary tumor offers the best chance of survival. However, many sites do not lend themselves to gross total resection without disfigurement or loss of organ function.[39] The use of intensive chemotherapy and radiation therapy has decreased the use of radical surgeries and has increased survival.[22,40] Accurate staging at the time of diagnosis is critically important, both as a guide to therapy and as probably the most significant determinant of prognosis.[1,17,33]

Table 25-5 shows the combined outcomes for patients treated on IRS III and the IRS IV pilot by the new NCI histology and clinical group. Histology is well known to be related to prognosis. In the past, the confusion in histologic classification made it difficult to plan risk-based therapy according to pathology. The current NCI histologic classification has been developed to establish a single classification system that incorporates prognostically useful parameters (Box 25-1). The best survival rate was observed for patients with botryoid rhabdomyosarcoma with a 95% survival at 5 years. The spindle cell variant of embryonal rhabdomyosarcoma was subsequently added to the classification because of the very favorable outcome for this group of patients. Alveolar tumors were consistently associated with poor prognosis, with only 54% of patients surviving 5 years. Patients with nonbotryoid embryonal tumors had survival in the intermediate range with 67% of patients surviving 5 years.[28]

Primary tumor site is also a significant prognostic factor. As a general rule, sarcomas arising in locations that produce symptoms early and offer relatively limited opportunities for spread (e.g., orbit) are associated with a better prognosis than are those that arise in deep, poorly confined areas (e.g., retroperitoneum).[1] Favorable sites include: (1) orbit, (2) superficial head and neck, and (3) genitourinary (e.g., vagina, bladder, and paratesticular—excluding prostate). The less favorable sites include: (1) parameningeal head and neck,[33] (2) prostate, (3) any extremity,[27,40] (4) retroperitoneal, and (5) trunk.[21,40]

Early data link the *PAX3* and *PAX7* fusion with prognosis, and 80% of alveolar tumors express these fusions. The *PAX7* fusion is seen in tumors in younger children. The tumors are less invasive and therefore have improved outcomes. *PAX3*, which is more common, has an even distribution over all ages, and the outcome is not as good. Even with metastatic disease, the children with *PAX7* fusion fared much better than those without the fusion.[23]

To a lesser degree, age and DNA ploidy are also prognostic indicators. Younger children seem to fare better in spite of extent of disease. Children under the age of 10 years with embryonal or botryoid histology and Clinical Group IV disease are treated as intermediate risk despite the fact that metastatic disease at diagnosis conveys such a poor prognosis to all other children with rhabdomyosarcoma.[4]

In a number of studies it has been learned that hyperdiploidy (1.1 to 1.8 times the normal cellular DNA content) was exclusively associated with embryonal histology, whereas near-tetraploidy (1.8 to 2.6 times the normal DNA content) was strongly

---

BOX 25-1

A PATHOLOGIC CLASSIFICATION FOR CHILDHOOD RHABDOMYOSARCOMA AND RELATED SARCOMAS BY PROGNOSIS

Superior Prognosis
  Botryoid rhabdomyosarcoma
  Spindle cell rhabdomyosarcoma
Intermediate Prognosis
  Embryonal rhabdomyosarcoma
Poor Prognosis
  Alveolar rhabdomyosarcoma
  Undifferentiated sarcoma
  Anaplastic rhabdomyosarcoma
Indeterminate
  Rhabdomyosarcoma with rhabdoid features

From Ruymann, F. B., & Grovas, A. C. (2000). Progress in the diagnosis and treatment of rhabdomyosarcoma and related soft tissue sarcomas. *Cancer Investigation, 18,* 223-241.

TABLE 25-5 IRS PATIENT OUTCOMES; IRSG III, IRSG IV PILOT		
Group	**3 Year EFS**	**Survival**
Embryonal at favorable site	88%	94%
Embryonal at unfavorable site, Clinical Group I/II	88%	93%
Embryonal at unfavorable site, Clinical Group III	76%	83%
Embryonal <10 yrs, Clinical Group IV	55%	59%
Alveolar, all sites, Clinical Group I-III	55%	—
Alveolar; Embryonal >10 yrs, Clinical Group IV	—	30%

Data from Anderson, J., Ruby, E., Link, M., et al. (1997). Identification of a favorable subset of patients (PTS) with metastatic (MET) rhabdomyosarcoma (RMS): A report from the Intergroup Rhabdomyosarcoma Study Group (IRSG). *Proceedings of American Society of Clinical Oncology, USA, 16,* 510a; Arndt, C., Tefft, M., Gehan, E., et al. (1997). A feasibility, toxicity, and early response study of etoposide, ifosfamide, and vincristine for the treatment of children with rhabdomyosarcoma: A report from the Intergroup Rhabdomyosarcoma Study (IRS) IV pilot study. *Journal of Pediatric Hematology/Oncology, 19,* 124-129; Ruymann, F. B., & Grovas, A. C. (2000). Progress in the diagnosis and treatment of rhabdomyosarcoma and related soft tissue sarcomas. *Cancer Investigation, 18,* 223-241.

associated with alveolar histology. Diploidy, seen in one third of patients and uncorrelated with histologic subtype, conferred the worst prognosis, whereas hyperdiploidy indicated a relatively good outcome.[1] The most meaningful prognostic variable is the response to treatment, because those who never achieve complete obliteration of the tumor do not survive. Early response to treatment correlates with a better outcome.[44]

NURSING IMPLICATIONS

The nursing care for a child with rhabdomyosarcoma is similar to that of any child with cancer undergoing aggressive multimodal therapy. Diligent supportive care is imperative given the high doses of chemotherapy and radiation therapy. The child and parents may need more time to understand the many intricacies of the detailed treatment plan. The therapy that is site-, group-, and response-based involves complicated road maps that can cause confusion among professionals and the family. Nurses will need to discuss the specifics for each child thoroughly with the physician to present a clear and concise plan to the family.[35] Frequent review and explanation will be necessary as the treatment progresses. Careful education about and assessment of the late effects of treatment are paramount for these children. Enrollment in comprehensive late effects follow-up programs is mandatory.

FUTURE DIRECTIONS

Although the cure rate for children with rhabdomyosarcoma has significantly improved over the last 25 years, there are still challenges in the treatment of this disease. Sixty-five percent of these children have either gross residual or metastatic disease, which responds poorly to current therapies. At present the plans for improving response include escalation of doses, addition of new drugs in up-front windows, and alternative sources of radiation therapy. These innovations will produce at best small gains in cure. It is likely that biologic studies exploring the basic molecular mechanisms of tumor genesis and metastases will lead to novel strategies that can be added to the current armamentarium.[25] Antiangiogenic agents or agents aimed at specific targets involved in metastatic behavior are potential modalities that are being explored.[14] Efforts to escalate drug and radiation doses may ultimately prove futile because none of the agents commonly used to treat rhabdomyosarcoma are tumor specific. These obstacles may be overcome if tumor-specific molecular targets such as the *PAX3-FKHR* oncogene could be identified and exploited in future therapies.[31]

For children with localized disease who respond well to therapy, risk-based planning will continue in an attempt to achieve cure while minimizing the undesirable effects of therapy and decreasing the risk of second malignancies. Changes may include further decrease in radiation doses, more refined surgical procedures, and the elimination of certain neoplasm-causing chemotherapeutic agents. All of these and newer approaches will require ongoing clinical evaluation to allow continued progress in the treatment of childhood rhabdomyosarcoma.

REFERENCES

1. Altman, A. J., & Quinn, J. J. (1998). Management of malignant solid tumors: Soft tissue sarcomas. In D. Nathan & S. Orkin (Eds.), *Nathan and Oski's hematology of infancy and childhood: Vol. 2* (pp. 1399-1410). Philadelphia: W. B. Saunders.
2. Anderson, J., Gordon, A., Pritchard-Jones, K., et al. (1999). Genes, chromosomes, and rhabdomyosarcoma. *Genes, Chromosomes and Cancer, 26,* 275-285.
3. Anderson, J. R., Link, M., Qualman, S., et al. (1998). Improved outcome for patients (PTS) with embryonal (EMB) histology (HIST) but not alveolar histology rhabdomyosarcoma (RMS): Results from Intergroup Rhabdomyosarcoma Study IV (IRS-IV). *Proceedings of American Society of Clinical Oncology, USA, 17,* 526a.
4. Anderson, J., Ruby, E., Link, M., et al. (1997). Identification of a favorable subset of patients (PTS) with metastatic (MET) rhabdomyosarcoma (RMS): A report from the Intergroup Rhabdomyosarcoma Study Group (IRSG). *Proceedings of American Society of Clinical Oncology, USA, 16,* 510a.
5. Arndt, C., Tefft, M., Gehan, E., et al. (1997). A feasibility, toxicity, and early response study of etoposide, ifosfamide, and vincristine for the treatment of children with rhabdomyosarcoma: A report from the Intergroup Rhabdomyosarcoma Study (IRS) IV pilot study. *Journal of Pediatric Hematology/Oncology, 19,* 124-129
6. Arndt, C., Womer, R., Sloan, J., et al. (1997). Alternating cycles of vincristine, doxorubicin, cyclophosphamide (VDC), and etoposide/ifosfamide (EI), for treatment of nonmetastatic rhabdomyosarcoma and undifferentiated sarcomas (US) of childhood. *Proceedings of American Society of Clinical Oncology, USA, 16,* 510a.
7. Arndt, C. A. S., & Crist, W. M. (1999). Common musculoskeletal tumors of childhood and adolescence. *The New England Journal of Medicine, 341,* 342-350.
8. Beech, T. R., Moss, R. L., Anderson, J. A., et al. (1999). What comprises appropriate therapy for children/adolescents with rhabdomyosarcoma (RMS) arising in the abdominal wall? A report from the Intergroup Rhabdomyosarcoma Study Group. *Journal of Pediatric Surgery, 34,* 668-671.
9. Blakely, M. L., Lobe, T. E., Anderson, J. R., et al. (1999). Does debulking improve survival in advanced stage retroperitoneal embryonal rhabdomyosarcoma? *Journal of Pediatric Surgery, 34,* 736-742.
10. Breneman, J. C. (1997). Genitourinary rhabdomyosarcoma. *Seminars in Radiation Oncology, 7,* 217-224.
11. Carli, M., Colombatti, R., Oberlin, O., et al. (1999). High-dose melphalan with autologous stem-cell rescue in metastatic rhabdomyosarcoma. *Journal of Clinical Oncology, 17,* 2796-2803.

12. Cecchetto, G., Carli, M., Sotti, G., et al. (2000). Importance of local treatment in pediatric soft tissue sarcomas with microscopic residual after primary surgery: Results of the Italian Cooperative Study RMS-88. *Medical and Pediatric Oncology, 34*, 97-101.

13. Chen, B., Liu, X., Savell, V. H., et al. (1999). Increased DNA methyltransferase expression in rhabdomyosarcoma. *International Journal of Cancer, 83*, 10-14.

14. Dagher, R., & Helman, L. (1999). Rhabdomyosarcoma: An overview. *The Oncologist, 4*, 34-44.

15. Daya, H., Chan, H. S., Sirkin, W., et al. (2000). Pediatric rhabdomyosarcoma of the head and neck: Is there a place for surgical management? *Archives of Otolaryngology— Head and Neck Surgery, 126*, 468-472.

16. Dias, P., Chen, B., Dilday, B., et al. (2000). Strong immunostaining for myogenin in rhabdomyosarcoma is significantly associated with tumors of the alveolar subclass. *American Journal of Pathology, 156*, 399-408.

17. Donaldson, S., & Anderson, J. (1997). Factors that influence treatment decisions in childhood rhabdomyosarcoma. *Radiology, 203*, 17-22.

18. Fiorillo, A., Migliorati, R., Vassallo, P., et al. (1999). Radiation late effects in children treated for orbital rhabdomyosarcoma. *Radiotherapy and Oncology, 53*, 143-148.

19. Kempf, B. E., & Vogt, P. K. (1999). A genetic analysis of PAX-3 FKHR, the oncogene of alveolar rhabdomyosarcoma. *Cell Growth and Differentiation, 10*, 813-818.

20. Koscielniak, E., Klingebiel, T. H., Peters, C., et al. (1997). Do patients with metastatic and recurrent rhabdomyosarcoma benefit from high-dose therapy with hematopoietic rescue? Report of the German/Austrian Pediatric Bone Marrow Transplantation Group. *Bone Marrow Transplantation, 19*, 227-231.

21. Lanzkowsky, P. (1995). *Manual of pediatric hematology and oncology.* New York: Churchill Livingstone.

22. Lobe, T. E., Wiener, R. J., Andrassy, R. J., et al. (1996). The argument for conservative, delayed surgery in the management of prostatic rhabdomyosarcoma. *Journal of Pediatric Surgery, 31*, 1084-1087.

23. Lynch, J. (2000, April). *Prognostic significance of PAX3-FKHR and PAX7-FKHR gene fusions in alveolar rhabdomyosarcoma.* Paper presented at the meeting of the Children's Oncology Group, Tampa, FL.

24. Merchant, T. E., Parsh, N., del Valle, P. L., et al. (2000). Brachytherapy for pediatric soft-tissue sarcoma. *International Journal of Radiation Oncology, Biology, Physics, 46*, 427-432.

25. Merlino, G., & Helman, L. J. (1999). Rhabdomyosarcoma—Working out the pathways. *Oncogene, 18*, 5340-5348.

26. Meyer, W. H. (2000, April). *The drug pair: Topotecan/cyclophosphamide, is active in previously untreated RMS.* Paper presented at the meeting of the Children's Oncology Group, Tampa, FL.

27. Neville, H. L., Andrassy, R. J., Lobe, T. E., et al. (2000). Preoperative staging, prognostic factors and outcome in extremity rhabdomyosarcoma: A preliminary report from the Intergroup Rhabdomyosarcoma Study IV (1991-97). *Journal of Pediatric Surgery, 35*, 317-321.

28. Newton, W. A., Gehan, E. A., Webber, B. L., et al. (1995). Classification of rhabdomyosarcomas and related sarcomas. *Cancer, 76*, 1073-1085.

29. Pappo, A. S. (2000, April). *Second malignant neoplasms (SMN) in IRS IV.* Paper presented at the meeting of the Children's Oncology Group, Tampa, FL.

30. Pappo, A. S., Anderson, J. R., Crist, W. M., et al. (1999). Survival after relapse in children and adolescents with rhabdomyosarcoma: A report from the Intergroup Rhabdomyosarcoma Study Group. *Journal of Clinical Oncology, 17*, 3487-3493.

31. Pappo, A. S., Shapiro, D. N., Crist, W. M., et al. (1997). Rhabdomyosarcoma: Biology and treatment. *Pediatric Clinics of North America, 44*, 953-969.

32. Pizzo, P., & Poplack, D. (1997). *Principles and practice of pediatric oncology* (3rd ed.). Philadelphia: Lippincott-Raven.

33. Raney, R. B. (2000, April). *Results of treatment of localized cranial parameningeal sarcoma in IRSG studies IRS II through IRS-IV, 1978-97.* Paper presented at the meeting of the Children's Oncology Group, Tampa, FL.

34. Raney, R. B., Asmar, L., Vassilopoulou-Sellin, R., et al. (1999). Late complications of therapy in 213 children with localized nonorbital soft-tissue sarcoma of the head and neck: A descriptive report from the Intergroup Rhabdomyosarcoma Studies (IRS)—II and III. *Medical and Pediatric Oncology, 33*, 362-371.

35. Rasco, C. (1998). Rhabdomyosarcoma. In M. Hockenberry-Eaton (Ed.), *Essentials of pediatric oncology nursing: A core curriculum* (pp. 45-48). Glenview, IL: Association of Pediatric Oncology Nurses.

36. Ruymann, F. B., Crist, W. M., Wiener, E., et al. (1997). Comparison of two doublet chemotherapy regimens and conventional radiotherapy in metastatic rhabdomyosarcoma: Improved overall survival using ifosfamide/etoposide compared to vincristine/melphalan in IRSG-IV. *Proceedings of American Society of Clinical Oncology, 16*, 521a.

37. Ruymann, F. B., & Grovas, A. C. (2000). Progress in the diagnosis and treatment of rhabdomyosarcoma and related soft tissue sarcomas. *Cancer Investigation, 18*, 223-241.

38. Spunt, S. L. (2000, April). *Routine brain imaging is unwarranted in asymptomatic patients with metastatic non-head-and-neck RMS.* Paper presented at the meeting of the Children's Oncology Group, Tampa, FL.

39. Spunt, S. L., Lobe, T. E., Pappo, A. S., et al. (2000). Aggressive surgery is unwarranted for biliary tract rhabdomyosarcoma. *Journal of Pediatric Surgery, 35*, 309-316.

40. Tabrizi, P., & Letts, M. (1999). Childhood rhabdomyosarcoma of the trunk and extremities. *The American Journal of Orthopedics, 28*, 440-446.

41. Tobar, A., Avigad, S., Zoldan, M., et al. (2000). Clinical relevance of molecular diagnosis in childhood rhabdomyosarcoma. *Diagnostic Molecular Pathology, 9*, 9-13.

42. Triche, T. J. (1997). Pathology and molecular diagnosis of pediatric malignancies. In P. A. Pizzo & D. G. Poplack (Eds.), *Principles and practice of pediatric oncology* (3rd ed., pp. 141-175). Philadelphia: Lippincott-Raven.

43. Vietti, T., Crist, W. M., Ruby, E., et al. (1997). Topotecan window in patients with rhabdomyosarcoma (RMS): An IRSG study. *Proceedings of American Society of Clinical Oncology, 16*, 510a.

44. Wexler, L. H., & Helman, L. J. (1997). Rhabdomyosarcoma and the undifferentiated sarcomas. In P. A. Pizzo & D. G. Poplack (Eds.), *Principles and practice of pediatric oncology* (3rd ed., pp. 799-824). Philadelphia: Lippincott-Raven.

45. Wharam, M. D., Jr. (1997). Rhabdomyosarcoma of parameningeal sites. *Seminars in Radiation Oncology, 7*, 212-216.

46. Wiener, E. (2000, April). *Staging retroperitoneal lymph node dissection is necessary for adolescents with resected paratesticular RMS: Results of IRS-III and IRS-IV.* Paper presented at the Children's Oncology Group Meeting, Tampa, FL.

47. Wolden, S. L., Anderson, J. R., Crist, W. M., et al. (1999). Indications for radiotherapy and chemotherapy after complete resection in rhabdomyosarcoma: A report from Intergroup Rhabdomyosarcoma studies I to III. *Journal of Clinical Oncology, 17*, 3468-3475.

26

Wilms Tumor

Rosemary Drigan
Arlene L. Androkites

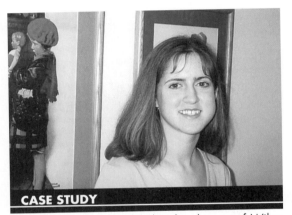

CASE STUDY

Jessica is a 15-year-old girl with a history of Wilms tumor. She is currently undergoing long-term follow-up for treatment of her disease. When Jessica was 2 years old, her parents noted fullness in her upper left abdomen. The pediatrician subsequently palpated an abdominal mass on the left side. An abdominal ultrasound examination, followed by computed tomography (CT) scan, revealed replacement of the left kidney with a mass. A left nephrectomy was performed, which confirmed Wilms tumor, stage II. Treatment consisted of vincristine and dactinomycin chemotherapy for 6 months. One year off therapy Jessica had a 4-day history of fever and cough. A chest x-ray revealed a left lower lobe infiltrate and a pleural effusion. A chest tube was inserted, and pleural fluid was diagnostic for tumor cells. A nodular density in the left lower lobe was seen on lung CT scan. For treatment of this relapse, Jessica received 6 months of chemotherapy consisting of etoposide, ifosfamide, doxorubicin, vincristine, and cisplatin, followed by whole lung radiation. She is currently 9 years off treatment and is without disease recurrence. Her physical examination is remarkable for scoliosis and decreased muscular growth in the radiation field. Pulmonary function tests reveal a decrease in total lung volume, and echocardiogram reveals an increase in afterload secondary to previous doxorubicin.

Wilms tumor (WT) is the most common primary malignant renal tumor affecting children.[10,19] The tumor is named after Max Wilms, a German surgeon who wrote one of the first descriptions of the tumor in 1899.[27] Prognosis has dramatically improved because of collaborative efforts among pediatric surgeons, pathologists, radiation therapists, and oncologists. Described as a paradigm for multimodal treatment of pediatric solid tumors, current management focuses on decreasing the acute and long-term morbidity of treatment for low-risk patients while reserving more intensive treatment for those with high-risk features.[23]

EPIDEMIOLOGY

Wilms tumor accounts for 6% of all childhood cancers in the United States with an annual incidence of 8.1 cases per million in white children less than 15 years of age.[5,6] There are approximately 460 new cases each year with 80% appearing before age 5.[15] The age at diagnosis peaks at 2 to 3 years with a slightly increased frequency in girls. Neither parental environmental exposures, maternal hormonal exposures during pregnancy, nor parental occupation has consistently been associated with the development of this tumor.[5,19]

Most commonly Wilms tumors arise in young children without any unusual physical features or family history and are considered sporadic.[19] Associations with a familial predisposition or as a feature of a specific genetic disorder are described in children with Wilms (Table 26-1).[7] Children with Wilms tumor may have associated anomalies, including aniridia (congenital absence of the iris); genitourinary malformations and mental retardation (WAGR syndrome); macroglossia, omphalocele, hemihypertrophy, and visceromegaly (Beckwith-Wiedemann syndrome); and pseudohermaphroditism and gonadal dysgenesis, especially in males (Denys-Drash syndrome) (Table 26-2).[9,14,15] Children with these syndromes are at high risk for developing Wilms tumor, and a surveillance program for early detection should be instituted (Table 26-3).[8]

Recent advances in cytogenetics suggest that there may be a hereditary and a sporadic form of Wilms tumor resulting from changes in one or more of several genes. Hereditary tumors occur more frequently in younger patients, those with aniridia, genitourinary anomalies, and bilateral disease. There is a 20% incidence of hereditary cases in 3000 patients in the National Wilms Tumor studies. One percent of these children have one or more family members with this tumor.[25] The reported risk of Wilms tumor in the offspring of children who had unilateral tumors is less than 2%.[14]

Chromosomal deletion at locus 11p13 is frequently present in patients with Wilms tumor. The *WT1* gene has been isolated from this region and is implicated in a predisposition to developing Wilms tumor.[25] A second WT locus, *WT2*, has been mapped to 11p15. Patients with Beckwith-Wiedemann syndrome have a predisposition to develop embryonic tumors including Wilms tumor. The gene associated with Beckwith-Weidemann also maps to 11p15 locus.[9] Approximately 20% of these tumors have loss of the long arm of chromosome 16. Loss of heterozygosity of 16q may have prognostic significance and has been associated with poor overall survival.[19] Mutations of *p53* have been found in tumors with favorable histology and anaplasia; currently, it is not known whether *p53* alterations are molecular markers for a poor outcome.[9] It is hoped that rapid progress in identifying both genetic and epigenetic alterations will provide a better understanding of the disease and identify significant prognostic factors.[14]

CLINICAL PRESENTATION

The most common initial presenting sign of Wilms tumor is an asymptomatic abdominal mass in a well-appearing child. A family member may detect the mass while dressing or bathing the child, or a physician or advanced practice nurse may palpate an abdominal mass during a routine visit.[19] Some children experience abdominal pain, microscopic or gross hematuria, malaise, fever, or hypertension. Hypertension is present in 25% of all cases and is attributed to an increase in renin activity.[11] Wilms tumor may also present with anorexia, vomiting, hemorrhage, abdominal enlargement, hypotension, and anemia.[14,19]

Wilms tumor is a firm flank mass, usually confined to one side of the abdomen. It is important to note the location and size of the abdominal mass and the presence of associated genitourinary abnormalities such as hypospadias or cryptorchidism, or other anomalies such as aniridia, macroglossia, or hemihypertrophy. A varicocele, secondary to obstruction of the spermatic vein, may be associated with tumor thrombosis in the renal vein or inferior vena cava.[19]

DIAGNOSTIC EVALUATION

Any child with a suspicious abdominal tumor needs an immediate and thorough evaluation. An abdominal ultrasound examination is generally the initial study used to detect a solid or cystic renal mass, tumor thrombus in renal veins, or abnormali-

TABLE 26-1	CONGENITAL ANOMALIES IN 3,442 PATIENTS REGISTERED BY THE NATIONAL WILMS TUMOR STUDY GROUP FROM 1969 TO 1985

Anomaly (per 1,000)	Number of Patients	Prevalence (per 1,000)
Aniridia	26	7.6
Hemihypertrophy	112	32.6
Cryptorchidism	53	32.7*
Hypospadias	37	22.8*
Other genital anomalies	24	7.0

From Pizzo, P. A., & Poplack, D. G. (Eds.). (1997). *Principles and practice of pediatric oncology* (3rd ed.). Philadelphia: Lippincott-Raven.
*Rates for males only.

TABLE 26-2	FAMILIAL VERSUS SPORADIC WILMS TUMOR	
	Percent Affected	
Patient Feature	Familial (N = 93)	Sporadic (N = 6438)
Female	49.5	52.3
Aniridia	3.2	0.7
Cryptorchidism	5.4	2.3
Beckwith-Wiedemann syndrome	3.2	0.9
Hemihypertrophy	5.4	3.1

From Breslow, N. E., Olson J., Mohsness J., et al. (1996). Familial Wilms' tumor: A descriptive study. *Medical and Pediatric Oncology, 27,* 398.

TABLE 26-3	SCREENING FOR WILMS TUMOR (WT) IN HIGH-RISK INDIVIDUALS		
Syndrome	Radiologic Evaluation	Physician Evaluation	Molecular Evaluation
Hemihypertrophy/ Beckwith-Wiedemann syndrome	Baseline CT scan at age 6 months Ultrasonography every 3 months until age 7 years	Physical examinations every 6 months through completion of growth	Uniparental disomy studies of 11p15
WAGR (Wilms tumor, aniridia, genitourinary abnormalities, mental retardation)	Baseline CT scan at diagnosis Ultrasonography every 3 months until age 7 years	Physical examinations every 6 months through completion of growth	Molecular evaluation of 11p13
DDS (Denys-Drash syndrome)	Baseline CT scan at 6 to 12 months of age Ultrasonography every 3 months until age 6 years	Physical examinations every 6 months until age 8 years	Molecular evaluation of 11p13
Aniridia	—	—	Molecular evaluation of the WAGR region of 11p13

From Clericuzio, O. L., D'Angio, G. L., Duncan, M., et al. (1993). Summary and recommendations: First International Conference on Clinical and Molecular Genetics of Childhood Renal Tumors. *Medical and Pediatric Oncology, 21*, 223.

ties of the inferior vena cava. The size of the mass, involvement of the contralateral kidney, and the presence of an extrarenal mass are also determined by ultrasonography.

Contrast-enhanced computed tomography (CT) and magnetic resonance imaging (MRI) of the abdomen will provide a more detailed picture of the extent of the Wilms tumor. Direct extension through the renal capsule and lymphatic vessels is a common route of extrarenal spread. Regional lymph nodes and the vena cava may be involved.[14] The most common site of distant metastasis is the lung, followed by the liver.[19] A chest x-ray is done preoperatively to detect any lung metastasis. However, a chest CT may reveal lesions not seen on chest x-ray. A lung biopsy may be obtained to confirm the presence of pulmonary disease.[17] A bone scan and skeletal survey are obtained in children with clear cell sarcoma of the kidney or in children suspected of having metastatic disease to bone. Brain imaging using CT scan or MRI is performed in all children with clear cell sarcoma or rhabdoid tumor of the kidney because metastasis to the brain is common.[14]

Laboratory work includes a complete blood count with differential and platelet count, liver and renal function tests, and urinalysis. Serum calcium levels may be elevated in patients with mesoblastic nephroma or rhabdoid tumor of the kidney.[15]

Wilms tumors are usually solitary, encapsulated, spherical masses that may reach considerable size before they are detected. The lesions are often vascular, gelatinous, and necrotic in the center with a bulging uniformly tan or gray-white appearance.[14,19] The majority of Wilms tumors are unicentric lesions, which may arise multifocally within the kidney. There are no data to suggest Wilms tumor occurs more frequently in the right or left kidney.[14]

Wilms tumor is characterized by histopathologic diversity. These tumors are thought to be composed of, or derived from, primitive metanephric blastema, a precursor of differentiated stromal and epithelial cells. Classic Wilms tumor is composed of persistent blastema, dysplastic tubules, and supporting mesenchyma or stroma.[19] *Nephroblastomatosis* is a term used to denote the diffuse or multifocal presence of nephrogenic rests or their recognized derivatives. A nephrogenic rest is a focus of abnormally persistent nephrogenic cells significant in the pathogenesis of Wilms tumor.[2] They take the form of small, usually microscopic clusters of blastemal cells, tubules, or stromal cells usually in the periphery of the kidney. When multifocal precursor lesions are found in both kidneys, there is an increased likelihood of subsequent Wilms tumor formation in the remaining parenchyma.[14] Following the discovery of nephroblastomatosis in a kidney removed for treatment of Wilms tumor, it is important to continue to assess the contralateral kidney for evidence of Wilms tumor.

There are two general histologic types of Wilms tumor: favorable and unfavorable. Favorable histology Wilms tumor is derived from or composed of blastema tissue that is undifferentiated and found in primitive development.[1] These tumors represent about 85% of all Wilms tumor cases and have an excellent prognosis for long-term survival.[19]

Unfavorable histology tumors include Wilms tumors with poor differentiation or anaplasia. These tumors are more aggressive and have a less favorable prognosis than tumors with favorable histology. Anaplasia is either focal or diffuse and is present when cells have a nuclear diameter at least three times that of adjacent cells, marked hyperchromatism, and abnormal mitotic figures.[3,4]

Anaplastic Wilms tumors are rare in the first 2 years of life with a subsequent increased incidence of 13% in patients 5 years of age and older.[14] These anaplastic tumors are more frequently seen in black children compared to white children and are not correlated with stage.[14,19]

Other unfavorable histology tumors include the anaplastic or sarcomatous features seen in clear cell sarcoma and rhabdoid tumor of the kidney. These tumors are not Wilms tumor variants but are important kidney tumors associated with significantly higher rates of relapse and death. Clear cell sarcomas of the kidney metastasize to lung, bone, and brain.[12,24] Histologically, there are distinct varieties such as epithelioid, spindling, and cystic patterns.[16] Rhabdoid tumor of the kidney is a monomorphous tumor characterized by eosinophilic cytoplasm and large nuclei.[19] It occurs more frequently in male infants and in children less than 5 years of age.[14] The tumor is highly aggressive and metastasizes to lung and brain.[22]

Congenital mesoblastic nephroma is a renal neoplasm occurring predominantly in infant boys.[20] The tumor is characterized by bundles of spindle cells resembling fibroblasts or smooth muscle cells.[14,19] Most cases do well following nephrectomy alone, with a low incidence of local recurrence or distant metastases.

Renal cell carcinoma can occur in children at any age. The histologic appearance and clinical evolution of this tumor are similar to that experienced in adult patients.[21]

The most important determinant of prognosis of Wilms tumor is the histologic type. Lymph node involvement remains an important predictor of treatment failure.[14] Age at diagnosis, tumor size, and capsular or vascular invasion are less important prognostic indicators for tumor recurrence or progression.

TREATMENT

The National Wilms Tumor Study Group (NWTSG), established in 1969, represents the major cooperative group involved in the treatment and research of Wilms tumor in children. The results of organized clinical trials have led to continued improvement in survival and cure rates. Treatment is currently based on histology and clinicopathologic stage.

Many centers in Europe and Canada routinely employ preoperative therapy for children with Wilms tumor.[14] In this country, preoperative therapy is reserved for patients with bilateral disease, unresectable tumors, or those with extensive vena caval thrombus or intravascular extension.[14,19] Although pretreatment makes tumor removal easier and decreases the risk of surgical complications, it does result in the loss of important staging information.[14]

Surgery plays a prominent role in the initial treatment and proper staging of Wilms tumor. The surgeon's responsibility is to completely remove the primary tumor without causing rupture of the capsule and to accurately assess tumor spread for proper staging.[19,25] A generous transabdominal-transperitoneal approach allows thorough inspection of the intraabdominal contents, including the contralateral kidney to rule out bilateral involvement. The liver, renal hilar, and paraaortic lymph nodes are inspected and a biopsy is performed if nodes appear suspicious. Lymph node sampling is imperative and suspicious nodes are excised, although radical lymph node dissection is not recommended. The walls of both the renal vein and artery are inspected for invasion or thrombosis. The tumor is removed entirely without disrupting the capsule.[19] The NWTS clinicopathologic staging system is detailed in Table 26-4.

Radiation therapy is not necessary for patients with stage I favorable histology, stage I anaplastic, or stage II favorable histology disease when chemotherapy includes vincristine plus dactinomycin. Stage III favorable histology patients benefit from the addition of doxorubicin to the two-drug combination of vincristine and dactinomycin and abdominal irradiation. Stage IV favorable histology patients receive vincristine, dactinomycin, and doxorubicin in addition to abdominal and whole lung irradiation. Adding cyclophosphamide may benefit patients with stage II to IV disease with diffuse anaplasia.[19] Patients with malignant rhabdoid tumor of the kidney have a poor prognosis despite three- or four-drug regimens.[18]

A clinical trial through the NWTSG evaluated treatment with either single or divided-dose administration of dactinomycin or doxorubicin, both given in combination with vincristine. The findings show that a single intensive dose of chemotherapy is just as effective as the standard 3- or 5-day regimen, when both are administered in combination

TABLE 26-4	NATIONAL WILMS TUMOR STUDY CLINICOPATHOLOGIC STAGING SYSTEM
Stage	**Characteristics**
Stage I	Tumor limited to kidney and completely excised. The surface of the renal capsule is intact. Tumor was not ruptured before or during removal. There is no residual tumor apparent beyond the margins of resection.
Stage II	Tumor extends beyond the kidney but is completely removed. There is regional extension of the tumor (i.e., penetration through the outer surface of the renal capsule into the perirenal soft tissues). Vessels outside the kidney substance are inflated or contain tumor thrombus. A biopsy of the tumor may have been taken or there has been local spillage of tumor confined to the flank. There is no residual tumor apparent at or beyond the margins of excision.
Stage III	Residual nonhematogenous tumor confined to the abdomen: 1. Lymph nodes on biopsy are found to be involved in the hilus, the periaortic chains, or beyond. 2. There has been diffuse peritoneal contamination by tumor, such as spillage of tumor beyond the flank before or during surgery or tumor growth that has penetrated through the peritoneal surface. 3. Implants are found on the peritoneal surface. 4. The tumor extends beyond the surgical margins either microscopically or grossly. 5. The tumor is not completely resectable because of local infiltration into vital structures.
Stage IV	Hematogenous metastases. Deposits beyond stage III (e.g., lung, liver, bone, and/or brain).
Stage V	Bilateral renal involvement at diagnosis. An attempt should be made to stage each side according to the previous criteria on the basis of the extent of disease before biopsy.

From Green, G. M., D'Angio, G. L., Beckwith, J. B., et al. (1996). Wilms' tumor. *CA: A Cancer Journal for Clinicians, 46,* 46.

with other chemotherapy agents. Studies also show that simultaneous administration of maximum tolerated doses of chemotherapy at more frequent intervals is less toxic and more efficacious, and that shorter maintenance therapy may be adequate.[19] Single-dose, intensive drug administration is now recommended as the new standard of treatment based on efficacy, dose intensity, less severe hematologic toxicity, and fewer outpatient visits.[13,14]

Radiation therapy, when used, begins when the patient is stable postoperatively and has a satisfactory blood count. Doses are delivered to the tumor bed and the field is extended to include areas of known residual disease. The port is extended to cross the midline covering the entire vertebrae to prevent scoliosis. Flank irradiation is sufficient for children with tumor spill confined to the flank, but whole abdomen irradiation is advisable when peritoneal seeding occurred during surgery.[15] The total dose administered to the liver, spleen, and remaining kidney is limited to safe levels and the femoral heads are shielded to prevent growth retardation. Radiotherapy may be used in conjunction with surgery and chemotherapy to treat metastatic disease.

Bilateral Wilms tumor occurs in approximately 5% of children with Wilms tumor.[23] The goal of therapy for children who have bilateral disease is to eradicate all tumor, preserve as much normal renal tissue as possible, and decrease chronic renal failure. Treatment needs to be individualized.[14] Initially bilateral renal biopsy and staging of each kid-

ney is recommended, followed by chemotherapy. Reevaluation is done in 5 weeks to determine the ability to resect the disease and preserve renal function.[14,19] Survival rates remain high, but long-term follow-up is essential, because relapses occur as late as 5 years following treatment and renal failure is seen in approximately 5% of patients.[25]

Wilms tumor can recur in several sites, including lung, liver, opposite kidney, original tumor bed, other intraabdominal sites, and rarely bone and brain. (Figure 26-1).[15] Most relapses occur within the first 2 years after nephrectomy. Prognosis and treatment depend on the site of recurrence, histology, length of time from diagnosis to recurrence, and previous treatment.[14]

Among patients who relapse, prognosis is better for those children with isolated lung lesions, those treated previously with only dactinomycin and vincristine, those with abdominal relapse without prior abdominal radiation, and those who relapse more than 12 months after diagnosis. Children in the more favorable group are treated with conventional agents such as doxorubicin, surgical excision, and radiation, because they generally have a good response to retrieval therapy.[14]

Adverse prognostic factors at the time of relapse include a recurrence within 12 months of diagnosis, or after initial treatment with doxorubicin, or an abdominal relapse following radiation therapy treatment. These children have a poor prognosis and need a more aggressive approach. Response

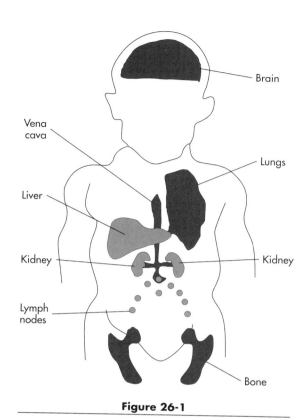

Brain

Vena cava

Lungs

Liver

Kidney

Kidney

Lymph nodes

Bone

Figure 26-1

Common sites of metastases associated with Wilms tumor. (From Rasco, C. [1998]. Tumors of the kidney. In M. J. Hockenberry-Eaton (Ed.), *Essentials of pediatric oncology nursing: A core curriculum* (pp. 41-45). Glenview, IL: Association of Pediatric Oncology Nurses.)

has been seen with single agents such as ifosfamide, etoposide, carboplatin, and cisplatin. Combination therapy with ifosfamide, mesna, and etoposide or combining cisplatin or carboplatin with etoposide is being evaluated. Very high dose chemotherapy followed by the infusion of autologous bone marrow is currently being studied. Referrals to centers conducting research on autologous bone marrow transplantation might be considered. If salvage attempts fail, patients may be offered treatment with available phase I or phase II studies or a no treatment option.[14]

PROGNOSIS

The NWTSG clinical trials have yielded therapeutic advances that have increased the long-term survival for children with Wilms tumor from 65% for those diagnosed in 1970 to 90% for those diagnosed in 1990.[19] Prognosis is related to the stage of disease, histopathologic features of the tumor, pa-

tient age, tumor size, and the team approach to treatment.[14,15] Children with nonmetastatic, favorable histology Wilms tumor and those patients with stage I anaplastic disease have survival rates of 90%.[19,28] Patients with either metastatic disease or unfavorable histology have survival rates of approximately 80% and patients with diffuse anaplasia and metastatic disease have a less favorable prognosis.[19] Children with rhabdoid tumor of the kidney have survival rates as high as 56%.[26]

NURSING IMPLICATIONS

Immediately after the initial diagnosis of Wilms tumor, parents are instructed to handle and bathe their child carefully to prevent trauma to the tumor. Additionally, health care professional abdominal examinations are kept to a minimum because manipulation of the tumor may cause the spread of malignant cells. Following the initial abdominal surgery, the potential for fatigue exists because chemotherapy is initiated immediately. Treatment-related nausea and vomiting can alter nutritional status, necessitating use of oral, nasogastric, or parenteral supplements.[22] Patients are monitored for liver function abnormalities during chemotherapy and radiation therapy, and for prolonged constipation and neuropathy during extended vincristine therapy. Families who have familial or inherited Wilms tumor are offered genetic counseling.

The evaluation of treatment-related toxicity is an integral part of long-term follow-up for children with Wilms tumor. Hepatomegaly, elevation of liver enzymes, and thrombocytopenia have been seen in patients treated with radiation therapy and chemotherapy.[14] Patients who receive 20 Gy of whole-lung irradiation may experience reductions in total lung capacity and vital capacity.[19] Patients who receive doxorubicin may develop cardiomyopathy and arrhythmias.[19] Scoliosis and soft tissue underdevelopment occur frequently in patients treated with trunk irradiation.[14] Decreased renal function and creatinine clearance are observed in patients following nephrectomy and abdominal irradiation. Proteinuria and hypertension are seen in patients 10 to 20 years after nephrectomy, local irradiation, and chemotherapy.[19]

There is a cumulative risk of 1.6% for the development of second malignant neoplasms such as bone, breast, and thyroid cancers up to 15 years from diagnosis among patients entered in the NWTS.[5] The relative risk for the occurrence of a second malignant neoplasm increased in patients treated with radiation. This risk increased further in those patients treated with both doxorubicin and radiation.[19]

FUTURE DIRECTIONS

Approximately 85% of children with Wilms tumor will be cured with modern multimodality treatment.[14] The efforts of the NWTSG (now part of the Children's Oncology Group) and other collaborative pediatric oncology groups are directed to intensifying treatment for patients with poor prognostic features and reducing treatment for those with standard risk features.[9] Gene identification conferring susceptibility to Wilms tumor, such as aniridia, cryptorchidism, and hypospadias will allow more precise genetic counseling and surveillance in the future.[9,14] The ability to detect chromosomal and molecular genetic abnormalities in tumor cells holds promise for identifying high-risk individuals. It is hoped this will provide more effective, less toxic treatment, and improve methods for prevention. Research in epidemiology and molecular biology will provide a better understanding of the malignant process and potential directions for future clinical trials.[15]

The progress that has been made in treating Wilms tumor is the very essence of the hopeful story of childhood cancer. Despite these advancements, the economic, physical, and psychosocial impacts of Wilms tumor during childhood remain substantial and have increased importance as more children are cured. Wilms tumor survivors must be carefully followed to address treatment-related effects of therapy and complications with immediate intervention to ensure the best quality of life.

REFERENCES

1. Beckwith, J. B. (1986). Wilms tumor and other renal tumors of childhood: An update. *Journal of Urology, 136,* 320-324.
2. Beckwith, J. B., Kiviat, N. B., & Bonadio, J. F. (1990). Nephrogenic rests nephroblastomatosis and the pathogenesis of Wilms tumor. *Pediatric Pathology, 10,* 1-36.
3. Beckwith, J. B., & Palmer, N. F. (1978). Histopathology and prognosis of Wilms tumor. *Cancer, 41,* 1937-1948.
4. Bonadio, J. F., Storer, B., Norkool, P., et al. (1985). Anaplastic Wilms' tumor: Clinical and pathologic studies. *Journal of Clinical Oncology, 3,* 513-520.
5. Breslow, N., Olshan, A., Beckwith, J. B., et al. (1993). Epidemiology of Wilms tumor. *Medical and Pediatric Oncology, 21,* 172-181.
6. Breslow, N., Olshan, A., Beckwith, J. B., et al. (1994). Ethnic variation in the incidence, diagnosis, prognosis and follow-up of children with Wilms tumor. *Journal of the National Cancer Institute, 86,* 49-51.
7. Breslow, N., Olson, J., Moksness, J., et al. (1996). Familial Wilms tumor: A descriptive study. *Medical and Pediatric Oncology, 27,* 398-403.
8. Clericuzio, C. L., D'Angio, G. L., Duncan, M., et al. (1993). Summary and recommendations: First International Conference on Clinical and Molecular Genetics of Childhood Renal Tumors. *Medical and Pediatric Oncology, 21,* 223-236.
9. Coppes, M. J., Haber, D. A., & Grundy, P. E. (1994). Genetic events in the development of Wilms tumor. *The New England Journal of Medicine, 331,* 586-590.
10. Crist, W. M., & Kun, L. E. (1991). Common solid tumors of childhood. *The New England Journal of Medicine, 324,* 461-471.
11. Ganguly, A., Gribble, J., Tune, B., et al. (1973). Renin secreting Wilms tumor with severe hypertension: Report of a case and brief review of renin-secreting tumors. *Annals of Internal Medicine, 79,* 835-837.
12. Green, D. M., Breslow, N. E., Beckwith, J. B., et al. (1994). The treatment of children with clear cell sarcoma of the kidney: A report from the National Wilms' Tumor Study Group. *Journal of Clinical Oncology, 12,* 2132-2137.
13. Green, D. M., Breslow, N. E., Beckwith, J. B., et al. (1998). Effect of duration of treatment on treatment outcome and cost of treatment for Wilms tumor: A report from the National Wilms Tumor Study Group. *Journal of Clinical Oncology, 16,* 3744-3751.
14. Green, D. M., Coppes, M. J., Breslow, N. E., et al. (1997). Wilms tumor. In P. A. Pizzo, & D. G. Poplack (Eds.), *Principles and practice of pediatric oncology* (3rd ed., pp. 733-759). Philadelphia: Lippincott-Raven.
15. Green, D. M., D'Angio, G. J., Beckwith, J. B., et al. (1996). Wilms tumor. *CA: A Cancer Journal for Clinicians, 46,* 46-63.
16. Haas, J. E., Bonadio, J. F., & Beckwith, J. B. (1984). Clear cell sarcoma of kidney with emphasis on ultrastructural studies. *Cancer, 54,* 2978-2987.
17. Meisel, J. A., Guthrie, K. A., Breslow, N. E., et al. (1999). Significance and management of computed tomography detected pulmonary nodules: A report from the National Wilms Tumor Study Group. *International Journal of Radiation Oncology and Biology Physicians, 44,* 579-585.
18. Palmer, N. F., & Sutow, W. (1983). Clinical aspects of the rhabdoid tumor of the kidney: A report from the National Wilms Tumor Study Group. *Medical and Pediatric Oncology, 11,* 242-245.
19. Petruzzi, M. J., & Green, D. M. (1997). Wilms Tumor. *Pediatric Clinics of North America, 44,* 939-952.
20. Pettinato, G., Manivel, J. C., Wick, M. R., et al. (1989). Classical and cellular (atypical) congenital mesoblastic nephroma: A clinicopathologic, ultrastructural, immunohistochemical, and flow cytometric study. *Human Pathology, 20,* 682-690.
21. Raney, R. B., Jr., Palmer, N., Sutow, W., et al. (1983). Renal cell carcinoma in children. *Medical and Pediatric Oncology, 11,* 91-98.
22. Rasco, C. (1998). Tumors of the kidney. In M. J. Hockenberry-Eaton (Ed.), *Essentials of pediatric oncology nursing: A core curriculum* (pp. 41-45). Glenview, IL: Association of Pediatric Oncology Nurses.
23. Ritchey, M. L., Haase, G. M., & Shochat, S. (1993). Current management of Wilms tumor. *Seminars in Surgical Oncology, 9,* 502-509.
24. Schmidt, D., & Beckwith, B. (1995). Histopathology of childhood renal tumors. *Hematology Oncology Clinics of North America, 9,* 1179-1199.
25. Shochat, S. (1993). Wilms tumor: Diagnosis and treatment in the 1990's. *Seminars in Pediatric Surgery, 2,* 59-68.
26. Weeks, D. A., Beckwith, J. B., Mierau, G. W., et al. (1989). Rhabdoid tumor of the kidney. *American Journal of Surgical Pathology, 13,* 439-458.
27. Wilms, M. (1899). Die Mischgeschwuelste der Niere. Leipzig: Verlag von A. Georgi.
28. Zuppan, C. W., Beckwith, J. B., & Luckey, D. W. (1988). Anaplasia in unilateral Wilms tumor: A report from the National Wilms Tumor Study Pathology Center. *Human Pathology, 19,* 1199-1209.

27

Bone Tumors

Donna L. Betcher
Pamela J. Simon
Kim M. McHard

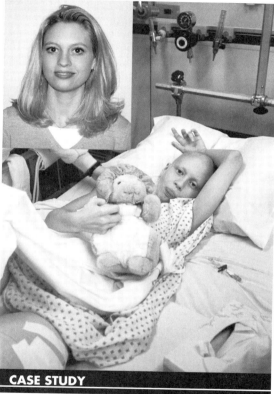

CASE STUDY

Sarah is a 14-year-old girl who experienced pain in her left knee for 3 months and swelling over the knee 1 month before diagnosis. She was an active teenager and first noticed the pain while participating in gym class. Neither she nor her parents could recall any specific injury related to the leg. When she could no longer participate in gym classes, Sarah went to see an orthopedic surgeon. An x-ray revealed a destructive lesion in the left proximal femur.

She was then referred to a specialist in musculoskeletal and orthopedic cancers. A magnetic resonance imaging (MRI) scan of the left femur, computed tomography (CT) exam of the chest, and bone scan were completed and correlated with the plain x-ray film. The tests revealed a 6×5×9 cm lesion of the left distal femur consistent with an osteosarcoma. No metastatic disease was detected. An open biopsy was performed that confirmed the diagnosis of osteoblastic osteosarcoma.

Sarah was referred to the pediatric oncology department as soon as the pathologist confirmed the final diagnosis. The multidisciplinary team consisted of physicians, advanced practice nurses, nurses, dieticians, social workers, child life specialists, physical therapists, educational specialists, and psychologists who followed Sarah and gave her and her family support as needed.

The pediatric oncologist and the orthopedic cancer specialist discussed the diagnosis and treatment with Sarah and her parents, beginning with surgery. Because Sarah was skeletally mature, a custom-made internal prosthesis was one surgical option. The other options for her included a rotationplasty or a high thigh amputation. These choices were discussed with her. Sarah indicated an interest in the custom-made internal prosthesis to replace her knee even though she would no longer be able to participate in activities that included running or jumping. The prosthesis took 6 to 8 weeks to manufacture. This process was started within the first week of the diagnosis. The advanced practice nurse showed Sarah videotapes of other patients who had these surgeries to help her make the decision.

The patient and family agreed to participate in the Children's Cancer Group protocol. Consent forms were signed, and chemotherapy was started after a central line was placed. The chemotherapy protocol consisted of high-dose methotrexate and doxorubicin with cyclophosphamide.

After the first 3 months of chemotherapy, the musculoskeletal oncologist and advanced practice nurse saw Sarah in preparation for surgery. An MRI of the left knee, bone scan, CT of the chest, and plain x-ray films were repeated. The lesion in the femur had decreased in size and the swelling of the left knee had resolved. No distant metastases were noted. The custom prosthesis was ready and surgery was planned when the blood counts recovered from week 12 chemotherapy.

Sarah's surgery was completed with no complications. Her postoperative physical therapy began immediately after surgery when she began using a continuous passive motion (CPM) machine. Transfer and weight-bearing activities were tolerated well. She was walking with no external aids 8 weeks after surgery.

Sarah resumed chemotherapy treatments 3 weeks after surgery when the incisions were healed. During the last 6 months of chemotherapy, she had problems with anorexia and was admitted for fever and neutropenia episodes. She had also previously experienced hair loss, nausea, vomiting, and decreased blood counts. She finished chemotherapy and her off therapy scans revealed no local recurrence, no metastases, and no complications with the prosthesis.

She has been followed closely since completing therapy with increasing intervals as each year passes. She volunteered to be videotaped so she could help other patients who are diagnosed with osteosarcoma in the future. She is engaged to be married and graduates from college this spring.

This chapter addresses primary malignant tumors that arise within or on bone surface, in contrast to metastatic or secondary bone tumors in which the primary cancer originates elsewhere and advances to bone. Metastatic bone lesions are uncommon in pediatrics,[5] but primary malignant bone tumors account for approximately 5% of all childhood malignancies. The majority of bone tumors occur in the decade between 10 and 20 years of age. The major bone tumors are osteogenic sarcoma, which accounts for 60% of the cases, and Ewing's sarcoma, which comprises 30%.[15] A variety of miscellaneous rare tumors make up the remaining 10%.

OSTEOGENIC SARCOMA

Osteogenic sarcoma, also known as *osteosarcoma*, is a malignant tumor of the bone derived from bone-forming mesenchyme. It is characterized by the production of osteoid tissue or immature bone by the malignant proliferating cellular stroma.[15] The most common primary sites are the long bones (usually at the metaphyses), although diaphyseal primary sites are well described. Osteogenic sarcoma is rare in the small bones of hands and feet, and rarely occurs distal to the elbow or ankle (Figure 27-1).

EPIDEMIOLOGY

Osteogenic sarcoma accounts for approximately 60% of the malignant bone tumors in children less than 15 years of age and occurs at a rate of 5.6 cases per million. There is a lower rate in blacks than in whites. It has a peak incidence during the second decade of life.[32] Although the etiology is unknown, there is a suggested causal relationship

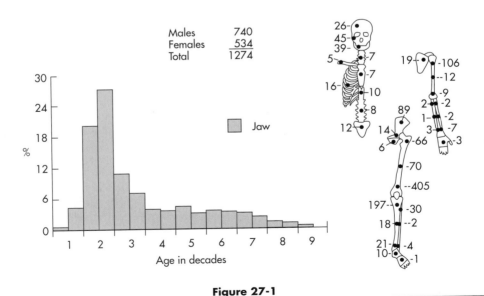

Figure 27-1

Age, sex, and skeletal site distribution of osteosarcomas. (From Dahlin, D. C., & Unni, K. K. [1986]. Osteosarcoma. In *Bone tumors* [4th ed.] Rochester, MN: Mayo Foundation.)

between adolescent growth spurts and other periods of rapid growth with the development of this malignancy. The evidence supporting this casual relationship includes: (1) children with osteogenic sarcoma are taller than their age peers and taller than patients with nonosseous malignancies, (2) osteogenic sarcomas occur at an earlier age in females corresponding to the more advanced skeletal age and earlier adolescent growth spurts in females than males, (3) before the adolescent years, the incidence of osteogenic sarcoma in boys and girls is equal, after which the incidence in males continues to increase but a plateau is reached in girls, and (4) large breeds of dogs have much greater chance of developing osteogenic sarcoma than do small breeds.[7] The increased risk of osteosarcoma in adolescent males may be related to the larger volume of bone formation during the longer growth spurt.[32] Osteogenic sarcomas occur most often in rapidly growing bones of the distal femur, proximal tibia, and proximal humerus[5] (Figure 27-1). Trauma has been associated with bone tumors in children, but rather than causing the tumor, the injury brings the patient to a medical facility where radiographs coincidentally reveal the neoplasm.

There are some genetic factors associated with osteogenic sarcoma, particularly the retinoblastoma gene *(RB)* and *p53*. It is well established that patients who have a germline mutation of the tumor suppressor *RB* have an increased risk of developing osteogenic sarcoma. Because of this association, investigators have assessed *RB* abnormalities in nonretinoblastoma, osteogenic sarcoma patients. Many abnormalities were identified with up to 63% of patients demonstrating loss of heterozygosity at the *RB* locus. This loss of heterozygosity coupled with DNA alterations of the gene are correlated with a poor prognosis.[33]

Abnormalities of another tumor suppressor gene, *p53,* have been identified in a wide range of malignancies, including osteogenic sarcoma. The presence of germline *p53* mutations is low in osteogenic sarcoma patients, about 3%. In some instances, these *p53* mutations occurred in patients with a history of cancer in first-degree relatives; occasionally osteogenic sarcoma was part of a family with Li-Fraumeni syndrome.[22]

Radiation-induced sarcoma may develop from exposure to dosages higher than 30 Gy.[7] This is the only environmental agent associated with the development of osteosarcoma and is implicated in 3% of cases.[7]

CLINICAL PRESENTATION

The patient with osteogenic sarcoma most frequently has pain over the affected area with or with-

out associated soft tissue mass. The pain is usually exacerbated with activity, and weight bearing may cause a limp. Irritability, crying, decreased movement, limping, or refusing to walk may indicate pain in the young child. Local edema, tenderness, decreased range of motion, redness, and occasionally a pulsation or bruits are found on examination. Older children are usually able to pinpoint the source of pain accurately. The duration of signs and symptoms may be short, although symptoms of 6 months duration or longer are not uncommon.

At diagnosis, 10% to 20% of patients will have metastases.[25] By far the most common site of metastatic disease is the lung, although a small fraction of patients may have bone, pleural, kidney, adrenal gland, brain, and pericardial metastases.

A number of distinct histologic subtypes have been noted. One subclassification of conventional osteosarcoma is based on the predominant cell type (osteoblastic, chondroblastic, fibroblastic)[32] (Box 27-1). Another subclassification is an unusual variant called *telangiectatic* and accounts for approximately 3% of all osteogenic sarcomas.[32] A third group of low grade, less aggressive osteosarcomas includes the parosteal and periosteal varieties, which arise on the surface of the bone without involvement of the marrow cavity. These are treated with surgical resection only and usually do not receive chemotherapy.[5]

DIAGNOSTIC EVALUATION

Evaluation of the child with a suspected bone tumor begins with a history, physical examination, and radiographic evaluations. Plain films of the primary site and the chest are initially obtained. The presence of metastases at diagnosis is an important prognostic variable.[19] Therefore, MRI and/or CT of the primary tumor are indicated to determine the extent of local disease. A total body bone scan and a CT of the chest are necessary to detect skip lesions and metastatic pulmonary nodules before biopsy. Skip lesions are tumor deposits in the affected bones

---

BOX 27-1

HISTOLOGIC SUBTYPES OF OSTEOGENIC SARCOMA

Conventional
  Osteoblastic
  Chondroblastic
  Fibroblastic
Telangiectatic
Parosteal and periosteal
Multifocal
Miscellaneous

that are separated from the primary tumor by several centimeters of normal bone. Although history, physical examination, and radiographic evaluations may suggest osteogenic sarcoma, an open biopsy is required to confirm the diagnosis and determine histologic features and the cell type.

Physiologic evaluation of cardiovascular, pulmonary, renal, hepatic, and auditory organ function will be done before the initiation of the intensive chemotherapy used to treat osteosarcoma. Studies will typically include a complete blood count with differential, erythrocyte sedimentation rate, liver chemistries to include alkaline phosphatase, lactate dehydrogenase (LDH), electrolytes, and glomerular filtration rate (GFR) or creatinine clearance to evaluate renal function. Patients will need a baseline cardiac evaluation to include multigaited angiography (MUGA) or echocardiogram. An audiogram to evaluate hearing is also obtained.

TREATMENT

Surgery, the mainstay of treatment, is discussed later in the chapter. Although surgery usually controls the primary tumor, more than 80% of patients with osteogenic sarcoma treated with surgery alone develop metastatic disease.[13,21] Chemotherapy plays an important role in the treatment of osteosarcoma. With the use of modern chemotherapy, survival rates of 65% to 75% are common.[19] The use of preoperative and postoperative chemotherapy has an irrefutably positive impact on the natural history of osteogenic sarcoma and is now a component of treatment for all children with these bone tumors.[25] The regimens contain combinations of the following drugs: high-dose methotrexate, doxorubicin, ifosfamide, and cisplatin (Box 27-2).

In the past decade, the role of preoperative chemotherapy has been evaluated. The amount of tumor necrosis at the time of definitive surgery is of prognostic significance and may influence dosages and length of postoperative chemotherapy.[16] After surgery it is important to balance the need to resume chemotherapy with wound healing require-

ments. Chemotherapy can usually be restarted 2 to 3 weeks after surgery.

With only 65% long-term survival, new chemotherapeutic agents and new methods to administer standard drugs must be evaluated to improve survival. Chemotherapy delivered intraarterially into the tumor, providing localized perfusion and producing maximal concentration of the drug to the tumor without the same degree of side effects of comparable intravenous chemotherapy, has been investigated. This method has been most effective using drugs with a short half-life such as doxorubicin and cisplatin, as single agents or in combination with intravenous therapy. Results indicate improved local control and better ability to use limb-sparing surgery than with intravenous therapy, but no increase in survival.[17]

Osteogenic sarcoma is highly radiation resistant and therefore unresponsive to conventional dose radiotherapy. High doses of radiation have been associated with only transient tumor control. If the tumor is judged unresectable because of its location, radiation may become part of the primary therapy, sometimes making resections possible. Radiation is useful for the palliation of pain from local recurrences or metastases.

PROGNOSIS

The prognosis for children with osteogenic sarcoma continues to improve. Two thirds of the patients who do not have metastases may be cured.[18] Improved chemotherapy regimens and advances in surgical techniques leading to less radical surgery have improved the quality of life for survivors of osteosarcoma. The most significant prognostic factors in children with osteosarcoma are the presence of metastases at diagnosis and the ability to completely resect the primary.[1,13] Only 10% to 20% of the children or adolescents who have metastatic disease at diagnosis will survive.[19] Tumors arising in certain axial skeletal sites (e.g., skull, vertebrae) have a poorer prognosis because they are not amenable to complete resection. In general, appendicular primary sites are associated with more favorable prognosis.[15]

Other characteristics associated with prognosis are tumor size, patient age, patient gender, alkaline phosphatase level, histology, and lactase dehydrogenase (LDH) level. The smaller the tumor is at diagnosis, the more favorable the prognosis, with a size greater than 15 cm in diameter associated with poor prognosis.[27] It also appears that children less than 10 years of age fare worse and patients older than 10 years have a better prognosis.[27] Females also have a more favorable outcome than males. Histologically the telangiectatic variant is associ-

BOX 27-2
CHEMOTHERAPY FOR BONE SARCOMAS

OSTEOGENIC SARCOMA	EWING'S SARCOMA
Doxorubicin	Doxorubicin
Cisplatin	Dactinomycin
Methotrexate— high dose	Vincristine
Ifosfamide	Ifosfamide
Etoposide	Etoposide
	Cyclophosphamide

ated with a worse outcome. An elevated LDH level can be considered a poor prognostic factor.[2] Four years from diagnosis, the projected disease-free survival for patients with an elevated LDH level at diagnosis was 32%, compared to 67% for patients with a normal LDH level at diagnosis.[1,19] Complete elimination of viable tumor after presurgical chemotherapy confers a very favorable prognosis.[18]

METASTASES

Osteogenic sarcoma most commonly metastasizes to the lungs. More unusually, other bones may be affected. Metastases can be detected at diagnosis, can be preceded by local disease recurrence, or can occur within the first 24 to 36 months after diagnosis. Rarely, metastatic disease appears 5 to 10 years posttreatment.[5]

The appearance of metastatic disease is often a grave prognostic sign, especially if disease is evident at presentation[26] or develops after initiation of chemotherapy.[21] Aggressive treatment is required to maximize opportunities for long-term control. Complete surgical resection of all overt metastatic lesions is essential. When the lung is the only site of recurrence, and the metastatic lesions are resectable, children may be cured by pulmonary resection alone.[18]

When widely metastatic disease is present, a systemic approach is necessary. The use of chemotherapy with or without radiotherapy is unlikely to produce a complete response, but the lesions may respond sufficiently to allow full resection at a later date with a chance of long-term control.

Patients with metastatic bone lesions have little hope of cure unless the bone lesions can be controlled with surgical removal. For patients with unresectable bone metastases, the approach is palliative. Radiation and chemotherapy rarely produce complete response; however, their treatments may shrink the tumor enough to allow surgical resection. The patient's quality of life may also be improved by reducing the size of the tumor and decreasing symptoms such as pain.

EWING'S SARCOMA

Originally described by James Ewing in 1921,[9] Ewing's sarcoma is a primitive malignant tumor of the bone characterized by uniform, densely packed small cells, with round nuclei but without distinctive cytoplasmic borders of the prominent nucleoli.[14] Ewing originally thought the tumor to be of endothelial origin but recent evidence suggests a neural origin.[14] Although Ewing's sarcoma is pri-

marily a tumor of the bone, it can also arise in soft tissue. The Ewing's family of tumors includes Ewing's sarcoma of the bone, extraosseous Ewing's sarcoma, and peripheral primitive neuroectodermal tumor (PPNET) or neuroepithelioma.[14]

EPIDEMIOLOGY

Ewing's sarcoma, a highly malignant tumor of the bone, can occur in any bone of the skeleton but is often seen in the extremities and pelvis with an associated infiltration of the soft tissue around the primary site. Ewing's sarcoma is rare in children less than 5 years of age and in adults older than 30 years. Ninety percent of all Ewing's sarcomas occur in patients less than 30 years of age, and 70% are diagnosed in patients less than 20 years of age[12] (Figure 27-2). There is a slight predominance in boys during adolescence; although there is no difference in incidence related to gender in prepubertal children. Ewing's sarcoma represents approximately 1% of all childhood cancers and 30% of all pediatric malignant bone tumors.[24] There is a very low incidence of Ewing's sarcoma in black and Chinese children.[12] White children younger than 15 years of age have an incidence of 1.7 cases per million per year in the United States.[14] There are no known patterns of hereditary transmission. Recent findings suggest that the reciprocal translocation of chromosomes 11 and 22 is common.[5] There may be a history of trauma, but as with osteosarcoma, the bone injury is the event that brings attention to the malignant lesion.

CLINICAL PRESENTATION

Although it may arise in any bone, Ewing's sarcoma most commonly affects bones of the femur, pelvis, tibia, and humerus. For example, a report of Ewing's sarcoma showed the primary site was the femur in 27%, the pelvis in 18%, and the tibia and fibula in 17% of cases.[28] Unlike osteogenic sarcoma, which most commonly arises in long bones in the extremities, Ewing's sarcoma more frequently involves the axial skeleton. Symptoms are often present for several months before diagnosis and may be intermittent, contributing to the difficulty in establishing a diagnosis.

The most common symptoms are pain and swelling with increasing intensity in the soft tissue around the affected bone. Patients with metastatic disease may exhibit systemic symptoms such as anorexia, fever, malaise, fatigue, and weight loss. Other symptoms are related to the site of the sarcoma. For example, patients with vertebral lesions may exhibit nerve root symptoms, and those with sacral lesions may exhibit a neurogenic bladder.

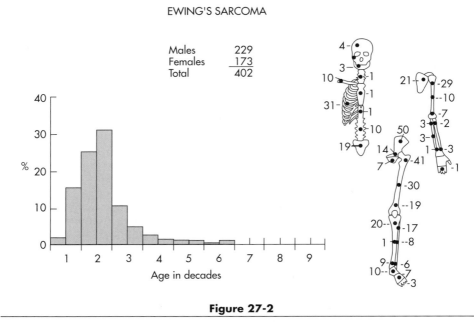

Figure 27-2

Age, sex, and skeletal site distribution of Ewing's sarcoma.   (From Dahlin, D. C., & Unni, K. K. [1986]. Osteosarcoma. In *Bone tumors* [4th ed.] Rochester, MN: Mayo Foundation.)

DIAGNOSTIC EVALUATION

The differential diagnosis of Ewing's sarcoma in the past included all common tumors in childhood that occur in a primitive or undifferentiated form. Small, round blue cell tumors of childhood include Ewing's sarcoma, primary bone tumors, rhabdomyosarcoma, lymphoma, metastatic neuroblastoma, and primitive neuroectodermal tumors. Ewing's sarcoma was therefore a diagnosis of exclusion. No unique morphologic markers were available. Recent evidence from cytogenetics, immunocytochemical, molecular genetics, and reverse transcriptase polymerase chain reaction investigations indicates a neural crest origin for Ewing's sarcoma.[14,27] Differences in histogenesis between Ewing's sarcoma and other tumors are now determined by cytogenetic protooncogene, histopathologic, ultrastructural, and immunophenotyping data. It has also been found that Ewing's sarcoma and other tumors in the Ewing's sarcoma family express a consistent reciprocal translocation t(11;22)(q24;q12).[24] This chromosomal translocation is present in 88% to 95% of tumors within the Ewing's sarcoma family.[24]

The initial diagnostic biopsy is a crucial component in the evaluation of Ewing's sarcoma because of the difficulties of establishing a correct diagnosis. Attention must be paid to obtaining sufficient histology and culture material because osteomy-elitis is part of the differential diagnosis.[8,28] Because 10% to 30% of patients have metastatic disease at the time of diagnosis, the initial workup includes evaluation for metastases. Ewing's tumors "easily breach compartmental barriers" and so the search for metastatic disease is broad.[5] Clinical evaluation includes MRI and CT imaging of the primary tumor, chest x-ray films, CT scan of the chest, bone scan, and bilateral bone marrow aspirates and biopsies. Metastases may be found in the lung, other bones, or the bone marrow. Physiologic evaluation of cardiovascular, pulmonary, renal, and hepatic organ function is done before the initiation of intensive chemotherapy and radiotherapy. Studies typically include complete blood count (CBC) with differential, erythrocyte sedimentation rate, liver chemistries to include alkaline phosphatase, LDH, electrolytes, and glomerular filtration rate (GFR) or creatinine clearance to evaluate renal function. Patients will need a baseline cardiac evaluation to include MUGA or echocardiogram.

TREATMENT

Chemotherapy is considered the cornerstone of treatment for Ewing's sarcoma.[1] Surgery and/or radiation therapy are important local control measures. Complete surgical removal of the primary tumor should be performed if feasible and if it will not cause an unacceptable loss of function.[1] Radiation therapy is highly effective for local control and thus is considered a standard part of care in many cases, especially in pelvic lesions, or in instances in which surgical resection is not possible. Irradiation should be used judiciously in young children because of the adverse effect on growth and because it is associated with secondary cancers. These cancers occur in approximately 10% of patients within 20 years of completion of radiation treatment.[7]

The first intergroup study of Ewing's sarcoma was conducted between 1973 and 1978 in patients with nonmetastatic disease. Patients received vincristine, dactinomycin, and cyclophosphamide alone or in combination with either pulmonary radiation or doxorubicin.[12] The second intergroup Ewing's sarcoma protocol was conducted between 1978 and 1982 and demonstrated that intermittent high-dose therapy with vincristine, doxorubicin, cyclophosphamide, and dactinomycin was superior to continuous moderate dose therapy with these agents for the treatment of localized extrapelvic tumors.[13,15] The third intergroup study of Ewing's sarcoma evaluated the addition of etoposide and ifosfamide to the four-drug regimen in a randomized trial and reported a significant improvement in survival among patients with localized disease. The survival rate at 3 years was 80% for patients who received the six-drug regimen as compared with only 56% for the patients who received the four-drug regimen.[14] A current intergroup study is now evaluating dose intensity among patients with localized disease, and a randomized trial of a five-drug regimen (vincristine, doxorubicin, cyclophosphamide, ifosfamide, and etoposide) that is given for either 30 weeks or 48 weeks[1] (see Box 27-2).

Surgical excision of the primary Ewing's sarcoma is considered whenever feasible. Complete resection of the tumor removes all obvious tumor burden and increases survival. Most current protocols use initial intensive chemotherapy followed by surgery and/or radiation. The timing of surgery and/or radiation is dependent on the radiographic response to chemotherapy and the accessibility of the lesion. Candidates for radiotherapy alone to provide local control include patients with bulky lesions in surgically difficult sites such as the spine, skull, paraacetabular pelvis, patients with a poor response to chemotherapy, and those in whom surgery would result in unacceptable loss of function. In summary, local control is provided either by surgery alone, surgery with radiation for close margins, or radiation alone. Many oncologists prefer to combine marginal resections with either preoperative or postoperative radiation on a routine basis, especially for bulky tumors in difficult sites.[1] Avoiding radiation completely is usually an option only when there is a good histologic response to chemotherapy and negative surgical margins. Not using radiation appears to offer some advantage because of the potential to develop secondary sarcomas caused by radiation. Also, radiation causes muscle wasting, instability of the bone, and extensive scarification in the tissues of the area.

PROGNOSIS

The extent of the disease at diagnosis is the most important prognostic factor. The presence of disseminated disease is an adverse prognostic factor regardless of the site of the primary lesion. The location and extent of the metastatic disease correlate with survival. For example, patients with metastatic bone or bone marrow disease have a poor prognosis. Patients with surgically resectable metastatic disease to the lung may fare better than those with unresectable metastases.[12] The Intergroup Ewing's Sarcoma Studies (IESS) have found that in patients with localized disease, the primary site was the most significant prognostic indicator, with pelvic and sacral lesions having the least favorable prognosis.[14] The most favorable sites were the bones of the distal extremities. Others have documented that the size, not the site of the primary, influences survival, with larger tumors faring worse.[15] Data from one study indicated that a primary tumor size greater than 8 cm in maximal diameter is an adverse prognostic factor.[12]

Histologic response to the chemotherapy correlates with prognosis. Patients with less than 10% of viable tumor during histologic examination of surgical specimens have a better prognosis than those with greater than 10% of viable tumor.[14] Other prognostic factors for patients with localized disease include age, leukocyte count, sedimentation rate, and serum LDH levels at diagnosis. IESS I found that younger patients had a more favorable prognosis.[14] Elevation of the serum LDH level at diagnosis is associated with metastatic disease and a poorer prognosis.[27]

ORTHOPEDIC SURGERY FOR BONE SARCOMAS

The most common surgical options available to the child and family are limb salvage or amputation. The goal of surgery is to facilitate cure by obtaining a clean, wide margin, which is defined as a zone of normal, healthy tissue around the tumor, while providing the patient with optimum function.[18,35] The advent of limb salvage and complex reconstruction has allowed more children and adolescents to have a functioning extremity rather than an amputation.

The initial biopsy is obtained as soon as possible after the diagnostic scans. The CT and/or the MRI will guide the surgeon to the best area to perform an open, incisional biopsy. Several institutions perform needle biopsy but most experts recommend an open procedure to obtain adequate tissue for diagnosis and to provide material for research study. Placement of the biopsy incision is critical. The biopsy should be performed along the line of the incision planned for the subsequent resection to limit contamination of surrounding tissue. If amputation is planned, the biopsy incision is made well distal to the planned incision site. The entire biopsy tract, including skin, fat, muscle, and bone, will need to be resected at the time of definitive surgery.[5]

Many factors are considered to determine the appropriate surgery for children and adolescents with bone sarcomas. First, the child must undergo preoperative staging with special studies. Most patients will require an MRI, CT, bone scan, and occasionally an arteriogram. These scans enable the surgeon to determine the extent and resectability of the tumor and response to chemotherapy, and are the blueprint for the surgical procedure.[17]

A second factor is the location of the tumor. Amputation is the choice for tumors in expendable bones such as fingers or ribs. Tumors in long bones and near joint spaces require a more complex surgery but amputation may still be an option. A child's age must also be considered. A child who has not reached skeletal maturity will require lengthening procedures of the affected limb or an epiphysiodesis, a surgery to cause early closure of the growth plate in the opposite limb to prevent leg length discrepancy.

Functional issues are also considered. Is the child active in sports or more comfortable with sedentary activities such as computer work or reading? Active children will wear out a total joint prosthesis and may have a better functional outcome with arthrodesis or amputation (Figure 27-3).

The ability of the patient and family to comply with care after the procedure is an important factor. If the family is unable to handle complex wound care and extensive physical therapy, then an amputation may be a better choice for the child and family. The appearance of one procedure, such as a rotationplasty, may be more offensive than that of another. Finally, the surgeon may have a preference for one type of procedure over another. All of these factors are taken into consideration to determine the final surgical procedure.

TYPES OF SURGERY

Limb salvage involves the wide resection of the tumor, including the biopsy tract, followed by bone

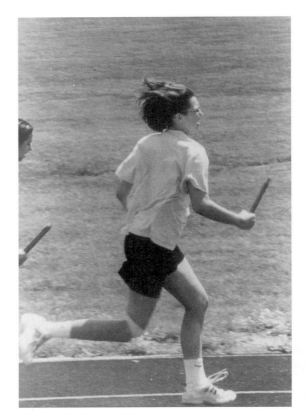

Figure 27-3

Adolescent after below the knee amputation who was originally diagnosed with clear cell sarcoma of the left ankle at age 7. (Courtesy James R. Neff, MD, and Pamela Simon, RN, MSN, PNP, Nebraska Health System.)

reconstruction with either an open reduction with internal fixation (ORIF) or arthroplasty.[30] An ORIF uses rods, plates, screws, and an allograft or autograft, whereas an arthroplasty uses a hinged or articulating internal prosthesis (Figure 27-4) (Table 27-1). Arthroplasty refers to surgeries including replacement of the total joint, hip or knee, with metallic implantation. An expandable internal prosthesis (with an arthroplasty) may be used in younger children to allow for bone growth, but this type of reconstruction will require surgery every 6 to 12 months to lengthen the internal prosthesis until full skeletal maturity is achieved.[10]

Arthrodesis is another type of limb salvage that fuses a joint, most commonly the knee or shoulder. The tumor is resected along with the surrounding bone and tissue and a rod is inserted and secured with locking screws.[17] The patient must be skeletally mature for this procedure. Full weight bearing is an advantage for this surgery, but activities may

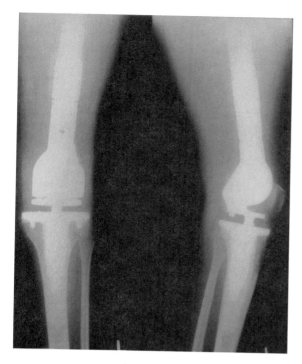

Figure 27-4

X-ray film of endoprosthesis of a 16-year-old with osteosarcoma of the left distal femur. (Courtesy James R. Neff, MD, and Pamela Simon, RN, MSN, PNP, Nebraska Health System.)

be limited because of the fusion of the joint (Figures 27-5, 27-6).

Rotationplasty is a surgical alternative combining amputation and limb salvage. It is used to remove malignant bone tumors arising above or below the knee. This procedure has also been called the *Van Ness* or *Winkleman's procedure.*[20] It involves a wide resection of the tumor involving the knee joint but leaving the nerves and vessels intact. The remaining lower portion of the leg is rotated 180 degrees and reattached. The ankle joint replaces the knee joint, which was removed with the resection of the tumor (Figures 27-7, 27-8). A plate is used for internal fixation of the tibia and femur.[4,11] An external prosthesis fits over the entire foot, ankle, and remaining extremity once the bones have healed (Figures 27-9, 27-10, p. 586). The rotated ankle joint now functions as a knee joint. The advantages of the procedure include improved limb function through retention of an effective knee joint, absence or reduction of phantom limb pain, and the unlimited weight capacity of the joint.[16,18] The disadvantages include the unusual appearance of the limb, which may cause body im-

TABLE 27-1	TYPES OF SURGERY
Amputation	Surgical removal of limb
Rotationplasty	Lower limb is rotated 180 degrees and reattached to thigh
	Ankle joint replaces knee joint
Arthrodesis	Fusion of joint
ORIF	Use of rods, screws, allograft, or autograft to reconstruct bone
Arthroplasty	Total joint, hip, knee replaced with metallic implant

age problems, and the additional time needed for the bone to heal before weight bearing as compared with an amputation.[10]

Amputation involves complete surgical removal of a diseased part of the body. This technique is used with expendable bones such as the fibula, ribs, toes, fingers, or ulna but may also be indicated for an arm or leg because of a complex tumor. If the tumor involves the vessels or nerves, or if poor patient compliance is anticipated, amputation may be necessary. The advantages of amputation include a wide resection margin and shorter healing time.[3]

COMPLICATIONS

Postoperatively the nurse will monitor the patient for a variety of potential complications. Individual surgeons will have procedures for wound care, mobilization, and treating postoperative complications. The wound is examined daily by the surgeon. The dressing is monitored for drainage every few hours. Complaints of excessive pain or tightness of the dressing are reported immediately to the surgeon, because the dressing may need to be split or removed. Evaluation of the child will include assessment of pain, wound healing, sensation, pulses, strength, temperature, and skin color. Any one or a combination of symptoms may signal failure of the graft, compromised circulation, and nerve impingement or compartment syndrome.

Infection can be both an immediate and long-term complication. Chemotherapy treatments continuing after the surgery increase the risk for infection. The hardware used for internal fixation can become infected. Antibiotics may be used during periods of neutropenia to lessen the risk of infection.[6] Systemic or central line infections can cause an infection to the hardware as the bacteria in the bloodstream attach to the internal metal components (screws, plates, rods, joints).

Another possible complication of limb salvage surgery is nonunion of the bones. When the tumor is removed, the portion of the bone resected may be

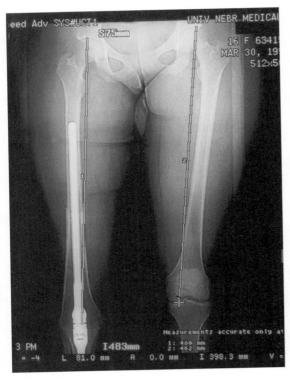

Figure 27-5

X-ray film of arthrodesis reconstruction of a 15-year-old with osteosarcoma of the left distal femur. (Courtesy James R. Neff, MD, and Pamela Simon, RN, MSN, PNP, Nebraska Health System.)

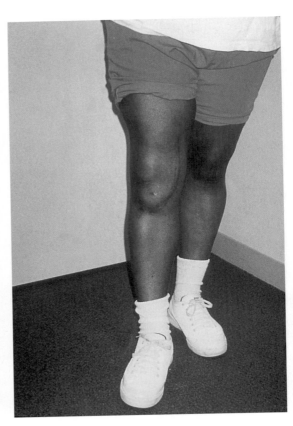

Figure 27-6

Fifteen-year-old with osteosarcoma (same patient as Figure 27-5) of the left distal femur showing left leg after arthrodesis reconstruction. (Courtesy James R. Neff, MD, and Pamela Simon, RN, MSN, PNP, Nebraska Health System.)

replaced with a graft of bone and/or hardware. Both ends of the graft must heal before weight bearing. Nonunion occurs when one or both ends of the replaced bone do not heal. Fractures can result from application of stress. When this occurs, the child may need to undergo surgery for additional bone grafting.

Certain chemotherapy agents, such as methotrexate, can cause osteoporosis resulting in a stress fracture through the grafted bone.[10] Other chemotherapy agents, such as ifosfamide and cisplatin, can cause long-term hypophosphatemia through renal damage, which can result in osteopenia or weakening of the bone. If a fracture occurs, the child cannot bear weight on the affected limb until ossification of the bone is seen on x-ray film.

Pain is expected following surgery. The acute postoperative pain usually lasts 2 to 4 days and can be controlled with a patient-controlled analgesia pump (PCA) and then by oral medications. Phan-

tom limb pain is a common consequence of an amputation. The intensity of phantom limb pain is often associated with the degree of pain in the extremity before the amputation.[23] The body perceives that the body part is still there. The frequency and intensity of pain decrease over time. Medication such as gabapentin (Neurontin) or amitriptyline (Elavil), biofeedback, and the use of local anesthetics at the time of surgery may lessen phantom limb pain.[31] Imagery, distraction, and hypnosis are other methods used to help alleviate phantom limb pain (refer to Chapter 12 for additional information).

Patients who have total joint replacement such as a total hip or knee replacement may develop joint instability. The instability may cause pain and limit activity. The total joint can also loosen and wear out, especially in active patients. These complications require further surgery to tighten or replace part or all of the prosthesis.

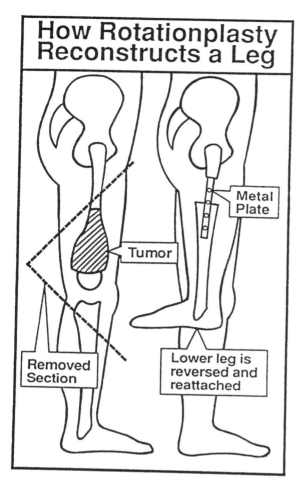

Figure 27-7

How rotationplasty reconstructs a leg. (Courtesy Kelly Grinnell, Marketing/Public Affairs, Nebraska Health System.)

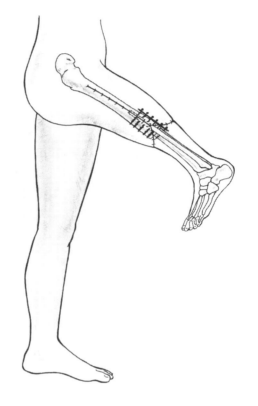

Figure 27-8

Final surgical outcome for child with rotationplasty. (Courtesy Kelly Grinnell, Marketing/Public Affairs, Nebraska Health System.)

REHABILITATION

Physical and occupational therapy are vital components of successful rehabilitation following orthopedic surgery. Patients will differ in their requirements for physical and occupational therapy. These services are introduced preoperatively and include the use of crutches; measurements for wheelchairs with elevated leg rests, and various types of braces; measurements for prosthesis; and the use of walkers, slings, and other supportive devices. The sooner patients and families adapt to use of special equipment and the new physical limitations of the surgery, the sooner patients can begin increasing their functional ability and improving their quality of life. Physical therapy can also teach the patient passive and active range-of-motion exercises to facilitate postoperative recovery. The physical thera-

pist instructs the patient and family how to mobilize safely in the hospital, at home, and at school. An in-home or school visit may be necessary preoperatively to plan for safe mobilization after surgery. The physical therapist and the occupational therapist play important roles in facilitating mobility and independence. Because most bone tumors occur in adolescence, enhancing independence may increase quality of life.

The primary goals following the surgical procedure are to support wound healing and increase patient mobility. Patients may be malnourished because of the previous chemotherapy. The use of a nutritional support team or dietary specialist needs to be implemented preoperatively. Dietary supplements and increasing protein intake can promote wound healing.[29]

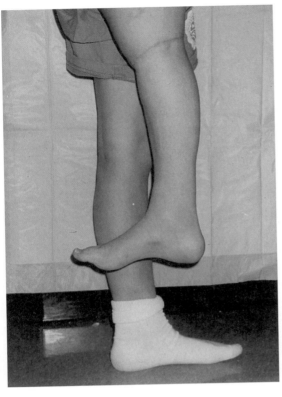

Figure 27-9

Nine-year-old with osteosarcoma of the right femur after rotationplasty. (Courtesy James R. Neff, MD, and Pamela Simon, RN, MSN, PNP, Nebraska Health System.)

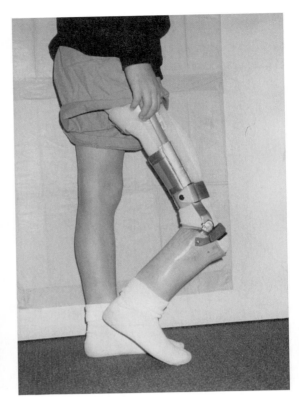

Figure 27-10

Nine-year-old with osteosarcoma of the right femur (same patient as Figure 27-9) after rotationplasty, with prosthesis in place. (Courtesy James R. Neff, MD, and Pamela Simon, RN, MSN, PNP, Nebraska Health System.)

LONG-TERM FOLLOW-UP

Patients undergoing a complex reconstruction are monitored closely on a weekly or biweekly basis until the wounds are healed, then monthly for the first 6 months to monitor the functional ability and recovery of the child. Periodic functional evaluations and x-ray examinations are performed to monitor healing and assist in early detection of local tumor recurrence. The follow-up intervals will be lengthened as the child progresses. However, these patients will require lifelong follow-up by an orthopedic surgeon because revisions may be required following limb salvage and amputation. These patients will also have lifelong follow-up by a medical oncologist to monitor for long-term effects of chemotherapy.

NURSING IMPLICATIONS

Children and adolescents with bone tumors present a complex and often challenging set of nursing care issues. The treatment may involve multiple modal-

ities including intensive chemotherapy, extensive surgery, and radiation therapy with all the education and coordination needs surrounding these therapies.

These patients require a multidisciplinary approach to care involving nursing, physical therapy, occupational therapy, radiation therapy, prosthetics and orthotics, social work, child life, as well as surgery and medical oncology. Often the patient will have two primary cancer physicians, the orthopedic surgeon and the pediatric oncologist. The majority of children who have bone tumors are adolescents. Issues related to adolescent growth and development will affect the patient's and family's needs and choices. Adolescents are striving for independence, and their psychologic issues will affect their consent, response to therapy, type of surgical resection and reconstruction chosen, and body image, in addition to other adolescent issues.

The patient and family need comprehensive education before and after surgery. The nurse plays an important role in helping children and families understand and accept the surgery. These surgeries can be difficult to visualize and comprehend. The use of x-ray films or videotapes of patients who have had these surgeries can be helpful to illustrate functional and cosmetic outcomes for these complicated procedures. The nurse can put families in contact with each other to discuss similar operations and their experiences. Photographs, models, and actual hardware components can help the family understand the procedure and encourage questions. A tour of a prosthesis center and meeting the prosthetist (the person who makes artificial limbs) can give the patient and family additional information important to their decision making about surgery. These surgical procedures are lengthy and support from a nurse well known to the family on the day of surgery can be very helpful. Education of the patient's teachers and peers can allow a smoother reentry into school for the patient following surgery.

FUTURE DIRECTIONS

As technology advances, so too will surgical techniques. The newer metals in the plates, screws, and internal prostheses that are now available last twice as long as previously used materials.[17] New models of expandable prostheses are now in limited use. These internal implants lengthen in response to an external electromagnetic field that causes activation of a spring within the implant. Return visits to the operating room are avoided, because the procedure is most often done in diagnostic imaging.[34]

Metastatic bone cancers remain a challenge. New developments in chemotherapy and other systemic modalities will be needed to extend the cure rate and improve the prognosis for all with bone tumors.

ACKNOWLEDGMENT

The authors acknowledge and express their appreciation to Stephanie Vitolano, RN, MS, CPON, Pediatric Nurse Practitioner, Memorial Sloan-Kettering Cancer Center, New York, for her thoughtful review of this chapter.

REFERENCES

1. Arndt, C. A. S., & Crist, W. M. (1999). Medical progress: Common musculoskeletal tumors of childhood and adolescence. *The New England Journal of Medicine, 341,* 342-352.
2. Bacci, G., Ferrari, S., Sangiorgi, L., et al. (1994). Prognostic significance of serum lactate dehydrogenase in patients with osteosarcoma of the extremities. *Journal of Chemotherapy, 6,* 204-210.
3. Bourne, B. A., & Kuthcher, J. L. (1985). Amputation: Helping a patient with the loss of a limb. *RN, 48*(2), 38-47.
4. Cammisa, F. P., Glasser, D. B., Otic, J. C., et al. (1990). The Van Ness tibial rotationplasty. *Journal of Bone, Joint and Tumor Surgery, 72-A,* 1541-1547.
5. Campanacci, M. (1999). *Bone and soft tissue tumors: Clinical features, imaging, pathology and treatment.* 2nd ed. New York: Springer, Verlag Wien.
6. DeBaun, B. J. (1998). Prevention of infection in the orthopedic surgery patient. *Nursing Clinics of North America, 33,* 4671-4684.
7. Dorfman, H. D., & Czerniak, B. (1998). Osteosarcoma. In *Bone tumors* (pp. 128-249). St. Louis, MO: Mosby.
8. Durbin, M., Randall, R. L., & James, M. (1998). Ewing's sarcoma masquerading as osteomyelitis. *Clinical Orthopaedic and Related Research, 357,* 176-185.
9. Ewing, J. (1921). Diffuse endothelioma of bone. *Proceedings of the New York Pathological Society, 21,* 17-19.
10. Gerrand, C. H., Curries, D., Grigoris, P., et al. (1999). Prosthetic reconstruction of the femur for primary bone sarcoma. *International Orthopaedics, 23,* 286-290.
11. Gottsauner-Wolf, F., Kotz, R., Knahr, K., et al. (1991). The rotation plasty for limb salvage in the treatment of malignant bone tumors of the knee region: The follow up of seventy cases. *Journal of Bone Joint Surgery [America], 73,* 1365-1369.
12. Grier, H. E. (1997). The Ewing family of tumors. *Pediatric Clinics of North America, 44,* 991-1002.
13. Hahn, M., & Dormans, J. P. (1996). Primary bone malignancies in children. *Current Opinions in Pediatrics, 8,* 71-74.
14. Horowitz, M. E., Malawer, M. M., Woo, S. Y., et al. (1997). Ewing's sarcoma family of tumors: Ewing's sarcoma of bone and soft tissue and the peripheral primitive neuroectodermal tumors. In P. A. Pizzo & D. G. Poplack (Eds.), *Principles and practice of pediatric oncology* (3rd ed., pp. 831-863). Philadelphia: Lippincott-Raven.
15. Hovos, A. (1991). *Tumors: Diagnosis, treatment, and prognosis.* Philadelphia: W. B. Saunders.
16. Kenan, S., Lewis, M. M., & Peabody, T. D. (1998). Special considerations for growing children. In M. A. Simon, & D. Springfield (Eds.), *Surgery for bone and soft-tissue tumors* (pp. 245-263). Philadelphia: Lippincott-Raven.
17. Lindner, N. J., Ramm, O., & Hillman, A. (1999). Limb salvage and outcome of osteosarcoma. *Clinical Orthopaedic and Related Research, 358,* 83-89.
18. Link, M. P., & Eilber, F. (1997). Osteosarcoma. In P. A. Pizzo, & D. G. Polack (Eds.), *Principles and practice of pediatric oncology* (3rd ed., pp. 889-915). Philadelphia: Lippincott-Raven.
19. Link, M. P., Goorin, A. M., Hornwitz, M., et al. (1991). Adjuvant chemotherapy of high-grade osteosarcoma of the extremity: Updated results of the Multi-Institutional Osteosarcoma Study. *Clinical Orthopedics, 270,* 8-14.
20. MacMillen, K., Morten, P., Quinlan, C., et al. (1987). The Van Ness rotation orthoplasty. *The Canadian Nurse, 83,* 23-28.
21. Marino, N., Pratt, C. B., Rao, B. N., et al. (1992). Improved prognosis of children with osteosarcoma metastatic to the lung(s) at the time of diagnosis. *Cancer, 70,* 2722-2727.
22. McIntyre, J. F., Smith-Sorenson, B. K., Friend, S. H., et al. (1994). Germ line mutation of the p53 tumor suppressor gene in children with osteosarcoma. *Journal of Clinical Oncology, 12,* 925-930.
23. Melzack, R. (1992). Phantom limbs. *Scientific American, 266,* 120-126.
24. Meyers, P. A. (1987). Malignant tumors in children: Ewing's sarcoma. *Hematology Oncology Clinics of North America, 1,* 667-673.

25. Meyers, P. A., & Gorlick, R. (1997). Osteosarcoma. *Pediatric Clinics of North America, 44,* 973-984.

26. Meyers, P. A., Heller, G., Healey, J. H., et al. (1993). Osteogenic sarcoma with clinically detectable metastasis at initial presentation. *Journal of Clinical Oncology, 11,* 449-453.

27. O'Connor, M. I., & Pritchard D. J. (1991). Ewing's sarcoma: Prognostic factors, disease control, and the re-emerging role of surgical treatment. *Clinical Orthopedics and Related Research, 262,* 78-87.

28. Pritchard, D. J. (1995). Malignant tumors of bone. In G. P. Murphy, W. Lawrence, & R. E. Lenhard (Eds.), *American Cancer Society textbook of clinical oncology* (2nd ed., pp. 428-434). Atlanta, GA: American Cancer Society.

29. Roberts, P. R., Black, K. W., Santamauro, J. T., et al. (1998). Dietary peptides improve wound healing following surgery. *Nutrition, 14,* 266-269.

30. Roughraff, B. T., Simon, M. A., Kneisl, J. S., et al. (1994). Limb salvage compared with amputation for osteosarcoma of the distal end of the femur. *Journal of Bone and Joint Surgery [American], 76,* 649-656.

31. Sherman, R. A. (1997). History of treatment attempts. In R. A. Sherman, M. Devor, & K. Heermann (Eds.), *Phantom pain* (pp. 143-147). New York: Plenum Press.

32. Unni, K. K. (1996). Osteosarcoma. In D. C. Dahlin & K. K. Unni (Eds.), *Dahlin's bone tumors: General aspects and data on 11,087 cases.* (5th ed., pp. 143-184). Philadelphia: Lippincott-Raven.

33. Wadayama, B., Toguchida, J., Shimizu, T., et al. (1994). Mutation spectrum of the retinoblastoma gene in osteosarcoma. *Cancer Research, 54,* 3042-3048.

34. Wilkins, R. M., & Soubeiran, A. (2000). The Phenix expandable prosthesis: Early American experience. *Clinical Orthopaedics and Related Research, 382,* 51-58.

35. Yaw, K. M. (1999). Pediatric bone tumors. *Seminars in Surgical Oncology, 16,* 173-183.

28

Retinoblastoma

Susan Dulczak
Barbara Frothingham

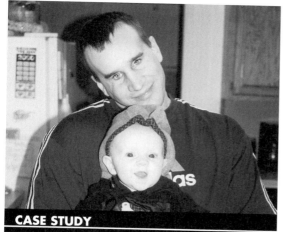

CASE STUDY

Dietrich is a 6-month-old boy diagnosed at 10 days of age with unilateral familial retinoblastoma involving the left eye. The prenatal and birth history were not contributory. His family history, however, is significant for his father being diagnosed and treated for bilateral sporadic retinoblastoma. The father's family history was negative for retinoblastoma, and he underwent bilateral enucleations, the first at 3 years of age and the second at 6 years of age after failure to control the local tumor.

Because of the family history, Dietrich was examined shortly after birth by an ophthalmologist. A single tumor was found in his left eye. At this time, he was referred for a more extensive ophthalmologic examination of both eyes under general anesthesia. The bilateral examination revealed a retinoblastoma of the left eye, measuring 3 × 3 × 2 mm involving the fundus, and two other smaller lesions located in the superior macular area. There was no evidence of heterochromia, cataracts, or vitreous seeding. The right eye was completely normal. The local ophthalmologist recognized the need for specialty care and referred the child to an ocular oncologist at a pediatric cancer center for treat-

ment planning including consideration of chemoreduction of the left eye tumor.

On presentation in the oncology clinic Dietrich was a well-appearing, active 10-day-old. Physical examination was unremarkable. His length, weight, and head circumference were at the 25th percentile for age. During this visit, the plan for chemotherapy was discussed. It was decided that he would receive full dose carboplatin, etoposide with a dose reduction, but because of his young age, vincristine would not be given. The protocol and potential toxicities were discussed with the parents, and both agreed and consented to treatment with chemotherapy. Laboratory data were all within normal limits.

At 3 months of age, before the third course of chemotherapy, another bilateral eye examination under general anesthesia was performed. The right eye remained normal. The two smaller tumors in the left eye had regressed but the largest tumor had increased. A fourth tumor was discovered. Vincristine was added to Dietrich's chemotherapy regimen along with transpupillary thermotherapy (the application of heat to the tumor bed).

Dietrich completed the fourth course of chemotherapy in November 2000. On reexamination of the eyes under anesthesia, Dietrich was found to have further progression of disease in the left eye. The right eye was still normal. Based on the findings in the left eye, plaque radiotherapy was recommended and chemotherapy was discontinued. The physicians were concerned that Dietrich was displaying either chemoresistance or inadequate delivery of the chemotherapy to the temporal macula area; therefore, the plaque would be designed to cover the temporal macular area and treat all tumors. The plaque treatment was successful in irradiating all the tumors.

Now at 6 months of age, Dietrich is happy and well appearing. Physical examination at his clinic visit was normal. Length, weight, and head circumference remain in the 25th percentile for age. The eye examination in clinic was attempted but was not successful. He does follow and appears to have normal vision in the right eye and decreased vision in the left eye.

Dietrich will have monthly bilateral eye examinations under general anesthesia to check for new tumors. Because he inherited the gene for this disease, every cell in his retina is susceptible to the development of a new lesion. It is hoped that new tumors can be detected early and treated with local therapy to avoid enucleation or external beam radiation.

Retinoblastoma is an infrequent malignancy that has played a critical role in advancing understanding of oncogenesis in adults and children. The identification of the retinoblastoma gene on chromosome 13q confirmed the theory that specific genes act to suppress cancer. The discovery of tumor suppressor genes ushered in a new and exciting era of cancer investigation. It is now known that abnormalities of the retinoblastoma gene are very common, occurring in a wide variety of malignancies. The still-unfolding story of the retinoblastoma tumor suppressor genes provides one of the most powerful examples of the contribution of pediatric cancer to the advancement of oncology.[34]

EPIDEMIOLOGY AND GENETICS

Retinoblastoma is the most common intraocular tumor of childhood, yet it is a rare malignancy. It accounts for approximately 1% to 3% of all childhood cancers and occurs in children at a rate of 1 : 18,000 live births with no predilection to race or sex.[10] In the United States, approximately 250 to 300 children per year are diagnosed with retinoblastoma.[34]

Retinoblastoma arises from embryonic retinal cells of one or both eyes. Approximately 25% of the cases occur in both eyes (bilateral) and are diagnosed at a young age, usually less than 1 year.[10] Unilateral retinoblastoma is more commonly diagnosed during the second and third years of life. Ninety percent of cases are diagnosed by 5 years of age[13] (Figure 28-1).

The recognized genetic patterns of retinoblastoma are hereditary (familial) and nonhereditary (sporadic). Accounting for all cases of retinoblastoma, about 60% are nonhereditary and unilateral, 15% are hereditary and unilateral, and 25% are hereditary and bilateral.[10] In the hereditary form of retinoblastoma, the initial mutation is in the germ cell line affecting all cells, with a second somatic mutation occurring after fertilization of the ovum affecting only the retinal cells. The hereditary form is transmitted as an autosomal dominant trait with 90% penetrance. Penetrance is the probability that

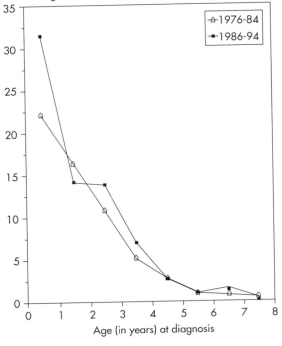

Average annual rate per million

Figure 28-1

Retinoblastoma age-specific incidence (from SEER). (From Young, J. L., Smith, M. A., Roffers, S. D., et al. [1999]. Retinoblastoma. In L. A. G. Reis, M. A. Smith, J. G. Gurney, et al. [Eds.], *Cancer incidence and survival among children and adolescents: United States SEER Program 1975-1995, National Cancer Institute, SEER Program* [p. 76]. Bethesda, MD: National Cancer Institute, NIH Pub. No. 99-4649.)

a person inheriting the mutation will have the disease. In hereditary retinoblastoma, 50% of the offspring of patients with a germinal mutation have the risk of carrying the retinoblastoma mutation. The risk of developing the disease is 45%.[15]

Fortunately, the majority of patients diagnosed with this disease have nonhereditary retinoblastoma. One series identified less than 25% of retinoblastoma patients as having a family history of the disease.[21] Approximately 60% of tumors develop sporadically (nonhereditary) and are associated with unilateral disease. In the nonhereditary form of retinoblastoma, both the first and second mutations occur in the retinal cells.

In 1971, Knudsen first described his "two hit" model to explain the hereditary and nonhereditary development of retinoblastoma. His model was further developed and with genetic and physical mapping, the retinoblastoma gene was located on chromosome 13 in band 14. It is now recognized that the development of retinoblastoma is due to the

TABLE 28-1	**CURRENT KNOWLEDGE OF CAUSES OF RETINOBLASTOMA**	
Exposure or Characteristic	**Comments**	
KNOWN RISK FACTORS		**References**
Parent with history of bilateral retinoblastoma	Each child has a 50% risk of inheriting the retinoblastoma gene. If the gene is inherited, the risk of retinoblastoma is over 90%. A small proportion of patients with unilateral disease also carry the gene and can pass it on to their children.	1, 2
13q deletion syndrome	Recognition of this syndrome led to the identification of the retino-blastoma gene.	2
FACTORS FOR WHICH EVIDENCE IS INCONSISTENT OR LIMITED		
Paternal occupation	There is a single report of association with employment in the military, metal manufacturing, and as welder, machinist, or related occupation.	3

Adapted from Young, J. L., Smith, M. A., Roffers, S. D., et al. (1999). Retinoblastoma. In L. A. G. Reis, M. A. Smith, J. G. Gurney, et al. (Eds.), *Cancer incidence and survival among children and adolescents: United States SEER Program 1975-1995,* (pp. 77). National Cancer Institute, SEER Program. Bethesda, MD: National Cancer Institute, NIH Pub. No. 99-4649.
[1]Knudson, A. G., Jr. (1971). Mutation and cancer: Statistical study of retinoblastoma. *Proceedings of the National Academy of Sciences, USA, 68,* 820-823.
[2]Li, F. (1996) Familial aggregation. In D. Schottenfeld & J. Fraumeni (Eds.). *Cancer epidemiology and prevention* (pp. 546-558). New York: Oxford University Press.
[3]Bunin, G. R., Petrakova, A., Meadows, A. T., et al. (1990). Occupations of parents of children with retinoblastoma: A report from the Children's Cancer Study Group. *Cancer Research, 50,* 7129-7133.

loss of genetic information on chromosome 13.[2,23] In the development of retinoblastoma as proposed by Knudson, the "hits" represent inactivation or loss of regulation genes at the 13q14 locus.[3] During cell replication, a mutation results in the loss of both copies of the retinoblastoma gene. As a result, a protein that regulates growth is not produced and normal barriers to cell growth are absent, leading to unregulated proliferation of cells and tumor development.

Most children with retinoblastoma have no intellectual impairments nor other congenital anomalies.[10] An association between bilateral retinoblastoma and 13q deletion syndrome has been noted in a small number of patients.[22] These patients have multiple congenital abnormalities such as growth delay, mental retardation, microcephaly, and bony defects. As these two extremes have been studied over the last decade, understanding has improved that there is a range of genetic mutations involved with the appearance of clinical disease. Further delination of this range may help target areas of future therapy.[14] Table 28-1 summarizes the current knowledge of causes of retinoblastoma.

CLINICAL PRESENTATION

In the majority of children, the diagnosis of retinoblastoma occurs within the first 2 years of life. Over 80% are diagnosed before the age of 3 years.[3] Children with a positive family history for retinoblastoma are often diagnosed before the de-velopment of clinical symptoms because of early, prospective screening that detects disease as early as possible.[14] Children without a family history are diagnosed as clinical symptoms develop. The most common presenting signs of retinoblastoma are leukokoria (56%) and strabismus (20%). A variety of other signs and symptoms occur in less than 10% of patients. These include glaucoma, a painful red eye, and orbital cellulitis.[14]

Leukokoria, or cat's eye reflex, is a white pupil (Figure 28-2). This "white pupil" is noted only at certain angles or lighting, when the tumor, pupil, and light source are in alignment. A parent may notice a "white spot" when the child's pupil is dilated in dim light or when a color photograph is taken and a white pupil seen.

Strabismus, either esotropia (eye turning in) or exotropia (eye turning out), is the second most common presenting sign. The presence of esotropia or exotropia is equally common in the diagnosis; however, exotropia is unusual in the first year of life. The presence of strasbismus should alert the practitioner to suspect the diagnosis of retinoblastoma.[14]

DIAGNOSTIC EVALUATION

Early diagnosis is of critical importance to achieve patient survival and to enhance opportunities for preserving vision. Most early signs and symptoms are initially noted by parents who then notify a health care professional. Unfortunately, delays in diagnosis may occur if the child's primary health

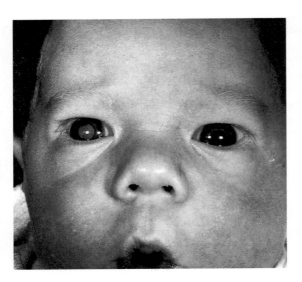

Figure 28-2

Leukokoria.

care providers do not pay full attention to parental reports.[14]

Retinoblastoma is an unusual malignancy in that diagnosis is clinically established by an ophthalmoscopic examination under general anesthesia. Biopsy is not performed because of the danger of spreading tumor to an extraocular location. Such spread seriously compromises patient outcome because metastatic retinoblastoma has a very low cure rate.[14] During the examination under anesthesia (EUA), the pupils are dilated, allowing the physician to fully visualize the retina. The examination determines tumor size and location. Retinal photography with imaging studies including computed tomography (CT) scanning, magnetic resonance imaging (MRI), and ultrasound and plain films of the orbit are used to determine extent of disease. The CT and/or MRI scan provides information about the presence of calcifications and extension of the tumor into the orbit, number and location of tumors, thickening of the optic nerve, and involvement of the central nervous system.[1]

Additional tests include measuring the level of lactic acid dehydrogenase in the aqueous humor, serum carcinoembryonic antigen (CEA), and serum α-fetoprotein. These levels can be elevated in the presence of retinoblastoma. A lumbar puncture and a bone marrow aspirate are performed in patients with signs and symptoms of hematogenous spread, central nervous system involvement, or with evidence of tumor extension beyond the globe.

Current recommendations for children with a family history of retinoblastoma include an ophthalmologic examination under anesthesia in the first few days of life, again at 6 weeks of age, every 2 to 3 months until 2 years of age, and every 4 months until 3 years of age.[24]

TREATMENT

Treatment for retinoblastoma is determined by the size of the tumor and the extent of the disease. The Reese-Ellsworth classification system has been the standard staging system for intraocular retinoblastoma.[8,10] This system categorizes the prognosis of patients with intraocular retinoblastoma from Group I (very favorable) through Group V (very unfavorable) (Box 28-1). The system predicts the probability of retaining vision and tumor control but does not predict survival. To date, there is no accepted standard for staging disease that has extended beyond the globe. Therefore, until a standard staging system is accepted for disease beyond the globe, the stages are subdivided to include: intraocular involvement, extension beyond the orbit, the optic nerve, brain and central nervous system, and hematogenous spread to distant sites.[24]

A second system developed at St. Jude Children's Research Hospital looks at classification differently. This system has proven useful to those investigators trying to incorporate factors influencing prognosis and therapy choices because it is based on the extent of extraocular involvement and metastic disease.[15]

The goal of treatment is to provide curative care for the patient while maximizing useful vision. Treatment considerations are based on whether the tumor is bilateral or unilateral; size, location, and number of lesions; and extent of disease. The treatment for retinoblastoma must be individualized, and for optimal results, treatment should be conducted at a childhood cancer center with expertise in treating children with ocular malignancies. In the case of bilateral disease, each eye is managed independently.

Treatment modalities for retinoblastoma include surgery (enucleation, cryotherapy, photocoagulation), radiation therapy, and chemotherapy. Enucleation is the treatment of choice if (1) there is no chance for vision; (2) glaucoma is present as a result of the formation of new vessels; (3) there has been failure to respond to other treatment; or (4) there is permanent damage to the retina.

Unilateral tumors most often have advanced disease with vitreous seeding and no chance for vision in the affected eye. Enucleation is the treatment of choice. However, early detection of unilateral disease expands the therapeutic options to include

BOX 28-1

REESE-ELLSWORTH STAGING FOR RETINOBLASTOMA

GROUP I: VERY FAVORABLE
A. Solitary tumor; <4 disc diameters (dd*) in size at or behind the equator
B. Multiple tumors; no tumor >4 dd in size at or behind the equator

GROUP II: FAVORABLE
A. Solitary tumor; 4 to 10 dd in size at or behind the equator
B. Multiple tumors; 4 to 10 dd in size at or behind the equator

GROUP III: DOUBTFUL
A. Any lesion anterior to the equator
B. Solitary tumors >10 dd in size behind the equator

GROUP IV: UNFAVORABLE
A. Multiple tumors; some >10 dd in size
B. Any lesion extending anteriorly to the ora serrata

GROUP V: VERY UNFAVORABLE
A. Tumors involving more than half the retina
B. Vitreous seeding

*1 dd = 1.5 mm

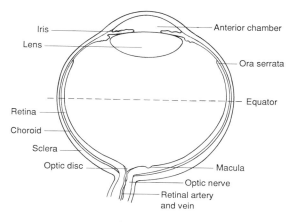

Figure 28-3

Diagram of the eye.

photocoagulation, cryotherapy, radiation therapy, or chemotherapy.

Management of bilateral disease is dependent on the extent of disease determined in each eye. Historically, the most affected eye was enucleated in patients with bilateral disease. Recently, if some vision is present in each eye, neither is enucleated and treatment to each eye is conservative. These patients require close follow-up.

When enucleation is performed, a segment of the optic nerve is removed and evaluated. If tumor is present at the cut end of the optic nerve, the disease is considered to be extraocular and radiation therapy will be required.[3] Enucleation can produce a "sunken" appearance of the socket; thus, an orbital implant is usually inserted during the operative procedure. A prosthetic eye can be fitted 6 weeks after surgery. A new prosthesis is needed about every 5 years or more depending on the age of the child.

Retinoblastoma is a radiosensitive tumor. Radiotherapy is considered when the eye has potential for useful vision. External beam radiation is employed with multifocal disease that may or may not have lesions close to the macula or optic nerve in an attempt to preserve vision and avoid enucleation.[17] Dosages range from 35 Gy over 3 weeks for stages I to III to 45 Gy over 4 weeks for stages IV and V. External beam radiation can be delivered using a D-shaped lateral field technique for unilateral disease.[19,24] Bilateral disease is treated with opposed lateral field technique. Radioactive applicators (plaques) are used in patients with unilateral disease and small tumors at diagnosis, and for small recurrent tumors after external beam radiation. The procedure involves surgery. An applicator is sutured to the sclera to deliver 35 to 40 Gy to the surface of the tumor for approximately 7 days.[16,24] During this time the patient remains in isolation to limit radiation exposure to others. Use of a lead eye patch may be appropriate depending on the child's age and ability to cooperate.

Photocoagulation and cryotherapy are valuable treatment options. Photocoagulation is the use of a laser to destroy the blood vessels that supply the tumor thus causing necrosis. It requires direct visualization and is most beneficial for tumors located posterior to the equator of the eye[24] (Figure 28-3). Cryotherapy involves the use of a freezing process that kills tumor cells in the involved area. This treatment interrupts the microcirculation by causing cellular damage during thawing. Indications for cryotherapy are the same as for photocoagulation, except it is more useful for tumors located in the anterior retina. It does not require direct visualization. A probe is placed directly on the conjunctiva or sclera and treatment is administered by a triple freeze thaw technique.[17,24] Complications of photocoagulation and cryotherapy include retinal detachment and hemorrhage.

Historically, chemotherapy was used in patients with extraocular or metastatic disease, or with radiation therapy to improve the response in children with advanced intraocular disease. It has been difficult to initiate clinical trials for chemotherapy in patients with intraocular disease because local control with surgery and radiation has produced an overall survival rate of 90%.[10] Currently, patients with intraocular disease receive chemotherapy in an attempt to reduce the initial tumor burden, improve vision preservation, and to avoid or postpone external beam radiation.[31] Chemotherapy regimens under study include carboplatin, etoposide, and vincristine. Additionally, the use of cyclosporine in combination with these drugs is also under investigation in an attempt to reverse multidrug resistance. The use of etoposide is being evaluated carefully because reports of etoposide-associated leukemia have begun to appear.[27]

After initial chemotherapy, patients then receive local therapy such as cryotherapy, photocoagulation, or plaque radiotherapy.[12] Such treatments may minimize the need for enucleation and external beam radiation, thereby reducing the incidence of second malignancy, cataracts, and growth disturbance of the bones in the face and orbit. Early data suggest that chemotherapy may be effective for specific children with intraocular retinoblastoma.[12]

The appearance of central nervous system (CNS) disease is an ominous sign. Central nervous system involvement is treated with intrathecal methotrexate, cytosine arabinoside, and hydrocortisone. Clinical trials are being developed using high-dose chemotherapy with autologous bone marrow rescue for patients with recurrent disseminated disease because present treatments are not effective.[24]

Trilateral retinoblastoma, a rare but well recognized syndrome, has serious consequences for the child. Typically 1% to 8% of patients with bilateral retinoblastoma develop a pineal tumor, a midline tumor that may spread in direct proximity to surrounding areas of the brain or spinal fluid. The syndrome was first described in the early 1980s.[4,5] It tends to appear within 5 years of the diagnosis of bilateral retinoblastoma and is associated with a high mortality rate. The name *trilateral retinoblastoma* is derived from the resemblance the pineal has to the retina histologically and the fact that in some animals the pineal is a photoreceptor organ.

PROGNOSIS

The overall prognosis for retinoblastoma is excellent (Figure 28-4). For many years, the 5-year survival rate for children with retinoblastoma stages I to IV has exceeded 90%.[8] Using the Reese-Ellsworth classification system that uses only orbital disease, survival in patients with Group V disease drops to 83% to 87%.[24] When extraocular disease is present, 30% to 35% are cured using orbital irradiation with or without chemotherapy.[24]

Sites of tumor invasion that signal a poor prognosis include the choroid, the scleral emisseric veins and episcleral tissues, and hematogenous spread through the choroidal vessels (invasion in 62% of cases). Optic nerve involvement beyond the lamina cribosa, if present, is a factor for orbit recurrence and CNS dissemination. Patients with tumor at the surgical margins of the optic nerve have a poor prognosis.[17] If CNS disease is present, the outlook is extremely grave. Recurrent disease carries a poor prognosis and radiotherapy is useful for palliation of masses, CNS disease, and distant metastases.[8,24,25,32]

FOLLOW-UP

Intense monitoring for disease recurrence continues for at least 3 years following treatment. Follow-up for the development of second malignancies continues indefinitely. A suggested schedule is ophthalmologic evaluation under general anesthesia 4 to 6 weeks after therapy ends, then every 2 to 3 months for the first year. During year 2, exams should be done every 3 to 4 months. Year 3 and future exams are recommended every 6 months until age 5, and then annually thereafter. It is recommended that surveillance for development of extraocular disease occur every 3 months for the first year, then annually thereafter.[24] If vision is spared, episodic evaluation of visual acuity and visual fields helps to maximize the child's potential for sight.[30]

LATE EFFECTS

When radiation is used to treat retinoblastoma there are both acute and long-term effects to the eye. These effects include erythema, epilation (the loss of eyelashes), conjunctivitis, scleral injection, dermatitis, keratitis (inflammation of the cornea), decreased corneal sensation, myopia, iritis, retinal edema, decreased tear production, and retarded bone growth.[28]

The long-term concerns following the diagnosis of retinoblastoma include second malignancies, decreased visual acuity, and altered body image. Five years after diagnosis, more patients die of second malignancies than of retinoblastoma. Sixty-five percent of the second malignancies occur in the irradiated field and include osteogenic sarcoma, fibrosarcoma, and other spindle cell sarcomas.[2,9,24] Second malignancies that occur outside of the field

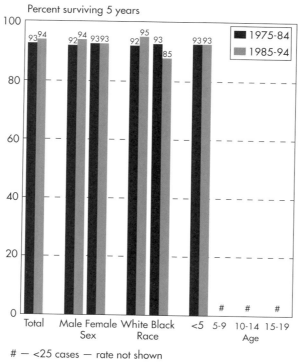

Percent surviving 5 years

Figure 28-4

Retinoblastoma 5-year survival rates (from SEER).   (From Young, J. L., Smith, M. A., Roffers, S. D., et al. [1999]. Retinoblastoma. In L. A. G. Reis, M. A. Smith, J. G. Gurney, et al. [Eds.], *Cancer incidence and survival among children and adolescents: United States SEER Program 1975-1995, National Cancer Institute, SEER Program* [p. 77]. Bethesda, MD: National Cancer Institute, NIH Pub. No. 99-4649.)

of irradiation include osteosarcoma, soft tissue sarcomas, melanoma, and thyroid carcinoma.[17] The incidence of second malignancies increases over time and reaches 70% at 30 years from diagnosis and treatment.[9]

Orbital bone growth retardation caused by external beam irradiation is a serious problem for the growing child. Radiation therapy given to an infant can produce marked bony abnormality and reduction of lacrimal function.[16] Orbital irradiation in a child younger than 6 months is more damaging than in an older child.[20] Other late complications of external beam orbital irradiation include cataract, retinopathy, vitreous hemorrhage, orbital deformities, glaucoma, ptisical eye (degenerative shrinkage of the eye), decreased corneal sensation, and chronic dry eye.[26,28]

Changes in peripheral vision pose difficulties for children treated for retinoblastoma. In one series, 10 patients successfully treated for retinoblastoma were evaluated for visual field deficits. All 10 had scotoma (areas of visual loss) in the affected eye. Reports of difficulties with schoolwork and reading need to be addressed and visual fields monitored as part of follow-up after treatment.[30] A pediatric opthamologist should evaluate the child's need for refraction at regular intervals.

NURSING IMPLICATIONS

Nurses from several disciplines contribute to the care of the patient diagnosed with retinoblastoma and the family. Nurses in pediatric oncology, ophthalmology, surgery, and radiation oncology may be involved, as well as the primary care nurse. It is helpful to consider the individual expertise and contribution of each specialty nurse. Obtaining a thorough family history early contributes to the identification of infants at risk for retinoblastoma. Parents may have prenatal genetic testing to determine the risk. Infants at risk need early examination under anesthesia by an ophthalmologist.

Ophthalmology, surgery, and radiation oncology nurses contribute expertise related to the specific treatment and procedures. Ophthalmology nurses perform visual field examinations and provide information related to peripheral vision and optimizing visual acuity. Oncology nurses are involved when chemotherapy is used. All disciplines contribute to the education of the patient and family and provide support and referral to appropriate resources.

The diagnosis of retinoblastoma is a significant life-altering event for the patient and family. The knowledge that heredity may play a related part in the child's disease leaves parents very vulnerable.[33] Other overwhelming emotions are evoked by the thought that their child may be without sight. The patient and family need information related to disease, treatment plan, monitoring, resources, and genetic counseling.[7,29] Siblings of patients with hereditary retinoblastoma should have an ophthalmology exam under anesthesia every 3 to 4 months for the first 2 years of life for early disease detection.[24]

The patient may have issues related to body image and coping. The use of humor and play provides mechanisms for the child to learn to cope with procedures.[11] Recommendations regarding protective eyewear, especially if the child has vision in only one eye, are important.[30] Referral to specific programs for visual devices and support is crucial. National resources are available (Box 28-2), and the nurse must seek out local and state resources.

FUTURE DIRECTIONS

The evolution of new and improved evaluation tools and treatments is directed at genetic screening, improving outcomes in orbital disease, and in-

creasing cure rates in patients with extraocular disease. Multiple approaches to the identification and eradication of extraocular disease are evolving. High-dose chemotherapy with autologous marrow rescue for advanced or recurrent disease is being used.[25] Strategies are being developed to overcome multidrug resistance.[24] Radiolabeled monoclonal antibodies are being investigated to treat cerebrospinal disease, which, in the past, has been incurable. Currently, too little data are available to know the impact of this treatment.[10,17] Idarubicin was used in a phase 2 window for extraocular retinoblastoma. Bone marrow disease cleared, but CNS disease progressed.[6]

Pathology studies are attempting to clarify whether second tumors are recurrent or new. Studies to identify retinoblastoma specific antigens and genetic markers are under way.[9] Understanding the cytogenetics of primary and second tumors will be helpful. Monoclonal F (ab1) 2-ricin-A conjugate in vitro has been found to be toxic to cultured retinoblastoma cells.[17,18]

Metaiodobenzylguanidine (MIBG) is under investigation as a possible tool to diagnose and identify disseminated disease. There is continuing discussion regarding the role of prophylactic radiotherapy for heritable retinoblastoma.[24,32]

Gene therapy is the transfer of new genetic material into cells of a patient resulting in therapeutic benefit. Several strategies are under development for malignant tumors including direct transfer of specific tumor-suppressor genes, transfer of genes that encode a particular toxic product, or the transfer of genes whose products induce cell death in the specific tumor cells. In very early research a suicide gene, herpes simplex virus thymidine kinase (*HSV-TK*), was used to demonstrate in vitro that the transfer of the *HSV-TK* gene was possible.[18] The model may be used to introduce a drug-sensitive gene into a retinoblastoma cell and could serve as a front-runner for gene therapy in retinoblastoma.[18]

Present-day treatment of retinoblastoma that is localized to the orbit yields excellent patient outcomes. Surgery and radiation therapy to localized tumors are well tested and effective strategies. The treatment goal of preserving sight while eradicating disease leads to an enhanced quality of life for children diagnosed with this disease. Early diagnosis and treatment are key to improved outcomes. Future challenges lie in the treatment of extraorbital disease, recurrent disease, and incorporating the evolving genetic applications to treatment of this disease. The study of this tumor has advanced understanding of tumor-suppressor genes and has led to an early genetic blueprint for a rare but important malignancy.

REFERENCES

1. Abramson, D. H. (1990). Retinoblastoma 1990: Diagnosis, treatment, and implications. *Pediatric Annals, 19,* 387-395.

2. Abramson, D. H., & Frank, C. M. (1998). Second nonocular tumors in survivors of bilateral retinoblastoma: Possible age effect on radiation-related risk. *Ophthalmology, 105,* 573-580.

3. Altman, A. J. (1993). Management of malignant solid tumors. In D. G. Nathan & F. A. Oski (Eds.), *Hematology of infancy and childhood* (4th ed., pp. 1420-1424). Philadelphia: W. B. Saunders.

4. Bader, J. L., Meadows, A. T., Zimmerman, L. E., et al. (1982). Bilateral retinoblastoma with ectopic intracranial retinoblastoma. *Cancer Genetics Cytogenetics, 5,* 203-213.

5. Bader, J. L., Miller, R. W., Meadows, A. T., et al. (1980). Trilateral retinoblastoma [letter]. *Lancet, 2,* 582-583.

6. Chantada, G. L., Fandino, A., Mato, G., et al. (1999). Phase II window of idarubicin in children with extraocular retinoblastoma. *Journal of Clinical Oncology, 17,* 1847-1850.

7. Cohen, D. G. (1992). Retinoblastoma: A hereditary tumor in children. *Seminars in Oncology Nursing, 8,* 235-240.

8. Crom, D. (1998). Retinoblastoma. In M. J. Hockenberry-Eaton (Ed.), *Essentials of pediatric oncology nursing: A core curriculum* (pp. 48-51). Glenview, IL: Association of Pediatric Oncology Nurses.

9. Dickman, P. S., Mandouha, B., Gollin, S. M., et al. (1997). Malignancy after retinoblastoma: Secondary cancer or recurrence? *Human Pathology, 28,* 200-205.

10. Donaldson, S. S., Egbert, P. R., Newsham, I., et al. (1997). Retinoblastoma. In P. A. Pizzo, & D. G. Poplack (Eds.), *Principles and practice of pediatric oncology* (3rd ed., pp. 699-715). Philadelphia: Lippincott-Raven.

11. Frankenfield, P. K. (1996). The power of humor and play as nursing interventions for a child with cancer: A case report. *Journal of Pediatric Oncology Nursing, 13,* 15-20.

12. Friedman, D. L., Himelstein B., Shields, C. L., et al. (2000). Chemoreduction and local ophthalmic therapy for intraocular retinoblastoma. *Journal of Clinical Oncology, 18,* 12-17.

13. Friedman, N. J., Pineda, R., II, & Kaiser, P. K. (1998). *The Massachusetts Eye and Ear Infirmary illustrated manual of ophthalmology.* Philadelphia: W. B. Saunders.

14. Gallie, B. L., & Moore, A. (1997). Retinoblastoma. In D. Taylor (Ed.), *Pediatric ophthalmology* (2nd ed., pp. 519-535). Malden, MA: Blackwell Science.

15. Green, D. M., Tarbell, N. J., & Shamberger, R. C. (1997). Retinoblastoma. In V. T. Devita, Jr., S. Hellman, & S. A. Rosenberg (Eds.) *Cancer: Principles and practice of oncology* (5th ed., pp. 2103-2107). Philadelphia: Lippincott-Raven.

16. Halperin, E. C. (2000). Neonatal neoplasms. *International Journal of Radiation Oncology, Biology and Physics, 47,* 171-178.

17. Halperin, E. C., Constine, L. S., Tarbell, N. J., et al. (1994). Retinoblastoma. *Pediatric radiation oncology,* (2nd ed., pp. 140-170). New York: Raven Press.

18. Hayashi, N., Ido, E., Ohtsuki, Y., et al. (1999). An experimental application of gene therapy for human retinoblastoma. *Investigative Ophthalmology & Visual Science, 40,* 265-272.

19. Imhof, S. M., Hofman, P., & Tan, K. E. (1993). Quantification of lacrimal function after D-shaped field irradiation for retinoblastoma. *British Journal of Ophthalmology, 77,* 482-484.

20. Imhof, S. M., Mourits, M. P., Hofman, P., et al. (1995). Quantification of orbital and mid-facial growth retardation after megavoltage external beam irradiation in children with retinoblastoma. *Ophthalmology, 103,* 263-267.

21. Jay, M., Cowell, J., & Hungerford, J. (1988). Register of retinoblastoma: Preliminary results. *Eye, 2,* 102-105.

22. Jensen, R. D., & Miller, R. W. (1971). Retinoblastoma: Epidemiologic characteristics (1971). *New England Journal of Medicine, 285,* 307-311.

23. Knudson, A. G. J. (1971). Mutation and cancer: Statistical study of retinoblastoma. *Proceedings of the National Academy of Sciences, USA, 68,* 620-623.

24. Lanzkowsky, P. (1999). Retinoblastoma. In *Manual of pediatric hematology and oncology,* (3rd ed., pp. 599-616). San Diego: Academic Press.

25. Nathan, D. G., & Orkin, S. H. (1998). Retinoblastoma. In D. G. Nathan & F. A. Oski (Eds.), *Hematology of infancy and childhood, Vol 2* (5th ed., pp. 1431-1434). Philadelphia: W. B. Saunders.

26. Pradhan, D. G., Sandridge, A. L., Mullaney, P., et al. (1997). Radiation therapy for retinoblastoma: A retrospective review of 120 patients. *International Journal of Radiation Oncology, Biology and Physiology, 39,* 3-13.

27. Pui, C.-H., Ribeiro, R. C., Hancock, M. L., et al. (1991). Acute myeloid leukemia in children treated with epipodophyllotoxins for acute lymphoblastic leukemia. *New England Journal of Medicine, 325,* 1682-1687.

28. Servodidio, C. A., & Abramson, D. H. (1993). Acute and long-term effects of radiation therapy to the eye in children. *Cancer Nursing, 16,* 371-381.

29. Servodidio, C. A., & Abramson, D. H. (1996). Genetic teaching for the retinoblastoma patient. *Insight: The Journal of the American Society of Ophthalmic Registered Nurses, 21,* 120-124.

30. Servodidio, C. A., Abramson, D. H., Boxrud, C., et al. (1993). Nursing implications of visual fields in successfully treated retinoblastoma patients. *Insight: The Journal of the American Society of Ophthalmic Registered Nurses, 281,* 10-16.

31. Shields, C. L., DePotter, P., Himelstein, B. P., et al. (1996). Chemoreduction in the initial management of intraocular retinoblastoma. *Archives of Ophthalmology, 114,* 1330-1338.

32. Shields, C. L., Shields, J. A., & DePotter, P. (1996). New treatment modalities for retinoblastoma. *Current Opinion in Ophthalmology, 7,* 20-26.

33. Thompson, D. G., & Cohen, D. G. (1996). Nursing management of the infant with a congenital malignancy. *Journal of Obstetrics, Gynecology and Neonatal Nursing, 25,* 32-38.

34. Young, J. L., Smith, M. A., Roffers, S. D., et al. (1999). Retinoblastoma. In L. A. G. Reis, M. A. Smith, J. G. Gurney, et al. (Eds.), *Cancer incidence and survival among children and adolescents: United States SEER Program 1975-1995, National Cancer Institute, SEER Program* (pp. 73-78). Bethesda, MD: National Cancer Institute, NIH Pub. No. 99-4649.

29

Rare Tumors

Jill E. Brace O'Neill

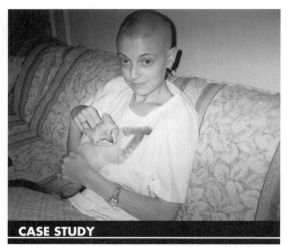

CASE STUDY

Amy is a 15-year-old girl who had been well until she came to her local pediatrician with an approximately 3-week history of scant bloody vaginal discharge and complaint of pelvic "fullness" with intermittent pain. Her past medical and surgical history was unremarkable. Amy had been having regular menses, every 28 days, since age 12; premenstrual symptoms and sexual activity were absent. The remainder of the review of systems was negative. She had never had an internal gynecologic examination at the time of presentation. Her pediatrician performed a physical examination that revealed a fixed, tender, lower right quadrant mass 5 to 7 cm in diameter. An internal gynecologic examination revealed the same, without other abnormalities or anomalies.

Amy was referred to the nearest major medical center that specialized in the treatment of pediatric malignancies. An ultrasound and computed tomography (CT) scan both confirmed the presence of an ovarian mass with solid characteristics, and calcifications attached to the right ovary. Metastatic evaluation by chest and abdominal CT scan was negative. A serum α-fetoprotein (AFP) level was obtained and was 8,000 ng/ml; β subunit of human chorionic gonadotropin (β-hCG) and lactate dehydrogenase (LDH) levels were within normal limits.

Amy was taken to surgery for resection of her ovarian mass. The surgeon was able to perform a gross total resection; however, two positive inguinal lymph nodes were found. Amy's ovarian germ cell tumor was classified as stage II (intermediate risk according to the newest Children's Oncology Group [C.O.G.] staging criteria) because of the positive lymph nodes smaller than 2 cm and a positive tumor marker. The surgeon reported that there was no visceral involvement (i.e., omentum, intestine, or bladder) or contralateral spread of the tumor, and peritoneal washings performed at the time of surgery were negative for malignant cells. Pathology review of the excised tumor and nodes confirmed that the histology of this ovarian tumor was yolk sac germ cell tumor (or endodermal sinus tumor).

Amy and her family consented to treatment that included four cycles of cisplatin, etoposide, and bleomycin every 3 weeks. She completed this treatment experiencing hematologic toxicities and intermittent nausea and vomiting controlled by lorazepam, dexamethasone, and ondansetron. The hematologic side effects were treated successfully with colony stimulating factor and transfusion support. Amy has remained without evidence of disease per follow-up evaluations for 18 months. She has returned to high school and plans to attend a local university next fall.

Rare tumors of childhood and adolescence comprise such diseases as germ cell tumor, thyroid carcinoma, nasopharyngeal carcinoma, malignant melanoma, and others. These diseases are rare in pediatric oncology because they originate in epithelial tissues, the source for most adult cancers, rather than embryonal tissue, the origin of most childhood cancer.[8] These rare cancers are diagnosed more commonly in the 15- to 19-year-old age-group and illustrate the differences in the spectrum of cancers that occur in this age-group as distinct from children younger than 15[73] (Figures 29-1 and 29-2).

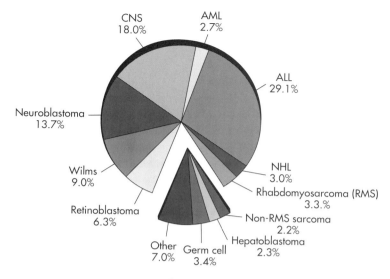

Figure 29-1

Distribution of cancer types, age <5, all races, both sexes, SEER, 1986-1995.   (Adapted from Smith, M. A., Gurney, J. G., & Ries, G. [1999]. Cancer among adolescents 15-19 years old. In L. A. G. Ries, M. A. Smith, J. G. Gurney, et al. [Eds.], *Cancer incidence and survival among children and adolescents: United States SEER Program 1975-1995* [p. 159]. Bethesda, MD: National Cancer Institute, NIH Pub. No. 99-4649.)

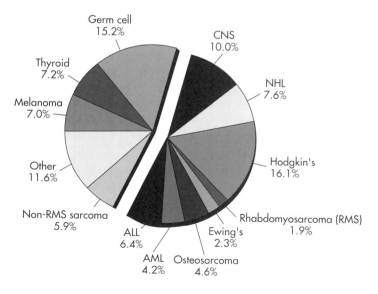

Figure 29-2

Distribution of cancer types, age 15 to 19, all races, both sexes, SEER, 1986-1995.   (Adapted from Smith, M. A., Gurney, J. G., & Ries, L. A. G. [1999]. Cancer among adolescents 15-19 years old. In L. A. G. Ries, M. A. Smith, J. G. Gurney, et al. [Eds.], *Cancer incidence and survival among children and adolescents: United States SEER Program 1975-1995* [p. 159]. Bethesda, MD: National Cancer Institute, SEER Program. NIH Pub. No. 99-4649.)

TABLE 29-1	TUMOR NODE METASTASIS (TNM) STAGING SYSTEM
T	The extent of the primary tumor
N	The presence or absence and extent of regional lymph node metastasis
M	The presence or absence of distant metastasis

The Addition of Numbers to the Three Components Indicates the Clinical Extent of Disease, Showing a Progressive Increase in Tumor Size, Regional Lymph Node Involvement, or Metastatic Spread

Tumor size	T_0	T_1	T_2	T_3	T_4
Nodal involvement	N_0	N_1	N_2	N_3	
Metastasis	M_0	M_1			

In essence, the system uses a shorthand notation for describing the clinical extent of malignant disease.

Data from Lenhard, R. E., Laurence, W., & McKenna, R. J. (1995). General approach to the patient. In G. P. Murphy, W. Lawrence, & R. E. Lenhard (Eds.), *American Cancer Society textbook of clinical oncology* (pp. 64-74). Atlanta, GA: American Cancer Society.

Patients and families who are affected by a diagnosis of a rare cancer need additional support because there is often little information available about the particular cancer diagnosed in the child. Families report a profound sense of isolation. This phenomenon has been described by adult patients with uncommon malignancies even though they may have thousands of counterparts.[21] For pediatric rare tumors, the numbers of cases diagnosed are more often only hundreds nationally or internationally. It is important for pediatric oncology nurses to recognize the importance of identifying resources, providing emotional support, and reducing the isolation felt by these children and families.

Understanding the staging systems used to describe rare tumors is an important objective for the pediatric oncology team. Whereas classification of tumors refers to the anatomic and histologic descriptions of the tumor, staging refers to the extent of the tumor at the time of diagnosis. Recommendations for treatment, and in some cases projections of survival, are based on disease staging. Many common childhood cancers have staging systems that have been developed specifically for the particular disease. Staging has an important role in predicting the clinical outcome and determining the most effective therapy for most pediatric tumors. As yet, no well-accepted staging system exists that is applicable to all childhood tumors.

The model most widely used, especially in adult oncology, is the tumor node metastasis (TNM) staging system developed by the International Union Against Cancer (UICC) and the American Joint Committee on Cancer Staging and Results Reporting (AJCCS). The three components are evaluated clinically by physical examination and the evaluations combined with radiology findings and tumor biopsy. The findings are confirmed histologically whenever possible, especially for lymph nodes, because visual inspection of nodes can be misleading.[43] Subscript numbers are added to describe the pretreatment extent of the patient's disease. The size of the tumor varies from T_0 to T_4 with higher numbers indicating a larger tumor. Nodal involvement ranges from N_0 to N_3, indicating regional lymph node involvement. Metastases are listed as M_0, no distant spread, or M_1, the presence of distant disease (Table 29-1). The appropriate use of the TNM staging system in adult oncology has taken decades to perfect. Pediatric team members have less experience with this system and with application to pediatric cancers, especially rare tumors.[43] Collaboration with nurse and physician colleagues in adult oncology may be useful in understanding application of TMN to pediatric patients.

LIVER TUMORS

Tumors of the liver are the third most common intraabdominal malignancies, after Wilms tumor and neuroblastoma. Thirty percent of childhood liver tumors are benign hemangiomas and hemangioendotheliomas.[60] Hepatoblastoma and hepatocellular carcinoma are the primary liver malignancies in children (Table 29-2).

HEPATOBLASTOMA

Epidemiology. Hepatoblastoma is associated with familial adenomatous polyposis (FAP), an inherited disorder that causes predisposition to multiple colonic adenomas and early-onset carcinomas.[29] The gene for this syndrome maps to chromosome 5q. Hepatoblastoma is also associated with syndromes involving organomegaly, like Beckwith-Wiedemann syndrome (BWS) and hemihypertrophy.[45] Periodic screening for elevated α-fetoprotein (AFP) levels and abdominal sonograms may be recommended for children of parents affected by FAP

TABLE 29-2	COMPARISON OF FEATURES BETWEEN HEPATOBLASTOMA AND HEPATOCELLULAR CARCINOMA	
Feature	**Hepatoblastoma**	**Hepatocellular Carcinoma**
Usual age at presentation	0-3 yr	5-18 yr
Associated congenital anomalies	Dysmorphic features Hemihypertrophy Beckwith-Wiedemann	Metabolic
Advanced disease at presentation	40%	70%
Usual site of origin	Right lobe	Right lobe-multifocal
Abnormal liver function tests	15%-30%	30%-50%
Jaundice	5%	25%
Elevated α-fetoprotein	80%-90%	50%
Positive hepatitis B serology	Absent	Present in some
Abnormal B_{12} binding protein	Absent	Absent
Distinctive radiographic appearance	None	None
Pathology	Fetal and/or embryonal cells ± mesenchymal component	Large pleomorphic tumor cells and tumor giant cells

From Greenberg, M. L., & Filler, R. M. (1997). Hepatic tumors. In P. A. Pizzo & D. G. Poplack (Eds.), *Principles and practice of pediatric oncology* (3rd ed., pp. 717-732). Philadelphia: Lippincott-Raven.

or those found to have inherited overgrowth syndromes. Other associations include renal anomalies, hernias, and Meckel's diverticulum.[13,25,31] At present, evidence is limited about whether associations exist between parental occupational exposures and subsequent development of hepatoblastoma.[15]

Hepatoblastoma can be subdivided into four types based on histology: pure fetal, epithelial-mesenchymal, small cell undifferentiated (anaplastic), and macrotrabecular. There is increasing evidence that pure fetal histology is associated with a better prognosis and that anaplasia is associated with a very poor prognosis.[57]

Clinical presentation.   The majority of children with hepatoblastoma present before 3 years of age with an enlarging asymptomatic abdominal mass; 10% of cases are first noted on routine physical exam.[13,31] Some children have anorexia, weight loss, vomiting, and abdominal pain, but these symptoms are typically associated with advanced disease and hepatocellular carcinoma.[31] Uncommonly, severe osteopenia with back pain, refusal to walk, and pathologic fractures of weight-bearing bones are a presenting clinical syndrome.[13] Some degree of osteopenia is present in the majority of patients, and severe osteopenia is present in 20% to 30% of patients.[13] This osteopenia regresses with tumor resection.

Serum AFP concentrations are elevated in approximately 70% of the cases.[13] Anemia, thrombocytopenia, and leukocytosis are also often found at diagnosis. However, liver function studies usually remain normal. Twenty percent of patients have

TABLE 29-3	CLINICAL GROUPING OF MALIGNANT HEPATIC TUMORS
Designation	**Criteria**
Group I	Complete resection of tumor by wedge resection lobectomy, or by extended lobectomy as initial treatment
Group IIA	Tumors rendered completely resectable by initial irradiation or chemotherapy
Group IIB	Residual disease confined to one lobe
Group III	Disease involving both lobes of the liver
Group IIIB	Regional node involvement
Group IV	Distant metastases, irrespective of the extent of liver involvement

From Greenberg, M. L., & Filler, R. M. (1997). Hepatic tumors. In P. A. Pizzo & D. G. Poplack (Eds.), *Principles and practice of pediatric oncology* (3rd ed., pp. 717-732). Philadelphia: Lippincott-Raven.

metastasis at diagnosis; most commonly to the lungs and porta hepatis and rarely to the bone, central nervous system (CNS), and bone marrow.[79,82]

Diagnostic evaluation.   At present, no clinical grouping system is universally accepted. The C.O.G. has adopted use of a pretreatment and presurgery system proposed by the International Society of Paediatric Oncology (SIOP) Study Group. This system is based on the extent of the tumor and of surgical resection (Table 29-3).

Abdominal ultrasound is the most useful screening technique for children who have an abdominal mass. The ultrasound identifies whether the mass is solid or cystic, and the extent of tumor within the liver. Doppler evaluation is used to assess the patency of the inferior vena cava and hepatic veins. Abdominal and chest CT are needed to assess resectability and identify the presence of pulmonary metastasis. Frequently, imaging reveals intratumoral calcification.[11,31] Ten percent to twenty percent of patients have pulmonary or nodal metastatic disease.[13]

AFP level is the most important biologic marker used to diagnose and follow hepatoblastoma. It is elevated in two thirds of patients with this disease to levels greater than 100 ng/ml and up to 1,000,000 ng/ml.[81] The levels usually decrease after tumor resection and effective therapy. The rate and magnitude of decline in AFP level may be a valuable predictor of outcome in metastatic or unresectable hepatoblastoma.[31,81] β-hCG is elevated in 3% of boys diagnosed with hepatoblastoma.[32] Serum ferritin, a form of iron stored in the liver, may be elevated in the presence of hepatoblastoma, as well.

Treatment. Surgical excision of the primary tumor is necessary for cure, but less than half of all patients have resectable disease.[13] If the tumor can be completely resected with low operative morbidity, chemotherapy is given postoperatively. If the disease is considered unresectable, the diagnosis is confirmed by biopsy and preoperative chemotherapy is given. Chemotherapy can cause enough necrosis and/or shrinkage of the tumor to allow subsequent resection in 70% of the patients.[61,68]

As much as 85% of the liver can be safely removed because of its regenerative capacity. Regeneration of liver cell mass will occur within 1 to 3 months following surgery.[31] The right lobe, which makes up about 70% of the hepatic cell mass, is the site of most hepatic tumors.[31] Mortality from hepatic lobectomy ranges from 10% to 25%, most commonly caused by bleeding intraoperatively and postoperatively.[31]

Hepatoblastoma is highly chemosensitive.[13,56] Effective chemotherapeutic agents include cisplatin, vincristine, fluorouracil, and doxorubicin. Carboplatin, etoposide, and topotecan have also been used to treat advanced stages of this disease.[31,52,82] Postoperative chemotherapy can begin approximately 4 weeks after hepatic resection when adequate regeneration of liver tissue has occurred.[31] Hepatic intraarterial coadministration of chemotherapy and vascular occlusive agents to treat liver tumors, hepatic arterial chemoembolization (HACE), may prove to be feasible, well tolerated, and effective in inducing surgical resectability of these tumors in children.[44] There is limited experience with intrahepatic chemotherapy in this population, but it has been shown to slow the progression of disease.[28] This therapy can also be used as a successful adjunct to liver transplantation.

Doses of radiation therapy used to treat hepatic tumors range between 12 and 20 Gy.[31] Radiation decreases liver regeneration after resection, and therefore has a limited role. Restricted localized-field irradiation may be used for microscopic residual disease at resection margins. However, with effective chemotherapy, residual disease is a rare occurrence.[31] With the encouraging results of preoperative chemotherapy for hepatoblastoma, liver transplantation is reserved for those patients whose primary tumors are still unresectable after preoperative chemotherapy.

Prognosis. Overall survival rates for children who have complete resection of their primary tumor exceeds 75%.[31,56] The following characteristics are correlated with a poor prognosis: tumor involvement of both liver lobes, multifocal disseminated growth pattern in the liver, distant metastases, vascular invasion, embryonal differentiation, and serum AFP value ($<$100 ng/ml or $>$1,000,000 ng/ml associated with a worse outcome than 100 to 1000 ng/ml).[81] The chance of achieving a response to therapy is improved if (1) the tumor does not recur until at least 6 months following primary resection, (2) the metastatic lesions are responsive to chemotherapy, (3) surgical resection of the pulmonary metastases occurs soon after the AFP starts to rise, and (4) the surgical resection is complete.[13] Recurrent disease most often appears in the liver and lungs.

HEPATOCELLULAR CARCINOMA

Epidemiology. Children with hepatocellular carcinoma (HCC) usually show symptoms after 5 years of age and the majority of patients are older than 10 years of age. Boys are affected more often than girls. Risk groups include patients with the chronic form of hereditary tyrosinemia, hepatic fibrosis and cirrhosis secondary to metabolic liver disease, glucose-6-phosphatase deficiency, viral hepatitis, extrahepatic biliary atresia, chemotherapy-induced liver fibrosis, Fanconi's anemia, neurofibromatosis, ataxia-telangiectasia, or FAP.[13,31] HCC in children younger than 15 years of age has the same strong association with the hepatitis B virus (HBV) seen in the adult population.[31,82]

Clinical presentation. Children with HCC often have abdominal discomfort from the size of the hepatic mass. Systemic manifestations may include weight loss, fever, and anorexia. Serum AFP levels are elevated in 50% of the cases and serum transaminase levels are frequently elevated as well.[13] The right lobe of the liver is involved most frequently; bilobar involvement occurs in 50% to 70% of the cases.[82] The tumor is resectable in less than 30% of cases because of multicentric, metastatic, or invasive disease.[83] Metastatic disease, present in 30% to 55% of the cases, is most often to the lymph nodes and lung.[82] Imaging of HCC is the same as with hepatoblastoma, but intratumoral calcification occurs less frequently.[13]

Treatment.   Treatment for HCC consists of chemotherapy and surgery. Complete surgical excision is the sole effective treatment, but it is only initially possible in one third of the cases.[13] Preoperative chemotherapy is seldom effective in converting an unresectable tumor. Most often, patients are treated on protocols for hepatoblastoma, but their overall survival rate is only approximately 15%.[13] Treatment with cisplatin and doxorubicin may be recommended as adjuvant therapy because these are active agents in the treatment of HCC.

Studies have demonstrated the safety and efficacy of transcatheter hepatic arterial chemoembolization (TACE) for the treatment of HCC.[27,65] This treatment option offers the possibility for tumor resection for patients whose tumors were initially thought to be unresectable. Furthermore, this treatment modality may help minimize the risk of tumor progression before liver transplant and when used in combination with other agents, may improve the overall survival time for patients with HCC. The role of liver transplantation in the management of hepatic malignancies is controversial. Results of liver transplantation have been poor but new protocols are being explored in an attempt to alter the dismal prognosis associated with this tumor.[13] In countries with high incidence of HCC, vaccination against the hepatitis virus is considered the best preventive measure.[80]

Prognosis.   In contrast to hepatoblastoma, combined chemotherapy and surgery has had little impact on the outcome for patients with HCC. Overall survival in HCC is between 10% to 20%.[82] The only exception is a variant form of HCC known as *fibrolamellar HCC* that is associated with a high rate of surgical resectability and improved overall survival compared with typical HCC.[36,82]

FUTURE DIRECTIONS

More research is necessary to improve treatment for the higher stage hepatoblastoma patient and for those with hepatocellular carcinoma. Future research will need to focus on the role of liver transplantation for these malignancies, as well as in-

traarterial chemotherapy administration and the effect of new or different chemotherapeutic agents. Determining the the impact of these treatments on survival in children with hepatic neoplasms will require larger series of patients evaluated in cooperative clinical trials.

FIBROSARCOMA

EPIDEMIOLOGY

Fibrosarcoma is one of the most common soft tissue sarcomas (non-rhabdomyosarcoma) in children and adolescents and is the most common soft tissue sarcoma occurring in children younger than 1 year of age.[74] No significant gender predominance can be clearly defined. Two peak incidences occur, the first in children younger than 5 years of age and the second in those 10 to 15 years of age.[49] The two types are referred to as congenital or infant and adult forms. Tumors in infants usually have a more benign course[17,49] and the incidence is highest in the first 6 months of life.[54] The adult form of fibrosarcoma has been associated with prior radiation exposure in some patients.[49]

CLINICAL PRESENTATION

Fibrosarcomas occur most frequently in the extremity, often in the distal segments (70%).[49] In a review of 182 children, 80% had localized disease, 8% had regional dissemination, and 12% had widespread disseminated disease.[51] Other sites include brain/spinal cord,[22,55] head and neck,[72] oral cavity,[33] or lung.[35] Presenting signs and symptoms are related to the location of the primary tumor or metastases.

DIAGNOSTIC EVALUATION

Myofibroblasts are cells of controversial origin that have immunohistochemical and ultrastructural features of both fibroblasts and smooth muscle.[72] They function in the pathophysiology of wound contracture and closure, and are found in abundance in granulation tissue. Histologically, fibrosarcoma cells appear spindle shaped with a herringbone or fascicular growth pattern.[54,72] Prominent mitoses and variable collagen formation may be observed. Characteristic dense cellularity, cellular anaplasia, high mitotic rates, and nuclear atypia are present, which are features shared with these tumors in the adult population.[54] A reliable method of distinguishing between high- and low-grade lesions is so far unknown.[49]

TREATMENT

The usual treatment for the infant with congenital fibrosarcoma is surgical excision,[49] but local recurrences have been reported in 17% to 43% of cases.[54] Because late local recurrences do not appear to affect overall survival, the preferred approach is conservative surgical management aimed at maintaining as much function as possible and avoiding amputation.[49] Chemotherapy is usually reserved for cases in which surgical removal is not possible or would be severely disfiguring. When preoperative chemotherapy is used, the agents include ifosfamide, vincristine, dactinomycin, and cyclophosphamide.[49,54] Radiation therapy has been successful in a small number of patients, but it is not generally recommended because of limited experience and the associated incidence of complications in infants.[54]

Fibrosarcoma is treated differently in the older child and young adult.[49] Preoperative chemotherapy is employed to reduce the tumor size and prevent metastatic disease, followed by an aggressive attempt to remove the tumor by wide local excision or amputation. Recent research has shown a margin of resection greater than 1 cm may reduce local recurrence.[10] After surgery, adjuvant chemotherapy is administered for approximately 6 months. Regimens include vincristine, doxorubicin, cyclophosphamide, dactinomycin, dacarbazine, ifosfamide, and etoposide in various combinations.[49,54]

PROGNOSIS

In fibrosarcoma the site of the primary lesion and the extent of disease at diagnosis significantly affect the prognosis.[51] A local recurrence of a congenital fibrosarcoma of an extremity does not herald systemic spread of the tumor.[49] Of the patients with congenital fibrosarcoma of the extremity, 92% were free of metastatic disease and 95% were alive despite a 32% local recurrence rate. This is in contrast to fibrosarcoma in adolescents and young adults in whom the 5-year survival rate is approximately 60%.[49] With the exception of infants with congenital fibrosarcoma, the prognosis for patients with recurrent or progressive disease is poor. The most common site of metastasis in the older patient is the lung. Local or isolated pulmonary recurrence is treated with complete surgical excision, followed by individualized therapy based on the site of recurrence and biologic characteristics (e.g., grade, invasiveness, and size) of the tumor.

FUTURE DIRECTIONS

For those patients with unresectable and metastatic fibrosarcoma, further research is necessary to determine the role of systemic chemotherapy in facilitating complete surgical resection of primary and metastatic sites. Furthermore, the relationship between cytogenetic traits and the course and re-

sponse to therapy of fibrosarcoma has yet to be determined, as well as the prognostic value of one grading system as opposed to another. Genetic events differentiating infant and adult forms of fibrosarcoma also need additional exploration and study.

NURSING IMPLICATIONS

Fibrosarcoma of the extremity in adolescents and young adults can necessitate amputation or limb-salvage procedures. The nurse provides education for the patient and family about disease and treatment and often helps them to adjust to the radical surgeries required to treat fibrosarcoma. Coordination of services may include surgery, pain service, and physical or occupational therapy.

GERM CELL TUMORS

EPIDEMIOLOGY

Germ cell tumors, occurring at a rate of 2.4 cases per million children, make up approximately 3% of cancers diagnosed in children under 15 years of age.[16,58] Because germ cell tumors can be benign or malignant, this number does not represent the total incidence. For example, the incidence of sacrococcygeal teratomas (80% of which are benign) has been estimated to be 1 in 35,000.[1]

The first germ cells develop in the human embryo yolk sac at approximately 4 weeks gestation, migrate to the gonadal ridge by 6 weeks, and then descend into the pelvis or scrotal sac, populating the developing ovary or testis.[1,16] As a result of this, germ cell tumors typically arise in the gonads or in tissues found along the midline migration path, which include sites such as intracranial, mediastinal, retroperitoneal, or sacrococcygeal.

Germ cell tumors arise from two regions, extragonadal and gonadal. Three distinct groups of pediatric germ cell tumors have been identified within these areas: tumors of the adolescent testis and ovary; extragonadal germ cell tumors of older children; and tumors of infants and young children.[16] Extragonadal tumors are more common in neonates and infants, whereas gonadal site tumors predominate in childhood and adolescence.[58] Extragonadal germ cell tumors most often occur in the following sites (in order of frequency): sacrococcygeal, mediastinal (including pericardium, heart, and lung), intracranial, and retroperitoneal.[16] At diagnosis, 5% will have metastases to the peritoneal cavity, liver, lungs, or brain.[3]

HISTOLOGY

The type of tumor that results depends on the degree of differentiation that has occurred in the migrated germ cell at the time of the malignant event.[1] There are multiple histologic classifications of germ cell tumors and it is not uncommon for one tumor to include more than one cell type. Histologic classifications of these tumors include: teratomas, germinomas (dysgerminomas, seminomas), endodermal sinus tumors (yolk sac tumors), choriocarcinomas, and embryonal carcinomas.[16]

Endodermal sinus tumor or yolk sac tumor is the most common malignant germ cell tumor in the pediatric age group.[1] The sacrococcygeal area is the major site in the newborn and infant, and the ovary in older children and adolescents. Less common sites include: mediastinum, retroperitoneum, pineal area, and vagina. Testicular endodermal sinus tumors have two peaks of incidence, one in infancy and the other in adolescence.[1]

Teratomas are considered the most controversial of the germ cell tumors. The majority (69%) of neonatal teratomas are found in the sacrococcygeal region.[1] Teratomas are classified as either benign (mature) or malignant (immature).

Germinomas can occur in the testis, ovary, or extragonadal sites. The ovary, anterior mediastinum, and pineal area are the most common sites in the pediatric age group.[1] Germinomas account for 10% of all ovarian tumors and approximately 15% of all germ cell tumors in all locations. These tumors are found more often in combination with other germ cell tumors than in the "pure" form and are the most usual malignancy found in dysgenetic (abnormally developed) gonads and undescended testes.[1] Embryonal carcinomas do not exhibit a definite histologic picture but instead are poorly differentiated or anaplastic carcinomas with extensive necrosis.[1]

Lastly, choriocarcinoma is an uncommon, highly malignant germ cell neoplasm. This tumor is seen after infancy most frequently in the mediastinum and gonads.[1] It may also occur in the young infant with disseminated metastases. Choriocarcinomas are rarely seen in the adolescent. Because of these histologic variants, germ cell tumors are each managed quite differently, and have different prognoses. It is therefore imperative to distinguish them before the initiation of treatment.

CLINICAL PRESENTATION

Extragonadal Tumors

Sacrococcygeal.   The clinical presentation of germ cell tumors in children varies according to the location and pathology of the tumor (Table 29-4). Thirty-nine percent of germ cell tumors arise from the sacrococcygeal region.[1] Forty-eight percent of these are benign, 29% are malignant, and 23% have immature components. Approximately 70%

of these occur in girls, and just over half occur in neonates.[1] Sacrococcygeal tumors are classified based on the amount of intrapelvic, abdominal, and external tumor (Figure 29-3).[3] Type I is the most common and the least likely to be malignant at diagnosis. The diagnosis for the first three types is made by physical examination. In type IV, constipation is a common complaint, in addition to urinary frequency or lower extremity weakness.[1] A rectal examination is important to detect a presacral mass indicating a germ cell tumor. In approximately 50% of teratomas, lateral and anteroposterior radiographs of the pelvis can reveal calcifications.[1]

Mediastinum.   The mediastinum is the second most frequent site of extragonadal germ cell tumors. They are almost always located in the anterior superior mediastinum, and occur predominantly in boys.[1] Bone scans may detect osseous metastases, and the levels of the markers AFP, β-hCG, and LDH may be elevated.

Abdominal.   Abdominal germ cell tumors are usually located in the retroperitoneum. This is the third most common extragonadal site.[1] Calcifications can be seen on radiologic studies.

Central Nervous System.   Germ cell tumors make up approximately 3% to 11% of brain tumors in children.[2] The sites of origin in the central nervous system (CNS) include 45% pineal, 35% suprasellar, 10% both, and 5% to 10% in other locations.[2] Chapter 21 provides a complete description of this CNS tumor.

Gonadal Tumors

Ovarian.   Ovarian tumors make up approximately 1% of childhood malignancies and usually appear toward the end of the first and throughout the second decade of life.[16] Ultrasonography initially determines cystic versus solid characteristics and detects calcifications. Assessment of serum tumor markers is critical before surgery to plan treatment and monitor disease activity.[16] Assessment of serum markers and ultrasonography serve as the basis for staging of these tumors. Metastatic evaluation includes an abdominal, pelvic, and/or chest CT scan (Table 29-5).

Testicular.   After birth, testicular germ cells begin mitosis at a slow rate until puberty, when rapid proliferation and spermatogenesis occur.[16] Approximately 7% of all germ cell tumors are testicular,[1] and about 75% of childhood testicular tumors are of a germ cell origin.[16] Ninety percent are localized. Metastatic disease most often occurs in

TABLE 29-4	AGE DISTRIBUTION AND CHARACTERISTICS OF GERM CELL TUMORS*		
Germ Cell Tumor	**Median Age**	**Pathology**	**Clinical Presentation**
EXTRAGONADAL			
Sacrococcygeal	Infancy	Endodermal sinus tumor (yolk sac) Embryonal Benign teratoma Immature Malignant	Variable, depending upon location and histology
Mediastinal (anterior, superior, posterior)	Children and adolescents	Teratoma Embryonal carcinoma Endodermal sinus tumor (yolk sac) Choriocarcinoma	Coughing, wheezing, dyspnea, or chest pain may occur with large tumors
Abdominal (retroperitoneum, stomach, omentum, liver)	Under 2 yr	Benign or malignant	Abdominal pain, constipation, or urinary difficulties
Intracranial (pineal, suprasellar, infrasellar)	Children	Germinomas Nongerminomatous (mixed with yolk sac, choriocarcinoma, or teratocarcinoma)	Headaches, visual disturbances, incoordination, diabetes insipidus, hypopituitarism, anorexia, and precocious puberty
Head and neck (oral cavity, pharynx, orbit, neck, upper jaw)	Infants	Usually benign	Variable, depending upon location
Vaginal	Under 3 yr	Usually malignant	Blood-tinged vaginal discharge
GONADAL			
Ovarian	Preadolescents and adolescents (10-14 yr)	Dysgerminomas Yolk sac tumors Immature teratomas Malignant mixed germ cell tumors Embryonal carcinomas	Palpable abdominal mass, abdominal distention, and varying degrees of acute or chronic abdominal pain, depending on age of the patient, histology, and the presence of ovarian torsion
Testicular	Infants and adolescents	Endodermal sinus tumor (yolk sac) Teratomas	Irregular, nontender scrotal mass

*In order of frequency of occurrence.

the retroperitoneal or chest lymph nodes.[16] As with ovarian germ cell tumors, assessment of serum markers and ultrasonography serve as the basis for staging of these tumors (Table 29-6).

The cryptorchid (undescended) testicle is the most significant risk factor for the development of testicular carcinoma.[53] Given that 10% of patients with testicular cancers are found to have undescended testicles, the potential risk for testicular cancer has been estimated to be 10 to 50 times higher in males with undescended testicles.[85] Because surgical relocation of the testes decreases the

TYPE I   TYPE II

TYPE III   TYPE IV

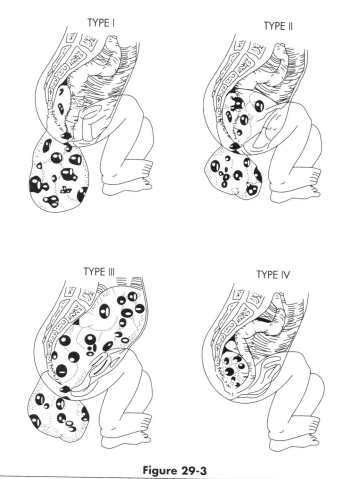

Figure 29-3

Anatomic categories of sacrococcygeal teratomas.   (From Altman, R. P., Randolph, J. G., & Lilly, J. R. [1974]. Sacrococcygeal teratoma: American Academy of Pediatrics Surgical Section survey—1973. *Journal of Pediatric Surgery, 9,* 389-398.)

incidence of histologic anomalies, orchidopexy is advised after 6 months and before 18 months of age.[53] However, orchidopexy may not prevent the subsequent development of testicular carcinoma, and, therefore, recommendations exist regarding surgical inguinal exploration, testicular biopsy, and follow-up for different patient age-groups.[16]

DIAGNOSTIC EVALUATION

The tumor markers AFP and β-hCG are of critical importance in the diagnosis of germ cell tumors. They are used to predict response or indicate the presence of residual or progressive disease.[16] AFP is almost always elevated with yolk sac tumors, but this can also occur with embryonic carcinoma.[1] The peak concentration of AFP is at 12 to 14 weeks gestation and it gradually reaches an adult normal level of less than 10 ng/dL at about 1 year of age.[86] Increasing levels of serum AFP, however, are not always indicative of tumor progression. Other conditions associated with elevated serum AFP include cell lysis secondary to chemotherapy, hepatoblastoma, pancreatic and gastrointestinal malignancies, lung cancers, and benign liver conditions, including hepatic dysfunction and cirrhosis[1,16,86] (Table 29-7).

Another clinical marker is β-hCG, which is a glycoprotein produced by the placenta during pregnancy to promote implantation of a fertilized egg. A normal level of β-hCG in a healthy, nonpregnant adult is less than 5 mIU/ml.[16] Germ cell tumors with trophoblastic elements (e.g., choriocarcinomas) can be identified by the production of β-hCG.[1] Other conditions in which modest elevations of serum β-hCG have been reported include cell lysis secondary to chemotherapy, multiple myeloma, and malignancies of the liver, pancreas, gastrointestinal tract, breast, lung, and bladder.[16] LDH also

TABLE 29-5	CHILDREN'S CANCER GROUP/PEDIATRIC ONCOLOGY GROUP STAGING OF OVARIAN GERM CELL TUMORS

Stage	Extent of Disease
I	Limited to ovary or ovaries; peritoneal washings negative for malignant cells
	No clinical, radiographic, or histologic evidence of disease beyond the ovaries
	Tumor markers normal after appropriate postsurgical half-life decline
	The presence of gliomatosis peritonei* does not upstage patient
II	Microscopic residual or positive lymph nodes (≤2 cm as measured by pathologist)
	Peritoneal washings negative for malignant cells
	Tumor markers positive or negative
	The presence of gliomatosis peritonei* does upstage patient
III	Lymph node with malignant metastatic nodule (>2 cm as measured by pathologist)
	Gross residual or biopsy only
	Contiguous visceral involvement (omentum, intestine, bladder)
	Peritoneal washings positive for malignant cells
	Tumor markers positive or negative
IV	Distant metastases, including liver

From Castleberry, R. P., Cushing, B., Perlman, E., et al. (1997). Germ cell tumors. In P. A. Pizzo & D. G. Poplack (Eds.), *Principles and practice of pediatric oncology* (3rd ed., pp. 921-945). Philadelphia: Lippincott-Raven.

*Peritoneal nodules composed entirely of mature glial tissue and with no malignant elements.

TABLE 29-6	CHILDREN'S CANCER GROUP/PEDIATRIC ONCOLOGY GROUP STAGING OF TESTICULAR TUMORS

Stage	Extent of Disease
I	Limited to testes
	Completely resected by high inguinal orchiectomy or transscrotal orchiectomy with no spill
	No clinical, radiographic, or histologic evidence of disease beyond the testes
	Tumor markers normal after appropriate postsurgical half-life decline; patients with normal or unknown markers at diagnosis must have a negative ipsilateral retroperitoneal node dissection to confirm stage I
II	Transscrotal orchiectomy with gross spill of tumor
	Microscopic disease in scrotum or high in spermatic core (≤5 cm from proximal end)
	Retroperitoneal lymph node involvement (≤2 cm)
	Increased tumor markers after appropriate half-life
III	Retroperitoneal lymph node involvement (<2 cm)
	No visceral or extraabdominal involvement
IV	Distant metastases, including liver

From Castleberry, R. P., Cushing, B., Perlman, E., et al. (1997). Germ cell tumors. In P. A. Pizzo & D. G. Poplack (Eds.), *Principles and practice of pediatric oncology* (3rd ed., pp. 921-945). Philadelphia: Lippincott-Raven.

can be elevated, although this is not specific for tumors of germ cell origin.

Present research is focused on identifying additional markers that would be beneficial in the classification of these tumors. Transcription factor GATA-4 regulates the differentiation and function of murine yolk sac endoderm, and its expression correlates with proliferation and cell survival in certain tissues.[71] It is a clinically useful marker of human yolk sac tumors and may play a role in the maintenance of the malignant phenotype.

TREATMENT

There is a need for individualized multimodal treatment because of the variety of pediatric germ cell tumors. The role of radiotherapy is not completely understood, except in the treatment of CNS germ cell tumors (refer to Chapter 21).

Surgical resection is the treatment of choice for benign germ cell tumors, such as teratoma.[23,47] In malignant tumors, removal is indicated if it does not sacrifice vital structures. Otherwise, debulking or biopsy only is appropriate. Chemotherapy can debulk some tumors initially, so that second-look surgery can occur. Surgical excision alone is safe and effective treatment for 80% to 100% of children with immature teratoma. Unfortunately, over 50% of immature teratomas actually have malignant components. It is recommended that malignant lesions with microscopic residual, lymph node disease, or metastatic disease receive platinum-based chemotherapy.[37,58]

Improvement in the cure rates for pediatric germ cell tumors has occurred in the past 20 years, especially with the addition of chemotherapy. Single agents such as dactinomycin, vinblastine, bleomycin, doxorubicin, cisplatin, and etoposide have proven activity in various tumors of germ cell origin, and combinations of these agents with synergistic activity have served as the basis for many mul-

TABLE 29-7	NORMAL RANGES OF SERUM α-FETOPROTEIN IN INFANTS	
Age	No. Pts.	Mean ± SD (ng/ml)
Premature	11	134,734 ± 41,444
Newborn	55	48,406 ± 34,718
Newborn-2 wk	16	33,113 ± 32,503
2 wk-1 mo	12	9,452 ± 12,610
2 mo	40	323 ± 278
3 mo	5	88 ± 87
4 mo	31	74 ± 56
5 mo	6	46.5 ± 19
6 mo	9	12.5 ± 9.8
7 mo	5	9.7 ± 7.1
8 mo	3	8.5 ± 5.5

From Wu, J. T., & Sudar, K. (1981). Serum AFP levels in normal infants. *Pediatric Research, 15*, 50-52.

tidrug regimens.[16] Vinblastine and bleomycin were considered the mainstays during the 1970s.[1,16] Disease-free survival (DFS) ranged from 22% to 74%. With the addition of cisplatin, a substantial increase in DFS to 68% to 92% occurred.[12,59] Cisplatin, etoposide, and bleomycin (PEB) is the standard treatment used in current studies.[16,19,30,46] Cisplatin has also improved the survival for recurrent or metastatic disease.[59]

Generally, in low-risk disease, no chemotherapy is indicated.[16,18] Patients with moderate-risk gonadal tumors or progression of disease in untreated tumors may be adequately managed with three to four courses of a platinum-containing regimen.[16,19] For higher-risk patients, 6 months of a platinum-based chemotherapy regimen is indicated.[30]

PROGNOSIS

Prognostic factors related to germ cell tumors vary. Pathologists differ regarding the prognostic importance of tumor grade vs. histologic category.[37] Other studies support that site, stage, and AFP level have prognostic significance for this disease.[39,46] Current survival for low-stage (stages I and II) gonadal sites approaches 100% and survival for higher stage (stages III and IV) gonadal sites is approximately 95%. Survival for extragonadal lesions is approximately 90% for stages I and II and 75% for stages III and IV. Retroperitoneal and testicular primary sites have been associated with a good outcome.[7] Sacrococcygeal and mediastinal tumors have a poorer prognosis.[7] A recent study of prognostic factors in children older than 1 year of age with extracranial localized malignant nonseminomatous germ cell tumors revealed the following three prognostic groups: (1) good prognosis patients had localized gonadal or retroperitoneal primary sites and AFP levels <10,000 ng/ml (3-year failure free survival [FFS] rate, 100%); (2) intermediate prognosis patients had extensive nonmetastatic primary sites and AFP levels <10,000 ng/ml or nongonadal nonretroperitoneal localized primary sites with AFP levels <10,000 ng/ml (3-year FFS rate, 81%); and (3) poor prognosis patients with AFP levels >10,000 ng/ml or advanced nonretroperitoneal nongonadal primary sites (3-year FFS rate, 43%).[7] Immature teratomas with microscopic foci of yolk sac tumor tend to have a worse prognosis, and elevations in AFP of greater than 100 ng/ml almost always indicate the presence of foci of yolk sac tumor.[37]

FUTURE DIRECTIONS

The national pediatric oncology research groups continue to develop treatment strategies for patients with germ cell tumors. A new classification schema based on stage and primary site has been developed. This new classification stratifies patients into three risk groups: low risk—patients with stage I malignant gonadal and extragonadal germ cell tumors, including stage I immature teratomas; intermediate risk—patients with stage II to IV gonadal and stage II extragonadal germ cell tumors; and high risk—patients with stage III and IV extragonadal germ cell tumors.[50] Under consideration is observation alone in the lowest stage patients after surgical resection, as well as decreasing the length and cost of treatment for the intermediate-risk group. In the high-risk population, decreasing the toxicities associated with present therapies while looking into new agents is also a goal.

The approach for treatment of relapsed germ cell tumors has not been standardized as yet. This may be partially due to the fact that these tumors are rare and treatment is effective; therefore the number of relapsed patients is small. This further emphasizes the need for all patients with germ cell tumors to be treated on a national research protocol, because long-term survival with chemotherapy has only been anecdotally reported.[50] Given this fact, further research is necessary regarding the role, if any, of stem cell transplant for this patient population.

NURSING IMPLICATIONS

The role of the nurse in preventive health care practices is important, especially with the male patient diagnosed with a gonadal germ cell tumor. Educational efforts focusing on the importance of testicular self-examination for these patients with a history of undescended testicles is essential. This is a subgroup that may need long-term follow-up.

A study documenting the incidence and types of late effects experienced by survivors of childhood or adolescent malignant germ cell tumors reported that more than two thirds of these long-term survivors had at least one complication, and half had greater than one organ system affected from their prior treatment.[34] The systems most often involved included musculoskeletal (41%), endocrine (42%), cardiovascular (16%), gastrointestinal (25%), genitourinary tract (23%), pulmonary (19%), and neurologic (16%) systems. This indicates that the survivors of germ cell tumors will continue to need follow-up for their potential late effects from treatment.

THYROID

EPIDEMIOLOGY

In the United States, approximately 1050 children and adolescents under 20 years of age are diagnosed with carcinomas each year, of which approximately 350 are thyroid carcinomas.[62] Thyroid tumors are divided into adenomas and carcinomas. Thyroid carcinomas are malignant; however, their clinical course is frequently relatively benign because of their slow growth.[76] They occur more commonly in girls (two thirds), with a peak incidence between 7 and 12 years of age.[62] Since the 1960s, the incidence of thyroid cancer has decreased because widespread use of radiotherapy to the neck has been discontinued. Doses of radiation exceeding 1.5 Gy have a carcinogenic effect with an average latency period of 7 to 8 years and a range of 3 to 33 years.[9,24]

Most thyroid carcinomas in childhood are differentiated and rarely anaplastic.[76] The four histologic types include papillary (mixed), follicular, anaplastic, and medullary, individually or in combination.[76] Papillary carcinoma is the most common of these and is characterized by disseminated cancer foci in the thyroid gland. It occurs in younger children. Follicular carcinoma is characterized by adenomatous, follicular formations of cells and occurs in older children. Anaplastic carcinomas are extremely rare in children and are undifferentiated, rapidly growing tumors. Medullary carcinomas are tumors composed of islets of regular, undifferentiated cells with abundant granular cytoplasm.[76] Medullary carcinomas may occur in isolation but more frequently are associated with one of the multiple endocrine neoplasia (MEN) syndromes.[42] The most common site for distant metastases is the lung, and recurrence rates range between 10% and 35%.[24,42] At least 20% of children with papillary thyroid cancer have pulmonary metastases at the time of diagnosis.[76]

CLINICAL PRESENTATION

The most common presenting symptom of thyroid carcinoma is anterior cervical adenopathy.[76] The second most common symptom is a firm, palpable thyroid nodule, isolated or associated with a cervical lymph node. Patients can have single or multiple nodules, but the risk of malignancy is lower with multiple nodules.[24] The incidence of lung metastases at diagnosis ranges from 5% to 28%.[24] Patients are more commonly euthyroid rather than hyperthyroid.[76]

DIAGNOSTIC EVALUATION

If a thyroid abnormality is palpated, a thorough evaluation is necessary, because thyroid nodules are uncommon in children. The patient's history includes questions regarding previous exposure to external radiation to the head and neck, goitrogen (substances that cause goiters and occur naturally in foods such as turnips and cabbage) ingestion, and the presence of local or systemic symptoms, hoarseness, or dysphagia. A thorough and complete physical examination is also warranted, as well as evaluation of thyroid function. Serum thyroglobulin levels can be elevated in thyroid carcinomas, as well as in patients with benign thyroid disorders.[76]

The most accurate diagnosis of thyroid carcinoma in the pediatric patient is based on surgical biopsy. Thyroid scintigrams with iodine-131 or technetium-99m can evaluate thyroid nodules, but discrepancies can occur. A thyroid ultrasound can assess the size of the thyroid and the presence and size of nodules, especially with very small nodules.[76]

TREATMENT

The long-term treatment results in well-differentiated thyroid carcinoma are excellent. Surgery is the initial treatment, though complete thyroidectomy is reserved for obvious bilateral disease or medullary cancer.[76] Disagreement exists over the extent of treatment required to adequately treat thyroid carcinomas. High complication rates follow total, or near total thyroidectomy, including the following complications: hypoparathyroidism, and unilateral and bilateral vocal cord palsies, with a small population of the patients requiring temporary tracheostomies postoperatively.[77] Because of this, others advocate for lobectomy or subtotal thyroidectomy to avoid the postoperative complications and achieve equal long-term cure rates.[77] A conservative, biopsy-only approach is recommended for lymph node evaluation.[76]

Postoperatively, patients are given replacement doses of thyroid to suppress thyroid-stimulating hormone (TSH) and eliminate the growth-promoting effects of this hormone on the tumor. Radioactive iodine, ^{131}I, can provide high levels of radiation to thyroid cancer cells. Treatment with this agent is generally recommended in the pediatric patient, because greater than 20% have lung metastases at the time of diagnosis.[76] Goals of this treatment include thyroid ablation and therapeutic treatment. Approximately 4 weeks after surgery or 6 weeks after discontinuation of T_4 replacement therapy, the patient is given a standard thyroid-ablation dose of [131]I.[76] Six weeks later, a standard scanning of ^{131}I is repeated. If less than 0.3% of the dose is found in the thyroid at 48 hours, ablation was successful.[76] Plasma TSH is elevated in these patients despite the fact that they are not hypothyroid; therefore, when no metastases are found, the patient is started on thyroid hormone replacement therapy.[76]

Iodine-131 therapy for metastatic disease is administered after successful thyroid ablation. Therapeutic doses are given every 3 months after scanning. Most patients achieve a cure after one or two doses, although some may require more.[76] Side effects of the radioactive iodine include bone marrow suppression, nausea and vomiting, adenitis, pain with metastatic disease, pulmonary fibrosis, and rarely leukemia.[41,87]

Treatment of thyroid carcinoma with chemotherapy and external beam radiation is reserved for local control of the anaplastic type. A combination of low-dose doxorubicin and external beam irradiation has been successful in the treatment of this disease.[76]

PROGNOSIS

The prognosis is excellent, and few children die from thyroid carcinomas (event free survival 93% to 100%).[77] The presence of involved neck nodes or distant metastases does not necessarily affect the long-term prognosis, so patients should not be overtreated with extensive surgery and radioactive iodine or external beam irradiation.[42,77] Because of the potential for long-term asymptomatic intervals after treatment, frequent monitoring is imperative including physical examination, chest radiographs, and annual measurement of plasma concentrations of thyroglobulin.[76]

NURSING IMPLICATIONS

Late relapses can occur with thyroid carcinoma, so long-term follow-up at a pediatric oncology center should continue for the patient's lifespan. Teaching patients about the signs and symptoms of thyroid cancer to monitor for a recurrence is the role of the nurse. Furthermore, a review of the symptoms associated with hypothyroidism and hyperthyroidism is necessary because replacement doses of thyroid hormones will be needed for life.

NASOPHARYNGEAL CARCINOMA

EPIDEMIOLOGY

Nasopharyngeal carcinomas are more common in adults and most cases diagnosed in childhood occur in adolescents 15 to 19 years of age. This tumor accounts for one third of all cancers of the upper airways.[50] There is a higher frequency of this tumor in North Africa and Southeast Asia. Although this disease predominates in males in the adult population, this has not been found in the pediatric experience. Nasopharyngeal carcinomas most commonly arise from the nasopharyngeal epithelium and initially spread to cervical lymph nodes.[20]

Cytogenetic abnormalities associated with nasopharyngeal carcinoma include an association with Epstein-Barr virus (EBV), with DNA from EBV found in biopsy specimens.[20] These cells also express the EBV nuclear antigen (EBNA), and patients with nasopharyngeal carcinoma have markedly elevated antibody titers to various EBV antigens. Most importantly, the titers of IgA and IgG antibodies to the viral capsid antigen (VCA) usually correlate with the total tumor burden and decrease with successful therapy.[20] Because these antibodies tend to increase before the actual appearance of recurrent disease, they are an important indicator of disease activity.

Three pathologic types of nasopharyngeal carcinoma exist: squamous cell carcinoma, nonkeratinizing carcinoma, and undifferentiated carcinoma.[20,50] Both nonkeratinizing and undifferentiated carcinoma are associated with elevated EBV titers and undifferentiated carcinoma is the most common in childhood.

CLINICAL PRESENTATION

Presenting signs and symptoms of nasopharyngeal carcinomas are related to the presence of tumor mass and its extension. Most often cervical lymphadenopathy is the initial and only clinical finding.[20] Nasal obstruction, epistaxis, trismus or lockjaw, hearing loss, earache, headache, and chronic otitis media can also occur.[40] Half the children have cranial nerve palsies involving the oculomotor (III), trigeminal (V), or abducens (VI) caused by tumor erosion at the base of the skull. A paraneoplastic syndrome of marked osteoarthropathy with joint swelling, clubbing, and bone and joint pain is most often associated with metastasis.[64]

DIAGNOSTIC EVALUATION

Frequently the diagnosis of nasopharyngeal carcinoma is made by lymph node biopsy. CT of the head and neck includes appropriate views of the brain, with special attention to the base of the skull.[20] Magnetic resonance imaging (MRI) may better define the extent of the primary tumor. CT of the chest and abdomen and a bone scan are performed to detect possible metastatic disease.[20] If invasion of the tumor through the base of the skull has occurred, evaluation of the cerebrospinal fluid (CSF) should also be considered.

A modified tumor node metastasis (TNM) classification system is used with pediatric patients to categorize nasopharyngeal carcinoma. However, with this system most children are classified as stage III or IV because of the high incidence of lymph node metastasis. Therefore this does not correctly assess prognosis or aid with planning therapy.[20] Nasopharyngeal carcinoma tends to be extensive and infiltrating at diagnosis, and subsequently to have a higher stage assigned (Table 29-8).

TREATMENT

The nasopharynx is a difficult area to approach surgically. Therefore, the goal of the initial surgery is to obtain an adequate biopsy specimen from the primary site or an involved lymph node.[20] Radiation therapy is the primary treatment for nasopharyngeal carcinoma. The volume given includes the nasopharynx, posterior nasal cavity, posterior maxillary sinus, base of the skull including the sphenoid and cavernous sinuses, and the cervical lymphatics, including the supraclavicular nodes.[20] The intent is cure, and total radiation doses are 54 to 72 Gy.[6,50,84] This disease is also responsive to several chemotherapy agents including cisplatin, fluorouracil, methotrexate, and bleomycin.[20,88] A multiinstitutional study of nasopharyngeal carcinoma in children and adolescents demonstrated improved survival with the use of neoadjuvant cisplatin plus fluorouracil, methotrexate, and leucovorin, for four courses before irradiation.[20] In addition, chemotherapy is appropriate for patients with recurrent disease. Often chemotherapy can be initiated to establish tumor responsiveness, followed by subsequent radiation therapy.

TABLE 29-8	MODIFIED TNM CLASSIFICATION OF NASOPHARYNGEAL CARCINOMA

PRIMARY TUMOR

T_0	No evidence of primary tumor
T_{is}	Carcinoma in situ
T_1	Tumor confined to nasopharyngeal mucosa or no tumor visible but biopsy positive
T_2	Tumor extended to the nasal fossa, oropharynx, or adjacent muscles or nerves below base of the skull
T_3	Tumor beyond T_2 limits and subclassified as follows:
	T_{3a} Bone involvement below base of the skull
	T_{3b} Involvement of base of skull
	T_{3c} Involvement of cranial nerves
	T_{3d} Involvement of orbit, laryngopharynx, or infratemporal fossa

NODAL INVOLVEMENT

N_0	No clinically positive node
N_1	Nodes wholly in the upper cervical level above larynx
N_2	Nodes between larynx and supraclavicular area
N_3	Nodes palpable in lower third of the neck or supraclavicular area

DISTANT METASTASIS

M	Distant metastasis present

THIS CLASSIFICATION HAS AN ACCOMPANYING STAGE GROUPING

I	T_1	N_0
II	T_2	and/or N_1
III	T_3	and/or N_2
IV	N_3	(any T)
V	M_1	

From Ho, J. H. C. (1979). Clinical staging recommendations. In G. de-Thé & Y. Ito (Eds.), *Nasopharyngeal carcinoma: Etiology and control* (p. 94). Lyon, France: International Agency for Research in Cancer.

Prognosis

No factors other than stage are correlated with prognosis for pediatric nasopharyngeal carcinoma. Patients with small (T_1 or T_2) tumors tend to have a more favorable prognosis than patients with tumors that extend outside the nasopharynx, invade the base of the skull, or cause cranial nerve dysfunction at diagnosis. No factors other than stage have correlated with prognosis for this disease. The most common sites of distant failure are the cervical spine, mediastinum, lung, bone, and liver.[78] An overall survival rate of 78% has been reported.[50]

Nursing Implications

Because of the radiation therapy and chemotherapy regimen necessary to treat this disease, complications (long- and short-term) can be common and extensive. Xerostomia is the most common side effect caused by radiotherapy and is most often permanent.[20] Severe mucositis can also occur during radiation therapy treatment, necessitating hospitalization and parenteral nutrition. Long-term effects of radiation to this region include fibrosis of the neck and trismus, cranial nerve palsies, and brachial plexus weakness.[20] Hypothryoidism may also occur secondary to the radiation. Specific to the chemotherapy regimen, long-term complications may include renal insufficiency, sterility, and pulmonary fibrosis.[20] Educating the patient and the family about these potential short- and long-term side effects will heighten awareness for their development and ensure immediate assessment with subsequent treatment.

MALIGNANT MELANOMA

Epidemiology

Of the 1050 children and adolescents under age 20 diagnosed with carcinomas each year, approximately 300 to 350 have melanomas.[62] The incidence is highest among the 15- to 19-year-olds, higher in females (1.65:1), and presently rising.[14,38] Melanoma is very rare in blacks, which may indicate a potential protective characteristic of skin pigmentation.[20] The primary risk factors for melanoma are sun exposure and an increased number of melanocytic and dysplastic nevi.[62,66] However, recent studies have demonstrated conflicting evidence surrounding whether the incidence of increased dysplastic nevi is related to sunscreen use.[5,26,63]

Relatives of melanoma patients are 1.7 times more likely to develop cutaneous melanoma than the general population.[20] It is estimated that 11% of melanomas may be hereditary, occurring 10 years earlier than the sporadic (also known as de novo)

melanoma.[20] There is also an association between dysplastic nevus syndrome and the occurrence of melanoma.[26] Dysplastic nevi have irregular and indistinct borders, range in size from 5 to 12 mm, and have variegated tan to dark brown coloring. Patients with large congenital nevi have an increased risk of melanoma and these lesions should be surgically removed.[20] For a person with dysplastic nevus syndrome who has one relative with melanoma, the risk of developing melanoma is 100%.[67]

Clinical Presentation/Diagnostic Evaluation

Melanomas are characterized by indolent, peripheral enlargement of relatively flat, complex-colored primary lesions.[20] Melanomas can be characterized by change in a pigmented lesion, including hypopigmentation or hyperpigmentation, scaling, size change, or texture change.[67] Metastasis is associated with penetration of the tumor into the deeper cutaneous tissues[20] and occurs in two thirds of children diagnosed with melanoma.[66] Surgical biopsy is the only method of definitive diagnosis. A biopsy should be performed on any irregularly pigmented lesion (> 2 cm) in a preadolescent individual.[67]

Treatment

Treatment for melanoma requires careful planning because of the potential for metastasis.[20] Definitive surgery depends on the site, size, level of invasion, and extent or stage of the tumor (Table 29-9). The surgical goal is wide excision, with skin grafting when necessary. When there is regional lymph node involvement, chemotherapy is indicated. Agents

TABLE 29-9	STAGING OF MELANOMAS IN RELATION TO DEPTH OF INVASION
Level I	All tumor cells are confined to epidermis with no invasion through basement membrane
Level II	Tumor cells penetrate through basement membrane into papillary dermis but do not extend to reticular dermis
Level III	Tumor cells fill papillary dermis and abut against reticular dermis without invasion of reticular dermis
Level IV	Extension of tumor cells between bundle of collagen characteristic of reticular dermis
Level V	Invasion into subcutaneous tissue

From Douglass, E. C., & Pratt, C. B. (1997). Management of infrequent cancers of childhood. In P. A. Pizzo & D. G. Poplack (Eds.), *Principles and practice of pediatric oncology* (3rd ed., pp. 977-1003). Philadelphia: Lippincott-Raven.

most commonly used include cyclophosphamide, dactinomycin, and vincristine.[20] Palliative radiation may be of benefit. Treatment with interferon-α2a and interleukin-2 has also demonstrated a response in metastatic disease, but without improved survival.[20] Presently cisplatin and etoposide are being evaluated,[20] as are vaccines and immunotherapy.[67]

The current recommendation for follow-up and monitoring is skin examinations every 3 to 6 months.[67] Patients are instructed to thoroughly examine their own skin on a weekly basis, as well.

PROGNOSIS

The 5-year overall survival rate is 91% for nonmetastatic malignant melanoma (females 93%, males 87%).[62] Spread to lymphatics or regional lymph nodes carries a less than 5% 5-year survival.[67] The key to curing melanoma is prevention: avoidance of blistering solar radiation, use of sunscreen, use of protective clothing, and shading as much as possible when exposure is unavoidable.[63,67] Of note is recent research suggesting that those exposed to occasional periods of intense sunlight may be at greater risk of melanoma than others who regularly spend long hours in the sun.[48]

NURSING IMPLICATIONS

Although skin malignancies in children are uncommon, a high index of suspicion is essential for prompt diagnosis and treatment. Late detection is believed to be a consequence of a low index of suspicion by medical providers because of the rarity of the condition.[66]

Nurses infrequently have the opportunity to prevent cancer, yet nurses can play an instrumental role in patient education surrounding sun exposure and preventing sunburn. Defining high-risk groups, prevention, and surveillance techniques are all important aspects of an educational program aimed to reduce the incidence of malignant melanoma. High-risk groups are those with a family history of dysplastic/melanocytic nevi, fair-skinned persons, and those living at higher latitudes. The regular and correct use of broad-spectrum sunscreens is a key part of a program to prevent sunburn, sun damage, and skin cancer; but it is only part of the solution. Other vital aspects of a comprehensive education program include limiting sun exposure and restricting it during the strongest times of day, covering exposed skin with clothing, and avoidance of sun lamps or beds.[4] Nurses can teach families not only prevention techniques, but also the importance of early diagnosis and skin surveillance.

Cancer in children and adolescents is rare. The previously described types of tumors are the least frequently seen of those cancers that occur in the pediatric population. Because of this, childhood and adolescent cancers must be referred to medical centers that have a multidisciplinary team of cancer specialists with experience treating these rare diseases and meeting the special needs of this population. The multidisciplinary team from such centers incorporates the skills of physicians, nurses, surgical specialists, social workers, psychologists, and others to ensure that children receive treatment, supportive care, and rehabilitation that will achieve optimal survival and quality of life. At these centers, there are clinical trials available for most of the types of cancer that occur in children and adolescents, and the opportunity to participate in these trials is offered to most eligible patients and their families.

For the rare group of tumors previously described, clinical trials may not be available or accrual to such studies may take a long time because of their low incidence, a frustrating reality for many patients and families. For example, pediatric cooperative groups enroll only 21% of these patients in protocols, and only 2.4% of patients are registered in adult cooperative group trials.[54a] Furthermore, the true incidence of these tumors can easily be underestimated with the lack of unified efforts to develop accurate databases. Although there are a variety of reasons that children and adolescents with rare tumors are not included in currently available databases tracking their incidence and are not enrolled in clinical trials, the Children's Oncology Group (C.O.G.) has initiated efforts to improve the study of these types of tumors. These efforts include establishment of a diagnostic registry, development of tumor banking protocols, participation in combined adult-pediatric trials when pediatric trials are not feasible, improving collaboration with adult oncologists, and, most importantly, providing information about rare tumors on the C.O.G. website for patients, families, and primary care practitioners.

The Internet is providing new means of education and support for cancer patients of all ages. This resource can be especially useful for those diagnosed with a rare cancer. A central role for the nurse is to educate patients and families about the use of medically oriented resources on the Internet, especially because some of the resources available for rare tumors are on established sites, whereas others are not.[69,70] Several general resources are available for rare tumors: Cancer Information and Support International (http://www.cancer-info.com/shonenos.html); Children's Cancer Association (http://www.childrenscancerassociation. org/resources.cfm); Cancer Index: A guide to internet resources for cancer (http://www.cancer index.org); Association of Cancer Online Resources (http://www.acor.org); Cancerlinks.org index (http://www.cancerlinks.org); or a stand-alone home page. These strategies help put the small numbers of persons with these diseases in touch with each other.

The challenges faced by pediatric cancer patients diagnosed with a rare tumor and by their families require that the pediatric oncology nurse use a wide array of resources to meet their diverse needs. Consultation with adult oncology nursing colleagues may be a useful intervention. Advances in treating the diseases encountered rarely in children and adolescents but more commonly in adults will likely come from clinical trials with adults. The pediatric oncology nurse who has established collegial ties with adult oncology nurse specialists will be better positioned to utilize this information to benefit pediatric populations.

REFERENCES

1. Ablin, A., & Isaacs, H., Jr. (1993). Germ cell tumors, In P. A. Pizzo & D. G. Poplack (Eds.), *Principles and practice of pediatric oncology* (2nd ed., pp. 867-890). Philadelphia: Lippincott-Raven.

2. Allen, J. C., Bruce, J., Kun, L. E., et al. (1996). Pineal region tumors. In V. A. Levin (Ed.), *Cancer in the nervous system* (pp. 171-185). New York: Churchill Livingstone.

3. Altman, R. P., Randolph, J. G., & Lilly, J. R. (1974). Sacrococcygeal teratomas: American Academy of Pediatrics Surgical Section survey-1973. *Journal of Pediatric Surgery, 9,* 389-398.

4. Austoker, J. (1994). Melanoma: Presentation and early diagnosis. *British Medical Journal, 306,* 1682-1686.

5. Autier, P., Dore, J. F., Cattaruzza, M. S., et al. (1998). Sunscreen use, wearing clothes, and number of nevi in 6- and 7-year-old European children. *Journal of the National Cancer Institute, 90,* 1873-1880.

6. Ayan, I., & Altun, M. (1996). Nasopharyngeal carcinoma in children: Retrospective review of 50 patients. *International Journal of Radiation Oncology, Biology, Physiology, 35,* 485-492.

7. Baranzelli, M. C., Kramar, A., Bouffet, E., et. al. (1999). Prognostic factors in children with localized malignant nonseminomatous germ cell tumors. *Journal of Clinical Oncology, 17,* 1212-1218.

8. Bernstein, L., & Gurney, J. G. (1999). Carcinomas and other malignant epithelial neoplasms. In L. A. G. Reis, M. A. Smith, J. G. Gurney, et al. (Eds.), *Cancer incidence and survival among children and adolescents: United States SEER Program 1975-1995* (pp. 139-147). Bethesda, MD: National Cancer Institute, SEER Program. NIH Pub. No. 99-4649.

9. Black, P., Straaten, A., & Gutjahr, P. (1998). Secondary thyroid carcinoma after treatment for childhood cancer. *Medical and Pediatric Oncology, 31,* 91-95.

10. Blakely, M. L., Spurbeck, W. W., Pappo, A. S., et. al. (1999). The impact of margin of resection on outcome in pediatric nonrhabdomyosarcoma soft tissue sarcoma. *Journal of Pediatric Surgery, 34,* 672-675.

11. Boechat, M. I., Kangarloo, H., Ortega, J., et al. (1988). Primary liver tumors in children: Comparison of CT and MR imaging. *Radiology, 169,* 727-732.

12. Bosl, G. J., Geller, N. L., Bajorin, D., et. al. (1988). A randomized trial of etoposide + cisplatin versus vinblastine + bleomycin + cisplatin + cyclophosphamide + dactinomycin in patients with good-prognosis germ cell tumors. *Journal of Clinical Oncology, 6,* 1231-1238.

13. Bowman, L. C., & Riely, C. A. (1996). Management of pediatric liver tumors. *The Surgical Oncology Clinics of North America, 5,* 451-459.

14. Bruce, A. J., & Brodland, D. G. (2000). Subspecialty clinics: Dermatology. Overview of skin cancer detection and prevention for the primary care physician. *Mayo Clinic Proceedings, 75,* 491-500.

15. Buckley, J. D., Sather, H., Ruccione, K., et. al. (1989). A case-control study of risk factors for hepatoblastoma: A report from the Childrens Cancer Study Group. *Cancer, 64,* 1169-1176.

16. Castleberry, R. P., Cushing, B., Perlman, E., et al. (1997). Germ cell tumors. In P. A. Pizzo & D. G. Poplack (Eds.), *Principles and practice of pediatric oncology* (3rd ed., pp. 921-945). Philadelphia: Lippincott-Raven.

17. Coffin, C. M. (1997). Fibroblastic-myofibroblastic tumors. In C. M. Coffin, L. P. Dehner, & P. A. O'Shea (Eds.), *Pediatric soft tissue tumors: A clinical, pathological, and therapeutic approach* (pp. 133-178). Baltimore, MD: Williams & Wilkins.

18. Cushing, B., Giller, R., Ablin, A., et. al. (1999). Surgical resection alone is effective treatment for ovarian immature teratoma in children and adolescents: A report of the Pediatric Oncology Group and the Children's Cancer Group. *American Journal of Obstetrics & Gynecology, 181,* 353-358.

19. Cushing, B., Giller, R., Lauer, S., et. al. (1998). Comparison of high dose or standard dose cisplatin with etoposide and bleomycin in children with stage I—IV extragonadal malignant germ cell tumors: A Pediatric Intergroup Report [meeting abstract]. *Proceeding of the Annual Meeting of the American Society of Clinical Oncology, 17,* A2017.

20. Douglass, E. C., & Pratt, C. B. (1997). Management of infrequent cancers of childhood. In P. A. Pizzo & D. G. Poplack (Eds.), *Principles and practice of pediatric oncology* (3rd ed., pp. 977-1003). Philadelphia: Lippincott-Raven.

21. Dow, K. H., Ferrell, B. R., & Anello, C. (1997). Balancing demands of cancer surveillance among survivors of thyroid cancer. *Cancer Practice, 5,* 289-295.

22. Duffner, P., Burger, P. C., Cohen, M. E., et al. (1994). Desmoplastic infantile gangliogliomas: An approach to therapy. *Neurosurgery, 34,* 583-589.

23. Ein, S. H., Mancer, K., & Alayemi, S. D. (1985). Malignant sacrococcygeal teratoma, endodermal sinus, yolk sac tumor in infants and children: A 32-year review. *Journal of Pediatric Surgery, 20,* 473-477.

24. Feinmesser, R., Lubin, E., Segal, K., et al. (1997). Carcinomas of the thyroid in children: A review. *Journal of Pediatric Endocrinology and Metabolism, 10,* 561-568.

25. Foley, G. V. (1997). Meeting the needs of the few. *Cancer Practice, 5,* 273.

26. Gallagher, R. P., Rivers, J. K., Lee, T. M., et al. (2000). Broad-spectrum sunscreen use and the development of new nevi in white children: A randomized controlled trial. *Journal of the American Medical Association, 283,* 2955-2960.

27. Gattoni, F., Cornalba, G., Brambilla, G., et al. (1998). Survival of 184 patients with hepatocellular carcinoma in cirrhotic liver treated with chemoembolization: A multicenter study. *Radiology Medicine, 95,* 362-368.

28. Gerber, D. A., Arcement, C., Carr, B., et al. (2000). Use of intrahepatic chemotherapy to treat advanced pediatric hepatic malignancies. *Journal of Pediatric Gastroenterology and Nutrition, 30,* 137-144.

29. Giardiella, F. M., Offerhaus, G. J., Krush, A. J., et al. (1991). Risk of hepatoblastoma in familial adenomatous polyposis. *Journal of Pediatrics, 119,* 766-768.

30. Giller, R., Cushing, B., Lauer, S., et al. (1998). Comparison of high dose or standard dose cisplatin with etoposide and bleomycin in children with stage III and IV malignant germ cell tumors at gonadal primary sites: A Pediatric Intergroup Trial [meeting abstract]. *Proceedings of the Annual Meeting of the American Society of Clinical Oncology, 17,* A2016.

31. Greenberg, M. L., & Filler, R. M. (1997). Hepatic tumors. In P. A. Pizzo & D. G. Poplack (Eds.), *Principles and practice of pediatric oncology* (3rd ed., pp. 717-732). Philadelphia: Lippincott-Raven.

32. Gregory, J. J., Jr., & Finlay, J. (1999). Alpha-fetoprotein and beta-human chorionic gonadotropin: Their clinical significance as tumour markers. *Drugs, 57,* 463-467.

33. Grundfast, K., Healy, G., & Richardson, M. (1991). Fibrosarcoma of the infratemporal fossa in an 8-year-old. *Head and Neck, 13,* 156-159.

34. Hale, G. A., Marina, N. M., Jones-Wallace, D., et al. (1999). Late effects of treatment for germ cell tumors during childhood and adolescence. *Journal of Pediatric Hematology/Oncology, 21,* 115-122.

35. Hancock, B. J., DiLorenzo, M., Youssef, S., et al. (1993). Childhood primary pulmonary neoplasms. *Journal of Pediatric Surgery, 28,* 1133-1136.

36. Hany, M. A., Betts, D. R., Schmugge, M., et al. (1997). A childhood fibrolamellar hepatocellular carcinoma with increased aromatase activity and a near triploid karyotype. *Medical and Pediatric Oncology, 28,* 136-138.

37. Heifetz, S. A., Cushing, B., Giller, R., et al. (1998). Immature teratomas in children—pathologic considerations: A report from the combined Pediatric Oncology Group/Children's Cancer Group. *American Journal of Surgical Pathology, 22,* 1115-1124.

38. Hoang, M. T., & Eichenfield, L. F. (2000). The rising incidence of melanoma in children and adolescents. *Dermatology Nursing, 12,* 192-193.

39. International Germ Cell Cancer Collaborative Group (IGCCCG). (2000). International germ cell consensus classification: A prognostic factor–based staging system for metastatic germ cell cancers. *Journal of Clinical Oncology, 15,* 594-603.

40. Komoroski, E. M. (1994). Nasopharyngeal carcinoma: Early warning signs and symptoms. *Pediatric Emergency Care, 10,* 284-286.

41. Kuefer, M. U., Moinuddin, M., Heideman, R. L., et al. (1997). Papillary thyroid carcinoma: Demographics, treatment, and outcome in eleven pediatric patients treated at a single institution. *Medical and Pediatric Oncology, 28,* 433-440.

42. LaQuaglia, M. P., & Telander, R. L. (1997). Differentiated and medullary thyroid cancer in childhood and adolescence. *Seminars in Pediatric Surgery, 6,* 42-49.

43. Lenhard, R. E., Lawrence, W., & McKenna, R. J. (1995). General approach to the patient. In G. P. Murphy, W. Lawrence, & R. E. Lenhard (Eds.), *American Cancer Society textbook of clinical oncology* (pp. 64-74). Atlanta, GA: American Cancer Society.

44. Malogolowkin, M. H., Stanley, P., Steele, D. A., et al. (2000). Feasibility and toxicity of chemoembolization for children with liver tumors. *Journal of Clinical Oncology, 18,* 1279-1284.

45. Mann, J. R., Kasthuri, N., Raafat, F., et al. (1990). Malignant hepatic tumours in children: Incidence, clinical features and aetiology. *Paediatric and Perinatal Epidemiology, 4,* 276-289.

46. Mann, J. R., Raafat, F., Robinson, K., et al. (2000). The United Kingdom Children's Cancer Study Group's second germ cell tumor study: Carboplatin, etoposide, and bleomycin are effective treatment for children with malignant extracranial germ cell tumors, with acceptable toxicity. *Journal of Clinical Oncology, 18,* 3809-3818.

47. Marina, N. M., Cushing, B., Giller, R., et al. (1999). Complete surgical excision is effective treatment for children with immature teratomas with or without malignant elements: A Pediatric Oncology Group/Children's Cancer Group Intergroup Study. *Journal of Clinical Oncology, 17,* 2137-2143.

48. Mayo Foundation for Medical Education and Research (MFMER). (1999, July). Sunbathing—protect your skin [19 paragraphs]. [On-line serial], January 10, 2001. Available e-mail: http://www.MayoClinic.com/home?id=HQ01462.

49. Miser, J. S., Tricher, T. J., Kinsella, T. J., et al. (1997). Other soft tissue sarcomas of childhood. In P. A. Pizzo & D. G. Poplack (Eds.), *Principles and practice of pediatric oncology* (3rd ed., pp. 865-888). Philadelphia: Lippincott-Raven.

50. National Cancer Institute's Physician Desk Query (PDQ) [electronic information]. (last modified 1/2001). Bethesda, MD.

51. Neifeld, J. P., Berg, J. W., Godwin, D., et al. (1978). A retrospective epidemiologic study of pediatric fibrosarcomas. *Journal of Pediatric Surgery, 13,* 735-739.

52. Nitschke, R., Parkhurst, J., Sullivan, J., et al. (1998). Topotecan in pediatric patients with recurrent and progressive solid tumors: A Pediatric Oncology Group phase II study, *Journal of Pediatric Hematology/Oncology, 20,* 315-318.

53. Palmer, J. M. (1991). The undescended testicle. *Endocrine Metabolism Clinics of North America, 20,* 231.

54. Palumbo, J. S., & Zwerdling, T. (1999). Soft tissue sarcomas of infancy. *Seminars in Perinatology, 23,* 299-309.

54a. Pappo, A. (2001). The Children's Oncology Group Rare Tumor Initiative: "Rare is relative," *Children's Oncology News, II*(2), 8-9.

55. Powers, T. A., Partain, C. L., Kessler, R. M., et al. (1988). Central nervous system lesions in pediatric patients: Gd-DTPA-enhanced MR imaging. *Radiology, 169,* 723-726.

56. Pritchard, J., Brown, J., Shafford, E., et al. (2000). Cisplatin, doxorubicin, and delayed surgery for childhood hepatoblastoma: A successful approach—results of the first prospective study of the International Society of Pediatric Oncology. *Journal of Clinical Oncology, 18,* 3819-3828.

57. Raney, B. (1997). Hepatoblastoma in children: A review. *Journal of Pediatric Hematology/Oncology, 19,* 418-422.

58. Rescorla, F. J. (1999). Pediatric germ cell tumors. *Seminars in Surgical Oncology, 16,* 144-158.

59. Rescorla, F. J., & Breitfeld, P. P. (1999). Pediatric germ cell tumors. *Current Problems in Cancer, 23,* 257-303.

60. Reynolds, M. (1999). Pediatric liver tumors. *Seminars in Surgical Oncology, 16,* 159-172.

61. Reynolds, M., Douglass, E. C., Finegold, M., et al. (1992). Chemotherapy can convert unresectable hepatoblastoma. *Journal of Pediatric Surgery, 27,* 1080-1084.

62. Ries, L. A. G., Smith, M. A., Gurney, J. G., et al. (Eds.). (1999). *Cancer incidence and survival among children and adolescents: United States SEER program 1985-1995,* Bethesda, MD: National Cancer Institute, SEER Program. NIH Pub. No. 99-4649.

63. Rigel, D. S., Naylor, M., & Robinson, J. (2000). What is the evidence for a sunscreen and melanoma controversy? *Issues in Dermatology, 136,* 1447-1449.

64. Roebuck, D. J. (1999). Skeletal complications in pediatric oncology patients. *Radiographics, 19,* 873-885.

65. Rose, D. M., Chapman, W. C., Brockenbrough, A. T., et al. (1999). Transcatheter arterial chemoembolization as primary treatment for heptocellular carcinoma. *American Journal of Surgery, 177,* 405-410.

66. Sasson, M., & Mallory, S. (1996). Malignant primary skin tumors in children. *Current Opinion in Pediatrics, 8,* 372-377.

67. Sealy, D. P. (2000). Melanoma. *Clinician Reviews, 10,* 130-131.

68. Seo, T., Ando, H., Watanabe, Y., et al. (1998). Treatment of hepatoblastoma: Less extensive hepatectomy after effective preoperative chemotherapy with cisplatin and adriamycin. *Surgery, 123,* 407-414.

69. Sharp, J. (1999). The Internet: Changing the way cancer survivors obtain information. *Cancer Practice, 7,* 266-269.

70. Sharp, J. (2000). The Internet: Changing the way cancer survivors receive support. *Cancer Practice, 8,* 145-147.

71. Siltanen, S., Anttonen, M., Heikkila, P., et al. (1999). Transcription factor GATA-4 is expressed in pediatric yolk sac tumors. *American Journal of Pathology, 155,* 1823-1829.

72. Smith, D. M., Mahmoud, H. H., Jenkins, J. J., et al. (1995). Myofibrosarcoma of the head and neck in children. *Pediatric Pathology & Laboratory Medicine, 15,* 403-418.

73. Smith, M. A., Gurney, J. G., & Reis, L. A. (1999). Cancer among adolescents 15-19 years old. In L. A. G. Reis, M. A. Smith, J. G. Gurney, et al. (Eds.), *Cancer incidence and survival among children and adolescents: United States SEER Program 1975-1995* (pp. 157-164). Bethesda, MD: National Cancer Institute, SEER Program. NIH Pub. No. 99-4649.

74. Soule, E. H., & Pritchard, D. J. (1977). Fibrosarcoma in infants and children: A review of 110 cases. *Cancer, 40,* 1711-1721.

75. Stocker, J. T. (1994). Hepatoblastoma. *Seminars in Diagnostic Pathology, 11,* 136-143.

76. Stratakis, C. A., & Chrousos, G. P. (1997). Endocrine tumors. In P. A. Pizzo & D. G. Poplack (Eds.), *Principles and practice of pediatric oncology* (3rd ed., pp. 947-976). Philadelphia: Lippincott-Raven.

77. Sykes, A. J., & Gattamaneni, H. R. (1997). Carcinoma of the thyroid in children: A 25-year experience. *Medical and Pediatric Oncology, 29,* 103-107.

78. Tom, L. W., Anderson, G. J., Womer, R. B., et al. (1992). Nasopharyngeal malignancies in children. *Laryngoscope, 102,* 509-514.

79. Uchiyama, M., Iwafuchi, M., Naito, M., et al. (1999). A study of therapy for pediatric hepatoblastoma: Prevention and treatment of pulmonary metastasis. *European Journal of Pediatric Surgery, 9,* 142-145.

80. Von Schweinitz, D. (1999). Treatment of liver tumors in children. In P. A. Clamien (Ed.), *Malignant liver tumors: Current and emerging therapies.* Malden, MA: Blackwell Science.

81. Von Schweinitz, D., Hecker, H., Schmidt-Von-Arndt, G., et al. (1994). Prognostic factors and staging systems in childhood hepatoblastoma. *International Journal of Cancer, 74,* 593-599.

82. Vos, A. (1995). Primary liver tumours in children. *European Journal of Surgical Oncology, 21,* 101-105.

83. Weinberg, A. G., & Finegold, M. J. (1983). Primary hepatic tumors of childhood. *Human Pathology, 14,* 512-537.

84. Wolden, S. L., Steinherz, P. G., Kraus, D. H., et al. (2000). Improved long-term survival with combined modality therapy for pediatric nasopharynx cancer. *International Journal of Radiation Oncology, Biology, and Physiology, 46,* 859-864.

85. Wright, J. E. (1986). Inpalpable testis: A review of 100 boys. *Journal of Pediatric Surgery, 21,* 151-153.

86. Wu, J. T., Book, L., & Sudar, K. (1981). Serum alpha fetoprotein (AFP) levels in normal infants. *Pediatric Research, 15,* 50-52.

87. Yeh, S. D., & LaQuaglia, M. P. (1997). [131]I therapy for pediatric thyroid cancer. *Seminars in Pediatric Surgery, 6,* 128-133.

88. Zubizarreta, P. A., D'Antonio, G., Raslawski, E., et al. (2000). Nasopharyngeal carcinoma in childhood and adolescence: A single-institution experience with combined therapy. *Cancer, 89,* 690-695.

Langerhans Cell Histiocytosis

Jacquie M. Toia
Danita Dumas
Susan L. Cohn

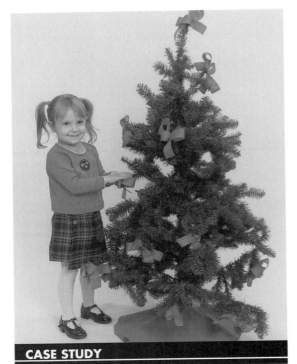

CASE STUDY

Jasmine is a 3½-year-old girl who at 1 year of age had a history of more than 30 "ear infections" with copious drainage, refractory "eczema," and poor growth. The child had been treated with many antibiotics with little effect. The rash was yellow with crust and seborrheic areas. The scalp was diffusely involved as were the ears, ear canals, axillae, groin, and umbilicus. The child was also thought to have vaginitis because of red swollen labia. She was treated with steroid creams, antifungal medications, antihistamines, and skin moisturizers, all to no avail. A skin biopsy confirmed the clinical suspicion of histiocytosis. Shortly after diagnosis she came to the doctor with excessive thirst and urination and had laboratory and magnetic resonance imaging (MRI)-

confirmed diabetes insipidus (DI) with destruction of the posterior pituitary gland.

Jasmine had been successfully managed on twice daily DDAVP therapy for her DI and, after nearly a year of weekly vinblastine and daily steroids, achieved clinical remission of her histiocytosis in June 2000. Since that time she has been maintained on weekly vinblastine as maintenance therapy and has had no recurrences. She will be treated for a total of 1 year following remission status.

After completion of therapy she will be followed closely for signs and symptoms of recurrence or late effects. Potential late effects could include short stature or thyroid failure secondary to her pituitary disease.

Langerhans cell histiocytosis (LCH) is a rare and clinically challenging disease that is characterized by a broad spectrum of clinical behaviors, ranging from lesions that will spontaneously regress to a multisystem, life-threatening disorder.[2,9] The true incidence of the disease is not known because isolated bone lesions may be asymptomatic, or mild skin disease may be mistaken for seborrheic eczema or dermatitis. Children with the more aggressive, disseminated forms of the disease are readily brought to the attention of specialists. Because the extent of disease correlates with outcome, therapy is tailored to the pattern of disease at presentation. Little, if any, therapy is needed when the disease occurs in a single site, whereas aggressive therapy is required for patients with multisystem LCH. Theories regarding the pathogenesis of this biologically complex disease, as well as recent advances in the diagnosis and treatment, are important to the understanding of LCH. LCH is not to be confused with the malignant histiocytic disorders, otherwise referred to as familial hemophagocytic lymphohistiocytosis. This chapter will focus on the diagnosis, treatment, and nursing care of children with LCH.

HISTORICAL PERSPECTIVE

The discovery of LCH dates back to the late 1800s when Paul Langerhan, then a medical student, identified dendritic cells in a layer of the epidermis.[20] However, these cells received little attention until 1961 when Birbeck and colleagues noted a specific structure in the cytoplasm of these dendritic cells with electron microscopy. In 1965 these cytoplasmic organelles were identified in the cells of patients with histiocytosis X. The Birbeck granule continues to be a distinct marker of the Langerhans cell and remains an important morphologic factor in the pathologic diagnosis of LCH.[20]

This disease has been given many names during the past decades,[12] and synonyms of LCH include the following: eosinophilic granuloma, Hand-Schüller-Christian disease, Letterer-Siwe disease, Hashimoto-Pritzker disease, histiocytosis X, self-healing histiocytosis X, self-healing histiocytosis, pure cutaneous histiocytosis, Langerhans cell granulomatosis, Langerhans cell (eosinophilic) granulomatosis, type II histiocytosis, and nonlipid reticuloendotheliosis.

Theories regarding the pathogenesis of LCH are as numerous as the names given to this condition. LCH was initially thought to be an infectious disease, and children were treated with antibiotics.[3] During the 1960s and 1970s, LCH was considered to be a malignant disease, and single-agent or multi-agent chemotherapy became the established treatment.[17] In the 1980s, Osband and colleagues described suppressor cell defects and thymic abnormalities in patients with LCH.[22] In addition, these investigators reported successful treatment with thymic extract, suggesting that the disease may be immunologic. The pathogenesis of LCH in the 1990s was challenged yet again with an enhanced understanding of the role of cytokines and the finding that lesional LCH cells show clonality.[16,27,28] However, despite these research advances, the pathogenesis of this disease remains an enigma, and treatment approaches continue to be based on clinical factors rather than disease biology.

EPIDEMIOLOGY

LCH is rare and sometimes undiagnosed, and therefore the actual incidence of LCH is difficult to establish. Case reporting or referral to pediatric oncology clinics is not mandatory, and in some cases LCH may not be clinically evident. Although LCH may occur at any age, 50% of the cases are diagnosed in children.[10] It is estimated that four to five children per million under the age of 15 years will be diagnosed with LCH each year. Peak occurrence is between 1 and 3 years of age. There is no significant gender difference. Clinical presentation is age dependent. Multisystem LCH frequently occurs in the first 2 years of life. Over 70% of cases with isolated bone lesions are seen in children during the first decade of life, with half of these occurring before age 5.[10]

Epidemiology data are limited. Three case-control studies have been performed, but different associations were found in each study.[4,15] Thus no definitive risk factors for LCH have been identified.

CLINICAL PRESENTATION

Symptoms of LCH vary significantly. Systemic symptoms include fever, weight loss, and/or fatigue. The symptoms associated with involvement of each organ can be defined separately; however, in many patients, the disease affects multiple organs.

SKIN

Skin is a common site of involvement, with skin rashes that are scaly, erythematous, seborrhea-like brown to red papules (Figure 30-1). These rashes are often pronounced in intertriginous areas such as behind the ears and in the axillary, inguinal, and perineal areas.[10] Skin lesions can present as petechial and purpuric lesions, papular xanthoma-like lesions, bronzing of the skin, and mucocutaneous ulcers.[2] Skin lesions may be the only presenting symptom of LCH.[21] However, a thorough physical examination is mandatory to ensure that there is not more extensive disease.

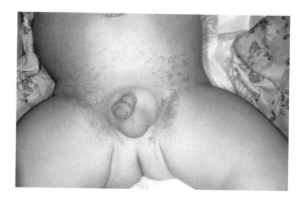

Figure 30-1

Classic skin rash associated with LCH.   (Courtesy Sharon B. Murphy, MD, Professor of Pediatrics, Northwestern University Medical School.)

BONE

The majority of LCH cases have osseous lesions. These lesions can be isolated or part of multisystem disease. The skull bones are affected most often (Figure 30-2). Other common locations include the femur, pelvis, tibia, scapula, jaw, humerus, vertebrae, and ribs. The small bones of the feet and hands are less likely to be involved.[2] Painful swelling is common, which may be accompanied by a dull aching pain, limited range of motion, or inability to bear weight. Orbital lesions may occur with proptosis.

Premature eruption of teeth, loss of teeth, and gingival infiltrates are associated with involvement of the mandible or maxilla (see Figure 30-2). Recurrent otitis media, with or without mastoid involvement, is a common problem for children with LCH. Extensive lesions of the middle ear can cause destruction of the ossicles and deafness. In the spine, the lytic process can cause compression and collapse of the vertebral body.

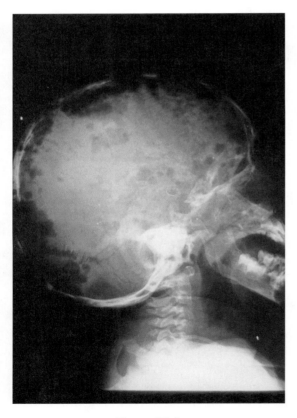

Figure 30-2

Plain skull x-ray demonstrating multiple skull defects associated with bone involvement of LCH. (Courtesy Sharon B. Murphy, MD, Professor of Pediatrics, Northwestern University Medical School.)

LYMPH NODES

Lymphadenopathy may occur from LCH infiltration or as a reaction to bone or skin lesions. Cervical nodes are most often affected, but inguinal, axillary, mediastinal, and retroperitoneal nodes can also be involved.

LIVER AND SPLEEN

Hepatosplenomegaly may result from primary LCH involvement, or as a secondary phenomenon related, for example, to enlarged lymph nodes in the porta hepatis. Ascites, jaundice, and/or a prolonged prothrombin time may be seen with severe liver disease.

LUNG

Symptoms of lung involvement include dyspnea, cough, and tachypnea. Pulmonary involvement in LCH may be isolated or disseminated. Primary pulmonary LCH in children is rare.[2]

GASTROINTESTINAL TRACT

Failure to thrive, caused by malabsorption, is the most common sign of gastrointestinal tract involvement. Other symptoms can include vomiting, diarrhea, and protein-losing enteropathy. Gastrointestinal tract involvement is uncommon, but can occur in generalized disease or as an extraordinary primary process.[2]

CENTRAL NERVOUS SYSTEM

The actual incidence of central nervous system (CNS) involvement is unknown, but it is estimated at 1% to 4% of patients.[14] Children with multisystem disease, skull and skull base lesions, and/or diabetes insipidus have a higher risk of developing neurologic complications. Symptoms most commonly occur 5 years after diagnosis. However, neurologic symptoms can develop 1 year before or up to 20 years after diagnosis.

Improved neuroimaging techniques have significantly increased the detection of CNS abnormalities. Magnetic resonance imaging (MRI) commonly reveals both white and gray matter changes, extraparenchymal and space occupying lesions, and atrophy. The majority of children display more than one type of change on MRI.

Children with neurodegeneration caused by LCH have a broad range of symptoms. Those with space-occupying lesions have site-dependent symptoms such as headaches or seizures. Progressive neurologic dysfunction follows the cerebellar pontine pathway, beginning with ataxia and nystagmus and progressing to dysarthria, dysphagia, and other cranial nerve deficits.[14]

Neuropsychologic assessments indicate significant deficits in memory, attention, verbal perform-ance, and full scale IQ.[25] There is no established treatment strategy for CNS disease. It is dependent on the disease type, site, and course, and on the disease status outside the nervous system.

ENDOCRINE

Approximately 30% of LCH patients develop diabetes insipidus (DI) with a reported range of 5% to 50%.[14] The pathogenesis is not clearly understood. Children with multisystem disease, temporal skull lesions, or orbital lesions with intracranial extension have a higher risk of DI development. DI can occur before, along with, or 1 to 5 years after the diagnosis of LCH. DI is confirmed by a water deprivation test and measurement of vasopressin. Partial DI does occur in LCH, and can spontaneously remit.[7]

MRI may reveal structural abnormalities of the hypothalamic-pituitary axis. The pituitary stalk is thickened, a normal pituitary bright signal on T2-weighted images is absent, and suprasellar mass lesions can also be present.[14]

Characteristic symptoms of DI are excessive thirst and frequent urination. There is no effective therapy for reversing or preventing DI. Unfortunately for patients and families, DI is a lifetime physical complication. The goal of treatment is to regulate fluids. DI is corrected by the administration of a synthetic vasopressin (DDAVP) intranasally.

Anterior pituitary function is often compromised in patients who develop DI. Growth hormone is the most affected. If a complete endocrine evaluation confirms growth hormone deficiency, growth hormone treatment is initiated early to maximize growth potential. Thyroid hormone deficiency is another component of anterior pituitary dysfunction and is treated with thyroid hormone replacement.[14]

DIAGNOSTIC EVALUATION

The Writing Group of the Histiocyte Society outlined an international standardized diagnostic approach to facilitate a common disease classification system.[29] Clinical evaluation includes a complete family and medical history with attention to pain, ear infections, loss of appetite, diarrhea, fever, polydipsia, polyuria, and activity level. The physical examination includes standing and sitting height, head circumference, and the presence of skin lesions, lymphadenopathy, orbital and dental abnormalities, or bone swelling. A complete neurologic evaluation is performed. Because LCH can mimic other diseases, such as Ewing's sarcoma or lymphoma, a

biopsy is mandatory to confirm the diagnosis.[4] Laboratory and radiographic evaluation of new patients includes a hematologic and endocrine evaluation, chest radiograph with posterior-anterior (PA) and lateral views, and a skeletal survey. A bone scan is not as sensitive as the skeletal survey in most patients. It may be performed optionally, but should not replace the skeletal survey.[4,6]

PATHOLOGY

The term *histiocyte* refers to two groups of immune cells: macrophages and dendritic cells. Histiocytes are derived from bone marrow and develop their characteristic phenotype under the influence of cytokines including granulocyte macrophage colony stimulating factor, tumor necrosis factor-α, interleukin-3, and interleukin-4.[24] LCH is classified as a dendritic cell–related disorder. It remains unclear whether dendritic cells arise from a lineage-specific marrow precurser cell or from a less specific immune cell influenced by a local paracrine cytokine effect. However, in support of the latter hypothesis, a single histiocytosis cell may manifest different phenotypes under different circumstances.[24]

The pathologic diagnosis of LCH is based on hematologic and histologic criteria established by the International Histiocyte Society in 1987.[29] The histopathology of LCH is generally uniform regardless of the clinical severity of the disease. The basic lesion is formed by collections of Langerhans cells and macrophages accompanied by T lymphocytes with variable numbers of multinucleated giant histiocytes and eosinophils. CD1a positivity and/or Birbeck granules by electron microscopy are required for a definitive diagnosis. Clonality of the CD1a+ cells is seen in all LCH lesions reported to date.[29] Although monoclonal proliferation of hematopoietic cells suggests that this disorder may be neoplastic, the clinical significance of this finding in LCH remains unclear because monoclonal histiocytes are detected in all forms of LCH. Furthermore, clonal cells have been detected in several nonmalignant disorders.

TREATMENT

Management of patients with LCH requires the collaboration of specialists using a multidisciplinary approach that encompasses a standardized diagnostic evaluation, treatment plan, and long-term follow-up. This team of health care providers should include hematology/oncology physicians, dermatologists, endocrinologists, orthopedic and neurosurgeons, radiologists, nurses, social workers, and neuropsychologists.

The approaches to the treatment of LCH vary

widely. Because some forms of LCH will regress without any therapy, whereas others are life-threatening, it is important to balance the extent of medical intervention with the severity of disease. General principles regarding treatment have emerged from clinical observation. A number of single-institutional studies demonstrated that age and severity of disease were major prognostic factors.[23] Disease confined to bone or lymph nodes was associated with a good prognosis, and little therapy was required. However, the outcome for patients with multisystem disease was poor regardless of the modality of treatment. Very young infants with extensive disease involving multiple organs had the worst outcome.[19] In addition, organ dysfunction was associated with an unfavorable prognosis.[19]

Although Lahey proposed criteria to define dysfunction of the liver, bone marrow, and lung, until recently, there was no uniformly accepted way of categorizing patients that would allow comparisons of disparate treatment regimens used at different institutions. However, with the publication of the Histiocyte Society's pathologic, diagnostic, clinical, and laboratory criteria, risk groups can now be clearly defined (Box 30-1).[4]

The criteria for response have also been difficult to define because spontaneous remission and fluctuations of disease activity are commonly seen. In the first international randomized therapy trial, LCH I,[17] the Histiocyte Society defined disease state as active or nonactive each time the patient was clinically assessed. In addition, response criteria were defined, and the disease was characterized as better, intermediate with or without complications, or worse.

SINGLE-SYSTEM DISEASE

A single bone lesion may resolve spontaneously during a period of months to years. The diagnostic biopsy of the lesion may initiate healing with or without curettage. Criteria for additional treatment include pain and the possibility of deformity or disability. Such lesions often respond to intralesional

---

BOX 30-1

LANGERHANS CELL HISTIOCYTOSIS RISK GROUPS

Single-system disease (low risk):
- Single site: single bone lesion, isolated skin disease, solitary lymph node
- Multiple sites: multiple bone lesions, multiple lymph node involvement

Multisystem disease (high risk):
- Multiple organ involvement, with or without dysfunction

---

steroid injection.[11] Polyostotic disease (multiple bone lesions) may require a short course of systemic steroids.

The role of radiotherapy in this disease is controversial. Because of possible late effects such as inhibition of growth and second malignancies, radiotherapy is generally reserved for disease that is not accessible to intralesional steroids or lesions that are compromising vital structures.

Single-system skin disease may respond to topical steroids.[5,21] However, severe cases may require topical nitrogen mustard applied in a 20% solution directly to the lesions.[21] For a solitary lymph node, excisional biopsy may be the only treatment required. A short course of systemic steroids may be needed to treat more extensive regional node disease. Resistant nodes may require systemic chemotherapy to induce a response. Although the optimal therapy for single-system disease remains unknown because it has not been carefully studied, it is important to remember that the treatment should not be worse than the disease.[5]

MULTISYSTEM DISEASE

For patients with multisystem disease, there is general agreement that systemic chemotherapy is beneficial. However, the optimal combination of chemotherapy agents and schedule is not known. Ongoing clinical trials, developed by the Histiocyte Society, are investigating these questions. During the 1980s some physicians advocated treating patients with multisystem disease with an intensive chemotherapy induction followed by maintenance therapy. Others, however, only treated patients during disease exacerbation.

The two largest cooperative clinical trials were those of the Italian group (AIEOP-CNR-HX 83)[8] and an Austrian/German group DAL-HX 83/90.[13] Although the regimens differed, induction therapy with multiple chemotherapy agents was administered in both trials, and some patients also received maintenance therapy. Overall mortality was low in both series (8% and 9%, respectively), but 54% mortality was observed in the poorest prognostic group in the Italian series and 38% was seen in the Austrian/German study.[13]

In LCH I, the first randomized chemotherapy trial, all patients with multisystem disease were randomly assigned to receive treatment with either etoposide or vinblastine.[18] Initially, a pulse of high-dose methylprednisolone was given in both arms. One hundred thirty-six patients were randomized. Interestingly, the evaluation of response at 6 weeks discriminated between responders and nonresponders, and failure to respond at 6 weeks was predictive of a poor outcome. Response did not correlate with age, number of organs affected, or the presence or absence of organ dysfunction. With a maximum follow-up of 2 years and 2 months, mortality for the cohort was 18%. Eight percent mortality was seen in the initial responder group of patients, 16% from the intermediate group, and 47% from the initial nonresponders. The risk of experiencing a reactivation in initial responders was 68%.[5,18]

Further analysis of the DAL-HX and LCH I studies revealed a subgroup of patients with multisystem disease with greater than 90% probability of survival. This "low-risk group" consisted of patients over 2 years of age at diagnosis without involvement of the hematopoietic system, liver, lungs, or spleen. Patients with multisystem disease with involvement of at least one of these systems were categorized as "risk group" patients. The results of LCH I and the DAL-HX studies formed the basis of the Histiocyte Society LCH II study, which opened in 1996.[5] This is a randomized trial to compare the effect of continuous oral prednisolone combined with vinblastine with or without the addition of etoposide in severely affected multisystem disease or "risk group" patients. The low-risk patients are excluded from the etoposide randomization. It is anticipated that this study will clarify the value of etoposide for patients with extensive multisystem disease.

SALVAGE THERAPY

There are few good treatment options for patients with extensive and/or progressive disease that does not respond to the conventional systemic chemotherapeutic agents. The recent use of 2-chlorodeoxyadenosine (2CdA) has shown some promising early results.[1] In addition, cyclosporine A has been shown to be an effective agent in resistant LCH.[1] Other agents that have been used in limited numbers of patients include deoxycoformycin, retinoic acid, thalidomide, interleukin-2, and FK506.[1] Bone marrow transplant has also been used to treat patients with progressive disease, and some children have achieved a complete remission. However, because only a small number of children have undergone transplantation, it remains unknown whether this approach will result in either improved survival or effect long-term cure.[1]

LATE EFFECTS

Survival for most patients with LCH is favorable. Complications from LCH are as variable as the disease. Late effects are more common in patients with multisystem disease, and in those that receive long treatment courses. In addition, children diagnosed at an early age have more late effects. The most common site for complications is the skeletal system, and many patients suffer from orthopedic, dental, and hearing abnormalities. Orthopedic defects include fractures, bony malformations, vertebral compressions, and scoliosis. Dental abnormalities manifest as missing or malformed teeth. Persistent middle ear disease can cause partial or complete hearing loss. Other common late effects are the previously discussed endocrinopathies. Growth failure is a late effect seen mostly in children with multisystem disease. This can result from a combination of factors including chronic illness, steroid therapy, and growth hormone deficiencies.[26] LCH can also affect the cognitive and psychosocial function of children, and neurologic changes can occur years after the disease has become inactive.[25]

A multiinstitutional international study investigating late effects is currently under way (e-mail: Histiosociety@aol.com). It is anticipated that this study will determine the incidence, severity, and prevalence of late effects in children with LCH.

NURSING IMPLICATIONS

A diagnosis of LCH presents a rare and confusing disease and treatment situation for parents. Parents have difficulty understanding and explaining to others whether LCH is a malignancy, despite the use of chemotherapy. Periods of remission followed by exacerbation of the disease requiring additional treatment can be frightening and frustrating for parents. Educational materials and support networks are available to parents from the Histiocytosis Association of America (www.histio.org).

Nurses are crucial members of the health care team involved in the care of patients with LCH. The role of the hematology/oncology nurse includes being a liaison for the multidisciplinary medical specialists, and providing ongoing education and support for patients and families. This requires effective communication skills and significant knowledge about the clinical and biologic aspects of the disease.[9] The Histiocytosis Nursing Network is an available resource, at the following address:

Histiocytosis Nursing Network
302 North Broadway
Pitman, NJ 08071

FUTURE DIRECTIONS

The formation of the Histiocyte Society has led to the establishment of standardized nomenclature, pathologic criteria, clinical groupings, and definitions of disease response. In addition, this international collaboration has resulted in the development of large-scale cooperative international studies of LCH. Studies are ongoing that will determine optimal primary and salvage treatment approaches. A clinical trial for the treatment of patients with CNS involvement is now open for patient enrollment, and another to treat multifocal bone lesions is under development. Although progress in the treatment of LCH has been made, more effective and less toxic therapy is still needed. Through basic research studies and rigorous clinical trials, such as those developed by the Histiocyte Society, it is likely that more effective therapeutic regimens will be developed, and outcomes for patients will continue to improve.

REFERENCES

1. Arceci, R. (2000). New treatment approaches for patients with LCH. *Histiocytosis Organization, 2,* 55-60.
2. Arico, M., & Egeler, R. M. (1998). Clinical aspects of Langerhans cell histiocytosis. *Hematology Oncology Clinics of North America, 12,* 247-258.
3. Aronson, R. P. (1951). Streptomycin in Letterer-Siwe disease. *Lancet, 1,* 889-890.
4. Broadbent, V., Egeler, R. M., & Nesbit, M. E. J. (1994). Langerhans cell histiocytosis: Clinical and epidemiological aspects. *British Journal of Cancer, 23* (Suppl.), S11-S16.
5. Broadbent, V., & Gadner, H. (1998). Current therapy for Langerhans cell histiocytosis. *Hematology Oncology Clinics of North America, 12,* 327-338.
6. Broadbent, V., Gadner, H., Komp, D. M., et al. (1989). Histiocytosis syndromes in children: II. Approach to the clinical and laboratory evaluation of children with Langerhans cell histiocytosis. Clinical Writing Group of the Histiocyte Society. *Medical and Pediatric Oncology, 17,* 492-495.
7. Broadbent, V., & Pritchard, J. (1997). Diabetes insipidus associated with Langerhans cell histiocytosis: Is it reversible? *Medical and Pediatric Oncology, 28,* 289-293.
8. de Ceci, A. T. M., Colella, R., Loiacono, G., et al. (1993). Langerhans cell histiocytosis in childhood: Results from the Italian cooperative AIEOP-CNR-HX '83 study. *Medical and Pediatric Oncology, 21,* 259-264.
9. Dumas, D. (2000). A vital link: The key role of the nurse in the team. *Histiocytosis Organization, 2,* 117-121.
10. Egeler, R. M., & D'Angio, G. J. (1995). Langerhans cell histiocytosis. *Journal of Pediatrics, 127,* 1-11.
11. Egeler, R. M., Thompson, R. C. J., Voute, P. A., et al. (1992). Intralesional infiltration of corticosteroids in localized Langerhans' cell histiocytosis. *Journal of Pediatric Orthopedics, 12,* 811-814.
12. Favara, B. E., Feller, A. C., Pauli, M., et al. (1997). Contemporary classification of histiocytic disorders. The WHO committee on histiocytic/reticulum cell proliferations. Reclassification working group of the Histiocyte Society. *Medical and Pediatric Oncology, 29,* 157-166.
13. Gadner, H., Heitger, A., Grois, N., et al. (1994). Treatment strategy for disseminated Langerhans cell histiocytosis. DAL HX-83 Study Group. *Medical and Pediatric Oncology, 23,* 72-80.
14. Grois, N. G., Favara, B. E., Mostbeck, G. H., et al. (1998). Central nervous system disease in Langerhans cell histiocytosis. *Hematology Oncology Clinics of North America, 12,* 287-305.
15. Hamre, M., Hedberg, J., Buckley, J., et al. (1997). Langerhans cell histiocytosis: An exploratory epidemiologic study of 177 cases. *Medical and Pediatric Oncology, 28,* 92-97.
16. Kannourakis, G., & Abbas, A. (1994). The role of cytokines in the pathogenesis of Langerhans cell histiocytosis. *British Journal of Cancer, 23* (Suppl.), S37-S40.
17. Komp, D. M., Vietti, T. J., Berry, D. H., et al. (1977). Combination chemotherapy in histiocytosis X. *Medical and Pediatric Oncology, 3,* 267-273.
18. Ladisch, S., Gadner, H., Arico, M., et al. (1994). LCH-I: A randomized trial of etoposide vs. vinblastine in disseminated Langerhans cell histiocytosis. The Histiocyte Society. *Medical and Pediatric Oncology, 23,* 107-110.
19. Lahey, M. E. (1975). Histiocytosis X: Comparison of three treatment regimens. *Journal of Pediatrics, 87,* 179-183.
20. Lampert, F. (1998). Langerhans cell histiocytosis. Historical perspectives. *Hematology Oncology Clinics of North America, 12,* 213-219.
21. Munn, S., & Chu, A. C. (1998). Langerhans cell histiocytosis of the skin. *Hematology Oncology Clinics of North America, 12,* 269-285.
22. Osband, M. E., Lipton, J. M., Lavin, P., et al. (1981). Histiocytosis-X: Demonstration of abnormal immunity, T-cell histamine H2-receptor deficiency and successful treatment with thymic extract. *New England Journal of Medicine, 304,* 146-153.
23. Raney, R. B. J., & D'Angio, G. J. (1989). Langerhans' cell histiocytosis (histiocytosis X): Experience at the Children's Hospital of Philadelphia, 1970-1984. *Medical and Pediatric Oncology, 17,* 20-28.
24. Schmitz, L., & Favara, B. E. (1998). Nosology and pathology of Langerhans cell histiocytosis. *Hematology Oncology Clinics of North America, 12,* 221-246.
25. Whitsett, S. F., Kneppers, K., Coppes, M. J., et al. (1999). Neuropsychologic deficits in children with Langerhans cell histiocytosis. *Medical and Pediatric Oncology, 33,* 486-492.
26. Willis, B., Ablin, A., Weinberg, V., et al. (1996). Disease course and late sequelae of Langerhans' cell histiocytosis: 25-year experience at the University of California, San Francisco. *Journal of Clinical Oncology, 14,* 2073-2082.
27. Willman, C. L. (1994). Detection of clonal histiocytes in Langerhans cell histiocytosis: Biology and clinical significance. *British Journal of Cancer, 23* (Suppl.), S29-S33.
28. Willman, C. L., Busque, L., Griffith, B. B., et al. (1994). Langerhans'-cell histiocytosis (histiocytosis X): A clonal proliferative disease. *New England Journal of Medicine, 331,* 154-160.
29. Writing Group of the Histiocyte Society (1987). Histiocytosis syndromes in children. *Lancet, 1,* 208-209.

V

Professional Practice Issues

31

Interdisciplinary Collaboration

Christina Rasco Baggott
Katherine Patterson Kelly

Publications concerning childhood cancer typically introduce the subject by referring to the amazing advances that have occurred over the past 30 to 40 years. This progress began with the early, multidisciplinary, collaborative research groups established by Dr. Sydney Farber in the early 1940s. Pediatric oncology cooperative research groups begun in the 1950s have provided a model for effective clinical medical research.[6,19] The collaboration consistently attained within these groups enabled development of national, interdisciplinary trials that led to improved outcomes (Figure 31-1). The original group participants were limited to the medical specialists involved in the care of children with cancer: pediatric oncologists, surgeons, radiation oncologists, and pathologists. More recently, disciplines outside of medicine have become well integrated within the cooperative group research structure, leading to effective implementation of complicated research protocol–based therapy.[28]

The study committees of the cooperative groups that develop research protocols now routinely include nurses, pharmacists, and clinical research associates as members. These disciplines bring their unique perspectives to the research conducted within a particular protocol. Multidisciplinary research efforts are also increasing in the areas of supportive care, end-of-life care, quality of life, late effects, and other areas. Nurse researchers in the pediatric cooperative group reach out to other disciplines to broaden and enrich the studies implemented.[16] These multidisciplinary research teams mirror the effective multidisciplinary treatment teams at each center providing childhood cancer care.

THE PEDIATRIC ONCOLOGY MULTIDISCIPLINARY TEAM

The multidisciplinary team is a necessary component of quality care for children with cancer and their families. Recently published standards for the development of childhood cancer centers formalized this mandate for multidisciplinary care,[1,2] and it will be a requirement for institutional membership in the newly formed Children's Oncology Group (C.O.G.).

Evaluation of treatment outcomes reveals that children who receive their care at childhood cancer centers have superior outcomes compared to those treated in a community setting.[20,24,25] The complexities of the medical treatment, combined with the psychosocial impact of a diagnosis of cancer for the child and family, create a mandate for a specialized approach to care that includes experts in all aspects of the child's needs.

The multidisciplinary team brings together care providers with a wide variety of expertise to provide care for children with cancer and their families. No single discipline can treat the complex physical and psychosocial needs of children with cancer and their families. The team must be multifaceted and flexible in devising individualized plans and implementing care. Pediatric oncology patients have complex needs. A disorganized multidisciplinary team may cause delays in discharge or ineffective symptom management. Professional roles must be clearly defined, with minimal areas of overlap, avoiding rivalry, particularly between nurses and physicians.[15] The roles must complement rather than duplicate one another. At times, care providers must adapt to new roles to meet a particular child's needs. Trust, respect, and open communication are essential elements of an effective multidisciplinary team. Patients and parents are considered essential members of the team, both while receiving cancer therapy[11] and in the off-therapy period.[7] Effective communication with patients and parents includes careful listening to their concerns, including those of very young children.[11] Educating team members regarding each other's roles and the process of teamwork can minimize group conflict and professional struggles. This education includes content on system and change theo-

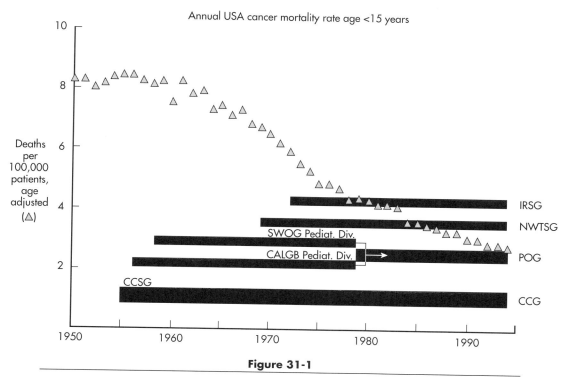

Figure 31-1

The pediatric cooperative groups and the national decline in rate of deaths before age 15 years among patients with cancer. *CALGB,* Cancer and Acute Leukemia Group B; *CCG,* Children's Cancer Group; *CCSG,* Children's Cancer Study Group; *IRSG,* Intergroup Rhabdomyosarcoma Study Group; *NWTSG,* National Wilms' Tumor Study Group; *POG,* Pediatric Oncology Group. (From Bleyer, W.A. [1997]. The U.S. pediatric cancer clinical trials programmes: International implications and the way forward. *European Journal of Cancer, 33,* 1442.)

ries, interpersonal communication skills, conflict resolution, and team building.[8]

In pediatric oncology, a large number of nursing roles exist. Within nursing, work settings include the pediatric oncology unit, surgical unit, intensive care unit, general medical ward, outpatient clinic, short-stay unit, research unit, case management department, or the patient's home. The role of a staff nurse varies, particularly related to the extent to which ancillary staff such as nursing assistants are used. Nursing roles focus on direct patient care including psychosocial support, case management, research, nursing leadership, quality management, nursing education, patient education, or any combination of these roles. Some nurses must function in the roles of the clinical research associate and the nurse. In most institutions, registered nurses must supervise and guide nursing assistants or other unlicensed assistive personnel. Nurses must learn to assess the care provided by the assistants and to promote quality care. Some institutions also use licensed vocational nurses, adding additional supervisory roles to the registered nurse. In centers with dedicated pediatric oncology units, the pediatric oncology nurse must often serve as a resource to nurses on other units, such as those in the pediatric intensive care unit.

Advanced practice nursing roles in pediatric oncology are also extremely diverse. Controversy exists when comparing and contrasting the roles of nurse practitioner (NP) and of clinical nurse specialist (CNS). Traditionally, the NP was described as providing patient care, whereas the CNS was described as improving patient care.[9] The impetus toward the development of the NP role was the lack of primary care physician coverage, whereas the impetus for CNS role development was the increasing complexity of health care. Both roles focus on theory, clinical practice, consultation, education, and research.[30] However, NPs reported spending 73% of their time in direct patient care, compared to 52% of time for the CNS.[10] Nurse practitioners in pediatric oncology work outside the traditional primary care setting of the NP, adding to the role confusion of advanced practice nursing. Roles for advanced practice nurses vary greatly between institutions, further blurring role boundaries.

In the past, educational preparation has differed for the two roles. The CNS role has always required master's preparation, whereas the NP role has only recently required a master's degree. Early in the history of the NP role, some NPs received preparation from 9- to 12-month certificate programs. There is a trend of CNSs returning to school for postmaster's NP programs. These programs tend to focus on the skills of history taking and physical examination, primary care, and the management of common ailments.[22] Additionally, many graduate programs now offer training for the combined role of CNS/NP. As early as 1986, the American Nurses Association (ANA) Council of Primary Health Care Nurse Practitioners and the Council of Clinical Nurse Specialists printed an editorial stating that the roles were more similar than different.[29] This is especially true in childhood cancer where the care needs of the child and family drive role definition for the advanced practice nurse.

Pediatric oncology patients interact with a wide range of physicians. Most pediatric oncology care is provided in teaching hospitals. In such centers, attending physicians are often faculty, employed by a university, who supervise and are ultimately responsible for all care provided by the medical team. Teaching hospitals also include fellows in pediatric oncology who have completed a residency program and are studying pediatric hematology/oncology. Fellowship training includes clinical,

teaching, and research responsibilities. In these settings, interns and residents often direct the children's care, with supervision by fellows and attending physicians. Most families are not familiar with this medical hierarchy. Thus, the roles of the team members should be clearly explained to patients and their families. Private pediatric oncologists treat some children with cancer, in community hospitals, without the assistance of interns or fellows, but often along with advanced practice nurses. Additionally, pediatric oncology patients interact with physicians from a variety of disciplines, such as radiation therapy, radiology, orthopedics, endocrinology, and neurology, to name a few.

Some of the practice domains of various health care providers are delineated in Table 31-1. Responsibilities for each type of professional vary greatly between institutions. For example, in one institution a member of the psychology team may be responsible for teaching families distraction techniques, whereas the child life specialist or nurse may perform this task at another institution.

TABLE 31-1	ROLES OF THE MULTIDISCIPLINARY TEAM MEMBERS IN PEDIATRIC ONCOLOGY	
Position/Preparation	**Role**	**Role Overlaps**
Staff Nurse: Bachelor's degree, associate's degree, or diploma. Staff nurse providing care may work on pediatric oncology unit, surgical unit, intensive care unit, general medical ward, outpatient clinic, short-stay unit, or research unit.	Identify family structure and assess coping styles Support positive coping behaviors Assess patient's general physical status Plan, administer, and evaluate direct patient care in hospital or clinic, based on nursing diagnoses and physician orders—involve patient and family in decision making Educate families (diagnosis and treatment, symptom management, hospital routines) Assist in informed consent process Support compliance with medical regimen Supervise care provided by nursing assistants and LVNs Provide psychosocial support Use behavioral interventions such as relaxation therapy, guided imagery Foster normalcy and support developmentally appropriate behaviors Act as patient advocate Coordinate patient's discharge Visit child's classroom to prepare for school re-entry Facilitate support groups Participate in quality improvement studies Develop research ideas from clinical experiences Collect research data	Home care nurse, case manager, advanced practice nurse, physician, social worker, psychologist, child life worker, teacher, pharmacist, dietitian, rehabilitation team, chaplain

TABLE 31-1	ROLES OF THE MULTIDISCIPLINARY TEAM MEMBERS IN PEDIATRIC ONCOLOGY—cont'd	
Position/Preparation	**Role**	**Role Overlaps**
Home Care Nurse: Bachelor's degree, associate's degree, or diploma.	Identify family structure and assess coping style Support positive coping behaviors Assess patient's general physical status Assess availability of community-based resources Plan, administer, and evaluate direct patient care in the home, based on nursing diagnoses and physician orders Educate families (diagnosis and treatment, symptom management, home care routines) Provide psychosocial support Use behavioral interventions such as relaxation therapy, guided imagery Foster normalcy and support developmentally appropriate behaviors Act as a patient advocate Relay information regarding home conditions, family's coping ability to hospital-based providers Support compliance with medical regimen	Staff nurse, case manager, advanced practice nurse, physician, social worker, psychologist, child life specialist, pharmacist, dietitian, rehabilitation team, chaplain
Hospital-Based Case Manager: Bachelor's degree, associate's degree, or diploma in nursing. Most often nurse role but some institutions use social workers.	Identify family structure and assess coping style Support positive coping behaviors Coordinate patient's discharge Inform families of financial resources Assess/secure payor authorization for home services Assist with development of institutional contracts with outside vendors	Staff nurse, home care nurse, insurance-based case manager, advanced practice nurse, physician, social worker, psychologist, child life specialist, rehabilitation team, chaplain
Insurance-Based Case Manager: Bachelor's degree, associate's degree, or diploma in nursing. Most often nurse role but some institutions use social workers.	Identify family structure and assess coping styles Support positive coping behaviors Coordinate patient's discharge Inform families of financial resources within insurance plan Expand services outside an insurance plan if deemed a lower cost alternative that provides better care for child	Staff nurse, home care nurse, hospital-based case manager, advanced practice nurse, physician, social worker, psychologist, child life specialist, rehabilitation team, chaplain
Advanced Practice Nurse (Nurse Practitioner or Clinical Nurse Specialist): Master's degree. (*Master's degree not required for nurse practitioners before or during 1980s.*)	Identify family structure and assess coping styles for areas of strength and dysfunction Recognize coping deficits and work to expand positive coping styles Assess patient's physical status through in-depth systems review Plan and evaluate direct patient care in hospital, clinic, or home Prescribe medications Perform lumbar punctures and bone marrow aspirates for diagnostic studies or treatments Educate families (diagnosis and treatment, symptom management, hospital routines) Assist in informed consent process Provide psychosocial support Use behavioral interventions such as relaxation therapy, guided imagery, and hypnosis if trained	Staff nurse, home care nurse, case manager, physician, social worker, psychologist, child life specialist, teacher, pharmacist, dietitian, rehabilitation team, chaplain

Continued

TABLE 31-1	ROLES OF THE MULTIDISCIPLINARY TEAM MEMBERS IN PEDIATRIC ONCOLOGY—cont'd	
Position/Preparation	**Role**	**Role Overlaps**
Advanced Practice Nurse—cont'd	Foster normalcy and support developmentally appropriate behaviors Support compliance with medical regimen Coordinate patient's discharge Visit child's classroom to prepare for school reentry Participate in quality improvement studies Initiate research studies Collect research data Facilitate support groups including staff nurse support groups Serve as a resource on pediatric oncology for the staff	
Physician: Medical degree plus residency and fellowship programs.	Assess patient's physical status through in-depth systems review Prescribe medications Perform lumbar punctures and bone marrow aspirates for diagnostic studies or treatment Assess family structure and coping behaviors Diagnose and classify patient's cancer Choose appropriate therapy for cancer Plan, implement, and evaluate direct patient care in hospital, clinic, or home by collaborating with other health care providers Make appropriate referrals to other health care providers Educate families (diagnosis and treatment, symptom management) Support compliance with medical regimen Initiate research studies Secure informed consent for tests, procedures, and research studies Participate in quality improvement studies	Staff nurse, home care nurse, case manager, advanced practice nurse, social worker, psychologist, child life specialist, teacher, pharmacist, dietitian, rehabilitation team, chaplain
Social Worker: Bachelor's or master's degree with training in human behavior and counseling skills.	Assess family structure and coping level for areas of strength and dysfunction Inform families of psychosocial resources Assess family financial resources Inform families of financial resources Assist in transportation and lodging needs Provide counseling services for patient and family members Foster normalcy and support developmentally appropriate behaviors Facilitate support groups Visit child's classroom to prepare for school reentry Support compliance with medical regimen Participate in quality improvement studies	Staff nurse, home care nurse, case manager, advanced practice nurse, physician, psychologist, child life specialist, teacher, pharmacist, dietitian, rehabilitation team, chaplain

TABLE 31-1	ROLES OF THE MULTIDISCIPLINARY TEAM MEMBERS IN PEDIATRIC ONCOLOGY—cont'd	
Position/Preparation	**Role**	**Role Overlaps**
Psychologist: Master's or doctoral degree with background in behavioral research methods. May have specialty in clinical, developmental, physiologic, or educational psychology.	Assess complex family structures and dysfunctional coping styles Provide counseling services for patient and family members Perform cognitive evaluation, such as neuropsychologic testing Promote behavior modification program Use behavioral interventions such as hypnosis if trained, relaxation therapy, guided imagery Foster normalcy and support developmentally appropriate behaviors Support compliance with medical regimen Educational psychologist may work with schools to formulate individualized education plan Initiate research studies Collect research data Facilitate support groups for patients, families, and/or staff Serve as resource to other staff on behavioral issues and interventions	Staff nurse, home care nurse, case manager, advanced practice nurse, physician, social worker, child life specialist, teacher, pharmacist, dietitian, rehabilitation team, chaplain
Child Life Specialist: Bachelor's or master's degree with specific training in child development.	Assess family structure and coping level Minimize adverse psychologic effects of chronic illness and treatment Provide medical play and expressive activities Promote age appropriate development in stressful environment for patient and siblings Use behavioral interventions such as relaxation therapy, guided imagery Provide health care team with information about normal developmental patterns Foster normalcy and support developmentally appropriate behaviors Orient volunteer staff Support compliance with medical regimen Visit child's classroom to prepare for school reentry Participate in quality improvement studies	Staff nurse, home care nurse, case manager, advanced practice nurse, physician, social worker, psychologist, teacher, pharmacist, dietitian, rehabilitation team, chaplain
Hospital-Based Teacher: Bachelor's or master's degree with teaching credentials.	Visit child's classroom to prepare for school reentry Work directly with child's teacher to integrate into regular classroom Provide health care team with information about intellectual progress and socialization skills Work with schools to formulate individualized education plan	Staff nurse, advanced practice nurse, social worker, psychologist, child life specialist, rehabilitation team
Clinical Pharmacist: Bachelor's (RPh) or doctoral degree (PharmD).	Dispense medications Provide pharmacologic information to health care team and families, including expected side effects, drug compatibilities and interaction information, serum drug levels, methods of administration	Staff nurse, home care nurse, advanced practice nurse, physician

Continued

TABLE 31-1	ROLES OF THE MULTIDISCIPLINARY TEAM MEMBERS IN PEDIATRIC ONCOLOGY—cont'd	
Position/Preparation	Role	Role Overlaps
Clinical Pharmacist—cont'd	Maintain investigational drug inventory Suggest therapy alternatives Support compliance with medical regimen Provide additional system of checks and balances for preventing drug errors Participate in quality improvement studies	
Clinical Dietitian: Bachelor's or master's degree.	Assess patient's nutritional status Provide information regarding appropriate nutritional supplements or guidelines Promote normalcy in eating patterns Participate in quality improvement studies	Staff nurse, home care nurse, advanced practice nurse, physician, rehabilitation team
Rehabilitation Team: Physical therapist, occupational therapist, speech therapist, rehabilitation physician, audiologist, prosthetic engineer.	Assess patient's physical status in focused dimensions Encourage exercises to promote attainment or maintenance of appropriate motor skills Prescribe rehabilitation plan/evaluate effectiveness of plan in hospital, outpatient, or home setting Participate in quality improvement studies	Staff nurse, home care nurse, advanced practice nurse, physician
Chaplain: Training varies by denomination.	Identify family structure and coping style Assess family's spiritual needs Arrange for spiritual care as desired Participate in quality improvement studies	Staff nurse, home care nurse, advanced practice nurse, physician, social worker, psychologist, child life specialist, teacher
Child and Family	Act as a partner with members of the health care team, advocating for the child's needs Maintain relationships within family and the broader community Provide accurate information during health assessments Report side effects experienced Make inquiries when clarification is needed Adhere to treatment plan Be open to assistance when needed Investigate resources available	

PROMOTING TEAMWORK

An interdisciplinary approach to patient care does not just happen by assigning people to work together. Teamwork depends on full use of the competencies of individual members. Many health care professionals are not experienced as part of an integrated team and often are not knowledgeable about specific roles and responsibilities of other professions. Consequently, people who work together do not necessarily function as a team. Although some degree of role confusion is unavoidable, professional territoriality hampers coordination attempts.

Members of the multidisciplinary team must respect all other members, and roles must be clearly defined and communicated. Ducanis and Golin state that when evaluating a multidisciplinary team's effectiveness, the viewpoint of the patient, professional, and organization must be considered.[8] Recommendations for evaluating a team are included in Box 31-1.

Collaboration is a key component to effective team functioning. Hanson and Spross define collaboration as: "An interpersonal process in which two or more individuals make a commitment to in-

BOX 31-1

HEALTH CARE TEAM EFFECTIVENESS: THE SEVEN C'S

1. Collaboration: Does the team include the child and family in making treatment plan decisions? Does the team meet regularly to discuss and plan for the physical and psychosocial needs for each child and family?
2. Continuity: Are specific team members identified to interact regularly with the child and family?
3. Consistency: Does the entire team facilitate the agreed on plan of care?
4. Communication: Does the team provide information in a timely manner to the child and family?
5. Coping: Does the team continually reassess the child's and family's perceived level of stress and wellness and intervene as needed?
6. Consultation: Does the team routinely refer the child and family to available resources within the treatment center and community?
7. Costs: Do the team's interventions affect the child's length of hospital stay or treatment charges?

Data from McMahon, L. W. (1993). Interdisciplinary management of the child or adolescent with cancer. In G. V. Foley, D. Fochtman, & K. H. Mooney (Eds.), *Nursing care of the child with cancer* (2nd ed., pp. 497-510). Philadelphia: W. B. Saunders.

teract constructively to solve problems and accomplish identified goals, purposes, or outcomes. The individuals recognize and articulate the shared values that make this commitment possible."[14]

The characteristics of successful collaboration include valuing and respecting diverse and complementary knowledge, a common purpose, clinical competence, interpersonal competence, humor, and trust. The processes that drive collaboration include recurring interactions between professionals, the ability to reorganize and rearrange boundaries within a practice setting, and consultation.[14]

Failure to collaborate has been associated with decreased patient and family satisfaction, unsatisfactory clinical outcomes, and clinician frustration.[3,12,14] Five criteria that promote collaborative practice in health care institutions were identified by a national joint practice committee: primary nursing, integrated patient records, encouraging nurse decision making, joint practice committees, and joint records review.[13] Unfortunately these recommendations have not been well accepted in our health care system.[12] Team meetings, joint projects such as research or writing projects and community service, and interdisciplinary education have been

identified as other methods to promote collaboration between disciplines. Additionally, collaboration within pediatric oncology has been promoted by the emergence of multidisciplinary continuous quality improvement (CQI) teams,[18] workgroups through the National Association of Children's Hospitals and Related Institutions (NACHRI),[23] the development of clinical paths,[5,23] and the evolution and ascendancy of the multidisciplinary pediatric cooperative groups now merged into a single voice for the care of children with cancer, the Children's Oncology Group.[26,28]

Emphasis on collaboration is demonstrated through increased funding for projects evaluating effective collaboration in health care and a recent emphasis within the Joint Commission on the Accreditation of Healthcare Organizations (JCAHO) on providing evidence and documentation of multidisciplinary assessment and care planning.[17] Figure 31-2 provides an example of a tool used to document care decisions made during daily multidisciplinary rounds.

INTERDISCIPLINARY ROUNDS: CONFERENCE SUMMARY

Amber is a 4-year-old girl diagnosed with B progenitor acute lymphocytic leukemia 3 weeks ago, currently in induction therapy. Her leukemia has been classified as high risk because of an initial white blood cell count of 178,000/mm^3. She was jaundiced on presentation, with a total bilirubin of 15.9 mg/dl, ammonia of 178 μ/100 ml, aspartate transaminase (AST) of 298 U/L and an alanine transaminase (ALT) level of 782 U/L at diagnosis. The liver dysfunction was possibly caused by multiple high doses of acetaminophen given to her by her mother in the week before diagnosis (20 mg/kg q 4 hours). She developed mental status changes with lethargy most likely because of elevated ammonia levels. Amber was scheduled to receive a four-drug induction with vincristine, prednisone, asparaginase, and daunorubicin, as well as intrathecal chemotherapy. The doses of vincristine, asparaginase, and daunorubicin were adjusted because of her liver dysfunction. She developed a deep vein thrombosis (DVT) in the left leg and required anticoagulants. She had severe leg weakness because of the DVT and was receiving physical therapy.

Amber's social situation was complex. Before the diagnosis, she was living with her mother and maternal aunt in a hotel room, because they were homeless. Amber's father was incarcerated. During Amber's initial hospitalization, her mother also became incarcerated. Amber's care was turned over to the aunt, although initially her mother did not

Interdisciplinary Rounds: Pediatric Hematology/Oncology				
Adm. date: **Primary PCP:**	**Adm. dx/reason:**		**Resident:** Notified: Y N	**Attending:** **Anticipated LOS:**

Date:	Date:	Date:
Members present: SN MD APN/NC Res MD RD CLAT SW CRA Others RPh Referrals needed: Peds Surg Home health _____ Peds ID DME _____ PCP f/u Home lab _____ Home lab Resource/$$ _____ Rehab Counseling Other _____	Members present: SN MD APN/NC Res MD RD CLAT SW CRA Others RPh Referrals needed: Peds Surg Home health _____ Peds ID DME _____ PCP f/u Home lab _____ Home lab Resource/$$ _____ Rehab Counseling Other _____	Members present: SN MD APN/NC Res MD RD CLAT SW CRA Others RPh Referrals needed: Peds Surg Home health _____ Peds ID DME _____ PCP f/u Home lab _____ Home lab Resource/$$ _____ Rehab Counseling Other _____

No new needs identified **Tasks**	DR	APN	SN	SW	DONE	No new needs identified **Tasks**	DR	APN	SN	SW	DONE	No new needs identified **Tasks**	DR	APN	SN	SW
1.						1.						1.				
2.						2.						2.				
3.						3.						3.				
Comments:						Comments:						Comments:				
Signature:						Signature:						Signature:				

MR 999B-8-85   © University of Missouri Health Care

Figure 31-2

Example of interdisciplinary documentation form.   (Courtesy Katherine Patterson Kelly and Children's Hospital at University of Missouri Health Care.)

complete the proper guardianship papers. The aunt has a seventh grade education level. With the help of a church group, Amber's aunt did find a home before her hospital discharge, located in a trailer park 50 miles from the hospital.

Amber was hospitalized for 26 days. By the end of her hospital stay, her liver function returned to normal, her mental status improved, and she was a playful child, yet extremely fearful of all medical procedures. For discharge, she required daily subcutaneous injections of low-molecular-weight heparin for treatment of her DVT, in addition to multiple oral medications. Amber became extremely agitated when injections were due. The nursing staff expressed concern regarding the competency of Amber's aunt in providing a complex regimen of medications because of her lack of education and her poor parenting skills observed during the hospitalization.

A care conference was called and the following actions occurred:

- Amber's primary nurse organized the care conference and made notes for the chart.
- The attending physician provided background information on the use of low-molecular-weight heparin for DVT, because the nursing staff had minimal experience with the drug. The attending physician also reviewed the pathophysiology of liver dysfunction and subsequent encephalopathy.
- The nurse practitioner developed a simple calendar and medication check sheet for the aunt and reviewed the medication plan with the home nurse.
- The social worker ensured that all guardianship papers were appropriately signed and connected the aunt with a local support group for chronically ill children. This support group helps with transportation, because the family's car is not reliable. The social worker also enrolled the aunt in a "Parents Helping Parents" group. These volunteers can serve as good role models for care providers with minimal parenting skills.
- The hospital-based case manager arranged for suitable home nursing and worked with the insurance case manager to get the low-molecular-weight heparin approved.
- The psychologist reviewed Amber's case with the group and determined that Amber's encephalopathy had resolved and that her anxiety is typical of many hospitalized 4-year-olds. He planned to provide on-going counseling sessions to Amber and her aunt on their many psychosocial issues.
- The child life specialist worked with Amber to blow bubbles during her injections as distraction and did hospital play focusing on her fears concerning injections. She also devised a sticker chart to encourage compliance with injections, oral medications, and other therapies and worked with Amber on how to swallow pills.
- The clinical pharmacist provided the aunt with a pillbox, with separate sections for each dose. She helped the aunt fill the box for the first week and instructed the aunt to bring all medications to the clinic at each visit.
- The visiting nurse inspected the newly found home and found it unsatisfactory, because it needed extensive cleaning. The chaplain spoke with the local minister to arrange for church members to clean the home.
- The home nurse agreed to monitor Amber's oral and subcutaneous medications and to assist with filling the pillbox. She also arranged for home physical therapy.

SUPPORT FOR THE CAREGIVER

Pediatric oncology nursing is undoubtedly a stressful field. Nurses and other professionals can easily become overwhelmed in providing care to pediatric cancer patients and their families. Researchers identified the following stressors when interviewing pediatric oncology nurses: death and dying, the professional image of the oncology nurse (view from others that pediatric oncology is a distressing field), the concept of the nurse as a fighter in the war against death, perceived isolation from the medical staff, and feeling professionally inferior.[21]

A recent investigation was undertaken into what pediatric oncology nurses with a median of 7 to 9.5 years' experience in the specialty define as meaningful about their work.[27] The researchers used a qualitative approach to determine the peak and nadir experiences of a convenience sample of 26 nurses employed at a large children's cancer center and 38 pediatric oncology nursing association members attending their national conference. Peak experiences, as described by these nurses, included times of emotional involvement with a child or family or in providing care that resulted in a positive difference for the child and family. The inability to meet the needs of a patient or family defined the most frequently reported nadir experiences.[27] Nurses who could articulate the meaning they derived from their work were more likely to report work satisfaction.[4] Table 31-2 summarizes the most frequently identified peak and nadir experiences, and the consequences of these experiences as reported by experienced pediatric oncology nurses who are still working in the specialty.

TABLE 31-2	PEAK AND NADIR EXPERIENCES REPORTED BY PEDIATRIC ONCOLOGY NURSES WITH A MEDIAN OF 7 TO 9.5 YEARS OF EXPERIENCE		
		Consequences	
Peak Experiences		**Short Term**	**Long Term**
1. Knowing my care/my presence made a positive difference 2. Witnessing a patient recover and continue to do well 3. Sharing closeness of dying with patient/family 4. Experiencing closeness with patient/family 5. Witnessing remarkable deaths		1. Getting a positive feeling 2. Having found my niche 3. Dying doesn't have to be awful 4. Experiencing spiritual renewal 5. Feeling empathy for parents 6. Learning more about myself and others 7. Being reminded than I am a good nurse	1. Finding pleasure in being a part 2. Practicing nursing differently 3. Learning more about myself and others 4. Reaffirming my faith 5. Knowing death can be good 6. Being reminded that I am a good nurse 7. Knowing that nursing makes a difference 8. Determination to help patients cope
		Consequences	
Nadir Experiences		**Short Term**	**Long Term**
1. Witnessing adverse effects of treatments and patient suffering 2. Facing a sudden and unexpected patient death 3. Not being able to give desired care 4. Working with uncooperative colleagues 5. Lacking administrative support 6. Concluding that we didn't do a good enough job		1. Feeling troubled 2. Being angry 3. Having guilt 4. Feeling frustrated 5. Crying	1. Coming to know own or team's strengths and weaknesses 2. Accepting that children die 3. Discovering negative experiences can be opportunities 4. Guilt 5. Attempting to be more perceptive 6. Knowing that I make a difference 7. Increased commitment to the specialty 8. Recognizing need to get more information

Data from Olson, M. S., Hinds, P. S., Euell, K., et al. (1998). Peak and nadir experiences and their consequences described by pediatric oncology nurses. *Journal of Pediatric Oncology Nursing, 15*, 13-24.

Members of the International Society of Pediatric Oncology (SIOP) formed a working committee on psychosocial issues in pediatric oncology and reported on burnout among staff members. The committee delineated five stages of burnout among pediatric oncology staff. The first stage is *mental and physical exhaustion,* involving feelings of emptiness and a lack of energy. The next phase is that of *indifference,* with individuals seeming cynical and disinterested. Individuals then move on to *a sense of failure as a professional,* which may be accompanied by a fear of committing serious errors. The next stage is that of *a sense of failure as a person.* The individual feels isolated and hopeless. These feelings intrude into the individual's personal life. The final stage is feeling *"dead inside."* The individual lacks affect and may leave the profession at this time.[31] Common causes of burnout

TABLE 31-3	CAUSES OF BURNOUT IN PEDIATRIC ONCOLOGY
Cause	**Characteristics**
The nature of the work	Dealing with life-threatening illness daily
	Seeing many ill young children
	Assuming emotional burdens of families
	Work culture that does not tolerate complaining
	Being "drained" by dissatisfied families
The work environment	Authoritarian administration
	Hostility among staff members
	No support among peers
	Too many demands; not enough time
	Not being heard by leadership
Characteristics of the individual	Poor preparation for this type of work
	High demands of oneself
	Expecting too much from one's work
	Difficulty in asking for help
	Difficulty in taking time off
	Difficulty in asking for counseling
	Not sharing thoughts
	Not using peers as support
	Fear, guilt, or helplessness that one did not do all that should have been done
	Becoming too involved with particular patients
	Difficulty in sharing work issues at home
	Not getting enough rest
	Wanting to change jobs, but feeling financially trapped
	Being unable to say "no" to families or staff
	Not having a healthy balance between work and outside life

Data from Spinetta, J. J., Jankovic, M., Ben Arush, M. W., et al. (2000). Guidelines for the recognition, prevention, and remediation of burnout in health care professionals participating in the care of children with cancer: Report of the SIOP Working Committee on Psychosocial Issues in Pediatric Oncology. *Medical and Pediatric Oncology, 35,* 122-125.

in pediatric oncology are listed in Table 31-3. Nursing leadership and hospital administration must assist the individual nurse in keeping prevention of burnout as a high priority.

Strategies to prevent or remediate burnout in pediatric oncology are listed in Table 31-4. These factors acknowledge the roles played by the nature of the work itself and the work environment, but more strongly emphasize characteristics of the individual. Being at peace with pediatric oncology nursing is a challenging journey for novice nurses and those experienced in the specialty. The individual nurse must be willing to examine her personal values, beliefs, and behaviors on a regular basis to determine her personal fit with the work and the work environment. Coping skills require continual reassessment for effectiveness. Developing insight is a difficult but crucial part of personal development. As the nurse moves toward greater self-knowledge,

the peer group assists the process through honest yet gentle feedback, consistent support, and a willingness to challenge destructive personal behavior such as drug or alcohol abuse. Nonnurse team members contribute positively when they recognize the contributions of the nurse, provide constructive feedback, and participate in educational programs designed to enhance knowledge and skills.

The complexities of childhood cancer require care from professional members of a highly skilled and smoothly functioning multidisciplinary team. The team members must strive to provide quality care in an efficient manner. They must take individual accountability and institutions must take collective responsibility to ensure effective team functioning. As a role model and patient advocate, the professional pediatric oncology nurse is well positioned to be an effective advocate for team functioning and coordination.

TABLE 31-4	STRATEGIES TO PREVENT OR REMEDIATE BURNOUT IN PEDIATRIC ONCOLOGY
Category	**Strategy**
The workplace environment—for administrators	Devise set of common goals for team
	Careful recruitment of staff
	Encourage staff to use informal support from co-workers
	Allow staff to have flexibility when possible
	Engage staff members in decision making
	Organize "debriefing" meetings at critical times of patient care (deaths, relapse, etc.)
	Organize staff retreats or educational leave days
	Have staff rotate outside the department when feasible and desired
	Allow short leaves on occasion
	Encourage parents to advocate on behalf of the staff when appropriate
Personal factors	Learn to set personal limits
	Avoid overinvolvement
	Let needs be known to both work peers and supervisors
	Engage in staff socials
	Keep communication open with colleagues
	Patch up minor differences as they occur
	Seek closure by attending funerals when feasible and appropriate
	Attend workshops on burnout
	Maintain a healthy balance between work and home life
	Find a relaxing hobby

Data from Spinetta, J. J., Jankovic, M., Ben Arush, M. W., et al. (2000). Guidelines for the recognition, prevention, and remediation of burnout in health care professionals participating in the care of children with cancer: Report of the SIOP Working Committee on Psychosocial Issues in Pediatric Oncology. *Medical and Pediatric Oncology, 35,* 122-125.

REFERENCES

1. American Academy of Pediatrics, Section on Hematology Oncology. (1997). Guidelines for the pediatric cancer center. Role of such centers in diagnosis and treatment. *Pediatrics, 99,* 139-141.
2. Arceci, R. J., Reaman, G. H., Cohen, A. R., et al. (1998). Position statement for the need to define pediatric hematology/oncology programs: A model of subspecialty care for chronic childhood diseases. Health Care Policy and Public Issues Committee of the American Society of Pediatric Hematology Oncology. *Journal of Pediatric Hematology Oncology, 20,* 98-103.
3. Baggs, J. G., Ruan, S. A., Phelps, C. E., et al. (1992). The association between interdisciplinary collaboration and patient outcomes in medical intensive care. *Heart and Lung, 21,* 18-24.
4. Clarke-Steffen, L. (1998). The meaning of peak and nadir experiences of pediatric oncology nurses: Secondary analysis. *Journal of Pediatric Oncology Nursing, 15,* 25-33.
5. Coffey, R. J., Richards, J. S., Remmert, C. S., et al. (1992). An introduction to critical paths. *Quality Management in Health Care, 1,* 45-54.
6. DeVita, V. T. (1989). Foreword. In P. A. Pizzo & D. G. Poplack (Eds.), *Principles and practice of pediatric oncology* (pp. xiii-xiv). Philadelphia: Lippincott.
7. Dow, K. H., Ferrell, B. R., Leigh, S., et al. (1997). The cancer survivor as coinvestigator: The benefits of collaborative research with advocacy groups. *Cancer Practice, 5,* 255-257.
8. Ducanis, A. J., & Golin, A. K. (1979). *The interdisciplinary health care team: A handbook.* Germantown, MD: Aspen.
9. Dunn, L. (1997). A literature review of advanced clinical nursing practice in the United States of America. *Journal of Advanced Nursing, 25,* 814-819.
10. Elder, R., & Bullough, B. (1990). Nurse practitioners and clinical nurse specialists: Are the roles merging? *Clinical Nurse Specialist, 4,* 78-84.
11. Ely, E. A. (1997). Collaborative practice with children and parents: Enhancing preparation for and management of cancer treatment. *Cancer Practice, 5,* 387-390.
12. Fagin, C. M. (1992). Collaboration between nurses and physicians: No longer a choice. *Nursing and Health Care, 13,* 354-363.
13. *Guidelines for establishing joint or collaborative practice in hospital: A demonstration project directed by the National Joint Practice Commission.* (1974). Chicago, IL: Nealy Printing.
14. Hanson, C. M., & Spross, J. A. (1996). Collaboration. In A. B. Hamric, J. A. Spross, & C. M. Hanson (Eds.), *Advanced nursing practice: An integrative approach* (pp. 229-248). Philadelphia: W. B. Saunders.
15. Hilderley, L. J. (1995). Physicians and nurses: Are we still playing games? *Cancer Practice, 3,* 114-116.
16. Hinds, P. S., & DeSwarte-Wallace, J. (2000). Positioning nursing research to contribute to the scientific mission of the pediatric cooperative group. *Seminars in Oncology Nursing, 16,* 251-252.

17. Joint Commission on Accreditation of Healthcare Organizations. (2000). *CAM H Comprehensive Accreditation Manual for Hospitals: The Official Handbook* (pp. TX-11-TX-12). Oakbrook Terrace, IL: Joint Commission on Accreditation of Healthcare Organizations.

18. Kibbe, D., Bentz, E., & McLaughlin, C. (1993). Continuous quality improvement for continuity of care. *Journal of Family Practice, 36,* 304-308.

19. Kolata, G., & Eichenwald, K. (1999). In pediatrics, a lesson on making use of experimental procedures. *New York Times,* October 3, 1999, p. 40.

20. Kramer, S., Meadows, A. T., Pastore, G., et al. (1984). Influence of place of treatment in diagnosis, treatment and survival in three pediatric solid tumors. *Journal of Clinical Oncology, 2,* 917-923.

21. Kushnir, T., Rabin, S., & Azulai, S. (1997). A descriptive study of stress management in a group of pediatric oncology nurses. *Cancer Nursing, 20,* 414-421.

22. Lindeke, L. L., Canedy, B. H., & Kay, M. M. (1997). A comparison of practice domains of clinical nurse specialists and nurse practitioners. *Journal of Professional Nursing, 13,* 281-287.

23. McMahon, L. W., Sealing, P. A., Mahoney, D. H., et al. (2000). Description of a multihospital process to develop a care path for the child with acute lymphoblastic leukemia. *Journal of Pediatric Oncology Nursing, 17,* 33-44.

24. Meadows, A. T., Kramer, S., Hopsin, R., et al. (1983). Survival in childhood acute lymphocytic leukemia: Effect of protocol and place of treatment. *Cancer Investigation, 1,* 49-55.

25. Murphy, S. B. (1995). The national impact of clinical cooperative group trials for pediatric cancer. *Medical and Pediatric Oncology, 24,* 279-280.

26. Murphy, S. B. (1998). POG, CCG, IRSG, NWTSG unanimously agree to form a single group: *Pediatric intergroup summit. POG Perspectives: Pediatric Oncology Group Quarterly Newsletter, Summer 1998,* 1-3.

27. Olson, M. S., Hinds, P. S., Euell, K., et al. (1998). Peak and nadir experiences and their consequences described by pediatric oncology nurses. *Journal of Pediatric Oncology Nursing, 15,* 13-24.

28. Ruccione, K., & Kelly, K. P. (2000). Pediatric oncology nursing in cooperative group clinical trials groups comes of age. *Seminars in Oncology Nursing, 16,* 253-260.

29. Sparacino, P., & Durand, B. A. (1986). Editorial on specialization in advanced nursing practice. Council of Primary Health Care Nurse Practitioners/Council of Clinical Nurse Specialists. American Nurses Association, Missouri, USA.

30. Sparacino, P., Cooper, D., & Minarik, P. (1990). *The clinical nurse specialist: Implementation and impact.* Norwalk, CT: Appleton & Lange.

31. Spinetta, J. J., Jankovic, M., Ben Arush, M. W., et al. (2000). Guidelines for the recognition, prevention, and remediation of burnout in health care professionals participating in the care of children with cancer: Report of the SIOP Working Committee on Psychosocial Issues in Pediatric Oncology. *Medical and Pediatric Oncology, 35,* 122-125.

32

Research

Pamela S. Hinds
Marilyn J. Hockenberry
Lisa Schum

Nursing research in pediatric oncology can strengthen the voices of seriously ill children and adolescents, their family members, and their health care providers. These voices—if carefully listened to—determine what is studied, when, and what methods are used. When this happens, the study findings will be relevant to current and future voices and can be used to improve the circumstances of patients, families, and the health care providers who work with children and adolescents who have cancer. Although each voice has unique needs and desires that can be addressed using research, the shared objective across these voices is to position children and adolescents for cure while decreasing their treatment and disease-related suffering, and to continually increase the competency of health care providers. A second shared objective is to promote the development and well-being of the children and adolescents and of their families so that the optimal level of functioning is achieved and maintained.

Cancer is a complex disease, and children and adolescents are complex developing beings who are raised in complex systems (families, communities, and other social groups). The research focus within these complexities may be as narrowly defined as a cell or as broadly defined as the impact of the child's treatment on a family system over time. The scope of nursing research in pediatric oncology is startlingly wide, reflecting the knowledge needs of nurses who are providing direct care to these patients and their complex systems. This wide scope reflects nursing's commitment to comprehensive care for the pediatric cancer patient but it also conveys the difficulty of building a body of knowledge when interests and needs are sizable and diverse, and the pool of nurse researchers is small. This small group of researchers has made notable progress in meeting wide-ranging and compelling care needs in pediatric oncology nursing. Their efforts have helped position patients for cure while decreasing their suffering and that of their families, and increasing the competency of their health care providers. This research-directed effort has contributed to the development of evidence-based nursing practice in pediatric oncology.

EVIDENCE-BASED NURSING PRACTICE

Evidence-based nursing practice is derived from the integration of findings and theoretical and research literature that together provide the foundation for clinical interventions.[20] A model for evidence-based nursing practice proposed by Rosswurm and Larrabee[19] includes six steps that begin with an assessment of the need for clinical practice change and end with integration of the evidence into patient care interventions (Figure 32-1). The first step involves problem assessment and identification of the need for change in nursing practice. Next, the problem is clearly defined and linked to possible interventions and likely outcomes that could serve as clinical indicators of more effective patient care. Third, relevant literature is searched and critiqued so that the potential risks and benefits of the new intervention can be weighed. Once the need for change is determined, the most appropriate process for implementing change is established, which may be in the format of a protocol, procedure, standard, or guideline that clearly defines the intervention. Next implementation and evaluation of the intervention occur to determine the influence of the change in practice on patient care outcomes. Finally, integration of evidence-based practice is completed through continuing education programs and written policies and procedures that maintain the changes in clinical practice. With the increasing numbers of published empirical studies, theoretical papers, and clinical case reports in pediatric oncology nursing, an evidence-based practice in this nursing specialty is now emerging. Evidence-based practice in pediatric oncology nursing requires nurses to develop and maintain skills to obtain, or create, interpret, and then in-

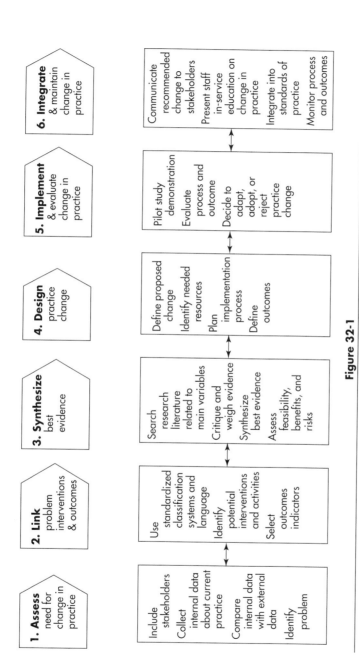

Figure 32-1

Model for evidence-based practice.   (Adapted from Rosswurm, M. A., & Larrabee, J. H. [1999]). A model for change to evidence-based practice, *Image, 31,* 317-322.)

tegrate the best available research into standards of care that reflect state-of-the-art technology and innovative methods of patient care delivery.[15] Often this process begins by identifying challenges or problems in clinical care that can best be addressed through a research process.

SOURCE OF RESEARCH IDEAS

The sources of ideas for research in pediatric oncology nursing are similar to those of other specialties and include: (1) nurses' direct observations or clinical experiences; (2) gaps in the practice literature; (3) discrepancies in research findings or current knowledge; and (4) applicability to practice of a published theory. In addition, our own work has suggested an additional source, that of careful listening to the musings ("How would the patient be different if we as nurses did this instead of that?") or the complaints ("I am never going to do that procedure again because it only has negative effects for patients") of co-workers.[10] This approach of lis-

tening to a co-worker may be formalized by soliciting the priorities for research from co-workers using a Delphi technique, an approach used repeatedly in pediatric oncology nursing.[2,12,13] Research priorities identified by pediatric oncology nurses in the 1990s indicated knowledge needs for decreasing pain, measuring quality of life during the acute treatment periods and after the completion of all treatment, maximizing coping efforts of patients and families, determining the most effective methods for delivery of certain medications or other therapeutic modalities, and minimizing care-related risks for pediatric oncology nurses (Box 32-1). Perhaps reflecting the improved survival of children and adolescents with cancer, the priorities identified at the end of the decade contained more research ideas related to late effects. These informal and formal strategies for identifying research priorities represent pediatric oncology nursing's efforts to determine what currently needs to be studied in an ongoing fashion that should be updated periodically.

BOX 32-1

RESEARCH PRIORITIES IDENTIFIED BY PEDIATRIC ONCOLOGY NURSES

APON DELPHI STUDY, 1992 (N = 227)

1. Measure quality of life and late effects in long-term survivors of childhood cancer.
2. Evaluate effectiveness of anesthesia, sedatives, or other supportive or educational techniques in reducing patients' anxiety about painful or diagnostic procedures.
3. Compare the safety and effectiveness of different pharmacologic (agent combinations, escalations, routes) and nonpharmacologic techniques used for pain control.
4. Document the effects on nurses of exposure to chemotherapeutic agents.
5. Identify factors that influence how children and adolescents comply with treatment regimens.
6. Evaluate interventions designed to help family members cope with the treatment process and its outcomes.
7. Identify strategies to minimize adverse effects of chemotherapy and radiation therapy.
8. Identify effective strategies for teaching patients and health care professionals effective pain management.
9. Document the safety and effectiveness of chemotherapy and/or other infusions given in the patient's home (administered by parent or nurse).
10. Compare the infection rates of bone marrow transplant patients by different isolation environments and techniques.

PEDIATRIC ONCOLOGY GROUP DELPHI STUDY, 2000 (N = 35)

1. Determine the most common treatment-related problems that patients and families experience at home.
2. Compare outcome variables of cost, quality of life, and disease response when therapy is given on an outpatient vs. inpatient basis.
3. Measure caregiver burdens for families receiving outpatient therapy vs. those families receiving primarily inpatient therapy.
4. Identify the impact of late treatment effects on the patient's subsequent educational efforts.
5. Identify most effective pain management strategies for use with terminally ill patients.
6. Identify effective interventions that promote optimal adjustment in survivors of childhood cancer.
7. Evaluate telephone-based interventions used by nurses in response to calls from patients and families.
8. Compare the quality of life among patients who receive care primarily as outpatients vs. inpatients.
9. Determine the impact of early screening and intervention on cognitive functioning of patients treated with cranial irradiation or intrathecal medications.
10. Determine the most cost-effective schedule of administration for differing antiemetics.

RESEARCH MILESTONES

Sure signs of nursing research becoming integrated into the specialty of pediatric oncology have been noted in the past 18 years. These include the creation of the *Journal of Pediatric Oncology Nursing,* research grants, preconference scientific sessions, and the State of the Science Summit for Pediatric Oncology Nursing Research.

JOURNAL OF PEDIATRIC ONCOLOGY NURSING

The *Journal of Pediatric Oncology Nursing (JOPON)* was created in 1984 with Dianne Fochtman as founding editor. This journal represented the commitment of the Association of Pediatric Oncology Nurses (APON) to research and clinical scholarship. The Research column, the responsibility of the APON Research Committee, which itself was established in 1981, has been a regular feature of the journal, as have original reports of research in this nursing specialty. In July 1989, one issue of *JOPON* was dedicated to advances in pediatric oncology nursing research (volume 6, number 3), and in July 1998, an issue was devoted to qualitative research in pediatric oncology (volume 15, number 3).

RESEARCH GRANTS

The APON Research Committee established its first research grant in 1986. This grant, initially sponsored by Davol, Inc., and subsequently by Bard Access Systems, has been awarded 10 times. A second grant, the Joanne Scungio Research grant, was created in 1988 in memory of Dr. Joanne Scungio who had served as the chair of the APON Research Committee.[3] That grant has been awarded eight times since 1989. The dollar value of both grants was initially $500 but subsequently increased to $1000 in 1997.

PRECONFERENCE SCIENTIFIC SESSIONS

Under the direction of the APON Research Committee, the first preconference scientific session was convened in 1997. The purpose of the session was to serve as a forum to feature pediatric oncology nursing research programs, to offer critical reviews of those programs, and to identify the implications of the research for clinical practice. The topics of the preconference sessions have included: treatment-related decision making (*JOPON* Supplement, 15[3], July 1998); the stress-response sequence in pediatric oncology nursing,[7] and fatigue in pediatric oncology patients.[11] These preconference sessions represented an important transition from a focus on reports of single and unrelated studies to research programs or clusters of related studies in pediatric oncology nursing.

THE STATE OF THE SCIENCE SUMMIT FOR PEDIATRIC ONCOLOGY NURSING RESEARCH

Advanced practice nurses, staff nurses, and nurse researchers from APON, the Pediatric Oncology Group (POG), and from the Children's Cancer Group (CCG) jointly planned the first State of the Science Summit for Pediatric Oncology Nursing Research. The recently initiated fusion of the pediatric oncology clinical trials groups prompted this coalition of nurses to examine their current research activities and to consider their future research contributions to the evolving pediatric oncology cooperative group, the Childrens Oncology Group (C.O.G.). The summit was convened in February 2000 at the National Institutes of Health. The overall intent was for nurses to outline a scientific agenda of highest relevance to the nursing discipline and to design the future scientific contributions from nursing to the C.O.G. The more specific objectives of the summit included:

1. To facilitate critique of four established nursing research programs in oncology for their potential usefulness to the research mission of the C.O.G.
2. To develop scientific hypotheses that represent nursing's scientific priorities, for incorporation into future clinical trials
3. To identify emerging pediatric oncology nursing research programs or research questions through a poster mechanism
4. To strengthen the working relationship between nurse researchers and advanced practice nurses in pediatric oncology through a shared responsibility for shaping the nursing scientific agenda and for contributing to the overall scientific agenda of C.O.G.

These objectives were achieved in part by the critiques of four established nursing research programs, three in pediatric oncology (fatigue, coping, and neurocognitive late effects of therapy)[6,14,17] and one in adult oncology. The latter program, self-care as developed by Dodd and colleagues,[1] was selected for inclusion because of its potential to improve symptom management in children and adolescents with cancer. Each program of research was critiqued by a nurse researcher and a nonnurse researcher. Then a working group composed of advanced practice nurses and researchers convened to consider the strengths of the research program and to identify strategies for incorporating the research into the scientific agenda of the cooperative group. The publication of the summit proceedings has been distributed to the leadership of the C.O.G. and to leaders of cancer-related and health policy setting organizations.[8]

TYPE OF NURSING RESEARCH STUDIES PUBLISHED IN PEDIATRIC ONCOLOGY

The number and type of studies completed by pediatric oncology nurse researchers have increased considerably during the past 3 decades.[5] The types of studies may be grouped by similarity into the following categories (Table 32-1):

1. Psychosocial care needs of patients and families: related to the emotions, coping, values, perceptions, decisions, and quality of life issues of the child or adolescent with cancer and the same for siblings, parents, and others
2. Biophysical processes in patients: related to the physiologic indicators of health or altered health and the connection between psychologic and biologic wellness in children and adolescents with cancer

3. Nursing care procedures: related to direct care actions by a nurse to respond to an immediate or potential need or changing status of a patient, and the results of those nursing actions
4. Professional development: related to the nurse's scope of responsibility and the unique knowledge required to practice in pediatric oncology and the stressors, coping strategies, and consequences for the nurse secondary to this role
5. Care delivery systems: related to management of health care resources and plans to effectively use those resources to benefit patients and their families[12,13]

A careful review of studies completed during the past 3 decades by nurse researchers in pediatric oncology who have published three or more studies of original research (Table 32-1) indicates that the

TABLE 32-1	TYPE OF STUDIES COMPLETED BY PEDIATRIC ONCOLOGY NURSES IN THE LAST 3 DECADES			
Author(s)	Title	Source/Year	Purpose	Design/Method
PSYCHOSOCIAL CARE NEEDS OF PATIENTS				
Haase	*Components of Courage in Chronically Ill Adolescents: A Phenomenological Study*	*Advances in Nursing Science, 9,* 1987	To determine the essential structure of the lived experience of courage in chronically ill adolescents	Phenomenological analysis of transcribed, unstructured interviews
Hinds, Martin, & Vogel	*Nursing Strategies to Influence Adolescent Hopefulness During Oncology Illness*	*Journal of the Association of Pediatric Oncology Nurses, 4,* 1987	To systematically investigate adolescents' perceptions of the nursing influence upon their hopefulness during an oncologic illness	Grounded theory method (interview, observations, and medical record review)
Martinson, Davies, & McClowry	*The Long-term Effects of Sibling Death on Self-concept*	*Journal of Pediatric Nursing, 2,* 1987	To examine the long-term effects of sibling bereavement on self-concept; to identify what factors may contribute to optimal levels of self-concept in bereaved siblings	Exploratory (interview and completion of the Piers-Harris Self-Concept Scale[a])

[a]Piers, E., & Harris, D. (1969). *The manual for the Piers-Harris Children's Self-Concept Scale.* Nashville, TN: Counselor Recordings and Tests.

majority of published studies (70%) are in the category of psychosocial care needs. Indeed, this category had six times as many studies as the next largest category (biophysical processes). Only 5.5% of the studies were on nursing care procedures, and less than 5% were on nursing professional issues. Only four studies on care delivery systems were found. Most studies (78.2%) were published in nursing journals and of those, 67% were published in cancer nursing journals. The most commonly used designs were descriptive or exploratory (86%), and most used a cross-sectional approach (83%). The participants in the studies were primarily patients in active treatment (30%), parents of patients (27%), or survivors (24%). Sources of funding for the studies were primarily private foundations (23%), the federal government

(17%), or the researcher's own work setting (17%). The majority of studies had multiple authors (87%). Finally, slightly more than half of the studies were completed at a single site (60.2%).

FUNDING SOURCES FOR PEDIATRIC ONCOLOGY NURSING RESEARCH

Multiple sources of funding have supported the research of pediatric oncology nurses. Examples include National Cancer Institute, National Institute of Nursing Research, American Cancer Society, Oncology Nursing Foundation, Milheim Foundation, Association of Pediatric Oncology Nurses, Project on Death in America, hospitals and other employers of pediatric oncology nurses, state nursing associations, universities, American Nurses

Text continued on p. 682

Sample	Findings	Funding	Single Site or Multisite
9 adolescents suffering from chronic illness, ages 14-21	Phenomenological analysis of subjective experiences of courage revealed 31 clusters in 9 categories from which an essential structure of courage in chronically ill adolescents was derived. Researchers define this structure (the lived experience of courage) as an interpersonally assigned attribute resulting from a gradual process of living through a health-related condition. Themes that emerged included heroism, fear, creativity, will, social support, time and consciousness, humor, and themes of transcendence.	—	Single
58 adolescent oncology patients, ages 12-18	Findings support the theorized nursing impact of hopefulness on adolescents experiencing cancer. Negative influence results when the nurse distances herself from the patient. Positive influence results when the nurse conveys commitment to the patient and an optimistic realism regarding the patient's situation and ability to deal with that situation.	American Nurses' Foundation	Single
29 children having experienced the loss of a sibling to childhood cancer, ages 8-18	Results indicated that bereaved siblings scored statistically higher on the Piers-Harris Self-Concept Scale as compared with the normative group of children. Although researchers suggest these findings may imply that sibling death does not necessarily inflict long-term negative consequences, other possible explanations for these surprising findings are presented.	American Cancer Society, California Division (Grant 2-210-PR-14)	Single

Continued

TABLE 32-1	TYPE OF STUDIES COMPLETED BY PEDIATRIC ONCOLOGY NURSES IN THE LAST 3 DECADES—cont'd

Author(s)	Title	Source/Year	Purpose	Design/Method
PSYCHOSOCIAL CARE NEEDS OF PATIENTS—cont'd				
Moore, Glasser, & Ablin	*The Late Psychosocial Consequences of Childhood Cancer*	*Journal of Pediatric Nursing, 3,* 1988	To investigate the late consequences of childhood cancer and treatment on overall psychosocial functioning	Comparative; Instrument used: the Deasy-Spinetta Behavioral Questionnaire (DSBQ[b])
Hinds & Martin	*Hopefulness and the Self-Sustaining Process in Adolescents with Cancer*	*Nursing Research, 37,* 1988	To explore, using grounded theory, the process through which adolescents with cancer move to achieve hopefulness	Grounded theory method (interview, observations, and medical record review)
Moore, Gilliss, & Martinson	*Psychosomatic Symptoms in Parents 2 Years After the Death of a Child with Cancer*	*Nursing Research, 37,* 1988	To investigate psychosomatic symptoms experienced by mothers and fathers 24 months after the death of a child with cancer	Exploratory (interview and completion of the Symptoms Checklist-90-Revised [SCL-90-R[c]])
Walker	*Stress and Coping in Siblings of Childhood Cancer Patients*	*Nursing Research, 37,* 1988	To identify and describe cognitive and behavioral coping strategies used by siblings of pediatric oncology patients	Exploratory; parent data were collected from open-ended interview and questionnaire. Sibling data included open-ended interviews and psychological assessments (including puppet play, kinetic family drawings, cartoon story telling, sentence completion)

[b]Spinetta, J. J., & Deasy-Spinetta, P. (1981). *Living with childhood cancer.* St. Louis, MO: Mosby.
[c]Derogatis, L. (1983). *SCL-90 (revised) manual.* Baltimore: Johns Hopkins University Press.

Sample	Findings	Funding	Single Site or Multisite
35 children previously treated for ALL or solid tumor not involving the CNS; 35 control children never diagnosed with or treated for cancer; children ranged from 3rd to 12th grade	Results indicate that children treated for leukemia function at a level below school peers. There were differences between parent and teacher appraisal of the cancer survivor suggesting a breakdown in ongoing communication. The results also indicate a possible relationship between cognitive and emotional problems.	National Research Service Award (NU 05625-03) funded under the Division of Nursing and the California Division of the American Cancer Society	Single
58 adolescent oncology patients, ages 12-18	Four sequential concepts (cognitive discomfort, distraction, cognitive comfort, and personal competence) emerged to represent the process adolescentsexperience to achieve hopefulness. The term *self-sustaining,* defined as a natural progression through which adolescents diagnosed with cancer move to comfort themselves and achieve competence in resolving health threats, emerged as the overall organizing construct.	American Nurses' Foundation	Single
70 parents having experienced the loss of a child to cancer, ages 22-61	Results indicated that 2 years following the death of a child from cancer, parents present a profile on the SCL-90-R that differs significantly from the normal, nonclinical, and psychiatric outpatient comparison groups. Researchers suggest that this indicates bereaved parents display a psychological pattern that is more symptomatic than normals, but less symptomatic than diagnosed outpatients. Similarly, researchers conclude that these findings suggest that the grieving process is incomplete at a year post-death.	National Cancer Institute (CA19490); American Cancer Society, California Division (Grant 2-210-PR-14)	Single
15 families of pediatric oncology patients with 26 siblings, ages 7-11	Content analysis of sibling data revealed major stressor themes of loss, fear of death, and change. Further analysis of sibling data pertinent to coping efforts led to the development of a taxonomy of cognitive and behavioral coping efforts. A 44% disagreement between what the parents thought their child's coping strategies were and what the children revealed as their coping strategies was found suggesting this information is best collected from the sibling directly.	—	Single

Continued

Author(s)	Title	Source/Year	Purpose	Design/Method
PSYCHOSOCIAL CARE NEEDS OF PATIENTS—cont'd				
Birenbaum	*The Relationship between Parent-Sibling Communication and Coping of Siblings with Death Experience*	*Journal of Pediatric Oncology Nursing, 6,* 1989	To investigate the effects of two types of terminal care on families who had a child dying of cancer, focusing specifically on parent-sibling communication	Longitudinal, prospective, repeated measures (measurements taken before death, at 2 weeks, 4 months, and 12 months postdeath of sibling); instruments used: Child Behavior Checklist (CBCL[d]) and the Parent-sibling Communication Instrument[e]
Birenbaum, Robinson, Phillips, Stewart, & McCown	*The Response of Children to the Dying and Death of a Sibling*	*OMEGA: Journal of Death and Dying, 20,* 1989-1990	To investigate patterns of behavioral responses of children during and after the terminal phase of their siblings' illness	Longitudinal, prospective, repeated measures (measurements taken before death, at 2 weeks, 4 months, and 12 months postdeath of sibling); instrument used: Child Behavior Checklist (CBCL[d])
Martinson, Gilliss, Colaizzo, Freeman, & Bossert	*Impact of Childhood Cancer on Healthy School-age Siblings*	*Cancer Nursing, 13,* 1990	To identify the emotional reactions of school-age siblings in response to childhood cancer in the family	Exploratory (open-ended, semistructured interview technique)
Birenbaum & Robinson	*Family Relationships in Two Types of Terminal Care*	*Social Science and Medicine, 32,* 1991	To investigate parents' perceptions of family relationships in 87 parents from 48 families during the terminal illness and first year following a child's death from cancer	Cross-sectional analyses of data obtained in a larger, prospective, longitudinal study; data were collected before death and 2 weeks, 4 months, and 1 year postdeath of child; instrument used: the Family Relations Index (FRI[f])

[d]Achenbach, T., & Edelbrock, D. (1983). *Manual for the child behavior checklist and revised child behavior profile.* Burlington, VT: University of Vermont.
[e]Friedrich W., Cohen, D., Pendergrass, T., et al. (1984). *Instruments to measure parent-child communication regarding pediatric cancer* [unpublished report]. Seattle: University of Washington.
[f]Birenbaum, L. K. (1987). *Effect of family nursing on sibling response to dying* (Final Report: Grant No. 5 RO1 NU00912 and 5 RO1 NU00912-02S). Division of Nursing, Health and Human Services. Portland, OR: Oregon Health Sciences University.

Sample	Findings	Funding	Single Site or Multisite
61 children (ages 4-17) whose sibling was in the terminal phase of cancer	Results indicated that parent-sibling communication was positively related to Social Competence before the ill child's death, and was inversely related to total Behavior Problems following the death. Parent-sibling communication was also inversely related to External Behavior Problems and to Internal Behavior Problems after the ill child's death. Researchers suggest that parent-sibling communication in connection with increased social competence may indicate a parental sensitivity to siblings' needs.	Human Health Service Division of Nursing (Grants No. 5 RO1 NU00912 and 5 RO1 NU00912-02S1)	Multi
61 children (ages 4-17) whose sibling was in the terminal phase of cancer	Results indicated that this sample of bereaved siblings had significantly increased incidence and severity of behavior problems as compared to the normal population. This sample also had significantly elevated scores on the Internalizing Behavior Problems scale at all four times of measurement. These behaviors include somatic complaints, depression, social withdrawal, obsession, anxiety, immaturity, obsessive compulsion, and uncommunicativeness. These siblings also displayed lower social competence than normal children.	Human Health Service Division of Nursing (Grants No. 5 RO1 NU00912)	Multi
16 siblings of childhood cancer patients, ages 6-12	Content analysis revealed themes in the siblings' feelings including experience of diagnosis and hospitalization, awareness of prognosis and mortality, need for information, continuing effect of disease or death on the well child, correct understanding of cancer, and hopes and desires for the future. Results were grouped as belonging to the "sibling with a living child" or the "sibling with a deceased child" category, and some contextual differences were seen between the groups of siblings.	Minnesota and California Divisions of the American Cancer Society; St. Paul Foundation, St. Paul, Minnesota; Home Care Research Fund, University of Minnesota, Minneapolis, Minnesota	Single
87 parents from 48 families with a child in the terminal phase of cancer	Results indicated that during the terminal care phase, families receiving home care were less cohesive and expressive and had more conflict than families whose child received care in the hospital. Similarly, families who received home care showed less expressiveness and cohesion while experiencing more conflict postdeath, at 2 weeks, and 4 months, than did families in hospital care. Researchers suggest that terminal care in the home may not be as beneficial to family functioning as hospital care.	—	Multi

Continued

Author(s)	Title	Source/Year	Purpose	Design/Method
PSYCHOSOCIAL CARE NEEDS OF PATIENTS—cont'd				
Martinson, Davies, & McClowry	*Parental Depression Following the Death of a Child*	*Death Studies, 15,* 1991	To determine whether the same parents continue to experience depression 7 years after the death of their child from cancer; to examine whether the gender of the parents or the length of the child's illness influenced parental depression	Exploratory (interview and completion of the Symptoms Check List [SCL-90][c])
Ruccione, Kramer, Moore, & Perin	*Informed Consent for Treatment of Childhood Cancer: Factors Affecting Parents' Decision Making*	*Journal of Pediatric Oncology Nursing, 8,* 1991	To identify influential circumstances surrounding the consent process in the pediatric setting; to describe the relationship of parental anxiety to these factors; to delineate related practice and research implications	Descriptive; instruments used: the State-Trait Anxiety Inventory (STAI[g]) and the Parent Informed Consent Questionnaire (PICQ[h])
Martinson & Liang	*The Reactions of Chinese Children Who Have Cancer*	*Pediatric Nursing, 18,* 1992	To explore how children in China react to cancer and how the experience affects their lives	Exploratory (data were collected by semi-structured interview)
Clarke-Steffen	*A Model of the Family Practice, Transition to Living with Childhood Cancer*	*Cancer Practice, 1,* 1993	To describe the family transition to living with childhood cancer, from the family's point of view, when a child is diagnosed with cancer with a favorable prognosis	Longitudinal, prospective, grounded theory design (data collected by semistructured interview and demographic questionnaire)

[g]Spielberger, C. D. (1983). *Manual for the State-Trait Anxiety Inventory.* Palo Alto, CA: Consulting Psychologists Press.
[h]Muss, H. B., White, D. R., Michielutte, R., et al. (1979). Written informed consent in patients with breast cancer. *Cancer, 43,* 1549-1556.

Sample	Findings	Funding	Single Site or Multisite
66 parents (ages 22-61) having experienced the loss of a child to cancer	Results showed no change in parental depression at 7 years as compared to 2 years following a child's death with 22% of the variance at 7 years accounted for by depression at 2 years. Parental depression was found to be unrelated to gender of parents or length of child's illness. Researchers suggest that parental depression resulting from a child's cancer-related death does not change significantly between the second and seventh years postdeath.	American Cancer Society, California Division (Grant No. 2-210-PR-14)	Single
28 parents (18 mothers, 10 fathers) of children entered on one of four protocols for the treatment of newly diagnosed ALL	Results confirmed clinical experience that parents are given complex information and asked to make decisions about their child's life in a highly anxious state. Subjects were generally satisfied with the informed consent process 48 hours after signing a consent form. Researchers suggest that further research is necessary to determine the adequacy of the consent process including the influence of time and the amount of information retained.	—	Multi
55 children in China diagnosed with cancer	Only one of the newly diagnosed children knew the correct name of her diagnosis as compared to 10 children undergoing treatment. All children had questions regarding the disease and treatment that they felt they were not allowed to ask under normal circumstances. None of the children claimed to know the cause of the cancer, yet some offered theories. Most had good relations with parents. Relationships with siblings depended on visitation to the hospital. Researchers suggest these interviews show the need for psychological and supportive care for Chinese children undergoing treatment.	National Academy of Science, Social and Behavioral Research Panel	Multi
40 members of 7 families with a child (ages 2-10) recently diagnosed with cancer with a favorable prognosis	A model of the family transition in response to the diagnosis of childhood cancer was developed. This transition was characterized by a fracturing of reality at the realization of the malignant nature of the illness; a period of limbo, characterized by uncertainty after the diagnosis; use of strategies to reconstruct reality; and construction of a "new normal" for the family, during which the nature of uncertainty changed but did persist. The transition process continued for the 4- to 5-month course of the study and extended beyond the study period.	D.H.H.S., P.H.S., National Center for Nursing Research (National Research Service Award #NR06157 Sigma Theta Tau, Beta Psi Chapter Research Award, Transitions Focal Area, Oregon Health Sciences University Small Grant, D.H.H.S., P.H.S., National Cancer Institute, and National Research Service Award #NR07036)	Single

Continued

	TABLE 32-1	TYPE OF STUDIES COMPLETED BY PEDIATRIC ONCOLOGY NURSES IN THE LAST 3 DECADES—cont'd

Author(s)	Title	Source/Year	Purpose	Design/Method
PSYCHOSOCIAL CARE NEEDS OF PATIENTS—cont'd				
Clarke-Steffen	*Waiting and Not Knowing: The Diagnosis of Cancer in a Child*	*Journal of Pediatric Oncology Nursing, 10,* 1993	To describe the experience families have during the period immediately surrounding the time of diagnosis of cancer in a child	Longitudinal, prospective, grounded theory design (data collected by semistructured interview and demographic questionnaire)
Hollen & Hobbie	*Risk Taking and Decision Making of Adolescent Long-Term Survivors of Cancer*	*Oncology Nursing Forum, 20,* 1993	To describe the prevalence of risk behaviors among adolescent long-term survivors of cancer; to describe these survivors' perceptions of the quality of their decision making; to test the hypothesis that the poorer the decision-making quality, the more risk behaviors exhibited; to examine the effects of CNS prophylactic leukemia therapy and academic achievement problems on quality of decision making and risk behaviors	Descriptive (semistructured interview and two behavioral instruments: Decision Making Quality Scale [DMQS[i]] and the Risk Behavior Interview Schedule[i])
Martinson, Chang, & Liang	*Chinese Families after the Death of a Child from Cancer*	*European Journal of Cancer Care, 2,* 1993	To describe the impact of losing a child to cancer in China	Descriptive (data were collected by interview)

[i]Hollen, P. J. (1994). Psychometric properties of two instruments to measure quality decision making. *Research in Nursing and Health, 17,* 137-148.

Sample	Findings	Funding	Single Site or Multisite
40 members of 7 families with a child (ages 2-10) recently diagnosed with cancer with a favorable prognosis	Constant comparative method analysis of the interviews revealed Waiting and Not Knowing as most distressing for families dealing with childhood cancer. Uncertainty, worry, preoccupation, vulnerability, and helplessness were identified as characterizing themes of Waiting and Not Knowing.	Public Service, National Center for Nursing Research (National Research Service Award #NR06157; the Sigma Theta Tau, Beta Psi Chapter Research Award; the Focal Area III, Oregon Health Sciences University School of Nursing Small Grant)	Single
36 long-term cancer survivors, ages 14-19	Although there was a trend toward higher experimental use of some risk behaviors, the prevalence rates were comparable to those of the general population. Some were good decision makers; however, the majority did not report quality decision-making skills. With better decision-making quality, fewer risk behaviors were exhibited. Prior CNS prophylactic leukemia therapy and academic achievement problems may be associated with poor quality decision making.	Nursing Research Seed Fund of the New York State Division of the American Cancer Society; University of Rochester Biomedical Research Support Grant (#1-160743209-A1)	Single
17 families who lost a child to cancer within a 5-year period	The majority of families stated that their children died of cancer without any knowledge of the disease. Eleven of the families remained at the hospital during the entire illness with the other six returning home rarely. Fifteen of the children died in the hospital. Six families paid for the entire treatment themselves, seven paid for 50% themselves, and the rest had between 70%-100% subsidized. Eight of the families rid themselves of all mementos of the child, including photos, with only five families keeping any pictures of the child. All families considered cancer the most serious of possible illnesses. Eleven of the families felt they could not talk of the deceased child because of grief.	National Academy of Science, Social and Behavioral Panel, the Committee for Scholarly Exchange with China	Multi

Continued

TABLE 32-1	TYPE OF STUDIES COMPLETED BY PEDIATRIC ONCOLOGY NURSES IN THE LAST 3 DECADES—cont'd			
Author(s)	**Title**	**Source/Year**	**Purpose**	**Design/Method**
PSYCHOSOCIAL CARE NEEDS OF PATIENTS—cont'd				
Martinson, Su-Xiao-Yin, & Liang	*The Impact of Childhood Cancer on 50 Chinese Families*	*Journal of Pediatric Oncology Nursing, 10,* 1993	To describe the impact of childhood cancer on Chinese families	Descriptive (data were collected by interview)
Thoma, Hockenberry-Eaton, & Kemp	*Life Change Events and Coping Behaviors in Families of Children with Cancer*	*Journal of Pediatric Oncology Nursing, 10,* 1993	To investigate life change events and coping behaviors in families of children with cancer compared with those who have physically healthy children	Between groups design; Instruments used included the Family Inventory of Life Events and Changes (FILE)[j] and the Family Crisis Oriented Evaluation Scales (F-COPES)[k]
Wright	*Parents' Perceptions of Their Quality of Life*	*Journal of Pediatric Oncology Nursing, 10,* 1993	To assess parents' perceptions of their quality of life after the diagnosis and treatment of cancer in their child	Descriptive study using Roy's Adaptation Model[l] as a theoretical framework. Data collection included parental completion of the Varricchio-Wright Impact of Cancer Questionnaire-Parents[m] and a demographic information form.
Finke, Birenbaum, & Chand	*Two Weeks Post-death Report by Parents of Siblings' Grieving Experience*	*Journal of Child and Adolescent Psychiatric Nursing, 7,* 1994	To explore the grieving of children who have experienced the death of a sibling; to describe the siblings' grieving experiences as identified by parents	Secondary analysis of a two-group repeated-measures design; data collection involved questionnaire and interview

[j]McCubbin, H. I., & Patterson, J. M. (1987). FILE: Family inventory of life events and changes. In H. I. McCubbin, & A. I. Thompson (Eds.), *Family assessment inventories for research and practice* (pp. 81-98) Madison, WI: University of Wisconsin.
[k]McCubbin, H. I., Olson, D. H., & Larsen, A. S. (1987). F-COPES: Family crisis oriented personal evaluation scales. In H. I. McCubbin & A. I. Thompson (Eds.), *Family assessment inventories for research and practice* (pp. 194-207) Madison, WI: University of Wisconsin.
[l]Roy, C. (1987). Roy's adaption model. In R. Parse (Ed.), *Nursing science, major paradigms, theories and critiques.* Philadelphia: W. B. Saunders.
[m]Varricchio, C., & Wright, P. (1986). Development of an instrument to measure the impact of cancer on quality of life. [unpublished data].

Sample	Findings	Funding	Single Site or Multisite
100 parents (50 mothers, 50 fathers) of pediatric oncology patients either newly diagnosed or undergoing treatment	The length of time between symptom onset and diagnosis ranged from 1 week to 2 years, with eight children experiencing symptoms for more than 8 months. 35 parents believed the affected child had little or no knowledge of the disease. The majority of families (76%) were paying the total cost of their child's care and treatment themselves with 14% reporting serious financial problems.	—	Multi
38 families (21 with children affected with cancer, 17 with physically healthy children)	Results indicate that families with a child who had cancer experienced significantly more stressful life change events (including intra-family strains, marital strains, and finance/business strains) as compared to families with healthy children. No significant differences were found in coping behaviors used by the two groups suggesting the possibility that both groups use effective coping strategies in dealing with problems.	American Cancer Society Nursing Scholarship	Single
30 parents of children with cancer; parents' ages 22-53; 93% female	Results indicate that parents perceive their quality of life as good, but not as good as before their child was diagnosed with cancer. These findings lead researchers to use a qualitative approach to probe the criteria by which parents judge their quality of life, to use a longitudinal approach to account for certain of the residual stimuli, and to limit studies to a single diagnosis so that prognosis may be quantified and factored into parental perceptions.	Joanne Scungio Award from the Association of Pediatric Oncology Nurses	Single
43 siblings from 31 families who had a child (age birth to 19 years) in the terminal phase of cancer	Results indicated that grieving behaviors of children were similar to those of adults, including crying, denial, avoidance, shock, and guilt, and such behaviors did not vary with age, gender, or family size. Grieving behaviors of children were similar to the behaviors of their parents. Most siblings maintained age-appropriate interaction with the dying child, and most parents maintained open communication with the siblings before and after the patient's death.	National Institutes of Health, Division of Nursing Research (Grant #5 RO1 NU00912 and NU00912-02S1)	Multi

Continued

	TABLE 32-1	**TYPE OF STUDIES COMPLETED BY PEDIATRIC ONCOLOGY NURSES IN THE LAST 3 DECADES—cont'd**			
Author(s)	**Title**	**Source/Year**	**Purpose**		**Design/Method**
PSYCHOSOCIAL CARE NEEDS OF PATIENTS—cont'd					
Haase & Rostad	*Experiences of Completing Cancer Therapy: Children's Perspectives*	*Oncology Nursing Forum, 21,* 1994	To explore the child's perspective of experiencing completion of cancer treatment		Descriptive, phenomenological (data were collected by open-ended interview and analyzed using Colaizzi's eight-step procedure)
Hockenberry-Eaton, Kemp, & DiIorio	*Cancer Stressors and Protective Factors: Predictors of Stress Experienced During Treatment for Childhood Cancer*	*Research in Nursing and Health, 17,* 1994	To explore the relationships among childhood cancer stressors, protective factors, and the physiological and psychological responses to stressors experienced during treatment of childhood cancer		Exploratory study; instruments used included the About My Illness Scale (AMIS), the Harter Self-Perception Profile for Children (HSPPC),[n] the Harter Social Support Scale for Children (HSSSC),[o] the State Anxiety Inventory for Children (SAIC),[p] the Family Environment Scale (FES),[q] the School-agers Coping Strategies Inventory (SCSI),[r] urinalysis
Hockenberry-Eaton & Minick	*Living with Cancer: Children with Extraordinary Courage*	*Oncology Nursing Forum, 21,* 1994	To gain an understanding of the personal experiences of school-age children with cancer		Phenomenological (data were collected by semistructured interview)
Martinson, McClowry, Davies, & Kuhlenkamp	*Changes Over Time: A Study of Family Bereavement Following Childhood Cancer*	*Journal of Palliative Care, 10,* 1994	To examine the familial changes over time following the death of a child with cancer		Longitudinal follow-up (data were collected by semistructured interview and questionnaire and analyzed qualitatively)

[n]Harter, S. (1985). *Manual for the Self-Perception Profile for Children.* Denver, CO: University of Denver Press.
[o]Harter, S. (1985). *Manual for the Social Support Scale for Children.* Denver, CO: University of Denver Press.
[p]Spielberger, C. D. (1972). Anxiety as an emotional state. In C. D. Spielberger (Ed.), *Anxiety: Current trends in theory and research, Vol. 1* (pp. 23-49). New York: Academic Press.
[q]Moos, R. (1974). *The social climate scales: An over-view.* Palo Alto, CA: Consulting Psychologists.
[r]Ryan, N. M. (1990). Development and psychometric properties of the school-agers' coping strategies inventory. *Nursing Research, 39,* 344-349.

Sample	Findings	Funding	Single Site or Multisite
7 children (ages 5-18) who have completed cancer therapy within the past year and who were in remission	Six themes emerged including: gradual realization of completion, hierarchical and cyclical recurrence fears, completion embedded within the cancer experience, seeking a new normal, modifying relationships, and resolution and moving on. Researchers suggest that these themes were developed into an essential structure indicating that the experience of completing cancer treatment has two faces—one of celebration and hope and one of uncertainty and fear.	Oncology Nursing Foundation and Bristol-Myers Oncology Division	Single
44 pediatric oncology patients receiving outpatient chemotherapy, ages 6-14	Results indicated increased physiologic responses to cancer stressors, the lack of correlation among physiologic and psychological responses to stressors, no difference in the response to stressors based on the type of clinic visit, and a difference in the models explaining the response to stressors at the first as compared to the second visit. Child's epinephrine was elevated during both clinic visits although norepinephrine and cortisol remained normal. Family environment and global self-worth were the best predictors of epinephrine levels, whereas social support from friends predicted norepinephrine levels. Family environment and social support from teachers predicted state anxiety.	NIH (NESA, NR06489-02); American Cancer Society predoctoral scholarship	Single
21 children undergoing cancer treatment, ages 7-13	Analysis of the interviews revealed common themes providing strength to these children during treatment including *knowing, caring, feeling special,* and *getting used to it.* Researchers suggest these interviews illustrate children can demonstrate patterns of strength and resilience in stressful situations, and health care professionals can help develop this strength.	Oncology Nursing Foundation Research Grant	Single
56 families having experienced the death of a child from cancer (included 46 mothers, 33 fathers/ stepfathers, 71 siblings)	Analysis indicated changes in the family structures including family reorganization, marital status, familial expansion, illness and other death, substance abuse, memories of the deceased child's illness and death, family priorities, and family attitudes to life and death.	California Division, American Cancer Society (Grant No. 2.210.PR.14)	Multi

Continued

Author(s)	Title	Source/Year	Purpose	Design/Method
PSYCHOSOCIAL CARE NEEDS OF PATIENTS—cont'd				
Martinson & Bossert	*The Psychological Status of Children with Cancer*	*Journal of Child and Adolescent Psychiatric Nursing,* 7, 1994	To examine the impact of treatment for cancer on the psychosocial well-being of a child	Descriptive/exploratory study (structured interview and administration of the Child Behavior Checklist [CBCL])[d]
Martinson, Bi-Hui, & Yi-Hua	*The Reaction of Parents to a Terminally Ill Child with Cancer*	*Cancer Nursing,* 17, 1994	To examine the reaction of Chinese parents to having a child dying from cancer	Descriptive/exploratory study (data were collected by structured interview)
Phipps, Hinds, Channell, & Bell	*Measurement of Behavioral, Affective, and Somatic Responses to Pediatric Bone Marrow Transplantation; Development of the BASES Scale*	*Journal of Pediatric Oncology Nursing,* 11, 1994	To refine the content of the Behavioral Affective and Somatic Experiences (BASES) and to establish its psychometric properties in terms of internal consistency, inter-rater reliability, and validity	Instrument development
Ruccione, Waskerwitz, Buckley, Perin, & Hammond	*What Caused my Child's Cancer? Parents' Responses to an Epidemiology Study of Childhood Cancer*	*Journal of Pediatric Oncology Nursing,* 11, 1994	To identify generic themes or concerns of parents related to the cause of their child's cancer that could be used in planning educational and supportive interventions, as well as further research	Descriptive/qualitative; involved parental completion of an epidemiology questionnaire including one open-answer question
Saiki, Martinson, & Inano	*Japanese Families Who Have Lost Children to Cancer: A Primary Study*	*Journal of Pediatric Nursing,* 9, 1994	To describe what happens in Japanese families who have lost children to cancer	Descriptive/qualitative (data were collected by semistructured interview)

Sample	Findings	Funding	Single Site or Multisite
16 pediatric cancer patients, ages 4-16 (10 male, 6 female)	Analysis indicated that 81% of the children were involved in age-appropriate social interactions and showed normal behavioral patterns. No significant differences were found by gender, tumor type, or behavior over time. Therefore, researchers concluded that these cancer patients seemed to be functioning normally, both psychologically and socially, 3 to 5 years after a diagnosis of cancer.	American Cancer Society, California and Minnesota divisions; St. Paul Foundation, St. Paul, MN	Single
22 families with children dying of childhood cancer	Descriptive analysis indicated that all families identified cancer as the most frightening aspect of their situations. Not having enough money for medicines and hospitalization was identified as the most difficult problem. Sixteen of the 22 families paid for the total cost of medical treatment and hospitalization by themselves. All but two of the families experienced a time when they could not work. The most common suggestion of these families to other parents in the same situation was to "treat the child as well as you can."	National Academy of Science, Social and Behavioral Panel, the Committee for Scholarly Exchange with China	Multi
Pilot 1: 17 nurses observed BMT patients for a total of 107 observations; Pilot 2: 17 nurses observed BMT patients for a total of 109 observations; Pilot 3: 7 parents completed a total of 10 parental observations	Results revealed an internal consistency (Chronbach's α) for the subscales ranging from 0.742 to 0.902. The inter-rater reliability had a median correlation between paired nurse observations of 0.866. There was also significant parent-nurse correlation providing preliminary evidence of the validity of the parent report version of the BASES. Overall, researchers suggest the BASES scale is an adequately reliable measure that is both brief and easy to complete.	American Lebanese Syrian Associated Charities (ALSAC); National Cancer Institute (Grants CA21765 and CA20810)	Single
500 parents of children treated at Children's Cancer Group member institutions	Twelve major themes included concern about environmental exposures, concern about family health history, specific causality attribution, puzzlement, specific feedback requests, myths/misconceptions, advocation of preventive education/screening, active information-seeking, and parental self-blame. The majority of respondents indicated environmental factors to be of greatest concern followed closely by family history.	Children's Cancer Group (CA13539) from the Division of Cancer Treatment; National Cancer Institute; National Institutes of Health; Department of Health and Human Service	Multi
13 Japanese families having lost one child to cancer within 3 years	The main caregiver for the sick child was the mother, and the mother was the leader whereas the father was a cooperator. The sick child was the center of the family, often leading to the isolation of siblings. The stable family structure reflected a strong mother-father relationship and a strong mother-child relationship whereas an unstable family lacked the mother-father connection. There was a general lack of communication concerning cancer and prognosis. The child was told little or nothing about the cancer, and the physician withheld cancer diagnosis.	—	Single

Continued

| TABLE 32-1 | **TYPE OF STUDIES COMPLETED BY PEDIATRIC ONCOLOGY NURSES IN THE LAST 3 DECADES—cont'd** |

Author(s)	Title	Source/Year	Purpose	Design/Method
PSYCHOSOCIAL CARE NEEDS OF PATIENTS—cont'd				
Cotanch, Hockenberry, & Herman	*Self-Hypnosis as Antietmeic Therapy in Children Receiving Chemotherapy*	*Oncology Nursing Forum, 12,* 1985	To examine the efficacy of the behavioral intervention of relaxation/self-hypnosis as antiemetic therapy in children receiving chemotherapy	Two-group, experimental design (nausea and vomiting was measured by staff nurses; psychophysical scaling was used for children to indicate the severity and intensity of the nausea)
Hockenberry-Eaton, Dilorio, & Kemp	*The Relationship of Illness Longevity and Relapse with Self-perception, Cancer Stressors, Anxiety and Coping Strategies in Children with Cancer*	*Journal of Pediatric Oncology Nursing, 12,* 1995	To investigate the relationship of the longevity of the cancer experience and the presence of a relapse to the child's self-perception, cancer stressors, anxiety, and use of coping strategies	Descriptive, correlational design; instruments used: Harter Self-Perception Profile for Children (HSPPC),[n] the State-Trait Anxiety Inventory for Children (STAIC),[p] the School-agers' Coping Strategies Inventory (SCSI),[r] and the About My Illness Scale (AMIS)[s]
Birenbaum, Stewart, & Phillips	*Health Status of Bereaved Parents*	*Nursing Research, 45,* 1996	To describe parents' health during the terminal illness of their child and during the first year following their child's death from cancer	Longitudinal, repeated measures design; instrument used: Duke-UNC Health Profile (Duke-UNC)[t]
Hinds, Birenbaum, Clarke-Steffen, Quargnenti, Kreissman, Kazak, Meyer, Mulhern, Pratt, & Wilimas	*Coming to Terms: Parents' Response to a First Cancer Recurrence in Their Child*	*Nursing Research, 45,* 1996	To explore, using grounded theory, the process experienced by parents who are dealing with the first recurrence of cancer in their child	Grounded theory method (interview, observations, and medical record review)

[s]Lewis, F. M., & Woods, N. F. (1986). *Final report: Family functioning in chronic illness.* Seattle, WA: University of Washington.
[t]Parkerson, G. R., Gehlback, S. H., Wagner, E. H., et al. (1981). The Duke-UNC Health Profile: An adult health status instrument for primary care. *Medical Care, 19,* 806-828.

Sample	Findings	Funding	Single Site or Multisite
12 children receiving chemotherapy on an inpatient basis and having "troublesome" nausea and vomiting, ages 10-18	In the experimental group, there was significant reduction in nausea and vomiting both in intensity and severity, and a significant increase in oral intake postchemotherapy. There was no change in antiemetic administration between groups. Researchers suggest that chemotherapy-related nausea and vomiting in children can be reduced and oral intake improved with the use of a behavioral intervention.	—	Single
44 pediatric outpatient oncology patients, ages 6.5-13.5; 15 of the patients had experienced a relapse of the disease either on or off therapy	Results indicated that the longevity of the cancer treatment and the presence of a relapse were negatively associated with the child's self-perception. Trait anxiety was positively associated with duration of the cancer experience and with the presence of a relapse. Children who reported lower self-perception and higher trait anxiety levels also reported experiencing more cancer stressors. Researchers suggest these results support the need for interventions designed to increase self-perception, increase feelings of self-worth, and decrease anxiety during the treatment process.	National Institutes of Health (National Research Service Award) Predoctoral Fellowship, and an American Cancer Society Predoctoral Scholarship	Single
80 parents of childhood oncology patients (47 mothers, 33 fathers)	Results indicated that parents' health is not adversely affected by the loss of a child to cancer. Mothers' social health before the child's death is adversely affected. Researchers suggest that parents are able to call upon their own resources to manage a profound ordeal.	Department of Health and Human Services (Grants #RO1 NU00912 and #RO1 NU00912 02S1)	Multi
33 guardians of pediatric oncology patients receiving active treatment for recurrent cancer; included 27 mothers, 1 grandmother, and 5 fathers	Four interactive components emerged: regulating shock, situation monitoring, alternating realizations, and eyeing care-limiting decisions. The overall organizing construct induced from these components was labeled "coming to terms," referring to parents' efforts to overcome shock/despair to make wise decisions about treatment while accepting that outcome is beyond their control.	Milheim Foundation for Cancer Research; Association of Pediatric Oncology Nurses; Cancer Center Support Core Grant (P30 CA21765); American Lebanese Syrian Associated Charities	Multi

Continued

Author(s)	Title	Source/Year	Purpose	Design/Method
PSYCHOSOCIAL CARE NEEDS OF PATIENTS—cont'd				
Hollen & Hobbie	*Decision Making and Risk Behaviors of Cancer-surviving Adolescents and Their Peers*	*Journal of Pediatric Oncology Nursing, 13,* 1996	To compare the quality of decision making of cancer-surviving adolescents and the prevalence of smoking, alcohol consumption, and illicit drug use with their most influential peers; to compare these relationships in a subset of survivors with threat of cognitive deficits caused by late effects of therapy to those without threat	Descriptive, comparative study; instruments used: the Decision Making Quality Scale (DMQS)[i] and the Periodic Assessment of Drug Use Among Youth (PADU)[u]
Neville	*Psychological Distress in Adolescents with Cancer*	*Journal of Pediatric Nursing, 11,* 1996	To investigate psychological distress among middle and late adolescents recently diagnosed with cancer	Exploratory/descriptive; instruments used: the Brief Symptom Inventory (BSI)[c] and the General Severity Index (GSI)[c]
Clarke-Steffen	*Reconstructing Reality: Family Strategies for Managing Childhood Cancer*	*Journal of Pediatric Nursing, 12,* 1997	To describe strategies used by the family in response to childhood cancer and to relate those strategies to two different conceptual frameworks	Longitudinal, prospective, grounded theory (data were collected through semi-structured interview and analyzed using the constant comparative method)
Gilliss, Moore, & Martinson	*Measuring Parental Grief After Childhood Cancer: Potential Use of the SCL-90R*	*Death Studies, 21,* 1997	To determine the applicability of the SCL-90R for assessing parental bereavement	Exploratory factor analysis; instrument used: Symptom Checklist-90-Revised (SCL-90-R)[c]

[u]Barnes, G. M., & Welte, J. W. (1986). Patterns and predictors of alcohol use among 7-12th grade students in New York State. *Journal of Studies on Alcohol, 47,* 53-62.

Sample	Findings	Funding	Single Site or Multisite
52 cancer-surviving adolescents, ages 14-19 and 44 survivors' peers (ages 14-19) served as the comparison group	Results indicated that the majority of teen survivors reported practicing poor-quality decision making for five of the seven criteria. There were no significant differences in decision making between teen survivors and their peers or between survivors with cognitive threat and those without. Peers were significantly more likely to engage in one or more risk behaviors than teen survivors, but comparisons with two normative samples revealed that cigarette smoking and alcohol use of the teen survivors were comparable with the general population. There was no significant difference in risk behaviors between survivors with a history of therapy with cognitive threat and those without. Survivors reporting higher adherence to quality decision criteria were less likely to report exhibiting risk behaviors than those with poorer decision making.	National Cancer Institute (1R29 CA55202)	Multi
60 adolescents diagnosed with cancer within the past 100 days, ages 14-22	No gender differences on the BSI or GSI were found. Scores on the BSI did not differ significantly from the healthy adolescent population. Adolescents with leukemia experienced the greatest psychological distress as compared with the other disease groups.	—	Multi
7 families with children diagnosed with cancer within the past 7-30 days (subjects included 7 mothers, 7 fathers, 6 ill children, 12 siblings)	Results indicated that the core process in which families engaged was reconstructing reality, using strategies of managing the flow of information, reorganizing roles, evaluating and shifting priorities, changing the future orientation, assigning meaning to the illness, and managing the therapeutic regimen. Researcher suggests these strategies fit a family management style of normalization in the population of families with a child with cancer, where the common goal for the family becomes creating a new normal or normalizing their lives.	D.H.H.S., P.H.S., National Center for Nursing Research National Research Service Award No. NR06157; Sigma Theta Tau Beta Psi Chapter Research Award; a Transitions Focal Area, Oregon Health Sciences University Small Grant	Single
97 parents who had children die of cancer 2 years earlier, ages 25-62 years	One predominant factor accounted for 34% of total variance and was labeled the grief factor. Many of the items on this factor reflected a somatic, rather than a behavioral, expression of distress. Four additional weak factors were identified.	Home Care for the Dying Child; National Cancer Institute; St. Paul Foundation; American Cancer Association (Minnesota Division); Home Care Research Fund (University of Minnesota School of Nursing); American Cancer Society California Division (Grant No. 2-210-PR-14)	Single

Continued

TABLE 32-1	TYPE OF STUDIES COMPLETED BY PEDIATRIC ONCOLOGY NURSES IN THE LAST 3 DECADES—cont'd			
Author(s)	**Title**	**Source/Year**	**Purpose**	**Design/Method**
PSYCHOSOCIAL CARE NEEDS OF PATIENTS—cont'd				
Hinds, Oakes, Furman, Foppiano, Olson, Quargnenti, Gattuso, Powell, Srivastava, Jayawardene, Sandlund, & Strong	*Decision Making by Parents and Health-care Professionals When Considering Continued Care for Pediatric Patients With Cancer*	*Oncology Nursing Forum, 24,* 1997	To better define the treatment-related decisions considered most difficult by parents of pediatric patients with cancer and the factors that influenced their final decisions	Retrospective-descriptive design (data were collected by open-ended interview and questionnaire)
Hockenberry-Eaton, Manteuffel, & Bottomley	*Development of Two Instruments Examining Stress and Adjustment in Children With Cancer*	*Journal of Pediatric Oncology Nursing, 14,* 1997	To evaluate the reliability and validity of the Childhood Cancer Stressors Inventory (CCSI) and the Children's Adjustment to Cancer Index (CACI)	Instrument development (item development, face and content validation, internal consistency reliability, and construct validity)
Hollen, Hobbie, & Finley	*Cognitive Late Effect Factors Related to Decision Making and Risk Behaviors of Cancer-surviving Adolescents*	*Cancer Nursing, 20,* 1997	To examine factors related to cognitive late effects of treatment that may be predictors of decision making and risk behaviors for cancer-surviving adolescents	Correlational; instruments used: the Decision Making Quality Scale (DMQS),[i] the Periodic Assessment of Drug Use Among Youth (PADU),[u] the Wechsler Intelligence Scale-Revised (WISC-R),[v] the Wechsler Adult Intelligence Scale-Revised (WAIS-R),[w] medical record review and semistructured interview

[v]Wechsler, D. (1981). *Manual for the Wechsler Intelligence Scale for Children-Revised.* New York: The Psychological Corporation.
[w]Wechsler, D. (1981). *WAIS-R Manual: Wechsler Adult Intelligence Scale-Revised.* New York: Psychological Corporation.

Sample	Findings	Funding	Single Site or Multisite
39 parents whose children died from cancer during the previous 6-24 months; 16 attending physicians, 3 nurses, and 2 chaplains at a pediatric oncology institution	Parents reported 15 types of difficult decisions, usually made late in the course of treatment. The three most frequently reported decisions included: deciding between a phase I drug study or no further treatment, maintaining or withdrawing life support, and giving more chemotherapy or withdrawing treatment. Parents rated "recommendations from health-care professionals" as the most important factor in their decisions, whereas health care professionals rated "discussion with the family" the most important.	Nellcor-AACN Mentorship Grant; a Beta Theta Tau Chapter Research Grant; National Cancer Institute (Grant #P30 CA 21765); the American Lebanese Syrian Associates Charities (ALSAC)	Single
75 patients receiving chemotherapy, ages 7-13	The CCSI consists of stressors that involve the physical, emotional, and psychosocial domains. Results of the reliability testing suggest that the instrument has a high degree of internal consistency for a true-false inventory where the internal coefficient reliability for the total was .82. The CACI concerns the school-age child's interactions with family, school peers, and friends, involvement in school and home activities, successful school performance and attendance, and positive feelings about self. Results indicate the CACI has a high degree of internal consistency for a new scale where the internal coefficient reliability for the total was .91. Hypothesis testing offered initial evidence for construct validity of both instruments.	—	Multi
52 cancer survivors, ages 14-19 without disease for 5 years or treatment for 2 years and never having had brain tumors	Results indicated that therapy type was a marginally significant predictor of quality decision making, where those survivors having a history of therapy threatening cognitive function showed poorer-quality decision making. Only poor-quality decision making was a predictor of one or more risk behaviors. Age at initial treatment and cognitive ability (full-scale IQ) were not significant predictors for either of the models. There were no significant differences for the Wechsler IQ subtests related to abstract and analytic ability by cognitive threat status, although post hoc analyses indicated that the test's lack of sensitivity to change might have affected these outcomes. Researchers suggest that these results support the need for interventions to improve adolescent decision making.	National Cancer Institute (Grant 1R29 CA55202)	Multi

Continued

Author(s)	Title	Source/Year	Purpose	Design/Method
PSYCHOSOCIAL CARE NEEDS OF PATIENTS—cont'd				
Hockenberry-Eaton, Hinds, Alcoser, O'Neill, Euell, Howard, Gattuso, & Taylor	*Fatigue in Children and Adolescents With Cancer*	*Journal of Pediatric Oncology Nursing, 15,* 1998	To define and describe fatigue experienced by children and adolescents receiving treatment for cancer	Focus group approach (data collected by group structured interview and coded independently)
Neville	*The Relationships Among Uncertainty, Social Support, and Psychological Distress in Adolescents Recently Diagnosed with Cancer*	*Journal of Pediatric Oncology Nursing, 15,* 1998	To describe the relationships among perceived social support, uncertainty, and psychological distress in adolescents recently diagnosed with cancer	Exploratory/descriptive; instruments used: the Mishel Uncertainty in Illness Scale (MUIS),[x] the Brief Symptom Inventory (BSI),[c] and the Personal Resource Questionnaire-84-Part-Two (PRQ-85-2)[y]
Hinds, Quargnenti, Fairclough, Bush, Betcher, Rissmiller, Pratt, & Gilchrist	*Hopefulness and Its Characteristics in Adolescents With Cancer*	*Western Journal of Nursing Research, 21,* 1999	To describe the degree and dynamism of hopefulness at four time points during the first 6 months of adolescents' treatment for newly diagnosed cancer; to identify and describe the adolescents' hoped-for objects; to evaluate potential relationships between the characteristics of hopefulness and patient gender, age, diagnosis, and time point in treatment	Longitudinal, experimental, two-group design; instruments used: the Hopefulness Scale for Adolescents (HSA),[z] Hopelessness Scale (HPLS),[aa] the Hopefulness Interview Question (HIQ)[z]
Hollen, Hobbie, & Finley	*Testing the Effects of a Decision-making and Risk-reduction Program for Cancer-surviving Adolescents*	*Oncology Nursing Forum, 26,* 1999	To test the effects of a decision-making and risk-reduction program for adolescent cancer survivors	Prospective clinical trial using a quasiexperimental pretest/posttest design with repeated measures; instruments used: Decision Making Quality Scale (DMQS),[i] the Risk Motivation Questionnaire (RMQ),[bb] and the Periodic Assessment of Drug Use Among Youth (PADU)[u]

[x]Mishel, M. (1981). The measurement of uncertainty in illness. *Nursing Research, 30,* 258-263.
[y]Weinert, C., & Tilden, V. P. (1990). Measures of social support: Assessment of validity. *Nursing Research, 39,* 212-216.
[z]Hinds, P. (1985). *Relationship among caring behaviors of nurses, adolescent hopefulness and adolescent health care outcomes* [unpublished doctoral dissertation] University of Arizona.
[aa]Kazdin, A., French, N., Unis, A., et al. (1983). Hopelessness, depression, and suicidal intent among psychiatrically disturbed inpatient children. *Journal of Consulting and Clinical Psychology, 51,* 504-510.
[bb]Ryan, R. M. (1990). [Risk Motivation Questionnaire]. Unpublished data.

Sample	Findings	Funding	Single Site or Multisite
29 children/adolescents receiving cancer treatment, ages 7-16	In focus groups, children (ages 7-12) produced eight descriptions of fatigue, both physical and mental. Adolescents generated 12 descriptions. Six codes were developed from children's groups and 12 from adolescents' groups describing the causes of fatigue. Three codes from children's groups and eight from adolescents' groups described ways to help fatigue. Researchers suggest that findings from this study will provide the foundation for developing a conceptual model for cancer-related fatigue in children and adolescents.	Oncology Nursing Foundation Grant	Multi
60 adolescents and young adults recently diagnosed with cancer, ages 14-22	Results indicated (1) an inverse relationship between perceived social support and uncertainty, (2) a positive relationship between uncertainty and psychological distress, and (3) an inverse relationship between perceived social support and psychological distress. No relationship between perceived social support and psychological distress was found when controlled for uncertainty. There was an interaction effect involving perceived social support and uncertainty.	—	Multi
78 adolescents with newly diagnosed cancer, ages 12-21	Results indicated that adolescents in this sample reported high hopefulness and low hopelessness relative to previously studied samples in the first 6 months of therapy. This sample also reported moderate to high specificity of the hoped-for objects, which combined with their apparent hopefulness, suggests these patients are focused on short- and immediate-term hopes with positive expectations of attaining the hoped-for objects. Adolescents identified a total of 57 different hopes. Differences by age, gender, and diagnosis were found.	National Cancer Institute (CA-48432); Cancer Center Support Core Grant (P30 CA-21765) from the National Cancer Institute; the American Lebanese Syrian Associated Charities (ALSAC)	Multi
64 adolescent cancer survivors, ages 13-21	The 5-hour intervention program designed to improve decision making and affect substance use in teen survivors showed significant effects for both decision making (at 1, 6, and 12 months postintervention) and alcohol use (at 1 and 6 months postintervention), while showing no effects for smoking behavior. Although these results were promising in regard to the potential to positively influence risk behaviors of adolescent cancer survivors, researchers suggest a larger sample size is needed to enhance the findings.	National Cancer Institute (I R29 CA55202)	Single

Continued

| TABLE 32-1 | TYPE OF STUDIES COMPLETED BY PEDIATRIC ONCOLOGY NURSES IN THE LAST 3 DECADES—cont'd |

Author(s)	Title	Source/Year	Purpose	Design/Method
PSYCHOSOCIAL CARE NEEDS OF PATIENTS—cont'd				
Kazak, Simms, Barakat, Hobbie, Foley, Golomb, & Best	*Surviving Cancer Competently Intervention Program (SCCIP): A Cognitive-Behavioral and Family Therapy Intervention for Adolescent Survivors of Childhood Cancer and their Families*	*Family Process, 38,* 1999	To develop and evaluate an intervention program for adolescent survivors of childhood cancer, their parents, and siblings to reduce symptoms of distress and improve family functioning	Evaluative (pilot study); instruments used: Post-Traumatic Stress Disorder Reaction Index,[cc] Impact of Event Scale (IES),[dd] State-Trait Anxiety Inventory (STAI),[p] Revised Children's Manifest Anxiety Scale (RCMAS),[ee] Family Life Scales (FLS)[ff]
Leavitt, Martinson, Liu, Armstrong, Hornberger, Zhang, & Han	*Common Themes and Ethnic Differences in Family Caregiving the First Year After Diagnosis of Childhood Cancer: Part II*	*Journal of Pediatric Nursing, 14,* 1999	To examine and compare caregiving patterns and practices of Chinese and white families for the first year after diagnosis of childhood cancer	Exploratory, longitudinal (data were collected by semistructured interview)
Neville	*The Impact of Cancer on Adolescent Development*	*European Journal of Oncology Nursing, 3,* 1999	To explore how the experience of cancer affects achievement of adolescent developmental tasks; to identify common themes regarding the impact of cancer on adolescent development	Exploratory (data collected through interviews and analyzed using constant comparison analyses)

[cc]Pynoos, R., Frederick, S., Nader, K., et al. (1987). Life threat and posttraumatic stress in school age children. *Archives of General Psychiatry, 44,* 1057-1063.

[dd]Horowitz, M., Wilner, N., & Alvarez, W. (1979). Impact of Event Scale: A measure of subjective stress. *Psychosomatic Medicine, 41,* 209-218.

[ee]Reynolds, D., & Richmond, B. (1985). *Manual for the Revised Children's Manifest Anxiety Scale.* Los Angeles: Western Psychological Services.

[ff]Fisher, P., Ransom, D. C., & Terry, H. E. (1993). The California Family Health Project: VII. Summary and integration of findings. *Family Process, 32,* 69-86.

Sample	Findings	Funding	Single Site or Multisite
19 families of adolescent patients who completed cancer treatment at least one year previously; subjects included 19 mothers, 13 fathers, 4 siblings; survivors' ages 10-17	Data were supportive of SCCIP's effectiveness and feasibility. Program evaluation data indicated that all family members found SCCIP helpful. Standardized measures showed symptoms of posttraumatic stress and anxiety decreased from pretest to posttest.	University of Pennsylvania Cancer Center; National Cancer Institute (63930)	Single
18 families (10 Chinese, 8 white) with a child with cancer	Results indicated the ill child remained the family priority. All children were physically well cared for, with strict adherence to Western medical protocols. Cultural differences and immigrant status contributed to lower verbal expression of distress, more isolation, and lower attention to emotional distress for the Chinese. Caregiving emphases were dietary for the Chinese and emotional for the whites. Differences over time in family caregiving and coping were determined by demands of care and evolving expertise. Care-inclusive routines were established by most families by the second interview, in spite of extent of continued difficulties. Emotional care demands, concern for needs of siblings, and marital conflict increased over time. At 1 year, all families complained of emotional and physical fatigue and the need to adapt to a tentative future with their child.	Academic Senate Research Grant	Single
7 former oncology patients off treatment for at least 5 years and considered "cured" of cancer, ages 23-30	Results indicate that having cancer in adolescence greatly affects development. Themes identified include catching-up, focused career direction, resilience, self-transcendence, return to preillness interests, and an intense connection with and gratitude for mother or spouse.	Kean University Office of Grants	Single

Continued

TABLE 32-1	TYPE OF STUDIES COMPLETED BY PEDIATRIC ONCOLOGY NURSES IN THE LAST 3 DECADES—cont'd			
Author(s)	**Title**	**Source/Year**	**Purpose**	**Design/Method**
PSYCHOSOCIAL CARE NEEDS OF PATIENTS—cont'd				
Wiley, Ruccione, Moore, McGuire-Cullen, Fergusson, Waskerwitz, Perin, Ge, & Sather	*Parents' Perceptions of Randomization in Pediatric Clinical Trials*	*Cancer Practice, 7,* 1999	To investigate parents' knowledge and perceptions about randomization in clinical trials for children with cancer; to determine whether parents' decisions are influenced by demographic factors, randomization circumstances, the clinical characteristics of the child with cancer, or a combination	Comparative case-control design; data collected through parental completion of the Clinical Investigation Randomization Scale (CIRS)[gg]
Hinds, Quargnenti, Bush, Pratt, Fairclough, Rissmiller, Betcher, & Gilchrist	*An Evaluation of the Impact of a Self-care Coping Intervention on Psychological and Clinical Outcomes in Adolescents with Newly Diagnosed Cancer*	*European Journal of Oncology Nursing, 4,* 2000	To determine the effects of a three-part educational intervention designed to facilitate coping on psychological (hopefulness, hopelessness, self-esteem, self-efficacy and symptom distress) and clinical outcomes (treatment toxicity) among adolescents newly diagnosed with cancer	Longitudinal, experimental, two-group design with random assignment; instruments used: Nowicki-Strickland Locus of Control Scale (NSLC),[hh] Hopefulness Scale for Adolescents (HSA), the Hopelessness Scale (HPLS),[ii] the Rosenberg Self-Esteem Scale (SE),[jj] the Self-Efficacy Scale (SES),[kk] the Symptom Distress Scale (SDS),[ll] and the Toxicity: The NCI Common Toxicity Criteria Scale (CTC)
BIOPHYSICAL PROCESSES				
Meadows & Hobbie	*The Medical Consequences of Cure*	*Cancer, 58,* 1986	To determine the long-term consequences of therapy for a representative group of children treated in the modern era	Data collected from a standardized physical examination of all patients with specific studies ordered based on the child's prior treatment

[gg]Moore, I. M., Wiley, F., Ruccione, K., et al. (1989). Development of an instrument to measure parents' perceptions of randomization. *Oncology Nursing Forum, 15,* 290-294.

[hh]Nowicki, S., & Strickland, B. (1973). A locus of control scale for children. *Journal of Consulting and Clinical Psychology, 40,* 148-154.

[ii]Kazdin, A., Rodgers, A., et al. (1986). The hopelessness scale for children: Psychometric characteristics and concurrent validity. *Journal of Consulting and Clinical Psychology, 54,* 241-245.

[jj]Rosenberg, M. (1979). *Conceiving the Self,* New York: Basic Books.

[kk]Sherer, M., Maddux, J., et al. (1982). The self-efficacy scale: Construction and validation. *Psychological Reports, 51,* 663-671.

[ll]McCorkle, R., & Young, K. (1978). Development of a symptom distress scale. *Cancer Nursing, 1,* 373-378.

Sample	Findings	Funding	Single Site or Multisite
192 parents of childhood cancer patients who either accepted (control) or refused (target) randomization	Parents' beliefs, values, and perceptions, rather than knowledge and information, about randomized clinical trials most accurately predicted acceptors and refusers. The predictor model developed from the data accurately predicted acceptance or refusal of randomization 87% of the time.	Division of Cancer Treatment; National Cancer Institute; National Institutes of Health; Department of Health and Human Services (CA-13539)	Multi
78 adolescents with a newly diagnosed malignancy, ages 12-21	No significant differences were found between the experimental and control groups or between male and female patients at any data point. Results indicate that adolescents began the cancer experience with high levels of hopefulness, self-esteem, and self-efficacy. Researchers suggest that the lack of difference from intervention may be due to insensitivity of measures, an ineffective program, or mistimed intervention.	National Cancer Institute (RO1 CA-48432, P30 CA-21765); American Lebanese Syrian Associated Charities (ALSAC)	Multi
200 former oncology patients previously diagnosed with childhood cancer and not having had treatment for the last 2 years	Results reveal a high proportion of severe sequelae secondary to radiation therapy in early childhood. Results also indicate that second malignant neoplasms may also be related to alkylating agent chemotherapy and to genetic conditions.	DHHA (CA 14489); Commonwealth of Pennsylvania (SPC 789311)	Single

Continued

Author(s)	Title	Source/Year	Purpose	Design/Method
BIOPHYSICAL PROCESSES—cont'd				
Moore, Kramer, & Ablin	*Late Effects of Central Nervous System Prophylactic Leukemia Therapy on Cognitive Functioning*	*Oncology Nursing Forum, 13,* 1986	To determine if CNS prophylactic therapy for ALL has late effects on cognitive functioning; to determine if the child is at greater risk for such sequelae if the treatment is administered during the period of the brain growth spurt	Comparative; data collected from medical record review, cognitive evaluation (assessing general intellectual potential, academic achievement, and visuomotor skills), and parent/teacher survey. Instruments included Wechsler Intelligence Scale for Children-Revised (WISC-R),[v] the Wide Range Achievement Test (WRAT),[mm] the Berry Test of Visuomotor Integration,[mm] and the Deasy-Spinetta Behavioral Questionnaire (DSBQ).[b]
Kramer, Norman, Brant-Zawadzki, Ablin, & Moore	*Absence of White Matter Changes on Magnetic Resonance Imaging in Children Treated with CNS Prophylaxis Therapy for Leukemia*	*Cancer, 61,* 1988	To investigate white matter damage in asymptomatic ALL patients using MRI; to evaluate the relationship between MRI findings and neuropsychological functioning measures	Data collected from magnetic resonance exams. Instrument used: Wechsler Intelligence Scale for Children-Revised (WISC-R)[v]
Hockenberry, Schultz, Bennett, Bryant, & Falletta	*Experience with Minimal Complications in Implanted Catheters in Children*	*The American Journal of Pediatric Hematology/ Oncology, 11,* 1989	To examine the efficacy of implanted catheters as a vascular access system in children/young adult hematology/oncology patients	Retrospective, exploratory (data collected included clinical assessments of bacteremia, inflammation, breakdown of the skin, occlusions, and needle dislodgement)
Moore, Kramer, Wara, Halberg, & Ablin	*Cognitive Function in Children with Leukemia: Effect of Radiation Dose and Time Since Irradiation*	*Cancer, 68,* 1991	To examine the effect of two cranial radiation doses and the time since radiation therapy on cognitive functioning	Patients were grouped according to cranial radiation dose and evaluated for general intelligence, academic achievement, and visual motor integration.

[mm]Lezak, M. D. (1983). *Neuropsychological Assessment.* New York: Oxford University Press.

Sample	Findings	Funding	Single Site or Multisite
31 long-term survivors of childhood cancer	Results indicate that CNS prophylaxis has a significant adverse effect on subsequent cognitive functioning in terms of general intelligence, academic achievement, school performance, and visuomotor skills. Also, children treated before 60 months (during the vulnerable period of brain development) performed worse than those who received the same therapy after this age.	National Research Service Award (NU 05625-03), funded under the division of nursing; California Division of the American Cancer Society, Graduate Nursing Research Grant; Patent Funds from the Graduate Division of the University of California, San Francisco; Century Club Funds from the School of Nursing, University of California, San Francisco; Computer Center, University of California, San Francisco	Single
10 former childhood ALL cancer patients currently in remission, ages 7-17	MRI exams were normal for nine of the ten children, and scans indicated white matter tracts normal in appearance for all ten subjects. Seven of the nine children with normal MR scans had IQ scores falling below the average range indicating below average intellectual functioning. These results suggest that children who received cranial radiation do not show white matter changes on MRI, despite evidence of cognitive impairment.	Radiology Research and Education Foundation	Single
82 patients needing long-term venous access for treatment of cancer or chronic hematologic disorder, ages 11 months to 24 years	The mean duration of catheter function was 168 days. Researchers reported complications as minimal with only four catheters requiring removal secondary to infection, infiltration, or tissue breakdown. Researchers report substantially reduced complication rates as compared to other studies using implanted central venous catheters. Researchers suggest that implanted central venous catheters were shown to be safe in patients with hematologic disorders.	—	Single
35 children having received treatment for ALL including radiation; 20 received radiation at 24 Gy and 15 received radiation at 18 Gy	Results indicated that patients scored significantly lower on verbal intelligence quotient, achievement tests of reading, spelling, and arithmetic as time since radiation therapy increased. The effect of cranial radiation dose was not found to be significant on those measures. The effect of dose and time on visual motor integration and performance intelligence quotient was not significant although both groups fell below the 33rd percentile. Researchers suggest that a larger study is needed to confirm the findings.	Affirmative Faculty Development Award, University of California at San Francisco; National Institutes of Health grant (MO1 RR01271) to the Pediatric Clinical Research Center, University of California at San Francisco	Single

Continued

Author(s)	Title	Source/Year	Purpose	Design/Method
BIOPHYSICAL PROCESSES—cont'd				
West, Oakes, Hinds, Sanders, Holden, Williams, Fairclough, & Bozeman	*Measuring Pain in Pediatric Oncology ICU Patients*	*Journal of Pediatric Oncology Nursing, 11,* 1994	To identify a clinically feasible and accurate method of measuring pain intensity in pediatric oncology patients in an ICU	Instrumentation study using a descriptive correlational design; instruments used: the Faces Pain Scale (FPS),[nn] the Poker Chip Tool (PCT),[oo] and the Objective Pain Scale (OPS)[pp]
Mollova, Moore, Hutter, & Schram	*Fast Atom Bombardment Mass Spectrometry of Phospholipids in Human Cerebrospinal Fluid*	*Journal of Mass Spectrometry, 30,* 1995	To describe the application of fast atom bombardment mass spectrometry (FABMS) and four sector machine tandem FABMS/MS in the analysis of phospholipids in human CSF; to determine if changes detected by FABMS of the CSF phospholipid composition following cancer treatment are markers of CNS cell damage	Lipid extracts of CSF collected from children with leukemia before and after treatment with chemotherapy and/or radiation were separated on normal-phase high-performance liquid chromatography and analyzed by FABMS and tandem FABMS/MS.
Hinds, Hockenberry-Eaton, Quargnenti, May, Burleson, Gilger, Randall, & Brace-O'Neill	*Fatigue in 7- to 12-year-old Patients with Cancer from the Staff Perspective: An Exploratory Study*	*Oncology Nursing Forum, 26,* 1999	To document and analyze the perspectives of staff members who provide direct care to pediatric cancer patients regarding the nature and characteristics of fatigue, causes and alleviators of fatigue for this population (ages 7-12)	Exploratory; responses to open-ended questions analyzed using content analysis techniques and a modified Wilson concept analysis technique[qq]

[nn]Robertson, J. (1993). Pediatric pain assessment: Validation of a multidimensional tool. *Pediatric Nursing, 19,* 209-213.

[oo]Hester, N. O., Foster R., & Kristensen, K. (1990). Measurement of pain in children: Generalizability and validity of the pain ladder. In D. C. Tyler, E. J. Krane (Eds.), *Advances in pain research and therapy, vol. 15* (pp. 79-84). New York: Raven.

[pp]Hanallah, R., Broadman, L., & Belman, A. (1987). Comparison of caudal and ilioinguinal/iliohypogastric nerve blocks for control of post-orchiopexy pain in pediatric ambulatory surgery. *Anesthesiology, 66,* 832-834.

[qq]Avant, K., & Abbott, D. (1993). *Wilsonian concept analysis: Applying the technique.* In B. Rogers & K. Knafl (Eds.), *Concept development in nursing: Foundations, techniques, and applications* (pp. 61-72). Philadelphia: W. B. Saunders.

Sample	Findings	Funding	Single Site or Multisite
30 pediatric oncology patients in the ICU (ages 5-13), their parents (28 mothers, 2 fathers), and 13 pediatric oncology nurses	Results indicated high intrarater reliability on the FPS and the PCT tools for both patients and parents suggesting a consistency in pain ratings. Patients' ratings on the FPS correlated significantly with the parents' ratings, but not on the PCT. Similarly, nurses' ratings on the OPS were moderately correlated with patients' FPS ratings, but were only weakly associated with PCT ratings. These results suggest that patients, parents, and nurses rate pain intensity differently. Patients, parents, and nurses preferred FPS to the PCT. Although limited only to those who can participate in self-report, the FPS appears to be a clinically useful and accurate approach for measuring the pain associated with childhood cancer in the ICU.	Cancer Center Support CORE Grant; the American Lebanese Syrian Associated Charities (ALSAC)	Single
13 children with ALL receiving chemo-therapy and/or radia-tion treatment	Results demonstrate the ability of the method to identify changes in the CSF phospholipid com-position resulting from the cancer treatment. Changes in the CSF phospholipid composition during treatment with chemotherapy included the presence of diacylglycerol (DAG) and lyso-phosphatidylcholine (LPC) molecular species and an increase in sphingomyelin (SM) relative to phosphatidylcholine. Also a predominance of the C18:1 SM was observed during radiation treatment. Researchers suggest that the pres-ence of DAGs and LPCs may be markers of CNS cell damage where changes in CSF SM may be associated with treatment-related damage to the white matter. Researchers con-clude that FABMS and FABMS/MS may be useful for direct analysis of total CSF lipid extracts in cancer patients.	National Institute of Nursing Research (NR0255705, NR0339902); Arizona Disease Control Commission; NIH shared Instru-mentation Program	Single
38 staff members in pediatric oncology including 8 advanced practice nurses, 23 staff nurses, 2 nurse managers, 3 nutrition-ists, 1 chaplain, 1 physician	Researchers determined that fatigue is a state of diminished to complete loss of energy or will that is influenced by environmental, biochemi-cal, personal, cultural, and treatment-related factors. This state, which may be acute, episodic, or chronic, can be accompanied by a changing emotional or mental state.	Completed as part of the Fatigue Clinical Scholar Program; Also supported by grants from the On-cology Nursing Foun-dation's Fatigue Initiative Through Research and Educa-tion, the Cancer Center Support CORE Grant (P30 CA2175), and the American Lebanese Syrian Associated Charities (ALSAC)	Multi

Continued

Author(s)	Title	Source/Year	Purpose	Design/Method
BIOPHYSICAL PROCESSES—cont'd				
Hockenberry-Eaton, Hinds, Brace-O'Neill, Alcoser, Bottomley, Kline, Euell, Howard, & Gattuso	*Developing a Conceptual Model for Fatigue in Children*	*European Journal of Oncology Nursing, 3*, 1999	To define fatigue experienced by children with cancer; to begin development of a conceptual model for fatigue in children	Content analysis of transcripts focus group yielded codes and definitions; concept analysis of codes and definitions resulted in basis of conceptual framework
NURSING CARE PROCEDURES				
Hinds, Wentz, Hughes, Pearson, Sims, Mason, Pratt, & Austin	*An Investigation of the Safety of the Blood Reinfusion Step Used With Tunneled Venous Access Devices in Children With Cancer*	*Journal of Pediatric Oncology Nursing, 8*, 1991	To determine if the usual clean nursing procedure used with the reinfusion step, compared with an exaggerated unclean alternate procedure, could contribute to new microbial pathogens being acquired during the interval between removal and reinfusion of the blood sample	Experimental, two-group design (blood samples were analyzed for the presence and type of organisms and the number of colony-forming units)
Oakes, Hinds, RAO, Bozeman, Taylor, Stokes, & Fairclough	*Chest Tube Stripping in Pediatric Oncology Patients: An Experimental Study*	*American Journal of Critical Care, 2*, 1993	To determine whether pediatric oncology patients whose chest tubes were not stripped would differ in frequency of pain, fever, or lung complications from patients who underwent routine tube stripping	Experimental, two-group design (clinical assessments were made by thermometer, stethoscope, and radiograph; pain was measured by the Faces Pain Scale[rr] and the Visual Analogue Scale)[ss]
Norville, Hinds, Wilimas, Fairclough, Kunkel, & Fischl	*The Effects of Infusion Methods on Platelet Count, Morphology, and Corrected Count Increment in Children with Cancer: In Vitro and In Vivo Studies*	*Oncology Nursing Forum, 21*, 1994	To determine whether infusion method influences the quality of platelets transfused	Linked in vitro and in vivo study; quasi-experimental design for in vitro and cross-over design with balanced randomization for in vivo
Norville, Hinds, Wilimas, Fischl, Fairclough, & Kunkel	*The Effects of Infusion Rate on Platelet Outcomes and Patient Responses in Children with Cancer: An In Vitro and In Vivo Study*	*Oncology Nursing Forum, 24*, 1997	To determine the influence of infusion rate on quality of transfused platelets and patients' physical and subjective responses	Linked in vitro and in vivo studies with repeated measures and crossover designs, respectively

[rr]Wong, D. L., & Baker, C. M. (1988). Pain in children: Comparison of assessment scales. *Pediatric Nursing, 14*, 9-17.
[ss]Abu-Saad, H., & Holzemer, W. L. Measuring children's self-assessment of pain. *Issues in Comprehensive Pediatric Nursing, 5*, 327-335.

Sample	Findings	Funding	Single Site or Multisite
14 pediatric cancer patients, ages 7-12	Analysis yielded eight codes defining fatigue, seven codes describing causes of fatigue, and three codes describing alleviating factors of fatigue. Data yielded a conceptual definition of fatigue. These findings led to the development of a conceptual model to demonstrate the relationship between fatigue and contributing and alleviating factors.	Oncology Nursing Foundation's Fatigue Initiative Through Research and Education	Multi
42 pediatric oncology patients with single-lumen Hickman catheters, ages 2-20	Analysis did not detect microbial organisms in any of the samples from either group. Researchers suggest these results indicate that the current institutional policy, requiring a reinfusion step, does not appear to create the conditions for infection.	—	Single
16 pediatric oncology patients receiving postoperative care in the ICU following thoracotomy, ages 3-21	Results indicated that the two groups did not differ significantly in frequency of pain, incidence of fever, breath sounds, or radiographic findings across measurement points. A strong correlation was found between pain scores from both instruments. Patients whose tubes were not stripped did not have an increased risk of infection or lung complications. Stripping did not increase reports of pain. Researchers suggest that because routine stripping did not show advantageous or deleterious effects, its need in clinical practice should be questioned in the absence of clots or drainage problems.	—	Single
26 pediatric cancer patients, ages 2-19	No significant differences noted in platelet count or morphology score among or across the three infusion methods in vitro. No significant differences noted between the two infusion methods in platelet count or corrected count increment in vivo.	IMED Corporation; Cancer Center Support CORE Grant P30 CA21765; American Lebanese Syrian Associated Charities (ALSAC)	Single
26 pediatric cancer patients, ages 3-20	No significant differences found with rate and outcome; concludes that faster infusion rate is appropriate, which cuts infusion time by half	IMED Corporation; Cancer Center Support CORE Grant P30 CA21765; American Lebanese Syrian Associated Charities (ALSAC)	Single

Continued

TABLE 32-1	TYPE OF STUDIES COMPLETED BY PEDIATRIC ONCOLOGY NURSES IN THE LAST 3 DECADES—cont'd				

Author(s)	Title	Source/Year	Purpose	Design/Method
PROFESSIONAL ISSUES FOR PEDIATRIC ONCOLOGY NURSES				
Hinds, Fairclough, Dobos, Greer, Herring, Mayhall, Arheart, Day, & McAulay	*Development and Testing of the Stressor Scale for Pediatric Oncology Nurses*	*Cancer Nursing, 13,* 1990	To develop and test an instrument that could accurately and sensitively measure the job-related stressors for pediatric oncology nurses	Instrument development (inductive development of scale from interviews of 30 pediatric oncology nurses)
Hinds, Sanders, Srivastava, Hickey, Jayawardene, Milligan, Olson, Puckett, Quargnetnti, Randall, & Tyc	*Testing the Stress-response Sequence Model in Paediatric Oncology Nursing*	*Journal of Advanced Nursing, 28,* 1998	To test the complete stress-response sequence model in a sample of pediatric oncology nurses by obtaining concurrent measures of the model's individual components: nurses' stressors, reactions, mediators, and consequences	Descriptive survey design; nurses completed six questionnaires; qualitative data were analyzed using a semantic content analysis technique
Hinds, Puckett, Donohoe, Milligan, Payne, Phipps, Davis, & Martin	*The Impact of a Grief Workshop for Pediatric Oncology Nurses on Their Grief and Perceived Stress*	*Journal of Pediatric Nursing, 9,* 1994	To determine the impact of a grief workshop on grief symptoms and perceived stress in two groups of pediatric oncology nurses who differ in years of experience in the specialty	Repeated measures; instruments used included Grief Experience Inventory (GEI),[tt] the Miller Behavior Style Scale (MBSS),[uu] and the Perceived Stress Scale (PSS)[vv]
CARE DELIVERY SYSTEMS				
Martinson, Armstrong, Geis, Anglim, Gronseth, Macinnis, Nesbit, & Kersey	*Facilitating Home Care for Children Dying of Cancer*	*Cancer Nursing,* Feb., 1978	To evaluate home care as an alternative for terminal childhood cancer patients	Descriptive (data were collected by chart review, interview of nurses and parents, and review of nurses' case notes)

[tt]Sanders, C., Mauger, P., & Strong, P. (1985). *A manual for the grief experience inventory.* Palo Alto, CA: Consulting Psychologists Press.
[uu]Miller, S., & Mangam, C. (1983). Interacting effects of information and coping style in adapting to gynecologic stress: Should the doctor tell all? *Journal of Personality and Social Psychology, 45,* 223-236.
[vv]Cohen, S., Kamarck, T., & Mermelstein, R. (1983). A global measure of perceived stress. *Journal of Health and Social Behavior, 24,* 385-396.

Sample	Findings	Funding	Single Site or Multisite
78 pediatric oncology nurses (length of practice from 6 months to 17 years)	Based on assessments of reliability, test-retest correlation, content validity, and construct validity, researchers suggest the Stressor Scale for Pediatric Oncology Nurses (SSPON) has adequate psychometric properties for a new instrument. The test-retest correlation coefficient for the total scale was 0.88, and the total scale α coefficient was 0.94.	American Cancer Society Grant IN-176; Department of Nursing at St. Jude Children's Research Hospital	Multi
126 pediatric oncology nurses; all female, ages 20+ (largest age group 30-39 years)	An important explanatory variable of the stress-response sequence model, role-related meaning, is missing in the model. The impact of stressors is somewhat mediated when a nurse finds her role in pediatric oncology fulfilling and meaningful.	Tennessee Nurses' Foundation grant; Cancer Center Support CORE Grant (P30 CA 21765); American Lebanese Syrian Associated Charities (ALSAC)	Single
27 nurses with 2-5 years of pediatric oncology experience and 22 nurses with 6 months to 2 years of experience	Results indicated that pediatric oncology nurses experience bereavement. Findings also indicate that one workshop intervention does not significantly lessen the nurses' grief symptoms of perceived stress. Researchers suggest that a carefully planned sequence of interventions may be needed.	Cancer Center Support CORE Grant (P30CA21765); American Lebanese Syrian Associated Charities (ALSAC)	Single
32 families with a child receiving home care for cancer in the terminal stages	Over 1 year, all children died, 27 at home and 5 after readmission to the hospital. Parents were principal providers of the child's care at home with a primary nurse coordinating home care and a backup nurse on call 24 hours a day. Pain care was a primary factor in successful home care. Nurse contact with the families included emotional support and reassurance. Researchers report home care recipients expenses were much less than those of a control group in the hospital for terminal care.	National Cancer Institute Grant CA 19490; Department of Health, Education, and Welfare	Multi

Continued

Author(s)	Title	Source/Year	Purpose	Design/Method
CARE DELIVERY SYSTEMS—cont'd				
Martinson, Moldow, Armstrong, Henry, Nesbit, & Kersey	*Home Care for Children Dying of Cancer*	*Research in Nursing and Health, 9,* 1986	To assess the feasibility of home care as an alternative to hospitalization for children dying of cancer including (1) the ability of the family to provide good sick care at home and to keep the child until death, (2) the willingness of the family to provide such care, (3) the degree of nurse and physician involvement in such care, and (4) the nurse and family abilities to procure adequate medication, medical equipment, and supplies	Observational/descriptive data were collected from children's medical records, records completed by home care nurses, questionnaires addressing standard demographic and personal characteristics, grief support lists, care ratings, and progress recordings by the project nurse coordinators
Jost & Haase	*At the Time of Death: Help for the Child's Parents*	*Child Health Care, 18,* 1989	To determine actions by health care personnel perceived as helpful and unhelpful to parents at the time of their child's death	Descriptive/qualitative (data were collected by semistructured interview and classified according to existing or emerging themes)
Birenbaum & Clarke-Steffen	*Terminal Care Costs in Childhood Cancer*	*Pediatric Nursing, 18,* 1992	To present a conceptualization of health care costs, to describe costs of health care in the terminal phase of childhood cancer, to present an exploratory comparison of the costs of terminal care in the hospital versus home care services, and to discuss the use of cost research in nursing practice	Retrospective within the context of a prospective longitudinal study (data were collected by phone interview and billing and insurance records)
Chen, Martinson, Chao, Lai, & Gau	*A Comparative Study of Health Care for Children with Cancer in 1981 and 1991 in Taiwan*	*Pediatric Nursing, 20,* 1994	To evaluate and compare the health care for children with cancer in 1981 and 1991 in Taiwan	Comparative (data were collected by semistructured interview)

Sample	Findings	Funding	Single Site or Multisite
58 families experiencing the death of a child from childhood cancer	Results indicated that home care was a feasible alternative for a wide range of children who had a variety of special needs and was satisfactory for families of diverse backgrounds. Results showed that physicians will refer patients, that children and parents will agree to participate, that home care nurses can be recruited, and that they can secure the necessary equipment, supplies, and medications.	DHEW, National Cancer Institute (Grant CA 19490)	Single
14 parents (ages 23-44) whose child had died of cancer 6 months to 3 years previously	Researchers suggest that the qualitative analysis shows the importance of the actions of health care personnel on the grieving process of bereaved parents. The classifying themes included: informing of the death, viewing the body, consent for autopsy, siblings, effects of health care personnel on the grieving process, supportive persons, chaplains, parents' states of mind at the time of death, attitudes of health care personnel, and closure.	—	Single
18 families who had a child die from childhood cancer	Results indicated that home care was less expensive for total costs than hospital care. Home care was more expensive for nonhealth care and indirect costs than hospital care. Researchers suggest that nurses, when advising on terminal care decisions, consider direct, nondirect, and indirect costs as related to home or hospital care.	Health and Human Services, Division of Nursing (5 RO1 NU00912 and 5 RO1 NU00912-0251)	Multi
75 children with cancer in 1981 and 121 children in 1991; children were divided into 5 groups: newly diagnosed, treated for 1-3 years, relapsed during treatment, received treatment and died within 1-1.5 years, discontinued treatment and remained healthy for more than 2 years	Results indicated that medical care improved over time: the length of time between symptom and diagnosis was shorter, the number of clinic visits before diagnosis decreased, and the length of time for hospitalization was much shorter with most children receiving their health care in the hospital near their home town. Also, pain control at the terminal stage showed improvement in 1991 with 70% of mothers stating that their child's pain had received appropriate care. Finally, the role and function of the physician and the nurse were more recognized by parents in 1991.	CAPCO Cultural and Educational Foundation of Taiwan	Multi

Foundation, Sigma Theta Tau International, and other general and specialty nursing organizations. The diversity of funding sources indicates the appeal of the research proposed by nurse researchers. The recent position taken at the federal level encouraging inclusion of children in research will likely increase the number of opportunities for children to be study participants and create an increased responsibility for nurses to ensure that the study designs and methods are appropriate for children and adolescents with cancer. As such, funding support for pediatric oncology nursing research could increase at the federal level.

CHALLENGES TO CONDUCTING NURSING RESEARCH IN PEDIATRIC ONCOLOGY

One challenge is access to adequate numbers of study participants to successfully achieve study aims. This challenge necessitates conducting multisite studies for certain kinds of research. Completing multisite studies requires particular coordination and administrative skills beyond typical research knowledge and abilities. Because these skills are not a routine part of a doctoral curriculum, current nurse researchers in pediatric oncology who have had the experience of coordinating multisite studies need to provide opportunities for other researchers to prepare for these demands.

The majority of children and adolescents who are receiving treatment for cancer are enrolled on a research protocol. Because of this, a nurse-initiated study needs to be carefully coordinated with the frontline therapeutic research protocol such that the nursing intervention does not create the possibility of influencing the therapeutic endpoints of the frontline protocol without being able to account for that influence. In addition, careful coordination of research could also lessen potential burdens related to participating in research for patients and their families and for the health care providers.

Given the intensity of treatment that children and adolescents experience for their cancer, nurses need to identify which patient care outcomes are most sensitive to nursing care and then study those in a consistent manner across studies. Adopting a conceptual framework that clarifies the outcomes and their relationship to nursing will be useful in guiding nursing research in pediatric oncology and in explaining this research to others. An example of such a framework is offered in Figure 32-2. This framework, the Environmental Care model, has guided nursing research at St. Jude Children's Research Hospital for the past 15 years[4] and was influenced by the work of Last and van Veldhuizen[16] and Rait and Holland.[18] In that model, three levels of environment interact to directly influence the quality of nursing care that can be given and the quality of the resulting care outcomes for patients and their families. It is also possible to consider di-

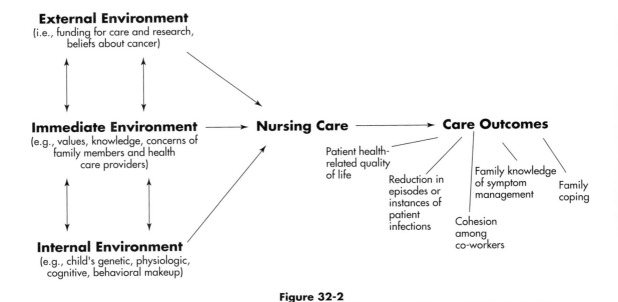

Figure 32-2

Example of a model that has been used to guide clinical nursing research at one pediatric cancer care setting.

rect and indirect influences on co-workers or the actual work environment as a care outcome. Examples of care outcomes are noted in Figure 32-2.

As with other nursing specialties, an ongoing challenge is to promote depth in our practice knowledge base. This is more difficult to do when single studies on a topic are completed rather than a series of related studies. Collaborative efforts may contribute to more study clusters because a team approach could be a more efficient use of limited resources (including the small number of patients diagnosed with cancer annually) and a way of distributing the responsibilities of initiating and conducting studies and disseminating study findings. The team may thus have the energy and momentum to conduct more than a single study.

A considerable number of nurses in pediatric oncology who are clinical experts in an aspect of care for pediatric oncology patients are prepared at the graduate level and thus have taken one or more advanced classes on research. Facilitating their involvement in research needs to be a priority of doctorally prepared nurse researchers and researchers from other disciplines.

A nursing research program that carefully incorporates the clinical research interests of advanced practice nurses is fully operational at the Texas Children's Cancer Center in Houston. Three research strands are included in the figure depicting the clinical research interest (Figure 32-3) and include symptom management, survivorship, and education. Symptom management reflects the belief that nurses who directly care for children with cancer can discover, design, and evaluate interventions designed to ameliorate untoward symptoms associated with cancer treatment. Symptom management research studies within this research strand include evaluation of fatigue, sleep, anemia, and the effects of dexamethasone during treatment for leukemia. Studies within the survivorship strand reflect the increasing number of children cured of cancer and include cancer survivors' concerns regarding the annual clinic visit, and body image and sexuality issues of bone marrow transplantation survivors. A third study evaluates the long-term effects of CNS treatment for leukemia. The education strand reflects the major role of nursing in providing education to patients, parents, and health care professionals. Two current projects designed to provide Web-based learning opportunities for health care professionals include pain management and end-of-life care for children with cancer.

At the same time, a greater commitment needs to also be made to foster the research involvement and interests of staff nurses who continually provide direct care to patients and their families. This kind of commitment can be demonstrated through research fellowship programs[9] and the instructional sessions offered annually at the Association of Pediatric Oncology Nurses Conference.

RECOMMENDATIONS FOR FUTURE NURSING RESEARCH

The efforts to develop evidence-based practice in pediatric oncology must continue and increase. The breadth of research interests needs to be respected and the conduct of series of related studies more actively encouraged. Purposeful, ongoing efforts to strengthen the joint involvement in all aspects of research by staff nurses, advanced practice nurses, and nurse researchers must be a priority for this specialty to create evidence-based practice. A second major focus needs to be on designing and maintaining research-focused collaborations with other disciplines in and beyond pediatric oncology. This focus will greatly facilitate the development and scientific credibility of nurse-initiated protocols or nurse-initiated study objectives for inclusion in the therapeutic protocols developed by oth-

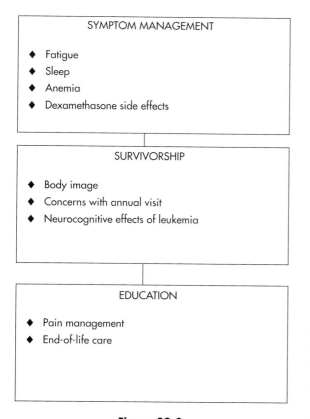

Figure 32-3

Texas Children's Cancer Center nursing research strands.

ers. More studies on nursing care procedures and their outcomes, and on nursing care delivery systems in pediatric oncology and professional issues that influence patient care also require more attention and financial support. Finally, the possibility of creating a national pediatric oncology nursing research program in alliance with the new cooperative group in pediatric oncology merits serious exploration.

ACKNOWLEDGMENTS

The authors express sincere appreciation to Flo Witte, Scientific Editor, for her careful review and to Linda Watts-Parker for her amazing abilities to format the contents of this chapter.

REFERENCES

1. Dodd, M., & Miakowski, C. (2000). The PRO-SELF Program: A self-care intervention program for patients receiving cancer treatment. *Seminars in Oncology Nursing, 16,* 300-308.
2. Fochtman, D., & Hinds, P. S. (2000). Identifying nursing research priorities in a pediatric clinical trials cooperative group: The Pediatric Oncology Group experience. *Journal of Pediatric Oncology Nursing, 17,* 83-87.
3. Heiney, S. P., & Wiley, F. M. (1996). Historical beginnings of a professional nursing organization dedicated to the care of children and adolescents with cancer and their families: The Association of Pediatric Oncology Nursing from 1974 to 1993. *Journal of Pediatric Oncology Nursing, 13,* 196-203.
4. Hinds, P. S. (1990). Quality of life in children and adolescents with cancer. *Seminars in Oncology Nursing, 6,* 285-291.
5. Hinds, P. S. (1994). Research in pediatric oncology nursing in the 1990's. *Canadian Oncology Nursing Journal, (4* Suppl.), 92-98.
6. Hinds, P. S. (2000). Facilitating hopefulness and coping in adolescents newly diagnosed with cancer. *Seminars in Oncology Nursing, 16,* 317-327.
7. Hinds, P. S. (2000). Testing the stress-response sequence in pediatric oncology nursing. *Journal of Pediatric Oncology Nursing, 17,* 59-69.
8. Hinds, P. S., & DeSwarte-Wallace, J. (2000). Positioning nursing research to contribute to the scientific mission of the Pediatric Oncology Cooperative Group. *Seminars in Oncology Nursing, 16,* 251-252.
9. Hinds, P. S., Gattuso, J. S., & Morrell, A. (2000). Creating a hospital-based nursing research fellowship program for staff nurses. *Journal of Nursing Administration, 30,* 317-324.
10. Hinds, P. S., Gattuso, J. S., Norville, R., et al. (1992). Bedside nursing research: A new category of research? *Clinical Nursing Research, 1,* 169-179.
11. Hinds, P. S., & Hockenberry-Eaton, M. (2001). Developing a research program on fatigue in children and adolescents with cancer. *Journal of Pediatric Oncology Nursing, 18*(2 Suppl 1), 3-12.
12. Hinds, P. S., Norville, R., Anthony, L. K., et al. (1990). Establishing pediatric cancer nursing research priorities: A Delphi study. *Journal of Pediatric Oncology Nursing, 7,* 101-108.
13. Hinds, P. S., Quargnenti, A., Olson, M. S., et al. (1994). The 1992 APON Delphi study to establish research priorities for pediatric oncology nursing. *Journal of Pediatric Oncology Nursing, 11,* 20-27.
14. Hockenberry-Eaton, M., & Hinds, P. (2000). Fatigue in children and adolescents: Evolution of a program of study. *Seminars in Oncology Nursing, 16,* 261-271.
15. Hockenberry-Eaton, M., Barrera, P., & Kline, N. E. (1998). Evidence-based practice: A role for nurse practitioners. *Journal of Pediatric Health Care, 12,* 338-339.
16. Last, B., & van Beldhuizen, A. (1987). Psychosocial research in childhood cancer. In N. Aaronson, & J. H. Beckmann (Eds.), *The quality of life of cancer patients* (pp. 127-134). New York: Raven.
17. Moore, I. M., Espy, K., Kaufmann, P., et al. (2000). A research program investigating cognitive consequences of treatment for childhood ALL: Cell membrane damage and intellectual and academic abilities in children receiving central nervous system treatment. *Seminars in Oncology Nursing, 16,* 279-290.
18. Rait, D., & Holland, J. (1986). Pediatric cancer: Psychosocial issues and approaches. *Mediguide to Oncology, 6,* 1-5.
19. Rosswurm, M. A., & Larrabee, J. H. (1999). A model for change to evidence-based practice. *Image—The Journal of Nursing Scholarship, 31,* 317-322.
20. Stotts, N. A. (1999). Evidence-based practice: What is it and how is it used in wound care? *Nursing Clinics of North America, 34,* vii-viii, 955-963.

33

Ethical Issues

Kathy Forte

Pediatric oncology nurses are often faced with ethical dilemmas. Technologic advances and scarce resources in health care have created an environment in which ethical issues frequently arise. The pediatric oncology nurse is in a position to advocate for patient rights and to identify and help resolve ethical conflicts. This chapter defines the basic principles of ethics and describes a tool for nurses to use when analyzing an ethical dilemma.

> *The teaching of ethics is not the process of giving "correct" answers. However, neither is it allowing everyone's opinions to stand unchallenged. It is the teaching of the process by which we test what we do against the reasons we do it and against the standards of society.*[10]

WHAT IS ETHICS?

Ethics is the study of the morals of a community. Ethics is not what an individual thinks is right or wrong, but rather what society deems as acceptable. In fact, the word *ethics* comes from the Greek word "ethos," which means spirit or values of a community. Clinical ethics can be described as a practical problem-solving discipline that provides a structured approach to decision making that can assist health care providers to identify, analyze, and resolve ethical issues.[15] What makes an issue an ethical issue, as opposed to a legal or social issue? If agreement about the facts alone does not resolve the conflict, then there may be a conflict in values. In general, values cannot be dismissed as inconsequential or debated as right or wrong. Individuals may have strong convictions based on an ethical principle that may conflict with the patient, members of the family, or the health care team. The overall goal in resolving a conflict is not to convince others that they are wrong, but rather to objectively communicate all the known facts of the case and the desires of the individuals involved, so that a compromise can be reached.

ETHICAL PRINCIPLES

Ethical principles are accepted as "rights" or "rules" that are generally used to direct conduct.[4] These principles help to outline rights that may be in conflict. They lay the groundwork for discussion, but do not in and of themselves lead to a resolution of a conflict. It is important to understand the principles that are described below to delineate which rule or right is being weighed as more or less important when trying to resolve an ethical dilemma.

Autonomy acknowledges one's right to "self-rule." Inherent in this principle is that each person has the right to self-determination, privacy, and confidentiality. These rights do not vary in the face of what may be perceived as social, cultural, or physical handicaps or differences. In the case of a minor, the parent or guardian is given the legal right to serve as the surrogate decision-maker. In this role the parent or guardian is given the authority to protect the autonomous interests of the child.

Beneficence evokes the duty to do what is most beneficial for the patient. It is often referred to as the "best interest" principle. It implies the obligation not just to treat persons with respect but to also contribute to their well-being.

Nonmaleficence asserts the obligation to do minimal or no harm to a patient. In the pediatric oncology setting this includes not only refraining from inflicting unnecessary pain, but also avoiding treatment that carries risks that outweigh the benefits. For example, proposing an intervention that could decrease a person's quality of life without a substantial benefit that meets the patient's goals is not in keeping with the principle of nonmaleficence.

Justice is the duty to give all persons fair and equal treatment. For the individual, this means that the same treatment or standard of care is given to everyone, regardless of age, race, financial status, and physical or cognitive abilities. In contrast, it could mean that allocation of resources should be fair and equal and the needs of one individual may or may not take precedence over the greater good of the community.

Veracity is the duty to tell the truth. Telling the truth means giving full disclosure about all the aspects of a person's medical care. Full disclosure means not only being factual about what is said to a patient, but also not withholding information that is pertinent to the patient's care and well-being.

A conflict in values arises when individuals disagree about whether one of these principles outweighs another. For example, parents may hold the principle of autonomy to be the most important and claim that as the surrogate decision-maker they have the ultimate right to decide to continue aggressive treatment. The health care team may disagree and believe that the treatment is futile and in the interest of minimizing harm, the principle of nonmaleficence should take priority. In some cases there may be no right or wrong answer, but a consensus may be achieved through communication. When there is a conflict in values it is vital that those in disagreement be brought together to communicate their individual and collective thoughts on the case. The ethical principles provide the background "rules" for discussion. In addition, a model or paradigm can be used to provide a framework to address the pertinent facts of the case and the opinions and feelings of the patient, family, and health care team.

ETHICAL ISSUES IN PEDIATRIC ONCOLOGY NURSING

Nurses frequently encounter ethical issues in the daily practice of caring for patients and families. A national survey of 136 adult oncology nurses identified priority ethical issues, including undertreatment of pain, truth telling, right to refuse treatment, informed consent, and withdrawing life support.[9] A second survey queried a similar group of nurses about their experiences with ethical issues in practice.[24] Responses were congruent with the previous study. Themes included suffering, truth telling (keeping secrets), and struggle (conflict). Pediatric oncology nurses may experience additional conflicts considering that most of the patients served are minors.

The topics discussed below illustrate some of the current ethical issues facing pediatric oncology nurses. Topics particularly significant to this field include informed consent, truth telling, minor assent, advanced directives, futility of treatment, undertreatment of pain, and scientific integrity in clinical trials.

INFORMED CONSENT

Ideally the process of informed consent is an ongoing two-way dialogue between the clinician or investigator and the patient, parent, or both, depending on the patient's level of understanding. This dialogue begins with the initial discussion of the diagnosis and consent for treatment, and possible involvement in a clinical trial, and should continue throughout the course of care.

The four key elements in this process include the following:[25]

Disclosure: the full revelation of the purpose, risks, benefits, and alternative options to the proposed therapy.

Comprehension: the subsequent understanding of the person who is receiving the information.

Competency: the person who is giving permission or consent must be aware of the risks and benefits and able to make a decision.

Voluntariness: the consenting individual must freely give permission and not be coerced in any way.

Despite the best intentions of the health care team, the informed consent process may be fraught with ethical issues. One may ask how any parent could be sufficiently informed and truly understand all the information presented during such a stressful event as a child being diagnosed with cancer. In addition to the difficulty of learning under stress, there are other barriers such as language, illiteracy, and cultural differences that may inhibit true comprehension. One could also argue that many parents do not feel as though they are truly "volunteering" for treatment, because they do not feel they have any other choice but to agree with the proposed therapy.

TRUTH TELLING

Inherent in the concept of obtaining true informed consent is the notion that the person giving the information is being completely truthful. This means presenting the facts and not withholding information that directly relates to the patient and the proposed treatment. The idea of being completely truthful when educating patients and families may become complicated as disclosing the "naked" truth may pose more harm than good. For example, when asking parents to consent for their child to undergo a bone marrow transplant, is it ethically necessary to show pictures of severe acute graft-versus-host disease of the skin? Some would argue that this potential complication should be explained in such detail. Others would state that showing such pictures could dissuade some parents from consenting at all, which would possibly decrease the child's best chance for cure.

Another example of an ethical dilemma related to truth telling is the withholding of information about the disease and treatment from a child at the parent's request. Parents may at the early stages of diagnosis of the disease or at the time of relapse wish to shield their child from the devastating news. The health care team is then put in the position of trying to honor the beneficent-based wishes of the parents while being truthful with the child. In most cases, given time and support, the parents will recognize the need to be truthful with their child.

MINOR ASSENT

A minor is considered anyone under the age of 18 years. A few states have enacted statutes that permit children under the age of 18 to consent to routine medical treatment. In most states there is no minimum age requirement for a minor to be able to consent for the treatment of sexually transmitted diseases, substance abuse, and pregnancy.[1] In addition, there are two categories recognized in some states that allow minors to consent to other treatments as well. These categories include the emancipated minor and the mature minor. Emancipated minors are children that live independent of their parents and provide self-support, thus demonstrating the ability to function as adults. A mature minor is a child who demonstrates the maturity and cognitive and emotional ability to make decisions about treatment. The age range for this category is usually between 15 and 17 years of age. However, this range could be broadened depending on the unique characteristics of the individual and the case.

For minors who do not fit into any of these categories, the right to give permission for treatment is given to a parent or guardian. However, federal regulations require that assent or permission is obtained from minors who are cognitively able (taking into account age, maturity, and psychologic state of the child). In the Code of Federal Regulations title 45 section 46, assent means a child's affirmative agreement to participate in research.[8] It also states that failure to object should not, absent affirmative agreement, be construed as assent. This means that minors must receive age-appropriate information about the treatment, including risks and benefits, and be given the opportunity to agree or disagree with the treatment plan.

MINORS AS HEMATOPOIETIC STEM CELL DONORS

The use of a minor as a hematopoietic stem cell donor has the potential to create ethical dilemmas.[6] First, the collection process is not in any way therapeutic for the donor; it is completely an altruistic endeavor. The donor may be too young to verbalize as-

sent for the procedure and older children who can verbalize assent may feel pressured to save the life of their sibling. In addition, although there are a few minimal physical risks involved with marrow collection, there is also the risk of psychologic harm if the sibling does not survive the transplant. For example, if the sibling develops severe graft-versus-host disease, the donor may feel at fault because the donor marrow is "attacking" the sibling's body. Second, the parents may feel a conflict of interest when making decisions for both the donor and the sick child. Do the parents feel any subtle pressure to protect the rights of the sick child over the rights of the child who is being asked to donate? In general, most cases involving a minor as a hematopoietic stem cell donor do not generate ethical conflicts. However, the rights of the minor donor must always be considered and subsequently protected.

ADVANCED DIRECTIVES

Health care facilities have, since the passage of the Patient Self-Determination Act in 1991, been required to give oral and written information to adult patients explaining their rights regarding accepting or refusing all types of treatment, including life-sustaining interventions.[9] It is widely accepted that persons 18 years of age and older need to be informed about these rights. The potential conflict in pediatrics is how age relates to cognitive development. Is there something magical about a person's eighteenth birthday that automatically makes one competent and able to make life and death decisions? It may make more sense to judge a person's competence on cognitive ability and level of maturity rather than age. However, because advanced directives are only legally recognized at the age of 18, it is from an ethical perspective that one would address these issues with younger children.

FUTILITY

Most members of the medical community would agree that the health care team is under no obligation to provide any medical intervention that is deemed futile. The question that is difficult to answer is, "What makes a treatment futile?" One definition is that "a treatment is futile if the intervention fails to reverse a physiologic disturbance that will lead to a patient's proximate death."[23] Once again the pertinent question remains, "What is a proximate death?" One person may believe that if a child cannot live well into adulthood or for a specific time such as a year, then the intervention is futile. Another may feel that if a child could live just one more day or long enough to attain a personal goal, then the treatment would not be in vain. The concept of futility is also important when a given intervention fails to achieve a specific goal.[29] It is imperative to first identify the goal and then ask the question, "What are the odds that this goal can be achieved and at what cost or benefit to the patient and family?"

It may also be helpful to consider the difference between quantitative and qualitative futility. Quantitative futility identifies how probable it is to systematically reproduce a result.[27] There are few situations in which a physician would say with absolute certainty that an intervention would be futile. However, based on experience and published reports it is reasonable to call an intervention futile if it did not produce the intended result in the last 100 cases. The problem with this approach is that fewer than 100 attempts may have occurred and each case may have unique variables that could affect the outcome. In contrast, qualitative futility considers whether an intervention will contribute to a better quality of life. For example, a child with renal failure may be treated with dialysis without the expectation that the kidneys will heal and the child will ultimately die. However, the dialysis has enabled the child to spend quality time with family and friends, play with favorite toys, and fulfill special requests or wishes. In this case dialysis would be considered futile in terms of a long-term cure but not at all futile in terms of meeting the goal to lengthen and improve the quality of this child's life.

UNDERTREATMENT OF PAIN

All children with cancer experience pain from the disease or treatment. Nurses are obligated to alleviate suffering, as long as the intervention does not lead to more harm. Patients may not receive adequate pain medication if parents are fearful of addiction. The ethical issue then arises, do the parents have the right to withhold pain medicine based on their beliefs, when their child is suffering and the pain could be relieved with adequate analgesia? Another example would be if a physician refused to escalate a dose of a pain medication for fear of respiratory depression. The nurse may be placed in the position of having to advocate for the patient's pain relief by challenging the physician's plan of care. Many cases related to the undertreatment of pain reflect the fear of legal retaliation if the patient has an adverse event related to the administration of pain medications. In contrast, there is the emerging concern that health care providers will be liable if a patient's pain is not relieved.

SCIENTIFIC INTEGRITY AND CLINICAL TRIALS

The Department of Health and Human Services has determined four categories of research for government funded trials that may be applied to children.[8] These categories include studies that (1) involve no more than minimal risk with the prospect of direct benefit to the child, (2) involve more than minimal risk with the prospect of direct benefit to the child, (3) involve more than minimal risk with no direct benefit, but offer the prospect of generalizable knowledge, and (4) could lead to understanding, preventing, or alleviating a serious problem affecting children's health or welfare. These categories permit children to be entered onto phase I through IV clinical trials, with the understanding that the parents and the child, if age appropriate, are fully informed about the risks and benefits of the study and consent to enrollment. However, concerns may arise if a child is asked to participate in a clinical trial that offers little benefit to the child, as is the case in most phase I studies. This situation is especially true if the child is not of the age to give assent. The principles of beneficence and nonmaleficence require investigators to produce benefits and as little harm as possible. The benefit of helping future children may be perceived as positive to some, but not to all. In addition, it is important to note that clinical research is uncertain and the risk/benefit analysis involves balancing the estimated probability of risks against the probability of benefits.[12]

There are many different issues to consider regarding scientific integrity in clinical trials. One question to ask is, does the principal investigator have a conflict of interest? If the investigator is paid for a patient's entry onto a clinical trial, is the patient or family informed of this payment? Are there any other incentives to enroll patients, such as the academic accolades of being the primary author on a paper because the investigator had the highest number of participants? Other facets to consider include the way in which the data are presented in the protocol or a publication. Are the data misleading or have the eligibility requirements been stretched to accommodate more patient entries? These questions are worth answering, particularly because clinical trials are vital in finding the treatments that will provide the best chance for cure with the fewest side effects. Clinical trials would be in jeopardy if the process lacked integrity and the public could not trust the intent or conduct of the investigators involved. The National Institutes of Health (NIH) mandated that all investigators submitting NIH grants involving human subjects must participate in a training program, effective in October 2000. This includes research nurses and clinical research associates or anyone else involved in conducting the research. Information regarding this program to promote integrity in research is available via the Internet.[21,22]

A MODEL FOR DECISION MAKING

There are many different tools, theories, or paradigms that can be used to analyze a case. For the purpose of this chapter one method will be described and subsequently used for analyzing the case studies that follow. This method identifies four topics that health care providers need to take into account when addressing the different aspects of a clinical case (Box 33-1). Analyzing the components of this four-part model helps those who are trying to resolve an ethical dilemma identify the different features that might bring the conflict to resolution.

MEDICAL INDICATIONS

This component is typically the first topic to be addressed in discussing any clinical case. It is simply the description of the patient's overall physical condition. Content to be covered in this component includes the diagnosis, the treatment, the patient's response to treatment, and the prognosis. The physician is usually the member of the health care team that summarizes this information and subsequently makes a medical recommendation about the course of treatment. This recommendation includes a description of the risks and benefits of the treatment, along with a clear explanation of the goals of care. This information is then shared with the patient and family. For most cases, the proposed treatment and subsequent action are straightforward. However, if there is disagreement about the prognosis or the proposed treatment plan on the part of the patient, family, or other members of the health care team, then an ethical conflict may arise.

PATIENT PREFERENCES

This component identifies the goals or the preferences of the patient. As discussed previously in this chapter, the patient or surrogate decision maker has the right to autonomy and can make decisions

---

BOX 33-1

A MODEL FOR ANALYZING CLINICAL CASES

MEDICAL INDICATIONS
1. What is patient's medical problem? history? diagnosis? prognosis?
2. Is problem acute? chronic? critical? emergent? reversible?
3. What are goals of treatments?
4. What are probabilities of success?
5. What are plans in case of therapeutic failure?
6. In sum, how can this patient be benefited by medical and nursing care, and how can harm be avoided?

PATIENT PREFERENCES
1. What has the patient expressed about preferences for treatment?
2. Has patient been informed of benefits and risks, understood, and given consent?
3. Is patient mentally capable and legally competent? What is evidence of capacity?
4. Has patient expressed prior preferences, e.g., advance directives?
5. If incapacitated, who is appropriate surrogate? Is surrogate using appropriate standards?
6. Is patient unwilling or unable to cooperate with medical treatment? If so, why?
7. In sum, is patient's right to choose being respected to extent possible in ethics and law?

QUALITY OF LIFE
1. What are the prospects, with or without treatment, for a return to patient's normal life?
2. Are there biases that might prejudice provider's evaluation of patient's quality of life?
3. What physical, mental, and social deficits is patient likely to experience if treatment succeeds?
4. Is patient's present or future condition such that continued life might be judged undesirable by him or her?
5. Any plan and rationale to forgo treatment?
6. What plans for comfort and palliative care?

CONTEXTUAL FEATURES
1. Are there family issues that might influence treatment decisions?
2. Are there provider (physicians and nurses) issues that might influence treatment decisions?
3. Are there financial and economic factors?
4. Are there religious, cultural factors?
5. Is there any justification to breach confidentiality?
6. Are there problems of allocation of resources?
7. What are legal implications of treatment decisions?
8. Is clinical research or teaching involved?
9. Any provider or institutional conflict of interest?

From Jonsen, A., Siegler, M., Winslade, W. J. (1998). *Clinical ethics: A practical approach to ethical decisions in clinical medicine* (4th ed.). New York: McGraw-Hill.

based on personal values, intentions, and goals. Questions to answer in this section include "What does the patient want?" and "Is the patient able to make decisions or express desires at this time?" Unfortunately in pediatrics there are many cases in which a child is too young to comprehend or verbalize specific preferences. In addition, even if the child is cognitively able to make decisions, there may be physical limitations that prevent discussion. In these cases parents are often the surrogate decision makers and may feel the heavy burden of making a decision that they feel is most in concert with what the child would want. In contrast, a child may have a preference that can be articulated that is in direct conflict with the desires of the parents. Members of the health care team may also disagree with the preferences of the patient and family, particularly if the family wants to continue treatment when the medical team feels that the treatment is futile. The goal in analyzing this section is to identify the preferences of the patient and parents (or surrogate) and to gain insight into any conflicts about these preferences that exist between the patient, parents, or health care team.

QUALITY OF LIFE

One of the most important goals of medical care is to maintain or improve the quality of life of the patient. This topic is often hard to define and analyze because quality of life may mean something different to any given person involved in a case. To some, quality of life means that a person can perform all the normal activities of daily life and enjoy them in the process. To others, these activities may be seriously curtailed but the experience of living day to day is worthwhile, even if discomfort is present. Determining the quality of someone's life is in fact a value judgment. This judgment, according to the principle of autonomy, must be left in the hands of the patient or surrogate decision maker. It is only the patient who can truly identify how the physical, psychologic, social, and personal effects of the disease and treatment affect the quality of life. If a patient lacks decision making capacity, the surrogate decision maker faces the challenge of identifying what the patient, if he or she could speak, would say about his or her quality of life. This may be accomplished by remembering what the patient has said or written prior to being incapacitated. Quality of life issues come to the forefront when making treatment decisions about patients who are developmentally delayed or have other concurrent serious illness. The benefits of the therapy must be considered along with the potential complications to determine the most appropriate care for the patient.

CONTEXTUAL FACTORS

Lastly, this topic addresses the social, legal, economic, and institutional circumstances that surround the case. Examples of these circumstances include the role of extended family members, the economics of health care (including insurance and the allocation of resources), the role of the law, and the welfare of society at large. These features do not, as a rule, take precedence over the medical indications, patient preferences, or quality of life. This component may become more integral in resolving a dilemma if the medical goals cannot be achieved, the patient preferences are not known, or the quality of life of the patient is perceived to be below minimal. In these cases a contextual feature may be brought forward as an important issue, particularly if there is perceived burden to someone or to society in general. Discussing the contextual features of any given case allows participants to think perhaps more globally, beyond the impact on the individual patient and family. It helps to identify the far-reaching implications of a case, but this part of the process may not be necessary if the conflict is resolved after analyzing the first three components.

CASE STUDIES

MINOR ASSENT

A 15-year-old girl with recurrent metastatic osteogenic sarcoma comes to the hospital with 20 pulmonary lesions, some of which are unresectable, 6 months after completing therapy. She states that she does not want to have surgery or salvage chemotherapy. Her parents are adamant that she agree to both treatment modalities.

Principle

Autonomy of the child versus rights of the parents to determine the best interests of the child

Medical Indications

Recurrent metastatic osteogenic sarcoma conveys a relatively poor prognosis, particularly if the patient has pulmonary disease in both lungs. The survival rate for children who have more than eight pulmonary lesions on initial diagnosis is estimated to be less than 25%.[13] Given that this patient has recurrent disease only 6 months off therapy, the estimated survival is lower. The physician recommended surgery, followed by salvage therapy with ifosfamide, because it could provide a small chance for cure and could prolong the child's life.

Patient Preferences

The child is very clear that she does not want surgery or salvage chemotherapy. She anticipates pain associated with the surgery and prolonged hospital stays associated with the chemotherapy regimen. She wants to be at home and socialize with friends. The parents are equally as adamant that she receive treatment, and they feel she is not able to make a mature decision about what is in her best interest.

Quality of Life

Given the side effects of this therapy, the child's short-term quality of life could be viewed as compromised. If the therapy minimized or removed the disease, in the long term her quality of life would be very much improved over what would be seen with progressive disease. The child and the parents are in agreement that quality of life means not having to go to the hospital and feeling well enough to enjoy day-to-day activities. What they do not agree on is whether the therapy is worth the risk of poor quality of life in the near term.

The Resolution

The parents in this case have the authority to make the decision to proceed with treatment. However, parents should consider that this authority should be shared as their child matures.[1] In some states this child may be considered a mature minor, because she can articulate well the risk and benefit of treatment and has experienced the side effects of previous therapies firsthand. After several discussions involving the parents, the child, and members of the multidisciplinary team, the parents were able to articulate that they are having a hard time accepting the poor prognosis. The parents decide to support their child's decision to not pursue aggressive chemotherapy.

Nursing Implications

In this case, the nurse can be instrumental in facilitating communication between the parents and the child. The parents needed time to accept the prognosis. The nurse was available to the parents to listen to their fears and concerns and answer their questions. This dialogue helped the parents to process their feelings and come to a decision. The nurse was also available in the same way to the child, who in turn felt as though her opinions were respected.

RELIGIOUS CONVICTION

An 11-year-old boy with newly diagnosed acute nonlymphocytic leukemia (ANLL) comes to the emergency room with a hemoglobin level of 5.0 g/dl and symptoms of impending cardiac failure. The parents and the patient are Jehovah's Witnesses and refuse a blood transfusion. In addition, the parents agree to comply with standard che-

motherapy but adamantly refuse to consider an allogeneic hematopoietic stem cell transplant (HSCT) as consolidation therapy for the disease.

Principle

Autonomy versus beneficence

Medical Indications

A child with ANLL has approximately a 30% to 45% chance of being cured with chemotherapy alone.[11] The proposed treatment for ANLL is intensive and blood transfusions are expected as a component of supportive care. Given the low hemoglobin of this patient, the physician recommended a blood transfusion right away and explained to the parents that intermittent transfusions would probably be necessary for several months. In addition, the proposed treatment protocol included the option to proceed with an allogeneic HSCT if there was a good match in the family. From the most current data, the physician explained that an HSCT from a matched sibling donor for a patient with ANLL in first remission yields a cure rate of about 50%.[11] The parents responded that they understood the risks and benefits of the proposed therapy and they would consent to chemotherapy, without blood transfusions or an HSCT.

Patient Preferences

Given the age of this child, the decision about treatment rests with the parents. When the diagnosis and treatment are explained to the child, he states that he agrees with his parents.

Quality of Life

Obviously the patient's quality of life would be compromised if the anemia led to serious morbidity or mortality. In the short term, the proposed treatment plan could decrease the patient's quality of life through the expenditure of time required for frequent clinic visits and hospital admissions, coupled with suffering associated with side effects, such as nausea, mouth sores, and infections.

Contextual Factors

There were few contextual features discussed in this case. Members of the church community were not involved in any treatment decisions. Other family members did not see any conflict in proceeding with the treatment plan.

The Resolution

Although religious freedom is considered a fundamental right, it does not necessarily mean a parent can exercise that right if it puts a child in substantial danger of harm. There is legal precedence for the court to intervene in such cases. In one landmark court case *(Prince v. Massachusetts)* the judge ruled that religious convictions may lead a parent to make a martyr of himself, but he is not free to make a martyr of his child.[14] In other words, children cannot be forced to adopt the religious convictions of their parents, but must be allowed to choose their own beliefs when cognitively mature enough to make such decisions. In the case being described in this chapter, the hospital obtained a court order for a blood transfusion. The parents and the child were comfortable with the decision, because the authority to transfuse did not come from the family. In addition, the health care team did not pursue legal intervention to mandate an HSCT. Parents may be legally required to choose a treatment option, but not necessarily the one with the best chance of success, if the chosen option has at least some chance of success.[1] Because the chance of survival with a matched sibling transplant is not overwhelmingly higher than with standard chemotherapy for ANLL and because an HSCT carries some additional risks, the health care team was content to continue with chemotherapy alone.

Nursing Implications

Nurses may frequently find themselves observing decisions made by families that are not congruent with their own values or beliefs. It is important to recognize the autonomous right of the patient and parents to make decisions. It may be necessary to identify one's own biases and consciously attempt to not allow these biases to compromise nursing care. In the event that a nurse has convictions that would impede care, the nurse may ask to be removed from direct care of the patient in question. On the other hand, it is vital that nurses do not ignore personal feelings that surface when something does not seem right. In this particular case the nurses helped to decrease the anxiety of the parents and patient during blood transfusion administration by covering the blood container with a brown bag.

INFORMED CONSENT

Parents of a 2-year-old child with newly diagnosed stage IV neuroblastoma tell the nurse that they feel relieved after the consult meeting with the physician because they understand the cure rate to be "good." The parents both have an eighth-grade education and admit that they had difficulty understanding the informed consent form. The nurse is concerned that the parents do not understand the risks and benefit of the proposed therapy. When the nurse asks the parents what they understand the

chances of cure to be, they respond with an enthusiastic 75% chance. The nurse conveys the concerns to the physician who provided the initial consult information and asked for consent. The physician responds that the parents were told a much lower number, between 30% to 40%.[18]

Principle

Autonomy

Medical Indications

The physician agreed to sit down with the parents and the nurse to review the child's diagnosis, proposed treatment plan, and prognosis. The nurse also provided the parents with a simple calendar that illustrated the treatment plan. The physician again recommended the child be entered on the current clinical trial for stage IV neuroblastoma. The parents were asked questions to ascertain their understanding of the information that was presented. The responses to the questions indicated a better understanding of the treatment plan and prognosis.

The Resolution

The parents, although less enthusiastic, gave permission to continue with treatment. The topics relating to patient preferences, quality of life, and contextual features did not need to be addressed, because the ethical issue was whether the parents were truly informed about the medical plan of care.

Nursing Implications

Nurses in pediatric oncology have many opportunities to make a difference in helping parents to be empowered to make decisions about their child's plan of care. The strategies that nurses can use to help improve the informed consent process include the following[25]:

- Be present with the family during consent meetings
- Improve the readability and format of written information that is given to parents
- Provide other mediums to reinforce the content (videos, audiotapes, and calendars)
- Ask questions using short words and sentences
- Assist parents in asking questions and encourage them to take notes
- Actively engage the parents in the process by discussing their perceptions

By listening to parents and answering their questions, the nurse is able to assess what the parents understand and perhaps bring to light concepts that may be unclear. The process of informed consent must be a mutual exchange of information that continues throughout the course of treatment.[5] This process communicates respect for the autonomy of others. Parents are in turn empowered with knowledge and can make decisions about their child's care from a position of strength.

FUTILE TREATMENT

A 4-year-old boy with acute lymphocytic leukemia (ALL) in second complete remission has had a matched unrelated hematopoietic stem cell transplant (HSCT). He was intubated following a pulmonary hemorrhage 2 weeks after the transplant and was extubated 2 days later after the bleeding stopped and his respiratory status improved. He also developed steroid-resistant grade IV graft-versus-host disease (GVHD). Several days later the bleeding in his lungs recurred and he was reintubated. The following day his kidneys failed and he needed dialysis. The parents wished to continue with aggressive treatment, but the health care team felt that, because of multisystem failure, further aggressive treatment would be futile. In addition, the staff was concerned that the patient was suffering.

Principle

Autonomy versus nonmaleficence versus beneficence

Medical Indications

It is important to step back and look at this child's overall prognosis in light of what is empirically accepted as the prognosis for a child with this particular diagnosis and treatment. A child with ALL in second complete remission after a matched unrelated transplant has a 45% chance of cure.[3] Acute GVHD grade IV that is unresponsive to steroid therapy carries a high mortality rate. Response rates to salvage therapy range from 17% to 75%, however, the responses are usually partial and brief and the majority of patients die from either GVHD or infection.[19] In addition, pulmonary hemorrhage carries a high mortality rate (70% to 90%).[20] Overall, this patient has an extremely poor prognosis. In fact the chance for survival is so small for a child with multiorgan system failure after an HSCT following intubation, that aggressive treatment should not be recommended.[16] In this case, the recommendation was made to the parents not to proceed with dialysis and to consider accepting a "do not resuscitate" order.

Patient Preferences

Because of the young age of this child, the parents are acting as surrogate decision makers. The parents agree that they want to continue with aggressive

therapy. They feel that God can work a miracle and they want their child to have every possible chance of surviving. However, they are both also committed to making their son as pain-free as possible.

Quality of Life

The boy's mother states that she is unsure if she wants her child to live if his quality of life will be significantly less than it was before his HSCT. She is concerned that he will have serious body image changes secondary to the severe skin GVHD, and pulmonary compromise from the hemorrhage.

Contextual Factors

Other family members were not concerned about the burden of caring for this child. The family and members of the health care team did not discuss the financial cost for complex treatment in the intensive care unit.

The Resolution

The parents met with the health care team to discuss dialysis. They agreed to forgo dialysis, but wished to continue ventilatory support. They agreed not to start cardiopulmonary resuscitation (CPR) or give cardiac medications if their son's heart stopped. Two days after this discussion the patient had a cardiac arrest and died. The parents felt comfortable that they did everything possible for their child.

It is vital to stay focused on the goals of care rather than the specific treatments that are available.[29] For example, when a physician asks a parent, "Would you like me to do everything I can to save your child, including CPR?" most reasonable parents would respond "Yes!" The response may be quite different if the physician first addresses the goals of care and then explains the risk and benefit inherent in performing CPR. Nurses can be instrumental in helping to educate patients and families about the risks and benefits of specific treatments. In addition it is vital that when discussing an "appropriate" goal it is both consistent with what the patient and/or parents want and is capable of being achieved.[7]

Nursing Implications

It is never easy to see a patient suffer, particularly if one is aware that the prognosis is poor. Perhaps one of the most difficult dilemmas for nurses is to witness suffering and feel the frustration that the family or other members of the health care team are not able to prevent or stop aggressive treatment. This scenario invokes the principle of doing no harm. It is important to first identify ways to relieve suffering if possible. The aggressive use of pain medications, sedatives, and other modalities can provide comfort, even in the worst of circumstances. Secondly, the nurse can strive to facilitate ongoing communication between the parents and members of the health care team with the intent to identify the goals of treatment. It is also essential to recognize that the decision to stop aggressive treatment is an extremely difficult one in most cases. Parents cannot be quickly forced into coming to terms with the prognosis before they are ready. Nurses must find the balance between comforting the patient and allowing the parents time to process the risk and benefit of each medical intervention and ultimately make decisions that are right for their child and their family.

It is the obligation of any nurse to apply ethical principles to practice. The nursing profession's current code of ethics requires that a nurse provide respect for human dignity, protect patient rights, provide competent nursing care, work to improve the quality of care, and protect the public from misinformation.[2] Implementing this code of ethics requires that nurses are educated about ethical principles and tools to help with moral reasoning.[26] It is not sufficient to rely on one's own values as the standard for ethical practice. It is the nurse's professional responsibility to learn about ethical principles in the context of society. This education begins in the undergraduate setting and continues into practice.

The pediatric oncology nurse is in a key position to identify and help resolve ethical conflicts. One approach is to identify the issue and constructively summarize the facts of the case or conflict.[28] The next step is to identify the ethical principles involved, because this will help one look at the situation from a more objective and less emotional viewpoint. Third, address the conflict with the persons involved, either through a family conference or a meeting between colleagues. Fourth, if the conflict is not resolved locally in the work setting, consult the institution's ethics committee. Strategies to help prevent ethical dilemmas include attending consent meetings; answering questions; facilitating communication; assessing patient and family values, perceptions, and experiences; and being willing to address any intervention, act, or policy that has the potential to violate patient rights.

Every nursing activity, however ordinary, must always be offered with dignity, honesty, and loving compassion. It is in the everyday exchanges between people that the best expressions of moral responsibility are recorded. In the higher task of nursing the sick, that is the ultimate measure of success.[17]

ACKNOWLEDGMENT

The author acknowledges and expresses thanks to Kathy Kinlaw, MDiv, Associate Director for the Emory University Center for Ethics in Public Policy and the Professions, for her careful review of this chapter.

REFERENCES

1. Ahronheim, J. C., Moreno, J., & Zuckerman, C. (1994). *Ethics in clinical practice.* Boston: Little, Brown.
2. American Nurses Association. (1985). *Code for nurses with interpretive statements.* Kansas City, MO: American Nurses Association.
3. Balduzzi, A., Gooley, T., Anasetti, C., et al. (1995). Unrelated donor marrow transplantation in children. *Blood, 86,* 3247-3256.
4. Beauchamp, T. L., & Children, J. F. (1994). *Principles of biomedical ethics* (4th ed.). New York: Oxford University Press.
5. Berry, D. L., Dodd, M. J., Hinds, P. S., et al. (1996). Informed consent: Process and clinical issues. *Oncology Nursing Forum, 23,* 507-512.
6. Chan, K. (1996). Use of minors as bone marrow donors: Current attitudes and management. *Journal of Pediatrics, 128,* 644-648.
7. Crawford, S. W. (1991). Decision making in critically ill patients with hematologic malignancy. *Western Journal of Medicine, 155,* 488-493.
8. Department of Health and Human Services. (1991). Code of Federal Regulations Title 45. Bethesda, MD: National Institutes of Health, 45 CFR 46.402, Subpart D: A4-47, 48.
9. Ersek, M., Scanlon, C., Glass, E., et al. (1995). Priority ethical issues in oncology nursing: Current approaches and future directions. *Oncology Nursing Forum, 22,* 803-807.
10. Freeman, J. M. (1992). Introduction and overview: Why another polemic on ethics? *Pediatric Annals, 21,* 279-286.
11. Golub, T. R., Weinstein, H. J., & Grier, H. E. (1997). Acute myelogenous leukemia. In P. A. Pizzo & D. G. Poplack (Eds.), *Principles and practice of pediatric oncology* (3rd ed., pp. 463-482). Philadelphia: Lippincott-Raven.
12. Grady, C. (1991). Ethical issues in clinical trials. *Seminars in Oncology Nursing, 7,* 288-296.
13. Harris, M. B., Gieser, P., Goorin, A. M., et al. (1998). Treatment of metastatic osteogenic sarcoma at diagnosis: A Pediatric Oncology Group study. *Journal of Clinical Oncology, 16,* 3641-3648.
14. Holder, A. R. (1985). *Legal issues in pediatrics and adolescent medicine.* New Haven, CT: Yale University Press.
15. Jonsen, A., Siegler, M., & Winslade, W. J. (1998). *Clinical ethics: A practical approach to ethical decisions in clinical medicine* (4th ed.). New York: McGraw-Hill.
16. Keenan, H. T., Bratton, S. L., Martin, L. D., et al. (2000). Outcome of children who require mechanical ventilation support after bone marrow transplant. *Critical Care Medicine, 28,* 830-835.
17. Levine, M. E. (1989). Ethical issues in cancer care: Beyond dilemma. *Seminars in Oncology Nursing, 5,* 124-128.
18. Matthay, K. K., O'Leary, M. C., Ramsey, N. K., et al. (1995). Role of myeloablative therapy in improved outcome for high risk neuroblastoma: A review of recent CCG results. *European Journal of Cancer, 31A,* 572-575.
19. McCaul, K. G., Nevill, T. J., Barnett, M. J., et al. (2000). Treatment of steroid-resistant acute graft-versus-host disease with rabbit antithymocyte globulin. *Journal of Hematotherapy and Stem Cell Research, 9,* 367-374.

20. Metcalf, J. P., Rennard, S. I., Reed, E. C., et al. (1994). Corticosteroids as adjunctive therapy for diffuse alveolar hemorrhage associated with bone marrow transplantation. *The American Journal of Medicine, 96,* 327-334.

21. National Institute of Health. (2000). Frequently asked questions for the requirement for education on the protection of human subjects. http://grants.nih.gov/grants/policy/hs_educ_faq.htm.

22. National Institute of Health. (2000). Required education in the protection of human research participants. http://grants.nih.gov/grants/guide/notice-files/NOT-OD-00-039.html.

23. Nelson, J. L., & Nelson, R. M. (1992). Ethics and the provision of futile, harmful, or burdensome treatment to children. *Critical Care Medicine, 20,* 427-433.

24. O'Connor, K. F. (1996). Ethical/moral experiences of oncology nurses. *Oncology Nursing Forum, 23,* 787-794.

25. Ruccione, K. S. (1994). Informed consent in pediatric oncology: A nursing perspective. *Journal of Pediatric Oncology Nursing, 11,* 128-133.

26. Scanlon, C., & Glover, J. (1995). A professional code of ethics: Providing a moral compass for turbulent times. *Oncology Nursing Forum, 22,* 1515-1521.

27. Schneiderman, L. J., Jecker, N. S., & Jonsen, A. R. (1990). Medical futility: Its meaning and clinical implications. *Annals of Internal Medicine, 112,* 949-954.

28. Winters, G., Glass, E., & Sakurai, C. (1993). Ethical issues in oncology nursing practice: An overview of topics and strategies. *Oncology Nursing Forum, 20,* 21-34.

29. Younger, S. J. (1996). Medical futility. *Critical Care Clinics, 12,* 165-178.

Index

Page numbers followed by f indicate figures; t, tables; b, boxes.